Feature Paper in Physiology and Pathology

Feature Paper in Physiology and Pathology

Stefanos Roumeliotis
Giuseppe Minervini

MDPI

Basel • Beijing • Wuhan • Barcelona • Belgrade • Novi Sad • Cluj • Manchester

Editors
Stefanos Roumeliotis
Division of Nephrology
and Hypertension
Aristotle University
Thessaloniki
Greece

Giuseppe Minervini
Multidisciplinary Department
of Medical-Surgical and
Dental Specialties
University of Campania
"Luigi Vanvitelli"
Naples
Italy

Editorial Office
MDPI AG
Grosspeteranlage 5
4052 Basel, Switzerland

This is a reprint of articles from the Special Issue published online in the open access journal *Life* (ISSN 2075-1729) (available at: www.mdpi.com/journal/life/special_issues/NMP2LMT8U1).

For citation purposes, cite each article independently as indicated on the article page online and as indicated below:

Lastname, A.A.; Lastname, B.B. Article Title. *Journal Name* **Year**, *Volume Number*, Page Range.

ISBN 978-3-7258-2176-1 (Hbk)
ISBN 978-3-7258-2175-4 (PDF)
doi.org/10.3390/books978-3-7258-2175-4

Contents

About the Editors

Stefanos Roumeliotis

Stefanos Roumeliotis graduated in Medicine (MD) from the Ioannina School of Medicine in 2007. During his early career, he completed his residency in Nephrology in 2016, passing his specialty exams with distinction. In 2019, he earned his PhD from the Democritus University of Thrace, focusing on Vascular Calcification in Diabetic Nephropathy. In 2020, he was awarded a Research Fellowship from the European Renal Association and completed his training at the CNR-IFC Research Unit in Italy, collaborating with renowned nephrologists and publishing 15 papers and 2 book chapters. Currently, he serves as an Academic Fellow in Nephrology at the Aristotle University of Thessaloniki and is the Chief Nephrologist at Achilleion Kalamaria. He is also a member of several scientific societies, including the Hellenic Nephrology Association and the European Renal Association. He has been recognized for his contributions to nephrology with an award for academic research and impact in 2024. Dr. Roumeliotis is an Editorial Board Member of *Frontiers in Physiology*, *Clinical Kidney Journal*, and *Life* (MDPI), and he serves as a Reviewer for over 50 journals. With 83 publications, an h-index of 23, and numerous invited lectures, his research focuses on cardiovascular disease, diabetic CKD, and oxidative stress in chronic kidney disease.

Giuseppe Minervini

Giuseppe Minervini graduated in Dental Medicine in July 2016 with honors. During his undergraduate studies, he participated in an Erasmus project at "Rey Juan Carlos Alcorcon" in Madrid, Spain, from September 2013 to June 2014. He received his Postgraduate Diploma in Orthodontics in December 2020 from the University of Campania, Luigi Vanvitelli, Naples, Italy, and later earned his PhD at the same institution (XXXIV cycle). In 2019, he attended the Tweed Study Course at the Charles H. Tweed International Foundation in Tucson, Arizona. Currently, he serves as an Adjunct Professor at Saveetha Dental College and Hospitals, Saveetha University, Chennai. Dr. Minervini is recognized as one of the top 10 experts worldwide in the field of "Temporomandibular disorders" according to Scopus' rankings. He is a Subject Expert in Dental Materials and a tutor at the Orthodontics Dentistry School at the University of Campania, Luigi Vanvitelli. His contributions include serving as an Editor for numerous dentistry journals (10 Editorial Boards, 14 Special Issues), and he is an active member of SIDO, EOS, and GSID. With over 188 publications, 70 posters, and an h-index of 32, he is a frequent speaker at national and international conferences. Dr. Minervini has received several awards for his contributions to the field. His research interests include biomedical and biomaterial applications in craniofacial, oral, and temporomandibular districts, as well as orthodontics, orofacial pain, temporomandibular joint disorders, and telemedicine.

Preface

Dear Colleagues,

This Special Issue aims to bring together groundbreaking research on natural molecules and their applications in pharmacology and biotechnology. It aims to highlight how these molecules can serve as bioactive compounds in drug discovery and therapeutic development. This collection features contributions from leading experts in the field, offering both original research and review articles. The goal is to provide readers with an in-depth understanding of the potential of natural products in advancing medical science. We express gratitude to the authors and reviewers for their valuable contributions.

Stefanos Roumeliotis and Giuseppe Minervini
Editors

life

MDPI

Review

Advancing Post-Stroke Depression Research: Insights from Murine Models and Behavioral Analyses

Mădălina Iuliana Mușat [1], Bogdan Cătălin [1,*], Michael Hadjiargyrou [2,*], Aurel Popa-Wagner [1,3] and Andrei Greșiță [1,4]

1 Experimental Research Centre for Normal and Pathological Aging, University of Medicine and Pharmacy of Craiova, 200349 Craiova, Romania; madalina.musat3@gmail.com (M.I.M.); aurel.popa-wagner@geriatrics-healthyageing.com (A.P.-W.)
2 Department of Biological and Chemical Sciences, New York Institute of Technology, Old Westbury, NY 11568, USA
3 Department of Neurology, Vascular Neurology and Dementia, University of Medicine Essen, 45122 Essen, Germany
4 Department of Biomedical Sciences, New York Institute of Technology, Old Westbury, NY 11568, USA
* Correspondence: bogdan.catalin@umfcv.ro (B.C.); mhadji@nyit.edu (M.H.)

Abstract: Post-stroke depression (PSD) represents a significant neuropsychiatric complication that affects between 39% and 52% of stroke survivors, leading to impaired recovery, decreased quality of life, and increased mortality. This comprehensive review synthesizes our current knowledge of PSD, encompassing its epidemiology, risk factors, underlying neurochemical mechanisms, and the existing tools for preclinical investigation, including animal models and behavioral analyses. Despite the high prevalence and severe impact of PSD, challenges persist in accurately modeling its complex symptomatology in preclinical settings, underscoring the need for robust and valid animal models to better understand and treat PSD. This review also highlights the multidimensional nature of PSD, where both biological and psychosocial factors interplay to influence its onset and course. Further, we examine the efficacy and limitations of the current animal models in mimicking the human PSD condition, along with behavioral tests used to evaluate depressive-like behaviors in rodents. This review also sets a new precedent by integrating the latest findings across multidisciplinary studies, thereby offering a unique and comprehensive perspective of existing knowledge. Finally, the development of more sophisticated models that closely replicate the clinical features of PSD is crucial in order to advance translational research and facilitate the discovery of future effective therapies.

Keywords: post-stroke depression; behavioral tests; cognition; social activity; motor function; antidepressants; murine models of depression

Citation: Mușat, M.I.; Cătălin, B.; Hadjiargyrou, M.; Popa-Wagner, A.; Greșiță, A. Advancing Post-Stroke Depression Research: Insights from Murine Models and Behavioral Analyses. *Life* **2024**, *14*, 1110. https://doi.org/10.3390/life14091110

Academic Editors: Stefanos Roumeliotis and Giuseppe Minervini

Received: 30 July 2024
Revised: 31 August 2024
Accepted: 2 September 2024
Published: 3 September 2024

1. Background

Studies estimate that annually, 15 million people are affected by a stroke worldwide. Roughly 5 million people die due to the ischemic event, while another 5 million survivors are permanently disabled [1,2]. Unfortunately, prevention cannot successfully reduce the stroke occurrence rate due to the high number of risk factors and comorbidities linked to its onset [3]. These include the most important factors, cardiovascular disease [4], high body mass index [5], chronic stress [6], and more importantly, aging [7]. Current therapeutic approaches are mostly focused on limiting the long-term multiple medical conditions of stroke survivors as well as the overall burden on the healthcare system and society [8].

Following stroke, motor complications, such as hemiparesis [9], hemiplegia, or postural instability [10], significantly challenge patient rehabilitation efforts [11]. Additionally, patients are faced with urinary and bowel incontinence [12], cognitive impairment and dementia [13], depression [14], anxiety [15], fatigue [16], and sleep disorders [17,18], all of which pose a significant challenge for successful diagnosis and treatment. While significant motor [11] and cognitive [19] dysfunction represent long-term consequences of ischemic injury, PSD represents the most frequent and challenging neuropsychiatric complication [20,21].

Estimating the exact prevalence of PSD is challenging, particularly due to methodological complexities, such as variations in the timing of patient evaluations after stroke onset and differences in instruments and criteria utilized in experimental settings [21]. However, recent findings suggest that PSD occurs in approximately 18–33% of cases [22,23], with the greatest number of occurrences observed within the first year following the ischemic insult [24]. Also, ~53% of individuals who were depressed within 3 months after stroke experienced persistent depression [21]. These results are concerning, especially because the mortality rate is higher among patients who suffer from PSD [22]. The risk of suicidal death is ~2 times higher for stroke patients compared to the general population [25], and in addition to suicidal ideation [26], cognitive deficits [27], long-term disability [28], and a substantially lower quality of life [29] are additional symptoms in patients who develop PSD.

Thus, it is of paramount importance to understand the underlying mechanisms of this disease and to accurately identify efficient screening tools and therapeutic modalities. However, studying the pathopsychological mechanisms underlying PSD, such as affected cellular plasticity [30], neuroinflammation, and neurodegeneration [31], as well as intrinsic recovery pathways (neurogenesis) [32], requires a highly accurate and performant experimental approach. But, establishing preclinical models can also pose challenges, particularly given the subjective nature of the psychological and physiological PSD symptoms [33]. Researchers have endeavored to create rodent models that capture key aspects of PSD, allowing for the evaluation of behavioral manifestations and underlying neurobiological changes [34–36]. One such approach involves inducing focal cerebral ischemia in rodents [37] and simulating the conditions of stroke observed in humans. Following a stroke, protocols for inducing depressive behavior [38] and behavioral tests tailored to assess depressive-like symptoms are used [39] and encompass a wide range of assays designed to evaluate various aspects of depressive behavior, including despair-like behavior [40], anhedonia [41], and alterations in locomotor activity and exploration [42,43].

Despite recent progress in PSD-related research, challenges persist in accurately reproducing the multifaceted nature of this condition in in vivo animal models. To advance translational research and the development of new therapeutic treatments for PSD, it is crucial to develop valid animal models that accurately replicate the complex symptomatology of the condition. According to the International Classification of Diseases, 11th Revision (ICD 11) criteria [44], psychiatrists diagnosing depression in patients typically confirm the presence of five or more symptoms from the depressive spectrum (i.e., depressed mood, anhedonia, appetite or weight changes, sleep disturbances, psychomotor agitation or retardation, fatigue, reduced concentration, feelings of worthlessness or excessive guilt, and recurrent thoughts of suicide or death) [45]. Accurate replication of the human condition in these models is crucial for understanding the pathology and to effectively test various therapeutic interventions. Variability in individual responses [46], differences in genetic backgrounds [47–51], and the subjective nature of depressive symptoms [52,53] all present challenges in interpreting the data effectively. Moreover, the environmental and social factors that can influence the onset and progression of PSD in humans [54,55] are difficult to replicate in murine models, limiting the validity and effectiveness of these studies. The complexity of stroke-induced brain injury, which involves not just the neural circuits traditionally associated with mood regulation [56,57] but also the broader neurological disruptions [58], complicates the accuracy of modeling PSD. Additionally, the lack of biomarkers or a valid genetic model for depression further contributes to the difficult task of studying neuropsychiatric disorders, including PSD, in a preclinical setting [59]. These challenges highlight the need for continued refinement of animal models and methodologies to enhance the translational potential of PSD preclinical research.

The purpose of this review was to conduct a thorough investigation of the current literature on murine models for PSD, highlighting both the strengths and weaknesses of these models, as well as the behavioral assessments employed. Our goal is to identify effective animal models and behavioral evaluations so that their inherent limitations can be overcome. Further, this review aims not only to underline the tools available for such studies but also discuss the challenges faced in translating these preclinical results into the clinic.

2. Materials and Methods

We have used PubMed and ClinicalTrials.gov in order to identify a thorough range of relevant scientific manuscripts. Importantly, our search extended to encompass animal models of PSD and various behavioral studies and provides a comprehensive overview of the methods used in exploring PSD. The search terms employed mostly included "post-stroke depression murine models" and "post-stroke depression murine behavioral studies". Also, to ensure thorough coverage, we used derived terms such as "vascular depression", "behavioral tests', "cognition in rodents", "social activity in rodents", "motor function in rodents", "stroke in rodents", "chronic mild stress", "depressive-like behavior", and "anxiety and depression assessments in murine models". Additionally, we manually reviewed the reference lists of all sourced articles to uncover further citations that the initial database search might have missed. Although additional searches yielded a large number of results, we focused on these specific terms to maintain the relevance and manageability of manuscripts. We specifically chose articles published within the past two decades, spanning from 2004 to 2024, thus ensuring the inclusion of up-to-date research findings. A language criterion was established to only consider articles written in English. This review primarily adopts a narrative approach and does not adhere to the Preferred Reporting Items for Systematic Reviews and Meta-Analysis (PRISMA) guidelines. However, the article selection process was meticulously structured, ensuring that included articles were scrutinized by a panel of three independent reviewers (Figure 1).

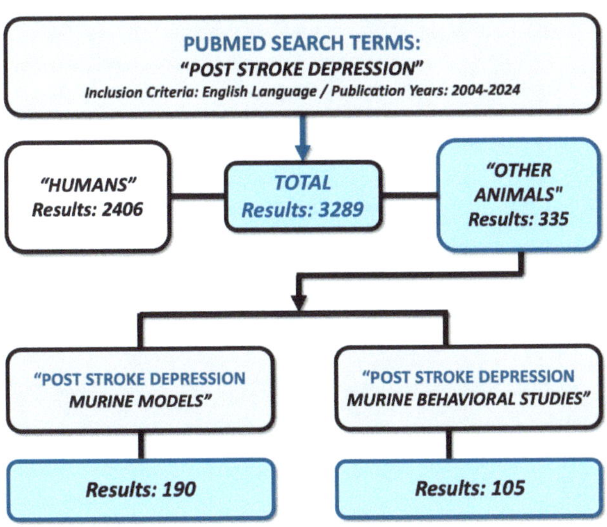

Figure 1. Flowchart of the literature search using PubMed.

3. Incidence and Prevalence of PSD

The incidence and prevalence of PSD exhibit considerable variability in the literature due to differences in methodology, population demographics, and stroke characteristics that underscore its recognition as a frequent consequence of cerebral ischemia [21]. Studies show that between 39% and 52% of stroke survivors experience symptoms of PSD within the first five years after the ischemic event [60]. Studies have also shown that the risk of developing depression is highest within the initial months following stroke [24], with a gradual decline over time [61]. This acute onset suggests a complex interplay of biological, psychological, and social factors, which includes inflammatory mechanisms, the hypothalamic–pituitary–adrenal (HPA) axis, limited capacity for independent living, economic status, negative life events, family burden, and social family support. Collectively, they all contribute to the development of PSD [51]. Additionally, the prevalence of PSD tends to be higher in individuals with more severe strokes, those with a history of depression, and those experiencing greater functional impairment post-stroke [60]. While certain studies suggest that the prevalence of depression after stroke does not significantly differ between sexes, it appears to vary depending on the individual's pre-stroke depression status [62]. But, other reports state that elderly female stroke patients are 20% more likely to develop PSD in comparison to males [63]. Collectively, all of the aforementioned point to the need for new, effective, and preventive therapeutic approaches [64].

4. Risk Factors Involved in PSD

4.1. Stroke Characteristics and Lesion Localization

Increased lesion volumes, cerebral atrophy, silent infarcts, and white matter lesions are factors that may correlate with an elevated risk of PSD [65] (Figure 2). Lesion location within the brain is a critical determinant of PSD risk, as specific brain regions play distinct roles in mood regulation and emotional processing. Previous studies have demonstrated that the site of stroke lesions (i.e., prefrontal cortex, limbic area, and basal ganglia) significantly influences the likelihood of developing PSD [56,66,67]. The neuroanatomical model proposed by Soares in 1997 also links mood disorders, including PSD, to specific brain regions such as the frontal lobe, basal ganglia, amygdala–hippocampus complex, and thalamus [68]. This model emphasizes the importance of the basal ganglia for the transmission of 5-HT and DA and how ischemic damage to brainstem monoaminergic nuclei or their projections can decrease monoamine levels, affecting mood and cognition. Damage to the left frontal cortex is also often linked to depressive symptoms; individuals with lesions in the left hemisphere may be particularly susceptible to developing depression and anxiety following a stroke [69]. Although there are data suggesting a significant risk for depression following right hemisphere strokes during the subacute phase [70], it appears that a higher risk is associated with left hemisphere lesions [71]. Overall, while the link between the lesion site and PSD is generally acknowledged, the exact relationship remains subject to ongoing research.

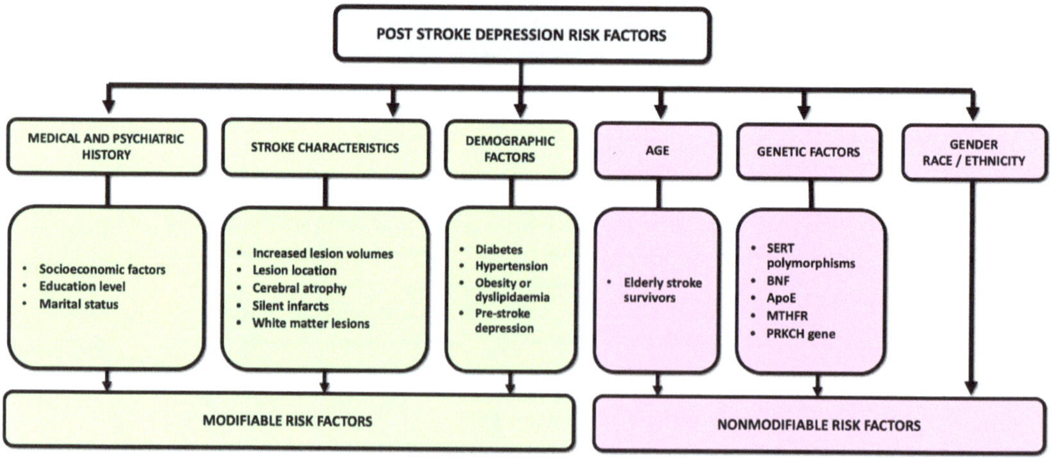

Figure 2. Diagram showing risk factors associated with PSD. Serotonin transporter (SERT), brain-derived neurotrophic factor (BNF), apolipoprotein E (ApoE), methylenetetrahydrofolate reductase (MTHFR), and Protein Kinase C Eta Gene (PRKCH).

4.2. Demographic Factors

Demographic factors play a significant role in influencing the risk and occurrence of PSD. Gender disparities exist in the prevalence of PSD, with women generally exhibiting higher rates of depression following a stroke compared to men [63,72,73]. Hormonal fluctuations, psychosocial factors, and differences in coping mechanisms may contribute to these gender differences observed [72]. Socioeconomic factors, including education level, income, and access to healthcare resources, also play a crucial role in the development and course of PSD [55]. Stroke survivors from lower socioeconomic backgrounds are more likely to experience financial strain, social isolation, and limited access to mental health services, exacerbating their risk of developing PSD [74]. Marital status is another factor associated with PSD risk, with unmarried individuals, including those who are divorced, widowed, or single, exhibiting higher rates of depression or suicidal ideations following a stroke [75].

4.3. Age

Studies have shown that the incidence and severity of PSD increase with advancing age, highlighting the importance of age-related considerations in its management [76,77]. The incidence of PSD is especially high in elderly stroke survivors [78], with 34% in stroke patients vs. 13% in the matched general population [79]. As most candidate therapies for PSD are being developed and studied on young animal models [34], age, which is proven to be detrimental to recovery, may aid in ushering a certain degree of accuracy to existing murine models, thus reducing the translational gap between preclinical and clinical studies [80]. Although a vast array of risk factors such as diabetes [81], hypertension [82], obesity, or dyslipidemia [83] are linked to ischemic brain injury, age represents a non-modifiable risk factor that is not only linked to an increased susceptibility to stroke but also to significantly decreased functional recovery [76,77,84]. It is, therefore, considered that age is a key modulatory factor for both stroke and PSD.

4.4. Genetic Factors

Genetic factors can also contribute to the complex interplay of biological and environmental determinants underlying PSD [85]. Polymorphisms within the serotonin transporter gene (SERT) are associated with PSD in stroke survivors [86], and BDNF is a significant contributor to the pathophysiological mechanisms underlying PSD [87]. Research also suggests that both apolipoprotein E (ApoE) and methylenetetrahydrofolate reductase (MTHFR) may contribute to an increased risk of major depressive disorder after a stroke. Interestingly, the catechol-O-methyltransferase (COMT) gene, crucial for DA degradation in the brain, along the 5-HT2A receptor gene that is crucial in serotonin signaling, were studied for their roles in ADHD, schizophrenia, mood regulation, and aggressive behavior [88]. Given their implications in such diverse neurological and behavioral conditions, it is particularly compelling to explore these genes within the context of PSD. The COMT and 5-HT2A genes, through their respective pathways in DA and 5-HT metabolism and signaling, could provide insightful connections to the neuropsychiatric and emotional challenges seen in PSD. While advancements in this area have been limited, certain genes such as protein kinase Cη (PRKCH), angiotensin-converting enzyme, and apolipoprotein may also play an important role in the development of vascular-related depression [89,90]. Additional investigations are ongoing to further delineate the precise genetic factors influencing genetic susceptibility to PSD [91].

4.5. Medical and Psychiatric History

The burden of comorbidities and the severity of pre-stroke functional impairment can influence the development and severity of PSD [81–83]. Additionally, a history of psychiatric disorders is a strong predictor of PSD [92]. It is concerning that one out of every six stroke patients has experienced PSD [93]. Attention to lifestyle factors, stress management, and social support networks can offer additional layers of prevention and therapeutic intervention, potentially mitigating the impact of pre-existing conditions and enhancing the overall wellbeing of stroke survivors. After-stroke rehabilitation programs, including progressive resistance training [94], modified cardiac rehabilitation [95], vocational rehabilitation [96], family-based programs [97], aquatic [98], music [99], cognitive behavioral therapy [100], repetitive transcranial magnetic stimulation [101], pet therapy [102], and robotic devices [103], can all significantly improve the quality of life and prevent or reduce PSD symptoms.

5. Valid Animal Models for PSD

PSD poses significant challenges in behavioral assessment due to the subjective nature of its psychological and physiological symptoms [33]. This subjectivity further complicates the development of accurate and reliable experimental animal models capable of capturing the full spectrum of human symptoms. Researchers seek to navigate this complexity by creating models that not only mimic the neuroanatomical and biochemical alterations following a stroke but also elicit behavioral changes consistent with depressive phenotypes. This endeavor extends to identifying and validating behavioral assays that can reliably quantify depressive-like behaviors in animals. However, the translation from animal models to the human condition is fraught with challenges, including differences in brain structure and function, the complexity of human emotions, and the influence of environmental and social factors on mental health [104]. Moreover, the heterogeneity of stroke in terms of location, severity [65], and individual patient factors, like pre-existing mental health conditions [93], further complicates the accuracy of modeling PSD. As such, ongoing research aims to refine these models, increase their translational value, and ultimately, enhance our understanding of PSD pathophysiology. Below, we outline several useful animal models that can contribute to PSD-related research (Figure 3).

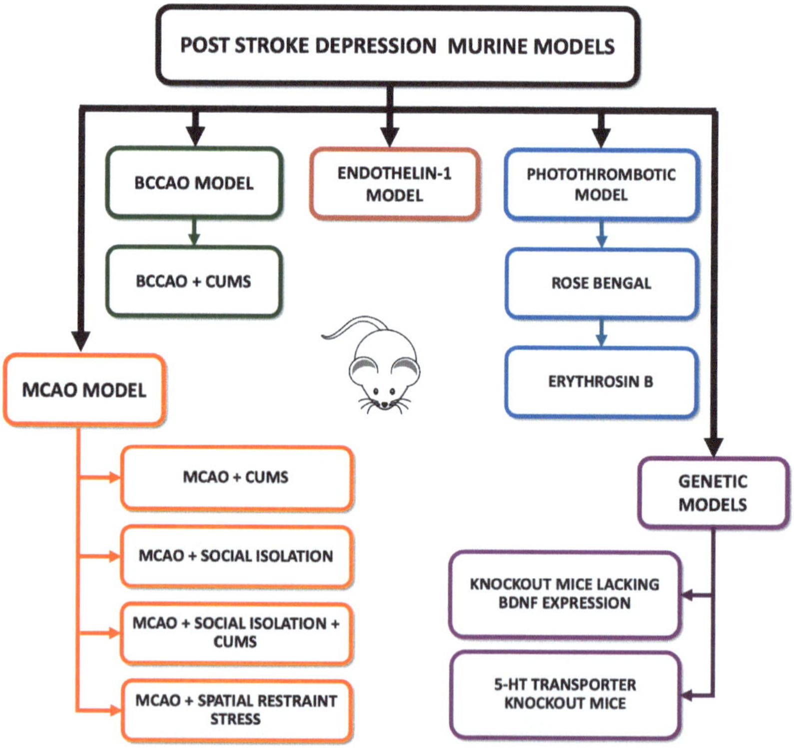

Figure 3. Diagram showing murine models of PSD. Bilateral Common Carotid Artery Occlusion (BCCAO), chronic unpredictable mild stress (CUMS), Middle Cerebral Artery Occlusion (MCAO), 5-Hydroxytryptamine (5-HT, serotonin), and brain-derived neurotrophic factor (BDNF).

5.1. Middle Cerebral Artery Occlusion (MCAO) Model

The MCAO model is one of the most widely used protocols to mimic stroke in rodents [105]. In this model, the middle cerebral artery is occluded either transiently or permanently [106], resulting in focal cerebral ischemia and subsequent stroke-like symptoms, including depressive-like behavior [107]. This model allows for precise quantitation of neurological deficits, infarct sizes, and the impact of therapeutic interventions. However, the MCAO model comes with its own set of challenges, one of them being the technical complexity of the procedure, which demands high surgical expertise to ensure consistency in ischemia severity and reduce variability among animals [108]. The procedure entails slowly lifting the right MCAO using a tungsten hook connected to a micromanipulator and then thermocoagulating it. Both common carotid arteries are subsequently ligated for 90 min. After this period, the common carotid arteries are reopened [109,110]. The muscle and soft tissue are then repositioned, and the skin is sutured. Initially, the occlusion is confirmed visually, followed by measuring and comparing the blood flow to normal levels. An 80% reduction in blood flow is deemed successful [111]. Researchers use various durations of MCAO to mimic different levels of stroke severity [112,113]. This approach allows them to investigate the underlying mechanisms of brain injury and assess potential therapeutic interventions. The occlusion periods can range from 20 [114], 30 [115], 45 [116], 50, 60, 70 [113], 90 [117], and 120 [118] minutes to permanent occlusion [119]. However, the success rate of PSD modeling using the MCAO model alone is limited. While some mice/rats with MCAO may exhibit depressive behaviors, these are often short lived and can include anxiety-like behaviors. To achieve more consistent and prolonged depressive behaviors, it is necessary to combine MCAO with other techniques, such as chronic unpredictable mild stress (CUMS). This combined approach enhances the validity and reliability of PSD models by more accurately replicating the complex pathophysiological and behavioral aspects of PSD. Such methodologies help to create a more comprehensive model, allowing for more in-depth studies and better understanding of PSD mechanisms [35].

5.2. MCAO Model Combined with CUMS

Animals undergoing MCAO followed by chronic mild stress exhibit a heightened severity of depression-like behavior compared to those undergoing MCAO alone [35]. This model is advantageous as it mimics the chronic stress often experienced by stroke survivors and allows for the study of PSD. This model was successfully demonstrated in both rats [120,121] and mice [122,123]. Stressors may include mild physical stress (electric shock, tail clamp, restraint stress, forced swim), social stress (isolation, overcrowding), and environmental stress (altered light–dark cycle, food or water deprivation, cage tilt or cage shaking, wet bedding). The stressors and duration for implementing CUMS can vary significantly, between 21 [124], 28 [125–127], 35 [128–130], 42 [131,132], 49 [133], and 56 days [134,135], involving both group and individual housing (Table 1).

Table 1. CUMS models of depression according to stressors and duration.

	Stressors and Duration													Days of CUMS/Mice Housing
Gaignier F., 2018 [124]	Alterations of the light-dark cycle	Cage tilt 1 h, 2 h, 15 h		Food deprivation overnight 15 h	Illumination at night 15 h		Small cage 1 h, 2 h	Soiled cage overnight 15 h	Paired housing 2 h					21 days Individually housing
Zhang M., 2023 [125]	Exposure to a stroboscope 12 h	Cage tilt 12 h	Traffic noise (70–90 dB) 6 h	Food deprivation 12 h	Illumination at night 12 h			Food and water deprivation 24 h	Crowding: ten mice per cage 12 h	Water deprivation 12 h	Level shaking 15 min			28 days Individually housing
Yan W., 2021 [126]	Ice water swimming 5 min	Cage tilt 5 min	Exposure to an empty bottle 1 h	Food deprivation 24 h	Illumination at night 12 h		Restraint stress 2 h	Soiled cage 24 h	Exposure to a foreign object 24 h	Water deprivation 24 h				28 days Group housing
Wu J., 2021 [128]	Ice water swimming 5 min	Cage tilt 24 h	Foot electric shock twice	Food deprivation 24 h	Continuous illumination 24 h		Restraint stress 2 h	Wet bedding 24 h	Tail-clamp 90 s	Water deprivation 24 h	Cage shaking 15 min			35 days Individually housing
Wang Y.I., 2021 [129]	Ice water swimming 5 min	Cage tilt 24 h		Food deprivation 24 h	Continuous illumination 24 h		Restraint stress 6 h	Wet bedding 24 h		Water deprivation 24 h	Cage shaking 30 min			35 days Individually housing
Wang G., 2019 [130]	Ice water swimming 5 min	Cage tilt 12 h	Plantar electrical stimulation 10 min	Food deprivation 12 h	Continuous illumination 36 h		White noise 12 h	Soiled cage 24 h	Tail nipping 2 min	Water deprivation 12 h	Exposure to a stroboscope 2 h			35 days Group housing
Wen G., 2019 [131]	Exposure to a stroboscope overnight	Cage tilt 4 h	120-dB noise overnight	Food deprivation 24 h	Alterations of the light-dark cycle		Restraint stress 4 h	Wet bedding 4 h		Water deprivation 24 h				42 days Individually housing
Li M., 2014 [132]	Alterations of the light-dark cycle	Cage tilt 12 h	Exposure to an empty bottle 10 min	Food deprivation 24 h	Overnight illumination	White noise 1 h	Overhang 10 min	Soiled cage 24 h	Exposure to a foreign object 12 h	Water deprivation 24 h	Tail pinch 1 min	Oscillation 5 min		42 days Group housing
Xie M., 2022 [133]	No bedding 24 h	Cage tilt 24 h		Food deprivation 24 h	Overnight illumination (twice per week)		Restraint stress 6 h	Wet bedding 24 h	Tail pinching 5 min	Water deprivation 24 h	Cage shaking 15 min			49 days Individually housing
Wassouf Z., 2019 [134]	Switched day/night-cycle 48 h	Cage tilt 2 h		Food deprivation 16 h	Illumination at night 12 h		Restraint stress 1 h		Rat confrontation 30 min	Water deprivation 16 h				56 days Individually housing
Wang Y., 2021 [135]	4 °C exposure 1 h	Cage tilt 12 h		Food deprivation 23 h	Day/night inversion		Restraint stress 1 h	Damp bedding 24 h		Water deprivation 23 h	Cage shaking 30 min			56 days Group housing

5.3. MCAO Model Combined with Social Isolation

Rodents are highly social mammals, and single housing, mimicking social isolation, can lead to various behavioral and physiological changes, including depressive-like behaviors [136]. Mice that underwent individual housing for 14 days following a stroke exhibited exacerbated depressive-like behavior compared to pair-housed mice [137].

5.4. MCAO + Social Isolation + CUMS Model

The MCAO + social isolation + CUMS protocol stands out as the most extensively utilized approach for modeling PSD in preclinical studies [38]. Following surgery, the animal is individually housed to facilitate postoperative recovery and, subsequently, it undergoes exposure to various stressors throughout the course of the CUMS procedure [138–141]. Previously, it was shown that even without a stroke procedure, social isolation is considered the most fitting housing condition during the CUMS regimen for studying depression [127,142]. This integrative model effectively mimics the human experience of PSD, incorporating both the physical impact of a vascular event and the psychological stress from environmental changes, thereby providing a comprehensive framework for exploring the complex interplay between physical and mental health and environmental factors in post-stroke outcomes.

5.5. MCAO Model Combined with Spatial Restraint Stress

Restraint stress has been demonstrated to impair sociability in rodents [143] and has also been successfully used as a stressor during the CUMS procedure for 2 h [126], 4 h [131], or 6 h [129]. Following MCAO, restraint stress-induced depressive-like behavior, as assessed through behavioral tests, was applied, which resulted in dull hair color and a poor general state [144].

5.6. Bilateral Common Carotid Artery Occlusion (BCCAO) Model

The BCCAO model, introduced as a stroke model, entails ischemic white matter and eye injury and is simpler to establish compared to MCAO [145]. Following BCCAO induction, depressive-like behavior was observed in 5-week-old Balb/c mice [146–148], albino mice [149], and Wistar rats [150] without the need for an additional method to induce PSD.

5.7. BCCAO Model Combined with CUMS

Recent research efforts have employed the BCCAO model, alongside a two-week CUMS protocol, in order to develop a murine (C57B16J) model of PSD [151]. While this model represents a significant advancement in replicating the complexities of PSD, it is important to acknowledge the inherent variability in response among different rodent strains and species.

5.8. Intracerebral Injection of Endothelin-1 (ET-1)

ET-1, a powerful vasoconstrictor produced internally during ischemic stroke, plays a crucial role in neuronal damage and subsequent disability [152]. The administration of ET-1 into the left medial prefrontal cortex (mPFC) of mice has been shown to cause a pronounced and lasting anxiety and depressive phenotype, establishing its potential as a murine model for PSD [153]. In contrast, experiments conducted in rats have demonstrated that ET-1 leads to anxiety-like behaviors but not depressive-like behaviors. This disparity suggests that additional damage to a secondary brain area might be necessary to elicit a depression phenotype in rats, highlighting the complications of modeling PSD across different rodent species [154].

5.9. Photothrombotic Model

Photothrombosis involves the induction of focal cerebral ischemia by illuminating a photosensitive dye in the presence of a light source, leading to thrombus formation and vascular occlusion [155]. One commonly used dye is Rose Bengal, which, when activated by green light (560 nm) [156], generates reactive oxygen species, leading to clot formation and vascular occlusion [157]. Another example is Erythrosin B, which operates in a similar manner but is activated by a different wavelength (near 660 nm) [158] and offers flexibility in experimental setups. These dyes are selected for their high quantum yield of singlet oxygen production, a key factor in inducing rapid and targeted vascular occlusion [159]. The photothrombosis model provides exceptional precision in dictating both the location and extent of ischemic lesions, a feature that has been instrumental in linking specific brain areas to behavioral outcomes. This level of control has facilitated research demonstrating that rodents subjected to ischemic lesions exhibit behavioral changes reminiscent of depression [38].

5.10. Genetic Models of PSD

Genetically modified animals with alterations in specific genes implicated in depression or stroke pathophysiology can also be valuable for studying PSD. For example, knockout mice lacking BDNF [160] and the 5-HT transporter [161] exhibit depressive-like behaviors and impaired neurogenesis. However, future research should aim to elucidate the complex interactions between genetic factors, environmental stressors, and stroke-induced neurobiological changes to enhance the understanding of PSD in these knockout murine models.

6. Assessing Symptoms and Behaviors: Key Tests for Studying PSD

This section outlines a range of behavioral tests crucial for investigating the pathophysiological impacts of stroke and for evaluating the accuracy of animal models and the efficacy of therapeutic interventions (Figure 4). These tests encompass motor function evaluations, assessing coordination and muscle strength, as well as cognition, which measures memory and learning capabilities. Additionally, social behavior tests are discussed, which are used to examine interaction patterns and anxiety levels among animals.

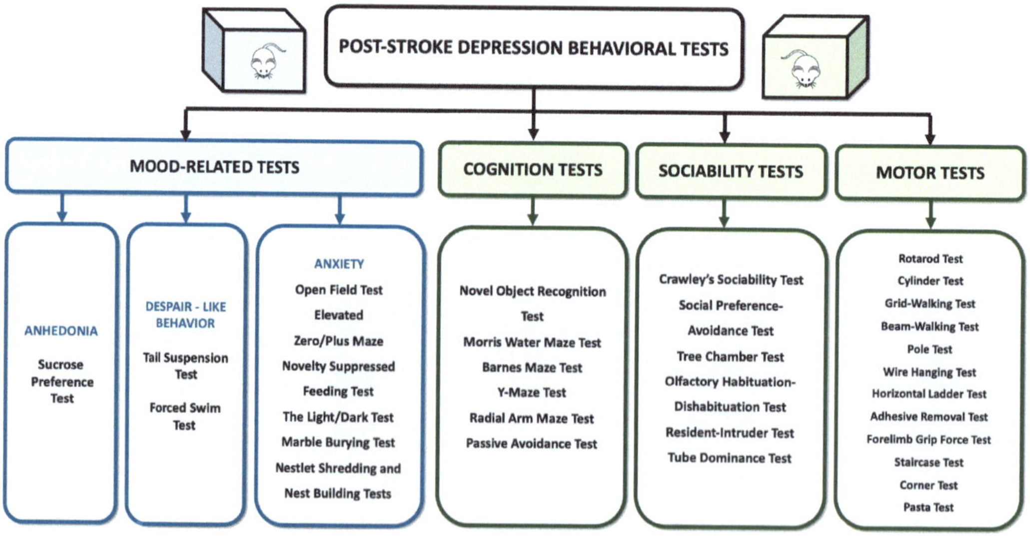

Figure 4. Behavioral assessment methods for post-stroke depression in rodent models.

6.1. Anhedonia Test: Sucrose Preference Test (SPT)

Anhedonia, defined as a diminished capacity to experience pleasure or interest in previously rewarding activities, is a hallmark symptom of depression that can significantly impact prognosis and complicate patient recovery [162]. In rodent models, the assessment of anhedonia primarily relies on measuring the preference for sucrose, a simple yet effective indicator of pleasure-seeking behavior. SPT involves providing each mouse with two identical bottles: one containing a sucrose solution and the other water. The animals are then allowed to choose freely between them [163]. A marked decrease in sucrose consumption is interpreted as an expression of anhedonia [164,165]. The test procedure encompasses several variables, including housing during the habituation, concentration of sucrose solution, period at which the experiments are performed (light/dark), type of habituation to the SPT procedure, type of food/water deprivation during the test, and test duration [166]. SPT has proven to have satisfactory results in various studies on different animal models of PSD. For example, it revealed severe anhedonia after MCAO and 18 consecutive days of CUMS [123]. Also, MCAO and spatial restraint stress led to a decreased percentage of sucrose consumption compared to stroke alone [113]. Lastly, MCAO followed by social isolation showed a significant increase in sucrose consumption for post-stroke pair-housed mice compared to those that were socially isolated [137].

6.2. Depression-like Behavior Tests: Forced Swim Test and Tail Suspension Test

Depression encompasses a complex array of symptoms, including profound feelings of hopelessness, persistent sadness, and thoughts of death or suicide [167]. The forced swim and tail suspension tests have been employed as a means to gauge aspects of despair and motivational withdrawal in rodents, which are considered analogs to the human experience of hopelessness and passive resignation.

The Forced Swim Test (FST) is widely utilized for evaluating despair-like behavior in animal models, quantifying the duration of immobility, except for the minimal movements necessary to maintain the animal's head above water. This behavior is interpreted as a sign of behavioral despair, mirroring aspects of depression [168]. Studies have shown that both MCAO and chronic mild stress can induce despair-like behavior in C57BL/6 mice [35], as well as in albino mice subjected to BCCAO [149].

The Tail Suspension Test (TST) is also used, but only in mouse models. In this test, animals are suspended by their tails, and the duration of immobility is recorded [169], with longer immobility times indicating a higher level of despair. The TST has demonstrated a significant increase in immobility time in C57BL/6 mice five days post-BCCAO [170], NMRI mice 72 h after permanent double ligation of the right common carotid artery [171], and ICR mice following MCAO and spatial restraint stress [172].

6.3. Anxiety Tests: Open Field/Elevated Zero Maze/Novelty Suppressed Feeding/The Light/Dark/Marble Burying

Before conclusively identifying PSD in animal models, it is critical to evaluate the presence of anxiety, as it often coexists with depression and can influence the overall behavior and response of the animal. Anxiety assessment in rodents can be integrated with social interaction tests or conducted through specific behavioral assays designed to measure anxiety levels, such as the ones outlined below.

The Elevated Zero Maze (EZM) [173,174] and Elevated Plus Maze (EPM) Tests [175] use an elevated apparatus designed to invoke anxiety-related behaviors by exploiting the rodent's aversion to open and elevated spaces. The EZM, a circular platform divided into open and closed sections, allows for the assessment of anxiety based on the animal's preference for the safer, enclosed areas over the exposed ones [173,174]. The EPM similarly measures anxiety by recording the time spent in the open arms of a plus-shaped apparatus, with decreased time indicating higher anxiety levels [175]. In experiments involving C57BL/6 mice, the administration of ET-1, a procedure used to mimic stroke conditions, was followed by an assessment using the EPM and indicated that post-ET-1 injection, mice exhibited a marked reduction in the time spent in the open arms of the EPM, suggesting heightened anxiety levels [153].

The Open Field Test (OFT) serves as a critical tool for assessing anxiety-like behavior in rodents by tracking the amount of time they spend in the center of an open arena [176].

Anxiety levels in this context are analyzed from the animal's exploration patterns, with a preference for the periphery over the center indicating higher anxiety [176]. Experiments using C57Bl/6 mice subjected to MCAO and 17 days of chronic mild stress revealed significant anxiety with OFT, as demonstrated by reduced central area exploration [35]. Similarly, MCAO followed by periods of social isolation also led to a noticeable decrease in the time these mice spent in the center [137].

The Novelty Suppressed Feeding Test (NSFT) is a behavioral assay designed to evaluate anxiety and depression-related behaviors by measuring both the amount of food intake and the delay before the animal engages with a new, highly palatable food item [177]. This test is predicated on the natural conflict between the fear of a novel environment and the motivation to eat, with increased latency and reduced food consumption indicating heightened anxiety or depressive states [177]. Studies involving C57BL/6 mice demonstrated that after microinjection of ET-1, mice exhibited a decreased interest in food and a significant delay before beginning to eat the novel food, suggesting an increase in anxiety or depressive-like behavior [153]. Similarly, following an MCAO procedure, mice showed increased latency to approaching and consuming the food pellet three weeks post-ischemia [178].

The Light/Dark Test (L/D Test) measures an animal's willingness to explore or avoid new environments [179,180]. This test utilizes a chamber divided into illuminated and dark sections and allows measurement of the time taken to enter the light compartment and the number of transitions between compartments, reflecting the animal's exploratory behavior and its aversion to brightly lit areas, respectively [179]. A preference for spending more time in the dark compartment is interpreted as an indication of anxiety. The L/D Test has been effectively employed in studying PSD in murine models [153].

In the Marble Burying Test, animals are placed into a cage layered with bedding, in which marbles or similar small objects are evenly distributed. Researchers then measure the number of marbles the rodent buries within a specified period. A tendency to bury more marbles is interpreted as an indication of heightened anxiety or compulsive tendencies, providing a straightforward method for assessing these behaviors [181,182].

Nestlet Shredding and Nest Building Tests also serve as valuable tools for determining stress levels in rodents [183]. These tests examine the natural nesting behavior, where rodents are provided with materials, like cotton nestlets, to build nests. The extent and quality of the nest constructed, along with the degree of shredding of the provided materials, are indicative of the animal's well-being, with poor nesting behavior suggesting elevated stress or discomfort [183].

6.4. Social Withdrawal Tests: Crawley's Sociability/Social Preference-Avoidance/Tree Chamber/Olfactory Habituation-Dishabituation/Resident-Intruder/Tube Dominance

Social withdrawal is a critical symptom observed in numerous psychiatric disorders, notably depression [184]. The array of behavioral tests deployed to study this condition in rodents not only sheds light on the underlying mechanisms but also holds significant value in assessing social withdrawal symptoms associated with PSD [185–187]. These tests, designed to evaluate interactions among rodents or their response to social stimuli, provide insight into changes in social behavior potentially indicative of PSD and are briefly described below.

Crawley's Sociability Test is a key method for evaluating social behavior and novelty preference in rodents [188]. This procedure involves an initial interaction phase where the test animal is given the opportunity to interact with a "stranger" mouse that it has not previously encountered. After a 10 min interaction period, a second, novel "stranger" mouse is introduced into the apparatus. The subject mouse is then observed to see whether it shows a preference for the already-investigated unfamiliar mouse or the new, novel unfamiliar mouse. This test provides valuable insights into the nuances of rodent social behavior, particularly after experiencing a stroke.

The Social Preference–Avoidance Test is used for both mice and rats and is designed to measure the dynamics of social interaction, specifically the speed of approach or avoidance displayed by the animal during the test [189,190]. This test provides insight into the social tendencies of rodents, offering a nuanced view of how they navigate social spaces and whether they show a propensity towards engaging with or avoiding other animals.

The Three Chamber Test is employed to assess sociability and social memory by evaluating a rodent's preference for an unfamiliar conspecific or an inanimate object and its preference for a new or a familiar conspecific [191]. This test effectively distinguishes between the animal's interest in social interactions and its ability to recognize and differentiate between familiar and unfamiliar individuals.

The Olfactory Habituation–Dishabituation Test, while initially utilized in evaluating autistic behaviors in mice, serves a broader purpose in assessing the olfactory system, which is vital for studying sensory processing in the brain [192]. Mice naturally exhibit a preference for novel scents over familiar ones [193]. Assessment of the olfactory system has proven useful for studying sensory processing in the brain [194] but also serves as a valuable tool for assessing social interaction, memory, and anxiety [195]. Social interaction is conditioned by the level of anxiety, while anxious behavior is often associated with depression [196].

The Resident–Intruder Test is another significant behavioral assay where a resident rodent is confronted with an unfamiliar "intruder" in its environment. The resultant behaviors, ranging from aggressive to affiliative, are observed and scored. This test is instrumental in evaluating behaviors such as territorial aggression, social dominance, and social recognition memory [197].

The Tube Dominance Test is primarily employed to measure social hierarchy and dominance in mice [198]. After a day of habituation and training, two mice enter a narrow tube from opposite sides and meet in the middle. The mouse that persuades the other to retreat is deemed the winner, respectively dominant. The test was successfully used in a mouse model of depression involving CUMS [199] and could provide additional insights regarding PSD.

6.5. Cognitive Impairments Tests: Morris Water Maze/Barnes Maze/Y-Maze/Novel Object Recognition/Radial Arm Maze/Passive Avoidance

When dealing with depression, individuals often experience cognitive impairments, including difficulties with memory and attention, loss of concentration, and problems with learning processes [200]. These cognitive symptoms are critical components of the overall clinical representation and can significantly affect the quality of life and daily functioning. Recognizing the importance of these symptoms, cognitive assessment in PSD has also been approached through various behavioral tests in research settings that are described below.

The Morris Water Maze Test is a widely recognized method for evaluating spatial learning and memory in rodents. Animals are placed in a sizable water pool with a platform submerged beneath the surface. Rodents must navigate using spatial cues in order to find the platform. Through repeated trials, they gradually learn and remember the platform's location, demonstrating spatial memory retention [201]. Pre-experimental learning trials are often conducted to familiarize rodents with the task [202,203]. Studies have shown an increased latency to find the platform in MCAO mice in the 3rd [178] and 6th week after stroke [35].

The Barnes Maze Test offers an alternative to the Morris Water Maze, utilizing a dry, less stressful environment for the rodent. This test involves a circular platform with multiple holes around its edge, one of which leads to an escape box. Rodents are required to navigate using spatial cues to find this escape route, providing insights into their spatial learning and memory capabilities [204].

The Y-Maze Test is another critical tool that measures the willingness of rodents to explore a new environment by recording the number of arm entries and the sequence of these entries to assess spontaneous alternation behavior [205]. This test is particularly useful for observing short-term memory by analyzing the percentage of correct alternations made by the rodent, reflecting its ability to remember previously visited arms [205]. Research involving C57BL/6 mice post-MCAO surgery and subsequent individual housing revealed a decrease in the percentage of correct alternations in the Y-maze, suggesting impairments in spatial working memory as compared to pair-housed mice [137].

The Novel Object Recognition Test (NORT) serves as a behavioral assay for evaluating memory capability, particularly recognition memory [206]. Initially, animals are allowed to familiarize themselves with an arena containing two identical objects [207]. Subsequently, one of the original objects is replaced with a novel object, and the animal's interaction with both objects is observed [208]. A preference for exploring the novel object over the familiar one is typically indicative of healthy recognition memory, as it suggests the animal remembers the original object and finds the new one more interesting [207,208]. Studies employing NORT have demonstrated its utility in detecting memory impairment. For example, socially isolated mice subjected to MCAO showed impairment in recognition memory, as evidenced by their equal interest in exploring both novel and familiar objects. This lack of preference for the novel object indicates a difficulty in recognizing or remembering the previously encountered object, underscoring the impact of social isolation and stroke on cognitive functions [137].

The Radial Arm Maze Test typically consists of a central platform with multiple arms extending outward, resembling the spokes of a wheel [209]. At the end of each arm, food rewards or other incentives are placed to motivate the rodent. The animal is placed in the central area and must efficiently navigate through the maze to collect the rewards. Successful navigation involves remembering which arms have already been visited to avoid unnecessary revisits, thereby demonstrating the animal's ability to learn and remember spatial information [210].

The Passive Avoidance Test is a specific behavioral assay used to assess learning and memory after stroke [211]. Rodents are typically placed into a two-compartment apparatus, one illuminated and one darkened. Initially, the animal is allowed to explore both compartments freely. After a predetermined period of time, usually during the training phase, the animal receives a mild aversive stimulus (i.e., foot shock) upon entering one of the compartments, typically the darkened compartment. This creates an association between the aversive stimulus and the compartment. During the testing phase, the animal is again placed in the apparatus and allowed to freely explore both compartments. The latency to enter the aversive compartment is recorded. Animals with intact memory will exhibit a longer latency to enter the aversive compartment due to their association with the stimulus [212].

6.6. Motor Function Tests: Rotarod/Cylinder/Grid-Walking/Beam-Walking/Pole/Wire Hanging/Horizontal Ladder/Adhesive Removal/Forelimb Grip/Staircase/Corner/Pasta

Assessing motor function in murine models of PSD is essential for comprehending the effects of stroke. Accordingly, a range of tests has been introduced to measure various aspects of motor skills, including coordination, balance, skilled locomotion, muscle strength, and forelimb functionality, and these are described below and shown in Figure 4.

The Rotarod Test stands as the benchmark for evaluating motor function, particularly coordination and balance in mice [43,213]. In this test, mice are placed on a rod that rotates at a controlled speed. The duration for which each mouse remains on the rod before falling is recorded, serving as a measure of its motor coordination and balance [214]. Additionally, a variation of the Rotarod, the RotaWheel, has emerged as a novel experimental tool for assessing locomotion in mice [215,216]. This apparatus offers a new dimension to the evaluation of motor skills, providing insights into locomotion abilities as well as endurance [215,216].

The Cylinder Test is a crucial assessment for evaluating forelimb asymmetry, particularly in the context of sensorimotor function following stroke [217]. In this test, mice are placed inside a transparent cylinder, and the use of their forelimbs during vertical exploration or rearing movements is carefully observed and recorded. Stroke-induced deficits can lead to a noticeable asymmetry in forelimb use, where the animal might predominantly use one limb over the other, reflecting the impairment of sensorimotor function to one side of the body. This test has frequently been adopted to assess motor function recovery or decline after stroke, providing valuable insights into the extent of motor rehabilitation or the effectiveness of therapeutic interventions aimed at mitigating motor function deficits [153]. The ability of this test to detect subtle changes in limb usage offers a sensitive measure of motor skills and recovery.

The Grid-Walking Test is specifically designed to evaluate skilled locomotion and motor coordination [217]. Mice are placed on a grid that features widely spaced holes. As the animals navigate across the grid, the incidence of foot slips through the holes is recorded [218]. This approach allows for precise quantification of motor deficits, particularly those affecting coordination and the ability to perform complex movements. Stroke-induced impairments are often manifested as an increase in the number of foot slips, indicating a loss of motor control or diminished spatial awareness [217,219].

The Beam-Walking Test assesses balance, coordination, and skilled locomotion [220], and it requires a raised-beam apparatus and training sessions for the subjects [221]. Animals have to traverse a narrow beam to reach a secure platform, with their performance providing insight into their motor capabilities. Both the time taken to cross the beam and the incidence of foot slips during the attempt are key metrics for assessing the presence and extent of motor deficits, particularly those resulting from stroke-induced damage. When the Beam-Walking Test was been applied to Sprague Dawley rats following MCAO, significant functional impairments were documented [222,223].

The Pole Test involves placing animals at the top of a vertical pole, where they are trained to perform a turnaround maneuver before descending the pole headfirst. Evaluation focuses on the time it takes for the animal to initiate and complete the turnaround maneuver, as well as the descent [43]. This approach allows researchers to assess motor coordination, agility, and the animal's overall ability to control and execute complex motor tasks. The test proved useful in the evaluation of mice after MCAO [224].

The Wire Hanging Test examines the forelimb motor strength of mice after stroke [224]. The mice undergo training to hang their bodies from a steel wire, which measures 2 mm in diameter, solely using their forelimbs. This training spans two days, including three trials per day. The average holding time across the three trials is calculated and analyzed [225]. A lower holding time is indicative of a decrease in motor strength.

The Horizontal Ladder Test is used to evaluate walking ability [226]. The animals are trained to cross the ladder from a neutral cage to reach their home cage [227]. During the test, the number of successful steps, slips, or missed steps is measured [228]. These assessments provide valuable insights into the animals' motor skills and coordination abilities.

The Adhesive Removal Test is another method for evaluating sensorimotor deficits and somatosensory function in rodent models after stroke [229,230]. Small adhesive stimuli, such as sticky tape or adhesive-backed dots, are placed on the forepaws of the animal, and their ability to detect, remove, and discriminate between the stimuli is assessed [231].

The Forelimb Grip Force Test is used to measure muscle strength, providing a quantitative assessment [223]. Studies have reported a decrease in grip force for both the right and left hind paws in C57BL mice 7 days following Distal Middle Cerebral Artery (DMCA) occlusion. Interestingly, this reduction in grip strength was not observed 28 days post-stroke, indicating some degree of recovery over time [232]. Additionally, rats subjected to MCAO combined with CUMS exhibited a significant decrease in grip force 22 days after the injury [223].

The Staircase Test is commonly used with rodents to assess skilled reaching and grasping abilities, particularly in the context of examining motor function and recovery after stroke. In this test, rodents are typically placed in a cage equipped with a staircase apparatus consisting of a series of steps with food rewards placed on each step. The animals' ability to navigate the staircase and retrieve the food rewards offers insight into their skilled reaching and grasping capabilities and overall motor recovery [233].

The Corner Test also provides valuable insights into motor asymmetry and sensorimotor function [43]. Following a stroke, the rodent is placed near a corner of a testing apparatus, typically a rectangular or triangular enclosure with two converging walls forming the corner. As the rodent approaches the corner, it tends to turn in the direction of its more impaired side, leading to a higher frequency of turns toward the affected side compared to the unaffected one. Researchers observe and record the direction of the turns as well as any asymmetry in movement patterns [234]. This method allows for the assessment of both the preference in turning direction and any motor deficits that might influence this preference, offering a direct indication of unilateral sensorimotor impairment.

The Pasta Test provides valuable insights into the motor abilities and functional recovery of rodents following neurological insults [235]. Animals are typically given a piece of pasta to manipulate and eat. The researchers then observe and analyze the rodent's behavior, focusing on the symmetry and effectiveness of its forepaw movements during the manipulation and consumption of the pasta. Impairments in fine motor skills or asymmetrical use of the forepaws can indicate deficits in manual dexterity, indicative of neurological damage or dysfunction [236].

Motor dysfunction and depressive symptoms frequently coexist in patients following a stroke, and there is evidence to suggest that these motor deficits can influence the onset and severity of depressive symptoms [237]. The DigiGait system provides detailed and quantitative assessments of gait and offers a unique opportunity to study these motor abnormalities in stroke models [43]. Although DigiGait has not been extensively used specifically for PSD research, its ability to precisely measure changes in gait and coordination could be invaluable in understanding the relationship between motor deficits and depressive behaviors post-stroke [238]. Incorporating DigiGait assessments in PSD studies could enhance our understanding of how motor impairments contribute to or exacerbate depressive symptoms. Future research may explore this intersection, potentially leading to more comprehensive therapeutic strategies that address both the motor and psychological aspects of post-stroke recovery.

7. Pathophysiological Mechanisms Involved in PSD

The pathophysiological mechanisms underlying PSD are multifactorial, involving biological, neurochemical, and psychosocial factors that interplay to reveal depressive symptoms following a cerebrovascular event. Stroke lesions in critical brain areas, notably the prefrontal cortex, limbic system, and basal ganglia, play a pivotal role in disrupting neurotransmission pathways essential for mood regulation, thus contributing to the onset of PSD [56]. Specifically, lesions in the left hemisphere (left frontal cortex and basal ganglia) are correlated with a higher incidence of depression, which is attributed to diminished levels of 5-HT and norepinephrine (NE) [56]. In contrast, another study also points to the right hemisphere's involvement in PSD, particularly during the subacute phase (1–6 months) [70]. This neurotransmitter hypothesis further underscores the role of monoamines (NE, 5-HT, DA) in mood regulation, as ischemic injury notably decreases their production and availability. Ischemic lesions can disrupt the axons containing biogenic amines that ascend from the brainstem to the cerebral cortex, resulting in reduced levels of monoamines in limbic structures found in the frontal and temporal lobes, as well as the basal ganglia. In turn, this influences motivation-related behaviors such as salience detection, reward and punishment learning, processing incentives, decision making, goal-directed actions, and regulation of anxiety levels [239]. Additionally, genetic predispositions, such as the 5-HTTLPR genotype, also modulate susceptibility to PSD [240–242].

Inflammatory cytokines also play significant roles in the pathophysiology of both stroke and depression. Specifically, the IL-10 -1082A/A genotype has been linked to PSD in general, while the IL-4 + 33C/C genotype has shown an association with major PSD [243]. These genetic variants highlight the interplay between immune response and psychiatric outcomes following stroke, suggesting potential genetic markers for susceptibility to PSD subtypes. Inflammation is a critical contributor, with elevated levels of pro-inflammatory cytokines (IL-1β, IL-4, IL-8, TNF-α) [244,245] and the activation of pathways, such as NLRP3, signifying an influence on PSD pathophysiology [246]. Neuroendocrine dysregulation, especially concerning the HPA axis and resultant elevated cortisol levels, also contributes significantly to PSD, highlighting the neuroendocrine system's critical role in mood regulation [247,248]. Poor post-stroke prognosis is linked to alterations in the HPA axis, elevated levels of catecholamines and natriuretic peptides, and reduced levels of melatonin and IGF-1 [249]. Moreover, neurotrophic factors, like brain-derived neurotrophic factor (BDNF) and glial cell line-derived neurotrophic factor (GDNF), essential for neuronal health and regeneration post-injury, are also linked to PSD development, with variations in their levels and methylation status closely associated with depressive outcomes post-stroke [250,251]. Together, these mechanisms offer a comprehensive insight into the intricate number of factors contributing to PSD [56].

8. Strain Differences in Rodents

Strain differences in rodents can significantly influence the manifestation and understanding of PSD [252]. The injection of ET-1 produced a pronounced and persistent anxiety and depression phenotype in C57/BL6 mice [153]. However, in Sprague Dawley rats, it resulted in anxiety-like behavior while it failed to induce depressive-like responses [154]. Even in various rat strains, distinct behavior patterns emerge following stroke. Lewis rats exhibited behavior indicative of depression but not fatigue, whereas Wistar and Sprague Dawley rats displayed behavior indicative of fatigue but not depression [252]. A future and comprehensive analysis of rodent strain-related differences should provide insight into symptom pathophysiology as well as guide researchers in choosing the appropriate mouse or rat strain. Additionally, the development of transgenic animals may also play a critical role in enhancing the translatability of preclinical tests for PSD. Introducing specific genetic modifications will enable researchers to generate animal models that more closely mimic the genetic and molecular aspects of human PSD.

9. Translatability of PSD Research

Examining clinical trial registries is essential in order to gain a broad understanding of the progress made in ongoing PSD research. An analysis of PSD research indicates a significant disparity between the abundance of preclinical studies and the relatively limited number of clinical trials. A PubMed search with the keyword "post stroke depression" over the past twenty years produces a total of 3273 entries. This includes 127 meta-analyses, 463 reviews, 180 systematic reviews, and 331 manuscripts related to clinical trials specifically focusing on PSD.

Further examination of the National Institutes of Health's (NIH) ClinicalTrials.gov registry (accessed up to and including 20 April 2024] revealed 68 clinical studies at various stages. This search encompassed studies marked both as completed and actively enrolling. Of these, only thirteen are actively recruiting patients, an additional three are not yet enrolling, and one is active but not recruiting. These trials, which primarily involve adult participants of both sexes, range from early Phase 1 to Phase 4, with 43 categorized as "Not applicable" regarding their phase. Fifty-three of these trials are interventional, with a focus on directly modifying participant treatment or behavior to assess efficacy and safety outcomes. There are also 15 observational studies, which typically gather data on PSD without altering the treatment regimen. Additionally, there are four patient registries that systematically collect information about patients with PSD to facilitate future research. None of the studies are classified under expanded access, intermediate-size populations, or treatment IND/Protocol categories, indicating a focus on controlled research settings rather than broad or emergency-use interventions. Remarkably, only four of these studies have reported results on ClinicalTrials.gov. This stark contrast to the abundance of preclinical studies highlights a significant translational gap. As such, there is a pressing need for innovative methodologies and testing that can bridge this divide, which are essential in accelerating the development of effective clinical PSD treatments.

10. Future Directions

PSD represents a prevalent and severe human neuropsychiatric complication that impacts a significant number of stroke survivors, presenting challenges not only for the patients but also for the healthcare system and support networks [60]. In this comprehensive review, we compiled and analyzed the current scientific literature on PSD, covering its epidemiological landscape, identifiable risk factors, and the biological and neurological underpinnings. We also explored the tools available for studying PSD in preclinical settings, including various animal (rodent) models and behavioral analyses. Our findings highlighted the complex nature of PSD and underscored the challenges associated with accurately modeling and evaluating its manifestations in preclinical settings. Recent studies have highlighted several pharmacological treatments for PSD. For example, selective serotonin reuptake inhibitors (SSRIs) are commonly prescribed and have demonstrated efficacy in alleviating depressive symptoms in stroke patients. Other antidepressants, such as trazodone and tricyclic antidepressants, like nortriptyline, have also been used with varying degrees of success [253,254]. These treatments work by modulating neurotransmitter levels, thereby reducing depressive symptoms and enhancing the overall quality of life. However, the selection of medication must be carefully considered due to the potential side effects and interactions with other drugs frequently prescribed to stroke patients. Neuromodulation techniques, such as repetitive transcranial magnetic stimulation and transcranial direct current stimulation, along with innovative psychosocial interventions, hold promise as effective treatments and warrant further investigations [254]. Furthermore, effective management of PSD necessitates a multidisciplinary approach that integrates pharmacological treatments with psychological, rehabilitative, and social interventions. This strategy ensures that all aspects of the patient's condition are addressed, promoting better overall outcomes. Concurrently, ongoing research is focused on developing novel therapeutic strategies, aiming to enhance the efficacy of treatments and minimize side effects [255].

The combination of MCAO with social isolation and CUMS has emerged as a prevalent murine model for studying PSD [38]. The duration of the CUMS procedure can vary for 3, 4, or 6 weeks, reflecting the different intensities and duration of stress exposure in studies that induce depressive-like behaviors [138–140,256,257]. Numerous studies utilizing the MCAO+CUMS model explored different aspects of PSD [120–123], indicating that social isolation on its own can significantly contribute to the induction of rodent depressive-like behavior [136]. This underscores the importance of social factors in the development of depressive symptoms post-stroke, suggesting that the most effective animal models of PSD must incorporate a multifaceted approach, mirroring the complex interplay of human symptoms. Animal models of PSD exhibit distinct pathophysiological changes, which are important for understanding the mechanisms underlying this condition. The MCAO model shows microglial activation [258,259] and elevated levels of pro-inflammatory cytokines in the brain [260,261] that are also involved in the neurodegenerative process [262]. The additional chronic restraint stress and foot shock stress have been observed to decrease BDNF levels [263]. The CUMS model induces the activation of the HPA axis [264], leading to elevated cortisol levels [134]. Finally, the combined models of PSD provide insights into the interaction between ischemia-induced brain damage and stress-induced neuroinflammation, offering a more complex understanding of PSD pathophysiology. By integrating findings from different models, researchers can better elucidate the complex biological processes contributing to PSD and develop more effective therapeutic strategies.

In order to develop a comprehensive animal model of PSD, it is imperative to thoroughly assess all depression-related aspects, such as the association between left hemisphere stroke lesions and the manifestation of depressive symptoms [56,265]. Approximately 40% of individuals who experience left hemispheric infarctions develop depression, typically exhibiting mild to moderate symptoms shortly after the stroke or after several months [266]. However, the hypothesis that the location of the brain lesion influences the risk of PSD is contested, with several studies challenging the notion that depression is more commonly associated with left-hemisphere strokes than with right-hemisphere strokes [70,267,268].

Age and gender also represent crucial factors that significantly impact the study of neurodegenerative diseases, including PSD. Research predominantly utilizes young animal models, which may not accurately reproduce the age-related complexities of PSD in humans [34,146–148]. Including older animals in these studies will enhance model validity, improve our understanding of age as a critical factor in disease progression and recovery [80], and hopefully reduce the translational gap in clinical applications. Moreover, the prevalence of studies focusing on male rodents [35,113,123,137] may overlook key sex-based dimorphic differences that could influence both the presentation and progression of PSD. Males and females may respond differently to stroke, with potential variations in motor function, mood, cognitive abilities, and memory tasks [269]. Notably, female rodents are more prone to weight loss during chronic social stress and may exhibit heightened anxious behaviors [270]. These differences are modulated by sex hormones, like estrogen and testosterone, which are also known to affect stroke responses and depressive behaviors [271]. For example, estrogen was shown to alleviate depressive symptoms post-stroke [272]; however, recent findings suggest that the estrous cycle in females does not significantly impact behavior or neurogenesis under basal conditions [273,274], indicating that sex differences might not drastically alter outcomes in commonly used behavioral tests. However, the inflammatory response to stroke, which is integral to PSD pathology, appears to vary between sexes, with females often showing a stronger anti-inflammatory response [275]. Future research should continue to address these variables, providing a deeper understanding of how age and sex influence the development, treatment, and ultimately, recovery from PSD. Such insights are vital for designing tailored neuro- or psychotherapeutic clinical approaches.

Behavioral tests play a crucial role in assessing depressive-like behaviors in animal models that aid our understanding of the multifaceted nature of PSD. These tests evaluate a range of symptoms, from mood disturbances and cognitive deficits to motor dysfunctions and social behavior changes. Commonly employed tests include the sucrose preference test for anhedonia, the forced swim and tail suspension tests for despair-like behavior, or social interaction tests for assessing social withdrawal. Additionally, motor function tests also help to gauge the physical aspects of depression, which are often impacted in post-stroke conditions [39]. Each test is designed to measure specific symptoms associated with PSD, providing a comprehensive view of the animal's emotional and cognitive state post-stroke. However, interpreting the results of these behavioral tests requires careful consideration and interpretation. The inherent variability in rodent behavior, the subjective nature of depressive symptoms, and the potential for human error in collecting data during the experiment or subsequent analyses necessitate a cautious approach [33,252]. Variations in test conditions, handling, and even the environment can influence the outcomes, potentially affecting the accuracy of the data [166]. Given these challenges, there is a pressing need for future research to focus on refining existing behavioral tests and also develop more sophisticated and direct methods for assessing PSD. This involves enhancing the objectivity, sensitivity, and specificity of behavioral assays to accurately capture the nuanced manifestations of PSD in animal models. Improvements in test design, execution, and data analysis can lead to more reliable and valid measurements of depressive-like behaviors, facilitating the identification of effective treatments and interventions for PSD.

In conclusion, this review summarized the complex and multifaceted nature of PSD, emphasizing the significant challenges involved in modeling and evaluating this condition in preclinical trials. Our exploration into the epidemiology, risk factors, underlying mechanisms, and the development of animal models for PSD has underscored the crucial need for advanced, nuanced approaches in preclinical research. Indeed, bridging the gap between animal studies and clinical applications requires focused efforts to refine and develop animal models and sophisticated behavioral assessments that more accurately mirror the human condition and behavior. Enhancing these models and assessments is essential for improving the translation of research findings into the clinic, resulting in more effective diagnostic tools and treatments for PSD. This includes addressing the variability in rodent responses, the challenge of extending the results to human pathology, and the integration of diverse biological, psychological, and social determinants of PSD. Additionally, considerations of age, gender differences, and strain variability among rodents highlight the importance of a custom-tailored approach in understanding and treating PSD. This approach will help ensure that the insights gained in the laboratory can be effectively applied in the clinic, ultimately improving patient outcomes and accelerating recovery. While most previous studies address these aspects individually, our aim was to integrate all recent developments in PSD pathology within both clinical and experimental contexts in order to provide a complete perspective, highlighting the gap between human clinical data and preclinical research.

11. Summary

PSD stands as a significant barrier to recovery from stroke and is defined by its complexity stemming from an interplay of physiological, psychological, and social factors. PSD research has expanded our understanding, revealing that risk factors such as age, gender, pre-stroke psychiatric history, and the physical location of the stroke significantly influence the likelihood and severity of PSD. Animal models, particularly those involving rodents, are pivotal for understanding the pathophysiological underpinnings of PSD. Models such as MCAO, BCAO, and various genetic models are utilized to mimic stroke in rodents, enabling the study of depressive-like behaviors subsequent to cerebrovascular insults. Techniques combining MCAO with CUMS or social isolation post-stroke have been particularly insightful and highlight the role of PSD environmental and social stressors. Further, behavioral assessments are crucial in measuring symptoms, like anhedonia, despair, hopelessness, and motor dysfunctions, which help evaluate the efficacy of potential treatments and the validity of the models themselves. Despite these advances, translating findings from animal models to human patients remains challenging. Variability in rodent responses, differences in stroke etiology, and the subjective nature of depressive symptoms complicate the direct application of preclinical results to the clinic. Moreover, the outcomes of these studies underline the need for a personalized approach to treatment, considering individual risk factors such as age, sex, comorbidities, social network, etc. While animal models and behavioral studies have greatly contributed to our understanding of PSD, the relatively limited number of clinical studies compared to the many preclinical studies underscores the complexity of this condition and the existing translational gap. Advancements in these areas are vital for developing targeted psychiatric, neuro-, or psychological interventions, ultimately improving the quality of life and recovery outcomes for stroke survivors worldwide.

Author Contributions: M.I.M., A.G., B.C., M.H. and A.P.-W.: methodology. B.C., M.H., A.G. and A.P.-W.: validation. M.I.M. and A.G.: formal analysis. M.I.M. and A.G.: investigation. A.G. and M.I.M.: resources. M.I.M. and A.G.: data curation. M.I.M. and A.G.: original draft. B.C., M.H. and A.P.-W.: final manuscript. B.C., M.H. and A.P.-W.: supervision. All authors contributed to editorial changes in the manuscript. All authors have read and agreed to the published version of the manuscript.

Funding: The Article Processing Charges were funded by the University of Medicine and Pharmacy of Craiova, Romania.

Institutional Review Board Statement: Not applicable.

Informed Consent Statement: Not applicable.

Data Availability Statement: No new data were created or analyzed in this study. Data sharing is not applicable to this article.

Conflicts of Interest: The authors declare no conflicts of interest. The funders had no role in the design of the study; in the collection, analyses, or interpretation of data; in the writing of the manuscript; or in the decision to publish the results.

References

1. Donkor, E.S. Stroke in the 21(st) Century: A Snapshot of the Burden, Epidemiology, and Quality of Life. *Stroke Res. Treat.* **2018**, *2018*, 3238165. [CrossRef] [PubMed]
2. Fekadu, G.; Adola, B.; Mosisa, G.; Shibiru, T.; Chelkeba, L. Clinical characteristics and treatment outcomes among stroke patients hospitalized to Nekemte referral hospital, western Ethiopia. *J. Clin. Neurosci.* **2020**, *71*, 170–176. [CrossRef]
3. Boehme, A.K.; Esenwa, C.; Elkind, M.S. Stroke Risk Factors, Genetics, and Prevention. *Circ. Res.* **2017**, *120*, 472–495. [CrossRef] [PubMed]
4. Arboix, A. Cardiovascular risk factors for acute stroke: Risk profiles in the different subtypes of ischemic stroke. *World J. Clin. Cases* **2015**, *3*, 418–429. [CrossRef] [PubMed]
5. Kernan, W.N.; Dearborn, J.L. Obesity increases stroke risk in young adults: Opportunity for prevention. *Stroke* **2015**, *46*, 1435–1436. [CrossRef]
6. Kotlęga, D.; Gołąb-Janowska, M.; Masztalewicz, M.; Ciećwież, S.; Nowacki, P. The emotional stress and risk of ischemic stroke. *Neurol. Neurochir. Pol.* **2016**, *50*, 265–270. [CrossRef]
7. Kelly-Hayes, M. Influence of age and health behaviors on stroke risk: Lessons from longitudinal studies. *J. Am. Geriatr. Soc.* **2010**, *58* (Suppl. 2), S325–S328. [CrossRef]
8. Platz, T. Evidence-Based Guidelines and Clinical Pathways in Stroke Rehabilitation-An International Perspective. *Front. Neurol.* **2019**, *10*, 200. [CrossRef]
9. Inatomi, Y.; Nakajima, M.; Yonehara, T.; Ando, Y. Ipsilateral hemiparesis in ischemic stroke patients. *Acta Neurol. Scand.* **2017**, *136*, 31–40. [CrossRef] [PubMed]
10. Yanohara, R.; Teranishi, T.; Tomita, Y.; Tanino, G.; Ueno, Y.; Sonoda, S. Recovery process of standing postural control in hemiplegia after stroke. *J. Phys. Ther. Sci.* **2014**, *26*, 1761–1765. [CrossRef]
11. Kim, Y.W. Update on Stroke Rehabilitation in Motor Impairment. *Brain Neurorehabil.* **2022**, *15*, e12. [CrossRef] [PubMed]
12. Chohan, S.A.; Venkatesh, P.K.; How, C.H. Long-term complications of stroke and secondary prevention: An overview for primary care physicians. *Singap. Med. J.* **2019**, *60*, 616–620. [CrossRef] [PubMed]
13. Rost, N.S.; Brodtmann, A.; Pase, M.P.; van Veluw, S.J.; Biffi, A.; Duering, M.; Hinman, J.D.; Dichgans, M. Post-Stroke Cognitive Impairment and Dementia. *Circ. Res.* **2022**, *130*, 1252–1271. [CrossRef]
14. Gaete, J.M.; Bogousslavsky, J. Post-stroke depression. *Expert. Rev. Neurother.* **2008**, *8*, 75–92. [CrossRef]
15. Li, W.; Xiao, W.M.; Chen, Y.K.; Qu, J.F.; Liu, Y.L.; Fang, X.W.; Weng, H.Y.; Luo, G.P. Anxiety in Patients With Acute Ischemic Stroke: Risk Factors and Effects on Functional Status. *Front. Psychiatry* **2019**, *10*, 257. [CrossRef]
16. Acciarresi, M.; Bogousslavsky, J.; Paciaroni, M. Post-stroke fatigue: Epidemiology, clinical characteristics and treatment. *Eur. Neurol.* **2014**, *72*, 255–261. [CrossRef] [PubMed]
17. Cai, H.; Wang, X.P.; Yang, G.Y. Sleep Disorders in Stroke: An Update on Management. *Aging Dis.* **2021**, *12*, 570–585. [CrossRef]
18. Guo, J.; Wang, J.; Sun, W.; Liu, X. The advances of post-stroke depression: 2021 update. *J. Neurol.* **2022**, *269*, 1236–1249. [CrossRef]
19. Al-Qazzaz, N.K.; Ali, S.H.; Ahmad, S.A.; Islam, S.; Mohamad, K. Cognitive impairment and memory dysfunction after a stroke diagnosis: A post-stroke memory assessment. *Neuropsychiatr. Dis. Treat.* **2014**, *10*, 1677–1691. [CrossRef]
20. Lee, C.H.; Jeon, S.H.; Kim, M.J.; Ra, G.D.; Lee, Y.H.; Hong, S.H.; Shin, B.S.; Kang, H.G. Factors Affecting Post-Stroke Depression in Acute Ischemic Stroke Patients after 3 Months. *J. Pers. Med.* **2021**, *11*, 1178. [CrossRef]
21. Liu, L.; Xu, M.; Marshall, I.J.; Wolfe, C.D.; Wang, Y.; O'Connell, M.D. Prevalence and natural history of depression after stroke: A systematic review and meta-analysis of observational studies. *PLoS Med.* **2023**, *20*, e1004200. [CrossRef]
22. Cai, W.; Mueller, C.; Li, Y.-J.; Shen, W.-D.; Stewart, R. Post stroke depression and risk of stroke recurrence and mortality: A systematic review and meta-analysis. *Ageing Res. Rev.* **2019**, *50*, 102–109. [CrossRef] [PubMed]
23. Shi, Y.; Xiang, Y.; Yang, Y.; Zhang, N.; Wang, S.; Ungvari, G.S.; Chiu, H.F.K.; Tang, W.K.; Wang, Y.; Zhao, X.; et al. Depression after minor stroke: Prevalence and predictors. *J. Psychosom. Res.* **2015**, *79*, 143–147. [CrossRef] [PubMed]
24. Bour, A.; Rasquin, S.; Aben, I.; Boreas, A.; Limburg, M.; Verhey, F. A one-year follow-up study into the course of depression after stroke. *J. Nutr. Health Aging* **2010**, *14*, 488–493. [CrossRef]
25. Hong, J.P.; Park, S.; Ahn, S.-H.; Kim, J.S. Factors associated with post-stroke suicidal death. *J. Psychiatr. Res.* **2018**, *96*, 135–137. [CrossRef] [PubMed]
26. Bartoli, F.; Pompili, M.; Lillia, N.; Crocamo, C.; Salemi, G.; Clerici, M.; Carrà, G. Rates and correlates of suicidal ideation among stroke survivors: A meta-analysis. *J. Neurol. Neurosurg. Psychiatry* **2017**, *88*, 498–504. [CrossRef]
27. Kauhanen, M.; Korpelainen, J.T.; Hiltunen, P.; Brusin, E.; Mononen, H.; Määttä, R.; Nieminen, P.; Sotaniemi, K.A.; Myllylä, V.V. Poststroke depression correlates with cognitive impairment and neurological deficits. *Stroke* **1999**, *30*, 1875–1880. [CrossRef]

28. Srivastava, A.; Taly, A.B.; Gupta, A.; Murali, T. Post-stroke depression: Prevalence and relationship with disability in chronic stroke survivors. *Ann. Indian. Acad. Neurol.* **2010**, *13*, 123–127. [CrossRef]
29. Kim, E.S.; Kim, J.W.; Kang, H.J.; Bae, K.Y.; Kim, S.W.; Kim, J.T.; Park, M.S.; Cho, K.H.; Kim, J.M. Longitudinal Impact of Depression on Quality of Life in Stroke Patients. *Psychiatry Investig.* **2018**, *15*, 141–146. [CrossRef]
30. Paparella, I.; Vandewalle, G.; Stagg, C.J.; Maquet, P. An integrated measure of GABA to characterize post-stroke plasticity. *NeuroImage Clin.* **2023**, *39*, 103463. [CrossRef]
31. Nagy, E.E.; Frigy, A.; Szász, J.A.; Horváth, E. Neuroinflammation and microglia/macrophage phenotype modulate the molecular background of post-stroke depression: A literature review. *Exp. Ther. Med.* **2020**, *20*, 2510–2523. [CrossRef]
32. Loubinoux, I.; Kronenberg, G.; Endres, M.; Schumann-Bard, P.; Freret, T.; Filipkowski, R.K.; Kaczmarek, L.; Popa-Wagner, A. Post-stroke depression: Mechanisms, translation and therapy. *J. Cell Mol. Med.* **2012**, *16*, 1961–1969. [CrossRef] [PubMed]
33. Zirk, M.; Storm, V. Subjective Stroke Impact and Depressive Symptoms: Indications for a Moderating Role of Health-Related Locus of Control. *Front. Psychiatry* **2019**, *10*, 918. [CrossRef] [PubMed]
34. Kronenberg, G.; Gertz, K.; Heinz, A.; Endres, M. Of mice and men: Modelling post-stroke depression experimentally. *Br. J. Pharmacol.* **2014**, *171*, 4673–4689. [CrossRef] [PubMed]
35. Kim, Y.R.; Kim, H.N.; Pak, M.E.; Ahn, S.M.; Hong, K.H.; Shin, H.K.; Choi, B.T. Studies on the animal model of post-stroke depression and application of antipsychotic aripiprazole. *Behav. Brain Res.* **2015**, *287*, 294–303. [CrossRef]
36. Wu, C.; Zhang, J.; Chen, Y. Study on the behavioral changes of a post-stroke depression rat model. *Exp. Ther. Med.* **2015**, *10*, 159–163. [CrossRef]
37. Braeuninger, S.; Kleinschnitz, C. Rodent models of focal cerebral ischemia: Procedural pitfalls and translational problems. *Exp. Transl. Stroke Med.* **2009**, *1*, 8. [CrossRef]
38. Tao, X.; Yang, W.; Zhu, S.; Que, R.; Liu, C.; Fan, T.; Wang, J.; Mo, D.; Zhang, Z.; Tan, J.; et al. Models of poststroke depression and assessments of core depressive symptoms in rodents: How to choose? *Exp. Neurol.* **2019**, *322*, 113060. [CrossRef]
39. Chen, D.; Wang, J.; Xing, Y.; Jia, P.; Zhang, Y.; Wang, J.; Ren, H.; Le, A.; Chen, X.; Wang, J. Behavioral assessment of post-stroke depression and anxiety in rodents. *Brain Hemorrhages* **2020**, *1*, 105–111. [CrossRef]
40. Can, A.; Dao, D.T.; Arad, M.; Terrillion, C.E.; Piantadosi, S.C.; Gould, T.D. The mouse forced swim test. *J. Vis. Exp.* **2012**, *59*, e3638. [CrossRef]
41. Liu, M.Y.; Yin, C.Y.; Zhu, L.J.; Zhu, X.H.; Xu, C.; Luo, C.X.; Chen, H.; Zhu, D.Y.; Zhou, Q.G. Sucrose preference test for measurement of stress-induced anhedonia in mice. *Nat. Protoc.* **2018**, *13*, 1686–1698. [CrossRef]
42. Kraeuter, A.K.; Guest, P.C.; Sarnyai, Z. The Open Field Test for Measuring Locomotor Activity and Anxiety-Like Behavior. *Methods Mol. Biol.* **2019**, *1916*, 99–103. [CrossRef] [PubMed]
43. Balkaya, M.; Kröber, J.M.; Rex, A.; Endres, M. Assessing post-stroke behavior in mouse models of focal ischemia. *J. Cereb. Blood Flow Metab.* **2013**, *33*, 330–338. [CrossRef] [PubMed]
44. Harrison, J.E.; Weber, S.; Jakob, R.; Chute, C.G. ICD-11: An international classification of diseases for the twenty-first century. *BMC Med. Inform. Decis. Mak.* **2021**, *21*, 206. [CrossRef] [PubMed]
45. Tolentino, J.C.; Schmidt, S.L. DSM-5 Criteria and Depression Severity: Implications for Clinical Practice. *Front. Psychiatry* **2018**, *9*, 450. [CrossRef] [PubMed]
46. Bos, E.H.; de Jonge, P.; Cox, R.F.A. Affective variability in depression: Revisiting the inertia-instability paradox. *Br. J. Psychol.* **2019**, *110*, 814–827. [CrossRef]
47. Liang, J.; Yue, Y.; Jiang, H.; Geng, D.; Wang, J.; Lu, J.; Li, S.; Zhang, K.; Wu, A.; Yuan, Y. Genetic variations in the p11/tPA/BDNF pathway are associated with post stroke depression. *J. Affect. Disord.* **2018**, *226*, 313–325. [CrossRef]
48. Zhou, Z.; Ding, X.; Yang, Q.; Hu, J.; Shang, X.; Huang, X.; Ge, L.; Zhou, T. Association between Single-Nucleotide Polymorphisms of the Tyrosine Kinase Receptor B (TrkB) and Post-Stroke Depression in China. *PLoS ONE* **2015**, *10*, e0144301. [CrossRef]
49. Zhao, F.; Yue, Y.; Jiang, H.; Yuan, Y. Shared genetic risk factors for depression and stroke. *Prog. Neuro-Psychopharmacol. Biol. Psychiatry* **2019**, *93*, 55–70. [CrossRef]
50. Okbay, A.; Baselmans, B.M.; De Neve, J.E.; Turley, P.; Nivard, M.G.; Fontana, M.A.; Meddens, S.F.; Linnér, R.K.; Rietveld, C.A.; Derringer, J.; et al. Genetic variants associated with subjective well-being, depressive symptoms, and neuroticism identified through genome-wide analyses. *Nat. Genet.* **2016**, *48*, 624–633. [CrossRef]
51. Wang, Z.; Shi, Y.; Liu, F.; Jia, N.; Gao, J.; Pang, X.; Deng, F. Diversiform Etiologies for Post-stroke Depression. *Front. Psychiatry* **2018**, *9*, 761. [CrossRef] [PubMed]
52. Caplan, S.; Alvidrez, J.; Paris, M.; Escobar, J.I.; Dixon, J.K.; Desai, M.M.; Whittemore, R.; Scahill, L.D. Subjective versus objective: An exploratory analysis of latino primary care patients with self-perceived depression who do not fulfill primary care evaluation of mental disorders patient health questionnaire criteria for depression. *Prim. Care Companion J. Clin. Psychiatry* **2010**, *12*, 26886. [CrossRef] [PubMed]
53. Perna, L.; Zhang, Y.; Matias-Garcia, P.R.; Ladwig, K.-H.; Wiechmann, T.; Wild, B.; Waldenberger, M.; Schöttker, B.; Mons, U.; Ihle, A.; et al. Subjective mental health, incidence of depressive symptoms in later life, and the role of epigenetics: Results from two longitudinal cohort studies. *Transl. Psychiatry* **2020**, *10*, 323. [CrossRef] [PubMed]
54. Dąbrowska-Bender, M.; Milewska, M.; Gołąbek, A.; Duda-Zalewska, A.; Staniszewska, A. The Impact of Ischemic Cerebral Stroke on the Quality of Life of Patients Based on Clinical, Social, and Psychoemotional Factors. *J. Stroke Cerebrovasc. Dis.* **2017**, *26*, 101–107. [CrossRef]

55. Paprocka-Borowicz, M.; Wiatr, M.; Ciałowicz, M.; Borowicz, W.; Kaczmarek, A.; Marques, A.; Murawska-Ciałowicz, E. Influence of Physical Activity and Socio-Economic Status on Depression and Anxiety Symptoms in Patients after Stroke. *Int. J. Environ. Res. Public Health* **2021**, *18*, 8058. [CrossRef]
56. Zhan, Q.; Kong, F. Mechanisms associated with post-stroke depression and pharmacologic therapy. *Front. Neurol.* **2023**, *14*, 1274709. [CrossRef]
57. Naghavi, F.S.; Koffman, E.E.; Lin, B.; Du, J. Post-stroke neuronal circuits and mental illnesses. *Int. J. Physiol. Pathophysiol. Pharmacol.* **2019**, *11*, 1–11.
58. Balami, J.S.; Chen, R.L.; Grunwald, I.Q.; Buchan, A.M. Neurological complications of acute ischaemic stroke. *Lancet Neurol.* **2011**, *10*, 357–371. [CrossRef]
59. Strawbridge, R.; Young, A.H.; Cleare, A.J. Biomarkers for depression: Recent insights, current challenges and future prospects. *Neuropsychiatr. Dis. Treat.* **2017**, *13*, 1245–1262. [CrossRef]
60. Ayerbe, L.; Ayis, S.; Wolfe, C.D.; Rudd, A.G. Natural history, predictors and outcomes of depression after stroke: Systematic review and meta-analysis. *Br. J. Psychiatry* **2013**, *202*, 14–21. [CrossRef]
61. Hackett, M.L.; Pickles, K. Part I: Frequency of depression after stroke: An updated systematic review and meta-analysis of observational studies. *Int. J. Stroke* **2014**, *9*, 1017–1025. [CrossRef]
62. Dong, L.; Sánchez, B.N.; Skolarus, L.E.; Stulberg, E.; Morgenstern, L.B.; Lisabeth, L.D. Sex difference in prevalence of depression after stroke. *Neurology* **2020**, *94*, e1973–e1983. [CrossRef] [PubMed]
63. Mayman, N.A.; Tuhrim, S.; Jette, N.; Dhamoon, M.S.; Stein, L.K. Sex Differences in Post-Stroke Depression in the Elderly. *J. Stroke Cerebrovasc. Dis.* **2021**, *30*, 105948. [CrossRef]
64. Driga, M.P.; Catalin, B.; Olaru, D.G.; Slowik, A.; Plesnila, N.; Hermann, D.M.; Popa-Wagner, A. The Need for New Biomarkers to Assist with Stroke Prevention and Prediction of Post-Stroke Therapy Based on Plasma-Derived Extracellular Vesicles. *Biomedicines* **2021**, *9*, 1226. [CrossRef] [PubMed]
65. Kim, J.S. Post-stroke Mood and Emotional Disturbances: Pharmacological Therapy Based on Mechanisms. *J. Stroke* **2016**, *18*, 244–255. [CrossRef] [PubMed]
66. Rupprechter, S.; Romaniuk, L.; Series, P.; Hirose, Y.; Hawkins, E.; Sandu, A.L.; Waiter, G.D.; McNeil, C.J.; Shen, X.; Harris, M.A.; et al. Blunted medial prefrontal cortico-limbic reward-related effective connectivity and depression. *Brain* **2020**, *143*, 1946–1956. [CrossRef]
67. Li, G.; Liu, Y.; Zheng, Y.; Wu, Y.; Li, D.; Liang, X.; Chen, Y.; Cui, Y.; Yap, P.T.; Qiu, S.; et al. Multiscale neural modeling of resting-state fMRI reveals executive-limbic malfunction as a core mechanism in major depressive disorder. *Neuroimage Clin.* **2021**, *31*, 102758. [CrossRef]
68. Soares, J.C.; Mann, J.J. The anatomy of mood disorders--review of structural neuroimaging studies. *Biol. Psychiatry* **1997**, *41*, 86–106. [CrossRef]
69. Barker-Collo, S.L. Depression and anxiety 3 months post stroke: Prevalence and correlates. *Arch. Clin. Neuropsychol.* **2007**, *22*, 519–531. [CrossRef]
70. Wei, N.; Yong, W.; Li, X.; Zhou, Y.; Deng, M.; Zhu, H.; Jin, H. Post-stroke depression and lesion location: A systematic review. *J. Neurol.* **2015**, *262*, 81–90. [CrossRef]
71. Klingbeil, J.; Brandt, M.L.; Wawrzyniak, M.; Stockert, A.; Schneider, H.R.; Baum, P.; Hoffmann, K.T.; Saur, D. Association of Lesion Location and Depressive Symptoms Poststroke. *Stroke* **2022**, *53*, e467–e471. [CrossRef]
72. Volz, M.; Ladwig, S.; Werheid, K. Gender differences in post-stroke depression: A longitudinal analysis of prevalence, persistence and predictive value of known risk factors. *Neuropsychol. Rehabil.* **2021**, *31*, 1–17. [CrossRef] [PubMed]
73. Poynter, B.; Shuman Hon, M.; Diaz-Granados, N.; Kapral, M.; Grace, S.L.; Stewart, D.E. Sex Differences in the Prevalence of Post-Stroke Depression: A Systematic Review. *Psychosomatics* **2009**, *50*, 563–569. [CrossRef]
74. Mirolovics, Á.; Bokor, M.; Dobi, B.; Zsuga, J.; Bereczki, D. Socioeconomic Factors Predicting Depression Differ in the Acute Stage and at 1 year After Ischemic Stroke or TIA. *J. Stroke Cerebrovasc. Dis.* **2020**, *29*, 105241. [CrossRef]
75. Gloria, M.U.; Jonah, O.E.; Olusanjo, A.C.; Chiebuka, O.E.; Nene, J.J.; Nwakego, A.U.; Chinyere, A.C. Post-Stroke Depression and Suicidal Ideations: Relationship with Gender and Marital Status: A Cross Sectional Study. *J. Prim. Care Community Health* **2024**, *15*, 21501319241233172. [CrossRef] [PubMed]
76. Tento, T.; Kume, A.; Kumaso, S. Risk factors for stroke-related functional disability and mortality at Felege Hiwot Referral Hospital, Ethiopia. *BMC Neurol.* **2023**, *23*, 393. [CrossRef]
77. Yoo, J.W.; Hong, B.Y.; Jo, L.; Kim, J.S.; Park, J.G.; Shin, B.K.; Lim, S.H. Effects of Age on Long-Term Functional Recovery in Patients with Stroke. *Medicina* **2020**, *56*, 451. [CrossRef] [PubMed]
78. Lökk, J.; Delbari, A. Management of depression in elderly stroke patients. *Neuropsychiatr. Dis. Treat.* **2010**, *6*, 539–549. [CrossRef]
79. Lindén, T.; Blomstrand, C.; Skoog, I. Depressive disorders after 20 months in elderly stroke patients: A case-control study. *Stroke* **2007**, *38*, 1860–1863. [CrossRef]
80. Wolf, V.L.; Ergul, A. Progress and challenges in preclinical stroke recovery research. *Brain Circ.* **2021**, *7*, 230–240. [CrossRef]
81. Chen, R.; Ovbiagele, B.; Feng, W. Diabetes and Stroke: Epidemiology, Pathophysiology, Pharmaceuticals and Outcomes. *Am. J. Med. Sci.* **2016**, *351*, 380–386. [CrossRef]
82. Johansson, B.B. Hypertension mechanisms causing stroke. *Clin. Exp. Pharmacol. Physiol.* **1999**, *26*, 563–565. [CrossRef] [PubMed]
83. Gajurel, B.P.; Gurung, A.; Ojha, R.; Rajbhandari, R.; Karn, R. Dyslipidemia and Obesity in Ischemic Stroke. *Cureus* **2023**, *15*, e45409. [CrossRef] [PubMed]

84. Popa-Wagner, A.; Petcu, E.B.; Capitanescu, B.; Hermann, D.M.; Radu, E.; Gresita, A. Ageing as a risk factor for cerebral ischemia: Underlying mechanisms and therapy in animal models and in the clinic. *Mech. Ageing Dev.* **2020**, *190*, 111312. [CrossRef] [PubMed]
85. Popa-Wagner, A.; Udristoiu, I.; Gresita, A.; Lledós, M.; Cadenas, I. *Post-Stroke Depression: Genetics, Mechanisms, and Treatment*; Springer International Publishing: Cham, Switzerland, 2022; pp. 4467–4478.
86. Kohen, R.; Cain, K.C.; Mitchell, P.H.; Becker, K.; Buzaitis, A.; Millard, S.P.; Navaja, G.P.; Teri, L.; Tirschwell, D.; Veith, R. Association of serotonin transporter gene polymorphisms with poststroke depression. *Arch. Gen. Psychiatry* **2008**, *65*, 1296–1302. [CrossRef]
87. Zhang, E.; Liao, P. Brain-derived neurotrophic factor and post-stroke depression. *J. Neurosci. Res.* **2020**, *98*, 537–548. [CrossRef]
88. Qayyum, A.; Zai, C.C.; Hirata, Y.; Tiwari, A.K.; Cheema, S.; Nowrouzi, B.; Beitchman, J.H.; Kennedy, J.L. The Role of the Catechol-o-Methyltransferase (COMT) GeneVal158Met in Aggressive Behavior, a Review of Genetic Studies. *Curr. Neuropharmacol.* **2015**, *13*, 802–814. [CrossRef]
89. Kwon, S.; Hartzema, A.G.; Duncan, P.W.; Min-Lai, S. Disability measures in stroke: Relationship among the Barthel Index, the Functional Independence Measure, and the Modified Rankin Scale. *Stroke* **2004**, *35*, 918–923. [CrossRef]
90. Notsu, Y.; Nabika, T.; Park, H.Y.; Masuda, J.; Kobayashi, S. Evaluation of genetic risk factors for silent brain infarction. *Stroke* **1999**, *30*, 1881–1886. [CrossRef]
91. Devereux, N.; Berns, A.M. Evaluation & Treatment of Psychological Effects of Stroke. *Dela J. Public. Health* **2023**, *9*, 62–69. [CrossRef]
92. Ladwig, S.; Werheid, K.; Südmeyer, M.; Volz, M. Predictors of post-stroke depression: Validation of established risk factors and introduction of a dynamic perspective in two longitudinal studies. *Front. Psychiatry* **2023**, *14*, 1093918. [CrossRef] [PubMed]
93. Taylor-Rowan, M.; Momoh, O.; Ayerbe, L.; Evans, J.J.; Stott, D.J.; Quinn, T.J. Prevalence of pre-stroke depression and its association with post-stroke depression: A systematic review and meta-analysis. *Psychol. Med.* **2019**, *49*, 685–696. [CrossRef] [PubMed]
94. Wist, S.; Clivaz, J.; Sattelmayer, M. Muscle strengthening for hemiparesis after stroke: A meta-analysis. *Ann. Phys. Rehabil. Med.* **2016**, *59*, 114–124. [CrossRef]
95. Cuccurullo, S.J.; Fleming, T.K.; Zinonos, S.; Cosgrove, N.M.; Cabrera, J.; Kostis, J.B.; Greiss, C.; Ray, A.R.; Eckert, A.; Scarpati, R.; et al. Stroke Recovery Program with Modified Cardiac Rehabilitation Improves Mortality, Functional & Cardiovascular Performance. *J. Stroke Cerebrovasc. Dis.* **2022**, *31*, 106322. [CrossRef] [PubMed]
96. Moore, N.; Reeder, S.; O'Keefe, S.; Alves-Stein, S.; Schneider, E.; Moloney, K.; Radford, K.; Lannin, N.A. "I've still got a job to go back to": The importance of early vocational rehabilitation after stroke. *Disabil. Rehabil.* **2023**, *46*, 2769–2776. [CrossRef]
97. Deepradit, S.; Powwattana, A.; Lagampan, S.; Thiangtham, W. Effectiveness of a family-based program for post-stroke patients and families: A cluster randomized controlled trial. *Int. J. Nurs. Sci.* **2023**, *10*, 446–455. [CrossRef]
98. Pérez-de la Cruz, S. Influence of an Aquatic Therapy Program on Perceived Pain, Stress, and Quality of Life in Chronic Stroke Patients: A Randomized Trial. *Int. J. Environ. Res. Public Health* **2020**, *17*, 4796. [CrossRef]
99. Dayuan, Z.; Lan, L.; Hui, C.; Huanjie, L.; Deliang, L.; Yihui, D. The effect of music as an intervention for post-stroke depression: A systematic review and meta-analysis. *Complement. Ther. Med.* **2022**, *71*, 102901. [CrossRef]
100. Wang, S.B.; Wang, Y.Y.; Zhang, Q.E.; Wu, S.L.; Ng, C.H.; Ungvari, G.S.; Chen, L.; Wang, C.X.; Jia, F.J.; Xiang, Y.T. Cognitive behavioral therapy for post-stroke depression: A meta-analysis. *J. Affect. Disord.* **2018**, *235*, 589–596. [CrossRef]
101. Gao, W.; Xue, F.; Yu, B.; Yu, S.; Zhang, W.; Huang, H. Repetitive transcranial magnetic stimulation for post-stroke depression: An overview of systematic reviews. *Front. Neurol.* **2023**, *14*, 930558. [CrossRef]
102. Machová, K.; Procházková, R.; Říha, M.; Svobodová, I. The Effect of Animal-Assisted Therapy on the State of Patients' Health After a Stroke: A Pilot Study. *Int. J. Environ. Res. Public Health* **2019**, *16*, 3272. [CrossRef] [PubMed]
103. Zulkifli, W.; Shamsuddin, S.; Lim, T.H. Animal Robot Assisted-therapy for Rehabilitation of Patient with Post-Stroke Depression. *IOP Conf. Ser. Mater. Sci. Eng.* **2017**, *210*, 012005. [CrossRef]
104. Remes, O.; Mendes, J.F.; Templeton, P. Biological, Psychological, and Social Determinants of Depression: A Review of Recent Literature. *Brain Sci.* **2021**, *11*, 1633. [CrossRef] [PubMed]
105. Liu, F.; McCullough, L.D. Middle cerebral artery occlusion model in rodents: Methods and potential pitfalls. *J. Biomed. Biotechnol.* **2011**, *2011*, 464701. [CrossRef] [PubMed]
106. Fluri, F.; Schuhmann, M.K.; Kleinschnitz, C. Animal models of ischemic stroke and their application in clinical research. *Drug Des. Devel Ther.* **2015**, *9*, 3445–3454. [CrossRef]
107. Kuts, R.; Melamed, I.; Shiyntum, H.N.; Frank, D.; Grinshpun, J.; Zlotnik, A.; Brotfain, E.; Dubilet, M.; Natanel, D.; Boyko, M. A Middle Cerebral Artery Occlusion Technique for Inducing Post-stroke Depression in Rats. *J. Vis. Exp.* **2019**, *147*, e58875. [CrossRef]
108. Liu, S.; Zhen, G.; Meloni, B.P.; Campbell, K.; Winn, H.R. RODENT STROKE MODEL GUIDELINES FOR PRECLINICAL STROKE TRIALS (1ST EDITION). *J. Exp. Stroke Transl. Med.* **2009**, *2*, 2–27. [CrossRef]
109. Gresita, A.; Mihai, R.; Hermann, D.M.; Amandei, F.S.; Capitanescu, B.; Popa-Wagner, A. Effect of environmental enrichment and isolation on behavioral and histological indices following focal ischemia in old rats. *GeroScience* **2022**, *44*, 211–228. [CrossRef]
110. Boboc, I.K.S.; Chirea, A.C.; Gheorman, V.; Gresita, A.; Balseanu, T.A.; Catalin, B.; Calina, D. Investigating the Neuroprotective and Neuroregenerative Effect of Trazodone Regarding Behavioral Recovery in a BL6C57 Mice Stroke Model. *Curr. Health Sci. J.* **2023**, *49*, 210–219. [CrossRef]

111. Pinosanu, L.R.; Boboc, I.K.S.; Balseanu, T.A.; Gresita, A.; Hermann, D.M.; Popa-Wagner, A.; Catalin, B. Beam narrowing test: A motor index of post-stroke motor evaluation in an aged rat model of cerebral ischemia. *J. Neural Transm.* **2024**, *131*, 763–771. [CrossRef]
112. Boboc, I.K.S.; Rotaru-Zavaleanu, A.D.; Calina, D.; Albu, C.V.; Catalin, B.; Turcu-Stiolica, A. A Preclinical Systematic Review and Meta-Analysis of Behavior Testing in Mice Models of Ischemic Stroke. *Life* **2023**, *13*, 567. [CrossRef] [PubMed]
113. Zhang, G.; Chen, L.; Yang, L.; Hua, X.; Zhou, B.; Miao, Z.; Li, J.; Hu, H.; Namaka, M.; Kong, J.; et al. Combined use of spatial restraint stress and middle cerebral artery occlusion is a novel model of post-stroke depression in mice. *Sci. Rep.* **2015**, *5*, 16751. [CrossRef]
114. Cunningham, C.J.; Wong, R.; Barrington, J.; Tamburrano, S.; Pinteaux, E.; Allan, S.M. Systemic conditioned medium treatment from interleukin-1 primed mesenchymal stem cells promotes recovery after stroke. *Stem Cell Res. Ther.* **2020**, *11*, 32. [CrossRef]
115. Kawai, H.; Yamashita, T.; Ohta, Y.; Deguchi, K.; Nagotani, S.; Zhang, X.; Ikeda, Y.; Matsuura, T.; Abe, K. Tridermal tumorigenesis of induced pluripotent stem cells transplanted in ischemic brain. *J. Cereb. Blood Flow. Metab.* **2010**, *30*, 1487–1493. [CrossRef]
116. Patkar, S.; Tate, R.; Modo, M.; Plevin, R.; Carswell, H.V. Conditionally immortalised neural stem cells promote functional recovery and brain plasticity after transient focal cerebral ischaemia in mice. *Stem Cell Res.* **2012**, *8*, 14–25. [CrossRef] [PubMed]
117. Sun, R.; Peng, M.; Xu, P.; Huang, F.; Xie, Y.; Li, J.; Hong, Y.; Guo, H.; Liu, Q.; Zhu, W. Low-density lipoprotein receptor (LDLR) regulates NLRP3-mediated neuronal pyroptosis following cerebral ischemia/reperfusion injury. *J. Neuroinflamm.* **2020**, *17*, 330. [CrossRef]
118. Cao, Z.; Balasubramanian, A.; Pedersen, S.E.; Romero, J.; Pautler, R.G.; Marrelli, S.P. TRPV1-mediated Pharmacological Hypothermia Promotes Improved Functional Recovery Following Ischemic Stroke. *Sci. Rep.* **2017**, *7*, 17685. [CrossRef] [PubMed]
119. Suenaga, J.; Hu, X.; Pu, H.; Shi, Y.; Hassan, S.H.; Xu, M.; Leak, R.K.; Stetler, R.A.; Gao, Y.; Chen, J. White matter injury and microglia/macrophage polarization are strongly linked with age-related long-term deficits in neurological function after stroke. *Exp. Neurol.* **2015**, *272*, 109–119. [CrossRef] [PubMed]
120. Ding, Z.; Gao, J.; Feng, Y.; Wang, M.; Zhao, H.; Wu, R.; Zheng, X.; Feng, X.; Lai, M. Electroacupuncture Ameliorates Depression-Like Behaviors in Post-Stroke Rats via Activating AMPK-Mediated Mitochondrial Function. *Neuropsychiatr. Dis. Treat.* **2023**, *19*, 2657–2671. [CrossRef]
121. Wang, S.; Sun, H.; Liu, S.; Wang, T.; Guan, J.; Jia, J. Role of hypothalamic cannabinoid receptors in post-stroke depression in rats. *Brain Res. Bull.* **2016**, *121*, 91–97. [CrossRef]
122. Qian, L.; Huang, S.; Liu, X.; Jiang, Y.; Jiang, Y.; Hu, Y.; Yang, Z. Morroniside improves the symptoms of post-stroke depression in mice through the BDNF signaling pathway mediated by MiR-409-3p. *Phytomedicine* **2024**, *123*, 155224. [CrossRef] [PubMed]
123. Xu, Y.; Liang, L. Vitamin D3/vitamin D receptor signaling mitigates symptoms of post-stroke depression in mice by upregulating hippocampal BDNF expression. *Neurosci. Res.* **2021**, *170*, 306–313. [CrossRef] [PubMed]
124. Gaignier, F.; Legrand-Frossi, C.; Stragier, E.; Mathiot, J.; Merlin, J.L.; Cohen-Salmon, C.; Lanfumey, L.; Frippiat, J.P. A Model of Chronic Exposure to Unpredictable Mild Socio-Environmental Stressors Replicates Some Spaceflight-Induced Immunological Changes. *Front. Physiol.* **2018**, *9*, 514. [CrossRef] [PubMed]
125. Zhang, M.; Li, A.; Yang, Q.; Li, J.; Zheng, L.; Wang, G.; Sun, Y.; Huang, Y.; Zhang, M.; Song, Z.; et al. Matrine alleviates depressive-like behaviors via modulating microbiota–gut–brain axis in CUMS-induced mice. *J. Transl. Med.* **2023**, *21*, 145. [CrossRef]
126. Yan, W.; Dong, Z.; Zhao, D.; Li, J.; Zeng, T.; Mo, C.; Gao, L.; Lv, Z. Xiaoyaosan Exerts Antidepressant Effect by Downregulating RAGE Expression in Cingulate Gyrus of Depressive-Like Mice. *Front. Pharmacol.* **2021**, *12*, 703965. [CrossRef] [PubMed]
127. Mușat, M.I.; Mitran, S.I.; Udriștoiu, I.; Albu, C.V.; Cătălin, B. The impact of stress on the behavior of C57BL/6 mice with liver injury: A comparative study. *Front. Behav. Neurosci.* **2024**, *18*, 1358964. [CrossRef]
128. Wu, J.; Li, J.; Gaurav, C.; Muhammad, U.; Chen, Y.; Li, X.; Chen, J.; Wang, Z. CUMS and dexamethasone induce depression-like phenotypes in mice by differentially altering gut microbiota and triggering macroglia activation. *Gen. Psychiatr.* **2021**, *34*, e100529. [CrossRef]
129. Wang, Y.-l.; Wu, H.-r.; Zhang, S.-s.; Xiao, H.-l.; Yu, J.; Ma, Y.-y.; Zhang, Y.-d.; Liu, Q. Catalpol ameliorates depressive-like behaviors in CUMS mice via oxidative stress-mediated NLRP3 inflammasome and neuroinflammation. *Transl. Psychiatry* **2021**, *11*, 353. [CrossRef]
130. Wang, G.; Lei, C.; Tian, Y.; Wang, Y.; Zhang, L.; Zhang, R. Rb1, the Primary Active Ingredient in Panax ginseng C.A. Meyer, Exerts Antidepressant-Like Effects via the BDNF-Trkb-CREB Pathway. *Front. Pharmacol.* **2019**, *10*, 1034. [CrossRef]
131. Wen, G.; Yao, H.; Li, Y.; Ding, R.; Ren, X.; Tan, Y.; Ren, W.; Yu, H.; Zhan, X.; Wang, X.; et al. Regulation of Tau Protein on the Antidepressant Effects of Ketamine in the Chronic Unpredictable Mild Stress Model. *Front. Psychiatry* **2019**, *10*, 287. [CrossRef]
132. Li, M.; Fu, Q.; Li, Y.; Li, S.; Xue, J.; Ma, S. Emodin opposes chronic unpredictable mild stress induced depressive-like behavior in mice by upregulating the levels of hippocampal glucocorticoid receptor and brain-derived neurotrophic factor. *Fitoterapia* **2014**, *98*, 1–10. [CrossRef] [PubMed]
133. Xie, M.; Wang, H.; Peng, J.; Qing, D.; Zhang, X.; Guo, D.; Meng, P.; Luo, Z.; Wang, X.; Peng, Q. Acacetin protects against depression-associated dry eye disease by regulating ubiquitination of NLRP3 through gp78 signal. *Front. Pharmacol.* **2022**, *13*, 984475. [CrossRef]
134. Wassouf, Z.; Hentrich, T.; Casadei, N.; Jaumann, M.; Knipper, M.; Riess, O.; Schulze-Hentrich, J.M. Distinct Stress Response and Altered Striatal Transcriptome in Alpha-Synuclein Overexpressing Mice. *Front. Neurosci.* **2018**, *12*, 1033. [CrossRef] [PubMed]

135. Wang, Y.; Gu, J.H.; Liu, L.; Liu, Y.; Tang, W.Q.; Ji, C.H.; Guan, W.; Zhao, X.Y.; Sun, Y.F.; Xu, D.W.; et al. Hippocampal PPARα Plays a Role in the Pharmacological Mechanism of Vortioxetine, a Multimodal-Acting Antidepressant. *Front. Pharmacol.* **2021**, *12*, 673221. [CrossRef]
136. Kalliokoski, O.; Teilmann, A.C.; Jacobsen, K.R.; Abelson, K.S.; Hau, J. The lonely mouse—Single housing affects serotonergic signaling integrity measured by 8-OH-DPAT-induced hypothermia in male mice. *PLoS ONE* **2014**, *9*, e111065. [CrossRef]
137. Zhang, Y.; Yu, P.; Liu, H.; Yao, H.; Yao, S.; Yuan, S.Y.; Zhang, J.C. Hyperforin improves post-stroke social isolation-induced exaggeration of PSD and PSA via TGF-β. *Int. J. Mol. Med.* **2019**, *43*, 413–425. [CrossRef] [PubMed]
138. Chen, H.H.; Zhang, N.; Li, W.Y.; Fang, M.R.; Zhang, H.; Fang, Y.S.; Ding, M.X.; Fu, X.Y. Overexpression of brain-derived neurotrophic factor in the hippocampus protects against post-stroke depression. *Neural Regen. Res.* **2015**, *10*, 1427–1432. [CrossRef]
139. Niu, L.; Jin, X.; Zhang, Y.; Liu, B.; Li, C. Feasibility of focal cerebral ischemia and reperfusion surgery combined with chronic unpredictable mild stress to simulate the post-stroke depressive state in rats. *Behav. Brain Funct.* **2015**, *11*, 39. [CrossRef]
140. Wang, A.R.; Mi, L.F.; Zhang, Z.L.; Hu, M.Z.; Zhao, Z.Y.; Liu, B.; Li, Y.B.; Zheng, S. Saikosaponin A improved depression-like behavior and inhibited hippocampal neuronal apoptosis after cerebral ischemia through p-CREB/BDNF pathway. *Behav. Brain Res.* **2021**, *403*, 113138. [CrossRef]
141. Aarsland, T.I.; Landaas, E.T.; Hegvik, T.A.; Ulvik, A.; Halmøy, A.; Ueland, P.M.; Haavik, J. Serum concentrations of kynurenines in adult patients with attention-deficit hyperactivity disorder (ADHD): A case-control study. *Behav. Brain Funct.* **2015**, *11*, 36. [CrossRef]
142. Pałucha-Poniewiera, A.; Podkowa, K.; Rafało-Ulińska, A. The group II mGlu receptor antagonist LY341495 induces a rapid antidepressant-like effect and enhances the effect of ketamine in the chronic unpredictable mild stress model of depression in C57BL/6J mice. *Prog. Neuropsychopharmacol. Biol. Psychiatry* **2021**, *109*, 110239. [CrossRef]
143. Zain, M.A.; Pandy, V.; Majeed, A.B.A.; Wong, W.F.; Mohamed, Z. Chronic restraint stress impairs sociability but not social recognition and spatial memoryin C57BL/6J mice. *Exp. Anim.* **2019**, *68*, 113–124. [CrossRef] [PubMed]
144. Zhi, L.; Zhang, F.; Liu, H.; Jiang, X.; Zhang, Y.; Yang, Q.; Zhang, X.; Liu, M.; Zhang, Z.; Song, J. CRS induces depression-like behavior after MCAO in rats possibly by activating p38 MAPK. *Behav. Brain Res.* **2023**, *437*, 114104. [CrossRef] [PubMed]
145. Tekam, C.S.; Shinde, S.; Ranjana, P.; Mahto, S. *Bilateral Common Carotid Artery Occlusion: Stroke Model*; Springer International Publishing: Cham, Switzerland, 2021; pp. 41–56.
146. Di Lorenzo, A.; Nabavi, S.F.; Sureda, A.; Moghaddam, A.H.; Khanjani, S.; Arcidiaco, P.; Nabavi, S.M.; Daglia, M. Antidepressive-like effects and antioxidant activity of green tea and GABA green tea in a mouse model of post-stroke depression. *Mol. Nutr. Food Res.* **2016**, *60*, 566–579. [CrossRef] [PubMed]
147. Daglia, M.; Di Lorenzo, A.; Nabavi, S.F.; Sureda, A.; Khanjani, S.; Moghaddam, A.H.; Braidy, N.; Nabavi, S.M. Improvement of Antioxidant Defences and Mood Status by Oral GABA Tea Administration in a Mouse Model of Post-Stroke Depression. *Nutrients* **2017**, *9*, 446. [CrossRef]
148. Nabavi, S.M.; Nabavi, S.F.; Sureda, A.; Caprioli, G.; Iannarelli, R.; Sokeng, A.J.T.; Braidy, N.; Khanjani, S.; Moghaddam, A.H.; Atanasov, A.G.; et al. The water extract of tutsan (Hypericum androsaemum L.) red berries exerts antidepressive-like effects and in vivo antioxidant activity in a mouse model of post-stroke depression. *Biomed. Pharmacother.* **2018**, *99*, 290–298. [CrossRef]
149. Aggarwal, A.; Gaur, V.; Kumar, A. Nitric oxide mechanism in the protective effect of naringin against post-stroke depression (PSD) in mice. *Life Sci.* **2010**, *86*, 928–935. [CrossRef] [PubMed]
150. Lee, S.R.; Choi, B.; Paul, S.; Seo, J.H.; Back, D.B.; Han, J.S.; Choi, D.H.; Kwon, K.J.; Shin, C.Y.; Lee, J.; et al. Depressive-like behaviors in a rat model of chronic cerebral hypoperfusion. *Transl. Stroke Res.* **2015**, *6*, 207–214. [CrossRef]
151. Hu, G.; Zhou, C.; Wang, J.; Ma, X.; Ma, H.; Yu, H.; Peng, Z.; Huang, J.; Cai, M. Electroacupuncture treatment ameliorates depressive-like behavior and cognitive dysfunction via CB1R dependent mitochondria biogenesis after experimental global cerebral ischemic stroke. *Front. Cell Neurosci.* **2023**, *17*, 1135227. [CrossRef]
152. Molcho, L.; Ben-Zur, T.; Barhum, Y.; Offen, D. DJ-1 based peptide, ND-13, promote functional recovery in mouse model of focal ischemic injury. *PLoS ONE* **2018**, *13*, e0192954. [CrossRef]
153. Vahid-Ansari, F.; Lagace, D.C.; Albert, P.R. Persistent post-stroke depression in mice following unilateral medial prefrontal cortical stroke. *Transl. Psychiatry* **2016**, *6*, e863. [CrossRef] [PubMed]
154. Happ, D.; Tasker, R.A.; Wegener, G.P. 2.038—Endothelin-1 injection into the left medial prefrontal cortex induces anxiety-like symptoms—A possible model for post-stroke anxiety? *Eur. Neuropsychopharmacol.* **2018**, *28*, S48–S49. [CrossRef]
155. Sommer, C.J. Ischemic stroke: Experimental models and reality. *Acta Neuropathol.* **2017**, *133*, 245–261. [CrossRef]
156. Kim, G.W.; Sugawara, T.; Chan, P.H. Involvement of oxidative stress and caspase-3 in cortical infarction after photothrombotic ischemia in mice. *J. Cereb. Blood Flow. Metab.* **2000**, *20*, 1690–1701. [CrossRef] [PubMed]
157. Talley Watts, L.; Zheng, W.; Garling, R.J.; Frohlich, V.C.; Lechleiter, J.D. Rose Bengal Photothrombosis by Confocal Optical Imaging In Vivo: A Model of Single Vessel Stroke. *J. Vis. Exp.* **2015**, *100*, e52794. [CrossRef]
158. Wester, P.; Watson, B.D.; Prado, R.; Dietrich, W.D. A photothrombotic 'ring' model of rat stroke-in-evolution displaying putative penumbral inversion. *Stroke* **1995**, *26*, 444–450. [CrossRef]
159. Lunardi Baccetto, S.; Lehmann, C. Microcirculatory Changes in Experimental Models of Stroke and CNS-Injury Induced Immunodepression. *Int. J. Mol. Sci.* **2019**, *20*, 5184. [CrossRef]

160. Lindholm, J.S.; Castrén, E. Mice with altered BDNF signaling as models for mood disorders and antidepressant effects. *Front. Behav. Neurosci.* **2014**, *8*, 143. [CrossRef]
161. Holmes, A.; Murphy, D.L.; Crawley, J.N. Abnormal behavioral phenotypes of serotonin transporter knockout mice: Parallels with human anxiety and depression. *Biol. Psychiatry* **2003**, *54*, 953–959. [CrossRef]
162. Craske, M.G.; Meuret, A.E.; Ritz, T.; Treanor, M.; Dour, H.J. Treatment for Anhedonia: A Neuroscience Driven Approach. *Depress. Anxiety* **2016**, *33*, 927–938. [CrossRef]
163. Sah, A.; Schmuckermair, C.; Sartori, S.B.; Gaburro, S.; Kandasamy, M.; Irschick, R.; Klimaschewski, L.; Landgraf, R.; Aigner, L.; Singewald, N. Anxiety- rather than depression-like behavior is associated with adult neurogenesis in a female mouse model of higher trait anxiety- and comorbid depression-like behavior. *Transl. Psychiatry* **2012**, *2*, e171. [CrossRef] [PubMed]
164. Labenz, C.; Huber, Y.; Michel, M.; Nagel, M.; Galle, P.R.; Kostev, K.; Schattenberg, J.M. Nonalcoholic Fatty Liver Disease Increases the Risk of Anxiety and Depression. *Hepatol. Commun.* **2020**, *4*, 1293–1301. [CrossRef] [PubMed]
165. Wu, H.H.; Wang, S. Strain differences in the chronic mild stress animal model of depression. *Behav. Brain Res.* **2010**, *213*, 94–102. [CrossRef]
166. Primo, M.J.; Fonseca-Rodrigues, D.; Almeida, A.; Teixeira, P.M.; Pinto-Ribeiro, F. Sucrose preference test: A systematic review of protocols for the assessment of anhedonia in rodents. *Eur. Neuropsychopharmacol.* **2023**, *77*, 80–92. [CrossRef]
167. Wang, L.; Cui, Q.; Liu, J.; Zou, H. Emotion Reactivity and Suicide Risk in Patients With Depression: The Mediating Role of Non-Suicidal Self-Injury and Moderating Role of Childhood Neglect. *Front. Psychiatry* **2021**, *12*, 707181. [CrossRef] [PubMed]
168. Busquet, P.; Nguyen, N.K.; Schmid, E.; Tanimoto, N.; Seeliger, M.W.; Ben-Yosef, T.; Mizuno, F.; Akopian, A.; Striessnig, J.; Singewald, N. CaV1.3 L-type Ca2+ channels modulate depression-like behaviour in mice independent of deaf phenotype. *Int. J. Neuropsychopharmacol.* **2010**, *13*, 499–513. [CrossRef]
169. Seo, J.S.; Wei, J.; Qin, L.; Kim, Y.; Yan, Z.; Greengard, P. Cellular and molecular basis for stress-induced depression. *Mol. Psychiatry* **2017**, *22*, 1440–1447. [CrossRef]
170. Sasaki, K.; Halder, S.K.; Matsunaga, H.; Ueda, H. Beneficial actions of prothymosin alpha-mimetic hexapeptide on central post-stroke pain, reduced social activity, learning-deficit and depression following cerebral ischemia in mice. *Peptides* **2020**, *126*, 170265. [CrossRef]
171. Partoazar, A.; Seyyedian, Z.; Zamanian, G.; Saffari, P.M.; Muhammadnejad, A.; Dehpour, A.R.; Goudarzi, R. Neuroprotective phosphatidylserine liposomes alleviate depressive-like behavior related to stroke through neuroinflammation attenuation in the mouse hippocampus. *Psychopharmacology* **2021**, *238*, 1531–1539. [CrossRef]
172. Wu, D.; Zhang, G.; Zhao, C.; Yang, Y.; Miao, Z.; Xu, X. Interleukin-18 from neurons and microglia mediates depressive behaviors in mice with post-stroke depression. *Brain Behav. Immun.* **2020**, *88*, 411–420. [CrossRef]
173. Weiss, S.M.; Wadsworth, G.; Fletcher, A.; Dourish, C.T. Utility of ethological analysis to overcome locomotor confounds in elevated maze models of anxiety. *Neurosci. Biobehav. Rev.* **1998**, *23*, 265–271. [CrossRef] [PubMed]
174. Li, X.; Zhang, J.; Niu, R.; Manthari, R.K.; Yang, K.; Wang, J. Effect of fluoride exposure on anxiety- and depression-like behavior in mouse. *Chemosphere* **2019**, *215*, 454–460. [CrossRef] [PubMed]
175. Sweeney, P.; O'Hara, K.; Xu, Z.; Yang, Y. HFD-induced energy states-dependent bidirectional control of anxiety levels in mice. *Int. J. Obes.* **2017**, *41*, 1237–1245. [CrossRef] [PubMed]
176. Pitzer, C.; La Porta, C.; Treede, R.D.; Tappe-Theodor, A. Inflammatory and neuropathic pain conditions do not primarily evoke anxiety-like behaviours in C57BL/6 mice. *Eur. J. Pain.* **2019**, *23*, 285–306. [CrossRef] [PubMed]
177. Blasco-Serra, A.; González-Soler, E.M.; Cervera-Ferri, A.; Teruel-Martí, V.; Valverde-Navarro, A.A. A standardization of the Novelty-Suppressed Feeding Test protocol in rats. *Neurosci. Lett.* **2017**, *658*, 73–78. [CrossRef]
178. Pietri, M.; Djillani, A.; Mazella, J.; Borsotto, M.; Heurteaux, C. First evidence of protective effects on stroke recovery and post-stroke depression induced by sortilin-derived peptides. *Neuropharmacology* **2019**, *158*, 107715. [CrossRef]
179. Bourin, M.; Hascoët, M. The mouse light/dark box test. *Eur. J. Pharmacol.* **2003**, *463*, 55–65. [CrossRef]
180. Takao, K.; Miyakawa, T. Light/dark transition test for mice. *J. Vis. Exp.* **2006**, *1*, e104. [CrossRef]
181. Njung'e, K.u.; Handley, S.L. Evaluation of marble-burying behavior as a model of anxiety. *Pharmacol. Biochem. Behav.* **1991**, *38*, 63–67. [CrossRef]
182. Bahi, A.; Dreyer, J.L. Hippocampus-specific deletion of tissue plasminogen activator "tPA" in adult mice impairs depression- and anxiety-like behaviors. *Eur. Neuropsychopharmacol.* **2012**, *22*, 672–682. [CrossRef]
183. Dorninger, F.; Zeitler, G.; Berger, J. Nestlet Shredding and Nest Building Tests to Assess Features of Psychiatric Disorders in Mice. *Bio Protoc.* **2020**, *10*, e3863. [CrossRef] [PubMed]
184. Teo, A.R.; Nelson, S.; Strange, W.; Kubo, H.; Katsuki, R.; Kurahara, K.; Kanba, S.; Kato, T.A. Social withdrawal in major depressive disorder: A case-control study of hikikomori in japan. *J. Affect. Disord.* **2020**, *274*, 1142–1146. [CrossRef] [PubMed]
185. Katayama, Y.; Nishiyama, M.; Shoji, H.; Ohkawa, Y.; Kawamura, A.; Sato, T.; Suyama, M.; Takumi, T.; Miyakawa, T.; Nakayama, K.I. CHD8 haploinsufficiency results in autistic-like phenotypes in mice. *Nature* **2016**, *537*, 675–679. [CrossRef]
186. Peça, J.; Feliciano, C.; Ting, J.T.; Wang, W.; Wells, M.F.; Venkatraman, T.N.; Lascola, C.D.; Fu, Z.; Feng, G. Shank3 mutant mice display autistic-like behaviours and striatal dysfunction. *Nature* **2011**, *472*, 437–442. [CrossRef]
187. Wilson, C.A.; Koenig, J.I. Social interaction and social withdrawal in rodents as readouts for investigating the negative symptoms of schizophrenia. *Eur. Neuropsychopharmacol.* **2014**, *24*, 759–773. [CrossRef] [PubMed]

188. Kaidanovich-Beilin, O.; Lipina, T.; Vukobradovic, I.; Roder, J.; Woodgett, J.R. Assessment of social interaction behaviors. *J. Vis. Exp.* **2011**, *48*, e2473. [CrossRef]
189. Ni, R.J.; Tian, Y.; Dai, X.Y.; Zhao, L.S.; Wei, J.X.; Zhou, J.N.; Ma, X.H.; Li, T. Social avoidance behavior in male tree shrews and prosocial behavior in male mice toward unfamiliar conspecifics in the laboratory. *Zool. Res.* **2020**, *41*, 258–272. [CrossRef]
190. Liu, Y.; Deng, S.L.; Li, L.X.; Zhou, Z.X.; Lv, Q.; Wang, Z.Y.; Wang, F.; Chen, J.G. A circuit from dorsal hippocampal CA3 to parvafox nucleus mediates chronic social defeat stress-induced deficits in preference for social novelty. *Sci. Adv.* **2022**, *8*, eabe8828. [CrossRef]
191. Piccin, A.; Contarino, A. Long-lasting pseudo-social aggressive behavior in opiate-withdrawn mice. *Prog. Neuropsychopharmacol. Biol. Psychiatry* **2020**, *97*, 109780. [CrossRef]
192. Alsaeed, I.; Al-Somali, F.; Sakhnini, L.; Aljarallah, O.S.; Hamdan, R.M.; Bubishate, S.A.; Sarfaraz, Z.K.; Kamal, A. Autism-relevant social abnormalities in mice exposed perinatally to extremely low frequency electromagnetic fields. *Int. J. Dev. Neurosci.* **2014**, *37*, 58–64. [CrossRef]
193. Bevins, R.A.; Besheer, J. Object recognition in rats and mice: A one-trial non-matching-to-sample learning task to study 'recognition memory'. *Nat. Protoc.* **2006**, *1*, 1306–1311. [CrossRef] [PubMed]
194. Takahashi, H.; Tsuboi, A. Olfactory Habituation-dishabituation Test (Mouse). *Bio Protoc.* **2017**, *7*, e2154. [CrossRef] [PubMed]
195. Zou, J.; Wang, W.; Pan, Y.W.; Lu, S.; Xia, Z. Methods to measure olfactory behavior in mice. *Curr. Protoc. Toxicol.* **2015**, *63*, 11.18.11–11.18.21. [CrossRef]
196. Choi, K.W.; Kim, Y.K.; Jeon, H.J. Comorbid Anxiety and Depression: Clinical and Conceptual Consideration and Transdiagnostic Treatment. *Adv. Exp. Med. Biol.* **2020**, *1191*, 219–235. [CrossRef]
197. Koolhaas, J.M.; Coppens, C.M.; de Boer, S.F.; Buwalda, B.; Meerlo, P.; Timmermans, P.J. The resident-intruder paradigm: A standardized test for aggression, violence and social stress. *J. Vis. Exp.* **2013**, *77*, e4367. [CrossRef]
198. Fan, Z.; Zhu, H.; Zhou, T.; Wang, S.; Wu, Y.; Hu, H. Using the tube test to measure social hierarchy in mice. *Nat. Protoc.* **2019**, *14*, 819–831. [CrossRef]
199. Yang, C.R.; Bai, Y.Y.; Ruan, C.S.; Zhou, H.F.; Liu, D.; Wang, X.F.; Shen, L.J.; Zheng, H.Y.; Zhou, X.F. Enhanced aggressive behaviour in a mouse model of depression. *Neurotox. Res.* **2015**, *27*, 129–142. [CrossRef]
200. Douglas, K.M.; Gallagher, P.; Robinson, L.J.; Carter, J.D.; McIntosh, V.V.; Frampton, C.M.; Watson, S.; Young, A.H.; Ferrier, I.N.; Porter, R.J. Prevalence of cognitive impairment in major depression and bipolar disorder. *Bipolar Disord.* **2018**, *20*, 260–274. [CrossRef] [PubMed]
201. Liu, X.; Zhang, M.; Liu, H.; Zhu, R.; He, H.; Zhou, Y.; Zhang, Y.; Li, C.; Liang, D.; Zeng, Q.; et al. Bone marrow mesenchymal stem cell-derived exosomes attenuate cerebral ischemia-reperfusion injury-induced neuroinflammation and pyroptosis by modulating microglia M1/M2 phenotypes. *Exp. Neurol.* **2021**, *341*, 113700. [CrossRef]
202. Balseanu, A.T.; Buga, A.M.; Catalin, B.; Wagner, D.C.; Boltze, J.; Zagrean, A.M.; Reymann, K.; Schaebitz, W.; Popa-Wagner, A. Multimodal Approaches for Regenerative Stroke Therapies: Combination of Granulocyte Colony-Stimulating Factor with Bone Marrow Mesenchymal Stem Cells is Not Superior to G-CSF Alone. *Front. Aging Neurosci.* **2014**, *6*, 130. [CrossRef]
203. Yang, K.; Tan, Y.; Wang, F.; Zhang, Q.; Sun, P.; Zhang, Y.; Yao, N.; Zhao, Y.; Wang, X.; Fan, A.; et al. The improvement of spatial memory deficits in APP/V717I transgenic mice by chronic anti-stroke herb treatment. *Exp. Biol. Med.* **2014**, *239*, 1007–1017. [CrossRef]
204. Pitts, M.W. Barnes Maze Procedure for Spatial Learning and Memory in Mice. *Bio Protoc.* **2018**, *8*, e2744. [CrossRef]
205. Kraeuter, A.K.; Guest, P.C.; Sarnyai, Z. The Y-Maze for Assessment of Spatial Working and Reference Memory in Mice. *Methods Mol. Biol.* **2019**, *1916*, 105–111. [CrossRef] [PubMed]
206. Huo, K.; Wei, M.; Zhang, M.; Wang, Z.; Pan, P.; Shaligram, S.S.; Huang, J.; Prado, L.B.D.; Wong, J.; Su, H. Reduction of neuroinflammation alleviated mouse post bone fracture and stroke memory dysfunction. *J. Cereb. Blood Flow. Metab.* **2021**, *41*, 2162–2173. [CrossRef]
207. Ahnstedt, H.; Patrizz, A.; Chauhan, A.; Roy-O'Reilly, M.; Furr, J.W.; Spychala, M.S.; D'Aigle, J.; Blixt, F.W.; Zhu, L.; Bravo Alegria, J.; et al. Sex differences in T cell immune responses, gut permeability and outcome after ischemic stroke in aged mice. *Brain Behav. Immun.* **2020**, *87*, 556–567. [CrossRef] [PubMed]
208. Toshkezi, G.; Kyle, M.; Longo, S.L.; Chin, L.S.; Zhao, L.R. Brain repair by hematopoietic growth factors in the subacute phase of traumatic brain injury. *J. Neurosurg.* **2018**, *129*, 1286–1294. [CrossRef] [PubMed]
209. Olton, D.S.; Collison, C.; Werz, M.A. Spatial memory and radial arm maze performance of rats. *Learn. Motiv.* **1977**, *8*, 289–314. [CrossRef]
210. Kohler, J.; Mei, J.; Banneke, S.; Winter, Y.; Endres, M.; Emmrich, J.V. Assessing spatial learning and memory in mice: Classic radial maze versus a new animal-friendly automated radial maze allowing free access and not requiring food deprivation. *Front. Behav. Neurosci.* **2022**, *16*, 1013624. [CrossRef]
211. Borlongan, C.V.; Cahill, D.W.; Sanberg, P.R. Locomotor and passive avoidance deficits following occlusion of the middle cerebral artery. *Physiol. Behav.* **1995**, *58*, 909–917. [CrossRef]
212. Senechal, Y.; Kelly, P.H.; Dev, K.K. Amyloid precursor protein knockout mice show age-dependent deficits in passive avoidance learning. *Behav. Brain Res.* **2008**, *186*, 126–132. [CrossRef]
213. Singh, N.; Ma, B.; Leonardo, C.C.; Ahmad, A.S.; Narumiya, S.; Doré, S. Role of PGE_2 EP1 receptor in intracerebral hemorrhage-induced brain injury. *Neurotox. Res.* **2013**, *24*, 549–559. [CrossRef] [PubMed]

214. Deacon, R.M. Measuring motor coordination in mice. *J. Vis. Exp.* **2013**, *75*, e2609. [CrossRef]
215. Jacobs, J.R.; Carey, M.R. Move Over Rotarod, Here Comes RotaWheel. *Neuroscience* **2021**, *466*, 258–259. [CrossRef]
216. Nguyen, K.P.; Sharma, A.; Gil-Silva, M.; Gittis, A.H.; Chase, S.M. Distinct Kinematic Adjustments over Multiple Timescales Accompany Locomotor Skill Development in Mice. *Neuroscience* **2021**, *466*, 260–272. [CrossRef]
217. Syeara, N.; Bagchi, S.; Al Shoyaib, A.; Karamyan, S.T.; Alamri, F.F.; Karamyan, V.T. The Finer Aspects of Grid-Walking and Cylinder Tests for Experimental Stroke Recovery Studies in Mice. *Methods Mol. Biol.* **2023**, *2616*, 345–353. [CrossRef]
218. Zalewska, K.; Pietrogrande, G.; Ong, L.K.; Abdolhoseini, M.; Kluge, M.; Johnson, S.J.; Walker, F.R.; Nilsson, M. Sustained administration of corticosterone at stress-like levels after stroke suppressed glial reactivity at sites of thalamic secondary neurodegeneration. *Brain Behav. Immun.* **2018**, *69*, 210–222. [CrossRef]
219. Modo, M.; Stroemer, R.P.; Tang, E.; Veizovic, T.; Sowniski, P.; Hodges, H. Neurological sequelae and long-term behavioural assessment of rats with transient middle cerebral artery occlusion. *J. Neurosci. Methods* **2000**, *104*, 99–109. [CrossRef]
220. Hayashi, K.; Hasegawa, Y.; Takemoto, Y.; Cao, C.; Mukasa, A.; Kim-Mitsuyama, S. Enhanced oxidative stress contributes to worse prognosis and delayed neurofunctional recovery after striatal intracerebral hemorrhage in 5XFAD mice. *Eur. J. Neurosci.* **2020**, *51*, 1806–1814. [CrossRef] [PubMed]
221. Carter, R.J.; Morton, J.; Dunnett, S.B. Motor coordination and balance in rodents. *Curr. Protoc. Neurosci.* **2001**, *15*, 8–12. [CrossRef]
222. Hu, M.Z.; Wang, A.R.; Zhao, Z.Y.; Chen, X.Y.; Li, Y.B.; Liu, B. Antidepressant-like effects of paeoniflorin on post-stroke depression in a rat model. *Neurol. Res.* **2019**, *41*, 446–455. [CrossRef]
223. Du, Y.; Liang, H.; Zhang, L.; Fu, F. Administration of Huperzine A exerts antidepressant-like activity in a rat model of post-stroke depression. *Pharmacol. Biochem. Behav.* **2017**, *158*, 32–38. [CrossRef]
224. Ji, S.; Kronenberg, G.; Balkaya, M.; Färber, K.; Gertz, K.; Kettenmann, H.; Endres, M. Acute neuroprotection by pioglitazone after mild brain ischemia without effect on long-term outcome. *Exp. Neurol.* **2009**, *216*, 321–328. [CrossRef]
225. Feng, L.; Han, C.-X.; Cao, S.-Y.; Zhang, H.-M.; Wu, G.-Y. Deficits in motor and cognitive functions in an adult mouse model of hypoxia-ischemia induced stroke. *Sci. Rep.* **2020**, *10*, 20646. [CrossRef] [PubMed]
226. Shi, X.; Bai, H.; Wang, J.; Wang, J.; Huang, L.; He, M.; Zheng, X.; Duan, Z.; Chen, D.; Zhang, J.; et al. Behavioral Assessment of Sensory, Motor, Emotion, and Cognition in Rodent Models of Intracerebral Hemorrhage. *Front. Neurol.* **2021**, *12*, 667511. [CrossRef] [PubMed]
227. Metz, G.A.; Whishaw, I.Q. The ladder rung walking task: A scoring system and its practical application. *J. Vis. Exp.* **2009**, *28*, e1204. [CrossRef]
228. Tamakoshi, K.; Ishida, A.; Takamatsu, Y.; Hamakawa, M.; Nakashima, H.; Shimada, H.; Ishida, K. Motor skills training promotes motor functional recovery and induces synaptogenesis in the motor cortex and striatum after intracerebral hemorrhage in rats. *Behav. Brain Res.* **2014**, *260*, 34–43. [CrossRef]
229. Sun, J.; Wei, Z.Z.; Gu, X.; Zhang, J.Y.; Zhang, Y.; Li, J.; Wei, L. Intranasal delivery of hypoxia-preconditioned bone marrow-derived mesenchymal stem cells enhanced regenerative effects after intracerebral hemorrhagic stroke in mice. *Exp. Neurol.* **2015**, *272*, 78–87. [CrossRef]
230. Beray-Berthat, V.; Delifer, C.; Besson, V.C.; Girgis, H.; Coqueran, B.; Plotkine, M.; Marchand-Leroux, C.; Margaill, I. Long-term histological and behavioural characterisation of a collagenase-induced model of intracerebral haemorrhage in rats. *J. Neurosci. Methods* **2010**, *191*, 180–190. [CrossRef] [PubMed]
231. Schaar, K.L.; Brenneman, M.M.; Savitz, S.I. Functional assessments in the rodent stroke model. *Exp. Transl. Stroke Med.* **2010**, *2*, 13. [CrossRef]
232. de Oliveira, J.L.; Ávila, M.; Martins, T.C.; Alvarez-Silva, M.; Winkelmann-Duarte, E.C.; Salgado, A.S.I.; Cidral-Filho, F.J.; Reed, W.R.; Martins, D.F. Medium- and long-term functional behavior evaluations in an experimental focal ischemic stroke mouse model. *Cogn. Neurodyn* **2020**, *14*, 473–481. [CrossRef]
233. Zarruk, J.; Garcia-Yebenes, I.; Romera, V.G.; Ballesteros, I.; Moraga, A.; Cuartero, M.; Hurtado, O.; Sobrado, M.; Pradillo, J.; Fernandez-Lopez, D.; et al. Neurological tests for functional outcome assessment in rodent models of ischaemic stroke. *Rev. Neurol.* **2011**, *53*, 607–618. [PubMed]
234. Hao, J.; Mdzinarishvili, A.; Abbruscato, T.J.; Klein, J.; Geldenhuys, W.J.; Van der Schyf, C.J.; Bickel, U. Neuroprotection in mice by NGP1-01 after transient focal brain ischemia. *Brain Res.* **2008**, *1196*, 113–120. [CrossRef]
235. Narayan, S.K.; Grace Cherian, S.; Babu Phaniti, P.; Babu Chidambaram, S.; Rachel Vasanthi, A.H.; Arumugam, M. Preclinical animal studies in ischemic stroke: Challenges and some solutions. *Anim. Model. Exp. Med.* **2021**, *4*, 104–115. [CrossRef] [PubMed]
236. Allred, R.P.; Adkins, D.L.; Woodlee, M.T.; Husbands, L.C.; Maldonado, M.A.; Kane, J.R.; Schallert, T.; Jones, T.A. The vermicelli handling test: A simple quantitative measure of dexterous forepaw function in rats. *J. Neurosci. Methods* **2008**, *170*, 229–244. [CrossRef] [PubMed]
237. Yoshida, H.M.; Lima, F.O.; Barreira, J.; Appenzeller, S.; Fernandes, P.T. Is there a correlation between depressive symptoms and motor skills in post-stroke patients? *Arq. Neuropsiquiatr.* **2019**, *77*, 155–160. [CrossRef]
238. Ritzel, R.M.; Lai, Y.J.; Crapser, J.D.; Patel, A.R.; Schrecengost, A.; Grenier, J.M.; Mancini, N.S.; Patrizz, A.; Jellison, E.R.; Morales-Scheihing, D.; et al. Aging alters the immunological response to ischemic stroke. *Acta Neuropathol.* **2018**, *136*, 89–110. [CrossRef]
239. Gu, S.; He, Z.; Xu, Q.; Dong, J.; Xiao, T.; Liang, F.; Ma, X.; Wang, F.; Huang, J.H. The Relationship Between 5-Hydroxytryptamine and Its Metabolite Changes With Post-stroke Depression. *Front. Psychiatry* **2022**, *13*, 871754. [CrossRef]

240. Sullivan, G.M.; Ogden, R.T.; Huang, Y.Y.; Oquendo, M.A.; Mann, J.J.; Parsey, R.V. Higher in vivo serotonin-1a binding in posttraumatic stress disorder: A PET study with [11C]WAY-100635. *Depress. Anxiety* **2013**, *30*, 197–206. [CrossRef]
241. Spasojevic, N.; Jovanovic, P.; Dronjak, S. Chronic fluoxetine treatment affects gene expression of catecholamine enzymes in the heart of depression model rats. *Indian. J. Exp. Biol.* **2012**, *50*, 771–775.
242. Starr, L.R.; Hammen, C.; Brennan, P.A.; Najman, J.M. Serotonin transporter gene as a predictor of stress generation in depression. *J. Abnorm. Psychol.* **2012**, *121*, 810–818. [CrossRef]
243. Kim, J.M.; Stewart, R.; Kim, S.W.; Shin, I.S.; Kim, J.T.; Park, M.S.; Park, S.W.; Kim, Y.H.; Cho, K.H.; Yoon, J.S. Associations of cytokine gene polymorphisms with post-stroke depression. *World J. Biol. Psychiatry* **2012**, *13*, 579–587. [CrossRef] [PubMed]
244. Ogłodek, E. Changes in the Serum Levels of Cytokines: IL-1β, IL-4, IL-8 and IL-10 in Depression with and without Posttraumatic Stress Disorder. *Brain Sci.* **2022**, *12*, 387. [CrossRef] [PubMed]
245. Wang, L.; Wang, R.; Liu, L.; Qiao, D.; Baldwin, D.S.; Hou, R. Effects of SSRIs on peripheral inflammatory markers in patients with major depressive disorder: A systematic review and meta-analysis. *Brain Behav. Immun.* **2019**, *79*, 24–38. [CrossRef] [PubMed]
246. Zhang, S.; Zong, Y.; Ren, Z.; Hu, J.; Wu, X.; Xiao, H.; Qin, S.; Zhou, G.; Ma, Y.; Zhang, Y.; et al. Regulation of indoleamine 2, 3-dioxygenase in hippocampal microglia by NLRP3 inflammasome in lipopolysaccharide-induced depressive-like behaviors. *Eur. J. Neurosci.* **2020**, *52*, 4586–4601. [CrossRef]
247. Holsboer, F. The corticosteroid receptor hypothesis of depression. *Neuropsychopharmacology* **2000**, *23*, 477–501. [CrossRef]
248. Pace, T.W.; Hu, F.; Miller, A.H. Activation of cAMP-protein kinase A abrogates STAT5-mediated inhibition of glucocorticoid receptor signaling by interferon-alpha. *Brain Behav. Immun.* **2011**, *25*, 1716–1724. [CrossRef]
249. El Husseini, N.; Laskowitz, D.T. The role of neuroendocrine pathways in prognosis after stroke. *Expert. Rev. Neurother.* **2014**, *14*, 217–232. [CrossRef]
250. Kim, J.M.; Stewart, R.; Kang, H.J.; Kim, S.Y.; Kim, S.W.; Shin, I.S.; Park, M.S.; Kim, H.R.; Shin, M.G.; Cho, K.H.; et al. A longitudinal study of BDNF promoter methylation and genotype with poststroke depression. *J. Affect. Disord.* **2013**, *149*, 93–99. [CrossRef]
251. Zhang, Y.; Jiang, H.; Yue, Y.; Yin, Y.; Zhang, Y.; Liang, J.; Li, S.; Wang, J.; Lu, J.; Geng, D.; et al. The protein and mRNA expression levels of glial cell line-derived neurotrophic factor in post stroke depression and major depressive disorder. *Sci. Rep.* **2017**, *7*, 8674. [CrossRef]
252. Kunze, A.; Zierath, D.; Drogomiretskiy, O.; Becker, K. Strain differences in fatigue and depression after experimental stroke. *Transl. Stroke Res.* **2014**, *5*, 604–611. [CrossRef]
253. Lavu, V.K.; Mohamed, R.A.; Huang, R.; Potla, S.; Bhalla, S.; Al Qabandi, Y.; Nandula, S.A.; Boddepalli, C.S.; Gutlapalli, S.D.; Mohammed, L. Evaluation and Treatment of Depression in Stroke Patients: A Systematic Review. *Cureus* **2022**, *14*, e28137. [CrossRef]
254. Starkstein, S.E.; Hayhow, B.D. Treatment of Post-Stroke Depression. *Curr. Treat. Options Neurol.* **2019**, *21*, 31. [CrossRef]
255. Medeiros, G.C.; Roy, D.; Kontos, N.; Beach, S.R. Post-stroke depression: A 2020 updated review. *Gen. Hosp. Psychiatry* **2020**, *66*, 70–80. [CrossRef] [PubMed]
256. Zhao, Z.; Zhang, W.; Zhang, Y.; Zhao, Y.; Zheng, C.; Tian, H.; Lei, J.; Liu, Y.; Zhao, R.; Tang, Q. Multimodal Magnetic Resonance Imaging and Therapeutic Intervention With Yi-nao-jie-yu Decoction in a Rat Model of Post-stroke Depression. *Front. Psychiatry* **2020**, *11*, 557423. [CrossRef]
257. Chen, C.; Dong, Y.; Liu, F.; Gao, C.; Ji, C.; Dang, Y.; Ma, X.; Liu, Y. A Study of Antidepressant Effect and Mechanism on Intranasal Delivery of BDNF-HA2TAT/AAV to Rats with Post-Stroke Depression. *Neuropsychiatr. Dis. Treat.* **2020**, *16*, 637–649. [CrossRef]
258. Ngwa, C.; Al Mamun, A.; Qi, S.; Sharmeen, R.; Xu, Y.; Liu, F. Regulation of microglial activation in stroke in aged mice: A translational study. *Aging* **2022**, *14*, 6047–6065. [CrossRef] [PubMed]
259. Morioka, T.; Kalehua, A.N.; Streit, W.J. Characterization of microglial reaction after middle cerebral artery occlusion in rat brain. *J. Comp. Neurol.* **1993**, *327*, 123–132. [CrossRef] [PubMed]
260. Lambertsen, K.L.; Biber, K.; Finsen, B. Inflammatory cytokines in experimental and human stroke. *J. Cereb. Blood Flow. Metab.* **2012**, *32*, 1677–1698. [CrossRef]
261. Kang, J.B.; Son, H.K.; Shah, M.A.; Koh, P.O. Retinoic acid attenuates ischemic injury-induced activation of glial cells and inflammatory factors in a rat stroke model. *PLoS ONE* **2024**, *19*, e0300072. [CrossRef] [PubMed]
262. Cojocaru, A.; Burada, E.; Bălșeanu, A.T.; Deftu, A.F.; Cătălin, B.; Popa-Wagner, A.; Osiac, E. Roles of Microglial Ion Channel in Neurodegenerative Diseases. *J. Clin. Med.* **2021**, *10*, 1239. [CrossRef]
263. Miao, Z.; Wang, Y.; Sun, Z. The Relationships Between Stress, Mental Disorders, and Epigenetic Regulation of BDNF. *Int. J. Mol. Sci.* **2020**, *21*, 1375. [CrossRef]
264. Wu, X.; Gu, J.; Zou, Z.; Yu, M.; Zhang, C.; Xiao, Q.; Chen, X.; Li, C. Suppressive Effects of Isofraxidin on Depressive-like Behaviors Induced by Chronic Unpredictable Mild Stress in Mice. *Brain Sci.* **2022**, *12*, 1376. [CrossRef] [PubMed]
265. Kim, J.S.; Choi-Kwon, S. Poststroke depression and emotional incontinence: Correlation with lesion location. *Neurology* **2000**, *54*, 1805–1810. [CrossRef]
266. Harciarek, M.; Mańkowska, A. Hemispheric stroke: Mood disorders. *Handb. Clin. Neurol.* **2021**, *183*, 155–167. [CrossRef]
267. Carson, A.J.; MacHale, S.; Allen, K.; Lawrie, S.M.; Dennis, M.; House, A.; Sharpe, M. Depression after stroke and lesion location: A systematic review. *Lancet* **2000**, *356*, 122–126. [CrossRef] [PubMed]
268. Singh, A.; Herrmann, N.; Black, S.E. The importance of lesion location in poststroke depression: A critical review. *Can. J. Psychiatry* **1998**, *43*, 921–927. [CrossRef] [PubMed]

269. Dockman, R.L.; Carpenter, J.M.; Diaz, A.N.; Benbow, R.A.; Filipov, N.M. Sex differences in behavior, response to LPS, and glucose homeostasis in middle-aged mice. *Behav. Brain Res.* **2022**, *418*, 113628. [CrossRef]
270. Furman, O.; Tsoory, M.; Chen, A. Differential chronic social stress models in male and female mice. *Eur. J. Neurosci.* **2022**, *55*, 2777–2793. [CrossRef]
271. Sohrabji, F.; Okoreeh, A.; Panta, A. Sex hormones and stroke: Beyond estrogens. *Horm. Behav.* **2019**, *111*, 87–95. [CrossRef]
272. Jiang, H.; Xiao, L.; Jin, K.; Shao, B. Estrogen administration attenuates post-stroke depression by enhancing CREB/BDNF/TrkB signaling in the rat hippocampus. *Exp. Ther. Med.* **2021**, *21*, 433. [CrossRef]
273. Zeng, P.Y.; Tsai, Y.H.; Lee, C.L.; Ma, Y.K.; Kuo, T.H. Minimal influence of estrous cycle on studies of female mouse behaviors. *Front. Mol. Neurosci.* **2023**, *16*, 1146109. [CrossRef] [PubMed]
274. Tsao, C.-H.; Wu, K.-Y.; Su, N.C.; Edwards, A.; Huang, G.-J. The influence of sex difference on behavior and adult hippocampal neurogenesis in C57BL/6 mice. *Sci. Rep.* **2023**, *13*, 17297. [CrossRef] [PubMed]
275. Tariq, M.B.; Lee, J.; McCullough, L.D. Sex differences in the inflammatory response to stroke. *Semin. Immunopathol.* **2023**, *45*, 295–313. [CrossRef] [PubMed]

life

Editorial

Feature Paper in Oral Physiology and Pathology

Giuseppe Minervini [1,2]

[1] Saveetha Dental College and Hospitals, Saveetha Institute of Medical and Technical Sciences, Saveetha University, Chennai 602105, Tamil Nadu, India; giuseppe.minervini@unicampania.it
[2] Multidisciplinary Department of Medical-Surgical and Odontostomatological Specialties, University of Campania "Luigi Vanvitelli", 80121 Naples, Italy

In the realm of life sciences, the journal *'Life'* has consistently served as a beacon for groundbreaking research and scientific discovery. This Special Issue continues this tradition, presenting a diverse array of studies that collectively underscore the intricate and multifaceted nature of biological research. The articles featured in this issue collectively enhance our comprehension of health and disease, with notable advancements in the realms of genetics, disease biomarkers, musculoskeletal health, therapeutic interventions, and beyond.

This Special Issue primarily concentrates on exploring the genetic and molecular pathways underlying various diseases. A notably important study examines the polymorphisms in the gene encoding heat shock factor 1 (HSF1) and their link to type 2 diabetes [1]. This research sheds light on the crucial role of protein folding and stress responses in diabetes pathogenesis, pinpointing specific genetic variations in HSF1 associated with an increased risk of the disease, especially in overweight and obese females [1–3]. This finding enhances our comprehension of the molecular mechanisms driving diabetes and proposes potential avenues for targeted genetic therapies.

The quest for dependable biomarkers continues to be a major research priority, especially for chronic and degenerative conditions like osteoarthritis (OA) [4]. The review of soluble and extracellular vesicle (EV)-associated biomarkers in knee OA pathology underscores the urgent need for early and precise diagnostic tools [5,6]. Scientists predict that developing non-invasive biomarkers capable of forecasting disease progression and identifying therapeutic targets will significantly enhance patient outcomes. Such biomarkers will change OA management by enabling early intervention and a more personalized approach to treatment [4,7–11].

This special edition also addresses the important topic of obesity and its effects on musculoskeletal health. A thorough study that looked at how cartilage works and how likely it is to break in the medial tibiofemoral compartment makes the link between having a higher body mass index and a higher risk of cartilage degradation very clear. This would imply that scientific research would more likely encourage weight control as a significant component of programs to prevent musculoskeletal diseases and how multidimensional lifestyle interventions can offset the effects on joint health [12–18].

Exercise functions as a crucial therapeutic intervention for mitigating chemotherapy-induced peripheral neuropathy (CIPN) [19]. Systematic reviews and meta-analyses detailed in this issue reveal that therapeutic exercise markedly alleviates peripheral neuropathy symptoms in cancer patients. These findings underscore the significance of exercise not only as an adjunctive treatment during chemotherapy but also as a strategy to enhance the overall quality of life for cancer patients [19,20]. This underscores the importance of integrating physical activity into standard cancer care protocols.

The intersection of autoimmune diseases and parasitic infections presents a unique and fascinating avenue for understanding disease mechanisms [21,22]. An intriguing study on the influence of intestinal nematode infections on growth factors in autoimmune models reveals how parasitic infections can modulate immune responses and angiogenesis. This research offers potential therapeutic insights, suggesting that manipulating parasitic

check for updates

Citation: Minervini, G. Feature Paper in Oral Physiology and Pathology. *Life* **2024**, *14*, 895. https://doi.org/10.3390/life14070895

Received: 5 July 2024
Accepted: 11 July 2024
Published: 19 July 2024

infections could lead to novel treatments for autoimmune diseases [22]. This kind of finding represents the complexity of interplay among various biological systems and the possibility of cross-disciplinary ways of disease treatment.

This emphasis on emerging breakthroughs is dynamic in the development of new insights into sepsis-induced coagulopathy. Understanding the prothrombotic states induced by severe infections is crucial for developing early-stage diagnostic markers and therapeutic strategies [23–25]. By identifying these markers, researchers aim to improve the management and outcomes of septic conditions, which remain a significant challenge in clinical settings.

This edition also advocates for the biomedical applications of platelet-derived extracellular vesicle (PEV) transfer. PEVs now elegantly transfer a diverse array of biomolecules, modifying numerous target cell functions and supporting processes like inflammation, coagulation, and tissue repair [26–28]. These findings indicate promising avenues for developing novel therapeutic regimens based on PEVs for various clinical contexts. Moreover, the potential of PEVs to serve as both diagnostic biomarkers and therapeutic tools represents a major advancement in translational medicine.

Cutting-edge research on chondrocyte biology further enriches this issue. Studies on the role of WNT16 in maintaining the articular chondrocyte phenotype bring new understandings to joint homeostasis and osteoarthritis [29,30]. Studies suggest that WNT16 stimulates proliferation and sustains chondrocytes at a crucial level for cartilage homeostasis [29]. The molecular mechanism by which WNT16 works basically helps to create a number of therapeutic interventions that can stop or at least slow the progression of OA [29]. Such advancements are particularly relevant given the aging global population and the increasing prevalence of joint-related disorders.

This issue also highlights the innovative use of dupilumab for treating dermatitis associated with immunoglobulin G4-related disease (IgG4-RD) [31]. The case study in this issue showcases how targeting specific interleukins can result in significant therapeutic benefits, underscoring the potential of personalized medicine. The patient dramatically improved in quality of life after treatment with dupilumab, thus reflecting how innovative therapeutic strategies can control complex and rare diseases [31,32].

Even more suggestively, the balance between genetic predisposition and added risk from environmental factors forms a constant undercurrent in this volume. Research on genetic susceptibility in various diseases takes into account both innate genetic makeup and exogenous ecological influences [33]. This holistic approach is crucial for developing more effective and comprehensive treatment strategies that address the multifactorial nature of most diseases.

In sum, this Special Issue of '*Life*' reflects the dynamic and interconnected nature of life sciences research. From genetic predispositions to innovative therapeutic interventions, the contributions within these pages highlight the relentless pursuit of knowledge aimed at understanding and ultimately improving human health. Each article, in addition to moving forward our scientific understanding, emphasizes the need for interdisciplinary collaboration in facing complex health and disease challenges. As we continue to explore new areas of biological research, the insights gained from these studies will undoubtedly aid in devising more effective strategies for improving human health and well-being.

Funding: This research received no external funding.

Conflicts of Interest: The authors declare no conflicts of interest in the data; in the writing of the manuscript; or in the decision to publish the results.

References

1. Chen, Z.; Ding, L.; Yang, W.; Wang, J.; Chen, L.; Chang, Y.; Geng, B.; Cui, Q.; Guan, Y.; Yang, J. Hepatic Activation of the FAM3C-HSF1-CaM Pathway Attenuates Hyperglycemia of Obese Diabetic Mice. *Diabetes* **2017**, *66*, 1185–1197. [CrossRef] [PubMed]
2. Purwana, I.; Liu, J.J.; Portha, B.; Buteau, J. HSF1 Acetylation Decreases Its Transcriptional Activity and Enhances Glucolipotoxicity-Induced Apoptosis in Rat and Human Beta Cells. *Diabetologia* **2017**, *60*, 1432–1441. [CrossRef] [PubMed]

3. Smith, R.S.; Takagishi, S.R.; Amici, D.R.; Metz, K.; Gayatri, S.; Alasady, M.J.; Wu, Y.; Brockway, S.; Taiberg, S.L.; Khalatyan, N.; et al. HSF2 Cooperates with HSF1 to Drive a Transcriptional Program Critical for the Malignant State. *Sci. Adv.* **2022**, *8*, eabj6526. [CrossRef] [PubMed]
4. Lin, X.; Li, L.; Liu, X.; Tian, J.; Zheng, W.; Li, J.; Wang, L. Genome-Wide Analysis of Aberrant Methylation of Enhancer DNA in Human Osteoarthritis. *BMC Med. Genom.* **2020**, *13*, 1. [CrossRef] [PubMed]
5. Øiestad, B.E.; Juhl, C.B.; Eitzen, I.; Thorlund, J.B. Knee Extensor Muscle Weakness Is a Risk Factor for Development of Knee Osteoarthritis. A Systematic Review and Meta-Analysis. *Osteoarthr. Cartil.* **2015**, *23*, 171–177. [CrossRef] [PubMed]
6. Bricca, A.; Struglics, A.; Larsson, S.; Steultjens, M.; Juhl, C.B.; Roos, E.M. Impact of Exercise Therapy on Molecular Biomarkers Related to Cartilage and Inflammation in Individuals at Risk of, or With Established, Knee Osteoarthritis: A Systematic Review and Meta-Analysis of Randomized Controlled Trials. *Arthritis Care Res.* **2019**, *71*, 1504–1515. [CrossRef]
7. Chahal, J.; Gómez-Aristizábal, A.; Shestopaloff, K.; Bhatt, S.; Chaboureau, A.; Fazio, A.; Chisholm, J.; Weston, A.; Chiovitti, J.; Keating, A.; et al. Bone Marrow Mesenchymal Stromal Cell Treatment in Patients with Osteoarthritis Results in Overall Improvement in Pain and Symptoms and Reduces Synovial Inflammation. *Stem Cells Transl. Med.* **2019**, *8*, 746–757. [CrossRef]
8. Minervini, G.; Franco, R.; Marrapodi, M.M.; Di Blasio, M.; Ronsivalle, V.; Cicciù, M. Children Oral Health and Parents Education Status: A Cross Sectional Study. *BMC Oral Health* **2023**, *23*, 787. [CrossRef] [PubMed]
9. Minervini, G.; Franco, R.; Marrapodi, M.M.; Almeida, L.E.; Ronsivalle, V.; Cicciù, M. Prevalence of Temporomandibular Disorders (TMD) in Obesity Patients: A Systematic Review and Meta-analysis. *J. Oral Rehabil.* **2023**, *50*, 1544–1553. [CrossRef]
10. Minervini, G.; Franco, R.; Marrapodi, M.M.; Di Blasio, M.; Isola, G.; Cicciù, M. Conservative Treatment of Temporomandibular Joint Condylar Fractures: A Systematic Review Conducted According to PRISMA Guidelines and the Cochrane Handbook for Systematic Reviews of Interventions. *J. Oral Rehabil.* **2023**, *50*, 886–893. [CrossRef]
11. Rapani, A.; Berton, F.; Tramontin, A.; Turco, G.; Marchesi, G.; Di Lenarda, R.; Stacchi, C. Surface Roughness of Enamel and Dentin after Preparation Finishing with Rotary Burs or Piezoelectric Instruments. *Prosthesis* **2023**, *5*, 711–720. [CrossRef]
12. Sekar, S.; Crawford, R.; Xiao, Y.; Prasadam, I. Dietary Fats and Osteoarthritis: Insights, Evidences, and New Horizons. *J. Cell Biochem.* **2017**, *118*, 453–463. [CrossRef] [PubMed]
13. Rosenberg, J.H.; Rai, V.; Dilisio, M.F.; Agrawal, D.K. Damage-Associated Molecular Patterns in the Pathogenesis of Osteoarthritis: Potentially Novel Therapeutic Targets. *Mol. Cell Biochem.* **2017**, *434*, 171–179. [CrossRef] [PubMed]
14. Chen, D.; Shen, J.; Zhao, W.; Wang, T.; Han, L.; Hamilton, J.L.; Im, H.-J. Osteoarthritis: Toward a Comprehensive Understanding of Pathological Mechanism. *Bone Res.* **2017**, *5*, 16044. [CrossRef] [PubMed]
15. Alkahtany, M.; Beatty, M.W.; Alsalleeh, F.; Petro, T.M.; Simetich, B.; Zhou, Y.; Feely, D.; Polyzois, G. Color Stability, Physical Properties and Antifungal Effects of ZrO2 Additions to Experimental Maxillofacial Silicones: Comparisons with TiO_2. *Prosthesis* **2023**, *5*, 916–938. [CrossRef]
16. Ghadirinejad, K.; Day, C.W.; Milimonfared, R.; Taylor, M.; Solomon, L.B.; Hashemi, R. Fretting Wear and Corrosion-Related Risk Factors in Total Hip Replacement: A Literature Review on Implant Retrieval Studies and National Joint Replacement Registry Reports. *Prosthesis* **2023**, *5*, 774–791. [CrossRef]
17. Pelivan, I.; Šeparović, I.; Vuletić, M.; Dulčić, N.; Gabrić, D. Radiological and Periodontal Evaluation of Stock and Custom CAD/CAM Implant Abutments—A One-Year Follow-Up Study. *Prosthesis* **2023**, *5*, 437–452. [CrossRef]
18. Tanaka, T.; Hara, S.; Hendawy, H.; El-Husseiny, H.M.; Tanaka, R.; Asakura, T. Development of Small-Diameter Artificial Vascular Grafts Using Transgenic Silk Fibroin. *Prosthesis* **2023**, *5*, 763–773. [CrossRef]
19. Chung, K.H.; Park, S.B.; Streckmann, F.; Wiskemann, J.; Mohile, N.; Kleckner, A.S.; Colloca, L.; Dorsey, S.G.; Kleckner, I.R. Mechanisms, Mediators, and Moderators of the Effects of Exercise on Chemotherapy-Induced Peripheral Neuropathy. *Cancers* **2022**, *14*, 1224. [CrossRef]
20. Nuñez de Arenas-Arroyo, S.; Cavero-Redondo, I.; Torres-Costoso, A.; Reina-Gutiérrez, S.; Lorenzo-García, P.; Martínez-Vizcaíno, V. Effects of Exercise Interventions to Reduce Chemotherapy-induced Peripheral Neuropathy Severity: A Meta-analysis. *Scand. J. Med. Sci. Sports* **2023**, *33*, 1040–1053. [CrossRef]
21. Matisz, C.E.; McDougall, J.J.; Sharkey, K.A.; McKay, D.M. Helminth Parasites and the Modulation of Joint Inflammation. *J. Parasitol. Res.* **2011**, *2011*, 942616. [CrossRef]
22. Everts, B.; Smits, H.H.; Hokke, C.H.; Yazdanbakhsh, M. Helminths and Dendritic Cells: Sensing and Regulating via Pattern Recognition Receptors, Th2 and Treg Responses. *Eur. J. Immunol.* **2010**, *40*, 1525–1537. [CrossRef] [PubMed]
23. Pons, S.; Fodil, S.; Azoulay, E.; Zafrani, L. The Vascular Endothelium: The Cornerstone of Organ Dysfunction in Severe SARS-CoV-2 Infection. *Crit. Care* **2020**, *24*, 353. [CrossRef] [PubMed]
24. Fletcher-Sandersjöö, A.; Bellander, B.-M. Is COVID-19 Associated Thrombosis Caused by Overactivation of the Complement Cascade? A Literature Review. *Thromb. Res.* **2020**, *194*, 36–41. [CrossRef] [PubMed]
25. Sokol, J.; Nehaj, F.; Mokan, M.; Lisa, L.; Stasko, J. COVID-19 Infection in a Patient with Paroxysmal Nocturnal Hemoglobinuria. *Medicine* **2021**, *100*, e25456. [CrossRef] [PubMed]
26. Antich-Rosselló, M.; Forteza-Genestra, M.A.; Monjo, M.; Ramis, J.M. Platelet-Derived Extracellular Vesicles for Regenerative Medicine. *Int. J. Mol. Sci.* **2021**, *22*, 8580. [CrossRef] [PubMed]
27. Zaldivia, M.T.K.; McFadyen, J.D.; Lim, B.; Wang, X.; Peter, K. Platelet-Derived Microvesicles in Cardiovascular Diseases. *Front. Cardiovasc. Med.* **2017**, *4*, 74. [CrossRef] [PubMed]

28. Taus, F.; Meneguzzi, A.; Castelli, M.; Minuz, P. Platelet-Derived Extracellular Vesicles as Target of Antiplatelet Agents. What Is the Evidence? *Front. Pharmacol.* **2019**, *10*, 1256. [CrossRef]
29. Yan, H.; Hu, Y.; Akk, A.; Rai, M.F.; Pan, H.; Wickline, S.A.; Pham, C.T.N. Induction of WNT16 via Peptide-MRNA Nanoparticle-Based Delivery Maintains Cartilage Homeostasis. *Pharmaceutics* **2020**, *12*, 73. [CrossRef]
30. Tong, W.; Zeng, Y.; Chow, D.H.K.; Yeung, W.; Xu, J.; Deng, Y.; Chen, S.; Zhao, H.; Zhang, X.; Ho, K.K.; et al. Wnt16 Attenuates Osteoarthritis Progression through a PCP/JNK-MTORC1-PTHrP Cascade. *Ann. Rheum. Dis.* **2019**, *78*, 551–561. [CrossRef]
31. Beck, L.A.; Thaçi, D.; Hamilton, J.D.; Graham, N.M.; Bieber, T.; Rocklin, R.; Ming, J.E.; Ren, H.; Kao, R.; Simpson, E.; et al. Dupilumab Treatment in Adults with Moderate-to-Severe Atopic Dermatitis. *N. Engl. J. Med.* **2014**, *371*, 130–139. [CrossRef]
32. Tameez Ud Din, A.; Malik, I.; Arshad, D.; Tameez Ud Din, A. Dupilumab for Atopic Dermatitis: The Silver Bullet We Have Been Searching For? *Cureus* **2020**, *12*, e7565. [CrossRef]
33. Rogler, G. Interaction between Susceptibility and Environment: Examples from the Digestive Tract. *Dig. Dis.* **2011**, *29*, 136–143. [CrossRef]

life

MDPI

Article

Alterations in Blood–Brain Barrier Integrity and Lateral Ventricle Differ in Rats Exposed to Space Radiation and Social Isolation

Austin M. Adkins [1], Zachary N. M. Luyo [1], Alayna J. Gibbs [2], Alea F. Boden [1], Riley S. Heerbrandt [1], Justin D. Gotthold [1], Richard A. Britten [3], Laurie L. Wellman [1] and Larry D. Sanford [1,*]

[1] Sleep Research Laboratory, Center for Integrative Neuroscience and Inflammatory Diseases, Pathology and Anatomy, Eastern Virginia Medical School, Norfolk, VA 23507, USA; adkinsam@evms.edu (A.M.A.); luyozn@evms.edu (Z.N.M.L.); bodenaf@evms.edu (A.F.B.); heerbrrs@evms.edu (R.S.H.); gotthojd@evms.edu (J.D.G.); wellmall@evms.edu (L.L.W.)

[2] Pathology and Anatomy, Eastern Virginia Medical School, Norfolk, VA 23507, USA; gibbsaj@evms.edu

[3] Center for Integrative Neuroscience and Inflammatory Diseases, Radiation Oncology, Eastern Virginia Medical School, Norfolk, VA 23507, USA; brittera@evms.edu

* Correspondence: sanforld@evms.edu; Tel.: +1-(757)-446-7081

Abstract: The proposed Mars missions will expose astronauts to long durations of social isolation (SI) and space radiation (SR). These stressors have been shown to alter the brain's macrostructure and microenvironment, including the blood–brain barrier (BBB). Breakdown of the BBB is linked to impaired executive functions and physical deficits, including sensorimotor and neurocognitive impairments. However, the precise mechanisms mediating these effects remain unknown. Additionally, the synergistic effects of combined exposure to SI and SR on the structural integrity of the BBB and brain remain unknown. We assessed the BBB integrity and morphology in the brains of male rats exposed to ground-based analogs of SI and SR. The rats exposed to SR had enlarged lateral ventricles and increased BBB damage associated with a loss of astrocytes and an increased number of leaky vessels. Many deficits observed in SR-treated animals were attenuated by dual exposure to SI (DFS). SI alone did not show BBB damage but did show differences in astrocyte morphology compared to the Controls. Thus, determining how single and combined inflight stressors modulate CNS structural integrity is crucial to fully understand the multiple pathways that could impact astronaut performance and health, including the alterations to the CNS structures and cell viability observed in this study.

Keywords: social isolation; space radiation; blood–brain barrier; lateral ventricle

check for updates

Citation: Adkins, A.M.; Luyo, Z.N.M.; Gibbs, A.J.; Boden, A.F.; Heerbrandt, R.S.; Gotthold, J.D.; Britten, R.A.; Wellman, L.L.; Sanford, L.D. Alterations in Blood–Brain Barrier Integrity and Lateral Ventricle Differ in Rats Exposed to Space Radiation and Social Isolation. *Life* **2024**, *14*, 636. https://doi.org/10.3390/life14050636

Academic Editor: Mengliang Zhang

Received: 4 April 2024
Revised: 3 May 2024
Accepted: 8 May 2024
Published: 16 May 2024

1. Introduction

The future of space exploration and planned NASA operations, such as the proposed Mars missions, will require crew members to log longer mission times and travel deeper into space than ever before. As such, crews will also experience increased exposure to multiple inflight stressors, including social isolation (SI) and space radiation (SR). Moreover, these missions will likely offer new challenges and obstacles that NASA and crews have not yet encountered [1].

SI and SR have been reported to alter immune system functionality. SI alone induces neuroinflammation and microglial overactivation [2]. SI can increase redox stress and levels of pro-inflammatory cytokines (e.g., TNF-α) [3]. Exposure to SR can induce neuroinflammation by elevating microglial activation [4]. Increases in neuroinflammation related to SI and SR can induce changes to the brain's macrostructure and microenvironment [5–7]. Significant alterations to CNS structural integrity have been associated with exposure to either SI and SR, including changes in tissue microenvironments [8] and regional morphology [9,10].

Individually, SI [11] and SR [8,12] have been reported to disrupt the blood–brain barrier (BBB). The BBB is an assembly of endothelial cells, blood vessels, astrocytes, and pericytes, which provides a semi-permeable border to regulate the movement of particles and cells into the CNS [13], thereby maintaining CNS homeostasis [14]. In contrast, the breakdown of the BBB leads to cognitive dysfunction and increases in neuroinflammation [15] and is associated with multiple neuropsychiatric disorders [16]. However, the precise mechanisms mediating these effects remain unknown. Therefore, alterations to immune functionality by exposure to SI and SR could reduce an astronaut's ability to maintain adequate levels of performance during missions that could not only affect crew health but mission success through several pathways.

Ultimately, SI and SR-induced immune system changes will likely result in significant alterations to the brain's structural integrity, which could lead to increases in anxiety, issues with memory processing, and impairments of cognitive and executive functions. However, the potential for SI and SR interactions to change immune system responses remains unknown. Given the dynamic environment of space missions, multiple stressors could have synergistic effects that interact in unknown ways that may result in differential outcomes. Thus, determining how single and compound inflight stressors interact to modulate the immune system and its relationship to structural alterations in the brain is crucial to fully understand the pathways impacting astronaut performance and health. In this experimental study, we investigated how SI and SR, and their combination, modified immune system function and its relevance to BBB integrity and brain homeostasis. Our goal was to assess how spaceflight stressors impact the BBB in ways that could alter brain function in astronauts.

2. Materials and Methods

2.1. Subjects

Male, outbred, Wistar strain rats (8–9 months old at the time of study, n = 4–5 per group) obtained from Hilltop Lab Animals, Inc. (Scottdale, PA, USA) were used in this study [17]. The rats were either subjected to SI (visual barriers between cages) or individually housed (as a Control group). SI began at least eight weeks prior to experimentation and was maintained throughout the study as previously described [17]. Separate groups of rats received a single dose of SR (15 cGy simplified 5-ion galactic cosmic radiation (GCRsim), Brookhaven National Laboratory (BNL); Long Island, NY) and were either individually housed or subjected to SI (dual flight stressors (DFS)). Other than irradiation, all the experimental manipulations and measures were conducted at Eastern Virginia Medical School in 2021–2022. Food and water were available ad libitum. The housing rooms were kept on a 12:12 light:dark cycle and the ambient temperature was maintained at 24.5 ± 0.5 °C. All the procedures were conducted in accordance with the National Institutes of Health Guide for the Care and Use of Experimental Animals and were approved by Eastern Virginia Medical School's Institutional Animal Care and Use Committee (Protocol#: 19-018).

2.2. Euthanasia

The rats were euthanized via isoflurane sedation (inhalant: 5%, $\leq$5 min duration) and cardiac perfusion with 1X PBS. Their brains were extracted and halved along the longitudinal fissure. The right hemisphere was used for analyses not discussed in this study. The left hemisphere was prepared as described in detail below.

2.3. Histology

The left hemisphere of the brain was fixed in 10% formalin solution at 4 °C for 24 h and then processed and paraffin-embedded for the subsequent histological analysis (n = 4–5 in each group). Five μm sagittal tissue sections through the limbic system were obtained via microtomy and mounted on glass slides (two sections per slide) for confocal or light microscopy.

2.4. Confocal Microscopy

Quadruple-label immunofluorescence staining was used to visually assess the potential effects of SI and SR on BBB integrity. The slides were first run through a deparaffinization/hydration sequence as follows: xylene 2 × 5 min each, 100% EtOH 2 × 2 min each, 95% EtOH 2 × 1 min each, 70% EtOH 2 × 1 min each, and dH_2O 2 × 1 min each. The slides were then quenched twice to reduce the fixative-induced auto-fluorescence by eliminating the free aldehyde groups using a 1% solution of $NaBH_4$ in 70% EtOH for 30 min at room temperature (RT) followed by a solution containing 0.375% glycine and 0.267% NH_4Cl in dH_2O for 10 min. Next, the tissue sections were soaked in the UltraCruz® blocking reagent for 30 min to eliminate potential background staining due to non-specific antibody binding. In between each solution, the tissue sections were quickly rinsed 3× each in 1X PBS. The tissue sections were then stained at RT for 1 h each with the following optimized concentrated antibodies: Fibrinogen (Diluted 1:600 in PBS. Biorbyt; Cat. #orb4255), Glut-1 (Diluted 1:200 in PBS. abcam; Cat. #ab195020), and GFAP (Diluted 1:400 in PBS. Novus Biologicals; Cat. #NBP2-34401AF488). In between each antibody incubation, the tissue sections were quickly rinsed 3× each in 1X PBS followed by a 5 min incubation in the glycine-containing quenching solution above. Following the final incubation, the tissue sections were covered in a Fluoroshield™ mounting medium containing DAPI (Abcam; Cat. #ab104139) and incubated for 5 min at RT and then cover-slipped and stored at 4 °C until imaged via confocal microscopy.

Stained tissue sections were imaged using a Zeiss Axio Observer Z.1 confocal microscope and ZEN Black acquisition software (version 2.1 SP3, Carl Zeiss, Inc.; Dublin, CA, USA) at 40× magnification. Eight 1024 × 1024 images including the basolateral amygdala, caudate putamen, hippocampus, and medial prefrontal cortex per treatment group were obtained. The acquired images were then uploaded to the ZEN Blue analysis software (version 3.7, Carl Zeiss, Inc.; Dublin, CA, USA) and the following parameters were assessed: total number of vessels, total number of astrocytes, total amount of fibrinogen extravasation, vesicular diameter, and astrocyte morphology (number of projections, distance of projections, and number of branches from projections).

The total number of vessels and astrocytes within each image were calculated using the cell counting tool within ImageJ (Version 2.14.0/1.54f) by manually "marking" each cell with the counter function. The counts were automatically tallied through ImageJ. The vesicular diameter was automatically calculated using the ImageJ measuring where a line was drawn across the width of the vessel. The number of astrocyte projections and branches within each image were calculated using the cell counting tool within ImageJ by manually "marking" each projection or branch with the counter function. Astrocyte projections were considered to be any protrusion that was directly connected to the cell body. Astrocyte branches were considered to be any outgrowth from a projection. The distance of each astrocyte projection was automatically calculated using the measuring tool within ImageJ, which was used to draw a line from the base of the astrocyte cell body to the furthest point of the projection.

2.5. Light Microscopy

H&E staining was used to assess the morphological changes in the brain. Following a deparaffinization/hydration sequence consisting of 60 dips in xylene, 20 dips in 100% EtOH, 10 dips 100% EtOH, 10 dips in 95% EtOH, 10 dips in 70% EtOH, and 10 dips in dH_2O, the slides were submerged for 2 min in filtered modified Harris hematoxylin. The slides were then briefly rinsed with tap water and dipped 10× each in bluing reagent followed by dH_2O. The slides were again briefly rinsed with tap water and then dipped 20× in eosin. Following a final dehydration sequence consisting of 10 dips in 95% EtOH, 20 dips in 100% EtOH, and 30 dips in xylene, the slides were cover-slipped.

The H&E-stained sagittal tissue sections (Lateral 1.4 mm, Bregma −0.45 mm) were imaged on a Nikon Eclipse E800 using the RT Slider SPOT Camera and SPOT acquisition software (version 3.1, Spot Imaging; Sterling Heights, MI, USA) light microscope at

2× magnification. Six 120 × 120 images per treatment group of the LV were obtained. All the images were then uploaded to ImageJ (Version 2.14.0/1.54f) software for analysis of the following parameters: LV total area, perimeter, width, and height, as well as number of endothelial cells.

The total area and perimeter of the LV for each image were automatically calculated using the ImageJ "freehand" selection tool to draw the area around the LV. The measuring tool was then used to draw a line within the area of the LV to automatically calculate the width and height for each image. The number of endothelial cells within the LV for each image were calculated using the cell counting tool within ImageJ by manually "marking" each cell with the counter function. The counts were automatically tallied through ImageJ.

2.6. Statistical Analyses

The data were analyzed with a one-way ANOVA with the treatment (Control, SI, SR, and DFS) as between factors. Tukey's post hoc multiple comparisons test was performed when indicated by a significant ANOVA. All the ANOVAs were generated using GraphPad PRISM software (Version 9.4.1).

3. Results

3.1. Blood–Brain Barrier (BBB) Integrity

Figure 1 provides representative images for each treatment group stained to examine the potential damage to the BBB. The rats exposed to SR (15cGy) had a reduction in astrocytes compared to the Control group (indicated by low GFAP staining (in green)). Astrocyte loss was also associated with increased fibrinogen extravasation (indicated in yellow) outside of the vasculature into the brain parenchyma. Interestingly, there was a rescue of astrocytes in the DFS animals, but this was still associated with increased fibrinogen extravasation. There was no apparent astrocyte loss or increase in fibrinogen extravasation in the SI group compared to the Controls. The Control animals did not exhibit any evident insults to the BBB. The quantification of these observations revealed no difference in the total vessel abundance ($p = 0.41$) (Figure 2A) or number of astrocytes ($p = 0.201$) (Figure 2B). However, the ANOVA revealed significant differences of treatment in the percent of leaky vessels (indicated by positive fibrinogen staining (in yellow) outside of the vessel) ($F_{3,28} = 29.49$; $p < 0.0001$). Tukey's post hoc test revealed that the SR and DFS groups had an increased percentage of leaky vessels compared to the Control and SI groups ($p < 0.0001$ and $p < 0.001$, respectively) (Figure 2C). The percentage of leaky vessels was also positively correlated with increased fibrinogen extravasation. The ANOVA revealed significant differences for the treatment group in the total amount of fibrinogen leaking from the vessels ($F_{3,28} = 15.17$; $p < 0.0001$). Tukey's post hoc tests revealed that the SR and DFS groups had increased fibrinogen extravasation compared to the Control and SI groups ($p < 0.0001$ and $p < 0.001$, respectively) (Figure 2D). Additional images showing separated color channels can be viewed in Supplementary Figure S1.

3.2. Astrocyte Morphology

Further investigation into the astrocytes between the groups also revealed morphological differences. The Control animals appeared to have a protoplasmic-like morphology with long, multi-branched radial projections [18,19]. The SI and DFS animals had a more fibrous morphology with an enlarged cell body and unilateral projections that were shorter, thinner, and less branched that showed increased GFAP staining intensity [18,19]. The astrocytes in the animals exposed to SR alone exhibited increased damage, including a dramatic loss of projections, or death (Figure 3). The quantification of these results via ANOVA revealed significant differences in the treatment group ($F_{3,78} = 27.65$; $p < 0.0001$). Tukey's post hoc comparisons revealed astrocytes in the SR ($p < 0.0001$ compared to Control and SI) and DFS ($p = 0.01$ compared to Control and $p < 0.001$ compared to SI) groups had fewer projections (Figure 4A).

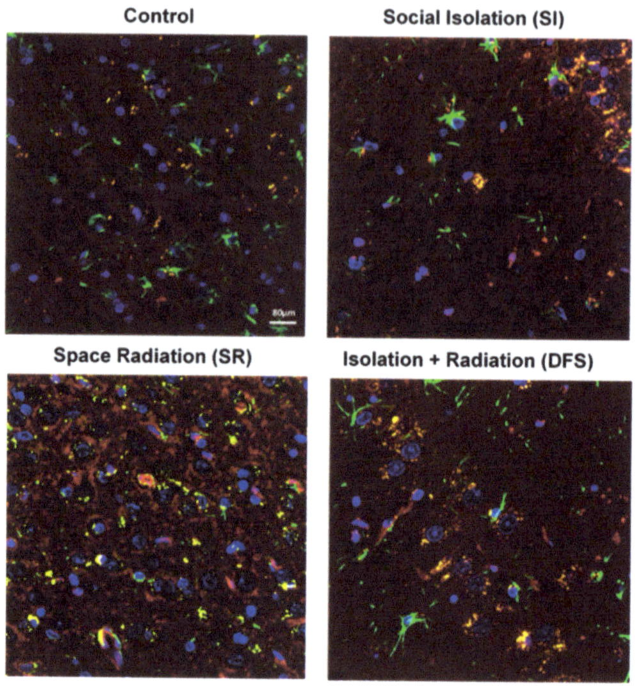

Figure 1. SR-induced BBB damage and astrocyte death was ameliorated by SI. Images of representative tissue slices within the limbic area of the brain showing quadruple-label immunofluorescence stained with GFAP (green), fibrinogen (yellow), Glut-1 (red), and DAPI (blue) displaying differences in vascular permeability in each treatment group. All images are at 40× magnification. Scale bar = 80 μm.

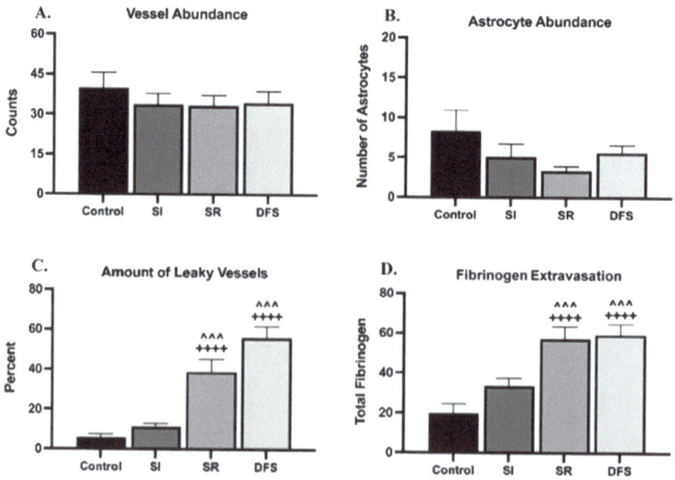

Figure 2. Irradiated animals had increased leaky vessels and fibrinogen extravasation in the brain. Graphs plotting the relative (**A**) vessel abundance (counts) ± SEM, (**B**) astrocyte abundance ± SEM, (**C**) % leaky vessels ± SEM, and (**D**) fibrinogen extravasation ± SEM based on quantified immunofluorescence staining amounts in the brain in each treatment group. Significant differences compared to Control: ++++ $p < 0.0001$. Significant differences compared to SI: ^^^ $p < 0.001$.

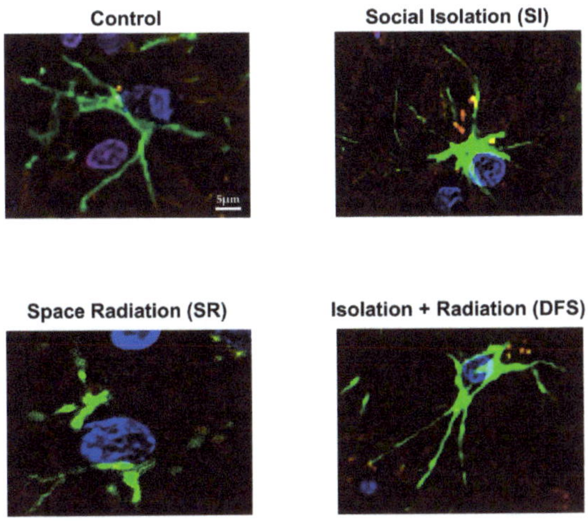

Figure 3. SI and SR differentially altered astrocyte morphology. Immunofluorescent images of individual astrocytes stained with GFAP (green) displaying differences in astrocyte morphology in each treatment group. Additional background staining includes fibrinogen (yellow), Glut-1 (red), and DAPI (blue). All images were acquired at 40× magnification and zoomed to focus on a single astrocyte. Scale bar = 5 μm.

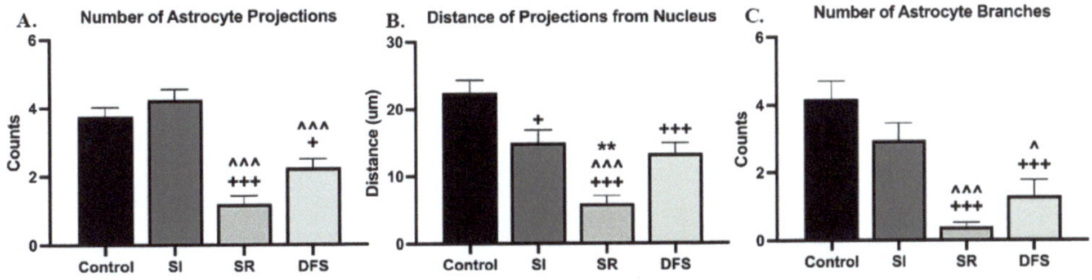

Figure 4. The average number of projections and branches from astrocytes differed between SI and SR exposure. Graphs plotting the (**A**) relative number (counts) of projections from an astrocyte soma ± SEM, (**B**) average distance from the soma of each projection ± SEM, and (**C**) relative number (counts) of branches off each projection ± SEM based on the quantified immunofluorescence staining amounts in each treatment group. Significant differences compared to Control: + $p < 0.05$, +++ $p < 0.001$. Significant differences compared to SI: ^ $p < 0.05$, ^^^ $p < 0.001$. Significant differences compared to DFS: ** $p < 0.01$.

The analyses of the projection length via the ANOVA revealed significant differences for the treatment group ($F_{3,95} = 19.88$; $p < 0.0001$). Tukey's post hoc tests revealed that the SI ($p = 0.02$), SR ($p < 0.0001$), and DFS ($p < 0.001$) groups had significantly shorter projections than the Control animals and fewer branches compared to the Control ($p < 0.001$) and SI ($p < 0.001$) groups, while the SR animals also had significantly shorter projections compared to the SI ($p < 0.0001$) and DFS ($p = 0.001$) groups (Figure 4B). Furthermore, the ANOVA analyses of the astrocyte branching revealed significant differences for the treatment group ($F_{3,78} = 22.56$; $p < 0.0001$). Tukey's post hoc tests revealed that compared to the Control and SI groups, the SR ($p < 0.0001$) and DFS ($p = 0.01$) groups had significantly fewer branches (Figure 4C). A summary of these results is provided in Supplementary Table S1.

3.3. Brain Morphology

When investigating the morphological differences between the treatment groups, we found that the SR animals had a 1.5- to 5.6-fold enlargement of the lateral ventricle (LV) compared to any other group (Figure 5). Interestingly, we found that these deficits were ameliorated when SR was combined with SI (DFS), similar to the findings for astrocytes discussed above. The quantification of these results analyzed by ANOVA did not reveal significant differences in the total area of the LV for any group ($F_{3,12}$ = 1.718; p = 0.2164) (Figure 6A). However, further investigation into the directionality of the LV enlargement revealed significant differences in the treatment group ($F_{3,12}$ = 8.116; $p < 0.01$). Tukey's post hoc tests that revealed significant differences in the LV size between the SR group compared to the other groups was in the medio-lateral direction ($p < 0.05$ compared to Control and $p < 0.01$ compared to SI, respectively) but not in the dorso-ventral direction ($p = 0.53$) (Figures 6B and 6C, respectively).

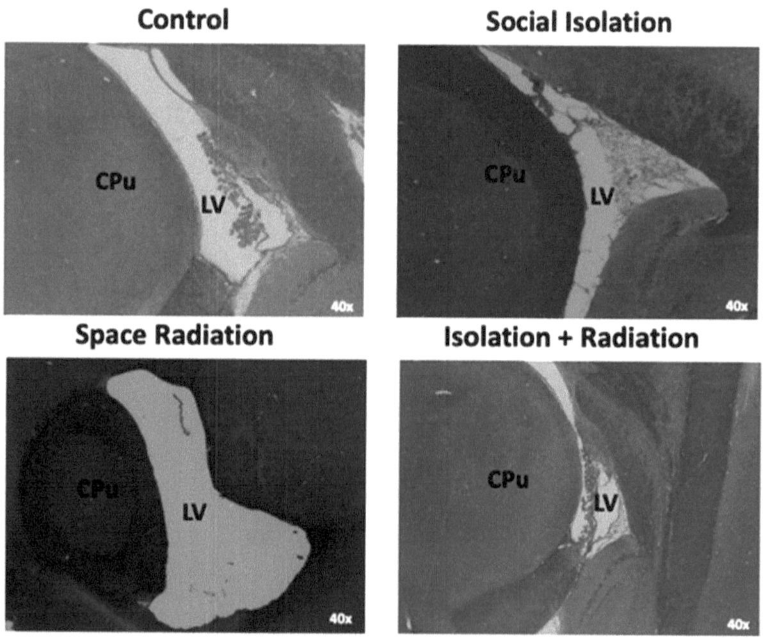

Figure 5. SR exposure resulted in an enlarged lateral ventricle (LV), which was ameliorated by a combined exposure to SI. Light microscopy images of sagittal brain sections (Lateral 1.4 mm, Bregma −0.45 mm) stained with H&E displaying morphological differences in LV area in each treatment group. Arrowheads point to endothelial cells within LV. CPu—caudate putamen. All images are at 2× magnification. Scale bar = 1 mm.

We also found that the SR animals had a 2.4- to 4.4-fold reduction in endothelial cells lining the LV compared to any other group. These deficits were also ameliorated when SR was combined with SI (DFS), similar to the findings for the astrocytes discussed above. The ANOVA analyses of the quantification of the number of endothelial cells within the LV revealed significant differences for the treatment group ($F_{3,12}$ = 17.15; p = 0.0001). Tukey's post hoc tests revealed that the SR animals had significantly fewer endothelial cells in the LV compared to the Control ($p < 0.0001$) and SI ($p < 0.01$) animals. The DFS animals also had significantly fewer endothelial cells in the LV compared to the Control animals ($p < 0.01$) (Figure 6D).

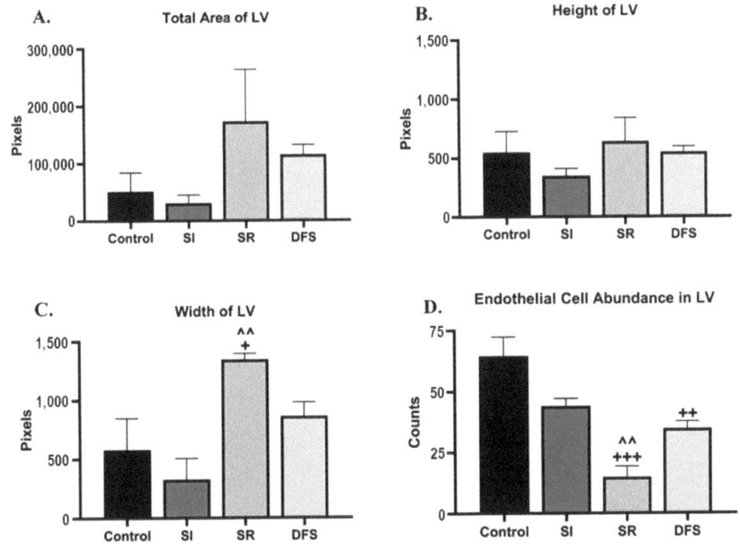

Figure 6. SR animals had an increased lateral ventricle (LV) size that was rescued by DFS. Graphs plotting the (**A**) average total area of LV ± SEM, (**B**) average height of LV ± SEM, (**C**) average width of LV ± SEM, and (**D**) average number of endothelial cells within LV ± SEM based on quantified H&E staining amounts in the brain for each treatment group. Significant differences compared to Control: + $p < 0.05$, ++ $p<0.01$, and +++ $p < 0.001$. Area measures are indicated in Pixels. Significant differences compared to SI: ^^ $p < 0.01$.

4. Discussion

The present study provides comparative data for the effects of SI, SR, and DFS relative to the Control on measures of BBB integrity and on astrocyte and gross brain morphology in rats. The Control and SI rats did not differ in astrocyte numbers or show differences in fibrinogen extravasation or in gross brain morphology but did differ in astrocyte morphology. The astrocytes in the Control animals had protoplasmic-like morphology with long, multi-branched radial projections [18,19], whereas the astrocytes in both the SI and DFS (which also experienced SI) animals had a fibrous morphology with an enlarged cell body and unilateral projections that were shorter, thinner, and less branched with increased GFAP staining intensity [18,19]. By comparison, the SR and DFS rats exhibited both an increased percentage of leaky vessels and fibrinogen extravasation relative to the Control and SI rats, and the astrocytes in the rats exposed to SR alone exhibited greater astrocyte damage, including a loss of projections and death. The SR rats also had an enlarged LV in the medial-to-lateral direction and both the SR and DFS rats had a reduction in endothelial cells lining the LV compared to the Control, and in SR rats was also reduced compared to SI rats. Together, these findings suggest that the greater loss of BBB integrity and structural changes in the brain were associated with greater astrocyte damage and loss.

Overall, these data indicate that SR exposure had a negative impact on the integrity of brain macro- and microstructures. The altered morphology induced by SR appeared to disrupt both the vascular and lymphatic systems, observed by increased BBB permeability and LV enlargement, and was associated with a loss of supporting cells, including astrocytes and endothelial cells. Interestingly, some of the deficits observed in the SR group were marginally rescued in the DFS group. We have also observed a similar effect in some behavioral tasks [17], though the mechanisms are not yet known. Despite this partial rescue, compared to the Control and SI groups, the DFS animals still had a significant reduction in structural integrity. The differences in the BBB morphology exhibited in the group that was exposed to SI alone were mainly related to altered astrocyte morphology compared to the Control group.

The breakdown of the BBB has been associated with cognitive dysfunction and increases in neuroinflammation [15]. Studies have shown the negative effects of singular SR [20,21] and SI [11,22,23] exposure on BBB integrity. Specifically, SR has been shown to target the microvascular system and disrupt endothelial barrier function by uncoupling important cell adhesion molecules (e.g., PECAM-1 and CD31) [8]. SI has been reported to increase levels of pro-inflammatory cytokines [22] and reactive oxygen species (ROS) [23] in the brain.

Our study found similar evidence for the disruption of the microvasculature system by SR. However, we also found that BBB permeability in this group was heavily associated with astrocyte viability and/or altered functionality (decrease in, or complete loss of, projections) in astrocytes that survived. These SR-induced changes were heavily associated with increased vessel leakage and fibrinogen relocation into the brain parenchyma. Other studies have reported that SR can induce astrocyte senescence [24]. In our study, it is possible that the SR-induced loss and/or senescence of astrocytes dysregulated the vascular endothelium, which led to increased BBB permeability. Interestingly, dual exposure to SI and SR (DFS) ameliorated the astrocyte loss observed in SR alone but was associated with an altered, fibrous-like astrocyte morphology and increased vessel leakage. The fibrous morphology was also found in the animals that experienced SI alone, but this was not coupled with fibrinogen extravasation. To our knowledge, this study is the first to report chronic individual or combination effects of SI and SR on astrocyte viability and morphology in association with BBB regulation in vivo [25].

Astrocytes are integral in maintaining CNS homeostasis by providing structural support, supplying energy and metabolites, participating in immune responses [26], and regulating vasculature endothelial responses [25,27]. The existence of two basic subtypes of astrocytes in rodents has been established [18]. Protoplasmic astrocytes possess highly branched projections that can extend to enwrap synapses, as well as blood vessels, to form the outermost layer of the BBB. This allows for the regulation of both synaptic functions and the regulation of blood flow/endothelium integrity. Fibrous astrocytes possess unilateral, thin projections that are less branched. While the function of this subtype is still not clear, its projections are mainly associated with blood vessel interactions similar to the protoplasmic subtype. However, they create fewer connections with vessels compared to the protoplasmic subtype [28] and are associated with increased GFAP staining [18,19]. This evidence could explain the increased BBB permeability that still occurred in the SI and DFS groups compared to the Control group. Previous studies have shown that SI alone can cause astrocytes to become hyperactive, and this change in astrocyte function by SI has been linked to suppressed memory formation [29]. In our previously published work [17], SI animals experienced blunted learning in sensorimotor tasks, though this was not a chronic impairment. Further investigation into these alterations is required to fully understand the effects of SI on astrocytes.

We also found that SR alone induced LV enlargement, which was also associated with a dramatic loss of endothelial cells within the LV. Unlike in the BBB, these deficits appeared to be rescued by DFS exposure. Previous studies have reported that prolonged spaceflight altered cerebrospinal fluid (CSF), specifically through an enlargement of the LV and decreased area of subarachnoid spaces [30]. The negative effects of SR on the endothelial barrier and vascular integrity have also been previously reported [31,32]. To our knowledge, this study is the first to report combination effects of SI and SR (DFS) on endothelial cell viability and LV morphology.

BBB dysfunction has been linked to the pathogenesis of multiple neuropsychiatric disorders [16,33,34] and to more severe anxiety symptoms [16,34]. Indeed, the SR and DFS animals in this study exhibited increased BBB damage as well as increased anxiety across multiple behavioral paradigms [17,35]. Elevated anxiety has been previously reported in animals exposed to GCR [4,36]. Anxiety-related disorders and symptoms have also been associated with endothelial dysfunction in multiple organ systems (e.g., in the LV) [37,38]. Additionally, altered CSF flow and brain lymphatics have been linked to multiple neurodegenerative and neuromuscular diseases [39,40]. Mechanistically, this may be through a loss of tight junction proteins, as previous studies have shown that a loss of these proteins (e.g., Cldn5) induced anxiety-like behaviors [41].

Alterations in immune system functionality could also be associated with these morphological changes as previously discussed. Immune system activation has been shown to negatively impact mood and behavior by increasing anxiety [42–44], fatigue, and emotional dysregulation [45]. Given that executive functions play an important role in regulating behavior, motivation, impulses, and arousal, astronauts with alterations in the BBB and LV may exhibit reduced motivation and possibly aberrant or impulsive behavior. However, further investigation into these mechanisms is necessary to understand fully how BBB and LV dysfunction leads to increased altered behaviors.

Interestingly, the reported effects of SI alone on tight junction proteins have varied across studies. Alshammari et al. [11] reported that SI increased Cldn5 and tight junction proteins in the hippocampus, which could result in a tighter BBB. However, other work has reported that SI beginning on post-natal day 21 decreased Cldn5 and increased BBB breakdown and microglial activation in the amygdala relative to group-housed female mice [46]. Other studies have reported similar decreases in BBB structural components [47] produced by SI, which would be consistent with greater deficits in combined stressor rats. Our results are consistent with these later findings, though we did not find additional significant increases in leaky vessels and fibrinogen extravasation in DFS rats.

Our study has limitations. We conducted analyses on a relatively small number of animals per condition. Thus, there is the possibility that we missed some alterations that could have achieved significance with larger sample sizes. However, even with a smaller n, we observed significant alterations in the BBB parameters in the SR and DFS rats. Our study also was primarily descriptive and did not assess the functional significance of the alterations that we observed. The changes we observed predict likely impairments in BBB function; however, additional studies will be needed to assess and quantify the extent of functional impairment.

The BBB serves a critical role in regulating the molecular exchange between peripheral blood and the central nervous system. Maintaining proper functioning of the BBB is essential for brain health, although the full pathological relevance of its dysfunction is poorly understood [48,49]. However, research has linked BBB dysfunction to cognitive dysfunction, increased neuroinflammation [15], and neuropsychiatric disorders [16], suggesting that SR and damage induced by SR and other spaceflight stressors could alter emotion and impair cognitive function in astronauts in ways that could impact their ability to complete their mission. Thus, determining how singular and combination inflight stressors interact to modulate the immune system and BBB is crucial to fully understand the multiple pathways that could impact astronaut performance and health, including the alterations to the CNS structures and cell viability observed in this study.

Supplementary Materials: The following supporting information can be downloaded at: https://www.mdpi.com/article/10.3390/life14050636/s1, Supplementary Figure S1: Stress Vulnerability Increased BBB Permeability and was Exacerbated by SR but Ameliorated by SI; Table S1: Summary of Results for Observed Differences in Astrocyte Morphology.

Author Contributions: Conceptualization, L.D.S., R.A.B. and L.L.W.; methodology, L.D.S., R.A.B., and L.L.W.; software, A.M.A.; validation, A.M.A.; formal analysis, A.M.A. and L.D.S.; investigation, A.M.A., A.J.G., Z.N.M.L., L.D.S., L.L.W., A.F.B., J.D.G. and R.S.H.; resources, L.D.S. and L.L.W.; data curation, A.F.B. and A.M.A.; writing—original draft preparation, A.M.A. and L.D.S.; writing—review and editing, L.D.S., L.L.W., R.A.B. and A.M.A.; visualization, A.J.G. and L.L.W.; supervision, L.D.S. and L.L.W.; project administration, L.D.S. and L.L.W.; funding acquisition, L.D.S. All authors have read and agreed to the published version of the manuscript.

Funding: This work was supported by the NASA CBS VNSCOR grant 80NSSC19K1582 and the NASA research grant NNX16AC40G.

Institutional Review Board Statement: This study was conducted according to the guidelines of the National Institutes of Health Guide for the Care and Use of Experimental Animals and were approved by Eastern Virginia Medical School's Institutional Animal Care and Use Committee (Protocol#: 19-018; approved 15 September 2019).

Informed Consent Statement: Not applicable.

Data Availability Statement: Experimental data available upon request.

Acknowledgments: We thank Diana Bohannon and Julian Hattler for their technical assistance.

Conflicts of Interest: The authors declare no conflicts of interest. The funders had no role in the design of the study; in the collection, analyses, or interpretation of data; in the writing of the manuscript; or in the decision to publish the results.

References

1. Mars, K.; Dunbar, B. 5 Hazards of Human Spaceflight. NASA. 2019. Available online: https://www.nasa.gov/hrp/5-hazards-of-human-spaceflight (accessed on 4 March 2023).
2. Al Omran, A.J.; Shao, A.S.; Watanabe, S.; Zhang, Z.; Zhang, J.; Xue, C.; Watanabe, J.; Davies, D.L.; Shao, X.M.; Liang, J. Social isolation induces neuroinflammation and microglia overactivation, while dihydromyricetin prevents and improves them. *J. Neuroinflammation* **2022**, *19*, 2. [CrossRef] [PubMed]
3. Filipović, D.; Stanisavljević, A.; Jasnić, N.; Bernardi, R.E.; Inta, D.; Perić, I.; Gass, P. Chronic Treatment with Fluoxetine or Clozapine of Socially Isolated Rats Prevents Subsector-Specific Reduction of Parvalbumin Immunoreactive Cells in the Hippocampus. *Neuroscience* **2018**, *371*, 384–394. [CrossRef] [PubMed]
4. Parihar, V.K.; Allen, B.D.; Caressi, C.; Kwok, S.; Chu, E.; Tran, K.K.; Chmielewski, N.N.; Giedzinski, E.; Acharya, M.M.; Britten, R.A.; et al. Cosmic radiation exposure and persistent cognitive dysfunction. *Sci. Rep.* **2016**, *6*, 34774. [CrossRef] [PubMed]
5. Allen, B.D.; Syage, A.R.; Maroso, M.; Baddour, A.A.D.; Luong, V.; Minasyan, H.; Giedzinski, E.; West, B.L.; Soltesz, I.; Limoli, C.L.; et al. Mitigation of helium irradiation-induced brain injury by microglia depletion. *J. Neuroinflammation* **2020**, *17*, 159. [CrossRef]
6. Tseng, B.P.; Giedzinski, E.; Izadi, A.; Suarez, T.; Lan, M.L.; Tran, K.K.; Acharya, M.M.; Nelson, G.A.; Raber, J.; Parihar, V.K.; et al. Functional Consequences of Radiation-Induced Oxidative Stress in Cultured Neural Stem Cells and the Brain Exposed to Charged Particle Irradiation. *Antioxid. Redox Signal.* **2014**, *20*, 1410–1422. [CrossRef]
7. Chakraborti, A.; Allen, A.; Allen, B.; Rosi, S.; Fike, J.R. Cranial Irradiation Alters Dendritic Spine Density and Morphology in the Hippocampus. *PLoS ONE* **2012**, *7*, e40844. [CrossRef] [PubMed]
8. Templin, T.; Sharma, P.; Guidab, P.; Grabhama, P. Short-Term Effects of Low-LET Radiation on the Endothelial Barrier: Uncoupling of PECAM-1 and the Production of Endothelial Microparticles. *Radiat. Res.* **2016**, *186*, 602–613. [CrossRef]
9. Pereda-Péreza, I.; Popović, N.; Otalora, B.B.; Popović, M.; Madrid, J.A.; Rol, M.A.; Venero, C. Long-term social isolation in the adulthood results in CA1 shrinkage and cognitive impairment. *Neurobiol. Learn. Mem.* **2013**, *106*, 31–39. [CrossRef]
10. Roberts, D.R.D.R.; Al, E.; Albrecht, M.H.; Collins, H.; Asemani, D. Effects of Spaceflight on Astronaut Brain Structure as Indicated by MRI. *N. Engl. J. Med.* **2017**, *377*, 1746–1753. [CrossRef]
11. Alshammari, T.K.; Alghamdi, H.M.; Alduhailan, H.E.; Saja, M.F.; Alrasheed, N.M.; Alshammari, M.A. Examining the central effects of chronic stressful social isolation on rats. *Biomed. Rep.* **2020**, *13*, 56. [CrossRef]
12. Bellone, J.A.; Gifford, P.S.; Nishiyama, N.C.; Hartman, R.E.; Mao, X.W. Long-term effects of simulated microgravity and/or chronic exposure to low-dose gamma radiation on behavior and blood–brain barrier integrity. *NPJ Microgravity* **2016**, *2*, 16019. [CrossRef] [PubMed]
13. Gupta, S.; Dhanda, S.; Sandhir, R. Anatomy and physiology of blood-brain barrier. In *Brain Targeted Drug Delivery System*; Academic Press: Cambridge, MA, USA, 2019; pp. 7–31.
14. Daneman, R.; Prat, A. The Blood-Brain Barrier. *Cold Spring Harb. Perspect. Biol.* **2015**, *7*, a020412. [CrossRef]
15. Bowman, G.L.; Dayon, L.; Kirkland, R.; Wojcik, J.; Peyratout, G.; Severin, I.C.; Henry, H.; Oikonomidi, A.; Migliavacca, E.; Bacher, M.; et al. Blood-brain barrier breakdown, neuroinflammation, and cognitive decline in older adults. *Alzheimer's Dement.* **2018**, *14*, 1640–1650. [CrossRef] [PubMed]
16. Wang, X.; Ma, L.; Luo, Y.; Yang, Y.; Upreti, B.; Cheng, Y.; Cui, R.; Liu, S.; Xu, J. Increasing of Blood Brain Barrier Permeability and the Association With Depression and Anxiety in Systemic Lupus Erythematosus Patients. *Front. Med.* **2022**, *9*, 852835. [CrossRef] [PubMed]
17. Adkins, A.M.; Colby, E.M.; Boden, A.F.; Gotthold, J.D.; Harris, R.D.; Britten, R.A.; Wellman, L.L.; Sanford, L.D. Differential Impact of Social Isolation and Space Radiation on Behavior and Motor Learning in Rats. *Life* **2023**, *13*, 826. [CrossRef] [PubMed]
18. Miller, R.H.; Raff, M.C. Fibrous and Protoplasmic Astrocytes are Biochemically and Developmentally Distinct. *J. Neurosci.* **1984**, *4*, 585–592. [CrossRef] [PubMed]
19. Tabata, H. Diverse subtypes of astrocytes and their development during corticogenesis. *Front. Neurosci.* **2015**, *9*, 114. [CrossRef]

20. Hart, E.; Odé, Z.; Derieppe, M.P.P.; Groenink, L.; Heymans, M.W.; Otten, R.; Lequin, M.H.; Janssens, G.O.; Hoving, E.W.; van Vuurden, D.G. Blood-brain barrier permeability following conventional photon radiotherapy—A systematic review and meta-analysis of clinical and preclinical studies. *Clin. Transl. Radiat. Oncol.* **2022**, *35*, 44–55. [CrossRef] [PubMed]
21. Trnovec, T.; Kállay, Z.; Bezek, S. Effects of ionizing radiation on the blood brain barrier permeability to pharmacologically active substances. *Int. J. Radiat. Oncol. Bioll Phys.* **1990**, *19*, 1581–1587. [CrossRef]
22. Wu, X.; Ding, Z.; Fan, T.; Wang, K.; Li, S.; Zhao, J.; Zhu, W. Childhood social isolation causes anxiety-like behaviors via the damage of blood-brain barrier in amygdala in female mice. *Front. Cell Dev. Biol.* **2022**, *10*, 943067. [CrossRef]
23. Schiavone, S.; Mhillaj, E.; Neri, M.; Morgese, M.G.; Tucci, P.; Bove, M.; Valentino, M.; Di Giovanni, G.; Pomara, C.; Turillazzi, E.; et al. Early Loss of Blood-Brain Barrier Integrity Precedes NOX2 Elevation in the Prefrontal Cortex of an Animal Model of Psychosis. *Mol. Neurobiol.* **2016**, *54*, 2031–2044. [CrossRef] [PubMed]
24. Turnquist, C.; Beck, J.A.; Horikawa, I.; Obiorah, I.E.; Von Muhlinen, N.; Vojtesek, B.; Lane, D.P.; Grunseich, C.; Chahine, J.J.; Ames, H.M.; et al. Radiation-induced astrocyte senescence is rescued by Δ133p53. *Neuro Oncol.* **2019**, *21*, 474–485. [CrossRef] [PubMed]
25. Verma, S.D.; Chapelle, E.P.; de la Malkani, S.; Juran, C.M.; Boyko, V.; Costes, S.V.; Cekanaviciute, E. Astrocytes regulate vascular endothelial responses to simulated deep space radiation in a human organ-on-a-chip model. *Front. Immunol.* **2022**, *13*, 864923. [CrossRef] [PubMed]
26. Kim, Y.; Park, J.; Choi, Y.K. The Role of Astrocytes in the Central Nervous System Focused on BK Channel and Heme Oxygenase Metabolites: A Review. *Antioxidants* **2019**, *8*, 121. [CrossRef] [PubMed]
27. Mishra, A. Binaural blood flow control by astrocytes: Listening to synapses and the vasculature. *J. Physiol.* **2017**, *595*, 1885–1902. [CrossRef] [PubMed]
28. Köhler, S.; Winkler, U.; Hirrlinger, J. Heterogeneity of Astrocytes in Grey and White Matter. *Neurochem. Res.* **2019**, *46*, 3–14. [CrossRef] [PubMed]
29. Cheng, Y.-T.; Woo, J.; Luna-Figueroa, E.; Maleki, E.; Harmanci, A.S.; Deneen, B. Social deprivation induces astrocytic TRPA1-GABA suppression of hippocampal circuits. *Neuron* **2023**, *111*, 1301–1315.e5. [CrossRef] [PubMed]
30. Barisano, G.; Sepehrband, F.; Collins, H.R.; Jillings, S.; Jeurissen, B.; Taylor, J.A.; Schoenmaekers, C.; De Laet, C.; Rukavishnikov, I.; Nosikova, I.; et al. The effect of prolonged spaceflight on cerebrospinal fluid and perivascular spaces of astronauts and cosmonauts. *Proc. Natl. Acad. Sci. USA* **2022**, *119*, e2120439119. [CrossRef] [PubMed]
31. Mao, X.W.; Boerma, M.; Rodriguez, D.; Campbell-Beachler, M.; Jones, T.; Stanbouly, S.; Sridharan, V.; Wroe, A.; Nelson, G.A. Acute effect of low-dose space radiation on mouse retina and retinal endothelial cells. *Radiat. Res.* **2018**, *190*, 45–52. [CrossRef]
32. Bouten, R.M.; Young, E.F.; Selwyn, R.; Iacono, D.; Rittase, W.B.; Day, R.M. Effects of radiation on endothelial barrier and vascular integrity. In *Tissue Barriers in Disease, Injury and Regeneration*; Elsevier: Amsterdam, The Netherlands, 2021; pp. 43–94.
33. Wen, J.; Chen, C.H.; Stock, A.; Doerner, J.; Gulinello, M.; Putterman, C. Intracerebroventricular administration of TNF-like weak inducer of apoptosis induces depression-like behavior and cognitive dysfunction in non-autoimmune mice. *Brain Behav. Immun.* **2016**, *54*, 27–37. [CrossRef]
34. Kamintsky, L.; Cairns, K.A.; Veksler, R.; Bowen, C.; Beyea, S.D.; Friedman, A.; Calkin, C. Blood-brain barrier imaging as a potential biomarker for bipolar disorder progression. *Neuroimage Clin.* **2020**, *26*, 102049. [CrossRef] [PubMed]
35. Adkins, A.M.; Colby, E.M.; Boden, A.F.; Gotthold, J.D.; Harris, R.D.; Britten, R.A.; Wellman, L.L.; Sanford, L.D. Effects of social isolation and galactic cosmic radiation on fine motor skills and behavioral performance. *Life Sci. Space Res.* **2024**, *41*, 74–79. [CrossRef] [PubMed]
36. Alaghband, Y.; Klein, P.M.; Kramár, E.A.; Cranston, M.N.; Perry, B.C.; Shelerud, L.M.; Kane, A.E.; Doan, N.-L.; Ru, N.; Acharya, M.M.; et al. Galactic cosmic radiation exposure causes multifaceted neurocognitive impairments. *Cell. Mol. Life Sci.* **2023**, *80*, 29. [CrossRef]
37. Sara, J.D.S.; Ahmad, A.; Toya, T.; Pardo, L.S.; Lerman, L.O.; Lerman, A. Anxiety Disorders Are Associated With Coronary Endothelial Dysfunction in Women With Chest Pain and Nonobstructive Coronary Artery Disease. *J. Am. Heart Assoc.* **2021**, *10*, e021722. [CrossRef] [PubMed]
38. Kheirabadi, G.R.; Toghani, F.; Kousha, M.; Hashemi, M.; Maracy, M.R.; Sharifi, M.R.; Bagherian-Sararoudi, R. Is there any association of anxiety-depressive symptoms with vascular endothelial function or systemic inflammation? *J. Res. Med. Sci.* **2013**, *18*, 979–983. [PubMed]
39. Louveau, A.; Da Mesquita, S.; Kipnis, J. Lymphatics in Neurological Disorders: A neuro-lympho-vascular Component of Multiple Sclerosis and Alzheimer's Disease. *Neuron* **2016**, *91*, 957–973. [CrossRef] [PubMed]
40. Eide, P.K.; Valnes, L.M.; Lindstrøm, E.K.; Mardal, K.A.; Ringstad, G. Direction and magnitude of cerebrospinal fluid flow vary substantially across central nervous system diseases. *Fluids Barriers CNS* **2021**, *18*, 16. [CrossRef] [PubMed]
41. Menard, C.; Pfau, M.L.; Hodes, G.E.; Kana, V.; Wang, V.X.; Bouchard, S.; Takahashi, A.; Flanigan, M.E.; Aleyasin, H.; LeClair, K.B.; et al. Social stress induces neurovascular pathology promoting depression. *Nat. Neurosci.* **2017**, *20*, 1752–1760. [CrossRef] [PubMed]
42. LeDoux, J. The Emotional Brain, Fear, and the Amydala. *Cell. Mol. Neurobiol.* **2003**, *23*, 727–738. [CrossRef]
43. Izquierdo, I.; Furini, C.R.G.; Myskiw, J.C. Fear Memory. *Physiol. Rev.* **2016**, *96*, 695–750. [CrossRef]
44. Davis, M. The Role of the Amygdala in Fear and Anxiety. *Annu. Rev. Neurosci.* **1992**, *15*, 353–375. [CrossRef] [PubMed]
45. Ravi, M.; Miller, A.H.; Michopoulos, V. The Immunology of Stress and the Impact of Inflammation on the Brain and Behavior. *BJPsych Adv.* **2021**, *27* (Suppl. S3), 158–165. [CrossRef] [PubMed]

46. Hong, H.; Guo, C.; Liu, X.; Yang, L.; Ren, W.; Zhao, H.; Li, Y.; Zhou, Z.; Lam, S.M.; Mi, J.; et al. Differential effects of social isolation on oligodendrocyte development in different brain regions: Insights from a canine model. *Front. Cell. Neurosci.* **2023**, *17*, 1201295. [CrossRef] [PubMed]
47. Quaegebeur, A.; Lange, C.; Carmeliet, P. The neurovascular link in health and disease: Molecular mechanisms and therapeutic implications. *Neuron* **2011**, *71*, 406–424. [CrossRef] [PubMed]
48. Rubio-Araiz, A.; Porcu, F.; Pérez-Hernández, M.; García-Gutiérrez, M.S.; Aracil-Fernández, M.A.; Gutierrez-López, M.D.; Guerri, C.; Manzanares, J.; O'Shea, E.; Colado, M.I. Disruption of blood-brain barrier integrity in postmortem alcoholic brain: Preclinical evidence of TLR4 involvement from a binge-like drinking model. *Addict. Biol.* **2017**, *22*, 1103–1116. [CrossRef]
49. Wolburg, H.; Noell, S.; Mack, A.; Wolburg-Buchholz, K.; Fallier-Becker, P. Brain endothelial cells and the glio-vascular complex. *Cell Tissue Res.* **2009**, *335*, 75–96. [CrossRef]

life

MDPI

Article

Impact of Patient Blood Management on Red Blood Cell Utilization in an Urban Community Teaching Hospital: A Seven-Year Retrospective Study

Ding Wen Wu [1,2], Mark T. Friedman [3,*], Daniel P. Lombardi [4], Richard Hwang [1], Joel Sender [4], Valdet Cobaj [1], Masooma Niazi [1], Yanhua Li [5] and Robert Karpinos [6]

1 Department of Pathology, SBH Health System, Bronx, NY 10457, USA; dingwen.wu@nyulangone.org (D.W.W.); vcobaj@sbhny.org (V.C.); mniazi@sbhny.org (M.N.)
2 Department of Pathology, New York University Grossman School of Medicine, New York, NY 10016, USA
3 Department of Pathology, New York University Grossman Long Island School of Medicine, Mineola, NY 11501, USA
4 Department of Medicine, SBH Health System, Bronx, NY 10457, USA; dlombardi@sbhny.org (D.P.L.); senderj@outlook.com (J.S.)
5 Division of Transfusion Medicine, Department of Medicine, UMass Chan Medical School, Worcester, MA 01655, USA; yanhua.li@umassmemorial.org
6 Department of Anesthesiology, SBH Health System, Bronx, NY 10457, USA; rkarpinos@sbhny.org
* Correspondence: mark.friedman@nyulangone.org; Tel.: +1-516-663-8307; Fax: +1-516-663-4581

Abstract: Objectives: This study aimed to showcase how implementing a patient blood management (PBM) program effectively cuts unnecessary red blood cell (RBC) transfusions in a New York City urban community teaching hospital. Methods: Analyzing seven years from 2013 to 2019, a retrospective review of RBC transfusions was conducted. Results: Following the introduction of PBM, considerable improvements were observed annually. These included a drop in mean pretransfusion hemoglobin levels from 7.26 g/dL (2013) to 6.58 g/dL (2019), a 34% reduction in yearly RBC unit transfusions, and fewer units given to patients with pre-Hgb levels $\geq$ 7 g/dL (from 1210 units in 2013 to 310 units in 2019). Furthermore, this study noted a decline in two-unit RBC orders when Hgb levels were $\geq$ 7 g/dL from 65 orders in 2013 to merely 3 in 2019. The estimated total cost savings attributed to the six-year PBM program duration after full implementation in 2014 amounted to USD 2.1 million. Conclusions: Overall, PBM implementation significantly decreased RBC transfusions and enhanced transfusion practices. The findings emphasize that successful PBM strategies do not always necessitate extensive resources or increased budgets but instead rely on the application of intuitive methods, as evidenced by this study.

Keywords: patient blood management; red blood cell; transfusion; hemoglobin; retrospective study

Citation: Wu, D.W.; Friedman, M.T.; Lombardi, D.P.; Hwang, R.; Sender, J.; Cobaj, V.; Niazi, M.; Li, Y.; Karpinos, R. Impact of Patient Blood Management on Red Blood Cell Utilization in an Urban Community Teaching Hospital: A Seven-Year Retrospective Study. *Life* **2024**, *14*, 232. https://doi.org/10.3390/life14020232

Academic Editor: Daniele Focosi

Received: 11 January 2024
Revised: 24 January 2024
Accepted: 5 February 2024
Published: 7 February 2024

1. Introduction

Introducing patient blood management (PBM) principles in a small hospital, despite the absence of a specific budget allocation, poses challenges. However, various strategic steps can be pursued to integrate PBM practices without relying on additional funding.

A 350-bed urban community teaching hospital serves an acute care trauma center in a sub-served area of New York City. The hospital provides a comprehensive array of residency training programs, covering specialties such as psychiatry, dentistry, surgery, podiatry, pediatrics, emergency medicine, osteopathic manipulative medicine, neuromusculoskeletal medicine, internal medicine, and dermatology.

Using an organized, evidence-based multidisciplinary approach [1] to transform blood transfusion practices to optimize patient care for the patients who might need a blood transfusion, a patient blood management (PBM) program was initiated in 2013 and fully implemented in 2014 at the hospital.

The PBM program was designed to promote better blood management practices, reduce transfusion rates, and improve patient outcomes. To achieve these goals, the implementation of the program required the cooperation of all healthcare professionals involved in the transfusion process, including physicians, nurses, laboratory technicians, and administrators.

One of our key strategies employed was the use of broad-based educational modules [2] for licensed practitioners. These modules were updated and provided annual education, especially for new attending physicians, residents, fellows, physician assistants, and nurse practitioners. The education was designed to improve practitioners' understanding of blood management principles and to promote best practices for the use of blood products. Transfusion guidelines and clinical transfusion protocols were adjusted to focus on symptomatic anemia rather than on hemoglobin triggers. This approach reduced the use of blood products in cases where transfusions were not clinically indicated.

Another critical aspect of the PBM program was the conversion of laboratory samples to low-volume testing. By using smaller samples, the laboratory was able to perform more efficient and cost-effective testing, reducing the need for unnecessary blood draws and minimizing the risk of iatrogenic anemia.

Furthermore, the program included a reduction in the critical-level reporting of hemoglobin (Hgb) from 7 g/dL to 6 g/dL. This change helped ensure that transfusions were only given when necessary, based on the patient's symptoms and clinical condition.

Finally, the initial orderable number of red blood cell (RBC) units in the electronic medical health record system was set to one unit instead of two units [3]. This change helped to reduce the number of unnecessary RBC transfusions and decreased the overall cost of the transfusion process.

Overall, the PBM program was effectively implemented without any specifically allocated budgetary support. The program's success was due in large part to the collaboration and dedication of all healthcare professionals involved in the transfusion process, as well as the commitment to evidence-based best practices for blood management.

2. Materials and Methods

We conducted a retrospective analysis of all RBC transfusions from 2013 to 2019 to examine the impact of this PBM program on RBC utilization in the hospital.

This retrospective study was given exempt status by the institutional review boards of St. Barnabas Health.

2.1. Hypothesis

The implementation of an evidence-based PBM program would effectively reduce unnecessary RBC transfusions in the hospital.

2.1.1. Aim

The goal of this study is to analyze the impact of this PBM program.

2.1.2. Data Selection Criteria

We retrospectively analyzed our health system's blood transfusion database from 1 January 2013 to 31 December 2019. RBC transfusion events without exclusion for all patients admitted during this seven-year period were identified, regardless of age, gender, race, or disease condition. However, certain exclusions were applied, such as emergency transfusion events involving the use of uncrossmatched RBC for trauma and acute severe bleeding cases, as well as events following the massive transfusion protocol. Outpatient transfusion events were excluded. Transfusion events with plasma products, platelet products, or cryoprecipitate were also excluded since this PBM study only focused on inpatient RBC transfusions.

2.1.3. Study Endpoints

To examine the impact of this restrictive PBM program, the following endpoints from 2014 to 2019 were analyzed and compared with baseline data from 2013:

1. Average (and median) of pre-transfusion Hgb levels that triggered the RBC transfusion orders.
2. Volume of RBC transfusion units.
3. Annual volume of RBC transfusion units when the pre-transfusion Hgb level was $\geq$ 7 g/dL (thereafter referred to as # Hb le7).
4. Annual percentage of RBC transfusion units when the pre-transfusion Hgb level was $\geq$ 7 g/dL (thereafter referred to as % Hb le7).

This comparison was used to show the reduction, if any, of unnecessary RBC transfusions since, in the context of the PBM program, orders for RBC transfusions in nonbleeding patients with Hgb $\geq$ 7 g/dL without symptomatic anemia or known cardiac disease are unnecessary. Thus, the impact on # Hb le7 and % Hb le7 reflect the effect on the reduction of unnecessary RBC transfusions.

5. The number of two-unit RBC transfusion orders.
6. When Hgb $\geq$ 7 g/dL, the number and percentage of two-unit orders of RBC transfusion.
7. Overall rate of RBC transfusions.

To remove the variations caused by the patient length of stay (LOS) and the number of admissions/discharges for the comparison, the annual overall rate of RBC transfusion is calculated and compared to the one in 2013.

The overall rate of RBC transfusions is calculated as follows: Overall rate of RBC transfusion = RBC transfusions without exclusions per 1000 patient days. Patient days = total number of discharges X average LOS (days).

8. Length of stay (LOS).

Since the goal of PBM is to optimize care for patients who might need a blood transfusion, the impact estimation was not limited to transfused patients only. The yearly LOS for all of the inpatients in 2014–2019 was analyzed and compared with the LOS for 2013.

9. Potential cost savings from reducing unnecessary RBC transfusions. This estimation is based on a reduction of % Hb le7. Calculation steps (see Table 1):
   (1) Number of transfused RBC units.
   (2) Number of RBC units transfused when Hgb triggers $\geq$ 7 g/dL.
   (3) % of RBC units transfused when Hgb trigger $\geq$ 7 g/dL.
   (4) Potential reduction of RBC units = ((3) of year 2013 (3) of year of interest (yi)) $\times$ (1) of yi.
   (5) Potential cost savings of yi = (4) potential reduced RBC units of yi $\times$ USD 1000/unit.

Per estimation [4], it costs about ~USD 1000 per unit of RBC transfusion.

The total potential cost saving of years 2014–2019 = the summary of potential cost saving from years 2014 to 2019.

2.1.4. Statistics

Quantitative data were expressed as the arithmetic mean $\pm$ standard deviation. The median of each group's data was also sometimes displayed as desired. Statistical analysis was conducted with the unpaired t-test using Excel 2019 (Microsoft Corp., Redmond, WA, USA) to evaluate the difference between each endpoint value mentioned above and the counterpart value for the year 2013. Values of $p < 0.05$ were considered statistically significant.

Table 1. RBC units transfused and potential cost savings.

Year	2013	2014	2015	2016	2017	2018	2019	Total
(1) Number of transfused RBC units	2061	1762 *	1460 *	1514 *	1251 *	1286 *	1350 *	
(2) Number of RBC units transfused when Hgb trigger ≥ 7 g/dL	1210	830 *	572 *	517 *	371 *	357 *	310 *	
(3) % of RBC units transfused when Hgb trigger ≥ 7 g/dL = (2) ÷ (1)	58.7	47.1	39.2	34.1	30.0	27.8	23.0	
(4) Potential reduction of RBC units = ((3) of year 2013 − (3) of this year) × (1) of the year) **	0	204	285	372	375	397	482	2115
(5) Potential cost saving (USD) = (4) × USD 1000/ unit	0	204K	285K	372K	375K	398K	482K	USD 2.1 million

* p-value < 0.0001 compared to the number in year 2013. ** Row (4) calculation example: potential reduction in RBC units in 2014 = (58.7% − 47.1%) × 1762 = 204 units.

3. Results

Our results show that significant improvements in RBC transfusion practices and usage have occurred since the implementation of the PBM program in 2014, as follows:

- Mean pre-transfusion Hgb for RBC transfusion orders consistently decreased year-over-year after PBM program implementation, comparing a nadir of 6.58 g/dL in 2019 to 7.26 g/dL in 2013 ($p < 0.0001$) (Figure 1).

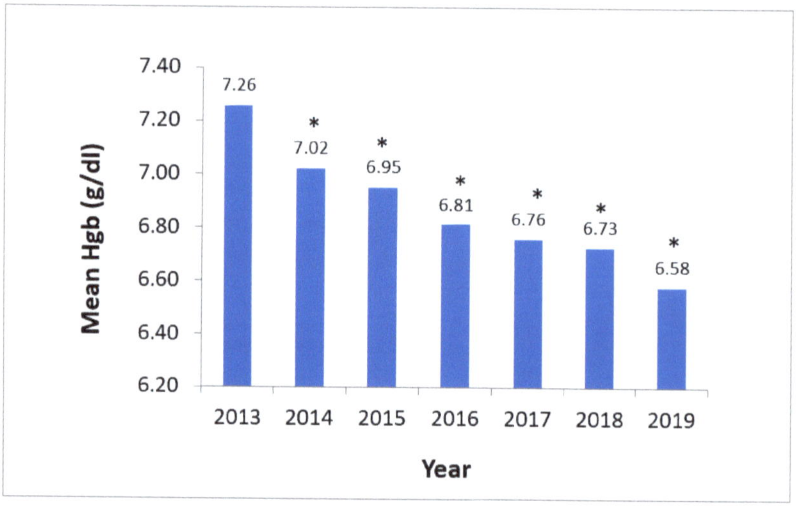

Figure 1. Average hemoglobin level for RBC transfusion orders. Note: * The p-value is < 0.0001 for the value of each year from 2014 to 2019 compared to the number for the year 2013.

- Median Hgb for RBC transfusion orders revealed the same trend (Supplementary Data Figure S1).
- During the same six-year period (2014–2019), the number of annual transfused RBC units showed a significant decrease of 34% compared to the one in 2013 (Table 1; (2061–1350) ÷ 2061 = 34%).
- Similarly, the absolute number and percentage of transfused RBC units with Hgb trigger ≥ 7 g/dL significantly decreased year-over-year, reaching a nadir in 2019 compared to 2013 (310 units vs. 1210 units, respectively, $p < 0.0001$, and 23.0% vs. 58.7%, respectively) (Table 1). This reflects a significant reduction (by 35.7%) of unnecessary RBC transfusions consistently year after year. 58.7% − 23.0% = 35.7%.

- The number of two-unit RBC transfusion orders decreased from 150 to 42 post-intervention (Figure 2).

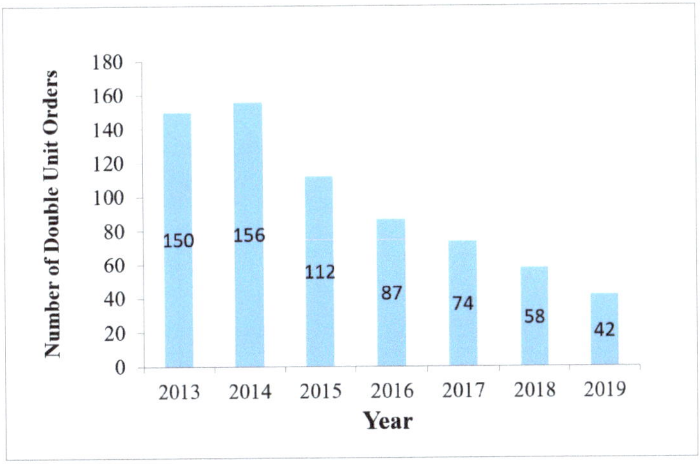

Figure 2. Number of double RBC orders.

- When Hgb trigger ≥ 7 g/dL, the number and percentage of two-unit orders for RBC transfusions decreased from 65 (3.4% of RBC transfusions) to 3 (0.2%) post-intervention ($p < 0.0001$), as shown in Figure 3.

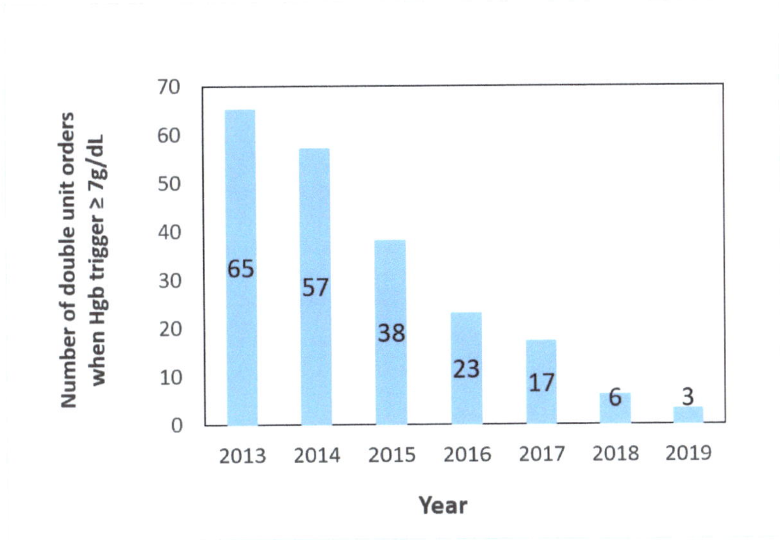

Figure 3. Number of double RBC orders when Hgb ≥ 7 g/dL.

- The annual overall rate of RBC transfusion without exclusion per 1000 patient days decreased from 21.9 in 2013 to 16.1 in 2019 (Figure 4), demonstrating a 26% reduction.

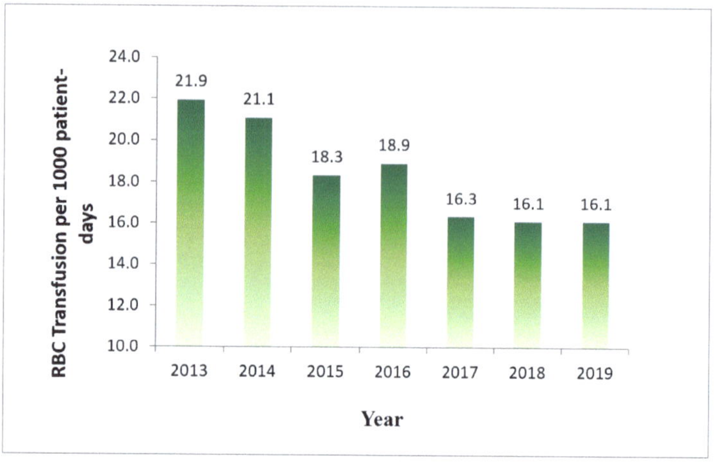

Figure 4. Annual inpatient RBC transfusion rate.

Overall rate of RBC transfusions = units of inpatient RBC transfusion without exclusions per 1000 inpatient days.

- Minimal change in the mean and median inpatient LOS over seven years suggested no hospital patient harm caused by the restrictive PBM program (Table 2).

Table 2. Hospital inpatients' length of stay (LOS).

LOS (Days)	2013	2014	2015	2016	2017	2018	2019
Mean (Days)	5.1	4.9	5.5	5.5	5.2	5.3	5.5
Standard deviation (Days)	13.1	9.3	12.5	8.7	10.8	10.5	11.2
Median (Days)	3.0	3.0	3.0	3.0	3.0	3.0	3.0

- This RBC usage reduction translates into approximately 2115 units of RBC saved during the six-year post-launch period (2014–2019). Based on a cost of ~USD 1000 per unit [4], the potential cost savings peaked at ~USD 482,000 in 2019, with total savings of ~USD 2.1 million during the six years of PBM implementation (Table 1).
- The data presented in this paper are original.

Remarkably, the advancement of this PBM program was achieved without any additional budget allocated to it.

4. Discussion

The scope of overtransfusion and the problems associated with it are significant in healthcare. Overtransfusion refers to the unnecessary or excessive administration of blood or blood products to patients. Some key issues associated with overtransfusion [5,6] are as follows:

- Transfusion reactions and complications: Receiving unnecessary blood transfusions increases the risk of adverse reactions, which can range from mild to severe transfusion-associated circulatory overload (TACO), transfusion-related acute lung injury (TRALI), allergic reactions, hemolytic reactions, and transfusion-transmitted infections, among others.
- Potential for adverse outcomes: Overtransfusion may not improve patient outcomes and can potentially lead to increased morbidity and mortality in certain cases [6].

- Increased healthcare costs: Blood transfusions are costly and can substantially contribute to healthcare expenses. Unnecessary transfusions lead to increased healthcare spending without providing commensurate benefits to the patient.
- Resource utilization: Inappropriate blood use leads to a strain on blood bank resources, potentially resulting in shortages for patients who genuinely require transfusions.

Shander et al. illustrated that the key strategies in PBM include support of hematopoiesis and improving hemoglobin level, optimizing coagulation and hemostasis, use of interdisciplinary blood conservation modalities, and patient-centered decision making throughout the course of care [1].

Patient blood management (PBM) aims to mitigate these problems by optimizing blood use, minimizing unnecessary transfusions, and improving patient outcomes through evidence-based practices tailored to individual patient needs. It emphasizes a personalized approach to care that prioritizes patient safety and well-being while conserving precious blood resources [1,7–9].

The primary pillars of PBM typically include:

(1) Optimizing red blood cell mass: Ensuring patients have adequate red blood cell levels before surgery or invasive procedures through treatments like iron supplementation, erythropoietin therapy, or other medications. (2) Minimizing blood loss: Employing surgical techniques, such as minimally invasive surgery, to reduce blood loss during procedures. Additionally, use specific medications or interventions to control bleeding. (3) Enhancing patients' tolerance to anemia: Some patients may tolerate lower blood levels without experiencing adverse effects. PBM involves identifying patients who can safely function with lower hemoglobin levels without the need for a transfusion. (4) Appropriate blood transfusion: Making evidence-based decisions on when to transfuse blood and ensuring that transfusions are only administered when necessary and beneficial.

Implementing PBM in a small hospital without a dedicated budget can be challenging, but there are several steps that can be taken to introduce PBM principles [5,6] without requiring significant additional funding.

The subsequent table encapsulates diverse approaches for executing PBM without the need for supplementary financial backing (Table 3).

Chau et al. reported that a successful multidisciplinary PBM program involved a series of educational lectures, consultations, and discussions with doctors, nurses, and theater staff [2].

By focusing on education, utilizing existing resources efficiently, implementing evidence-based guidelines, and fostering an interdisciplinary culture of responsible blood utilization, a hospital can implement PBM practices without a dedicated budget.

Our study validates the principle that successful implementation of practical PBM strategies is achievable without budgetary support and no funds allocated toward the PBM program in a small urban community teaching hospital. Main outcome measures across the seven-year study period showed that statistically significant (i.e., $p < 0.05$) improvements in RBC utilization occurred marked by reductions in the overall number of transfused RBC units, transfusion rate per 1000 patient days, two vs. single unit transfusions, transfusions with a Hgb trigger greater than 7 g/dL, and blood product wastage. In addition, PBM implementation led to significant cost savings. These beneficial study outcomes were realized despite the inclusion of all inpatient populations, including trauma and neonatal patients; larger reductions in blood utilization and cost savings may have resulted had these patient populations been excluded from the study. The observational nature of this study is a noted limitation, though.

Jenkins et al. implemented a restrictive transfusion strategy with a typical quality improvement framework and, based on education and computerized physician order entry (CPOE) enhancements, significantly reduced off-protocol and total blood transfusions [7]. Our keys to successful implementation included ongoing PBM education via online learning modules targeted for licensed practitioners, along with the use of PBM tools such as restrictive transfusion guidelines, computerized physician order entry alerts with clinical decision choices in the hospital EMR system to guide physicians in transfusion decisions, the use of low-volume test sample tubes to reduce hospital-acquired anemia, and the reduction in the critical Hgb alert value from 7 g/dL to 6 g/dL. The calculation method of the overall RBC transfusion rate by Jenkins et al. was utilized in this study.

Table 3. Ways to Introduce PBM without Additional Funding.

Education and training	Start by educating staff, including physicians, nurses, and other healthcare professionals, about the principles and benefits of PBM. Utilize internal expertise that may offer free or low-cost educational materials and training sessions.
Clinical guidelines and pathways	Develop and implement evidence-based clinical guidelines and pathways that emphasize conservative blood management strategies. These guidelines can include practices such as minimizing unnecessary blood tests, optimizing hemoglobin levels pre-operatively, and employing blood conservation techniques during surgery.
Utilize existing resources	Assess and optimize the use of existing resources within the hospital. Work with the laboratory and clinical staff to reduce unnecessary blood tests, adopt restrictive transfusion thresholds, and explore alternatives to transfusions, such as iron supplementation or medications that reduce bleeding.
Quality improvement initiatives	Implement quality improvement initiatives aimed at reducing blood product waste, improving blood utilization practices, and ensuring that transfusions are given based on the established clinical criteria rather than routine practice.
Collaboration and partnerships	Collaborate with blood banks, regional blood centers, or other healthcare facilities in the area to explore cost-sharing opportunities, joint training programs, or information sharing related to best practices in blood management.
Utilize data and analytics	Leverage data analytics to monitor blood utilization patterns, transfusion rates, and associated costs. This information can help identify areas for improvement and guide decision making to optimize blood utilization without requiring additional funds.
Engage stakeholders	Involve stakeholders across different departments and specialties in discussions about PBM. Encourage collaborative efforts to implement changes and promote a culture of responsible blood use throughout the hospital.
Adopt technology solutions	Implement electronic health record (EHR) systems or clinical decision support tools that can help clinicians adhere to evidence-based transfusion guidelines, thereby reducing unnecessary blood transfusions.
Evaluate and Adjust	Continuously monitor the impact of PBM initiatives on patient outcomes, transfusion rates, and associated costs. Use these data to refine strategies and make the necessary adjustments to improve the effectiveness of PBM practices.
Seek Grants or collaborative opportunities	Look for grants or collaborative opportunities within the healthcare community that support PBM initiatives or projects aimed at improving blood management. Participating in such programs can provide additional resources and support without requiring a separate budget allocation.

In comparison, Warner et al. published observational data from an eight-year study to support the successful implementation of PBM in a large U.S. academic medical center without evidence of patient harm. Their data, which included 400,998 admissions, showed a 33% reduction of allogenic transfusions per 1000 admissions, an absolute risk reduction for transfusion of 6%, and a 22% decrease in the rate of transfusions over projected [8].

PBM has emerged as a crucial aspect of healthcare, seeking to optimize patient outcomes, enhance safety, and achieve cost savings. In the study conducted by Hofmann et al., the implementation of PBM was explored across 12 nations through in-depth, semi-structured interviews. The findings revealed a unanimous consensus among healthcare professionals on the potential benefits of PBM, including improved patient outcomes, enhanced safety measures, and financial savings. However, despite this agreement, several barriers to successful PBM implementation were identified. One of the primary obstacles highlighted by this study was the limited experience with PBM among healthcare practitioners. The lack of familiarity with PBM practices posed a significant challenge, emphasizing the need for comprehensive education and training initiatives. Additionally, this study identified the necessity for a shift in work practices and emphasized the crucial roles of collaboration and communication in facilitating successful PBM integration. To address these challenges and enhance the implementation of PBM, this study proposed six intervention levels. These levels encompassed various stakeholders, including government entities, healthcare providers, educational institutions, funders, research organizations, and patients [9].

Recognizing the significance of education in fostering better patient care, the focus of our PBM project was on educating healthcare providers. In alignment with the findings of the broader study, the PBM project underscored the importance of healthcare providers adopting dual roles. Providers were encouraged not only to serve as front-line care providers but also as leaders in quality improvement initiatives. This approach aimed to empower healthcare professionals with the knowledge and skills needed to effectively implement and practice PBM within their clinical settings. By fostering a culture of continuous learning and quality improvement, the PBM project sought to overcome barriers to implementation. The dual role of healthcare providers as both caregivers and quality improvement leaders was envisioned as a pivotal strategy for creating sustainable change. Through education, training, and the cultivation of leadership skills among healthcare providers, the PBM project aimed to contribute to broader efforts to enhance patient care, safety, and the overall effectiveness of healthcare delivery.

The "Why give 2 when 1 will do?" Choosing Wisely campaign, inspired by Podlasek et al. and Warner et al. [3,10], further exemplifies the commitment to sustaining positive changes. We launched a "Why give 2 when 1 will do?" Choosing Wisely campaign, and we have been sustaining it using education and computer-physician-order entry alerts with clinical decision support (CPOE-CDS). We witnessed an overall decrease of 2-unit orders for Hgb ≥ 7 g/dL progressively from 65 orders per year (3.4% of total orders) to 3 orders (0.2%) from 2013 to 2019.

Fischer et al. studied the effect of PBM implementation on physicians' risk perception, clinical knowledge, and perioperative practice across four German university hospitals. Key implementation strategies targeted knowledge (i.e., development and distribution of PBM educational materials and local guidelines; standardization of performance metrics and data collection to allow valid benchmarking within organizations, etc.); attitude (i.e., fostering team spirit and corporate identity; aggressive marketing, etc.); and behavior (i.e., changing the infrastructure and preoperative flow of patients; preoperative anemia assessment; measurement of individual physician transfusion practice, etc.). Utilizing pre- and post-implementation questionnaires, Fischer et al. demonstrated significant positive shifts in physicians' attitudes toward preoperative anemia treatment and patient assessment after each single-unit RBC transfusion. Moreover, there was a noteworthy reduction in the percentage of physicians routinely using Hgb < 6 g/dL as an indicator for transfusion. This reduction was coupled with an increase in those favoring physiological transfusion triggers, such as electrocardiogram changes or lactic acidosis [11].

In parallel, the strategies implemented in response to the "Why give 2 when 1 will do?" Choosing Wisely campaign aligns with Fischer et al.'s findings. The educational efforts and the integration of CPOE local guidance in the original text are reflected in the success story of improved clinicians' knowledge, attitude, and behavior regarding RBC transfusion orders. The progressive and substantial decrease in RBC transfusions observed further reinforces the positive impact of these combined strategies. These parallel successes underscore the universality of certain principles in optimizing blood transfusion practices. Both the campaign and Fischer et al.'s study emphasize the importance of education, attitude change, and behavioral modification in achieving positive outcomes in the realm of patient blood management. The amalgamation of these principles, as evident in the original text, stands as a testament to the multifaceted and comprehensive approach needed to bring about meaningful change in healthcare practices.

Our strategies of education and CPOE local guidance successfully improved clinicians' knowledge, attitude, and behavior toward RBC transfusion orders, with evidence of a progressively substantial decrease in RBC transfusions.

Finally, in its policy brief calling for the urgent implementation of PBM, the World Health Organization [12] highlighted data from the largest study on PBM outcomes to date published by the Western Australia PBM Program. This study included over 600,000 patients admitted to Western Australia's four major adult hospitals during a six-year study period and showed significant reductions in mortality, infection, acute myocardial infarction and stroke, and hospital length of stay. Improved key indicators showed reductions in preoperative anemia, pre-transfusion Hgb, and transfused blood products. Meanwhile, single-unit RBC transfusions increased. This program resulted in an estimated product cost savings of USD 18.5 million and activity cost savings of USD 80–USD 100 million [13]. Our study demonstrated that our PBM was successful in reducing unnecessary blood products with a total cost savings of 2.1 million US dollars over 6 years (2014–2019). Our experience also showed that the PBM can be achieved in a community hospital without budgetary support. Lowering the hemoglobin trigger for blood transfusion may reduce the amount of blood transfused to patients, which could result in lower risks of transfusion reactions, infections, and other adverse events associated with blood transfusions. On the other hand, a lower hemoglobin trigger may increase the risk of patient harm, especially in patients with cardiac disease or other medical conditions where a higher hemoglobin level may be required to maintain adequate oxygen delivery. The decision to lower the hemoglobin trigger from 7 g/dL to 6 g/dL for non-cardiac patients was made in conjunction with an interdisciplinary team of healthcare providers, taking into account the patient's individual needs, the clinical context, and the best available evidence.

The minimal change in the mean and no change in the median of the inpatient length of stay over a 7-year period indicates that the restrictive PBM program did not result in harm to hospital patients.

Another limitation in our PBM implementation is that although the initial orderable RBC units were set to one unit per order in our EMR, the full impact of computerized physician order entry with clinical decision support (CPOE-CDS) may not have been realized to its maximum potential. Goodnough and Hollenhorst [14] demonstrated a 42% reduction in RBC transfusions using a targeted CPOE-CDS to promote restrictive blood transfusion practices in their institution through smart best practice alerts (SBPA's) that are triggered for RBC orders above 7 g/dL or 8 g/dL for patients with acute coronary syndrome or post-cardiothoracic procedure. The inclusion of CPOE-CDS with SBPA's could potentially have impacted further reductions in RBC transfusions in our institution.

The study authors believe that this report demonstrates that successful PBM can be achieved without the allocation of significant additional resources or budgetary support through the implementation of a few common-sense strategies. It should serve as a source of inspiration for other healthcare facilities that have yet to embark on their journey toward successful PBM implementation.

To further enhance the impact of PBM, future directions should focus on continuous improvement and adaptation to evolving healthcare landscapes. This includes ongoing education and training programs, updates to clinical guidelines based on emerging evidence, using targeted CPOE-CDS with smart best practice alerts to promote restrictive blood transfusion practices, and the integration of advanced technologies such as artificial intelligence to optimize decision-making processes.

Continuous monitoring and evaluation of PBM initiatives are essential for identifying areas for improvement and ensuring sustained positive outcomes. Collaboration with other healthcare institutions and participation in national and international initiatives can facilitate the sharing of best practices, fostering a global community committed to advancing patient blood management.

5. Conclusions

This retrospective seven-year study demonstrated that this multidiscipline PBM program in an urban community teaching hospital using education and restrictive tools effectively reduced total RBC usage without specific budgetary support. In particular, the PBM program markedly reduced the unnecessary RBC transfusion for Hgb $\geq$ 7 g/dL (by 35.7%) and total RBC transfusion (by 28%) and reduced unnecessary 2-unit RBC orders for Hgb $\geq$ 7 g/dL (from 3.4% to 0.2%). The potential cost savings is estimated at 2.1 million US dollars. This research underscores how effective PBM implementation can occur without the need for substantial extra resources or increased budgetary support by adopting a handful of practical strategies.

Supplementary Materials: The following are available online at https://www.mdpi.com/article/10.3390/life14020232/s1, Figure S1: Median hemoglobin level for RBC transfusion orders * p value < 0.0001 comparing to the number in year 2013.

Author Contributions: Conceptualization, R.K., D.W.W. and M.T.F.; study methodology, D.W.W.; validation, D.W.W.; study analysis, D.W.W.; data curation, R.K., D.P.L., R.H., J.S. and V.C.; writing—original draft preparation, D.W.W., M.T.F. and Y.L.; writing—review and editing, M.T.F., D.W.W. and M.N. All authors have read and agreed to the published version of the manuscript.

Funding: This research received no external funding or internal budget allocation.

Institutional Review Board Statement: This retrospective study was given exempt status by the institutional review boards of St. Barnabas Health.

Informed Consent Statement: Patient consent was waived due to the nature of a retrospective study, which was initially designed to monitor the impact of the PBM program for quality improvement.

Data Availability Statement: Data are unavailable due to privacy and ethical restrictions.

Acknowledgments: The authors express their gratitude to Zane Last, IT Director, for timely providing the essential data files required for our study's analysis.

Conflicts of Interest: All the authors have no relevant conflicts of interest.

References

1. Shander, A.; Lobel, G.P.; Javidroozi, M. Anesthesia for Patients with Anemia. *Anesth. Clin.* **2016**, *34*, 711–730. [CrossRef]
2. Chau, M.; Cohil, D.; Schofield, N.; Abevsiri, S.; Klein, A.; Richards, T. Development and feasibility of a Patient Blood Management implementation programme in vascular surgery. *Vasc. Med.* **2020**, *25*, 41–46. [CrossRef] [PubMed]
3. Warner, M.A.; Schaefer, K.K.; Madde, N.; Burt, J.M.; Higgins, A.A.; Kor, D.J. Improvements in red blood cell transfusion utilization following implementation of a single-unit default for electronic ordering. *Transfusion* **2019**, *59*, 2218–2222. [CrossRef] [PubMed]
4. Blumberg, N.; Kirkley, S.A.; Heal, J.M. A cost analysis of autologous and allogeneic transfusions in hip-replacement surgery. *Am J Surg.* **1996**, *171*, 324–330. [CrossRef] [PubMed]
5. Shander, A.; Hofmann, A.; Ozawa, S.; Theusinger, O.M.; Gombotz, H.; Spahn, D.R. Activity-based costs of blood transfusions in surgical patients at four hospitals. *Transfusion* **2010**, *50*, 753–765. [CrossRef] [PubMed]
6. Shander, A. Transfusion Overuse Exposing an International Problem and Patient Safety Issue. Available online: https://www.sabm.org/assets/pdfs/SABM-Transfusion-Overuse-2019.pdf (accessed on 12 April 2022).
7. Jenkins, I.; Doucet, J.J.; Clay, B.; Kopko, P.; Fipps, D.; Hemmen, E.; Paulson, D. Transfusing Wisely: Clinical Decision Support Improves Blood Transfusion Practices. *Jt. Comm. J. Qual. Patient Saf.* **2017**, *43*, 389–395. [CrossRef] [PubMed]
8. Warner, M.A.; Schulte, P.J.; Hanson, A.C.; Madde, N.R.; Burt, J.M.; Higgins, A.A.; Andrijasevic, N.M.; Kreuter, J.D.; Jacob, E.K.; Stubbs, J.R.; et al. Implementation of a Comprehensive Patient Blood Management Program for Hospitalized Patients at a Large United States Medical Center. *Mayo Clin. Proc.* **2021**, *96*, 2980–2990. [CrossRef] [PubMed]
9. Hofmann, A.; Spahn, D.R.; Holtorf, A.P. Making patient blood management the new norm(al) as experienced by implementors in diverse countries. *BMC Health Serv. Res.* **2021**, *21*, 634. [CrossRef] [PubMed]
10. Podlasek, S.J.; Thakkar, R.N.; Rotello, L.C.; Fleury, T.A.; Demski, R.J.; Ness, P.M.; Frank, S.M.; Thakkar, R.D. Implementing a "Why give 2 when 1 will do?" Choosing Wisely campaign. *Transfusion* **2016**, *56*, 2164. [CrossRef] [PubMed]
11. Fischer, D.P.; Zacharowski, K.D.; Müller, M.M.; Geisen, C.; Seifried, E.; Müller, H.; Meybohm, P. Patient blood management implementation strategies and their effect on physicians' risk perception, clinical knowledge and perioperative practice—The frankfurt experience. *Transfus. Med. Hemother.* **2015**, *42*, 91–97. [CrossRef] [PubMed]
12. WHO. The Urgent need to implement patient blood management: Policy brief. 19 October 2021. Available online: https://www.who.int/publications/i/item/9789240035744 (accessed on 3 March 2022).

13. Leahy, M.F.; Hofmann, A.; Towler, S.; Trentino, K.M.; Burrows, S.A.; Swain, S.G.; Hamdorf, J.; Gallagher, T.; Koay, A.; Geelhoed, G.C.; et al. Improved outcomes and reduced costs associated with a health-system-wide patient blood management program: A retrospective observational study in four major adult tertiary-care hospitals. *Transfusion* **2017**, *57*, 1347–1358. [CrossRef] [PubMed]
14. Goodnough, L.T.; Hollenhorst, M.A. Clinical decision support and improved blood use in patient blood management. *Hematol. Am. Soc. Hematol. Educ. Program* **2019**, *2019*, 577–582. [CrossRef] [PubMed]

life

MDPI

Article

Pilot Lipidomics Study of Copepods: Investigation of Potential Lipid-Based Biomarkers for the Early Detection and Quantification of the Biological Effects of Climate Change on the Oceanic Food Chain

Paul L. Wood [1,*], Michael D. Wood [2] and Stan C. Kunigelis [3]

[1] Metabolomics Unit, College of Veterinary Medicine, Lincoln Memorial University, 6965 Cumberland Gap Pkwy., Harrogate, TN 37752, USA
[2] Child and Adolescent Psychiatry, BC Children's and Women's Hospital & Provincial Health Services Authority, Vancouver, BC V5Z 4H4, Canada; michael.wood@ubc.ca
[3] Imaging and Analysis Center, DeBusk College of Osteopathic Medicine, Lincoln Memorial University, 6965 Cumberland Gap Pkwy., Harrogate, TN 37752, USA; stan.kunigelis@lmunet.edu
* Correspondence: paul.wood@lmunet.edu

Abstract: Maintenance of the health of our oceans is critical for the survival of the oceanic food chain upon which humanity is dependent. Zooplanktonic copepods are among the most numerous multicellular organisms on earth. As the base of the primary consumer food web, they constitute a major biomass in oceans, being an important food source for fish and functioning in the carbon cycle. The potential impact of climate change on copepod populations is an area of intense study. Omics technologies offer the potential to detect early metabolic alterations induced by the stresses of climate change. One such omics approach is lipidomics, which can accurately quantify changes in lipid pools serving structural, signal transduction, and energy roles. We utilized high-resolution mass spectrometry ($\leq$2 ppm mass error) to characterize the lipidome of three different species of copepods in an effort to identify lipid-based biomarkers of copepod health and viability which are more sensitive than observational tools. With the establishment of such a lipid database, we will have an analytical platform useful for prospectively monitoring the lipidome of copepods in a planned long-term five-year ecological study of climate change on this oceanic sentinel species. The copepods examined in this pilot study included a North Atlantic species (*Calanus finmarchicus*) and two species from the Gulf of Mexico, one a filter feeder (*Acartia tonsa*) and one a hunter (*Labidocerca aestiva*). Our findings clearly indicate that the lipidomes of copepod species can vary greatly, supporting the need to obtain a broad snapshot of each unique lipidome in a long-term multigeneration prospective study of climate change. This is critical, since there may well be species-specific responses to the stressors of climate change and co-stressors such as pollution. While lipid nomenclature and biochemistry are extremely complex, it is not essential for all readers interested in climate change to understand all of the various lipid classes presented in this study. The clear message from this research is that we can monitor key copepod lipid families with high accuracy, and therefore potentially monitor lipid families that respond to environmental perturbations evoked by climate change.

Keywords: copepods; lipidomics; climate change; oceanic food chain; sentinel species

check for updates

Citation: Wood, P.L.; Wood, M.D.; Kunigelis, S.C. Pilot Lipidomics Study of Copepods: Investigation of Potential Lipid-Based Biomarkers for the Early Detection and Quantification of the Biological Effects of Climate Change on the Oceanic Food Chain. *Life* **2023**, *13*, 2335. https://doi.org/10.3390/life13122335

Academic Editor: Joseph Neigel

Received: 14 November 2023
Revised: 30 November 2023
Accepted: 11 December 2023
Published: 13 December 2023

1. Introduction

Oceans contain the largest ecosystem on our planet, dominated by phytoplankton [1]. Primary producing phytoplankton play an important role in the regulation of global temperature through the seeding of low-lying clouds with volatile sulfur-based organics. In turn, phytoplankton are a major component of the diet of copepods, the dominant zooplankton in the pelagic food chain [2]. As primary consumers, copepods feed heavily on phytoplankton, thereby influencing their role in climate regulation. In this regard, copepods are a keystone species in marine food webs and have been referred to as the singing canaries of the ocean due to their sensitivity to the physiochemical conditions of the oceans [3]. Copepods serve both as a food source for marine fish larvae, including a variety of commercially harvested fish, and they also are critical players in carbon sequestration. In studies of climate change, it has been shown that copepods are intrinsic to the carbon cycle, which involves fixation of atmospheric CO_2 by photosynthetic algae and the export of this carbon via detrital debris from copepods and other predators to deeper depths of oceans [4,5]. With climate change resulting in elevated oceanic temperatures and pCO_2 (i.e., ocean acidification), populations of phytoplankton are projected to increase, while those of copepods are projected to decrease [6–10] or shift with regard to dominant copepod species, since *Calanus finmarchicus* (*C. finmarchicus*) is most sensitive to warmer temperatures [11]. Monitoring the numbers of these species is important, but there are limitations to observational methods. It is therefore important to obtain early biomarkers of the viability/health of phyto- and zoo-plankton populations.

"Omics" technologies, which monitor mRNA (transcriptomics), proteins (proteomics), and metabolites (metabolomics), offer a solution to this current problem. Lipidomics is a subfield of metabolomics which provides an in-depth evaluation of lipids involved in structural, signal transduction, and energy functions. High-resolution mass spectrometry (HR-MS) provides a high-capacity workflow which acquires high-precision data that allows for the identification and quantification of a broad range of individual lipid members of a diverse array of lipid families. In the case of our analytical platform, we monitor over 12,000 potential lipids across 181 lipid families. The platform also monitors organic soluble non-lipids from 12 different chemical families. Direct flow infusion analysis (FIA) reduces the risk of sample alteration during processing, reduces the variation introduced by manipulative steps, significantly reduces the sample preparation time, and provides a stable ionization via the supply of a constant lipid concentration during the FIA [12].

In studies of the nutritional quality of phytoplankton, lipidomics evaluations have monitored isoprostanoids, glycerophospholipids (GPL), diacylglycerols (DG), triacylglycerols (TG), monogalactosyl-DG (MGDG), digalactosyl-DG (DGDG), and diacylglycyceryl-trimethylhomoserine (DGTS) lipid families [13–22]. In addition, tandem mass spectrometry has been used in a number of these studies to define the fatty acid substitutions of lipids. Definition of fatty acid substituents in complex lipids supplies information on the availability and flux of free fatty acids involved in the dynamic and critical processes of lipid remodeling [23]. These processes include altered deacylation/reacylation mechanisms, changes in the utilization of biosynthetic precursors, and altered lipid degradation. Monitoring the fatty acid constituents of complex lipids has a proven track record of utility in the study of responses in the lipidome to environmental changes [24–27]. It is already established that remodeling of membrane lipids, to maintain membrane fluidity, is a critical process in cellular stability. Work from a number of laboratories has already established that one of the major effects of ocean acidification is to decrease the quality of the lipidome in microalgae [28,29]. The domino effects of this are projected to affect copepods which utilize microalgae as a major nutrient source, and subsequently on fish which feed on copepod populations. Defining these climate-dependent lipid alterations in copepods is our long-term research goal.

The lipidome of *Gammarus fossarum* has been characterized to monitor environmental effects on this freshwater crustacean sentinel species [30]. Lipidomics studies of copepods have been more limited, but have characterized fatty acids and fatty alcohols [31–33], wax esters [34–36], carotenoids [37–39], and copepodamides [40–42]. Our goal is to utilize this published data and expand on it to obtain a more detailed picture of the lipidomes of three different copepod species and compare that to the lipidome of a marine alga. With this database, we will next be positioned to move into a longer-term ecological study of the effects of climate change on copepod health and viability. Our data will also provide information on the health of phytoplankton, since these marine organisms represent a major source of nutrition for copepods that are filter feeders. These speculations are based on prior research that has shown large alterations in membrane lipids with environmental stressors on fungi [43], bacteria [44], and algae [45]. Having the first highly quantitative longitudinal data of copepod viability will ultimately be of incredible value to agencies involved in regulatory decision-making.

2. Materials and Methods

2.1. Copepods

Freeze-dried zooplankton copepods (*Calanus finmarchicus*) were purchased from Brine Shrimp Direct (sales@brineshrimpdirect.com; accessed on 4 April 2022). *Acartia tonsa* (*A. tonsa*) and *Labidocerca aestiva* (*L. aestiva*) were both harvested via netting from the Gulf of Mexico in May of 2022. Sea water was filtered in a plankton net with a 200 μm mesh, and the copepods were identified and separated under 400× magnification light microscopy. Copepods were washed in distilled water and frozen at −20 °C for future analysis. Microalgae (*Isochrysis galbana*) were obtained from Algae Research & Supply (Carlsbad, CA, USA) for comparison to copepods, since microalgae are a major source of lipids and lipid precursors for copepods. This is only one of many species of microalgae consumed by copepods.

2.2. Lipidomics

The copepod and algal samples (n = 5) were sonicated in 2 mL of methanol:water (1:1) containing stable isotope internal standards. These included 2 nmoles $[^{2}H_5]$DHA and 2 nmoles $[^{13}C_3]$diacylglycerol 36:2. Next, 2 mL of methyl-tert-butyl ether were added prior to vigorous shaking at room temperature for 30 min. To attain phase separation, the samples were centrifugated at 4000× g for 30 min. at room temp. One mL of the upper organic layer was isolated and dried by centrifugal vacuum evaporation. The lower layer was dried at 80 °C overnight, and the resulting dried pellets weighed to obtain the dry weight for each sample.

The dried organic extracts were dissolved in infusion solution (2-propanol: methanol: chloroform: H_2O (160:80:80:1) with the water containing 15 mg of NH_4Cl) for mass spectrometric analyses. For flow infusion analysis (FIA), the samples were infused at 12 μL per min into the ESI source for high-resolution data acquisition (140,000, <2 ppm mass error), with an orbitrap mass spectrometer (Thermo Q Exactive). The specific adducts monitored are listed in data Tables [12,46,47]. Between injections, the transfer line was washed with successive 800 μL washes of methanol and hexane/ethyl acetate/chloroform/H_2O (3:2:1:0.1). Structural validation was achieved via tandem mass analyses (MS^2). Product ions were monitored with <2 ppm mass error. For MS^2 analyses, an isolation window of 0.4 amu and collision energies of 15, 25, and 35 NCE (arbitrary units) were used.

2.3. Data Analysis

HR-MS provides high quality data with <2 ppm mass error, and in the majority of cases <1 ppm. Within a given lipid family, this allows for clear separation of family members with similar but not identical masses. In the case of isobars, lipids with the same exact mass but different chemical structures, tandem mass spectrometry (MS^2) often allows differentiation, since product ions are collected with high resolution. In cases where HR-MS is insufficient to resolve compounds, chromatographic methods prior to HR-MS are required.

We have built an Excel spreadsheet database of over 12,000 unique lipids which includes exact masses and calculated ion adducts. Based on our infusion solvent, the predominant ions were $[M+H]^+$, $[M-H_2O+H]^+$, or $[M+NH_4]^+$ in positive electrospray ionization (PESI), while they were $[M-H]^-$ or $[M+Cl]^-$ in NESI. For lipids forming a chloride adduct, the Cl^{37} isotope was also monitored to validate the lipid identity. The HR-MS scan data were imported into this Excel spreadsheet, and any mass with less than 2 ppm mass error for the calculated ion adduct was recorded as a hit; the peak intensity for each hit was imported into the spreadsheet if greater than 100,000 integrated counts (S/N > 3). The exact masses used to build our database were obtained (December 2022) from LipidMaps

(lipidmaps.org), Human Metabolome Database (https//hmdb.ca), Mycobacterium Lipid Database (mrl.colostate.edu/mtb), Chemspider (https://www.chemspider.com), Seaweed Metabolite Database (SWMD), and PubChem (https://pubchem.ncbi.nlm.nih.gov). Since these databases are not all inclusive or always up-to-date with regard to invertebrate lipids, we also extensively used scientific publications to expand the database. This is essential for copepod and microalgal lipids.

For relative quantitation, the peak intensities of individual lipids were divided by the peak intensity of the appropriate internal standard. The internal standard for negative ESI (NESI; 2 nmoles [$^2H_5$]DHA) or for positive ESI (PESI; 2 nmoles [$^{13}C_3$]diacylglycerol 36:2) were used in these calculations. The values obtained were corrected for the sample dry weight, which ranged from 5 to 20 mg, and are presented as mean $\pm$ standard deviation (SD) in Tables and as a summary Figure with bar plots created in R Version 4.2.3 (R Core Team, 2023, R: A language and environment for statistical computing. R Foundation for Statistical Computing, Vienna, Austria. URL https://www.R-project.org/), to visualize lipid ratio trends across copepod species.

For MS^2 studies, parent ions were selected with a 0.4 amu window and product ions monitored with 140,000 resolution (<2 ppm mass error). The HCD energies used were 15, 25, and 35 arbitrary units [46,47].

2.4. Nomenclature

Lipid nomenclature adheres to the guidelines of Lipid Maps [48]. Carbon positions are counted from the terminal carboxy group. Lipid notation such as 20:5 indicates 20 carbons and 5 double bonds. Lyso is shorthand for loss of a fatty acid substitution.

3. Results and Discussion

3.1. Overview

The following section integrates the background, our findings, and relevance of these observations to a planned long-term prospective study of the consequences of climate change on the lipidome of oceanic copepods.

3.2. Carotenoid Pigments

Carotenoids are organic pigments synthesized from lipid precursors by algae, bacteria, fungi, and plants [49]. The long hydrocarbon chains of these pigments span membranes with the terminal ring groups residing at the interior and exterior surfaces of membranes. These terminal ring groups act as antioxidants at the membrane surfaces. Copepods utilize carotenoids, which they ingest with phytoplankton [50], as protective pigments against the oxidative stress of short-wavelength solar radiation [51,52].

In copepods and microalgae (*Isochrysis galabana*), we found high levels of the carotenoids phoenicoxanthin and astaxanthin, along with fatty acyl esters of astaxanthin in copepods (Table 1). These included myristyl (14:0), behenyl (22:0), and cervonyl (22:6) esters, which have previously been reported for krill, another crustacean [53,54]. Red carotenoid pigments are generated by metabolism of yellow dietary precursors from microalgae [38,40]. Dietary pigments include 3-hydroxyechinenone, canthaxanthin, zeaxanthin, adonirubin, and adonixanthin. We did not observe any of these carotenoids or apocarotenoids [55] in copepods. We therefore speculate that dietary pigments are rapidly converted to astaxanthin and phoenicoxanthin by mitochondrial metabolism in copepods [42]. Therefore, at this time, we anticipate that astaxanthin levels in copepods may have the potential to be biomarkers of the health of the microalgal community that provides a food reservoir to copepods, which are filter feeders, and of copepod mitochondrial function. These future data will supply valuable information regarding the interplay of these oceanic species.

Carotenoid identities were validated by MS^2 of the $[M+H]^+$ cations. In all cases, the product ions were monitored with less than 1 ppm mass error for $[\text{Toluene}–H_2]^+ = [91.0542]^+$ and $[\text{MH-Toluene}]^+ = [\text{MH } 92.0526]^+$. While these data validate that the monitored lipids were carotenoids, it cannot distinguish between potential isobaric carotenoids.

Table 1. Relative levels of carotenoids and carotenoid fatty esters in copepods and microalga. Levels are presented as a ratio of the peak intensity of each lipid to the peak intensity of the internal standard (2 nanomoles [$^{13}C_3$]triacylglycerol 48:0), corrected for the sample dry weight. Results are presented as Mean ± SD (*n* = 5). -, not detected.

Carotenoids	[M+H]$^+$	*Isochrysis galbana*	*Acartia tonsa*	*Calanus finmarchicus*	*Labidocerca aestiva*
Phoenicoxanthin	581.3989	566.9 ± 124.8	3.34 ± 1.23	32.8 ± 15.3	1.04 ± 0.72
Astaxanthin	597.3938	18.56 ± 4.32	2.46 ± 1.07	3854.0 ± 200.8	16.5 ± 7.0
Astaxanthin-14:0	807.5922	-	0.99 ± 0.12	-	10.2 ± 3.6
Astaxanthin-22:0	919.7174	-	-	-	2.34 ± 1.34
Astaxanthin-22:6	907.6235	-	-	-	3.63 ± 0.66

3.3. Copepodamides

Copepodamides are polar isoprenoid fatty acids with a terminal amide linkage to the amino acid taurine. These amino lipids are produced and released into the water solely by copepods, where they stimulate toxin production by phytoplankton to evade predation [40,56,57]. Copepodamides (=CH_2 at C2) and dihydrocopepodamides (-CH_3 at C2) possess a fatty acid acyl linkage at C3 [40,58].

In our study we only monitored copepodamides in *C. finmarchicus* (Table 2). High levels of the lyso forms were measured, along with lower levels of the palmitoyl (16:0) and gaidyl (16:1) acyl esters. The lack of copepodamides in *A. tonsa* and *L. aestiva* may relate to the Gulf of Mexico environment, which possesses a much richer food source for copepods. It is more essential to synthesize copepodamides to protect less-rich food sources from predation by other species [56]. The high levels of lysocopepodamide measured in *C. finmarchicus* suggest that this may be a storage pool of this precursor of copepodamides that are synthesized for secretion.

Table 2. Relative levels of copepodamides in *C. finmarchicus*. Levels are presented as a ratio of the peak intensity of each lipid to the peak intensity of the internal standard (2 nanomoles [$^2H_5$]DHA), corrected for the sample dry weight. Results are presented as Mean ± SD (*n* = 5).

Copepodamides	[M-H]$^-$	*Calanus finmarchicus*
Lysocopepodamide	448.2739	1240 ± 329
Lysodihydrocopepodamide	450.2895	59 ± 13
Copepodamide-16:0	686.5035	2.11 ± 1.20

Copepodamide structures were validated by MS^2 of the [M-H]$^-$ anions (Supplementary File). In all cases, the product ions were monitored with less than 1 ppm mass error for the terminal taurine [124.0074]$^-$ and for the base scaffold [$C_{22}H_{41}NO_5S$]$^-$ = [430.2633]$^-$, with loss of the acyl substitutions at position C5.

Since copepodamides are lipids that are unique to copepods, monitoring this lipid family will provide biomarkers of *C. finmarchicus* viability and ability to participate in the maintenance of their major food source, marine phytoplankton.

3.4. Wax Esters and Triacylglycerols

The two major lipid families that serve as energy reservoirs are triacylglycerols (TG) and wax esters (WE). In the case of copepods, wax esters are generally stored at higher concentrations [32,35,36,59–61]. WE are generated by acylation of a fatty alcohol [62]. First, fatty-acyl-CoA reductase (FAR; EC 1.2.1.84) converts a fatty acyl-CoA to the corresponding fatty aldehyde, which in turn is converted to the fatty alcohol by fatty aldehyde reductase (FALR; EC 1.1.1.2). Acylation of the fatty alcohol involves acyl-CoA wax alcohol acyltransferase (AWAT1; EC 2.3.1.75), which has been reported for algae [63] but requires confirmation in copepods. Wax ester metabolism occurs via wax ester hydrolase (WEH; EC 3.1.1.50), which has been characterized in plants but not in copepods at this time.

Our analyses demonstrated high levels of wax esters in copepods and microalgae (*Isochrysis galabana*) (Table 3). The higher molecular weight wax esters and triacylglycerols possessed significant levels of the fatty acids 20:4, 20:5, 22:5, and 22:6 (Table 3), suggesting that these lipids also function as storage pools of this critical polyunsaturated fatty acid (PUFA). *C. finmarchicus* was unique in that wax esters were the dominant lipid storage pool. This may be the result of the cold-water environment of *C. finmarchicus*. Previous work has demonstrated that cold-water copepods like *Tigriopus kingsejongensis* have greater lipid metabolism than Pacific Ocean copepods like *Tigriopus japonicus* [64].

Table 3. Relative levels of wax esters (WE) and triacylglycerols (TG) in copepods and microalga. Levels are presented as a ratio of the peak intensity of each lipid to the peak intensity of the internal standard (2 nanomoles [$^{13}C_3$]triacylglycerol 48:0), corrected for the sample dry weight. Results are presented as Mean ± SD (n = 5). -, not detected.

Wax Esters	**[M+NH$_4$]$^+$**	***Isochrysis galbana***	***Acartia tonsa***	***Calanus finmarchicus***	***Labidocerca aestiva***
WE 32:1	496.5088	-	-	4318 ± 2414	-
WE 32:2	494.4932	-	-	2516 ± 1392	0.058 ± 0.017
WE 34:4	518.4932	-	0.54 ± 0.25	10,686 ± 5960	1.50 ± 0.28
WE 38:2	578.5871	18.35 ± 4.84	-	8009 ± 4530	-
WE 38:3	576.5714	2.67 ± 0.77	0.091 ± 0.008	2835 ± 1618	-
WE 38:5	572.5401	2.41 ± 1.23	0.13 ± 0.019	22,497 ± 12,673	0.16 ± 0.017
WE 38:6	570.5245	-	-	11,219 ± 6374	0.018 ± 0.006
WE 40:2	606.6184	0.20 ± 0.026	-	6865 ± 3916	-
WE 40:3	604.6027	0.16 ± 0.024	0.71 ± 0.062	2042 ± 1423	-
WE 40:6	598.5558	1.21 ± 0.034	-	11,687 ± 6611	-
WE 42:2	634.6497	0.31 ± 0.051	-	5028 ± 2764	-
WE 42:5	628.6027	0.038 ± 0.008	4.63 ± 2.25	7584 ± 4321	2.64 ± 0.065
WE 42:6	626.5871	1.20 ± 0.23	1.08 ± 0.23	10,882 ± 6056	0.66 ± 0.18
Triacylglycerols	**[M+NH$_4$]$^+$**	***Isochrysis galbana***	***Acartia tonsa***	***Calanus finmarchicus***	***Labidocerca aestiva***
TG 46:1	780.7076	-	1.51 ± 0.75	-	5.81 ± 3.00
TG 47:0	810.7545	-	0.57 ± 0.26	-	1.70 ± 0.88
TG 47:1	808.7389	-	0.29 ± 0.15	-	3.24 ± 1.57
TG 48:3	818.7232	-	-	-	2.01 ± 1.00
TG 48:4	816.7076	-	-	-	1.28 ± 0.65
TG 50:1	850.7858	-	1.02 ± 0.17	-	5.29 ± 2.89
TG 50:2	848.7702	-	0.15 ± 0.05	-	-
TG 50:3	846.7545	-	0.042 ± 0.021	-	2.79 ± 1.45
TG 50:5	842.7232	-	-	-	1.68 ± 1.02
TG 51:1	864.8015	-	-	-	2.20 ± 1.01
TG 52:2	876.8015	-	-	-	3.19 ± 1.66
TG 52:3	874.7858	-	-	-	1.75 ± 0.090
TG 52:6	868.7389	-	-	-	8.97 ± 3.12

Table 3. *Cont.*

Triacylglycerols	$[M+NH_4]^+$	*Isochrysis galbana*	*Acartia tonsa*	*Calanus finmarchicus*	*Labidocerca aestiva*
TG 54:6	896.7702	-	-	-	1.63 ± 0.83
TG 56:4	928.8328	-	-	-	0.51 ± 0.15
TG 56:6	924.8015	-	-	-	3.31 ± 1.53

TGs were not detected in *C. finmarchicus*, which had the highest levels of WE (Table 3). WE serve as a rich energy resource pool in the copepods *C. finmarchicus*, *Calanus helgolanicus*, and *Gaussia princeps* [34,65]. In contrast, in the hunter copepod species *L. aestiva*, TGs predominated, presumably a biomarker of the more complex diet of this species. As with WEs, TGs also were found to have PUFA constituents (Table 3).

3.5. Monoacylglycerols (MG) and Modified MGs

Monoacylglycerols (MG) have diverse functions that include storage pools of fatty acids, membrane structure, and signal transduction. We monitored MGs with saturated fatty acid and PUFA substituents in copepods and microalgae (*Isochrysis galabana*) (Table 4).

We also report, for the first time, alanyl-MGs (Table 4) in copepods and microalga (*Isochrysis galabana*). This finding was validated via monitoring the product cation of 90.0550 for alanine in MS^2 experiments. Alanyl-phosphatidylglycerols (Ala-PG) and alanyl-phosphatidyl-ethanolamines (Ala-PE) have been reported for many Gram-positive bacterial strains, but not alanyl-MGs [66–68]. These aminoacylations modify the membrane charge in bacteria. It remains to be determined if the alanyl-MGs we monitored are synthesized by copepods or their gut bacteria, or if they are degradation products of Ala-PG and Ala-PE. However, we did not monitor Ala-PGs or Ala-PEs in our analysis.

There are also a number of betaine lipids that have been reported for bacteria, fungi, and microalgae [69,70]. Monoacylglyceryl trimethylhomoserine (MGTS) is one of these betaine lipids which we monitored in copepods and microalga. Structural validation was obtained with the product cation of 104.1075 for choline in MS^2 experiments (Supplementary File), however, monoacylglyceryl hydroxymethyltrimethyl-β-alanine (MGTA) is a structural isomer of MGTS that we cannot rule out at this time. It is important to note that all previous publications of algae have monitored only MGTS and not MGTA. While MGTSs may be acquired via the diet, the biosynthetic pathway for these lipids may well be present in copepods. This involves the initial formation of an aminolipid by the reaction of S-adenosylmethionine with either an MG or a DG. Next, the homoserine addition to the glycerol backbone is sequentially methylated to generate MGTSs. In the green alga *Chlamydomonas reinhardtii*, a single DGTS synthase protein (BTA1Cr) co-ordinates all of these reactions [71].

MGTSs, like phosphatidylcholines (PC), are quaternary amines, making them zwitterionic membrane lipids. However, they are connected to the glycerol backbone via an ether linkage, which is more flexible than the phosphodiester linkage of a PC, more chemically stable, and more stable against degradation by phospholipases, presumably improving membrane stability in an aquatic environment [71].

The third betaine lipid family in algae and plants is monoacylglyceryl carboxyhydroxymethylcholine (MGCC) which is present in the non-plasmid membrane fraction where it also can substitute for PCs [72]. We monitored, and report for the first time, high levels of MGCCs in C. finmarchicus (Table 4). MGCC structures were validated via identification of the product cation of 104.1070 for choline in MS^2 experiments. It remains to be determined if these MGCCs are dietary or synthesized by copepods.

Table 4. Relative levels of monoacylglycerols (MG) and modified MGs in copepods and microalga. Levels are presented as a ratio of the peak intensity of each lipid to the peak intensity of the internal standard (2 nanomoles [$^{2}H_{5}$]DHA for NESI and 2 nanomoles [$^{13}C_{3}$]triacylglycerol 48:0 for PESI), corrected for the sample dry weight (Mean ± SD; n = 5). -, not detected.

Monoacylglycerols	**[M+Cl]$^{-}$**	***Isochrysis galbana***	***Acartia tonsa***	***Calanus finmarchicus***	***Labidocerca aestiva***
MG 16:0	365.2469	1.76 ± 0.094	24.09 ± 14.64	21.70 ± 3.08	-
MG 18:0	393.2782	0.73 ± 0.079	177.7 ± 88.2	28.43 ± 6.91	-
MG 18:1	391.2625	3.31 ± 0.061	5.07 ± 0.79	19.07 ± 8.00	10.11 ± 4.78
MG 18:3	387.2312	0.29 ± 0.011	9.35 ± 4.64	9.42 ± 1.95	13.26 ± 4.20
MG 20:4	413.2469	1.20 ± 0.13	1.59 ± 0.58	5.45 ± 1.49	7.28 ± 3.73
MG 22:6	437.2469	1.32 ± 0.10	9.26 ± 0.26	52.88 ± 12.05	42.74 ± 20.38
Alanyl-monoacyl-glycerols	**[M+H]$^{+}$**	***Isochrysis galbana***	***Acartia tonsa***	***Calanus finmarchicus***	***Labidocerca aestiva***
Ala-MG 16:1	400.3057	0.20 ± 0.063	3.55 ± 0.57	2.24 ± 0.81	0.34 ± 0.012
Ala-MG 18:1	428.3370	0.27 ± 0.084	5.77 ± 0.35	1.14 ± 0.26	0.30 ± 0.11
Ala-MG 20:1	456.3683	0.029 ± 0.013	3.31 ± 1.72	-	0.13 ± 0.070
Ala-MG 20:4	450.3214	-	0.20 ± 0.11	17.8 ± 7.10	0.18 ± 0.051
MGTS	**[M+H]$^{+}$**	***Isochrysis galbana***	***Acartia tonsa***	***Calanus finmarchicus***	***Labidocerca aestiva***
MGTS 20:4	522.3789	-	0.19 ± 0.028	3.74 ± 2.56	1.26 ± 0.58
MGTS 22:2	554.4415	1.77 ± 0.71	0.86 ± 0.51	14.01 ± 4.07	1.29 ± 0.85
MGTS 22:4	550.4102	-	0.044 ± 0.021	11.37 ± 3.32	0.52 ± 0.20
MGTS 24:2	582.4728	0.83 ± 0.38	0.48 ± 0.21	19.88 ± 5.12	0.59 ± 0.20
MGCC	**[M+H]$^{+}$**	***Isochrysis galbana***	***Acartia tonsa***	***Calanus finmarchicus***	***Labidocerca aestiva***
MGCC 16:0	490.3738	-	0.95 ± 0.03	0.22 ± 0.23	0.83 ± 0.40
MGCC 18:0	518.4051	-	-	293.0 ± 69.6	-
MGCC 20:0	546.4364	-	-	1504 ± 1002	-
MGCC 22:0	574.4677	-	-	2100 ± 66	-
MGCC 22:6	562.3738	0.18 ± 0.12	-	1781 ± 798	-
MGCC 24:0	602.4990	-	-	1498 ± 516	-
MGCC 24:2	598.4677	-	-	1534 ± 424	-

Ala, Alanine; MGCC, Monoacylglyceryl carboxyhydroxymethylcholine; MGTS, Monoacylglyceryl trimethylhomoserine.

3.6. Diacylglycerols (DG) and Modified DGs

We monitored high levels of DGs in copepods but much lower levels in *Isochrysis galabana* (Table 5). DGs are essential for membrane function both as structural lipids and as precursors for structural GPLs. DGs are also important lipids in the membranes of the nuclear envelope, endoplasmic reticulum [73], and in the Golgi for transport carrier biogenesis [74]. DGs are involved in signal transduction pathways via activation of protein kinases and by direct modulation of nuclear signal transduction [75].

As with the MGs, we also monitored the trimethylhomoserine modification of DGs (DGTS) in copepods and microalga (*Isochrysis galabana*) (Table 5). DGTSs have been reported for microalgae [64,69–71], but this is the first report of these lipids in copepods. As with MGTSs, structural validation for DGTSs was obtained with the product cation of 104.1075 for choline in MS^{2} experiments. However, DGTAs are possible isobars. In microalgae, DGTSs substitute for glycerophospholipids in membranes, thereby conserving phosphate but also function as a source for triacylglycerols under stress conditions, thereby maintaining a major energy source [76].

Table 5. Relative levels of diacylglycerols (DG) and modified DGs in copepods and microalga. Levels are presented as a ratio of the peak intensity of each lipid to the peak intensity of the internal standard (2 nanomoles [$^2H_5$]DHA) for NESI and 2 nanomoles [$^{13}C_3$]triacylglycerol 48:0 for PESI), corrected for the sample dry weight. Results are presented as Mean ± SD (n = 5). -, not detected.

Diacylglycerols	$[M+Cl]^-$	*Isochrysis galbana*	*Acartia tonsa*	*Calanus finmarchicus*	*Labidocerca aestiva*
DG 34:0	631.5078	0.12 ± 0.022	28.1 ± 14.6	4.94 ± 1.35	8.26 ± 4.40
DG 34:1	629.4922	1.14 ± 0.14	2.45 ± 1.24	1.99 ± 0.20	4.25 ± 1.29
DG 34:5	621.4296	0.18 ± 0.039	-	3.38 ± 0.92	2.81 ± 0.64
DG 36:0	659.5391	-	45.1 ± 5.24	2.37 ± 1.01	28.8 ± 10.1
DG 38:4	679.5078	0.012 ± 0.005	0.022 ± 004	1.19 ± 0.46	0.78 ± 0.44
DG 38:6	675.4765	0.37 ± 0.04	0.54 ± 0.10	0.52 ± 0.11	5.81 ± 2.12
DGTS	$[M+H]^+$	*Isochrysis galbana*	*Acartia tonsa*	*Calanus finmarchicus*	*Labidocerca aestiva*
DGTS 28:0	656.5460	1.99 ± 0.64	0.019 ± 0.009	41.6 ± 22.5	0.16 ± 0.025
DGTS 30:0	684.5773	0.67 ± 0.23	1.29 ± 0.67	44.8 ± 21.9	029 ± 0.18
DGTS 32:1	710.5929	39.7 ± 5.8	0.63 ± 0.075	67.6 ± 23.7	0.069 ± 0.033
DGTS 32:2	708.5773	1.97 ± 0.37	0.024 ± 0.004	27.7 ± 6.2	-
DGCC	$[M+H]^+$	*Isochrysis galbana*	*Acartia tonsa*	*Calanus finmarchicus*	*Labidocerca aestiva*
DGCC 32:0	728.6035	0.81 ± 0.045	6.74 ± 2.12	-	2.12 ± 1.2
DGCC 32:1	726.5878	4.23 ± 0.94	0.86 ± 0.51	-	2.66 ± 1.37
DGCC 32:2	724.5722	2.18 ± 1.0	-	-	0.93 ± 0.13
DGCC 34:0	756.6348	-	1.72 ± 0.91	-	1.84 ± 1.00
DGCC 36:6	772.5722	5.41 ± 1.05	-	-	-
DGCC 40:6	828.6348	0.18 ± 0.051	-	-	0.51 ± 0.11
Monogalactosyl DG	$[M+Cl]^-$	*Isochrysis galbana*	*Acartia tonsa*	*Calanus finmarchicus*	*Labidocerca aestiva*
MGDG 32:1	763.5137	12.31 ± 3.91	-	-	-
MGDG 32:2	761.4981	4.07 ± 1.12	-	-	-
MGDG 32:3	759.4824	2.04 ± 0.65	-	-	-
MGDG 32:4	757.4668	3.90 ± 1.26	-	-	-
MGDG 32:5	755.4511	1.22 ± 0.42	-	-	-
MGDG 34:1	791.5450	4.25 ± 1.29	-	-	-
MGDG 34:2	789.5294	3.96 ± 1.16	-	-	-
MGDG 34:6	781.4668	1.57 ± 0.48	-	-	-
MGDG 36:2	817.5607	11.13 ± 3.40	-	-	-
MGDG 36:3	815.5450	1.92 ± 0.51	-	-	-
MGDG 36:4	813.5294	1.39 ± 0.39	-	-	-
MGDG 36:5	811.5137	2.55 ± 0.86	-	-	-
MGDG 36:6	809.4981	2.64 ± 0.76	-	-	-

Table 5. *Cont.*

Digalactosyl DG	[M+Cl]$^-$	*Isochrysis galbana*	*Acartia tonsa*	*Calanus finmarchicus*	*Labidocerca aestiva*
DGDG 30:1	897.5352	1.11 ± 0.60	-	-	-
DGDG 30:2	895.5196	0.49 ± 0.16	-	-	-
DGDG 32:1	925.5665	0.51 ± 0.04	-	-	-
DGDG 32:4	919.5196	0.33 ± 0.01	-	-	-
DGDG 34:3	949.5665	0.22 ± 0.11	-	-	-
DGDG 34:5	945.5396	2.79 ± 1.25	-	-	-
DGDG 36:3	977.5978	3.96 ± 1.16	-	-	-
DGDG 36:4	975.5822	0.64 ± 0.17	-	-	-
DGDG 36:5	973.5665	0.42 ± 0.19	-	-	-
DGDG 36:6	971.5509	0.22 ± 0.05	-	-	-

DGCC, Diacylglyceryl carboxyhydroxymethylcholine; DGTS, Diacylglyceryl trimethylhomoserine.

We also monitored the carboxyhydroxymethylcholine modification of MGs (MGCC) and DGs (DGCC) in copepods and microalgae (*Isochrysis galabana*) (Table 5). DGCCs which were detected at higher levels than MGCCs in the microalga *I. galabana* and the copepods *A. tonsa* and *L. aestiva* (Table 5), suggesting that MGCCs may be deacylation products (i.e., lyso) of DGCCs. *C. finmarchicus* lacked detectable DGCCs.

Major saccharolipids that are integral to photosynthetic membranes are mono- and di-galactosyl DGs (MGDG and DGDG, respectfully). In the case of microalga (*Isochrysis galabana*), we monitored both MGDGs and DGDGs (Table 5). In this regard, previous studies have demonstrated that MGDG levels in microalgae are decreased with exposure to ocean acidification [20]. As expected, these lipids were not monitored in copepods since they lack chloroplasts.

3.7. Docosahexaenoic Acid (DHA)

Copepods have the enzyme machinery [34] required for the biosynthesis of docosahexaenoic acid (DHA; FA 22:6n-3). Our data (Table 6) validate that copepods maintain very high levels of DHA and hydroxy-DHA isoforms, oxylipin metabolites of DHA [77–81]. Oxylipins are also synthesized by closely related krill [80]. We monitored these oxylipins in copepods, where they may come from their diet but are more likely synthesized by the copepods. Our data cannot distinguish the many isoforms of hydroxy-DHA. The complex roles of oxylipins in cellular regulation in copepods require further study. In contrast to copepods, low levels of DHA and hydroxy DHA were monitored in microalga (*Isochrysis galabana*).

3.8. Sterols: Cholesterol

Cholesterol is the most abundant sterol in the membranes of copepods [82–84]. This sterol is critical for the formation of a liquid-ordered phase in membranes, thereby providing membrane stabilization/fluidity and maintenance/restriction of membrane permeability across a range of body temperatures [84]. Cholesterol is also contained within lipid rafts, regulating the integration of receptor, enzyme, transporter, and ion channel proteins. In our samples, we, like previous researchers [83], observed that copepods have high levels of cholesterol and cholesterol esters (Table 6). It should be cautioned that, without chromatography, our cholesterol measurements may also include other sterol isobars at the same monitored mass; however, chromatography of copepod lipid extracts support the identity of cholesterol [83]. We also report, for the first time, that microalgae (*Isochrysis galabana*) have high levels of galactosyl/glucosyl cholesterol.

Table 6. Relative levels of docosahexaenoic acid (DHA; PUFA 22:6), cholesterol, and cholesterol esters (CE) in copepods and microalga. Levels are presented as a ratio of the peak intensity of each lipid to the peak intensity of the internal standard (2 nanomoles [$^2H_5$]DHA for NESI and 2 nanomoles [$^{13}C_3$]triacylglycerol 48:0 for PESI), corrected for the sample dry weight. Results are presented as Mean ± SD (n = 5). -, not detected.

PUFA	**[M-H]$^-$**	*Isochrysis galbana*	*Acartia tonsa*	*Calanus finmarchicus*	*Labidocerca aestiva*
DHA	327.2330	0.57 ± 0.055	394 ± 153	696 ± 149	2090 ± 769
Hydroxy-DHA	343.2279	0.36 ± 0.10	333 ± 67	1139 ± 278	712 ± 310
Cholesterol	**[MH-H$_2$O]$^+$**	*Isochrysis galbana*	*Acartia tonsa*	*Calanus finmarchicus*	*Labidocerca aestiva*
Cholesterol	369.3516	-	34.58 ± 15.34	4.59 ± 2.12	12.98 ± 2.43
Cholesterol Esters	**[M+NH$_4$]$^+$**	*Isochrysis galbana*	*Acartia tonsa*	*Calanus finmarchicus*	*Labidocerca aestiva*
Hexosyl-Cholesterol *	566.4415	591 ± 252	-	-	-
CE 12:0	586.5558	-	0.66 ± 0.13	-	0.11 ± 0.04
CE 14:0	614.5871	-	4.11 ± 1.83	-	1.51 ± 0.74
CE 15:0	628.6027	-	4.63 ± 2.24	7584 ± 4521	2.64 ± 0.66
CE 15:1	626.5871	-	1.08 ± 0.40	-	0.66 ± 0.18
CE16:0	642.6184	-	1.76 ± 0.89	12.44 ± 4.75	0.90 ± 0.22
CE 16:1	640.6027	-	4.31 ± 0.23	-	3.63 ± 0.69
CE 17:0	656.6340	-	0.30± 0.99	20.70 ± 1.78	1.03 ± 0.26
CE 18:2	668.6340	-	4.94 ± 1.26	-	2.90 ± 0.10
CE 22:6	714.6184	-	2.28 ± 0.93	-	1.71 ± 0.84

*, hexosyl = glucosyl and/or galactosyl.

In contrast to copepods, hopanoids are the major membrane sterols in eubacteria, but not archaebacteria. Both sterols and hopanoids are polycyclic triterpene products of the metabolic precursor squalene. Archaebacteria are conjectured to utilize polyterpenes (polyprenols, carotenoids, and quinones) as membrane regulators [84].

3.9. Glycerophospholipids (GPL)

The chemical skeleton of glycerophospholipids (GPL) includes a glycerol back bone with one (i.e., Lyso-GPL) or two (i.e., diacyl, also termed phosphatidyl) fatty acid substituents and a polar phosphodiester head group. In the case of this study, we detected GPL with headgroups of phosphocholine, phosphoethanolamine, and phosphoglycerol.

Copepods were found to contain choline and ethanolamine GPL with the rank order of *C. finmarchicus* >> *L. aestiva* > *A. tonsa* (Table 7). In the cases of PCs and PEs, PUFAs were present in a large number of these GPLs (Table 7). This profile for PCs is similar to that previously reported for krill [85]. No phosphatidylcholines were detected in the microalgae (*Isochrysis galabana*), along with low levels of phosphatidylethanolamines. However, phosphatidylglycerols were only monitored in the microalgae (*Isochrysis galabana*) (Table 7) and did not contain PUFAs. Previous work has demonstrated that ocean acidification results in elevated levels of both phosphatidylglycerols and phosphatidylethanolamines in microalgae [86]. These data demonstrate the sensitivity of lipidomics analyses in monitoring the effects of climate change on marine organisms.

Table 7. Relative levels of glycerophospholipids in copepods and microalga. Levels are presented as a ratio of the peak intensity of each lipid to the peak intensity of the internal standard (2 nanomoles [$^2H_5$]DHA) for NESI and 2 nanomoles [$^{13}C_3$]triacylglycerol 48:0 for PESI), corrected for the sample dry weight. Results are presented as Mean ± SD (n = 5). -, not detected.

Phosphatidylcholine (PC)	**[M+H]$^+$**	***Isochrysis galbana***	***Acartia tonsa***	***Calanus finmarchicus***	***Labidocerca aestiva***
PC 28:0 (14:0/14:0)	678.5068	-	3.44 ± 1.23	-	5.91 ± 2.34
PC 28:1	676.4912	-	-	-	0.39 ± 0.21
PC 28:4	670.4442	-	-	2134 ± 658	3.03 ± 0.75
PC 30:5	696.4599	-	-	1037 ± 324	-
PC 34:1 (16:0/18:1)	760.5851	-	0.92 ± 0.21	995 ± 473	2.24 ± 0.90
PC 34:4	754.5381	-	-	360 ± 114	-
PC 34:5	752.5225	-	-	116 ± 56	-
PC 36:4	782.5694	-	0.73 ± 0.11	806 ± 52	1.60 ± 0.87
PC 36:5	780.5538	-	2.70 ± 0.34	1416 ± 745	1.37 ± 0.29
PC 38:6 (18:1/20:5)	806.5694	-	-	1984 ± 868	-
Phosphatidylethanolamine (PE)	**[M-H]$^-$**	***Isochrysis galbana***	***Acartia tonsa***	***Calanus finmarchicus***	***Labidocerca aestiva***
PE 32:0 (16:0/16:0; 18:0/14:0)	690.5079	-	0.35 ± 0.05	-	4.27 ± 2.1
PE 32:1	688.4923	0.14 ± 0.04	0.19 ± 0.06	11.70 ± 1.25	0.29 ± 0.12
PE 34:1	716.5236	0.025 ± 0.011	-	-	0.17 ± 0.08
PE 36:0	746.5705	-	-	-	1.94 ± 0.93
PE 36:2	742.5392	0.051 ± 0.020	0.68 ± 0.21	-	-
PE 38:3	768.5549	-	-	-	2.07 ± 0.88
PE 40:4	794.5702	-	-	114 ± 51	2.59 ± 0.11
PE 42:5	820.5862	-	-	-	1.69 ± 0.79
PE 42:6 (20:0/22:6)	818.5705	-	-	13.99 ± 3.81	-
PE 44:6	846.6018	-	-	-	0.67 ± 0.33
Phosphatidylglycerol (PG)	**[M-H]$^-$**	***Isochrysis galbana***	***Acartia tonsa***	***Calanus finmarchicus***	***Labidocerca aestiva***
PG 30:0 (15:0/15:0)	693.4712	1.23 ± 0.62	-	-	-
PG 32:1	719.4869	0.63 ± 0.23	-	-	-
PG 34:1 (16:0/18:1)	747.5182	3.51 ± 1.35	-	-	-
PG 34:2	745.5025	2.51 ± 0.99	-	-	-
PG 36:2 (18:1/18:1)	773.5338	7.58 ± 3.06	-	-	-
PG 36:3	771.5182	1.27 ± 0.51	-	-	-

PCs were the predominant GPL in all three copepod species (Table 7), and relative levels were higher than what we monitored with DGTSs (Table 5), lipid substitutes for PCs.

PC and PE are isobaric with, for example, PC 36:0 = PE 39:0. Since PCs do not form [M-H]$^-$ ions, reliable measurement of PEs in negative ESI is possible. We also performed MS^2 analyses of the observed PEs and monitored the expected product [PE headgroup]$^-$ = [140.0118]$^-$. In positive ESI, the PEs could contribute to the PC signals; however, this contribution would come from odd-carbon PCs, which are rare. In addition, we performed MS^2 analyses of the PCs and monitored the expected product [Phosphocholine]$^+$ = [184.0739]$^+$.

Since our analytical platform accurately quantitates both PCs and DGTSs, calculating a ratio of the levels of PCs to DGTSs could be a future useful index of phosphorous under- or over-supply with environmental stressors, based on prior studies of fungi [43], bacteria [44], and algae [86,87].

3.10. Sphingolipids: Ceramides

The basic skeleton of a ceramide is a sphingolipid base with an amide-linked fatty acid. For all but one class of sphingolipids, the sphingolipid base is sphingosine or sphinganine, both generated by addition of a long-chain CoA to the carboxy function of serine. In contrast, in the case of deoxyceramides, the addition of the long-chain CoA is to alanine, which lacks a hydroxy group, hence they are termed deoxyceramides. In the biosynthesis of both ceramides and deoxyceramides, a second fatty acid undergoes N-acylation to the amine group of serine or alanine, respectfully. With the absence of the 1-hydroxyl group in the sphingolipid base, deoxyceramides cannot be converted into ceramide phosphates, hexosylceramides, or sphingomyelins (SM). In the case of *C. finmarchicus*, which had the highest levels of deoxyceramides, this copepod species had the smallest variety of SM variants (Table 8).

Table 8. Relative levels of sphingolipids (ceramides and sphingomyelins) in copepods and microalga. Levels are presented as a ratio of the peak intensity of each lipid to the peak intensity of the internal standard (2 nanomoles [$^2H_5$]DHA for NESI and 2 nanomoles [$^{13}C_3$]triacylglycerol 48:0 for PESI), corrected for the sample dry weight. Results are presented as Mean ± SD (n = 5). -, not detected.

Deoxyceramides	**[M+H]$^+$**	***Isochrysis galbana***	***Acartia tonsa***	***Calanus finmarchicus***	***Labidocerca aestiva***
Cer 34:0; O	524.5401	-	-	12,363 ± 6942	-
Cer 34:1; O	522.5245	-	-	3871 ± 2188	-
Cer 34:2; O	520.5088	-	-	5258 ± 2970	0.42 ± 0.064
Cer 34:3; O	518.4932	-	-	10,686 ± 5960	1.50 ± 0.28
Cer 34:4; O	516.4775	-	-	4711 ± 1458	0.70 ± 0.17
Cer 34:5; O	514.4619	-	-	978 ± 562	-
Cer 36:0; O	552.5714	-	-	16,760 ± 9450	-
Cer 36:1; O	550.5558	-	-	5883 ± 3285	-
Cer 36:2; O	548.5401	-	0.14 ± 0.04	3146 ± 1805	0.11 ± 0.05
Cer 36:3; O	546.5245	-	0.11 ± 0.06	6435 ± 3759	0.25 ± 0.13
Cer 36:4; O	544.5088	-	0.61 ± 0.31	12,199 ± 6893	0.76 ± 0.02
Cer 36:5; O	542.4932	-	0.058 ± 0.023	9800 ± 5450	0.11 ± 0.02
Cer 38:0; O	580.6027	-	-	11,112 ± 6221	-
Cer 38:1; O	578.5871	-	-	8009 ± 4500	-
Cer 38:2; O	576.5714	-	0.091 ± 0.008	2835 ± 1618	-
Cer 38:3; O	574.5558	-	-	5059 ± 2750	0.079 ± 0.039
Cer 38:4; O	572.5401	-	0.13 ± 0.01	22,497 ± 12,676	0.16 ± 0.01
Cer 38:5; O	570.5245	-	-	11,220 ± 6341	0.018 ± 0.006
Cer 40:1; O	606.6184	-	-	6865 ± 3716	-
Cer 40:5; O	598.5558	-	-	11,687 ± 6211	-
Cer 42:4; O	628.6027	-	4.63 ± 2.25	7584 ± 4012	2.64 ± 0.66

Table 8. *Cont.*

Deoxyceramides	[M+H]$^+$	*Isochrysis galbana*	*Acartia tonsa*	*Calanus finmarchicus*	*Labidocerca aestiva*
Cer 42:5; O	626.5871	-	1.08 ± 0.22	10,822 ± 6156	0.66 ± 0.18
Cer 44:4; O	656.6340	-	0.21 ± 0.11	20.7 ± 1.7	1.03 ± 0.26
Cer 44:5; O	654.6184	-	0.094 ± 0.01	3289 ± 1642	0.18 ± 0.04
Ceramides	**[M+Cl]$^-$**	***Isochrysis galbana***	***Acartia tonsa***	***Calanus finmarchicus***	***Labidocerca aestiva***
Cer 34:0; O2	574.49758	0.69 ± 0.09	2.33 ± 0.10	8.17 ± 3.2	12.16 ± 6.31
Cer 34:1; O2	572.48193	0.25 ± 0.09	43.45 ± 5.56	0.86 ± 0.23	60.3 ± 23.0
Cer 34:2; O2	570.46628	8.93 ± 0.28	32.91 ± 15.17	43.8 ± 10.4	145 ± 43
Cer 34:3; O2	568.45063	-	17.50 ± 6.56	132.4 ± 29.0	77.9 ± 19.7
Cer 34:4; O2	566.43498	-	4.75 ± 1.22	37.5 ± 7.6	13.7 ± 6.63
Cer 34:5; O2	564.41933	-	1.22 ± 0.34	9.00 ± 1.31	1.38 ± 0.52
Cer 36:0; O2	602.52888	1.93 ± 0.37	0.63 ± 0.24	8.38 ± 2.56	2.67 ± 1.89
Cer 36:3; O2	596.48193	-	17.25 ± 6.59	151 ± 30	86.8 ± 28.0
Cer 36:4; O2	594.46628	-	7.18 ± 3.77	91.5 ± 20.5	26.03 ± 14.63
Cer 36:5; O2	592.45063	-	3.44 ± 1.56	42.5 ± 8.4	11.69 ± 4.96
Cer 38:3; O2	568.45063	-	8.28 ± 1.86	375 ± 86	27.03 ± 8.33
Cer 38:4; O2	566.43498	-	1.80 ± 0.34	85.9 ± 22.5	6.63 ± 2.21
Cer 38:5; O2	564.41933	-	2.12 ± 0.45	18.6 ± 3.0	6.72 ± 3.23
Cer 40:4; O2	622.49758	-	3.98 ± 1.45	68.5 ± 16.4	6.62 ± 3.78
Cer 42:3; O2	652.54453	-	4.00 ± 1.10	421 ± 104	326 ± 54
Cer 42:4; O2	650.52888	-	18.81 ± 5.84	771 ± 210	66.3 ± 4.1
Cer 42:5; O2	648.51323	-	0.92 ± 0.26	24.2 ± 6.1	2.26 ± 1.0
Cer 44:3; O2	680.57583	-	16.76 ± 8.49	12.9 ± 3.7	130 ± 2
Cer 44:4; O2	678.56018	-	6.32 ± 2.30	274 ± 72	44.30 ± 1.05
Cer 44:5; O2	676.54453	-	-	9.77 ± 2.04	0.45 ± 0.17
Cer 46:4; O2	706.59148	-	-	19.5 ± 5.7	0.16 ± 0.09
Sphingomyelins (SM)	**[M+H]$^+$**	***Isochrysis galbana***	***Acartia tonsa***	***Calanus finmarchicus***	***Labidocerca aestiva***
SM 32:0; O2	677.5592	-	0.42 ± 0.17	-	1.55 ± 0.38
SM 34:0; O2	705.5905	-	4.04 ± 2.03	-	0.44 ± 0.06
SM 34:2; O2	701.5592	-	-	-	0.81 ± 0.37
SM 36:3; O2	727.5749	-	-	44.83 ± 21.90	1.23 ± 0.60
SM 42:3; O2	811.6688	-	5.31 ± 1.89	15.76 ± 5.39	12.35 ± 5.62
SM 42:4; O2	809.6531	-	0.96 ± 0.48	-	2.51 ± 0.79
SM d18:1/25:3	823.6688	-	2.87 ± 1.21	-	20.21 ± 10.39
SM d18:1/25:4	821.6531	-	0.47 ± 0.14	-	1.45 ± 0.72
SM d18:1/26:2	839.7001	-	-	-	5.72 ± 2.39
SM d18:1/26:3	837.6844	-	0.40 ± 0.15	19.04 ± 8.32	1.46 ± 0.47

The loss of the hydroxy function in deoxyceramides results in a significant reduction in the ability of deoxyceramides to hydrogen bond, making them more hydrophobic [88,89]. Ceramides function as structural components of membranes and in signal transduction pathways. In this regard, a number of studies indicate that ceramides [89] and deoxyceramides [89] are activators of autophagy and mitophagy. Specifically, deoxyceramides augment the autophagic flux via inducing the accumulation of phagosomes and lysosomes, thereby regulating cellular proliferation/differentiation and programmed cell death.

High levels of deoxyceramides were detected in copepods but not microalgae (*Isochrysis galabana*), with the rank order of *C. finmarchicus* >>> *L. aestiva* $\approx$ *A. tonsa* (Table 8). This is the first report of these sphingolipids in copepods. The identity of deoxyceramides was validated by monitoring the dehydrated deoxybases in MS^2 experiments. These bases included m18:2 (264.2686) for deoxyceramides 34:2 and 36:2, m18:3 (262.2529) for deoxyceramides 34:3 and 36:3, and m18:4 (260.2373) for deoxyceramides 34:4 and 36:4.

The functions of deoxyceramides in copepods remain to be defined, but the greater lipophilicity of these unique lipids may be important for their roles in membrane function in species with lower GPL content. In the study of climate change effects on microalgae, sphingolipid levels (ceramides) were augmented [90].

3.11. Sphingolipids: Sphingomyelins

Copepods and closely related krill possess significant levels of sphingomyelins (SM) [91–93]. This is a result of the unique feature of these invertebrates possessing myelinated axons [92,93]. In contrast to mammals, the dominant sphingomyelin was not SM 42:5;O2. We monitored a variety of sphingomyelins, with each copepod species possessing a unique fingerprint for these sphingolipids (Table 8). No hydroxy-sphingomyelins were detected in copepods and no sphingomyelins were detected in microalgae (*Isochrysis galabana*). Since SM are isobaric with ceramide phosphoethanolamines [94], we performed MS^2 analyses and monitored the expected SM product ion $[\text{Phosphocholine}]^+ = [184.0739]^+$ with < 1 ppm mass error. Monitoring SMs in future studies may be useful, since these lipids represent a nervous system biomarker.

3.12. Copepod Heterofibrins

Lipid droplets are cellular organelles that store cholesterol, cholesterol esters, and acylglycerols (mainly TGs). These organelles are critical in energy metabolism via regulation of the cellular levels of free lipids. This involves a complex integration of lipid storage, hydrolysis, and transport [95]. The levels of lipid droplets have been shown to vary with the reproductive cycle in *C. finmarchicus* [96]. Heterofibrins have been described as small molecule modulators of lipid droplet formation [96]. Heterofibrins encompass two families of 18 and 19 carbon fatty acids possessing a unique diyne-ene moiety. Analogs within each family have a carboxy-terminal monolactyl or dilactyl substitution [96]. These complex lipids were initially isolated from *Spongia (Heterofibria)*. Ours is the first data to demonstrate the presence of heterofibrins in the copepod *C. finmarchicus* (Table 9). We monitored both heterofibrin A2 (HF-A2) and heterofibrin B2 (HF-B2); the structures were validated by MS^2 of the $[M\text{-}H]^-$ anions (Supplementary File). Both heterofibrins generated product ions for lactic acid $[89.0244]^-$ and propionic acid $[73.0294]^-$ of the carboxy terminal. Both heterofibrins also had product ions that resulted from cleavage at the diyne-ene moiety closest to the carboxy terminal, resulting in product ions of $[173.1336]^-$ for HF-A2 and $[187.1492]^-$ for HFB2. All product ions were monitored with less than 1 ppm mass error.

These data support a complex regulation of lipid droplet storage in cold-water copepods. Hence, heterofibrins may prove to be useful as biomarkers of the complex effects of climate change on energy metabolism in *C. finmarchicus*.

Table 9. Relative levels of heterofibrins in *C. finmarchicus* and chlorophylls in *I. galabana*. Levels are presented as a ratio of the peak intensity of each lipid to the peak intensity of the internal standard (2 nanomoles $[^2H_5]$DHA for NESI and 2 nanomoles $[^{13}C_3]$triacylglycerol 48:0 for PESI), corrected for the sample dry weight. Results are presented as Mean ± SD (n = 5).

Heterofibrins (HF)	$[M-H]^-$	*Calanus finmarchicus*
HF-A2	345.2071	6.40 ± 1.33
HF-A3	417.2283	4.50 ± 1.54
HF-B1	287.2017	0.82 ± 0.15
HF-B2	359.2228	495 ± 105
HF-B3	431.2439	1.10 ± 0.58
Chlorophylls	**$[M+H]^+$**	***Isochrysis galbana***
Chlorophyll a	911.5532	0.40 ± 0.12
Pheophytin a	872.5765	12.6 ± 3.7

3.13. Microalgal Chlorophylls

Microalgae are a large photosynthetic biomass that represents a significant feedstock for many aquatic inhabitants [90]. In our analysis of *I. galabana*, we demonstrated that pheophytin a [97] is the major chlorophyll in this microalgae (Table 9), which are known to utilize pheophytin a and chlorophyll a for photosynthesis [97]. In contrast, chlorophylls were not detected in copepods, which do not utilize photosynthesis as an energy source. These data also suggest that any dietary chlorophylls are presumably rapidly digested after ingestion.

3.14. Bacillariolides

Bacillariolides are heterocyclic (hydroxycyclopentafuranone) oxylipins with a 13 carbon isopentyl sidechain that have only previously been reported in diatoms [98]. This is the first report of these oxylipins in copepods, with none being detected in algae (*Isochrysis galabana*). Bacillariolide II and its methoxymethyl derivative were monitored in all three copepod species (Table 10). Presumably, the 13-carbon isoprenoid chain inserts into membranes and the terminal cyclopentafuranone ring contributes to membrane charge.

Table 10. Relative levels of bacillariolides in *copepods*. Levels are presented as a ratio of the peak intensity of each lipid to the peak intensity of the internal standard (2 nanomoles $[^2H_5]$DHA) corrected for the sample dry weight. Results are presented as Mean ± SD (n = 5). -, not detected.

Bacillariolides	$[M-H]^-$	*Isochrysis galbana*	*Acartia tonsa*	*Calanus finmarchicus*	*Labidocerca aestiva*
Bacillariolide II	315.1966	-	10.7 ± 4.8	27.6 ± 6.2	10.7 ± 3.1
Methoxymethyl-Bacillariolide II	359.2228	-	70.4 ± 38.4	494.8 ± 105.1	120.8 ± 60.2

Product ions of the $[M-H]^-$ molecular ions were fragments of the lipid sidechain (Supplementary File). These included $[C_{10}H_{16}]^-$ = $[135.1179]^-$ and $[C_{12}H_{18}]^-$ = $[161.1336]^-$, all monitored with less than 1 ppm mass error. The function(s) of these novel marine oxylipins remains to be determined.

4. Summary

Our lipidomics analytical platform, with the desired characteristics of high precision and accuracy, will allow for quantitation of lipid adaptations to the stressors of climate change. In fact, lipidomics has already been shown to quantify the effects of herbicide exposure, as an experimental stressor, on microalgae [99] and lipid changes in heat-stressed mussels [100]. The lipidomics platform we have established provides the technology required to monitor copepod species-specific lipid adaptations to climate change as well as shifts in their food sources [101]. This is essential for the quantification of long-term multigenerational responses of this oceanic sentinel species to altering climate conditions. As presented in Figure 1, the lipidome of each copepod species is very unique, and our data clearly indicate that detailed lipidomics analyses will be required to evaluate the effects of climate stressors on the lipidome of each copepod species.

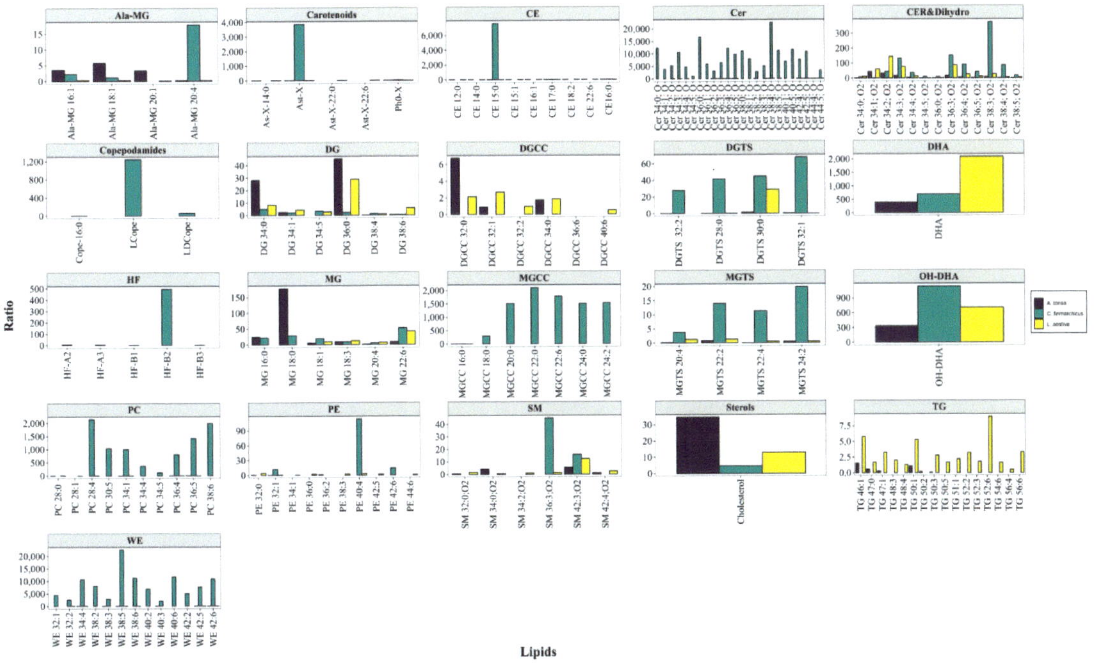

Figure 1. Relative levels (R) of lipids in copepods. Levels are presented (mean values) as a ratio of the peak intensity of each lipid to the peak intensity of the internal standard (2 nanomoles $[^2H_5]$DHA) corrected for the sample dry weight. (n = 5). Ala, alanine; ASt-X, astaxanthin; CE, cholesterol ester; Cer, ceramide; Cope, copepodamide; DG, diacylglycerol; DGCC, diacylglyceryl carboxyhydroxymethylcholine; DGTS, diacylglyceryl trimethylhomoserine; DHA, FA 22:6; HF, heterofibrin; L, lyso; MG, monoacylglycerol; OH-DHA, hydroxy FA 22:6; PC, phosphatidylcholine; PE, phosphatidylethanolamine; SM, sphingomyelin; TG, triacylglycerol; WE, wax ester.

5. Conclusions

While lipid biochemistry and nomenclature are extremely complex, it is not essential for all readers interested in climate change to understand all of the various lipid classes presented in this study. The clear message from this research is that we can monitor key copepod lipid families with high accuracy and, therefore, potentially monitor lipid families that respond to environmental perturbations evoked by climate change. Ultimately, it is the goal of this research to identify sensitive lipid biomarkers of climate change.

Study Limitations

Biological: Copepods have complex life cycles and their lipidomes will vary with those cycles and the seasons. We have only taken a snapshot of one point in time with this probe study. However, these analyses have established the major lipid families to monitor in our longitudinal studies. Larger sample sets from different seasons of the year will be crucial to build a lipid database for a long-term climate change study.

Technical: Our HR-MS analytical platform (<2 ppm mass error), that utilizes both PESI and NESI, significantly reduces the risk of lipid misassignments. However, there are a number of lipid structural isobars that require MS^2 and/or TLC evaluations for full structural validation. Over the last 10 years, our Metabolomics Unit has built a database of a number of these specific issues and optimal technical solutions. Specific issues include our inability to distinguish between: (i) a cyclopropyl group and a double bond in a fatty acid chain, and (ii) an added methyl group vs. addition of a CH_2 in a fatty acid chain. Again, MS^2 and/or TLC evaluations will be our first strategies with lipids of high interest. NMR may be considered if required, but this involves significant scale-up and purification methods due to the low sensitivity of NMR.

Supplementary Materials: The following supporting information can be downloaded at: https://www.mdpi.com/article/10.3390/life13122335/s1, Supplementary Figure S1. The MS^2 product spectra for novel lipid observations.

Author Contributions: P.L.W. and S.C.K. were responsible for study conceptualization and conduct; P.L.W., S.C.K. and M.D.W. for methodology, software, validation, data curation and formal analysis; P.L.W. and S.C.K. for resources; P.L.W. wrote the original draft; all authors were involved in review and editing. All authors have read and agreed to the published version of the manuscript.

Funding: This study was funded by Lincoln Memorial University.

Data Availability Statement: All data is included in the manuscript and Supplementary Materials.

Conflicts of Interest: The authors declare no conflict of interest.

References

1. Field, C.B.; Behrenfeld, M.J.; Randerson, J.T.; Falkowski, P. Primary production of the biosphere: Integrating terrestrial and oceanic components. *Science* **1998**, *281*, 237–240. [CrossRef] [PubMed]
2. Turner, J.T. The importance of small planktonic copepods and their roles in pelagic marine food webs. *Zool. Stud.* **2004**, *43*, 255–266.
3. Marmorek, D.R.; Korman, J. The use of zooplankton in a biomonitoring program to detect lake acidification and recovery. *Water Air Soil* **1993**, *69*, 223. [CrossRef]
4. Mayor, D.J.; Gentleman, W.C.; Anderson, T.R. Ocean carbon sequestration: Particle fragmentation by copepods as a significant unrecognised factor?: Explicitly representing the role of copepods in biogeochemical models may fundamentally improve understanding of future ocean carbon storage. *Bioessays* **2020**, *42*, e2000149. [CrossRef] [PubMed]
5. Iversen, M.H. Carbon Export in the Ocean: A Biologist's Perspective. *Ann. Rev. Mar. Sci.* **2023**, *15*, 357–381. [CrossRef] [PubMed]
6. Wang, M.; Jeong, C.B.; Lee, Y.H.; Lee, J.S. Effects of ocean acidification on copepods. *Aquat. Toxicol.* **2018**, *196*, 17–24. [CrossRef] [PubMed]
7. Doan, N.X.; Vu, M.T.T.; Pham, H.Q.; Wisz, M.S.; Nielsen, T.G.; Dinh, K.V. Extreme temperature impairs growth and productivity in a common tropical marine copepod. *Sci. Rep.* **2019**, *9*, 4550. [CrossRef] [PubMed]
8. Engström-Öst, J.; Glippa, O.; Feely, R.A.; Kanerva, M.; Keister, J.E.; Alin, S.R.; Carter, B.R.; McLaskey, A.K.; Vuori, K.A.; Bednaršek, N. Eco-physiological responses of copepods and pteropods to ocean warming and acidification. *Sci. Rep.* **2019**, *9*, 4748. [CrossRef]
9. Benedetti, F.; Vogt, M.; Elizondo, U.H.; Righetti, D.; Zimmermann, N.E.; Gruber, N. Major restructuring of marine plankton assemblages under global warming. *Nat. Commun.* **2021**, *12*, 5226. [CrossRef]
10. McGinty, N.; Barton, A.D.; Record, N.R.; Finkel, Z.V.; Johns, D.G.; Stock, C.A.; Irwin, A.J. Anthropogenic climate change impacts on copepod trait biogeography. *Glob. Change Biol.* **2021**, *27*, 1431–1442. [CrossRef]
11. Montero, J.T.; Lima, M.; Estay, S.A.; Rezende, E.L. Spatial and temporal shift in the factors affecting the population dynamics of Calanus copepods in the North Sea. *Glob. Change Biol.* **2021**, *27*, 576–586. [CrossRef] [PubMed]
12. Wood, P.L. Non-targeted lipidomics utilizing constant infusion high resolution ESI mass spectrometry. In *Lipidomics*; Wood, P.L., Ed.; Humana Press: New York, NY, USA, 2017; Volume 125, pp. 13–19. ISBN 978-1-0716-0863-0; 978-1-0716-0864-0.
13. Nuzzo, G.; Gallo, C.; d'Ippolito, G.; Cutignano, A.; Sardo, A.; Fontana, A. Composition and quantitation of microalgal lipids by ERETIC ^{1}H NMR method. *Mar. Drugs* **2013**, *11*, 3742–3753. [CrossRef] [PubMed]
14. Stonik, V.; Stonik, I. Low-Molecular-Weight Metabolites from Diatoms: Structures, Biological Roles and Biosynthesis. *Mar. Drugs* **2015**, *13*, 3672–3709. [CrossRef] [PubMed]
15. Da Costa, E.; Silva, J.; Mendonça, S.H.; Abreu, M.H.; Domingues, M.R. Lipidomic approaches towards deciphering glycolipids from microalgae as a reservoir of bioactive lipids. *Mar. Drugs* **2016**, *14*, 101. [CrossRef] [PubMed]
16. Hunter, J.E.; Brandsma, J.; Dymond, M.K.; Koster, G.; Moore, C.M.; Postle, A.D.; Mills, R.A.; Attard, G.S. Lipidomics of Thalassiosira pseudonana under phosphorus stress reveal underlying phospholipid substitution dynamics and novel diglycosylceramide substitutes. *Appl. Environ. Microbiol.* **2018**, *84*, e02034-17. [CrossRef] [PubMed]

17. Vigor, C.; Oger, C.; Reversat, G.; Rocher, A.; Zhou, B.; Linares-Maurizi, A.; Guy, A.; Bultel-Poncé, V.; Galano, J.M.; Vercauteren, J.; et al. Isoprostanoid profiling of marine microalgae. *Biomolecules* **2020**, *10*, 1073. [CrossRef] [PubMed]
18. Řezanka, T.; Řezanka, M.; Mezricky, D.; Vítová, M. Lipidomic analysis of diatoms cultivated with silica nanoparticles. *Phytochemistry* **2020**, *177*, 112452. [CrossRef] [PubMed]
19. Yang, Y.; Du, L.; Hosokawa, M.; Miyashita, K. Total lipids content, lipid class and fatty acid composition of ten species of microalgae. *J. Oleo Sci.* **2020**, *69*, 1181–1189. [CrossRef]
20. Oishi, Y.; Otaki, R.; Iijima, Y.; Kumagai, E.; Aoki, M.; Tsuzuki, M.; Fujiwara, S.; Sato, N. Diacylglyceryl-*N*,*N*,*N*-trimethylhomoserine-dependent lipid remodeling in a green alga, *Chlorella kessleri*. *Commun. Biol.* **2022**, *5*, 19. [CrossRef]
21. Pinger, C.; Copeman, L.; Stowell, M.; Cormack, B.; Fugate, C.; Rogers, M. Rapid measurement of total lipids in zooplankton using the sulfo-phospho-vanillin reaction. *Anal. Methods* **2022**, *14*, 2665–2672. [CrossRef]
22. Rey, F.; Melo, T.; Lopes, D.; Couto, D.; Marques, F.; Domingues, M.R. Applications of lipidomics in marine organisms: Progress, challenges and future perspectives. *Mol. Omics* **2022**, *18*, 357–386. [CrossRef] [PubMed]
23. Wood, P.L. Lipidomics of Alzheimer's disease: Current status. *Alzheimer's Res. Ther.* **2012**, *4*, 5. [CrossRef] [PubMed]
24. Liang, J.; Wen, F.; Liu, J. Transcriptomic and lipidomic analysis of an EPA-containing *Nannochloropsis* sp. PJ12 in response to nitrogen deprivation. *Sci. Rep.* **2019**, *9*, 4540. [CrossRef] [PubMed]
25. McLaskey, A.K.; Keister, J.E.; Schoo, K.L.; Olson, M.B.; Love, B.A. Direct and indirect effects of elevated CO_2 are revealed through shifts in phytoplankton, copepod development, and fatty acid accumulation. *PLoS ONE* **2019**, *14*, e0213931. [CrossRef] [PubMed]
26. Graeve, M.; Boissonnot, L.; Niehoff, B.; Hagen, W.; Kattner, G. Assimilation and turnover rates of lipid compounds in dominant Antarctic copepods fed with ^{13}C-enriched diatoms. *Philos. Trans. R. Soc. B* **2020**, *375*, 20190647. [CrossRef]
27. Imbs, A.B.; Ermolenko, E.V.; Grigorchuk, V.P.; Sikorskaya, T.V.; Velansky, P.V. Current progress in lipidomics of marine invertebrates. *Mar. Drugs* **2021**, *19*, 660. [CrossRef] [PubMed]
28. Rossoll, D.; Bermúdez, R.; Hauss, H.; Schulz, K.G.; Riebesell, U.; Sommer, U.; Winder, M. Ocean acidification-induced food quality deterioration constrains trophic transfer. *PLoS ONE* **2012**, *7*, e34737. [CrossRef] [PubMed]
29. Jin, P.; Liang, Z.; Lu, H.; Pan, J.; Li, P.; Huang, Q.; Guo, Y.; Zhong, J.; Li, F.; Wan, J.; et al. Lipid Remodeling Reveals the Adaptations of a Marine Diatom to Ocean Acidification. *Front. Microbiol.* **2021**, *12*, 748445. [CrossRef]
30. Fu, T.; Knittelfelder, O.; Geffard, O.; Clément, Y.; Testet, E.; Elie, N.; Touboul, D.; Abbaci, K.; Shevchenko, A.; Lemoine, J.; et al. Shotgun lipidomics and mass spectrometry imaging unveil diversity and dynamics in *Gammarus fossarum* lipid composition. *iScience* **2021**, *24*, 102115. [CrossRef]
31. Hiltunen, M.; Strandberg, U.; Keinänen, M.; Taipale, S.; Kankaala, P. Distinctive lipid composition of the copepod *Limnocalanus macrurus* with a high abundance of polyunsaturated fatty acids. *Lipids* **2014**, *49*, 919–932. [CrossRef]
32. Yamada, Y.; Nishida, S.; Graeve, M.; Kattner, G. Lipid and fatty acid/alcohol compositions of the subarctic copepods *Neocalanus cristatus* and *Eucalanus bungii* from various depths in the Oyashio region, western North Pacific. *Comp. Biochem. Physiol. Part B Biochem. Mol. Biol.* **2016**, *198*, 57–65. [CrossRef] [PubMed]
33. Kabeya, N.; Ogino, M.; Ushio, H.; Haga, Y.; Satoh, S.; Navarro, J.C.; Monroig, Ó. A complete enzymatic capacity for biosynthesis of docosahexaenoic acid (DHA, 22:6n-3) exists in the marine Harpacticoida copepod *Tigriopus californicus*. *Open Biol.* **2021**, *11*, 200402. [CrossRef] [PubMed]
34. Lee, R.F.; Nevenzel, J.C.; Paffenhöfer, G.A. Wax esters in marine copepods. *Science* **1970**, *167*, 1510–1511. [CrossRef] [PubMed]
35. Lee, R.F.; Paffenhöfer, G.A.; Nevenzel, J.C.; Benson, A.A. The metabolism of wax esters and other lipids by the marine copepod, Calanus helgolandicus. *J. Lipid Res.* **1970**, *11*, 237–240. [CrossRef] [PubMed]
36. Lee, R.F.; Barnes, A.T. Lipids in the mesopelagic copepod, *Gaussia princeps*. Wax ester utilization during starvation. *Comp. Biochem. Physiol. B* **1975**, *52*, 265–268. [CrossRef] [PubMed]
37. Caramujo, M.J.; de Carvalho, C.C.; Silva, S.J.; Carman, K.R. Dietary carotenoids regulate astaxanthin content of copepods and modulate their susceptibility to UV light and copper toxicity. *Mar. Drugs* **2012**, *10*, 998–1018. [CrossRef] [PubMed]
38. Mojib, N.; Amad, M.; Thimma, M.; Aldanondo, N.; Kumaran, M.; Irigoien, X. Carotenoid metabolic profiling and transcriptome-genome mining reveal functional equivalence among blue-pigmented copepods and appendicularia. *Mol. Ecol.* **2014**, *23*, 2740–2756. [CrossRef] [PubMed]
39. Powers, M.J.; Martz, L.D.; Burton, R.S.; Hill, G.E.; Weaver, R.J. Evidence for hybrid breakdown in production of red carotenoids in the marine invertebrate *Tigriopus californicus*. *PLoS ONE* **2021**, *16*, e0259371. [CrossRef]
40. Selander, E.; Kubanek, J.; Hamberg, M.; Andersson, M.X.; Cervin, G.; Pavia, H. Predator lipids induce paralytic shellfish toxins in bloom-forming algae. *Proc. Natl. Acad. Sci. USA* **2015**, *112*, 6395–6400. [CrossRef]
41. Powers, M.J.; Baty, J.A.; Dinga, A.M.; Mao, J.H.; Hill, G.E. Chemical manipulation of mitochondrial function affects metabolism of red carotenoids in a marine copepod (*Tigriopus californicus*). *J. Exp. Biol.* **2022**, *225*, jeb244230. [CrossRef]
42. Hansen, B.H.; Sørensen, L.; Størseth, T.R.; Altin, D.; Gonzalez, S.V.; Skancke, J.; Rønsberg, M.U.; Nordtug, T. The use of PAH, metabolite and lipid profiling to assess exposure and effects of produced water discharges on pelagic copepods. *Sci. Total Environ.* **2020**, *714*, 136674. [CrossRef] [PubMed]
43. Riekhof, W.R.; Naik, S.; Bertrand, H.; Benning, C.; Voelker, D.R. Phosphate starvation in fungi induces the replacement of phosphatidylcholine with the phosphorus-free betaine lipid diacylglyceryl-*N*,*N*,*N*-trimethylhomoserine. *Eukaryot. Cell* **2014**, *13*, 749–757. [CrossRef] [PubMed]

44. Geske, T.; Vom Dorp, K.; Dörmann, P.; Hölzl, G. Accumulation of glycolipids and other non-phosphorous lipids in *Agrobacterium tumefaciens* grown under phosphate deprivation. *Glycobiology* **2013**, *23*, 69–80. [CrossRef] [PubMed]
45. Murakami, H.; Nobusawa, T.; Hori, K.; Shimojima, M.; Ohta, H. Betaine Lipid Is Crucial for Adapting to Low Temperature and Phosphate Deficiency in *Nannochloropsis*. *Plant Physiol.* **2018**, *177*, 181–193. [CrossRef] [PubMed]
46. Wood, P.L.; Woltjer, R.L. Electrospray ionization high resolution mass spectrometry of the chloride adducts of steroids, mono- and oligo-saccharides, xyloglucans, ceramides, gangliosides, and phenols. In *Metabolomics*; Wood, P.L., Ed.; Neuromethods; Humana Press: New York, NY, USA, 2021; Volume 159, pp. 69–76. ISBN 978-1-0716-0863-0; 978-1-0716-0864-0.
47. Wood, P.L.; Hauther, K.A.; Scarborough, J.H.; Craney, D.J.; Dudzik, B.; Cebak, J.E.; Woltjer, R.L. Human brain lipidomics: Utilities of chloride adducts in flow injection analyses (FIA). *Life* **2021**, *11*, 403. [CrossRef]
48. Liebisch, G.; Fahy, E.; Aoki, J.; Dennis, E.A.; Durand, T.; Ejsing, C.S.; Fedorova, M.; Feussner, I.; Griffiths, W.J.; Köfeler, H.; et al. Update om LIPID MAPS classification, nomenclature, and shorthand notation for MS-derived lipid structures. *J. Lipid Res.* **2020**, *61*, 1539–1555. [CrossRef]
49. Fernandes, A.S.; Petry, F.C.; Mercadante, A.Z.; Jacob-Lopes, E.; Zepka, L.Q. HPLC-PDA-MS/MS as a strategy to characterize and quantify natural pigments from microalgae. *Curr. Res. Food Sci.* **2020**, *3*, 100–112. [CrossRef]
50. Andersson, M.; Van Nieuwerburgh, L.; Snoeijs, P. Pigment transfer from phytoplankton to zooplankton with emphasis on astaxanthin production in the Baltic Sea food web. *Mar. Ecol. Prog. Ser.* **2003**, *254*, 213–224. [CrossRef]
51. Hairston, N.C., Jr. Photoprotection by carotenoid pigments in the copepod *Diaptomus nevadensis*. *Proc. Natl. Acad. Sci. USA* **1976**, *73*, 971–974. [CrossRef]
52. Schneider, T.; Herzig, A.; Koinig, K.A.; Sommaruga, R. Copepods in turbid shallow soda lakes accumulate unexpected high levels of carotenoids. *PLoS ONE* **2012**, *7*, e43063. [CrossRef]
53. Takaichi, S.; Matsui, K.; Nakamura, M.; Muramatsu, M.; Hanada, S. Fatty acids of astaxanthin esters in krill determined by mild mass spectrometry. *Comp. Biochem. Physiol. B Biochem. Mol. Biol.* **2003**, *136*, 317–322. [CrossRef] [PubMed]
54. Grynbaum, M.D.; Hentschel, P.; Putzbach, K.; Rehbein, J.; Krucker, M.; Nicholson, G.; Albert, K. Unambiguous detection of astaxanthin and astaxanthin fatty acid esters in krill (*Euphausia superba Dana*). *J. Sep. Sci.* **2005**, *28*, 1685–1693. [CrossRef] [PubMed]
55. Zoccali, M.; Giuffrida, D.; Salafia, F.; Socaciu, C.; Skjånes, K.; Dugo, P.; Mondello, L. First apocarotenoids profiling of four microalgae strains. *Antioxidants* **2019**, *8*, 209. [CrossRef] [PubMed]
56. Selander, E.; Berglund, E.C.; Engström, P.; Berggren, F.; Eklund, J.; Harðardóttir, S.; Lundholm, N.; Grebner, W.; Andersson, M.X. Copepods drive large-scale trait-mediated effects in marine plankton. *Sci. Adv.* **2019**, *5*, eaat5096. [CrossRef] [PubMed]
57. Hansen, B.H.; Nordtug, T.; Altin, D.; Booth, A.; Hessen, K.M.; Olsen, A.J. Gene expression of GST and CYP330A1 in lipid-rich and lipid-poor female *Calanus finmarchicus* (Copepoda: Crustacea) exposed to dispersed oil. *J. Toxicol. Environ. Health A* **2009**, *72*, 131–139. [CrossRef] [PubMed]
58. Grebner, W.; Berglund, E.C.; Berggren, F.; Eklund, J.; Harðadóttir, S.; Andersson, M.X.; Selander, E. Induction of defensive traits in marine plankton—New copepodamide structures. *Limnol. Oceanogr.* **2019**, *61*, 820–831. [CrossRef]
59. Patton, S.; Leen, R.F.; Benson, A.A. The presence of unusually high levels of lysophosphatidylethanolamine in a wax ester-synthesizing copepod (*Calanus plumchrus*). *Biochim. Biophys. Acta* **1972**, *270*, 479–488. [CrossRef]
60. Holtz, R.B.; Marquez, E.D.; Benson, A.A. Wax ester biosynthesis by isolated membrane fractions from calanoid copepods. *Comp. Biochem. Physiol. B* **1973**, *45*, 585–591. [CrossRef]
61. Thor, P.; Vermandele, F.; Bailey, A.; Guscelli, E.; Loubet-Sartrou, L.; Dupont, S.; Calosi, P. Ocean acidification causes fundamental changes in the cellular metabolism of the Arctic copepod Calanus glacialis as detected by metabolomic analysis. *Sci. Rep.* **2022**, *12*, 22223. [CrossRef]
62. Benson, A.A.; Lee, R.F. Wax esters: Major marine metabolic energy sources. *Biochem. J.* **1972**, *128*, 10P. [CrossRef]
63. Tomiyama, T.; Kurihara, K.; Ogawa, T.; Maruta, T.; Ogawa, T.; Ohta, D.; Sawa, Y.; Ishikawa, T. Wax ester synthase/diacylglycerol acyltransferase isoenzymes play a pivotal role in wax ester biosynthesis in *Euglena gracilis*. *Sci. Rep.* **2017**, *7*, 13504. [CrossRef] [PubMed]
64. Kim, H.S.; Lee, B.Y.; Han, J.; Lee, Y.H.; Min, G.S.; Kim, S.; Lee, J.S. De novo assembly and annotation of the Antarctic copepod (*Tigriopus kingsejongensis*) transcriptome. *Mar. Genom.* **2016**, *28*, 37–39. [CrossRef] [PubMed]
65. Höper, A.C.; Salma, W.; Sollie, S.J.; Hafstad, A.D.; Lund, J.; Khalid, A.M.; Raa, J.; Aasum, E.; Larsen, T.S. Wax esters from the marine copepod *Calanus finmarchicus* reduce diet-induced obesity and obesity-related metabolic disorders in mice. *J. Nutr.* **2014**, *144*, 164–169. [CrossRef] [PubMed]
66. Atila, M.; Luo, Y. Profiling and tandem mass spectrometry analysis of aminoacylated phospholipids in *Bacillus subtilis*. *F1000Res.* **2016**, *5*, 121. [CrossRef] [PubMed]
67. Sohlenkamp, C.; Geiger, O. Bacterial membrane lipids: Diversity in structures and pathways. *FEMS Microbiol. Rev.* **2016**, *40*, 133–159. [CrossRef] [PubMed]
68. Slavetinsky, C.; Kuhn, S.; Peschel, A. Bacterial aminoacyl phospholipids—Biosynthesis and role in basic cellular processes and pathogenicity. *Biochim. Biophys. Acta Mol. Cell Biol. Lipids* **2017**, *1862*, 1310–1318. [CrossRef] [PubMed]
69. Cañavate, J.P.; Armada, I.; Ríos, J.L.; Hachero-Cruzado, I. Exploring occurrence and molecular diversity of betaine lipids across taxonomy of marine microalgae. *Phytochemistry* **2016**, *124*, 68–78. [CrossRef]
70. Conde, T.A.; Couto, D.; Melo, T.; Costa, M.; Silva, J.; Domingues, M.R.; Domingues, P. Polar lipidomic profile shows *Chlorococcum amblystomatis* as a promising source of value-added lipids. *Sci. Rep.* **2021**, *11*, 4355. [CrossRef]

71. Rickhof, W.R.; Sears, B.B.; Benning, C. Annotation of genes involved in glycerolipid biosynthesis in *Chlamydomonas reinhardtii*: Discovery of the betaine lipid synthase BTA1$_{Cr}$. *Eukaryot. Cell* **2005**, *4*, 242–252. [CrossRef]
72. Eichenberger, W.; Gribi, C. Lipids of *Pavlova lutheri*: Cellular site and metabolic role of DGCC. *Phytochemistry* **1997**, *45*, 1561–1567. [CrossRef]
73. Domart, M.C.; Hobday, T.M.; Peddie, C.J.; Chung, G.H.; Wang, A.; Yeh, K.; Jethwa, N.; Zhang, Q.; Wakelam, M.J.; Woscholski, R.; et al. Acute manipulation of diacylglycerol reveals roles in nuclear envelope assemb ly & endoplasmic reticulum morphology. *PLoS ONE* **2012**, *7*, e51150.
74. Sarri, E.; Sicart, A.; Lázaro-Diéguez, F.; Egea, G. Phospholipid synthesis participates in the regulation of diacylglycerol required for membrane trafficking at the Golgi complex. *J. Biol. Chem.* **2011**, *286*, 28632–28643. [CrossRef] [PubMed]
75. Carrasco, S.; Mérida, I. Diacylglycerol, when simplicity becomes complex. *Trends Biochem. Sci.* **2007**, *32*, 27–36. [CrossRef] [PubMed]
76. Popko, J.; Herrfurth, C.; Feussner, K.; Ischebeck, T.; Iven, T.; Haslam, R.; Hamilton, M.; Sayanova, O.; Napier, J.; Khozin-Goldberg, I.; et al. Metabolome analysis reveals betaine lipids as major source for triglyceride formation, and the accumulation of sedoheptulose during nitrogen-starvation of *Phaeodactylum tricornutum*. *PLoS ONE* **2016**, *11*, e0164673. [CrossRef] [PubMed]
77. Lauritano, C.; Romano, G.; Roncalli, V.; Amoresano, A.; Fontanarosa, C.; Bastianini, M.; Braga, F.; Carotenuto, Y.; Ianora, A. New oxylipins produced at the end of a diatom bloom and their effects on copepod reproductive success and gene expression levels. *Harmful Algae* **2016**, *55*, 221–229. [CrossRef] [PubMed]
78. Meyer, N.; Rettner, J.; Werner, M.; Werz, O.; Pohnert, G. Algal oxylipins mediate the resistance of diatoms against algicidal bacteria. *Mar. Drugs* **2018**, *16*, 486. [CrossRef] [PubMed]
79. Jagusch, H.; Baumeister, T.U.H.; Pohnert, G. Mammalian-like inflammatory and pro-resolving oxylipins in marine algae. *Chembiochem* **2020**, *21*, 2419–2424. [CrossRef] [PubMed]
80. Zhou, L.; Wu, X.; Yang, F.; Zhang, M.; Huang, R.; Liu, J. Characterization of molecular species and anti-inflammatory activity of purified phospholipids from antarctic krill oil. *Mar. Drugs* **2021**, *19*, 124. [CrossRef]
81. Nelson, M.M.; Phleger, C.F.; Mooney, B.D.; Nichols, P.D. Lipids of gelatinous Antarctic zooplankton: Cnidaria and Ctenophora. *Lipids* **2000**, *35*, 551–559. [CrossRef]
82. Hassett, R.P.; Crockett, E.L. Habitat temperature is an important determinant of cholesterol contents in copepods. *J. Exp. Biol.* **2009**, *212*, 71–77. [CrossRef]
83. Graeve, M.; Janssen, D. Improved separation and quantification of neutral and polar lipid classes by HPLC-ELSD using a monolithic silica phase: Application to exceptional marine lipids. *J. Chromatogr. B* **2009**, *877*, 1815–1819. [CrossRef] [PubMed]
84. Salvador-Castell, M.; Tourte, M.; Oger, P.M. In search for the membrane regulators of Archaea. *Int. J. Mol. Sci.* **2019**, *20*, 4434. [CrossRef] [PubMed]
85. Winther, B.; Hoem, N.; Berge, K.; Reubsaet, L. Elucidation of phosphatidylcholine composition in krill oil extracted from *Euphausia superba*. *Lipids* **2011**, *46*, 25–36. [CrossRef]
86. Jiménez-Rojo, N.; Sot, J.; Busto, J.V.; Shaw, W.A.; Duan, J.; Merrill, A.H., Jr.; Alonso, A.; Goñi, F.M. Biophysical properties of novel 1-deoxy-(dihydro)ceramides occurring in mammalian cells. *Biophys. J.* **2014**, *107*, 2850–2859. [CrossRef] [PubMed]
87. Lone, M.A.; Santos, T.; Alecu, I.; Silva, L.C.; Hornemann, T. 1-Deoxysphingolipids. *Biochim. Biophys. Acta Mol. Cell Biol. Lipids* **2019**, *1864*, 512–521. [CrossRef] [PubMed]
88. Jiang, W.; Ogretmen, B. Autophagy paradox and ceramide. *Biochim. Biophys. Acta* **2014**, *1841*, 783–792. [CrossRef] [PubMed]
89. Lauterbach, M.A.; Saavedra, V.; Mangan, M.S.J.; Penno, A.; Thiele, C.; Latz, E.; Kuerschner, L. 1-Deoxysphingolipids cause autophagosome and lysosome accumulation and trigger NLRP3 inflammasome activation. *Autophagy* **2021**, *17*, 1947–1961. [CrossRef]
90. Grobbelaar, J.U. Microalgal biomass production: Challenges and realities. *Photosynth. Res.* **2010**, *106*, 135–144. [CrossRef]
91. Zhou, L.; Zhao, M.; Ennahar, S.; Bindler, F.; Marchioni, E. Liquid chromatography-tandem mass spectrometry for the determination of sphingomyelin species from calf brain, ox liver, egg yolk, and krill oil. *J. Agric. Food Chem.* **2012**, *60*, 293–298. [CrossRef]
92. Wilson, C.H.; Hartline, D.K. Novel organization and development of copepod myelin. I. ontogeny. *J. Comp. Neurol.* **2011**, *519*, 3259–3280. [CrossRef]
93. Wilson, C.H.; Hartline, D.K. Novel organization and development of copepod myelin. II. nonglial origin. *J. Comp. Neurol.* **2011**, *519*, 3281–3305. [CrossRef] [PubMed]
94. Panevska, A.; Skočaj, M.; Križaj, I.; Maček, P.; Sepčić, K. Ceramide phosphoethanolamine, an enigmatic cellular membrane sphingolipid. *Biochim. Biophys. Acta Biomembr.* **2019**, *1861*, 1284–1292. [CrossRef] [PubMed]
95. Olzmann, J.A.; Carvalho, P. Dynamics and functions of lipid droplets. *Nat. Rev. Mol. Cell Biol.* **2019**, *20*, 137–155. [CrossRef] [PubMed]
96. Salim, A.A.; Rae, J.; Fontaine, F.; Conte, M.M.; Khalil, Z.; Martin, S.; Parton, R.G.; Capon, R.J. Heterofibrins: Inhibitors of lipid droplet formation from a deep-water southern Australian marine sponge, *Spongia (Heterofibria)* sp. *Org. Biomol. Chem.* **2010**, *8*, 3188–3194. [CrossRef] [PubMed]
97. Fernandes, A.S.; Nascimento, T.C.; Pinheiro, P.N.; de Rosso, V.V.; de Menezes, C.R.; Jacob-Lopes, E.; Zepka, L.Q. Insights on the intestinal absorption of chlorophyll series from microalgae. *Food Res. Int.* **2021**, *140*, 110031. [CrossRef] [PubMed]
98. Seo, S.Y.; Jung, J.K.; Paek, S.M.; Lee, Y.S.; Kim, S.H.; Lee, K.O.; Suh, Y.G. Asymmetric total synthesis of bacillariolide III, a marine oxylipin. *Org. Lett.* **2004**, *6*, 429–432. [CrossRef] [PubMed]

99. Shanta, P.V.; Li, B.; Stuart, D.D.; Cheng, Q. Lipidomic profiling of algae with microarray MALDI-MS toward ecotoxicological monitoring of herbicide exposure. *Environ. Sci. Technol.* **2021**, *55*, 10558–10568. [CrossRef] [PubMed]
100. Facchini, L.; Losito, I.; Cataldi, T.R.; Palmisano, F. Ceramide lipids in alive and thermally stressed mussels: An investigation by hydrophilic interaction liquid chromatography-electrospray ionization Fourier transform mass spectrometry. *J. Mass Spectrom.* **2016**, *51*, 768–781. [CrossRef]
101. Strack, T.; Jonkers, L.; CRillo, M.; Hillebrand, H.; Kucera, M. Plankton response to global warming is characterized by non-uniform shifts in assemblage composition since the last ice age. *Nat. Ecol. Evol.* **2022**, *6*, 1871–1880. [CrossRef]

life

MDPI

Article

Depressive Disorders, Cognitive and Physical Function of Older People in Early Dementia Detection

Beata Pietrzak [1], Jolanta Kujawa [1] and Anna Lipert [2,*]

[1] Department of Medical Rehabilitation, Medical University of Lodz, 92-213 Lodz, Poland; beata.pietrzak@umed.lodz.pl (B.P.); jolanta.kujawa@umed.lodz.pl (J.K.)
[2] Department of Sports Medicine, Medical University of Lodz, 92-213 Lodz, Poland
* Correspondence: anna.lipert@umed.lodz.pl

Abstract: Background: Aging is associated with cognitive decline, leading to cognitive and physical impairments, which are risk factors for loss of independence and dementia development. Early diagnosis is beneficial for both, the patient and their family, to avoid long-term consequences. The aim of this study was to analyze the frequency of depressive disorders and their influence on cognitive and physical function of older people in early dementia detection. Methods: There were 852 patients, aged at least 60 years, from the Central Teaching Hospital. The study was conducted between September 2022 and June 2023. The qualified participants were examined using four tools: Geriatric Depression Scale (GDS), Instrumental Activities of Daily Living (IADL), Timed Up and Go (TUG) and Schulman's Clock-Drawing Test. Results: Over one-third had depressive disorders. A relationship with $p < 0.05$ was observed between GDS and IADL: r = −0.61. A relationship with $p > 0.05$ was observed between GDS and TUG: r = −024. A relationship with $p < 0.05$ was observed between GDS and CDT: r = 0.74. Conclusions: The first signs of depressive disorders in older people may be considered an indication for further diagnosis of dementia.

Keywords: depressive disorders; cognitive function; physical function; dementia; older people

Citation: Pietrzak, B.; Kujawa, J.; Lipert, A. Depressive Disorders, Cognitive and Physical Function of Older People in Early Dementia Detection. *Life* **2023**, *13*, 2010. https://doi.org/10.3390/life13102010

Academic Editor: Wenceslao Peñate

Received: 4 September 2023
Revised: 29 September 2023
Accepted: 1 October 2023
Published: 4 October 2023

1. Introduction

Aging of societies is a global phenomenon, especially in highly developed countries [1]. Aging is associated with the deterioration of cognitive functions, leading to their impairment and dementia, which, together with the impairment of physical functions, leads to a loss of independence [2]. The search for effective solutions to prevent the loss of independence of the elderly by detecting emerging physical, mental and social dysfunctions as soon as possible is the theme of many studies [3]. The mutual relationship between the deterioration of cognitive functions, physical functions, mental functions and independence in everyday life should be emphasized.

Many reports emphasize that a common problem is the lack of screening for cognitive decline. Meanwhile, early diagnosis of dementia allows for avoiding long-term consequences [4], such as deterioration of thinking skills leading to loss of independence and deterioration of physical functions. It is important to note that cognitive impairment affects tens of millions of people worldwide, not only patients but also their caregivers, placing a financial burden on families and healthcare systems. It is interesting to study cognitive and physical functions at the same time, as both are associated with the risk of loss of independence and a higher risk of dementia [5]. The limited success of current treatments has led to the search for early markers of dementia that could predict future progression or improve the quality of life of people already suffering from the disease [6].

The risk of cognitive impairment increases with age due to physical disability [5,7]. This risk increases if it is accompanied by a noticeable decrease in walking speed [8]. In addition, a slower gait is associated with worse results in tests of attention, executive function, and memory [9]. Identifying early physical decline in older adults is important, but individuals who experience decline can usually ignore early changes in physical functioning and therefore do not report them [10]. The lack of adequate epidemiological studies on comprehensive measurements of physical fitness in the elderly also makes it difficult to compare functional status across countries and cultures [11,12]. Physical fitness is a key indicator of the health status of older people. According to gerontological studies, physical fitness may be an important predictor of later disability, significant morbidity and mortality, or may help predict future health needs and the use of social care [6]. The research also confirms the hypothesis that the loss of physical fitness may be an additional risk factor for the clinical onset of Alzheimer's disease [7,13].

The deteriorating condition of the elderly leads to dependence, i.e., the inability to live independently and requires constant or long-term care and assistance from third parties in the performance of everyday activities [14]. For some people, it becomes necessary to use care facilities. In turn, institutionalization in older people deepens the process of loss of adaptive abilities that occurs with age, and resistance to adversity, as does the diagnosis of mental disorders. A relationship was also found between the decline in adaptive abilities of psychiatric patients staying in nursing homes, especially in psychotic and mentally disabled patients [15]. One of the confirmed actions reducing the risk of institutionalization of older people is the introduction of regular adapted physical activity (APA) that improves physical and mental functions [16]. APA should be treated as a prevention against loss of independence, especially since the vast majority of older people do not meet the minimum requirements for the level of physical activity necessary to maintain health, leading to the premature onset of frailty [17].

In the case of evaluating the functioning of the elderly, many studies have shown a significant impact of age on the daily functioning of seniors in terms of complex everyday activities, stating a decrease in functional efficiency with increasing age [18–21]. Researchers' opinions on the relationship between gender and independence in everyday activities are divided, in some of the studies women were more often disabled in these activities than men [19,22], and others did not find any significant differences between the sexes [18,23]. In terms of instrumental activities of daily living (IADL), financial capacity is of great importance for older people. It covers a variety of activities and specific skills, including executive skills (such as coin/currency arithmetic, paying bills, etc.) and decision-making and judgment skills. It is clearly related to general cognitive and neuropsychological efficiency [24].

The coexistence of depressive symptoms reduces the financial capacity of both older adult men and women with mild Alzheimer's disease [25], vascular dementia [26], as well as older adults with depression without a diagnosis of neurocognitive disorders [27]. Cognitive dysfunction combined with depressive disorders also significantly impairs the financial capacity of patients [28]. Financial deficits in patients with mixed dementia and coexisting depression require a thorough neuropsychological assessment to prevent financial exploitation [29].

The relationship between failure in daily activities and the occurrence of depressive disorders has been confirmed in numerous studies. People with disabilities in basic and complex activities and with reduced efficiency of cognitive functions, more dependent on others and with greater deficits in self-care were more likely to be depressed. Research results confirm that older people with greater functional impairment were more likely to experience depressive symptoms, similarly demonstrated by other researchers [18,30–32].

Elderly depression is a serious and growing social problem, although in practice it seems to be diagnosed too rarely. It increases mortality rates, is associated with the unfavorable course of somatic diseases, intensifies disability and leads to loss of independence, affecting the quality of life of patients and their relatives. This disorder is a challenge at the stage of diagnosis due to the masking of depressive symptoms by other psychological and health problems occurring in this period of life [33]. The diagnosis of depression in the elderly is a challenge for researchers. Ailments reported by the patient or his family may be both symptoms of dementia and depression. Dementia may also intensify the occurrence of depression and be its mask [34]. Frequent coexistence of depressive disorders and somatic diseases may delay the entire diagnostic process and accelerate the evolution of both disorders [35]. When examining the prevalence of depressive disorders in Poland in the WOBASZ study, symptoms of depression were confirmed in over 25% of the examined population on the basis of the Beck Depression Scale [36]. On the other hand, in the PolSenior study, in which the Geriatric Depression Rating Scale (GDS) was used, the incidence of age-related depressive disorders ranged from 20% to 33%, depending on the age of the respondents [31].

In another study, the prevalence of major depression in the elderly population ranged from 30 to 45%, with 10–12% of these patients admitted to an intensive care unit and 12–14% to a nursing home [37]. Some researchers confirm the thesis that age is an important factor influencing the increased risk of depression [30,31,38,39]. Others have not observed such a relationship [18,40].

Depressive symptoms may be part of the clinical picture of dementia, which has led to a debate about the direction of causality: whether depression is a prodromal symptom or an independent risk factor for dementia. Cohort studies with longer follow-ups indicate a relationship between the number of depressive episodes and the risk of dementia, which confirms the thesis that depression is a risk factor for dementia [41]. The incidence of cognitive decline in combination with depression in the elderly is high and both factors influence each other [42]. It has been documented that cognitive impairment occurs in 85–94% of cases of an acute depressive episode and 39–44% of the time after a depressive episode has subsided [43]. On the other hand, neurodegenerative dementia is accompanied by depression in 15–23% of cases [44].

Few studies report differences between men and women in the observed relationship between depression and dementia [45]. Current knowledge and conducted scientific research prove that the prognosis is equally good for the treatment of depressive syndrome, regardless of age [46]. However, a big problem is the lack of screening tests, more than 82% of the surveyed patients declared that primary care physicians omit the issue of mental well-being during the general examination. Taking into account the prevalence of depression in the elderly and the risks it entails, this situation requires rapid changes [47]. The lack of a systemic examination of the state of cognitive, physical and mental functions and the ability to function independently in order to implement prompt treatment and prevention of further impairments was described by many Polish researchers [31,33,36].

In Poland, from January 2022, the National Health Fund (NFZ) introduced a mandatory assessment of patients aged 60+, referred to hospitalization [48]. Until now, it was only applicable to patients in geriatric wards. The healthcare provider is required to document the geriatric assessment performed by a geriatric physician or geriatric consultative team. On the day of admission, the doctor performs a screening assessment using the Vulnerable Elders-13 Survey (VES-13). If the patient scores at least 3 points, he/she is qualified for the Comprehensive Geriatric Assessment (CGA). It is a widely recognized and repeatedly validated research tool used to assess the health and functioning of the elderly. It consists of questionnaires assessing the severity of depression, independence in everyday life, physical condition and cognitive abilities. The results obtained in the questionnaires, together with the assessment of the patient's health condition and the degree of nutrition, are assessed by a geriatrician, who directs patients in need to specialist geriatric care.

Currently, the Polish medical literature lacks current reports on the results of the CGA, which has been in force since January 2022, therefore the aim of the study was to analyze the incidence of depressive disorders and their impact on the cognitive and physical functioning of the elderly and independence in the field of daily activities based on the results of the CGA conducted in patients of a multi-profile hospital.

2. Materials and Methods

2.1. Participants

The study involved 852 patients aged 60 years at the Central Teaching Hospital of the Medical University of Lodz. The study was conducted between September 2022 and June 2023. The inclusion criteria for the participants were: (1) age of at least 60 years; (2) a score of at least 3 or more points in the Vulnerable Elders-13 Survey (VES-13) scale performed during admission to the hospital. The VES-13 scale is used to assess the health of the older people. It aims to identify people at risk of a sudden deterioration in health or death in the course of age-related diseases. The subjects were patients of the following clinics: cardiology, cardio surgery, electrocardiology, internal medicine, diabetology, endocrinology, surgery, nephrology, gastrology and rehabilitation. These were people admitted on a scheduled basis for diagnostic tests, surgical and conservative treatment or in an emergency due to a sudden deterioration—health status.

2.2. Desing and Procedure

The participants who were qualified for the study were examined using four different tools: the Geriatric Depression Scale (GDS), Instrumental Activities of Daily Living (IADL), The Timed Up and Go (TUG) and Schulman's Clock-Drawing Test. The Comprehensive Geriatric Assessment was carried out on the second or third day of hospitalization, which in the case of patients after surgical procedures, invasive diagnostics or in the state of persistent symptoms of health deterioration sometimes made it impossible to conduct a full examination. The results of the questionnaires together with diagnostic tests and the assessment of the patient's general health were the basis for the geriatrician to qualify the patient for permanent specialist geriatric care.

The study was approved by the Institutional Review Board, approval Ref: RNN/200/23/KE.

2.3. Instruments

The Geriatric Depression Rating Scale (GDS) according to Yesavage is used for screening depressive disorders in older people. The person can get a maximum of 15 points by answering the questions. The interpretation of the results is as follows: a score between 0–5 means no depression; a score between 6–10 means moderate depression and a score between 11–15 means severe depression. Based on the current literature, many studies reported that the mean internal consistency coefficient was 85 and the test-retest coefficient was 83. [49].

Activities of Daily Living (IADL) questionnaire is used to assess the level of physical disability in older people. The person is asked to define his/her abilities in the scope of 8 daily activities. For every activity performed independently, the patient receives 1 point. The interpretation of the results is as follows: the total score between 5–6 points means no disability, a score between 3–4 points means moderate disability and a score between 0–2 points means severe disability. Based on the study on the Polish population, the reliability coefficients of the scale measured with the internal consistency method and test-retest were $\geq$0.80 [50].

Test Time Up and Go (TUG) is used to assess the physical fitness of the elderly. The course of the test is as follows: a person gets up from the chair on time, walks a distance of 3 m, turns around, returns and sits on the chair as quickly as possible. The interpretation of the results is as follows: time of the covered distance below 10 s means a correct functional efficiency; time between 10–19 s means that the person can go outside on his/her own, does not need any walking aids, is independent in most activities of daily living, but has a low risk of falls; time over 19 s means that the person has a significantly limited functional capacity, cannot go outside on his/her own and has a high risk of falls. Here, the walking aids are recommended.

Clock Drawing Test (CDT) allows for quick detection of cognitive and executive function deterioration. The patient draws a clock face on a blank sheet of paper, marking the time "11.10". In our study the person gets a point from 1 to 5 according to the correctness of the task: 1 point means a correctly drawn clock; 2 points mean minor visual-spatial errors; 3 points mean a wrong designation 10 after 11 with a generally good visuo-spatial organization; 4 points mean the visuospatial difficulties, correct marking of 10 after 11 is impossible; 5 points mean inability to fill the clock face in a clock-like manner and 6 points refers to 'no reasonable attempt of a clock'. There are several different well-validated scales to interpret the result of CDT. However, there is no consensus about which of them is the most reliable. The methods by Shulman et al. demonstrated the best diagnostic accuracy, therefore the results were analyzed according to the Shulman protocol [51].

2.4. Statistical Analysis

Statistical analyses were performed using Statistical version 13.1 software (StatSoft, Tulsa, OK, USA). The Shapiro–Wilk test was used to check whether the data had a normal distribution. Normally distributed measurement data were expressed as mean ± standard deviation (SD) and the enumeration data were expressed in numbers and percentages. The Chi^2 test was performed to analyze the differences between and inside the groups. Multivariance ANOVA was used for comparison of measurement data between groups, and post-doc least significant difference (LSD) was used for comparison of data between and within groups. Spearman correlation test was used to analyze the relationship between GDS, IADL, TUG and CDT. Significant differences were accepted for all analyses at the level of $p < 0.05$.

3. Results

3.1. Characteristics of the Study Group

Half of the study participants, both females and males, did not have any depressive disorders and were not disabled. However, almost 30% of the female and male participants were characterized by a moderate level of depressive disorders or severe disability. Most of the participants had a correct functional efficiency, but if not, their physical fitness was characterized by a low risk of falls. One-third of the participants, both males and females, were not able to obtain satisfying results from CDT (Table 1). Based on the mean values of GDS, IADL, TUG and CDT, there were statistically significant differences between females and males in the results. Generally, females had worse results in GDS and TUG tests than males, but slightly better in CDT (Table 2).

Analysing the IADL results, it was observed that half of the study participants had problems with doing shopping, preparing meals, cleaning or washing, both males and females. In opposition to males, the study females more often were noticed to have problems with different forms of transport (Table 3).

3.2. Spearman Correlation Test

Spearman's correlation test identified a relationship between the results of IADL, TUG, CDT and GDS. A strong negative relationship statistically significant ($p < 0.05$) was observed between GDS related to depressive disorders and IADL results related to disability level. Additionally, a strong positive relationship statistically significant ($p < 0.05$) was observed between GDS and CDT related to cognitive disorders. There was observed a negative small relationship between GDS and TUG results related to physical fitness, but with no statistical significance. In contrast, there was a small, but positive relationship between IADL and TUG results A moderate negative relationship was also observed between IADL and CDT with $p < 0.05$ (Table 4). Similar correlations were observed in males and females (Tables 5 and 6).

Table 1. Characteristics of the study group.

	ALL	MALES	FEMALES
		N (%)	
GDS			
No depression	452 (52.99) *	177 (57.65) *	275 (50.37) *
Moderate depression	250 (29.31) *	84 (27.36) *	166 (30.40) *
Severe depression	53 (6.21)	15 (4.88)	38 (6.96)
Impossible to do	98 (11.49)	31 (10.10)	67 (12.27)
IADL			
Severe disability	255 (29.89) *	88 (28.66)	167 (30.59)
Moderate disability	146 (17.12)	49 (15.96)	97 (17.76)
No disability	452 (52.99) *	170 (55.37)	282 (51.65)
TUG			
Correct functional efficiency	436 (51.11) *	163 (53.09) *	273 (50.00) *
Low risk of falls	281 (32.94) *	105 (34.20) *	176 (32.23) *
High risk of fall	136 (15.94)	39 (12.70)	97 (17.76)
CDT			
Correct drawing	186 (21.80)	53 (17.26)	133 (24.36)
Minor visual-spatial errors	86 (10.08)	17 (5.54)	69 (12.64)
Wrong designation 10 after 11	128 (15.01)	38 (12.38)	90 (16.48)
Visuospatial difficulties	111 (13.01	53 (17.26)	58 (10.62)
Inability to draw a clock	258 (30.25) *	119 (38.76) *	139 (25.46) *
Impossible to do	83 (9.73)	27 (8.77)	57 (10.44)

* $p < 0.05$.

Table 2. The mean values of the results obtained by the study participants.

	ALL (N = 853)	MALES (N = 307)	FEMALES (N = 546)	t	df	p
		Mean (±SD)				
Geriatric Depression Scale (GDS)	7.02 ± 6.18	6.32 ± 6.03	7.41 ± 6.24	−2.47	853	0.014 *
Instrumental Activities of Daily Living (IADL)	4.53 ± 2.98	4.75 ± 3.01	4.41 ± 2.96	1.57	853	0.116
The Timed Up And Go (TUG)	10.36 ± 14.97	9.01 ± 10.32	11.13 ± 17.00	−1.98	853	0.048 *
Clock-Drawing Test (CDT)	5.02 ± 5.74	5.16 ± 5.34	4.94 ± 5.96	−2.17	853	0.030 *

* $p < 0.05$.

Table 3. The analysis per item of the IADL scale in the study sample.

	ALL (N = 853)		MALES (N = 307)		FEMALES (N = 546)	
			N (%)			
	Yes	No	Yes	No	Yes	No
IADL 1 ACTIVITY: USING A PHONE	716 (83.94)	137 (16.06) *	258 (84.04)	49 (15.96) *	458 (83.88)	88 (16.12) *
IADL 2 ACTIVITY: DOING SHOPPING	350 (41.03)	503 (58.97)	156 (50.81)	151 (49.18)	194 (35.53)	352 (64.47) *
IADL 3 ACTIVITY: PREPARING MEALS	446 (52.29)	407 (47.71)	154 (50.16)	153 (48.84)	292 (53.48)	254 (46.52)
IADL 4 ACTIVITY: CLEANING	405 (47.48)	448 (52.52)	153 (49.84)	154 (50.16)	256 (46.15)	290 (53.85)

Table 3. *Cont.*

	ALL (N = 853)		MALES (N = 307)		FEMALES (N = 546)	
IADL 5 ACTIVITY: WASHING	456 (53.46)	397 (46.54)	151 (49.18)	156 (50.81)	305 (55.86)	241 (44.14)
IADL 6 ACTIVITY: USING DIFFERENT FORMS OF TRANSPORT	303 (35.52)	550 (64.48) *	144 (46.90)	163 (53.09)	159 (29.12)	387 (70.88) *
IADL 7 ACTIVITY: USING MEDICATIONS	574 (67.29)	279 (32.71) *	206 (67.10)	101 (32.90) *	368 (67.40)	178 (32.60) *
IADL 8 ACTIVITY: USING MONEY	621 (72.80)	232 (27.20) *	235 (76.55)	72 (23.45) *	386 (70.70)	160 (29.30) *

* $p < 0.05$.

Table 4. Correlations between the results of GDS, IADL, TUG and CDT test results in the whole study group.

	GDS	IADL	TUG	CDT
GDS	1.00	−0.61 *	−0.24	0.74 *
IADL	−0.61 *	1.00	0.28	−0.54 *
TUG	−0.24	0.28	1.00	−0.25
CDT	0.74 *	−0.54 *	−0.25	1.00

* $p < 0.05$.

Table 5. Correlations between the results of GDS, IADL, TUG and CDT test results in males.

	GDS	IADL	TUG	CDT
GDS	1.00	−0.62 *	−0.34	0.75 *
IADL	−0.62 *	1.00	0.34	−0.53 *
TUG	−0.34	0.34	1.00	−0.28
CDT	0.75 *	−0.53 *	−0.28	1.00

* $p < 0.05$.

Table 6. Correlations between the results of GDS, IADL, TUG and CDT test results in the whole study group in females.

	GDS	IADL	TUG	CDT
GDS	1.00	−0.61 *	−0.22	0.73 *
IADL	−0.61 *	1.00	0.27	−0.54 *
TUG	−0.22	0.27	1.00	−0.25
CDT	0.73 *	−0.54 *	−0.25	1.00

* $p < 0.05$.

The Spearman correlation test was provided to identify a relationship between the results of GDS and instrumental activities assessed by IADL. Generally, a negative relationship was observed between GDS related to depressive disorders and every IADL activity. A statistically significant relationship was observed especially among the activities related to using a phone, medications and money. In females, also a negative statistically significant relationship was observed between GDS results and the activity related to using transport (Table 7).

Table 7. The analysis of the relationship between the depressive symptomatology measured and instrumental activities.

	GDS		
	ALL	MALES	FEMALES
IADL 1	−0.46 *	−0.48 *	−0.45 *
IADL 2	−0.42	−0.45	−0.38 *
IADL 3	−0.40	−0.43	−0.40
IADL 4	−0.41	−0.42	−0.40
IADL 5	−0.41	−0.42	−0.43
IADL 6	−0.42 *	−0.47	−0.37 *
IADL 7	−0.47 *	−0.46 *	−0.49 *
IADL 8	−0.51 *	−0.53 *	−0.49 *

* $p < 0.05$.

3.3. Relationship between the Level of Depressive Disorders and Cognitive and Physical Function

Figures 1 and 2 present the association between the TUG test related to physical fitness and the CDT test related to cognitive function. It can be observed that the results of the tests depended significantly on the severity of the diagnosed depressive disorders (Figures 1 and 2).

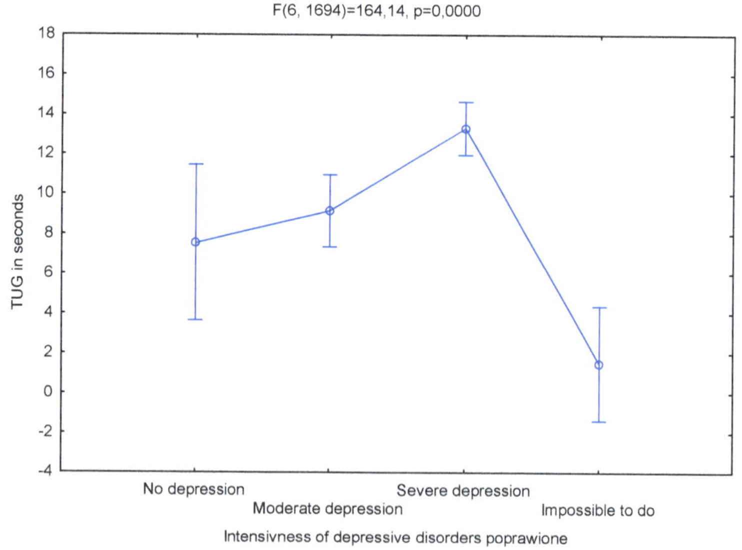

Figure 1. The relationship between the level of depressive disorders and physical fitness.

No relationship between the GDS test results and sex was observed. There was an observed relationship between GDS test results, TUG and CDT test results, but it was not statistically significant. There was also observed the statistically significant relationship between GUS and IDAL results with $p < 0.001$ and the interaction between GDS, IDAL and sex with $p < 0.05$ (Table 8).

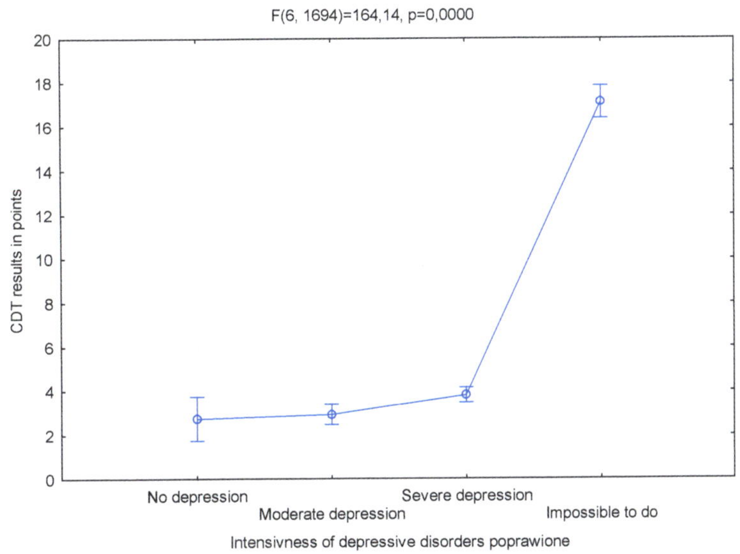

Figure 2. The relationship between the level of depressive disorders and cognitive impairment.

Table 8. Multivariate analysis of variance (MANOVA) comparing the results of GDS with other variables.

	Value	F	df	Mean Square	p
SEX	0.979	4.32	4	841.000	0.002 *
GDS	0.293	109.38	12	2225.368	0.001 *
GDS × SEX	0.993	0.47	12	2225.368	0.934
GDS × TUG	0.975	1.12	18	1624	0.320
GDS × IDAL	0.922	3.82	18	2370.707	0.001 *
GDS × CDT	0.975	1.12	18	1624	0.319
GDS × SEX × TUG	0.974	1.17	18	1624	0.280
GDS × SEX × IADL	0.974	1.78	12	2190.974	0.046 *
GDS × SEX × CDT	0.974	1.17	18	1624	0.279

* $p < 0.05$.

4. Discussion

Dementia is a neurodegenerative disease that results mostly in a decline in cognition abilities due to neuron death affecting the independent functioning of older people [52]. The primary risk factor for dementia development is age. Research shows that more than 50% of 90-year-olds have a dementia disorder and according to WHO, there are nearly 10 million new cases every year. It is also estimated that the total number of people with dementia will reach 82 million in 2030 and 152 million in 2050 [53]. WHO recognizes dementia as a public health priority [54]. Currently, there is no reliable test or sufficiently developed diagnostic tools for the early identification of dementia or screening of its first symptoms. Although there are different scales or indices that can be used to measure the severity of symptoms, such as cognitive deterioration, functional decline and behavioral changes which can be the predictors of dementia development, studies are lacking that have combined different types of testing and showing which approaches are most effective [52,55]. Apart from dementia, depression is one of the most challenging mental health problems in late life which is even more common among older people than in adolescents [56]. There were identified several risk factors for dementia and among them, depression seems to have an important role [57]. Therefore, the present study was to analyze the frequency of depressive disorders among older people and notice its relationship with cognitive and physical impairment in older people. Previous studies have indicated that it is of great importance to examine the association between cognitive impairment in older patients with depressive disorder for early diagnosis and timely treatment intervention [58].

The results of the study showed that over 35% of the participants were diagnosed with depressive symptoms. Moreover, most of them were characterized by the moderate level of depressive symptoms and it was similar among males and females. It is in line with the meta-analysis in which it was found that over a third of elderly populations globally were diagnosed with depression symptoms [59]. In turn, in the PolSenior study, in which the Geriatric Depression Rating Scale (GDS) was used, it was noted that the prevalence of depressive disorders increases with age (20% in the 55–59 age group; 25% in the 65–79 age group; 33% in the age group of 80 and more years) [31]. In the study of the prevalence of depressive symptoms in 202 people aged 65 and over in treatment and care facilities in the Bielsko district in Poland, the mean values of the GDS test for the entire study population were 11.7 ± 6.5 points. The absence of a depressive mood was found in 45.6% of the subjects, mild symptoms of depression in 43.6%, and severe depression in 10.9% of the subjects. A statistically significant positive relationship between the GDS results and the sex of the subjects was demonstrated [60]. In turn, in a study of 151 people over 65 who are patients of the Geriatrics Clinic of Collegium Medi-cum im. Ludwik Rydygiera in Bydgoszcz, using the Geriatric Depression Rating Scale in the extended version, depressive symptoms were found in 41.72% of the respondents (of which 77.78% were mild depression). Of these, 5 people were patients with depression diagnosed earlier—treated during the study, while the rest were cases of newly diagnosed depressive disorders. A relationship between the occurrence of depressive symptoms and the advancing age of the subjects and the female gender was found [47].

In China's population study, it was noticed that the depression tendency in the elderly was associated with the cognitive function change trajectory, so attention should be paid to the mental health of older people to prevent the development of dementia [61]. In the present study, one-third of the participants, both males and females, were not able to obtain satisfying results of CDT which means that their cognitive function was impaired. Unfortunately, it is evidenced that people with cognitive impairment, especially the mild level of CI, are 3 to 4 times more likely to develop dementia in comparison to those with normal cognitive function [62].

According to the test results, about one-third of the participants were noticed to have severe impairment of physical fitness with a high risk of falls. However, almost one-fifth of the study participants were characterized with a physical impairment which enabled them to go outside on his/her own with no walking aids, they felt independent in most activities of daily living and had a low risk of falls. The rest of the participants had a correct functional efficiency. Reppermund S. et al. study confirmed no relationship between current depression with functional abilities, although it was observed with poorer cognitive performance [63]. In contrast, in the cross-sectional study among elder people aged over 65 years and with diagnosed MCI or dementia, there was observed a significant relationship between physical fitness and cognition, except the components such as flexibility [64].

There were statistically significant differences between females and males in the results. Generally, females had worse results related to depressive disorders and those results characterized physical fitness. However, their cognitive function seemed to be slightly better than males. Evidence shows that there are differences between the sexes in the rate of cognitive decline with aging [65], which is explained by estrogens which can be helpful in maintaining cognitive function, especially in women who are current users of hormone therapy [66].

Depression disorders were related to greater impairment of cognitive function of the study participants which has been confirmed in previous research [67]. In Bellou et al. study it was reported that over half of patients who were diagnosed with depressive disorder also met the diagnosis of cognitive dysfunction [68]. In the present study, depressive disorders had an impact on the activities of daily living of the participants and the level of perceived physical disability. Moreover, in the present study, there was observed a relationship between the severity of the diagnosed depressive disorders and the physical fitness and cognitive function test results. Some other studies indicated also the inverse relationship, namely that physical function may influence the course of depressive disorders [69].

To sum up, the study showed that depressive disorders are frequent among the older population and affect 1 in 3 people. The cognitive impairment of older people and physical fitness can be associated with the degree of severity of depressive disorders. There is a need to examine if effective treatment of depressive disorders has any effect in reducing the prevalence of dementia. In addition, it is important to be vigilant with the clinicians for depression development indicating also the possible development of dementia in older people, and therefore carefully following up these individuals for future cognitive impairment.

There are several strengths of the present study, including large sample size, simultaneous use of several tests enabling a multi-aspect assessment of the patient and the use of methods which are internationally recognized standardized tools. It is also worth to underline that the tests for older people were conducted by the same researcher, so the results were not influenced by the subjective assessment of different people. However, some limitations should be acknowledged. Firstly, the study population was only from one medical center in the country which may affect the incidence of depression. The incidence of the phenomenon may vary depending on the region of the country, so the results cannot be generalized to the whole elderly people and treated with caution. Further, multi-centered studies would be recommended. Secondly, we did not make a direct analysis of depression, but it can be carried out by a professional psychiatrist and not by a self-reported questionnaire. Our study also does not take into account the time of occurrence of the first symptoms of depression, which can help to differentiate subtypes of depression in old age. In addition, the results could be supplemented with additional morphological and biochemical tests or other information related to the health status of the older people which could be cofounders influencing the study results.

5. Conclusions

Observing the first signs of depression among older people may be considered an indication for further diagnosis of dementia. Therefore, mandatory screening of older people for dementia should be introduced, and extended by tools diagnosing depressive disorders. This will allow for early diagnosis and appropriate preventive measures to slow down the development of the disease and maintain independence and good quality of life for older people as long as possible.

Author Contributions: Conceptualization, B.P. and J.K.; methodology, B.P. and J.K.; software, A.L.; validation, A.L.; formal analysis, A.L.; investigation, B.P.; resources, B.P. and J.K.; data curation, B.P.; writing—original draft preparation, A.L. and B.P.; writing—review and editing, A.L. and B.P.; visualization, A.L.; supervision, J.K. and A.L.; project administration, A.L.; funding acquisition, A.L. and J.K. All authors have read and agreed to the published version of the manuscript.

Funding: This research received no external funding.

Institutional Review Board Statement: The study was conducted according to the guidelines of the Declaration of Helsinki, and approved by the Institutional Review Board, approval Ref: RNN/200/23/KE.

Informed Consent Statement: Informed consent was obtained from all subjects involved in the study.

Data Availability Statement: The data presented in this study are available on request from the corresponding author.

Conflicts of Interest: The authors declare no conflict of interest.

References

1. Rasińska, R.; Nowakowska, I. Obraz ludzi starszych w raportach i zestawieniach. *Now. Lek.* **2012**, *81*, 84–88.
2. Gallou-Guyot, M.; Mandigout, S.; Combourieu-Donnezan, L.; Bherer, L.; Perrochon, A. Cognitive and physical impact of cognitive-motor dual-task training in cognitively impaired older adults: An overview. *Neurophysiol. Clin.* **2020**, *50*, 441–453. [CrossRef] [PubMed]
3. Reher, D.S. Baby booms, busts, and population aging in the developed world. *Popul. Stud.* **2015**, *69*, S57–S68. [CrossRef] [PubMed]
4. Wright, A.E.H.; Harrell, H.E. Physical Examination in the Evaluation of Dementia. *Med. Clin. N. Am.* **2022**, *106*, 471–482. [CrossRef] [PubMed]
5. Jacobs, J.M.; Cohen, A.; Ein-Mor, E.; Maaravi, Y.; Stessman, J.E. Frailty, cognitive impairment and mortality among the oldest old. *J. Nutr. Health Aging* **2011**, *15*, 678–682. [CrossRef] [PubMed]
6. Johnson, N.E. The racial crossover in comorbidity, disability, and mortality. *Demography* **2000**, *37*, 267–283. [CrossRef]
7. Ávila-Funes, J.A.; Amieva, H.; Barberger-Gateau, P.; Le Goff, M.; Raoux, N.; Ritchie, K.; Carrière, I.; Tavernier, B.; Tzourio, C.; Gutiérrez-Robledo, L.M.; et al. Cognitive impairment improves the predictive validity of the phenotype of frailty for adverse health outcomes: The Three-City Study. *J. Am. Geriatr. Soc.* **2009**, *57*, 453–461. [CrossRef]
8. Montero-Odasso, M.M.; Barnes, B.; Speechley, M.; Muir Hunter, S.W.; Doherty, T.J.; Duque, G.; Gopaul, K.; Sposato, L.A.; Casas-Herrero, A.; Borrie, M.J.; et al. Disentangling cognitive-frailty Results from the Gait and Brain Study. *J. Gerontol. A Biol. Sci. Med. Sci.* **2016**, *71*, 1476–1482. [CrossRef]
9. McGough, E.L.; Cochrane, B.B.; Pike, K.C.; Logsdon, R.G.; McCurry, S.M.; Teri, L. Dimensions of physical frailty and cognitive function in older adults with amnestic mil cognitive impairment. *Ann. Phys. Reabil. Med.* **2013**, *56*, 329–341. [CrossRef]
10. Brach, J.S.; Van Swearingen, J.M.; Newman, A.B.; Kriska, A.M. Identifying early decline of physical function in community-dwelling older women: Performance-based and self-report measures. *Phys. Ther.* **2002**, *82*, 320–328. [CrossRef]
11. Dong, X.; Chang, E.S.; Wong, E.; Wong, B.; Skarupski, K.A.; Simon, M.A. Assessing the Health Needs of Chinese Older Adults: Findings from a Community-Based Participatory Research Study in Chicago's Chinatown. *J. Aging Res.* **2011**, *2010*, 124246. [CrossRef] [PubMed]
12. Dong, X.; Chang, E.S.; Wong, E.; Simon, M. The perceptions, social determinants, and negative health outcomes associated with depressive symptoms among U.S. Chinese older adults. *Gerontologist* **2012**, *52*, 650–663. [CrossRef] [PubMed]
13. Robertson, D.A.; Savva, G.M.; Kenny, R.A. Frailty and cognitive impairment—A review of the evidence and causal mechanisms. *Ageing Res. Rev.* **2013**, *12*, 840–851. [CrossRef]
14. Wdowiak, L.; Ćwikła, S.; Bojar, I.; Kapka, L.; Woźnica, I. Starość jako problem społeczno—Demograficzny oraz zdrowotny. *Med. Ogólna* **2009**, *15*, 451–462.
15. Callegari, C.; Bertù, L.; Caselli, I.; Isella, C.; Ielmini, M.; Bonalumi, C.; Ferrario, M.; Vender, S. Resilience in older adults: Influence of the admission in nursing home and psychopathology. *Neuropsychiatry* **2016**, *6*, 117–123. [CrossRef]
16. Panella, L.; Incorvaia, C.; Caserta, A.V.; Amata, O.; Consonni, D.; Pessina, L.; Leo, G.; Caselli, I.; Callegari, C. A bio-psycho-social approach in elderly population: Outcome of adapted physical activity in patients with osteoarthritis. *Clin. Ter.* **2019**, *1*, e74–e77.
17. McPhee, J.S.; French, D.P.; Jackson, D.; Nazroo, J.; Pendleton, N.; Degens, H. Physical activity in older age: Perspectives for healthy ageing and frailty. *Biogerontology* **2016**, *17*, 567–580. [CrossRef]
18. Starczewska, M.E.; Prociak, L.; Rybicka, A.; Stanisławska, M.; Grochans, E. Ocena sprawności funkcjonalnej i występowania ryzyka depresji wśród seniorów. *Pol. Nurs. Pielegniarstwo Pol.* **2019**, *73*, 258–264.
19. Gureje, O.; Ogunniyi, A.; Kola, L.; Afolabi, E. Functional disability in elderly Nigerians: Results from the Ibadan Study of Aging. *J. Am. Geriatr. Soc.* **2006**, *54*, 1784–1789. [CrossRef]
20. Liang, J.; Wang, C.N.; Xu, X.; Hsu, H.C.; Lin, H.S.; Lin, Y.H. Trajectory of functional status among older Taiwanese: Gender and age variations. *Soc. Sci. Med.* **2010**, *71*, 1208–1217. [CrossRef]
21. Chen, S.W.; Chippendale, T. Factors associated with IADL independence: Implications for OT practice. *Scand. J. Occup. Ther.* **2017**, *24*, 109–115. [CrossRef] [PubMed]
22. Wysokiński, M.; Fidecki, W.; Gębala, S. Ocena samodzielności osób starszych hospitalizowanych na oddziałach internistycznych. *Gerontol. Pol.* **2013**, *21*, 89–97.
23. Teixeira-Leite, H.; Manhães, A.C. Association between functional alterations of senescence and senility and disorders of gait and balance. *Clinics* **2012**, *67*, 719–729. [CrossRef] [PubMed]
24. Giannouli, V.; Stamovlasis, D.; Tsolaki, M. Exploring the role of cognitive factors in a new instrument for elders' financial capacity assessment. *J. Alzheimer's Dis.* **2018**, *62*, 1579–1594. [CrossRef] [PubMed]
25. Giannouli, V.; Tsolaki, M. Mild Alzheimer Disease, financial capacity, and the role of depression: Eyes wide shut? *Alzheimer Dis. Assoc. Disord.* **2021**, *35*, 360–362. [CrossRef] [PubMed]
26. Giannouli, V.; Tsolaki, M. Vascular dementia, depression, and financial capacity assessment. *Alzheimer Dis. Assoc. Disord.* **2021**, *35*, 84–87. [CrossRef]
27. Giannouli, V.; Tsolaki, M. Are left angular gyrus and amygdala volumes important for financial capacity in mild cognitive impairment? *Hell. J. Nucl. Med.* **2019**, *22*, 160–164.
28. Giannouli, V.; Tsolaki, M. Unraveling Ariadne's Thread Into the Labyrinth of aMCI: Depression and Financial Capacity. *Alzheimer Dis. Assoc. Disord.* **2021**, *35*, 363–365. [CrossRef]

29. Giannouli, V.; Tsolaki, M. Beneath the Top of the Iceberg: Financial Capacity Deficits in Mixed Dementia with and without Depression. *Healthcare* **2023**, *11*, 505. [CrossRef]
30. Maqsood, F.; Flatt, J.D.; Albert, S.M.; Maqsood, S.; Nizamuddin, M. Correlates of self-reported depressive symptoms: A study of older persons of Punjab, Pakistan. *J. Cross Cult. Gerontol.* **2013**, *28*, 65–74. [CrossRef]
31. Broczek, K.; Mossakowska, M.; Szybalska, A.; Kozak-Szkopek, E.; Ślusarczyk, P.; Wieczorkowska-Tobis, K.; Parnowski, T. Występowanie objawów depresyjnych u osób starszych. In *Aspekty Medyczne, Psychologiczne, Socjologiczne i Ekonomiczne Starzenia Się Ludzi w Polsce*; Mossakowska, M., Więcek, A., Błędowski, P., Eds.; Termedia: Poznan, Poland, 2012; pp. 123–136.
32. Busch, T.A.; Duarte, Y.A.; Nunes, D.P.; Lebrão, M.L.; Naslavsky, M.S.; dos Santos Rodrigues, A.; Amaro, E., Jr. Factors associated with lower gait speed among the elderly living in a developing country: A cross-sectional population-based study. *BMC Geriatr.* **2015**, *15*, 35. [CrossRef] [PubMed]
33. Domańska, Ł. Depresja wieku podeszłego–wyzwania diagnostyczne. *Ann. Univ. Mariae Curie Skłodowska Sect. J. Paedagog. Psychol.* **2019**, *31*, 327–338. [CrossRef]
34. Bidzan, L. Depresyjne zaburzenia nastroju u osób w wieku podeszłym. *Med. Wieku Podeszłego* **2011**, *1*, 31–41.
35. Rzewuska, M. Leczenie zaburzeń psychicznych. *Wydaw. Lek. PZWL* **2003**, 257–264.
36. Piwoński, J.; Piwońska, A.; Głuszek, J.; Bielecki, W.; Pająk, A.; Kozakiewicz, K.; Wyrzykowski, B.; Rywik, S. Ocena częstości występowania niskiego poziomu wsparcia społecznego oraz objawów depresji w populacji polskiej. *Wyniki Programu WOBASZ Kardiol. Pol.* **2005**, *63*, 645–648.
37. Sekhon, S.; Patel, J.; Sapra, A. Late-Life Depression. In *StatPearls*; StatPearls Publishing: Treasure Island, FL, USA, 2023.
38. Shin, J.M.; Sims, R.C.; Bradley, D.L.; Pohlig, R.T.; Harrison, B.E. Prevalence of depressive symptoms and associated factorsin older adult public housing residents. *Res. Gerontol. Nurs.* **2014**, *7*, 249–255. [CrossRef]
39. Bhamani, M.A.; Karim, M.S.; Khan, M.M. Depression in the elderly in Karachi, Pakistan: A cross sectional study. *BMC Psychiatry* **2013**, *13*, 181. [CrossRef]
40. Płaszewska-Żywko, L.; Brzuzan, P.; Malinowska-Lipień, I.; Gabryś, T. Sprawność funkcjonalna u osób w wieku podeszłym w domach pomocy społecznej. *Probl. Hig. Epidemiol.* **2008**, *89*, 62–66.
41. Livingston, G.; Sommerlad, A.; Orgeta, V.; Costafreda, S.G.; Huntley, J.; Ames, D.; Ballard, C.; Banerjee, S.; Burns, A.; Cohen-Mansfield, J.; et al. Dementia prevention, intervention, and care. *Lancet* **2017**, *390*, 2673–2734. [CrossRef]
42. Zou, C.; Yu, Q.; Wang, C.; Ding, M.; Chen, L. Association of depression with cognitive frailty: A systematic review and meta-analysis. *J. Affect. Disord.* **2023**, *320*, 133–139. [CrossRef]
43. Perini, G.; Cotta Ramusino, M.; Sinforiani, E.; Bernini, S.; Petrachi, R.; Costa, A. Cognitive impairment in depression: Recent advances and novel treatments. *Neuropsychiatr. Dis. Treat.* **2019**, *15*, 1249–1258. [CrossRef] [PubMed]
44. Kang, H.; Zhao, F.; You, L.; Giorgetta, C.D.V.; Sarkhel, S.; Prakash, R. Pseudo-dementia: A neuropsychological review. *Ann. Indian Acad. Neurol.* **2014**, *17*, 147–154. [PubMed]
45. Mirza, S.S.; de Bruijn, R.F.A.G.; Direk, N.; Hofman, A.; Peter, J.; Koudstaal, P.J.; Ikram, M.A.; Tiemeier, H. Depressive symptoms predict incident dementia during short- but not long-term follow-up period. *Alzheimer's Dement.* **2014**, *10*, S323–S329. [CrossRef] [PubMed]
46. Steffens, D.C.; Skoog, I.; Norton, M.C.; Hart, A.D.; Tschanz, J.T.; Plassman, B.L.; Wyse, B.W.; Welsh-Bohmer, K.A.; Breitner, J.C. Prevalence of depression and its treatment in an elderly population. The Cache County Study. *Arch. Gen. Psychiatry* **2000**, *57*, 601–607. [CrossRef]
47. Weterle, K.; Sołtysiak, J. Objawy depresji i ich wykrywalność przez lekarzy podstawowej opieki zdrowotnej u pacjentów po 65. roku życia. *Now. Lek.* **2006**, *75*, 433–437.
48. The National Health Fund Organization. The Order of the President of the National Health Fund of 3 January 2022 on Defining the Conditions for Concluding and Implementing Contracts such as Hospital Treatment and Hospital Treatment—Highly Specialized Services. Available online: https://www.nfz.gov.pl/zarzadzenia-prezesa/zarzadzenia-prezesa-nfz/zarzadzenie-nr-32022dsoz,7476.html (accessed on 3 August 2023).
49. Pedraza, O.; Dotson, V.M.; Willis, F.B.; Graff-Radford, N.R.; Lucas, J.A. Internal Consistency and Test-Retest Stability of the Geriatric Depression Scale-Short Form in African American Older Adults. *J. Psychopathol. Behav. Assess.* **2009**, *31*, 412–416. [CrossRef]
50. Kroemeke, A. Perceived Autonomy in Old Age scale: Factor structure and psychometric properties of the Polish adaptation. *Psychiatr. Pol.* **2015**, *49*, 107–117. [CrossRef]
51. Shulman, K.I.; Gold, D.P.; Cohen, C.A.; Zucchero, C.A. Clock-drawing and dementia in the community: A longitudinal study. *Int. J. Geriatr. Psychiatry* **1993**, *8*, 487–496. [CrossRef]
52. Gale, S.A.; Acar, D.; Daffner, K.R. Dementia. *Am. J. Med.* **2018**, *131*, 1161–1169. [CrossRef]
53. World Health Organization. Risk Reduction of Cognitive Decline and Dementia: WHO Guidelines. 2019. Available online: https://www.who.int/publications/i/item/9789241550543 (accessed on 3 August 2023).
54. World Health Organization. Dementia. Available online: https://www.who.int/health-topics/dementia#tab=tab_3 (accessed on 3 August 2023).
55. Swedish Council on Health Technology Assessment. *Dementia—Caring, Ethics, Ethnical and Economical Aspects: A Systematic Review*; SBU Assessment No. 172; Swedish Council on Health Technology Assessment (SBU): Stockholm, Sweden, 2008.

56. Kasa, A.S.; Lee, S.C.; Chang, H.R. Prevalence and factors associated with depression among older adults in the case of a low-income country, Ethiopia: A systematic review and meta-analysis. *BMC Psychiatry* **2022**, *22*, 675. [CrossRef]
57. Fernández Martínez, M.; Castro Flores, J.; Pérez de Las Heras, S.; Mandaluniz Lekumberri, M.; Gordejuela Menocal, M.; Zarranz Imirizaldu, J.J. Risk factors for dementia in the epidemiological study of Munguialde County (Basque Country-Spain). *BMC Neurol.* **2008**, *8*, 39. [CrossRef] [PubMed]
58. Rajtar-Zembaty, A.; Sałakowski, A.; Rajtar-Zembaty, J.; Starowicz-Filip, A. Executive dysfunction in late-life depression. *Psychiatr. Pol.* **2017**, *51*, 705–718. [CrossRef] [PubMed]
59. Cai, H.; Jin, Y.; Liu, R.; Zhang, Q.; Su, Z.; Ungvari, G.S.; Tang, Y.L.; Ng, C.H.; Li, X.H.; Xiang, Y.T. Global prevalence of depression in older adults: A systematic review and meta-analysis of epidemiological surveys. *Asian J. Psychiatr.* **2023**, *80*, 103417. [CrossRef] [PubMed]
60. Babiarczyk, B.; Schlegel-Zawadzka, M.; Turbiarz, A. Ocena częstości występowania objawów depresji w populacji osób powyżej 65 roku życia. *Med. Og. Nauk. Zdr.* **2013**, *19*, 453–457.
61. Han, Y.F.; Yang, Y.T.; Fang, Y. Association between depression tendency and cognitive trajectory in the elderly in rural area in China. *Zhonghua Liu Xing Bing Xue Za Zhi* **2022**, *43*, 1491–1496. (In Chinese) [CrossRef]
62. Chippa, V.; Roy, K. *Geriatric Cognitive Decline and Polypharmacy*; StatPearls Publishing: Treasure Island, FL, USA, 2023.
63. Reppermund, S.; Brodaty, H.; Crawford, J.D.; Kochan, N.A.; Slavin, M.J.; Trollor, J.N.; Draper, B.; Sachdev, P.S. The relationship of current depressive symptoms and past depression with cognitive impairment and instrumental activities of daily living in an elderly population: The Sydney Memory and Ageing Study. *J. Psychiatr. Res.* **2011**, *45*, 1600–1607. [CrossRef]
64. Hesseberg, K.; Bentzen, H.; Ranhoff, A.H.; Engedal, K.; Bergland, A. Physical Fitness in Older People with Mild Cognitive Impairment and Dementia. *J. Aging Phys. Act.* **2016**, *24*, 92–100. [CrossRef]
65. Li, R.; Singh, M. Sex differences in cognitive impairment and Alzheimer's disease. *Front. Neuroendocrinol.* **2014**, *35*, 385–403. [CrossRef]
66. Doraiswamy, P.M.; Bieber, F.; Kaiser, L.; Krishnan, K.R.; Reuning-Scherer, J.; Gulanski, B. The Alzheimer's Disease Assessment Scale: Patterns and predictors of baseline cognitive performance in multicenter Alzheimer's disease trials. *Neurology* **1997**, *48*, 1511–1517. [CrossRef]
67. Pitts, B.L.; Wen, V.; Whealin, J.M.; Fogle, B.M.; Southwick, S.M.; Esterlis, I.; Pietrzak, R.H. Depression and cognitive dysfunction in older U.S. military veterans: Moderating effects of BDNF Val66Met polymorphism and physical exercise. *Am. J. Geriatr. Psychiatry* **2020**, *28*, 959–967. [CrossRef]
68. Bellou, V.; Belbasis, L.; Tzoulaki, I.; Middleton, L.T.; Ioannidis, J.P.; Evangelou, E. Systematic evaluation of the associations between environmental risk factors and dementia: An umbrella review of systematic reviews and meta-analyses. *Alzheimers Dement.* **2017**, *13*, 406–418. [CrossRef] [PubMed]
69. van Milligen, B.A.; Vogelzangs, N.; Smit, J.H.; Penninx, B.W. Physical function as predictor for the persistence of depressive and anxiety disorders. *J. Affect. Disord.* **2012**, *136*, 828–832. [CrossRef] [PubMed]

life

Article

Assessment of Ileal Crohn's Disease Activity by Gastrointestinal Ultrasound and MR Enterography: A Pilot Study

Răzvan-Cristian Statie [1], Sevastiţa Iordache [2,*], Lucian Mihai Florescu [3,*], Ioana-Andreea Gheonea [3], Victor-Mihai Sacerdoţianu [2], Bogdan Silviu Ungureanu [2], Ion Rogoveanu [2], Dan-Ionuţ Gheonea [2], Tudorel Ciurea [2] and Dan Nicolae Florescu [2]

1 Doctoral School, University of Medicine and Pharmacy of Craiova, 200349 Craiova, Romania; statierazvan@gmail.com
2 Department of Gastroenterology, University of Medicine and Pharmacy of Craiova, 200349 Craiova, Romania
3 Department of Radiology and Medical Imaging, University of Medicine and Pharmacy of Craiova, 200349 Craiova, Romania
* Correspondence: sevastita@gmail.com (S.I.); lucian.florescu@umfcv.ro (L.M.F.)

Abstract: Introduction: In some cases, there may be a discrepancy between the symptomatology alleged by Crohn's disease (CD) patients and the results of laboratory tests or imaging investigations. Ileocolonoscopy with biopsy is the primary investigation for diagnosing and monitoring CD patients. Cross-sectional imaging techniques such as CT or MR enterography (MRE) and intestinal ultrasonography (IUS) have been proposed as complementary methods to colonoscopy for a complete evaluation of this category of patients. This study aims to identify the role of IUS, contrast-enhanced ultrasound (CEUS) and MRE in evaluating ileal CD activity, using clinical severity scores (Crohn's disease activity index—CDAI, Harvey–Bradshaw index—HBI) and faecal calprotectin or C-reactive protein (CRP) levels as reference methods. Materials and Methods: A total of 44 adult patients with ileal CD confirmed using an ileocolonoscopy with biopsy and histopathological examination were assessed by IUS, CEUS and MRE. The evaluation of the disease activity based on the results obtained from the cross-sectional imaging tests was carried out by using some severity scores available in the literature. The sensitivity and specificity of IUS + CEUS and MRE for differentiating active from inactive forms of CD were determined using CDAI, HBI, faecal calprotectin and CRP as reference methods. The accuracy of the results was assessed by the receiver operating characteristics method. The Pearson correlation coefficient was used to determine the types of correlation. A p-value less than 0.05 suggested a statistically significant relationship. Results: Compared to CDAI, the best correlation was identified for Limberg score ($r = 0.667$, 95% confidence interval (CI) [0.46, 0.8], $p < 0.001$), followed by MaRIAs score ($r = 0.614$, 95% CI [0.39, 0.77], $p < 0.001$). A sensitivity of 93.33% and a specificity of 71.43% (AUC = 0.98) were demonstrated in the case of Limberg score for differentiating patients with active disease from those in remission and for MaRIAs score a sensitivity of 100.00% and a specificity of 57.14% (AUC = 0.97). Regarding HBI, the best correlation was observed for MaRIAs score ($r = 0.594$, 95% CI [0.36, 0.76], $p < 0.001$). Also, faecal calprotectin showed the best correlation with MaRIAs score ($r = 0.697$, 95% CI [0.46, 0.84], $p < 0.001$), but in the case of CRP, there was only a weak correlation for all evaluated scores. Conclusions: Although magnetic resonance imaging does not appear to be superior to ultrasonography in terms of accuracy for differentiating active forms of CD from those in remission, the results of our study suggest that MRE associates a better correlation with clinical severity scores and faecal calprotectin levels compared to ultrasonography. More studies are needed to validate these results.

Keywords: Crohn's disease; intestinal ultrasonography; contrast-enhanced ultrasound; MR enterography

Citation: Statie, R.-C.; Iordache, S.; Florescu, L.M.; Gheonea, I.-A.; Sacerdoţianu, V.-M.; Ungureanu, B.S.; Rogoveanu, I.; Gheonea, D.-I.; Ciurea, T.; Florescu, D.N. Assessment of Ileal Crohn's Disease Activity by Gastrointestinal Ultrasound and MR Enterography: A Pilot Study. *Life* **2023**, *13*, 1754. https://doi.org/10.3390/life13081754

Academic Editors: Nicole D. Bouvy and Saulius Svagzdys

Received: 18 May 2023
Revised: 15 July 2023
Accepted: 14 August 2023
Published: 16 August 2023

1. Introduction

Crohn's disease (CD) is one of the primary forms of inflammatory bowel disease (IBD). The characteristic inflammatory process of CD is transmural, can affect all layers of the bowel wall and can spread to adjacent tissues. Regarding location, CD may interest any segment of the digestive tract. A predilection for the terminal ileum and proximal colon is noted [1]. Approximately 40% of CD patients present with ileocolonic localisation, 30% have a localisation at the colon level and 25% at the small bowel level [2]. Cases with extensive lesions in the small bowel seem to be associated with a less favourable outcome, with reduced response to drug therapy and requiring surgery and higher healthcare costs [1,3]. For this reason, properly managing these patients requires a more complex evaluation of the entire digestive tract with the correct establishment of the extent of the disease.

Ileocolonoscopy with biopsy is the primary investigation for diagnosing and monitoring CD patients [4]. The limitations of this method refer to the fact that it does not always allow endoscopic exploration of the terminal ileum, and the examination is limited to the appearance of the mucosa without providing information on the deeper layers of the bowel wall. Moreover, it is not an investigation accepted by patients to be repeated frequently [5].

Imaging evaluation of the small bowel is required in all patients in whom the diagnosis of CD is suspected [4]. Thus, cross-sectional imaging techniques such as CT enterography (CTE) or MR enterography (MRE) and intestinal ultrasonography (IUS) have been proposed as complementary methods to colonoscopy for a complete evaluation of this category of patients [6]. The computed tomography (CT) scan of the small bowel allows for obtaining high-resolution images in a shorter time compared to MRE, reducing the discomfort created for certain patients (e.g., those with claustrophobia); this method uses ionising radiation, which is why it cannot be performed repeatedly, especially in young patients [6]. MRE shows superior sensitivity and specificity to IUS in evaluating CD extension in the small bowel [4,7]. Therefore, MRE is considered the best non-ionising imaging investigation for evaluating CD patients [6,8,9]. But this method is not widely available, involves relatively high costs and sometimes patients hardly tolerate the examination [10]. Furthermore, a series of meta-analyses revealed no significant differences in diagnostic accuracy in CD between MRE, CTE or IUS [4,11–15]. Based on these results, IUS could represent an effective alternative to MRE for evaluating CD patients. Ultrasonography is widely available, relatively inexpensive and does not use ionising radiation, and is, thus, of great interest, especially for young patients who require frequent monitoring. But it is an operator-dependent method, which can associate difficulties in obtaining quality images in the case of obese patients and the experience in evaluating the digestive tract is limited. However, despite these impediments, recent years have seen an increase in the popularity of ultrasonography for evaluating patients with IBD.

Over time, several methods have been proposed for evaluating CD activity. Among these, we mention clinical severity scores, such as Crohn's disease activity index (CDAI) [16] and the Harvey–Bradshaw index (HBI) [17], or laboratory tests, such as faecal calprotectin or C-reactive protein (CRP) levels [18–20]. The assessment of inflammation with the help of cross-sectional imaging techniques can be achieved by measuring the thickness of the bowel wall [10,11,21,22] and evaluating the mural blood flow using the colour Doppler during US examination [10,23–25] or by the bowel wall enhancement of the contrast agent in the case of CT or magnetic resonance imaging (MRI) [26,27]. Another parameter with an essential role in the imaging assessment of inflammation severity is the appearance of mesenteric fat [28]. Using contrast agents during US examination (contrast-enhanced ultrasound—CEUS) allows the evaluation of the microcirculation at the level of the bowel wall [10,29]. According to the EFSUMB guidelines [30], CEUS can be used to assess the activity of IBD and also allows the differentiation of inflammatory stenoses from fibrous ones in the case of CD; it can also be used to monitor treatment response in CD. Several scores have been proposed to evaluate CD activity using CEUS [10,31,32] or MRE [33], which seem to show excellent correlations with disease severity assessed by colonoscopy [34]. However, in some instances, there is a contradiction between the symptomatology alleged by the patient and the results of laboratory tests or imaging investigations.

Thus, this study aims to identify the role of IUS, CEUS and MRE in evaluating ileal CD activity, using clinical severity scores (CDAI, HBI) and faecal calprotectin or CRP levels as reference methods.

2. Materials and Methods

2.1. Study Population

This prospective study was conducted over a period of 27 months. From November 2020 to January 2023, a total of 44 adult patients with ileal CD confirmed by ileocolonoscopy with biopsy and histopathological examination were included in the study.

Inclusion criteria for patients: (1) over 18 years of age; (2) known ileal CD confirmed by histopathological examination; and (3) signed written informed consent.

Patients with general contraindications for MRE (e.g., claustrophobia, presence of metal implants); those with contraindications for contrast agents used for US or MRE; patients in whom difficulties were encountered in obtaining high-quality images during the US examination; patients who associated other diseases that could have influenced the results of laboratory tests; pregnant women; and patients who refused to participate in the study were excluded.

The interval between the two cross-sectional imaging examinations, US and MRE, was a maximum of 7 days.

The study was performed according to the principles of the Declaration of Helsinki. The local ethics committee approved the study protocol, and written informed consent was obtained for all patients before inclusion in the study.

2.2. Clinical Activity Scores and Laboratory Tests

When patients presented for ultrasonographic examination, they were assessed by CDAI (<150—remission) and HBI (<5—remission) activity scores. Blood and stool samples were also collected from the patients to determine hematocrit levels (necessary for CDAI calculation), CRP and faecal calprotectin. We used threshold values of 10 mg/L for CRP, respectively, and 250 μg/g for faecal calprotectin to differentiate inactive forms of the disease from active ones [35,36].

2.3. Ultrasound

The examination was performed by a gastroenterologist with about 15 years of experience in IUS using a Hitachi Arietta V70 ultrasonography system (Hitachi Ltd., Tokyo, Japan) and the L34 linear transducer with a frequency of 7.5 MHz. Patients were instructed to fast for at least 6 h before the procedure. The ultrasound examination was performed at the level of the terminal ileum. The assessed parameters included: maximum bowel wall thickness (BWT), parietal stratification, mural blood flow on colour Doppler imaging (CDI), mesenteric fatty proliferation and the presence of lymph nodes (Appendix A Figure A1). Considering BWT and relying on a classification proposed by Rigazio et al. [37], CD could be divided as follows: inactive, BWT < 4 mm; mild, BWT 4 mm-6 mm; moderate, BWT 6.1 mm–8 mm; and severe, BWT $\geq$ 8.1 mm. To assess the mural blood flow at the CDI, we used the Limberg score [23].

Next, an intravenous bolus injection of 4.8 mL of a second-generation contrast agent (SonoVue, Bracco S.p.A., Milan, Italy) was administered, followed by an infusion of 5 mL sodium chloride 0.9%. CEUS examinations (T0-T180s) were evaluated in real-time (Appendix A Figure A2) and then recorded on an external storage drive for quantitative analysis of the obtained images.

The quantitative analysis of the vascular pattern at the level of the wall of the terminal ileum was performed using a dedicated software called VueBox® (Bracco Suisse SA, Plan-les-Ouates, Switzerland). Images recorded during CEUS were converted to DICOM format. Afterward, they were analysed through the mentioned dedicated software. Three regions of interest (ROI) were selected at the level of the terminal ileum wall—Figure 1. The time-intensity curve (TIC) was analysed with the automatic generation of the following parameters—Figure 2, as follows:

- Peak Enhancement (PE)—Figure 3b;
- Wash-in Area Under the Curve (WiAUC);
- Rise Time (RT);
- Mean Transit Time Local (mTTl);
- Time To Peak (TTP);
- Wash-in Rate (WiR);
- Wash-in Perfusion Index (WiPI);
- Wash-out AUC (WoAUC);
- Wash-in and Wash-out AUC (WiWoAUC);
- Fall Time (FT);
- Wash-out Rate (WoR);
- Quality Of Fit between the echo-power signal and f(t) (QOF).

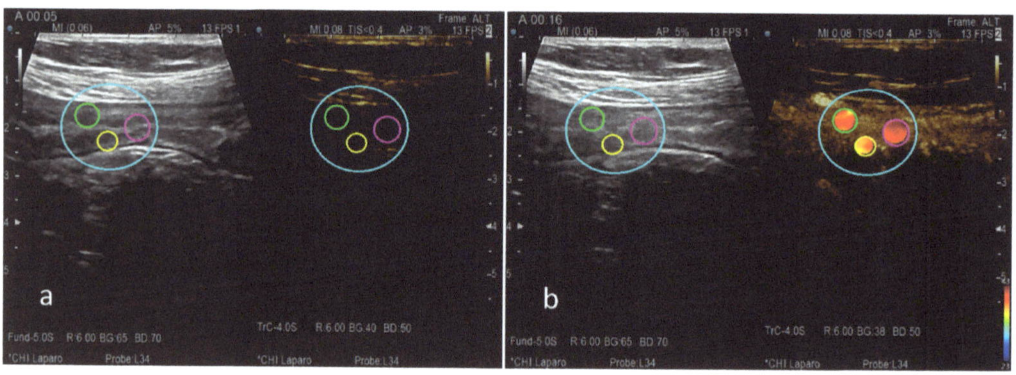

Figure 1. (**a**) Quantitative analysis of vascular pattern by manually choosing specific regions of interest (the three small circles) in the terminal ileum using dedicated software, Vuebox® (https://www.bracco.com/en-se/product/vuebox), resulting in TIC parameters. (**b**) An example of one of the automatically calculated parameters, peak enhancement.

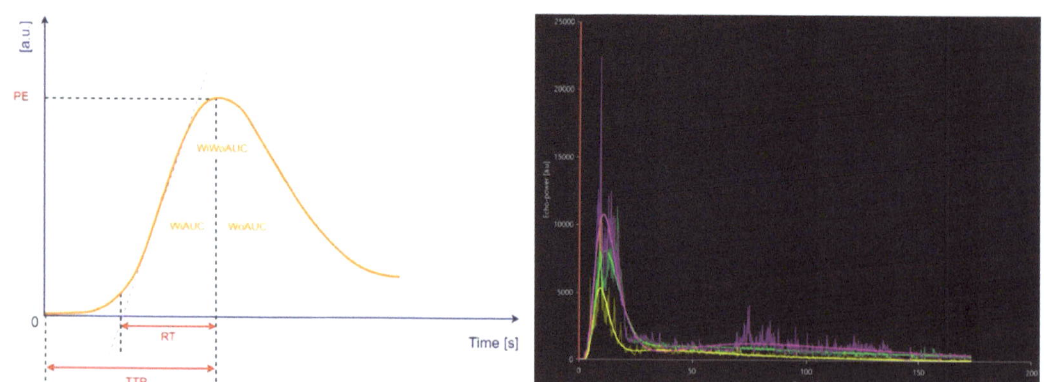

Figure 2. Time-intensity curve with generated parameters: peak enhancement (PE); wash-in area under the curve (WiAUC); rise time (RT); time to peak (TTP); wash-out area under the curve (WoAUC); wash-in and wash-out area under the curve (WiWoAUC). a.u., arbitrary units; s, seconds. Adapted from VueBox® Quantification Toolbox User Manual, Copyright© 2019 Bracco Suisse SA.

The quality of this process was assessed based on the value of the QOF parameter, which is considered appropriate if it exceeded the 50% threshold. The results of the generated parameters were expressed in arbitrary units [a.u] and seconds [s]. To convert [a.u.] to decibels [dB], we used the following formula suggested by the developer: value_dB = 10 × log10 (value_au/1).

The evaluation of the disease activity based on the results obtained from the ultrasonographic examination was carried out by using some severity scores available in the literature. These scores used colonoscopy as a reference method, resulting in good correlations. The first score used was proposed by Medellin-Kowalewski et al. [10] and evaluates the PE parameter obtained following CEUS quantification. Thus, a value of PE < 18.2 dB seems to associate with an inactive form of the disease, values between 18.2–22.8 dB seem to characterise mild to moderate forms, and a value above 22.8 dB suggests moderate to severe forms. Ripollés et al. [31] developed an ultrasonographic score based on grey-scale ultrasound and CEUS parameters. It uses the BWT, the colour Doppler grade based on the Limberg score and the WiR parameter (expressed in [a.u]) obtained after CEUS quantification, according to the following formula (parietal thickness × 0.957) + (colour Doppler grade × 0.859) + (wash-in × 0.036). A cut-off value of 8.38 was established to distinguish inactive from active forms of the disease. They also proposed a simplified variant—simple CEUS score: thickness (mm) + colour Doppler grade + (wash-in × 0.036) (with the same cut-off value of 8.38) or a score based only on the BWT and colour Doppler grade—simple US score: parietal thickness (mm) + colour Doppler grade, using a cut-off value of 5.5. The PE and WiR values we introduced in the formulas mentioned above were represented by the average of these parameters obtained at the level of each ROI.

2.4. Magnetic Resonance Enterography

MRE examinations were performed using a Philips Ingenia 3.0T device (Philips Medical Systems International, Best, Noord-Brabant, The Netherlands). Patients were instructed to fast for at least 6 h before the examination. In addition, they were given 1.5 L of 2.5% mannitol water-based oral solution, which they had to consume 60 min before the actual procedure. No particular preparation of the colon was performed before the examination.

A radiologist with experience in the field of IBD analysed the images obtained at MRE. He was blinded to the results of clinical activity scores, laboratory tests or those obtained from US and CEUS. The assessed parameters included: BWT, the presence of parietal edema, mesenteric fatty proliferation, the existence of bowell wall ulcers, the presence of complications such as stenoses, fistulas or abscesses and the bowel wall enhancement after the administration of gadolinium (Appendix A Figure A3).

Quantification of CD severity by MRE was performed using a score proposed by Ordás et al. [33], called Simplified Magnetic Resonance Index of Activity for Crohn's Disease (MaRIAs). This score evaluates 4 parameters and gives 1 point each for bowel wall thickness > 3 mm, the presence of bowel wall edema and perienteric fat stranding, and 2 points for the existence of bowel wall ulcers.

A MaRIAs score greater than 1 has been shown to identify intestinal segments with an active CD with 90% sensitivity and 81% specificity, and a score greater than 2 indicates the presence of severe lesions with 85% sensitivity and 92% specificity [33].

2.5. Statistical Analysis

The obtained data were analysed using Microsoft Excel (Microsoft Corp., Redmond, WA, USA). The utility of IUS + CEUS and MRE for differentiating active from inactive forms of CD was evaluated by determining the sensitivity, specificity and positive and negative predictive values, using the results of clinical activity scores (CDAI, HBI) and laboratory tests (calprotectin faecal, CRP) as reference methods. Next, we created receiver operating characteristics (ROC) curves using this data and calculated the area under the curve (AUC) for accuracy assessment.

According to the data obtained from the studies of Swets [38], an AUC value between 0.50–0.70 suggests poor accuracy, values between 0.70–0.90 indicate good accuracy, and values above 0.90 offer excellent accuracy.

The Pearson correlation coefficient was used to determine the type of correlation between cross-sectional imaging findings, clinical activity scores, and laboratory tests. To identify the statistical significance of the correlation coefficient obtained after comparing the data, we used the *t*-test (*t*-test). A *p*-value less than 0.05 suggested a statistically significant relationship.

3. Results

During a time interval of 27 months, 44 patients with confirmed ileal CD were included in the study (18 men, 26 women; mean age 43 years, standard deviation (STDEV)—10.34). One female patient was excluded because she could not tolerate the MRE examination due to claustrophobia. The clinical characteristics of the patients are shown in Table 1. From a total of 44 patients, according to the Montreal classification, 8 were known to have a stenotic form of CD. Four patients from this group required surgical intervention for intestinal obstruction before the study. Using the IUS, we could highlight the presence of intestinal stenoses in the case of four patients, the results being later confirmed by the MRE (Appendix A Figure A4). The mean values of the clinical severity scores were 210.54 (STDEV = 84.61) for CDAI, respectively, and 7.04 (STDEV = 3.25) for HBI.

Table 1. Clinical characteristics of the patients (n = 44).

Age [mean (range)]	43 (23–66)	
Gender (male/female)	18/26	
Disease behaviour		
Non-stricturing/non-penetrating		36
Stricturing		8
Penetrating		0
- Perianal disease		2
Crohn's Disease Activity Index [mean (STDEV)]	210.54 (84.61)	
Harvey–Bradshaw Index [mean (STDEV)]	7.04 (3.25)	

STDEV—standard deviation.

Based on clinical activity scores, CDAI identified 14 patients (31.81%) in clinical remission and 30 patients with active disease (Appendix A Table A1); according to HBI, there were 8 patients (18.18%) with inactive disease and 36 patients with active forms of the disease. The faecal calprotectin and CRP levels revealed 28 (63.63%), respectively, and 25 (56.81%) patients with active disease. Regarding the information obtained at CDI, the Limberg score classified 12 patients (27.27%) as having inactive disease and 32 patients with active disease. At CEUS, the scores proposed by Medellin-Kowalewski et al. [10] and Ripollés et al. [31] identified 4 (9.09%), respectively, 8 (18.18%), patients with inactive disease and 40, respectively, 36 patients with active disease. MaRIAs score, used to quantify the results obtained after MRE, detected 8 patients (18.18%) with inactive disease and 36 patients with active disease, of which 26 patients (59.09%) had severe lesions (Figure 3).

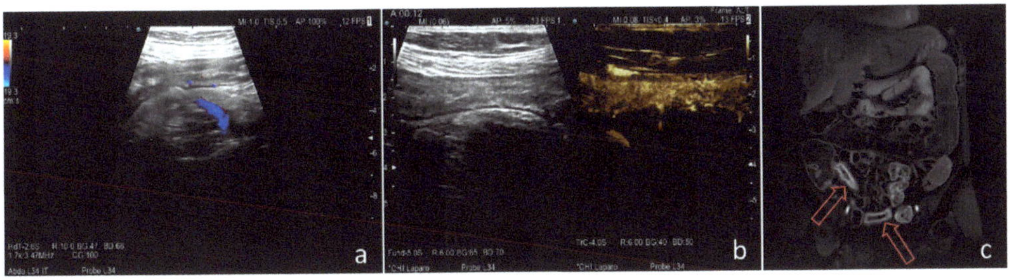

Figure 3. Comparison between the different scores for evaluating disease activity using IUS + CEUS or MRE in the case of a patient with a mild form of Crohn's disease (CDAI = 152; HBI = 5; fecal calprotectin = 390 µg/g; CRP = 1.42 mg/L). (**a**) Colour Doppler imaging shows intermittent increases in vascularity—Limberg score = 2. (**b**) CEUS highlights transmural enhancement (Peak Enhancement = 38.86 dB, Wash-in Rate = 1750.75 [a.u], after the quantitative analysis of vascular pattern using VueBox®)—Ripollés score = 72.31, Medellin-Kowalewski score = 38.86. (**c**) MRE—T1 postcontrast phase (venous phase), coronal plane: the arrows indicate an increased wall thickness affecting the terminal ileum continuously, mainly with a mucosal contrast enhancement pattern in this phase and engorged vasa recta in the affected region—MaRIAs score = 3. In this case, we notice a discrepancy between the results of the imaging tests that suggest a severe form of CD and the results of the clinical activity scores and laboratory tests.

Using CDAI as the reference method, the Limberg score presented a sensitivity of 93.33% and a specificity of 71.43% (AUC = 0.98) for differentiating active from inactive forms of the disease (Table 2—a more detailed table version can be consulted in the Appendix A, Tables A2 and A3). For the score proposed by Ripollés et al. [31] and MaRIAs score, the sensitivity and specificity results were similar, 100.00% and 57.14%, respectively, with an AUC value for Ripollés score of 0.847 and 0.971 for MaRIAs score (Figure 4).

Table 2. Assessment of the quality of IUS + CEUS and MRE in detecting active forms of Crohn's disease using Crohn's disease activity index, Harvey–Bradshaw Index, fecal calprotectin test and C-reactive protein test as reference methods.

	US—Maximal Wall Thickness			Limberg Score			Ripollés Score			MaRIAs Score		
	Sen (%)	Spe (%)	AUC	Sen (%)	Spe (%)	AUC	Sen (%)	Spe (%)	AUC	Sen (%)	Spe (%)	AUC
Crohn's disease activity index	100	14.29	0.87	93.33	71.43	0.98	100	57.14	0.84	100	57.14	0.97
Harvey–Bradshaw Index	100	25	0.88	83.33	75%	0.95	88.89	50	0.80	88.89	50	0.88
Faecal calprotectin	100	16.67	0.9	100	83.33	1	100	66.67	0.86	100	66.67	1
C-reactive protein	100	12.50	0.72	90.91	50	0.88	100	37.50	0.71	100	37.50	0.88

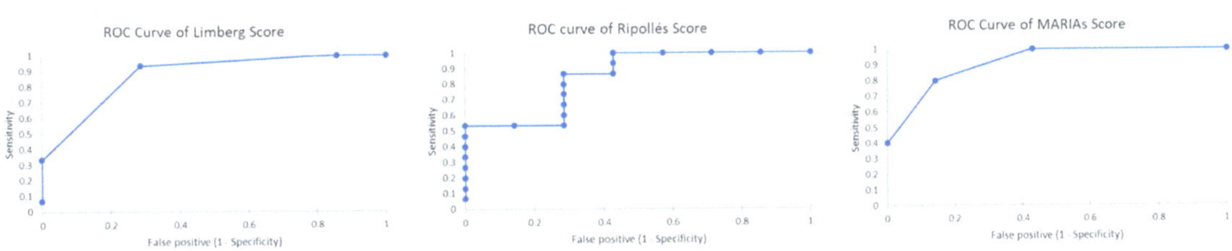

Figure 4. Receiver operating characteristic curves of Limberg score, Ripollés score and MaRIAs score for the diagnosis of active CD using Crohn's disease activity index as reference method.

Compared to HBI (Table 2), Limberg score presented a sensitivity of 83.33% and a specificity of 75.00% (AUC = 0.958) for the evaluation of CD activity and Ripollés and MaRIAs scores had a sensitivity of 88.89% and a specificity of 50.00% (AUC = 0.805 for Ripollés score, respectively, 0.888 for MaRIAs score). In comparison, the score proposed by Medellin-Kowalewski et al. [10] had a sensitivity of 100.00% and a specificity of 50.00% (AUC = 0.805) (Figure 5).

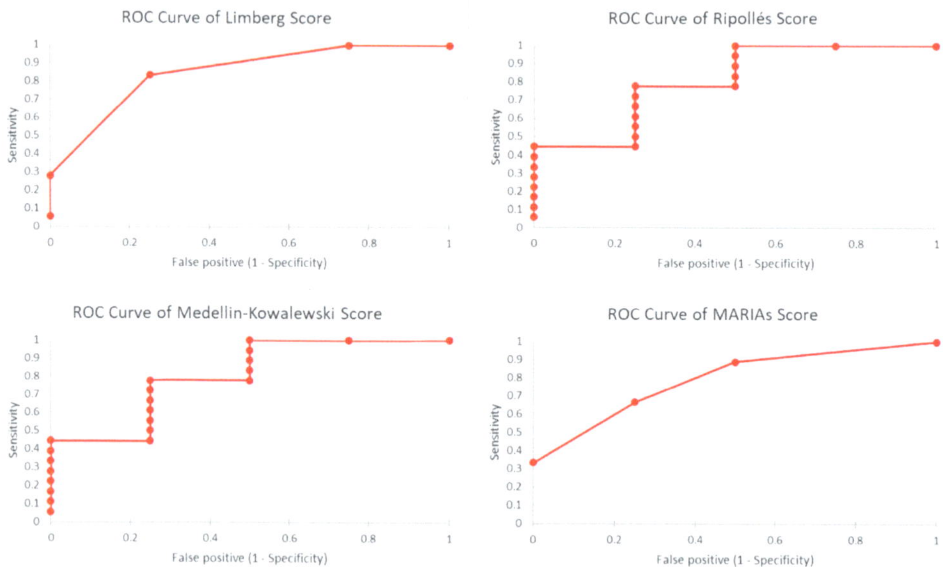

Figure 5. Receiver operating characteristic curves of Limberg score, Ripollés score and MaRIAs score for the diagnosis of active CD using Harvey–Bradshaw Index as reference method.

Regarding the use of laboratory tests as reference methods, based on the results of faecal calprotectin (Table 2), the Limberg score was characterised by a sensitivity of 100.00% and a specificity of 83.33% (AUC = 1), and in the case of MaRIAs score, a sensitivity of 100.00% and a specificity of 66.67% (AUC = 1) were achieved for the differentiation of active forms of the disease. The results of the sensitivity and specificity of the imaging tests for assessing CD activity using the CRP levels as the reference method are shown in Table 2 (Appendix A Table A3).

Pearson correlation coefficient values between clinical severity scores, laboratory tests and results of cross-sectional imaging techniques are shown in Table 3 (a more detailed table version can be consulted in the Appendix A, Tables A4 and A5). Our study demonstrated a good correlation between CDAI and Limberg score (r = 0.667, 95% confidence interval (CI) [0.46, 0.8], $p < 0.001$) and between CDAI and MaRIAs score (r = 0.614, 95% CI [0.39, 0.77], $p < 0.001$) and a reasonable correlation between CDAI and Medellin-Kowalewski score (r = 0.537, 95% CI [0.29, 0.72], $p < 0.001$). Between HBI and imaging investigations, the results demonstrated reasonable correlations for most of the evaluated scores, the highest Pearson correlation coefficient value being obtained for HBI and MaRIAs score (r = 0.594, 95% CI [0.36, 0.76], $p < 0.001$). In addition, the study identified a good correlation between faecal calprotectin values and MaRIAs score (r = 0.697, 95% CI [0.46, 0.84], $p < 0.001$). In the case of CRP, only weak correlations with the scores assessed were demonstrated.

Table 3. Correlation values and significance of results in comparison between clinical activity scores (Crohn's disease activity index/Harvey–Bradshaw Index), laboratory tests (fecal calprotectin/C-reactive protein), IUS + CEUS and MRI.

	US—Maximal Wall Thickness		Limberg Score		Medellin-Kowalewski Score		MaRIAs Score	
	r	*p*-Value	r	*p*-Value	r	*p*-Value	r	*p*-Value
Crohn's disease activity index	0.502	<0.001	0.667	<0.001	0.537	<0.001	0.614	<0.001
Harvey–Bradshaw Index	0.352	<0.05	0.468	<0.01	0.459	<0.01	0.594	<0.001
Faecal calprotectin	0.419	<0.05	0.446	<0.05	0.159	>0.05	0.697	<0.001
C-reactive protein	0.195	>0.05	0.238	>0.05	0.298	>0.05	0.395	<0.05

r—Pearson correlation coefficient.

4. Discussion

A consensus has yet to be established regarding the treatment goals in CD. Both achieving clinical remission and mucosal healing are discussed. There is often a discrepancy between the symptoms reported by CD patients and the results of laboratory tests or imaging investigations. Colonoscopy is currently an indispensable method for monitoring patients with CD. One of the most used endoscopic scores in clinical practice is represented by the Simple Endoscopic Score for Crohn's Disease (SES-CD) (a score between 0–2 suggests inactive disease) [39]. Results are conflicting regarding the correlation of SES-CD with various clinical severity scores, such as the CDAI, with some studies suggesting a weak correlation between the two methods [40,41]. The levels of some inflammatory biomarkers, such as CRP and faecal calprotectin, seem to show good correlations with the endoscopic activity of colonic or ileocolonic CD, but not in patients with lesions limited to the ileum [19,42–44]. Therefore, such biomarkers should be used as initial methods to identify patients who require more complex investigations but often find utility in monitoring disease activity and response to drug treatment [5]. A meta-analysis that included 13 studies (1471 patients with IBD) demonstrated that a faecal calprotectin threshold value of 250 μg/g presents a specificity of 82% for identifying active forms of IBD, which is superior to values corresponding to a threshold of 100 μg/g or 50 μg/g (specificity of 66% and 60%, respectively) [45]. However, faecal calprotectin appears to be associated with a more remarkable ability to assess disease activity in ulcerative colitis than CD [45].

The ileum cannot always be explored endoscopically. A study evaluating 189 patients with CD using ileocolonoscopy and CTE found that 53.7% of patients with normal endoscopic aspects had an active CD of the small bowel [46]. For this reason, all newly diagnosed CD patients should benefit from small bowel evaluation by complementary radiological methods, such as MRE, CTE or IUS, to assess the disease's extent, activity and the presence of complications [47].

Cross-sectional imaging techniques provide information on the bowel wall and surrounding tissues, thus supplying a superior disease phenotype classification [4]. Studies have demonstrated similar sensitivity and specificity for CT and MRI to diagnose small bowel lesions [14,48,49]. Since most CD patients are diagnosed at young ages due to the lack of ionising radiation, MRI is preferable if this investigation is available [4,47]. The MRI examination of the pelvis is instrumental in describing the anatomy of perianal fistulas as an auxiliary method to the examination under anaesthesia (EUA) of the anorectal region by an experienced surgeon, currently representing the method of choice for the evaluation of perianal CD [4]. In addition to the diagnostic role, MRI can also be used to assess CD activity. In this regard, several scores have been developed, some of which have been validated in clinical practice [50–53]. Among the most used is the Magnetic Resonance Index of Activity (MaRIA), which shows a good correlation with the Crohn's Disease Endoscopic Index of Severity (CDEIS) [51,54].

In recent years there has been a growing interest in using IUS and CEUS as alternatives to MRI for evaluating CD patients. IUS is a non-irradiating method, being particularly useful in the case of young patients. In addition, it is cheap and widely available, readily accepted by patients, and thus can be repeated as often as needed. It has the disadvantage of being operator-dependent, and experience in evaluating the digestive tract is limited [55]. A study evaluating the learning curve of IUS for the evaluation of patients with IBD concluded that at least 150 supervised examinations are required to acquire proficiency in IUS, with physicians already experienced in abdominal ultrasonography developing these skills more quickly than those without experience [56]. Most patients prefer IUS to MRE. MRE examination is associated with more significant discomfort and longer post-procedural recovery than IUS, especially in young or emotional patients [57]. However, the discomfort associated with the procedure seems to matter less than the diagnostic accuracy of the investigation [57]. Several meta-analyses have demonstrated similar results between IUS, CTE or MRE, with sensitivity and specificity between 85–95% regarding the diagnosis of CD [11–15]. IUS seems inferior to MRI for establishing the extension of the disease in the small bowel and characterising proximal lesions or lesions localised in the pelvis [7,14]. Still, the diagnostic accuracy of complications such as stenoses, fistulas or abscesses is similar between the methods [7,14]. In our study, most patients had lesions limited to the terminal ileum, which is why no great difficulties were identified in evaluating the segments affected by the inflammatory process by ultrasonography. CD's most frequent and constant ultrasonographic feature is the thickening of the intestinal wall above the threshold value of 3–4 mm, directly proportional to the disease severity [58]. A meta-analysis by Fraquelli et al. [59] demonstrated that, although the BWT threshold of 4 mm has a lower sensitivity than the value of 3 mm, it is associated with a higher specificity for Crohn's disease. Numerous studies have demonstrated a good correlation between BWT assessed by ultrasonography and disease activity assessed by colonoscopy [37,59,60]. Increased BWT and loss of parietal layering, identified via IUS, appear to be associated with a higher risk of surgery in CD patients [37,61,62].

Recently, there has been increasing talk of transmural healing (TH) as a therapeutic goal in CD [63]. Achieving TH appears to be associated with a more favourable long-term outcome than mucosal healing [64]. For this reason, some authors propose that TH represents the main therapeutic target in CD [63]. At the moment, there is yet to be a universally valid definition of this term. TH can be assessed through MRE, CTE or IUS. Parameters used to define TH could include BWT and parietal vascularisation assessed by CDI or bowel wall enhancement of contrast agents [63]. However, using BWT as the sole criterion for defining TH seems insufficient, as this could result from fibrosis, which is why additional evaluation of the vascular pattern is recommended [63,65]. CDI can evaluate the inflammatory activity of the bowel wall by assessing the vascular signal provided by the larger blood vessels [23,25,66]. According to the classic Limberg classification, the degree of the colour Doppler signal is usually measured at the level of the thickened bowel wall (stage ≥ 2), but modified versions of this score have been proposed that evaluate the presence of the signal also at the level of the normal looking bowel wall, considering punctiform Doppler signal as non-pathological or uncertain [67–70]. In our study, the colour Doppler signal was identified only in association with bowel wall thickening of >4 mm, consistent with the classic Limberg score. Most likely, these modified variants of the classification were proposed to be adapted to modern ultrasonographic systems that associate a better image resolution. Using contrast agents during CEUS allows a superior evaluation of the inflammation by assessing the bowel wall vascularisation at the microcirculatory level, the neoangiogenesis of the bowel wall is characteristic of the active inflammation associated with CD [10,29,71,72].

Numerous studies, including those that provided the scores used in our research, have demonstrated a good correlation between disease severity assessed by cross-sectional imaging techniques and endoscopic CD activity [10,26,29,31–34,73,74]. Ripollés et al. [31] confirm that the primary ultrasonographic criterion for evaluating CD activity is represented by the bowel wall enhancement after intravenous administration of contrast agents, describing a sensitivity of 92% and a specificity of 86.4% for this parameter. In addition, TH also seems to show a good correlation with faecal calprotectin and CRP levels [63]. Cerrillo et al. [75] described a sensitivity of 90% and a specificity of 74%, corresponding to a faecal calprotectin cut-off level of 166.50 μg/g for the diagnosis of inflammation in ileal CD, using MRE as the reference method. Regarding the correlation with clinical activity scores, the results available in the literature are contradictory. Recently, Yamanashi et al. [76] described a strong correlation between an ultrasonographic score (based on BWT, parietal stratification, presence of stenoses, colour Doppler signal and mesenteric fat appearance) proposed for assessing the severity of CD and CDAI, even superior to the correlation established for SES-CD and CDAI. Also, Yiğit et al. [74] identified a good correlation between Limberg score, bowel wall thickness and mesenteric inflammation assessed through IUS or CTE and clinical activity scores (CDAI and HBI). However, other studies have suggested that quantitative measurement of bowel wall vascularisation utilising CEUS or MRI shows a weak or no correlation with clinical activity scores or laboratory tests, such as CRP levels [77,78].

Our study aimed to identify the correlation between various scores proposed in the literature for assessing CD activity by IUS + CEUS or MRI and clinical activity scores (CDAI, HBI) or specific laboratory tests (faecal calprotectin, CRP). The scores were selected according to the degree of difficulty of their calculation, the simplicity and the quickness of obtaining a result being essential elements in everyday clinical practice. Time optimisation could be achieved by integrating dedicated quantitative analysis software, such as the one used in our study, in ultrasonography systems, without the need for image recording and subsequent processing on other devices. Compared to CDAI, the best correlation was identified for the Limberg score, followed by MaRIAs score, the simple US score and then the score proposed by Medellin-Kowalewski and colleagues. A sensitivity of 93.33% and a specificity of 71.43% (AUC = 0.98) were demonstrated in the case of the Limberg score for differentiating patients with active forms of CD from those in remission and for MaRIAs score a sensitivity of 100.00% and a specificity of 57.14% (AUC = 0.97). BWT showed a reasonable correlation with CDAI but was still inferior to the Limberg score, reinforcing the idea that the additional assessment of the vascular pattern provides superior information for the evaluation of disease activity. Regarding HBI, the best correlation was observed for MaRIAs score, followed by the Limberg score, the Medellin-Kowalewski score, and the simple US score. Faecal calprotectin showed the best correlation also with MaRIAs score. Still, in the case of CRP, there was only a weak correlation for all evaluated scores, which shows that more than this investigation is needed to assess the disease activity.

Other authors also confirmed similar results for MaRIAs score. Roseira et al. [79] demonstrated a strong correlation between this score and faecal calprotectin ($R = 0.88$, $p < 0.001$) in patients with ileal CD. Regarding CEUS, in our study, the score proposed by Medellin-Kowalewski et al. which uses the PE parameter showed reasonable correlations with clinical activity scores but only a weak correlation with inflammatory biomarkers. Also, Freitas et al. [80] reported a good correlation between PE and HBI, with PE being significantly different in patients with clinically active disease (HBI $\geq$ 5) compared to those with inactive forms. In contrast, no statistically significant correlations were identified with CRP or faecal calprotectin levels. For that reason, although CEUS appears to be a promising method, there are currently insufficient data to recommend its use as a first-line investigation.

Taking an overview, we can see that the assessment of CD activity by MRI using MaRIAs score shows overall the best correlations with clinical severity scores and inflammatory biomarkers, especially CDAI and faecal calprotectin. Favourable results were also obtained for the ultrasonographic scores, particularly the Limberg score, which is even superior to MaRIAs score in terms of specificity for diagnosing active forms of CD, according to the reference methods used. Therefore, following international guidelines, we suggest using MRI for the initial evaluation of patients and, subsequently, IUS for their follow-up.

The main limitation of our study concerns the small number of patients evaluated, so the results obtained may not be reliable in the case of larger groups. Thus, additional multicenter studies that include more subjects are needed. At the same time, another limitation could be that we used only one type of contrast agent during CEUS, especially since in the study conducted by Medellin-Kowalewski et al., another contrast agent was used. Thus, there could be a discrepancy between the PE values obtained in our research and the cut-off value proposed by the authors of the score. It should also be emphasised that this threshold could be a device-dependent parameter, possibly obtaining different results when using different settings and ultrasound systems. Ileocolonoscopy remains the gold standard for diagnosing and monitoring patients with CD. Therefore, another limitation of our study is that we could not compare the results of the assessed imaging investigations with the endoscopic activity scores in the case of all patients included. It should be noted that only 26 of 44 patients agreed to be evaluated by ileocolonoscopy. Referring to this number of patients, the best correlation with SES-CD was identified for MaRIAs score (r = 0.562, 95% CI [0.22, 0.78], $p < 0.01$), then for the Limberg score (r = 0.382, 95% CI [−0.0056, 0.67], $p > 0.05$), but only a very weak correlation was observed for the other evaluated scores. Regarding the accuracy of diagnosing active forms of the disease using SES-CD as a reference method, for MaRIAs score, a sensitivity of 100.00% and a specificity of 66.67% (AUC = 0.933) were established. In comparison, the Limberg score had a sensitivity of 90.00% and a specificity of 66.67% (AUC = 0.667).

Considering that more and more authors propose transmural healing as the primary goal of Crohn's disease therapy, we can conclude that cross-sectional imaging techniques represent viable methods for evaluating disease activity. Thus, the prognosis of patients with Crohn's disease could be improved by monitoring with the help of non-invasive imaging investigations, widely available and easily tolerated by patients, such as ultrasonography. Although magnetic resonance does not appear to be superior to ultrasonography in terms of accuracy for differentiating active forms of Crohn's disease from those in remission, the results of our study suggest that magnetic resonance associates a better correlation with clinical severity scores and faecal calprotectin levels compared to ultrasonography. However, more studies are needed to validate these results.

Author Contributions: Conceptualization, R.-C.S., S.I., D.N.F. and L.M.F.; methodology, R.-C.S., S.I., D.N.F., D.-I.G., L.M.F. and I.-A.G.; software, R.-C.S., V.-M.S. and B.S.U.; validation, S.I., D.-I.G., I.-A.G., I.R. and T.C.; formal analysis, R.-C.S., V.-M.S., D.N.F., B.S.U. and L.M.F.; investigation, R.-C.S., S.I. and L.M.F.; resources, S.I., D.-I.G., I.-A.G. and T.C.; data curation, R.-C.S., D.N.F., V.-M.S., B.S.U. and L.M.F.; writing—original draft preparation, R.-C.S. and L.M.F.; writing—review and editing, S.I., D.N.F. and B.S.U.; visualization, R.-C.S., S.I. and L.M.F.; supervision, D.-I.G., I.-A.G., I.R. and T.C.; project administration, S.I., D.-I.G. and I.-A.G. All authors have read and agreed to the published version of the manuscript.

Funding: The article processing charges were funded by the University of Medicine and Pharmacy of Craiova, Romania.

Institutional Review Board Statement: The study was conducted in accordance with the Declaration of Helsinki and approved by the Ethics Committee of the University of Medicine and Pharmacy of Craiova, Romania (No. 93/28.09.2020).

Informed Consent Statement: Informed consent was obtained from all subjects involved in the study.

Data Availability Statement: The data used to support the findings of this study are available from the corresponding author upon reasonable request.

Conflicts of Interest: The authors declare no conflict of interest.

Appendix A

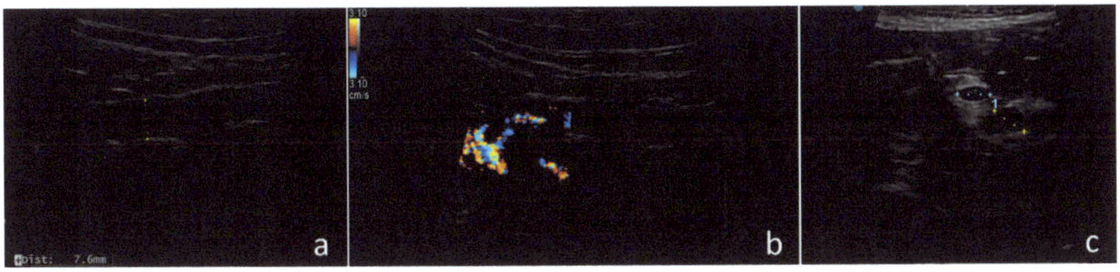

Figure A1. (**a**) Thickened wall (7.6 mm) with normal bowel wall stratification loss. (**b**) Colour Doppler imaging of affected segment shows abundant mural blood flow—Limberg score = grade 3. (**c**) The presence of enlarged lymph nodes.

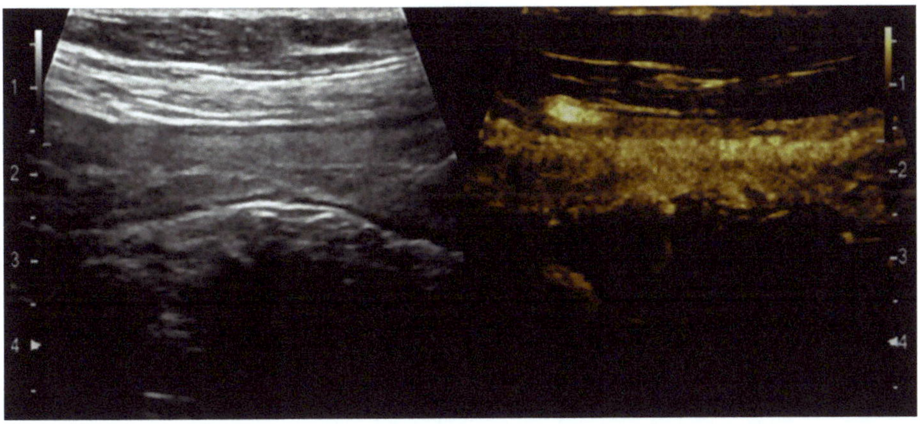

Figure A2. Dual-screen ultrasound representation of an abnormal segment of bowel, in grey-scale imaging (B-mode) (**left**) and contrast-enhanced ultrasound (CEUS) of the matching segment (**right**). CEUS shows transmural enhancement.

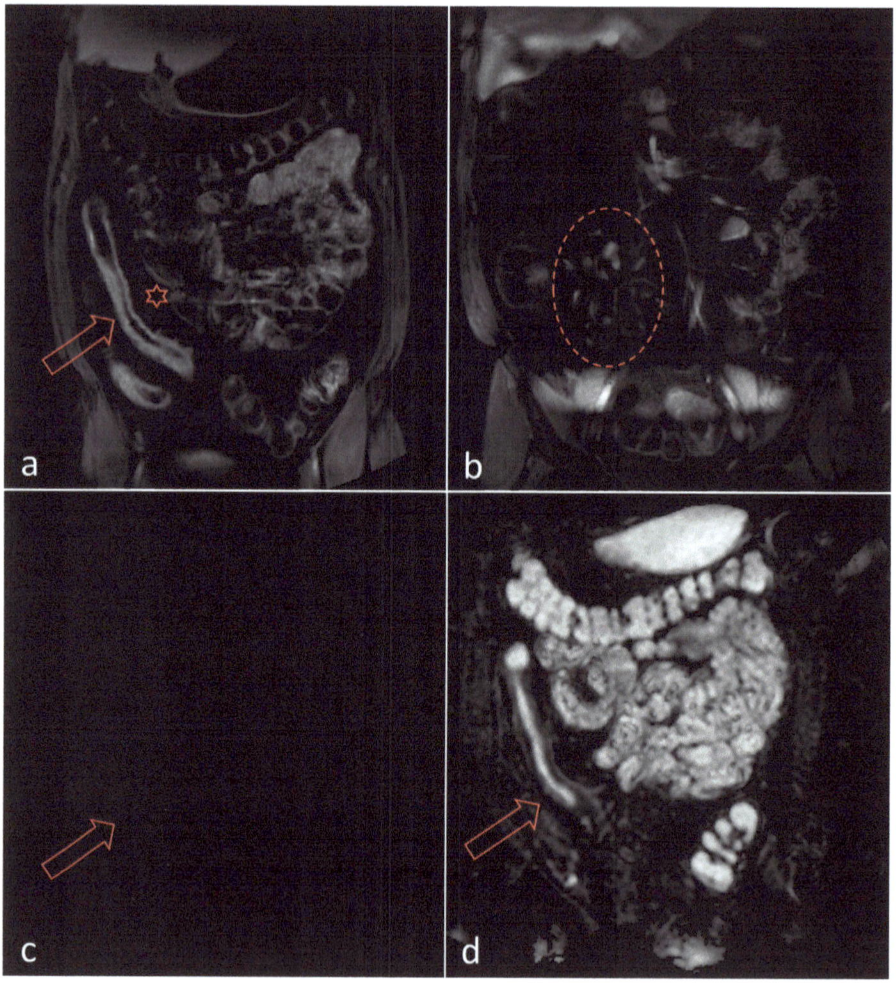

Figure A3. MRE—T1 postcontrast phase (venous phase), coronal plane: (**a**) the arrow indicates an increased wall thickness affecting the terminal ileum continuously, with increased homogeneous contrast uptake and engorged vasa recta in the affected region (star). (**b**) The area inside the circle highlights the presence of multiple enlarged lymph nodes located near the affected terminal ileum. The terminal ileum wall demonstrates restricted diffusion, seen as high signal intensity on the DWI sequence (**c**) and low signal intensity on the ADC map (**d**).

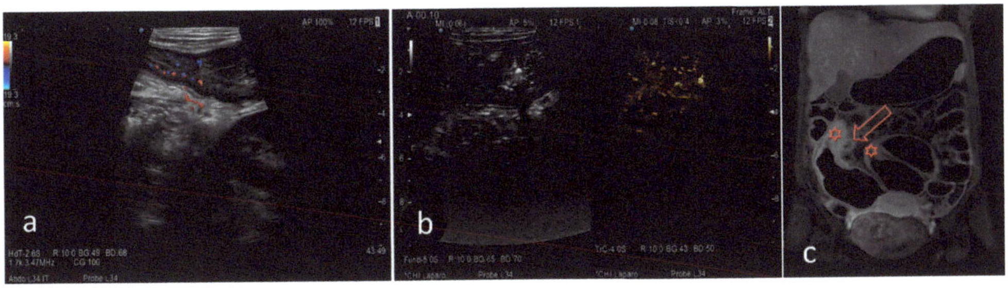

Figure A4. IUS and MRE aspects in a patient with a moderate form of stricturing Crohn's disease (CDAI = 339; HBI = 9; faecal calprotectin = 2190 µg/g; CRP = 30.51 mg/L). (**a**) IUS: Thickened wall, with typical bowel wall stratification loss, resulting in stenosis with dilation of the intestinal lumen upstream of the obstruction. Colour Doppler imaging highlights the presence of the colour flow signal in both the bowel wall and surrounding mesenteric fat—Limberg score = 4. (**b**) CEUS shows transmural enhancement, suggesting an inflammatory stricture. (**c**) MRE: T1 postcontrast phase (venous phase), coronal plane—the stars highlight stenotic areas with an increased wall thickness affecting the ileum discontinuously, resulting in dilated normal ileum segments between the affected areas. The arrow indicates a possible abscess near one of the affected ileum segments.

Table A1. Disease activity based on results of clinical activity scores, laboratory tests and imaging techniques.

Parameters Evaluated	Disease's Activity—No. of Patients (%)			
	Inactive	Active		
Maximal wall thickness (mm)	<4 mm: 2 (4.54%)	Mild (4.0–6.0): 10 (22.73%)	Moderate (6.1–8.0): 26 (59.09%)	Severe (≥8.1): 6 (13.63%)
Limberg Score	Grade 0 and Grade 1: 12 (27.27%)	Grade 2: 22 (50%)	Grade 3: 8 (18.18%)	Grade 4: 2 (4.54%)
Ripollés Score	Inactive disease < 8.38: 8 (18.18%)	Active disease > 8.38: 36 (81.81%)		
Simple CEUS Score	Inactive disease < 8.38: 6 (13.63%)	Active disease > 8.38: 38 (86.36%)		
Simple US score	Inactive disease < 5.5: 2 (4.54%)	Active disease > 5.5: 42 (95.45%)		
Medellin-Kowalewski Score	Inactive < 18.2 dB: 4 (9.09%)	Mild to moderate 18.2–22.8 dB: 8 (18.18%)	Moderate to severe >22.8 dB: 32 (72.72%)	
MaRIAs	Inactive < 1: 8 (18.18%)	Active disease ≥ 1: 10 (22.72%)	Severe lesions ≥ 2: 26 (59.09%)	
Crohn's disease activity index	Remission (<150): 14 (31.81%)	Mild (150–220): 10 (22.72%)	Moderate (220–450): 20 (45.45%)	Severe (>450): 0 (0%)
Harvey–Bradshaw Index	Remission (<5): 8 (18.18%)	Mild (5–7): 16 (36.36%)	Moderate (8–16): 20 (45.45%)	Severe (>16): 0 (0%)
Faecal calprotectin (µg/g)	Inactive (<250 µg/g): 16 (36.36%)	Active (> 250 µg/g): 28 (63.63%)		
CRP (mg/L)	Inactive (<10 mg/L): 19 (43.18%)	Active (>10 mg/L): 25 (56.81%)		

Table A2. Assessment of the quality of IUS + CEUS and MRE in detecting active forms of Crohn's disease using Crohn's disease activity index and Harvey–Bradshaw Index as reference methods.

Parameters	Sensitivity (%)	Specificity (%)	AUC	Positive Predictive Value (%)	Negative Predictive Value (%)
US—maximal wall thickness vs. CDAI	100%	14.29%	0.876	71.43%	100%
Limberg Score vs. CDAI	93.33%	71.43%	0.980	87.50%	83.33%
Ripollés Score vs. CDAI	100%	57.14%	0.847	83.33%	100%
Simple CEUS Score vs. CDAI	100%	42.86%	0.847	78.95%	100%
Simple US Score vs. CDAI	100%	14.29%	0.895	71.43%	100%
Medellin-Kowalewski Score vs. CDAI	100%	28.57%	0.828	75%	100%
MaRIAs Score vs. CDAI	100%	57.14%	0.971	83.33%	100%
US—maximal wall thickness vs. HBI	100%	25%	0.888	85.71%	100%
Limberg Score vs. HBI	83.33%	75%	0.958	93.75%	50%
Ripollés Score vs. HBI	88.89%	50%	0.805	88.89%	50%
Simple CEUS Score vs. HBI	94.44%	50%	0.805	89.47%	66.67%
Simple US Score vs. HBI	100%	25%	0.916	85.71%	100%
Medellin-Kowalewski Score vs. HBI	100%	50%	0.805	90%	100%
MaRIAs Score vs. HBI	88.89%	50%	0.888	88.89%	50%

Table A3. Assessment of the quality of IUS + CEUS and MRE in detecting active forms of Crohn's disease using faecal calprotectin test and C-reactive protein test as reference methods.

Parameters	Sensitivity (%)	Specificity (%)	AUC	Positive Predictive Value (%)	Negative Predictive Value (%)
US—maximal wall thickness vs. FC	100%	16.67%	0.9	66.67%	100%
Limberg Score vs. FC	100%	83.33%	**1**	90.91%	100%
Ripollés Score vs. FC	100%	66.67%	0.866	83.33%	100%
Simple CEUS Score vs. FC	100%	50%	0.866	76.92%	100%
Simple US Score vs. FC	100%	16.67%	0.9	66.67%	100%
Medellin-Kowalewski Score vs. FC	100%	33.33%	0.833	71.43%	100%
MaRIAs Score vs. FC	100%	66.67%	**1**	83.33%	100%
US—maximal wall thickness vs. CRP	100%	12.50%	0.727	61.11%	100%
Limberg Score vs. CRP	90.91%	50%	0.886	71.43%	80%
Ripollés Score vs. CRP	100%	37.50%	0.715	68.75%	100%

Table A3. *Cont.*

Parameters	Sensitivity (%)	Specificity (%)	AUC	Positive Predictive Value (%)	Negative Predictive Value (%)
Simple CEUS Score vs. CRP	100%	25%	0.715	25%	100%
Simple US Score vs. CRP	100%	12.50%	0.750	61.11%	100%
Medellin-Kowalewski Score vs. CRP	100%	12.50%	0.715	61.11%	100%
MaRIAs Score vs. CRP	100%	37.50%	0.886	68.75%	100%

FC—faecal calprotectin; CRP—C-reactive protein.

Table A4. Correlation values and significance of results in comparison between clinical activity scores (Crohn's disease activity index/Harvey–Bradshaw Index), IUS + CEUS and MRI.

Parameters	Pearson Correlation Coefficient	95% Confidence Interval	*p*-Value
CDAI vs. US—maximal wall thickness	0.502	[0.24, 0.7]	<0.001
CDAI vs. Limberg score	0.667	[0.46, 0.8]	<0.001
CDAI vs. Ripollés score	0.320	[0.026, 0.56]	<0.05
CDAI vs. Simple CEUS score	0.324	[0.031, 0.57]	<0.05
CDAI vs. Simple US score	0.598	[0.37, 0.76]	<0.001
CDAI vs. Medellin-Kowalewski score	0.537	[0.29, 0.72]	<0.001
CDAI vs. MaRIAs	0.614	[0.39, 0.77]	<0.001
HBI vs. US—maximal wall thickness	0.352	[0.062, 0.59]	<0.05
HBI vs. Limberg score	0.468	[0.2, 0.67]	<0.01
HBI vs. Ripollés score	0.184	[−0.12, 0.46]	>0.05
HBI vs. Simple CEUS score	0.186	[−0.12, 0.46]	>0.05
HBI vs. Simple US score	0.420	[0.14, 0.64]	<0.01
HBI vs. Medellin-Kowalewski score	0.459	[0.19, 0.67]	<0.01
HBI vs. MaRIAs	0.594	[0.36, 0.76]	<0.001

Table A5. Correlation values and significance of results in comparison between laboratory tests (faecal calprotectin/C-reactive protein), IUS + CEUS and MRI.

Parameters	Pearson Correlation Coefficient	95% Confidence Interval	*p*-Value
FC vs. US—maximal wall thickness	0.419	[0.083, 0.67]	<0.05
FC vs. Limberg score	0.446	[0.12, 0.69]	<0.05
FC vs. Ripollés score	0.076	[−0.28, 0.41]	>0.05
FC vs. Simple CEUS score	0.079	[−0.28, 0.42]	>0.05
FC vs. Simple US score	0.395	[0.054, 0.65]	<0.05
FC vs. Medellin-Kowalewski score	0.159	[−0.2, 0.48]	>0.05

Table A5. *Cont.*

Parameters	Pearson Correlation Coefficient	95% Confidence Interval	p-Value
FC vs. MaRIAs	0.697	[0.46, 0.84]	<0.001
CRP vs. US—maximal wall thickness	0.195	[−0.13, 0.48]	>0.05
CRP vs. Limberg score	0.238	[−0.088, 0.52]	>0.05
CRP vs. Ripollés score	0.030	[−0.29, 0.35]	>0.05
CRP vs. Simple CEUS score	0.031	[−0.29, 0.35]	>0.05
CRP vs. Simple US score	0.213	[−0.11, 0.5]	>0.05
CRP vs. Medellin-Kowalewski score	0.298	[−0.023, 0.56]	>0.05
CRP vs. MaRIAs	0.395	[0.087, 0.64]	<0.05

FC—faecal calprotectin; CRP—C-reactive protein.

References

1. Freeman, H.J. Natural history and long-term clinical course of Crohn's disease. *World J. Gastroenterol.* **2014**, *20*, 31–36. [CrossRef] [PubMed]
2. Freeman, H.J. Application of the Montreal classification for Crohn's disease to a single clinician database of 1015 patients. *Can. J. Gastroenterol. Hepatol.* **2007**, *21*, 363–366. [CrossRef] [PubMed]
3. Odes, S.; Vardi, H.; Friger, M.; Wolters, F.; Hoie, O.; Moum, B.; Bernklev, T.; Yona, H.; Russel, M.; Munkholm, P.; et al. Effect of phenotype on health care costs in Crohn's disease: A European study using the Montreal classification. *J. Crohns Colitis.* **2007**, *1*, 87–96. [CrossRef] [PubMed]
4. Lamb, C.A.; Kennedy, N.A.; Raine, T.; Hendy, P.A.; Smith, P.J.; Limdi, J.K.; Hayee, B.; Lomer, M.C.E.; Parkes, G.C.; Selinger, C.; et al. British Society of Gastroenterology consensus guidelines on the management of inflammatory bowel disease in adults. *Gut* **2019**, *68* (Suppl. S3), s1–s106, Erratum in *Gut* **2021**, *70*, 1. [CrossRef] [PubMed]
5. D'Incà, R.; Caccaro, R. Measuring disease activity in Crohn's disease: What is currently available to the clinician. *Clin. Exp. Gastroenterol.* **2014**, *7*, 151–161. [CrossRef]
6. Dambha, F.; Tanner, J.; Carroll, N. Diagnostic imaging in Crohn's disease: What is the new gold standard? *Best. Pract. Res. Clin. Gastroenterol.* **2014**, *28*, 421–436. [CrossRef]
7. Taylor, S.A.; Mallett, S.; Bhatnagar, G.; Baldwin-Cleland, R.; Bloom, S.; Gupta, A.; Hamlin, P.J.; Hart, A.L.; Higginson, A.; Jacobs, I.; et al. Diagnostic accuracy of magnetic resonance enterography and small bowel ultrasound for the extent and activity of newly diagnosed and relapsed Crohn's disease (METRIC): A multicentre trial. *Lancet Gastroenterol. Hepatol.* **2018**, *3*, 548–558. [CrossRef]
8. Fiorino, G.; Bonifacio, C.; Malesci, A.; Balzarini, L.; Danese, S. MRI in Crohn's disease--current and future clinical applications. *Nat. Rev. Gastroenterol. Hepatol.* **2011**, *9*, 23–31. [CrossRef]
9. Lichtenstein, G.R.; Hanauer, S.B.; Sandborn, W.J. Practice Parameters Committee of American College of Gastroenterology. Management of Crohn's disease in adults. *Am. J. Gastroenterol.* **2009**, *104*, 465–484. [CrossRef]
10. Medellin-Kowalewski, A.; Wilkens, R.; Wilson, A.; Ruan, J.; Wilson, S.R. Quantitative Contrast-Enhanced Ultrasound Parameters in Crohn Disease: Their Role in Disease Activity Determination With Ultrasound. *AJR Am. J. Roentgenol.* **2016**, *206*, 64–73. [CrossRef]
11. Horsthuis, K.; Bipat, S.; Bennink, R.J.; Stoker, J. Inflammatory bowel disease diagnosed with, U.S.; MR, scintigraphy, and CT: Meta-analysis of prospective studies. *Radiology* **2008**, *247*, 64–79. [CrossRef] [PubMed]
12. Dong, J.; Wang, H.; Zhao, J.; Zhu, W.; Zhang, L.; Gong, J.; Li, Y.; Gu, L.; Li, J. Ultrasound as a diagnostic tool in detecting active Crohn's disease: A meta-analysis of prospective studies. *Eur. Radiol.* **2014**, *24*, 26–33. [CrossRef]
13. Liu, W.; Liu, J.; Xiao, W.; Luo, G. A Diagnostic Accuracy Meta-analysis of CT and MRI for the Evaluation of Small Bowel Crohn Disease. *Acad. Radiol.* **2017**, *24*, 1216–1225. [CrossRef] [PubMed]
14. Panés, J.; Bouzas, R.; Chaparro, M.; García-Sánchez, V.; Gisbert, J.P.; de Guereñu, B.M.; Mendoza, J.L.; Paredes, J.M.; Quiroga, S.; Ripollés, T.; et al. Systematic review: The use of ultrasonography, computed tomography and magnetic resonance imaging for the diagnosis, assessment of activity and abdominal complications of Crohn's disease. *Aliment. Pharmacol. Ther.* **2011**, *34*, 125–145. [CrossRef] [PubMed]
15. Greenup, A.J.; Bressler, B.; Rosenfeld, G. Medical Imaging in Small Bowel Crohn's Disease-Computer Tomography Enterography, Magnetic Resonance Enterography, and Ultrasound: "Which One Is the Best for What?". *Inflamm. Bowel Dis.* **2016**, *22*, 1246–1261. [CrossRef]
16. Best, W.R.; Becktel, J.M.; Singleton, J.W.; Kern, F., Jr. Development of a Crohn's disease activity index. National Cooperative Crohn's Disease Study. *Gastroenterology* **1976**, *70*, 439–444. [CrossRef]

17. Harvey, R.F.; Bradshaw, J.M. A simple index of Crohn's-disease activity. *Lancet* **1980**, *1*, 514. [CrossRef] [PubMed]
18. Vermeire, S.; Van Assche, G.; Rutgeerts, P. Laboratory markers in IBD: Useful, magic, or unnecessary toys? *Gut* **2006**, *55*, 426–431. [CrossRef]
19. Chen, P.; Zhou, G.; Lin, J.; Li, L.; Zeng, Z.; Chen, M.; Zhang, S. Serum Biomarkers for Inflammatory Bowel Disease. *Front. Med.* **2020**, *7*, 123. [CrossRef]
20. Chamouard, P.; Richert, Z.; Meyer, N.; Rahmi, G.; Baumann, R. Diagnostic value of C-reactive protein for predicting activity level of Crohn's disease. *Clin. Gastroenterol. Hepatol.* **2006**, *4*, 882–887. [CrossRef]
21. Panes, J.; Bouhnik, Y.; Reinisch, W.; Stoker, J.; Taylor, S.; Baumgart, D.; Danese, S.; Halligan, S.; Marincek, B.; Matos, C.; et al. Imaging techniques for assessment of inflammatory bowel disease: Joint ECCO and ESGAR evidence-based consensus guidelines. *J. Crohns Colitis.* **2013**, *7*, 556–585. [CrossRef]
22. Parente, F.; Greco, S.; Molteni, M.; Cucino, C.; Maconi, G.; Sampietro, G.M.; Danelli, P.G.; Cristaldi, M.; Bianco, R.; Gallus, S.; et al. Role of early ultrasound in detecting inflammatory intestinal disorders and identifying their anatomical location within the bowel. *Aliment. Pharmacol. Ther.* **2003**, *18*, 1009–1016. [CrossRef] [PubMed]
23. Limberg, B. Diagnostik von chronisch-entzündlichen Darmerkrankungen durch Sonographie [Diagnosis of chronic inflammatory bowel disease by ultrasonography]. *Z. Gastroenterol.* **1999**, *37*, 495–508. [PubMed]
24. Esteban, J.M.; Maldonado, L.; Sanchiz, V.; Minguez, M.; Benages, A. Activity of Crohn's disease assessed by color Doppler ultrasound analysis of the affected loops. *Eur. Radiol.* **2001**, *11*, 1423–1428. [CrossRef]
25. Spalinger, J.; Patriquin, H.; Miron, M.-C.; Marx, G.; Herzog, D.; Dubois, J.; Dubinsky, M.; Seidman, E.G. Doppler US in patients with crohn disease: Vessel density in the diseased bowel reflects disease activity. *Radiology* **2000**, *217*, 787–791. [CrossRef]
26. Bodily, K.D.; Fletcher, J.G.; Solem, C.A.; Johnson, C.D.; Fidler, J.L.; Barlow, J.M.; Bruesewitz, M.R.; McCollough, C.H.; Sandborn, W.J.; Loftus, E.V.; et al. Crohn Disease: Mural attenuation and thickness at contrast-enhanced CT Enterography—Correlation with endoscopic and histologic findings of inflammation. *Radiology* **2006**, *238*, 505–516. [CrossRef] [PubMed]
27. Taylor, S.A.; Punwani, S.; Rodriguez-Justo, M.; Bainbridge, A.; Greenhalgh, R.; De Vita, E.; Forbes, A.; Cohen, R.; Windsor, A.; Obichere, A.; et al. Mural Crohn disease: Correlation of dynamic contrast-enhanced MR imaging findings with angiogenesis and inflammation at histologic examination–pilot study. *Radiology* **2009**, *251*, 369–379. [CrossRef]
28. Maconi, G.; Greco, S.; Duca, P.; Ardizzone, S.; Massari, A.; Cassinotti, A.; Radice, E.; Porro, G.B. Prevalence and clinical significance of sonographic evidence of mesenteric fat alterations in Crohn's disease. *Inflamm. Bowel Dis.* **2008**, *14*, 1555–1561. [CrossRef]
29. Romanini, L.; Passamonti, M.; Navarria, M.; Lanzarotto, F.; Villanacci, V.; Grazioli, L.; Calliada, F.; Maroldi, R. Quantitative analysis of contrast-enhanced ultrasonography of the bowel wall can predict disease activity in inflammatory bowel disease. *Eur. J. Radiol.* **2014**, *83*, 1317–1323. [CrossRef] [PubMed]
30. Sidhu, P.S.; Cantisani, V.; Dietrich, C.F.; Gilja, O.H.; Saftoiu, A.; Bartels, E.; Bertolotto, M.; Calliada, F.; Clevert, D.-A.; Cosgrove, D.; et al. The EFSUMB Guidelines and Recommendations for the Clinical Practice of Contrast-Enhanced Ultrasound (CEUS) in Non-Hepatic Applications: Update 2017 (Long Version). Die EFSUMB-Leitlinien und Empfehlungen für den klinischen Einsatz des kontrastverstärkten Ultraschalls (CEUS) bei nicht-hepatischen Anwendungen: Update 2017 (Langversion). *Ultraschall Med.* **2018**, *39*, e2–e44. [CrossRef]
31. Ripollés, T.; Poza, J.; Suarez Ferrer, C.; Martínez-Pérez, M.J.; Martín-Algíbez, A.; de Las Heras Paez, B. Evaluation of Crohn's Disease Activity: Development of an Ultrasound Score in a Multicenter Study. *Inflamm. Bowel Dis.* **2021**, *27*, 145–154. [CrossRef] [PubMed]
32. Paredes, J.M.; Ripollés, T.; Cortés, X.; Moreno, N.; Martínez, M.J.; Bustamante-Balén, M.; Delgado, F.; Moreno-Osset, E. Contrast-enhanced ultrasonography: Usefulness in the assessment of postoperative recurrence of Crohn's disease. *J. Crohns Colitis.* **2013**, *7*, 192–201. [CrossRef]
33. Ordás, I.; Rimola, J.; Alfaro, I.; Rodríguez, S.; Castro-Poceiro, J.; Ramírez-Morros, A.; Gallego, M.; Giner, À.; Barastegui, R.; Fernández-Clotet, A.; et al. Development and Validation of a Simplified Magnetic Resonance Index of Activity for Crohn's Disease. *Gastroenterology* **2019**, *157*, 432–439.e1. [CrossRef] [PubMed]
34. Horjus Talabur Horje, C.S.; Bruijnen, R.; Roovers, L.; Groenen, M.J.; Joosten, F.B.; Wahab, P.J. Contrast Enhanced Abdominal Ultrasound in the Assessment of Ileal Inflammation in Crohn's Disease: A Comparison with MR Enterography. *PLoS ONE* **2015**, *10*, e0136105. [CrossRef] [PubMed]
35. Sachar, D.B. Biomarkers Task Force of the IOIBD. Role of biomarkers in the study and management of inflammatory bowel disease: A "nonsystematic" review. *Inflamm. Bowel Dis.* **2014**, *20*, 2511–2518. [CrossRef]
36. D'haens, G.; Ferrante, M.; Vermeire, S.; Baert, F.; Noman, M.; Moortgat, L.; Geens, P.; Iwens, D.; Aerden, I.; Van Assche, G.; et al. Fecal calprotectin is a surrogate marker for endoscopic lesions in inflammatory bowel disease. *Inflamm. Bowel Dis.* **2012**, *18*, 2218–2224. [CrossRef]
37. Rigazio, C.; Ercole, E.; Laudi, C.; Daperno, M.; Lavagna, A.; Crocellà, L.; Bertolino, F.; Viganò, L.; Sostegni, R.; Pera, A.; et al. Abdominal bowel ultrasound can predict the risk of surgery in Crohn's disease: Proposal of an ultrasonographic score. *Scand. J. Gastroenterol.* **2009**, *44*, 585–593. [CrossRef]
38. Swets, J.A. Measuring the accuracy of diagnostic systems. *Science* **1988**, *240*, 1285–1293. [CrossRef]
39. Daperno, M.; D'Haens, G.; Van Assche, G.; Baert, F.; Bulois, P.; Maunoury, V.; Sostegni, R.; Rocca, R.; Pera, A.; Gevers, A. Development and validation of a new, simplified endoscopic activity score for Crohn's disease: The SES-CD. *Gastrointest. Endosc.* **2004**, *60*, 505–512. [CrossRef]

40. Sipponen, T.; Nuutinen, H.; Turunen, U.; Färkkilä, M. Endoscopic evaluation of Crohn's disease activity: Comparison of the CDEIS and the SES-CD. *Inflamm. Bowel Dis.* **2010**, *16*, 2131–2136. [CrossRef]
41. Schoepfer, A.M.; Beglinger, C.; Straumann, A.; Trummler, M.; Vavricka, S.R.; E Bruegger, L.; Seibold, F. Fecal calprotectin correlates more closely with the Simple Endoscopic Score for Crohn's disease (SES-CD) than CRP, blood leukocytes, and the CDAI. *Am. J. Gastroenterol.* **2010**, *105*, 162–169. [CrossRef]
42. Solem, C.A.; Loftus, E.V., Jr.; Tremaine, W.J.; Harmsen, W.S.; Zinsmeister, A.R.; Sandborn, W.J. Correlation of C-reactive protein with clinical, endoscopic, histologic, and radiographic activity in inflammatory bowel disease. *Inflamm. Bowel Dis.* **2005**, *11*, 707–712. [CrossRef] [PubMed]
43. Sipponen, T.; Savilahti, E.; Kolho, K.L.; Nuutinen, H.; Turunen, U.; Färkkilä, M. Crohn's disease activity assessed by fecal calprotectin and lactoferrin: Correlation with Crohn's disease activity index and endoscopic findings. *Inflamm. Bowel Dis.* **2008**, *14*, 40–46. [CrossRef] [PubMed]
44. Sipponen, T.; Kärkkäinen, P.; Savilahti, E.; Kolho, K.-L.; Nuutinen, H.; Turunen, U.; Färkkilä, M. Correlation of fecal calprotectin and lactoferrin with an endoscopic score for Crohn's disease and histological findings. *Aliment. Pharmacol. Ther.* **2008**, *28*, 1221–1229. [CrossRef]
45. Lin, J.-F.; Chen, J.-M.; Zuo, J.-H.; Yu, A.; Xiao, Z.-J.; Deng, F.-H.; Nie, B.; Jiang, B. Meta-analysis: Fecal calprotectin for assessment of inflammatory bowel disease activity. *Inflamm. Bowel Dis.* **2014**, *20*, 1407–1415. [CrossRef]
46. Samuel, S.; Bruining, D.H.; Loftus, E.V., Jr.; Becker, B.; Fletcher, J.G.; Mandrekar, J.N.; Zinsmeister, A.R.; Sandborn, W.J. Endoscopic skipping of the distal terminal ileum in Crohn's disease can lead to negative results from ileocolonoscopy. *Clin. Gastroenterol. Hepatol.* **2012**, *10*, 1253–1259. [CrossRef]
47. Maaser, C.; Sturm, A.; Vavricka, S.R.; Kucharzik, T.; Fiorino, G.; Annese, V.; Calabrese, E.; Baumgart, D.C.; Bettenworth, D.; Borralho Nunes, P.; et al. European Crohn's and Colitis Organisation [ECCO] and the European Society of Gastrointestinal and Abdominal Radiology [ESGAR]. ECCO-ESGAR Guideline for Diagnostic Assessment in IBD Part 1: Initial diagnosis, monitoring of known IBD, detection of complications. *J. Crohns Colitis.* **2019**, *13*, 144–164. [CrossRef]
48. Fiorino, G.; Bonifacio, C.; Peyrin-Biroulet, L.; Minuti, F.; Repici, A.; Spinelli, A.; Fries, W.; Balzarini, L.; Montorsi, M.; Malesci, A.; et al. Prospective comparison of computed tomography enterography and magnetic resonance enterography for assessment of disease activity and complications in ileocolonic Crohn's disease. *Inflamm. Bowel Dis.* **2011**, *17*, 1073–1080. [CrossRef]
49. Puylaert, C.A.; Tielbeek, J.A.; Bipat, S.; Stoker, J. Grading of Crohn's disease activity using, CT, MRI, US and scintigraphy: A meta-analysis. *Eur. Radiol.* **2015**, *25*, 3295–3313. [CrossRef] [PubMed]
50. Steward, M.J.; Punwani, S.; Proctor, I.; Adjei-Gyamfi, Y.; Chatterjee, F.; Bloom, S.; Novelli, M.; Halligan, S.; Rodriguez-Justo, M.; Taylor, S.A. Non-perforating small bowel Crohn's disease assessed by MRI enterography: Derivation and histopathological validation of an MR-based activity index. *Eur. J. Radiol.* **2012**, *81*, 2080–2088. [CrossRef]
51. Rimola, J.; Ordás, I.; Rodriguez, S.; García-Bosch, O.; Aceituno, M.; Llach, J.; Ayuso, C.; Ricart, E.; Panés, J. Magnetic resonance imaging for evaluation of Crohn's disease: Validation of parameters of severity and quantitative index of activity. *Inflamm. Bowel Dis.* **2011**, *17*, 1759–1768. [CrossRef]
52. Tielbeek, J.A.; Makanyanga, J.C.; Bipat, S.; Pendsé, D.A.; Nio, C.Y.; Vos, F.M.; Taylor, S.A.; Stoker, J. Grading Crohn disease activity with MRI: Interobserver variability of MRI features, MRI scoring of severity, and correlation with Crohn disease endoscopic index of severity. *AJR Am. J. Roentgenol.* **2013**, *201*, 1220–1228. [CrossRef]
53. Rimola, J.; Alvarez-Cofiño, A.; Pérez-Jeldres, T.; Ayuso, C.; Alfaro, I.; Rodríguez, S.; Ricart, E.; Ordás, I.; Panés, J. Comparison of three magnetic resonance enterography indices for grading activity in Crohn's disease. *J. Gastroenterol.* **2017**, *52*, 585–593. [CrossRef] [PubMed]
54. Mary, J.Y.; Modigliani, R. Development and validation of an endoscopic index of the severity for Crohn's disease: A prospective multicentre study. Groupe d'Etudes Therapeutiques des Affections Inflammatoires du Tube Digestif (GETAID). *Gut* **1989**, *30*, 983–989. [CrossRef] [PubMed]
55. Calabrese, E.; Maaser, C.; Zorzi, F.; Kannengiesser, K.; Hanauer, S.B.; Bruining, D.H.; Iacucci, M.; Maconi, G.; Novak, K.L.; Panaccione, R.; et al. Bowel Ultrasonography in the Management of Crohn's Disease. A Review with Recommendations of an International Panel of Experts. *Inflamm. Bowel Dis.* **2016**, *22*, 1168–1183. [CrossRef]
56. Monteleone, M.; Friedman, A.; Furfaro, F.; Dell'Era, A.; Bezzio, C.; Maconi, G. P139 The learning curve of intestinal ultrasonography in assessing inflammatory bowel disease—Preliminary results. *J. Crohn Colitis* **2013**, *7*, S64. [CrossRef]
57. Miles, A.; Bhatnagar, G.; Halligan, S.; Gupta, A.; Tolan, D.; Zealley, I.; Taylor, S.A. METRIC investigators. Magnetic resonance enterography, small bowel ultrasound and colonoscopy to diagnose and stage Crohn's disease: Patient acceptability and perceived burden. *Eur. Radiol.* **2019**, *29*, 1083–1093. [CrossRef] [PubMed]
58. Maconi, G.; Nylund, K.; Ripolles, T.; Calabrese, E.; Dirks, K.; Dietrich, C.F.; Hollerweger, A.; Sporea, I.; Saftoiu, A.; Maaser, C.; et al. EFSUMB Recommendations and Clinical Guidelines for Intestinal Ultrasound (GIUS) in Inflammatory Bowel Diseases. *Ultraschall Med.* **2018**, *39*, 304–317. [CrossRef] [PubMed]
59. Fraquelli, M.; Colli, A.; Casazza, G.; Paggi, S.; Colucci, A.; Massironi, S.; Duca, P.; Conte, D. Role of US in detection of Crohn disease: Meta-analysis. *Radiology* **2005**, *236*, 95–101. [CrossRef]
60. Miao, Y.M.; Koh, D.M.; Amin, Z.; Healy, J.C.; Chinn, R.J.; Zeegen, R.; Westaby, D. Ultrasound and magnetic resonance imaging assessmentof active bowel segments in Crohn's disease. *Clin. Radiol.* **2002**, *57*, 913–918. [CrossRef]

61. Kunihiro, K.; Hata, J.; Manabe, N.; Mitsuoka, Y.; Tanaka, S.; Haruma, K.; Chayama, K. Predicting the need for surgery in Crohn's disease with contrast harmonic ultrasound. *Scand. J. Gastroenterol.* **2007**, *42*, 577–585. [CrossRef] [PubMed]
62. Rosenbaum, D.G.; Conrad, M.A.; Biko, D.M.; Ruchelli, E.D.; Kelsen, J.R.; Anupindi, S.A. Ultrasound and MRI predictors of surgical bowel resection in pediatric Crohn disease. *Pediatr. Radiol.* **2017**, *47*, 55–64. [CrossRef] [PubMed]
63. Geyl, S.; Guillo, L.; Laurent, V.; D'Amico, F.; Danese, S.; Peyrin-Biroulet, L. Transmural healing as a therapeutic goal in Crohn's disease: A systematic review. *Lancet Gastroenterol. Hepatol.* **2021**, *6*, 659–667. [CrossRef] [PubMed]
64. Ma, L.; Li, W.; Zhuang, N.; Yang, H.; Liu, W.; Zhou, W.; Jiang, Y.; Li, J.; Zhu, Q.; Qian, J. Comparison of transmural healing and mucosal healing as predictors of positive long-term outcomes in Crohn's disease. *Ther. Adv. Gastroenterol.* **2021**, *14*, 17562848211016259. [CrossRef]
65. Lafeuille, P.; Hordonneau, C.; Vignette, J.; Blayac, L.; Dapoigny, M.; Reymond, M.; Rouquette, O.; Sollelis, E.; Boube, M.; Magnin, B.; et al. Transmural healing and MRI healing are associated with lower risk of bowel damage progression than endoscopic mucosal healing in Crohn's disease. *Aliment. Pharmacol. Ther.* **2021**, *53*, 577–586. [CrossRef]
66. Sasaki, T.; Kunisaki, R.; Kinoshita, H.; Kimura, H.; Kodera, T.; Nozawa, A.; Hanzawa, A.; Shibata, N.; Yonezawa, H.; Miyajima, E.; et al. Doppler ultrasound findings correlate with tissue vascularity and inflammation in surgical pathology specimens from patients with small intestinal Crohn's disease. *BMC Res. Notes* **2014**, *7*, 363. [CrossRef]
67. Novak, K.L.; Nylund, K.; Maaser, C.; Petersen, F.; Kucharzik, T.; Lu, C.; Allocca, M.; Maconi, G.; de Voogd, F.; Christensen, B.; et al. Expert Consensus on Optimal Acquisition and Development of the International Bowel Ultrasound Segmental Activity Score [IBUS-SAS]: A Reliability and Inter-rater Variability Study on Intestinal Ultrasonography in Crohn's Disease. *J. Crohns Colitis.* **2021**, *15*, 609–616. [CrossRef]
68. De Voogd, F.; Wilkens, R.; Gecse, K.; Allocca, M.; Novak, K.; Lu, C.; D'Haens, G.; Maaser, C. A Reliability Study: Strong Inter-Observer Agreement of an Expert Panel for Intestinal Ultrasound in Ulcerative Colitis. *J. Crohns Colitis.* **2021**, *15*, 1284–1290. [CrossRef]
69. Dolinger, M.T.; Kayal, M. Intestinal ultrasound as a non-invasive tool to monitor inflammatory bowel disease activity and guide clinical decision making. *World J. Gastroenterol.* **2023**, *29*, 2272–2282. [CrossRef]
70. Muñoz, F.; Ripollés, T.; Poza Cordón, J.; de Las Heras Páez de la Cadena, B.; Martínez-Pérez, M.J.; de Miguel, E.; Zabana, Y.; Mañosa Ciria, M.; Beltrán, B.; Barreiro-de Acosta, M. Recommendations of the Spanish Working Group on Crohn's Disease and Ulcerative Colitis (GETECCU) on the use of abdominal ultrasound in inflammatory bowel disease. *Gastroenterol. Hepatol.* **2021**, *44*, 158–174, (In English and Spanish). [CrossRef]
71. Danese, S.; Sans, M.; De La Motte, C.; Graziani, C.; West, G.; Phillips, M.H.; Pola, R.; Rutella, S.; Willis, J.; Gasbarrini, A.; et al. Angiogenesis as a novel component of inflammatory bowel disease pathogenesis. *Gastroenterology* **2006**, *130*, 2060–2073. [CrossRef] [PubMed]
72. Deban, L.; Correale, C.; Vetrano, S.; Malesci, A.; Danese, S. Multiple pathogenic roles of microvasculature in inflammatory bowel disease: A Jack of all trades. *Am. J. Pathol.* **2008**, *172*, 1457–1466. [CrossRef] [PubMed]
73. Sævik, F.; Gilja, O.H.; Nylund, K. Gastrointestinal Ultrasound Can Predict Endoscopic Activity in Crohn's Disease. Gastrointestinaler Ultraschall zur Prädiktion der endoskopischen Krankheitsaktivität bei Morbus Crohn. *Ultraschall Med.* **2022**, *43*, 82–89. [CrossRef] [PubMed]
74. Yigit, B.; Sezgin, O.; Yorulmaz, E.; Erturk, M.S.; Erdem, U.; Yanc, U.; Oyman, G.B.; Yorulmaz, H. Effectiveness and Power of Abdominal Ultrasonography in the Assessment of Crohn's Disease Activity: Comparison with Clinical, Endoscopic, and CT Enterography Findings. *Turk. J. Gastroenterol.* **2022**, *33*, 294–303. [CrossRef]
75. Cerrillo, E.; Beltrán, B.; Pous, S.; Echarri, A.; Gallego, J.C.; Iborra, M.; Pamies, J.; Nos, P. Fecal Calprotectin in Ileal Crohn's Disease: Relationship with Magnetic Resonance Enterography and a Pathology Score. *Inflamm. Bowel Dis.* **2015**, *21*, 1572–1579. [CrossRef] [PubMed]
76. Yamanashi, K.; Katsurada, T.; Nishida, M.; Onishi, R.; Omotehara, S.; Otagiri, S.; Sakurai, K.; Nagashima, K.; Kinoshita, K.; Takagi, R.; et al. Crohn's Disease Activity Evaluation by Transabdominal Ultrasonography: Correlation with Double-Balloon Endoscopy. *J. Ultrasound Med.* **2021**, *40*, 2595–2605. [CrossRef]
77. Pauls, S.; Gabelmann, A.; Schmidt, S.A.; Rieber, A.; Mittrach, C.; Haenle, M.M.; Brambs, H.-J.; Kratzer, W. Evaluating bowel wall vascularity in Crohn's disease: A comparison of dynamic MRI and wideband harmonic imaging contrast-enhanced low MI ultrasound. *Eur. Radiol.* **2006**, *16*, 2410–2417. [CrossRef]
78. Malagò, R.; D'onofrio, M.; Mantovani, W.; D'alpaos, G.; Foti, G.; Pezzato, A.; Caliari, G.; Cusumano, D.; Benini, L.; Mucelli, R.P. Contrast-enhanced ultrasonography (CEUS) vs. MRI of the small bowel in the evaluation of Crohn's disease activity. *Radiol. Med.* **2012**, *117*, 268–281. [CrossRef]

79. Roseira, J.; Ventosa, A.R.; de Sousa, H.T.; Brito, J. The new simplified MARIA score applies beyond clinical trials: A suitable clinical practice tool for Crohn's disease that parallels a simple endoscopic index and fecal calprotectin. *United Eur. Gastroenterol. J.* **2020**, *8*, 1208–1216. [CrossRef]
80. Freitas, M.; de Castro, F.D.; Macedo Silva, V.; Arieira, C.; Cúrdia Gonçalves, T.; Leite, S.; Moreira, M.J.; Cotter, J. Ultrasonographic scores for ileal Crohn's disease assessment: Better, worse or the same as contrast-enhanced ultrasound? *BMC Gastroenterol.* **2022**, *22*, 252. [CrossRef]

life

MDPI

Article

The Effects of the Combination of Rhein and Platelet-Rich Plasma on Human Articular Chondrocytes

Mario Simental-Mendía [1], Sonia Amelia Lozano-Sepúlveda [2], Marsela Garza-Tapia [3], Jorge Lara-Arias [1], Carlos Alberto Acosta-Olivo [1], Félix Vilchez-Cavazos [1] and Víctor Manuel Peña-Martínez [1,*]

1 Orthopedic Trauma Service, "Dr. José Eleuterio González" University Hospital, Universidad Autónoma de Nuevo León, Monterrey 66455, Mexico; mario.simentalme@uanl.edu.mx (M.S.-M.); jorge.larars@uanl.edu.mx (J.L.-A.); carlos.acostalv@uanl.edu.mx (C.A.A.-O.); jose.vilchezcvz@uanl.edu.mx (F.V.-C.)

2 Department of Biochemistry and Molecular Medicine, School of Medicine, Universidad Autónoma de Nuevo León, Monterrey 66455, Mexico; sonia.lozanosp@uanl.edu.mx

3 Department of Analytical Chemistry, School of Medicine, Universidad Autónoma de Nuevo León, Monterrey 66455, Mexico; marsela.garzatp@uanl.edu.mx

* Correspondence: victor.penam@uanl.mx; Tel.: +52-81-8347-6698

Abstract: Background: The presence of side effects and low bioavailability of rhein has limited its use in the treatment of osteoarthritis. We aimed to evaluate the in vitro response of human articular chondrocytes to the presence of the combination of platelet-rich plasma (PRP) and rhein. Methods: Solutions of rhein were prepared to assess solubility and select a working concentration. A stimulus with interleukin-1β (IL-β, 10 ng/mL) was induced for 24 h on human chondrocytes. Five treatment groups were established: control, IL-β control, PRP, rhein, and PRP + rhein. Cell viability, cell migration, nitric oxide (NO) production, tumor necrosis factor-α (TNF-α), and gene expression analyses were carried out. Results: A concentration of 50 mg/L was selected after a dose–response curve assay. Both NO and tumor TNF-α production significantly decreased after PRP and PRP + rhein treatments at 24 and 48 h. The wound healing assay revealed a significant stimulation of migration after 72 h with the PRP and PRP + rhein treatments. Expression of IL-1β, IL-6, MMP-13, and ADAMTS-5 was significantly downregulated, particularly after treatment with the combination of PRP + rhein. Conclusions: Much of the determinations denoted a better performance of the combination of PRP and rhein in decreasing the levels of the different targets evaluated; however, this was not great enough to detect a significant difference in comparison with the PRP treatment alone.

Keywords: chondrocytes; platelet-rich plasma; rhein; knee osteoarthritis

Citation: Simental-Mendía, M.; Lozano-Sepúlveda, S.A.; Garza-Tapia, M.; Lara-Arias, J.; Acosta-Olivo, C.A.; Vilchez-Cavazos, F.; Peña-Martínez, V.M. The Effects of the Combination of Rhein and Platelet-Rich Plasma on Human Articular Chondrocytes. *Life* **2023**, *13*, 1723. https://doi.org/10.3390/life13081723

Academic Editors: Michela Battistelli, Stefanos Roumeliotis and Giuseppe Minervini

Received: 26 June 2023
Revised: 24 July 2023
Accepted: 9 August 2023
Published: 11 August 2023

1. Introduction

Osteoarthritis (OA) is a chronic degenerative disorder mostly characterized by joint pain and stiffness which leads to a progressive decline in joint function and a deterioration in quality of life [1,2]. The prevalence of OA increases with age, with an estimated almost twice as many cases in women than in men over 60 years of age [3]. Particularly, obesity (BMI ≥ 30 kg/m^2) represents an increased risk factor for the development of symptomatic knee OA (19.7% versus 10.9% of nonobese persons) [4]. As OA progresses, the joint undergoes a series of structural changes as part of the pathophysiological process, such as cartilage degradation, bone remodeling, osteophyte formation, and synovial inflammation [5].

Despite the high prevalence of OA worldwide, the therapeutic options initially recommended by the main clinical treatment guidelines continue to be topical and oral nonsteroidal anti-inflammatory drugs (NSAIDs) [6]. This occurs in the absence of approved pharmacological agents that may interfere with the progression of the disease.

As an alternative to NSAIDs, other molecules such as glucosamine, chondroitin sulfate, and diacerein have been considered as secondary interventions that may improve or control OA-associated symptomatology [7]. Diacerein, of which the active metabolite is rhein, is an anthraquinone derivative that has been shown to inhibit the production and activity of the proinflammatory cytokine interleukin-1β (IL-1β) [8,9]. Rhein has been also credited with different biological properties, including anti-inflammatory and chondroprotective activities [10]. Diacerein can improve pain and joint function, but its oral administration is associated with gastrointestinal secondary effects [11].

Intra-articular injections of platelet-rich plasma (PRP) have served as an effective emerging therapeutic alternative in the improvement of symptoms caused by OA [12]. This fact has also been supported by the beneficial effects that PRP exerts on certain tissues and cell types within the joint (particularly cartilage and chondrocytes), such as promoting cell proliferation, anti-inflammatory, antiapoptotic, anabolic, and anticatabolic effects [13].

This study aimed to evaluate the response in vitro of human articular chondrocytes in the presence of the combination of PRP and the active metabolite of diacerein (rhein), in search of a therapeutic alternative with a potential synergistic effect.

2. Materials and Methods

2.1. Patients and Samples

Articular cartilage was obtained from patients undergoing total knee replacement surgery. Tissue handling and procurement of human tissues was approved by the Institutional Research Ethics Committee (approval No. OR 18-00004). Informed consent was obtained from all patients. Cartilage samples were obtained from nine patients (six female and three male) with a median of 70 years and an interquartile range of 61–79 years. Samples from infected joints were excluded, and samples from patients in whom the tissue sample was insufficient or not presenting viable tissue for processing were also eliminated. To recover viable cartilage, the procured joint tissue was cut using an Osteochondral Autograft Transfer System (OATS®, Arthrex Inc., Naples, FL, USA). Precise circular samples measuring 6–8 mm in diameter were meticulously extracted. The goal was to obtain cartilage specimens free from erosion or any exposure of the subchondral bone. These samples were specifically taken from non-weight-bearing regions located at the periphery of the femoral condyles.

2.2. Isolation and Culture of Articular Chondrocytes

Isolation of articular chondrocytes was carried out through several cycles of enzymatic digestion. Briefly, cartilage was mechanically disrupted into small pieces (1 mm^3 approximately) using a scalpel, and subsequently subjected to enzymatic breakdown (30 min at 37 °C with constant stirring at 90 rpm) with trypsin without EDTA (GIBCO®-BRL Life Technologies, Grand Island, NY, USA). Then, digestion continued with at least two cycles of type II collagenase 2 mg/mL at 37 °C with constant stirring at 90 rpm. Cells contained in the supernatant were pelleted via centrifugation at 1800 rpm for 5 min for each digestion cycle. Chondrocytes were suspended in complete DMEM/F12 (GIBCO®-BRL Life Technologies, Grand Island, NY, USA) culture medium supplemented with 10% fetal bovine serum (FBS, GIBCO®-BRL Life Technologies, Grand Island, NY, USA) and gentamicin (0.05 mg/mL, Laboratorios Química SON'S, Puebla, Mexico), and transferred to 75 cm^2 culture flasks at 37 °C in a 5% CO_2 environment and relative humidity of 100%. Cells with less than three passages were used.

2.3. Rhein Solubility Determination

Solubility tests were performed by following the OECD (Organisation for Economic Cooperation and Development) guidelines for the testing of chemicals No. 107 (shake flask method) at a constant temperature [14]. Briefly, a saturated rhein solution was left under constant stirring for 24 h at 25 °C, followed by 24 h of rest at the same temperature, and finally centrifuged at 3500 rpm at 25 °C for 5 min to separate the solution from the undissolved solid. The tests were performed on pooled human PRP samples activated with 10% calcium gluconate in a ratio of 0.15 mL for each mL of serum (to simulate the combination of PRP and rhein if injected in an OA knee). For rhein quantification, a high-performance liquid chromatography (HPLC) method was developed using a Waters 3695 chromatograph with a diode array detector (Waters Corporation, Milford, MA, USA). The developed method was validated considering ICH (International Council for Harmonisation of Technical Requirements for Pharmaceuticals for Human Use) recommendations [15]. The parameters evaluated were linearity, precision, accuracy, limit of detection, and limit of quantification. To validate the method, a 200 μg/mL concentrated solution of rhein was prepared in a mixture of 100 mM ammonium/ammonia buffer (pH 9) and methanol (60:40). Working solutions were prepared in a range of 0.25 to 16 μg/mL [16–19] in the same mixture of solvents.

2.4. Determination of Rhein Working Concentration

Once the rhein solubility in human plasma was determined, we aimed to establish the working concentration of rhein by evaluating the cell viability of cultured human chondrocytes with a dose–response assay (5, 10, 25, 50, 75 mg/L), considering previous data from the literature [16–20]. Chondrocyte viability was evaluated through an ATP quantitation assay of metabolically active cells (CellTiter-Glo® Luminescent Cell Viability Assay, Promega, WI, USA). This assay is ideal for automated high-throughput screening and cell proliferation and cytotoxicity examinations. Chondrocytes were cultivated in 96-opaque-walled plates suitable for luminescence measurements (Thermo Fisher Scientific, Nunc, Denmark) at a cellular density of 2×10^5 cells per well with complete DMEM/F12 for 24 h. Mono-oxygenation of luciferin is catalyzed by luciferase in the presence of Mg^{2+}, ATP and molecular oxygen. There is a direct relationship between the luminescent signal and the number of cells in the culture.

2.5. Establishment of Experimental Groups

Chondrocytes were cultivated in 24-well plates (Costar® Corning Incorporated, Corning, NY, USA) at a density of 5×10^5 cells/well with complete DMEM/F12 (10% FBS and gentamicin). After the cells were attached, a stimulus with interleukin-1β (IL-β, 10 ng/mL) for 24 h was induced. Then, five treatment groups were established: (1) negative control (chondrocytes without IL-1β stimulus), (2) IL-1β (control of inflammation), (3) PRP (10% PRP), (4) rhein (50 mg/L), and (5) PRP + rhein (10% PRP + 50 mg/L). Samples were obtained from each group at different time points (0–72 h) of culture for total RNA extraction or supernatant culture medium storage at −80 °C for subsequent analysis.

2.6. Cell Migration

The migration of chondrocytes was evaluated using a wound healing assay technique by creating a cell-free vertical wound area in the confluent monolayer through mechanical damage using a pipette tip [21,22]. The tip was placed firmly and perpendicular to the surface at 90° to produce a vertical wound. Then, the cell debris was aspirated, and a new culture medium was added. The gap generated was evaluated with microphotographs at 0, 24, 48, and 72 h. The wound healing size tool plugin for ImageJ was used to estimate the area (percentage) devoid of cells through densitometric analysis [23]. The color parameters, distribution, saturation, and luminance were established in the software, and were the same for all the images obtained. The images were transformed to a gray scale and the percentage of the area devoid of chondrocytes was estimated. The images obtained were analyzed with the ImageJ program version 1.49 (National Institutes of Health).

2.7. Total RNA Extraction and Gene Expression Analysis

Total RNA was isolated from chondrocytes at the described time intervals and in the described culture conditions with the RNeasy Mini Kit (QIAGEN, Hilden, Germany) following the manufacturer's specifications. The yield and purity of the RNA were measured spectrophotometrically with NanoDrop 2000 equipment (Thermo Fisher Scientific Inc., Waltham, MA, USA). Complementary DNA (cDNA) synthesis and quantitative polymerase chain reaction (qPCR) reactions were performed using a GoTaq Probe 2-Step RT-qPCR System (Promega Corporation, Madison, WI, USA). Chondrocytes were examined for their gene expression concerning inflammatory response and extracellular matrix (ECM) synthesis. Specific probes were used for each gene (Integrated DNA Technologies, Inc., Coralville, IA, USA), and the evaluation was conducted in triplicate for each tested condition and experimental group. A 7500 Fast Real-Time PCR System (Applied Biosystems; Thermo Fisher Scientific, Inc., Foster City, CA, USA) was utilized for gene expression assays. The list of genes assessed can be found in Table 1. Data analysis involved the ΔΔCq method for relative expression, with β-2-microglobulin (B2M) serving as the endogenous gene for normalization [24].

Table 1. Gene symbols and assay ID of the genes evaluated using RT-qPCR.

Gene	Symbol	Probe Assay ID [1]
Interleukin-1 β	IL-1β	Hs.PT.58.1518186
Interleukin-6	IL-6	Hs.PT.58.40226675
Matrix metallopeptidase 13	MMP13	Hs.PT.58.40735012
ADAM metallopeptidase with thrombospondin type 1 motif 4	ADAMTS4	Hs.PT.58.4659383
β-2-microglobulin	B2M	Hs.PT.58v.18759587

[1] Integrated DNA Technologies (IDT), Inc.

2.8. Quantification of Nitric Oxide Production

The levels of nitric oxide (NO) in the culture supernatants were assessed using the Griess reagent (Promega Corporation, Madison, WI, USA). This reagent converts available nitrate into nitrite with the aid of nitrite reductase. Absorbance at 540 nm was measured in 96-well plates using a Cytation3 HT multimodal plate reader (BioTek Instruments Inc., Winooski, VT, USA). A standard curve was generated using sodium nitrate to determine the concentrations of the samples being evaluated. The production of NO was evaluated five times for each culture condition and experimental group (five groups).

2.9. Quantification of Tumor Necrosis Factor-α

Tumor necrosis factor-α (TNF-α) production, released into the culture medium, was measured using a Human TNF-α Quantikine ELISA Kit (R&D Systems, Minneapolis, MN, USA), following the manufacturer's instructions. All measurements were conducted in duplicate, employing a quantitative sandwich enzyme immunoassay technique in a 96-well plate format in all the experimental conditions previously mentioned. The optical density of each well was determined at 450 nm using a Cytation3 HT multimodal plate reader (BioTek Instruments Inc., Winooski, VT, USA).

2.10. Statistical Analysis

The data are expressed as the mean ± standard deviation (SD) from nine independent experiments, each performed in triplicate unless otherwise stated. Normality testing was conducted using a Shapiro–Wilk test. For numerical variables, a parametric one-way ANOVA test with Tukey's post hoc test was utilized to identify potential differences between the experimental groups. Statistical significance was determined by p-values less than 0.05. Data analysis was performed using GraphPad Prism software version 5.00 for Windows (GraphPad Software, Inc., San Diego, CA, USA).

3. Results

3.1. Determination of Rhein Working Concentration

The average solubility of rhein in human serum samples supplemented with 10% calcium gluconate was 1.8 mg/mL, as determined by the HPLC method. Rhein serum solubility along with previous concentration reported in the literature was considered for the construction of the dose–response assay to determine an optimal working concentration. The dose–response assay revealed that the highest concentration of rhein tested (75 mg/L) reduced chondrocyte viability by more than 20%. The working concentration selected was the highest in which cell proliferation surpassed 90% with respect to the control. The concentration of 50 mg/L was chosen for further experiments (Figure 1).

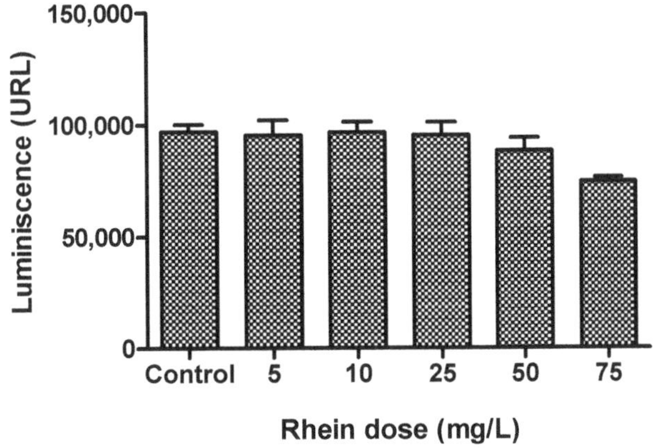

Figure 1. Graphical representation of the dose–response assay to determine the rhein working concentration based on chondrocyte viability.

3.2. Effects of Rhein and PRP on Cell Migration

The effect of the selected rhein working concentration was evaluated on the migration of human chondrocytes under different conditions, based on the chondrocytes' capability to fill the wound created in the monolayer culture. The effect of the rhein by itself was not capable of inducing wound closure after 72 h (Figure 2), though the area that remained cell-free was smaller compared to the IL-1β group (rhein 18.8 ± 1.8% vs. IL-1β 25.4 ± 5.4%; $p < 0.05$; Figure 3). The combination of PRP + rhein (11.3 ± 1.2%) induced a greater chondrocyte migration than the rhein alone (rhein 18.8 ± 1.8%; $p < 0.05$; Figure 3), as reflected by the wound area, while the gap could not be entirely filled after 72 h as with control and PRP groups (Figure 2). In all cases, the treatments were able to improve the delay in wound closure caused by IL-1β at 72 h of culture (Figure 3).

3.3. Effect of Rhein and PRP on Inflammation- and Matrix Degradation-Related Genes

The normalized gene expression of IL-1β was significantly increased in all experimental groups after incubation with recombinant IL-1β. This effect was counteracted by both PRP alone and PRP + rhein, inducing an mRNA downregulation (Figure 4A). Likewise, IL-6 mRNA levels were upregulated after inflammatory stimulation, and this effect was reversed after PRP and PRP + rhein treatments. At 48 h, the rhein by itself showed a decrease in IL-6 gene expression (Figure 4B). Although IL-1β mRNA levels were lower in the presence of PRP + rhein combination compared to the PRP group, the difference was not statistically significant.

The expression of MMP-13 was significantly influenced by recombinant IL-1β. After 48 h, culture conditions with PRP and the PRP + rhein combination showed a significant decrease in MMP-13 mRNA levels as compared to the inflammation control (Figure 4C). Furthermore, the expression of ADAMTS-4 was similarly downmodulated after the treatment with PRP and PRP + rhein. For this marker, the sole stimulation with rhein also decreased the ADAMTS-4 expression at 48 h (Figure 4D). Despite the combination of PRP + rhein inducing lower expression levels, the difference from the levels of the PRP group was not significant.

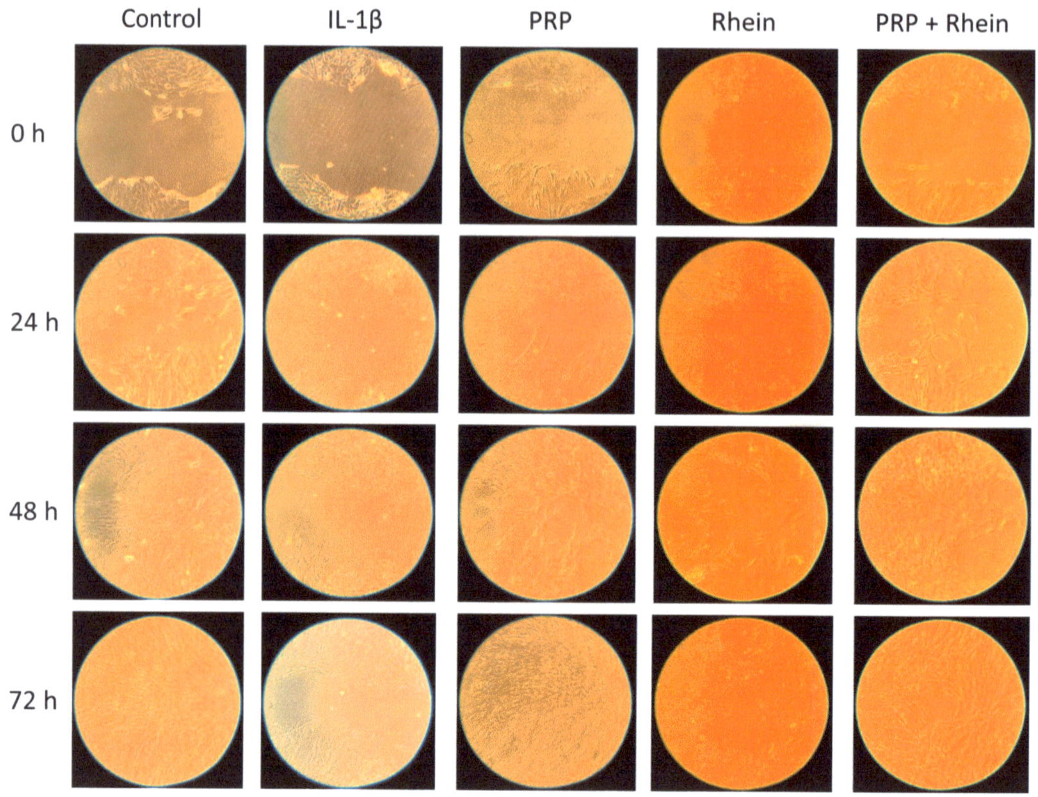

Figure 2. Example of images acquired at 0, 24, 48, and 72 h to assess chondrocyte migration in the wound healing assay under different conditions.

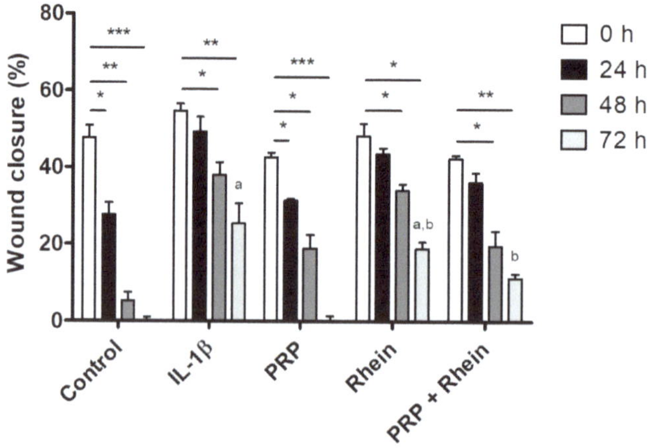

Figure 3. Graphical representation of the gap closure in the wound healing assay for chondrocyte migration. * $p < 0.05$, ** $p < 0.01$, *** $p < 0.001$; [a] $p < 0.05$ for IL-1β vs. Rhein, [b] $p < 0.05$ for Rhein vs. PRP + Rhein.

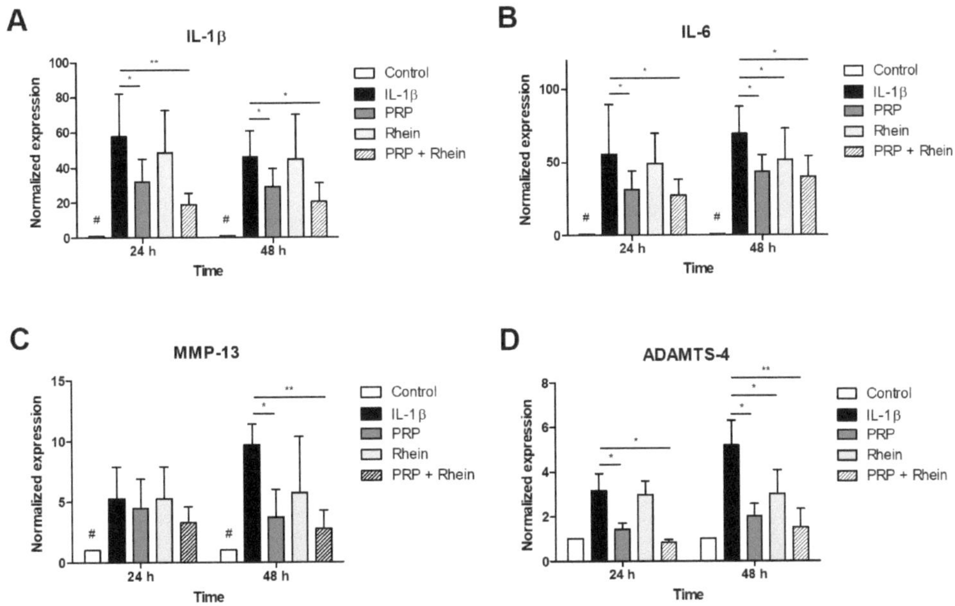

Figure 4. Normalized expression of inflammation− and matrix degradation−related genes in articular human chondrocytes exposed to rhein or PRP after IL-1β stimulation. (**A**) Relative expression of IL-1β. (**B**) Relative expression of IL-6. (**C**) Relative expression of MMP13. (**D**) Relative expression of ADAMTS-5. Data represent the analysis of nine different experiments performed with three replicates. Data are expressed as the mean ± SD. * $p < 0.05$ and ** $p < 0.01$; # $p < 0.05$ vs. all experimental groups. IL-1β, interleukin-1β; IL-6, interleukin 6; MMP-13, matrix metallopeptidase 13; ADAMTS-4, ADAM metallopeptidase with thrombospondin type 1 motif 4.

3.4. *Effect of Rhein and PRP on NO Production*

Nitrite concentrations were determined as an index of NO production, increasing markedly in the groups in which inflammation with IL-1β was induced, compared to the control group at 24 and 48 h ($p < 0.01$; Figure 5). A decrease in the production of NO was especially observed in the groups treated with PRP and the combination of PRP + rhein with respect to the IL-1β group at 24 and 48 h ($p < 0.05$; Figure 5). The effect of rhein alone was not enough to detect a significant reduction after 48 h.

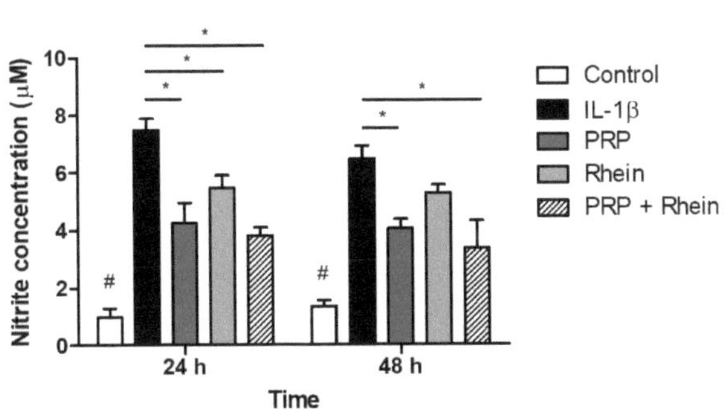

Figure 5. Effect of rhein and PRP on NO production. Data represent the analysis of nine different experiments carried out with five replicates. Data are expressed as mean ± SD. * $p < 0.05$; # $p < 0.01$ vs. all experimental groups. PRP, platelet-rich plasma; NO, nitric oxide.

3.5. Effect of Rhein and PRP on TNF-α Production

The TNF-α levels produced by chondrocytes stimulated with IL-1β were investigated using an ELISA assay. As shown in Figure 6, the results showed that the concentration of TNF-α in the supernatant increased significantly after IL-1β treatment. However, in the presence of both the PRP and the PRP + rhein, the IL-1β-induced TNF-α production was suppressed at 24 and 48 h ($p < 0.01$).

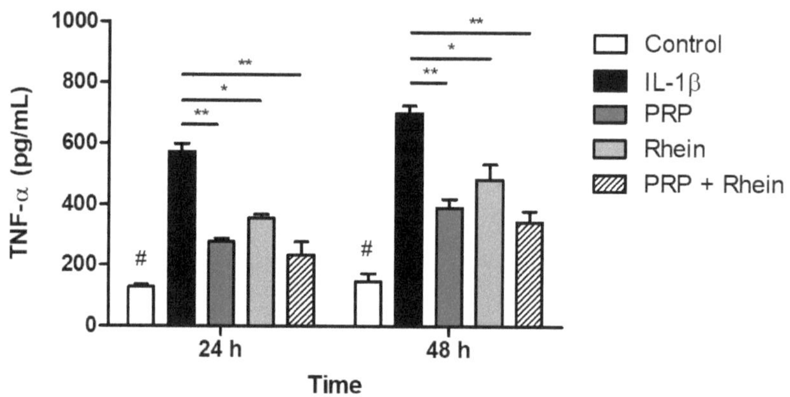

Figure 6. Effect of rhein and PRP on TNF-α production. Data represent the analysis of nine different experiments carried out with three replicates. Data are expressed as the mean ± SD. * $p < 0.05$; ** $p < 0.01$; # $p < 0.05$ vs. all experimental groups. PRP, platelet-rich plasma; TNF-α, tumor necrosis factor-α.

4. Discussion

The main results of this study showed that rhein concentrations lower than 50 mg/L do not affect human chondrocyte viability, and rhein exerts a mild chondroprotective effect by itself. In combination with PRP, no evident synergistic effect was observed; however, in some determinations, this combination produced the greatest reduction in inflammatory and catabolic markers. Due to the poor systemic availability of rhein after diacerein is metabolized, and its gastrointestinal side effects [8], alternative delivery systems for rhein have been studied [25]. We wanted to explore the possibility of combining rhein and PRP as an intra-articular administration alternative. The intra-articular administration of rhein has not been explored before; however, we first wanted to evaluate the chondrocyte response to the rhein + PRP combination.

IL-1β plays a significant role in the development of OA by promoting inflammation and breaking down cartilage. It exerts a strong catabolic influence on cartilage by enhancing the production and function of crucial enzymes involved in the degradation of the extracellular matrix [26]. Therefore, IL-1β can be used to simulate an OA model in vitro in chondrocytes. This was evidenced by the marked increase in TNF-α, NO, IL-1β, IL-6, MMP-13, and ADAMTS-4, as well as a decrease in the chondrocyte migration capacity. The treatments employed in the different experimental conditions were able to counteract or ameliorate the IL-1β-induced changes. Chondrocyte migration was significantly improved in the presence of PRP, which was not surpassed by rhein or PRP + rhein. Evidence on the effect of PRP or rhein specifically on chondrocyte migration is scarce; nevertheless, PRP has been previously shown to stimulate the migration of chondral progenitor cells [27]. In our study, the capability of chondrocytes to fill the area wounded might be directly related to a proliferative effect. In this regard, the proliferative effect of PRP on articular chondrocytes is well documented [28], even when these cells are in the presence of proinflammatory cytokines such as IL-1β [27,29,30]; this is in agreement with our results. On the other hand, rhein did not show the ability to improve gap filling after IL-1β stimulation. Previous studies have shown that rhein can affect chondrocytes' and synoviocytes' proliferation in vitro, probably by targeting the cyclin-dependent kinase inhibitor p21, which is active in the cell-cycle regulation of chondrocytes [31,32]. This might help to explain the incomplete wound closure observed after 72 h in the PRP + rhein group.

We further investigated the effect of PRP and rhein on the expression of pro-inflammatory and ECM-related genes. PRP was shown to decrease IL-1β-induced MMP-13, ADAMTS-4, IL-6, and IL-1β mRNA levels. Several reports indicate that PRP has demonstrated the ability to decrease the gene expression of certain proteinases, such as MMP-13, disintegrin, ADAMTS-4, and ADAMTS-5 in animal and human OA chondrocytes [33–37], as well as reducing gene expression of pro-inflammatory markers IL-1β, COX-2, IL-6, IL-8, and IL-18 [34,38,39], thereby reversing the pro-inflammatory and extracellular matrix-degrading effect caused by pro-inflammatory cytokines. Furthermore, rhein has been shown to counteract some of the deleterious effects of IL-1β, including the downregulation of ADAMTS-4, MMP-1, MMP-3, and MMP-13 gene expression in bovine chondrocytes [32]. Moreover, it hinders the expression of genes associated with MMP-1 and MMP-3 (which encode for enzymes involved in cartilage degradation), while promoting the production of aggrecan and collagen, which help maintain cartilage health and prevent joint deterioration [40]. Our data also indicate that rhein was able to reduce ADAMTS-4 and MMP-13 mRNA levels after IL-1β induction. A previous report has shown that inhibition of IL-1β stimulated transcription factors such as NF-κB, which can induce a downregulation of MMPs gene expression in articular chondrocytes [41]. This may help to explain the positive effect on gene expression that we observed. However, rhein did not significantly downmodulate expression of IL-1β and IL-6. Interestingly, the combination of PRP + rhein did not produce an additive effect in modulating the gene expression of the targets evaluated, as the mRNA levels remained with slight decreases with respect to those observed in the PRP group, while maintaining a positive effect. The chondroprotective effect of PRP on chondrocytes exposed to IL-1β has been documented [29,42–44].

Rhein exhibits chondroprotective properties by suppressing various substances that contribute to cartilage breakdown, including IL-1β and NO [45,46]. There is a close relationship between these two proinflammatory mediators, since IL-1β has been shown to induce the production of reactive oxygen species such as NO through inducible NO synthase [47]. The induction of this signaling pathway becomes important, because it has been documented that it leads to the inhibition of the synthesis of cartilage ECM [48]. We detected inhibition of NO production after exposure to both rhein and PRP; the combination of PRP + rhein did not have an additive effect on the reduction of NO, reaching levels very similar to those of the PRP group. The inhibition of NO production by rhein and PRP on articular chondrocytes has been reported elsewhere [17,46,49]. Since it was earlier established that NO mediates the stimulatory effect of IL-1β on MMPs synthesis [46,50], it is possible that the effects of rhein and PRP on MMPs' production result from the inhibition of NO synthesis.

As with NO, the production of TNF-α was also reduced by the effect of both PRP and rhein. This inhibitory effect can be directly related to the counteracting effect of rhein and PRP on IL-1β. Previous research has proposed that the effect of rhein on IL-1β is a result of the inhibition of the NF-κB pathway, resulting in the decrease of transcription factors for different pro-inflammatory mediators such as IL-1β and TNF-α [45,51,52]. The reduction of TNF-α has also been reported in IL-1β articular chondrocytes stimulated by activated PRP, which can be attributed to the bioactive molecules encapsulated in exosomes [53].

Some of the limitations of this study include that some determinations were evaluated within a short period, looking for an immediate effect after an inflammatory stimulation through this first approach. However, since chondrocytes are exposed to chronic inflammatory conditions in knee OA, it would be interesting to determine the activity of PRP + rhein or rhein alone in longer periods. In addition, the effects of PRP and rhein were tested on chondrocytes derived from OA cartilage, instead of chondrocytes derived from healthy tissue. We intended to evaluate the response of chondrocytes under conditions similar to what we expect to find in an OA knee. Both rhein and PRP have been tested in healthy chondrocytes without reporting any kind of harmful effect [29,32,54–56]. The selection of the rhein working concentration was based on a dose-dependent viability assay, because we were not certain whether the active metabolite of diacerein would affect the viability of chondrocytes due to the little information available in the literature. An assay of this type evaluating the activity of chondrogenic or inflammatory markers could help to clarify whether a concentration other than the one determined in this study (probably a lower one) would provide a better additive effect for PRP.

5. Conclusions

A potential chondroprotective effect of the combination of PRP and rhein was observed in chondrocytes subjected to pro-inflammatory stimulation. Although many of the determinations denoted a better performance of the combination in decreasing the levels of the different targets evaluated, this was not greater enough to detect a significant difference in comparison with PRP treatment alone. It would be convenient to evaluate lower concentrations of rhein with PRP in search of a potential synergistic effect.

Author Contributions: Conceptualization, M.S.-M. and V.M.P.-M.; methodology, S.A.L.-S. and M.G.-T.; software, M.S.-M.; validation, J.L.-A., S.A.L.-S. and M.G.-T.; formal analysis, M.S.-M. and J.L.-A.; investigation, C.A.A.-O. and F.V.-C.; resources, F.V.-C.; data curation, S.A.L.-S. and M.G.-T.; writing—original draft preparation, C.A.A.-O. and F.V.-C.; writing—review and editing, M.S.-M., C.A.A.-O. and S.A.L.-S.; visualization, M.G.-T.; supervision, F.V.-C.; project administration, V.M.P.-M.; funding acquisition, V.M.P.-M. All authors have read and agreed to the published version of the manuscript.

Funding: This research received no external funding.

Institutional Review Board Statement: The study was conducted according to the guidelines of the Declaration of Helsinki, and approved by the Institutional Ethics Committee of the SCHOOL OF MEDICINE AND UNIVERSITY HOSPITAL "DR. JOSÉ ELEUTEERIO GONZÁLEZ" (approval No. OR 18-00004, 6 July 2018).

Informed Consent Statement: Informed consent was obtained from all subjects involved in the study.

Data Availability Statement: Data are contained within the article.

Conflicts of Interest: The authors declare no conflict of interest.

References

1. Murray, C.J.L.; Vos, T.; Lozano, R.; Naghavi, M.; Flaxman, A.D.; Michaud, C.; Ezzati, M.; Shibuya, K.; Salomon, J.A.; Abdalla, S.; et al. Disability-Adjusted Life Years (DALYs) for 291 Diseases and Injuries in 21 Regions, 1990–2010: A Systematic Analysis for the Global Burden of Disease Study 2010. *Lancet* **2012**, *380*, 2197–2223. [CrossRef] [PubMed]
2. Woolf, A.D.; Pfleger, B. Burden of Major Muskuloskeletal Conditions. *Bull. World Health Organ* **2003**, *81*, 646–656. Available online: https://apps.who.int/iris/handle/10665/269026 (accessed on 8 June 2022). [PubMed]
3. Glyn-Jones, S.; Palmer, A.J.R.; Agricola, R.; Price, A.J.; Vincent, T.L.; Weinans, H.; Carr, A.J. Osteoarthritis. *Lancet* **2015**, *386*, 376–387. [CrossRef]
4. Losina, E.; Weinstein, A.M.; Reichmann, W.M.; Burbine, S.A.; Solomon, D.H.; Daigle, M.E.; Rome, B.N.; Chen, S.P.; Hunter, D.J.; Suter, L.G.; et al. Lifetime Risk and Age at Diagnosis of Symptomatic Knee Osteoarthritis in the US. *Arthritis Care Res.* **2013**, *65*, 703–711. [CrossRef] [PubMed]
5. Kolasinski, S.L.; Neogi, T.; Hochberg, M.C.; Oatis, C.; Guyatt, G.; Block, J.; Callahan, L.; Copenhaver, C.; Dodge, C.; Felson, D.; et al. 2019 American College of Rheumatology/Arthritis Foundation Guideline for the Management of Osteoarthritis of the Hand, Hip, and Knee. *Arthritis Rheumatol.* **2020**, *72*, 220–233. [CrossRef]
6. Overton, C.; Nelson, A.E.; Neogi, T. Osteoarthritis Treatment Guidelines from Six Professional Societies: Similarities and Differences. *Rheum. Dis. Clin. N. Am.* **2022**, *48*, 637–657. [CrossRef]
7. Bruyère, O.; Cooper, C.; Pelletier, J.P.; Branco, J.; Luisa Brandi, M.; Guillemin, F.; Hochberg, M.C.; Kanis, J.A.; Kvien, T.K.; Martel-Pelletier, J.; et al. An Algorithm Recommendation for the Management of Knee Osteoarthritis in Europe and Internationally: A Report from a Task Force of the European Society for Clinical and Economic Aspects of Osteoporosis and Osteoarthritis (ESCEO). *Semin. Arthritis Rheum.* **2014**, *44*, 253–263. [CrossRef]

8. Panova, E.; Jones, G. Benefit-Risk Assessment of Diacerein in the Treatment of Osteoarthritis. *Drug Saf.* **2015**, *38*, 245–252. [CrossRef]
9. Solignac, M. Mechanisms of Action of Diacerein, the First Inhibitor of Interleukin-1 in Osteoarthritis. *Presse Med.* **2004**, *33*, S10–S12.
10. Zhou, Y.X.; Xia, W.; Yue, W.; Peng, C.; Rahman, K.; Zhang, H. Rhein: A Review of Pharmacological Activities. *Evid.-Based Complement. Altern. Med.* **2015**, *2015*, 578107. [CrossRef]
11. Li, G.; Zhang, Z.; Ye, Y.; Li, H.; Luo, H.; Tang, K.; Lai, Y. Efficacy, Residual Effectiveness and Safety of Diacerein in the Treatment of Knee Osteoarthritis: A Meta-Analysis of Randomized Placebo-Controlled Trials. *Medicine* **2022**, *101*, e31700. [CrossRef] [PubMed]
12. Siddiq, M.A.B.; Clegg, D.; Jansen, T.L.; Rasker, J.J. Emerging and New Treatment Options for Knee Osteoarthritis. *Curr. Rheumatol. Rev.* **2022**, *18*, 20–32. [CrossRef]
13. Rodríguez-Merchán, E.C. Intra-Articular Platelet-Rich Plasma Injections in Knee Osteoarthritis: A Review of Their Current Molecular Mechanisms of Action and Their Degree of Efficacy. *Int. J. Mol. Sci.* **2022**, *23*, 1301. [CrossRef] [PubMed]
14. *OECD Test No. 107: Partition Coefficient (n-Octanol/Water): Shake Flask Method*; OECD Guidelines for the Testing of Chemicals, Section 1; OECD: Paris, France, 1995; ISBN 9789264069626.
15. International Conference On Harmonisation of Technical Requirements for Registration of Pharmaceuticals for Human Use. Validation of Analytical Procedures: Text and Methodology Q2(R1). Available online: https://database.ich.org/sites/default/files/Q2%28R1%29Guideline.pdf (accessed on 8 June 2022).
16. Nicolas, P.; Tod, M.; Padoin, C.; Petitjean, O. Clinical Pharmacokinetics of Diacerein. *Clin. Pharmacokinet.* **1998**, *35*, 347–359. [CrossRef] [PubMed]
17. Sanchez, C.; Mathy-hartert, M.; Deberg, M.A.; Ficheux, H.; Reginster, J.L.; Henrotin, Y.E. Effects of Rhein on Human Articular Chondrocytes in Alginate Beads. *Biochem. Pharmacol.* **2003**, *65*, 377–388. [CrossRef]
18. Zhu, W.; Wang, X.-M.; Li, X.-Y.; Wang, B.-X. Pharmacokinetic of Rhein in Healthy Male Volunteers Following Oral and Retention Enema Administration of Rhubarb Extract: A Single Dose Study. *Am. J. Chin. Med.* **2005**, *33*, 839–850. [CrossRef]
19. Mandawgade, S.D.; Kulkarni, S.; Pal, A.; Srivastava, S.; Padhi, B.K.; Raghuvanshi, R.S. Development and Pharmacokinetic Evaluation of New Oral Formulations of Diacerein. *Curr. Drug Deliv.* **2016**, *13*, 83–89. [CrossRef]
20. Sun, H.; Yin, Q.; Zhang, A.; Wang, X. UPLC-MS/MS Performing Pharmacokinetic and Biodistribution Studies of Rhein. *J. Sep. Sci.* **2012**, *35*, 2063–2068. [CrossRef]
21. Justus, C.R.; Leffler, N.; Ruiz-Echevarria, M.; Yang, L. V In Vitro Cell Migration and Invasion Assays. *J. Vis. Exp.* **2014**, *88*, e51046. [CrossRef]
22. Jonkman, J.E.N.; Cathcart, J.A.; Xu, F.; Bartolini, M.E.; Amon, J.E.; Stevens, K.M.; Colarusso, P. An Introduction to the Wound Healing Assay Using Live-Cell Microscopy. *Cell Adhes. Migr.* **2014**, *8*, 440–451. [CrossRef]
23. Suarez-Arnedo, A.; Torres Figueroa, F.; Clavijo, C.; Arbeláez, P.; Cruz, J.C.; Muñoz-Camargo, C. An Image J Plugin for the High Throughput Image Analysis of in Vitro Scratch Wound Healing Assays. *PLoS ONE* **2020**, *15*, e0232565. [CrossRef]
24. Pfaffl, M.W. A New Mathematical Model for Relative Quantification in Real-Time RT-PCR. *Nucleic Acids Res.* **2001**, *29*, e45. [CrossRef]
25. Ebada, H.M.K.; Nasra, M.M.A.; Elnaggar, Y.S.R.; Nassra, R.A.; Solaiman, A.A.; Abdallah, O.Y. Novel Rhein Integrate Transphytosomes as Non-Invasive Local Therapy for Osteoarthritis to Ameliorate Cartilage Deterioration in MIA-Arthritic Rats. *Colloids Surf. B Biointerfaces* **2021**, *202*, 111713. [CrossRef]
26. Chow, Y.Y.; Chin, K.-Y. The Role of Inflammation in the Pathogenesis of Osteoarthritis. *Mediat. Inflamm.* **2020**, *2020*, 8293921. [CrossRef] [PubMed]
27. Smyth, N.A.; Murawski, C.D.; Fortier, L.A.; Cole, B.J.; Kennedy, J.G. Platelet-Rich Plasma in the Pathologic Processes of Cartilage: Review of Basic Science Evidence. *Arthrosc.-J. Arthrosc. Relat. Surg.* **2013**, *29*, 1399–1409. [CrossRef]
28. Szwedowski, D.; Szczepanek, J.; Paczesny, Ł.; Zabrzyński, J.; Gagat, M.; Mobasheri, A.; Jeka, S. The Effect of Platelet-Rich Plasma on the Intra-Articular Microenvironment in Knee Osteoarthritis. *Int. J. Mol. Sci.* **2021**, *22*, 5492. [CrossRef]
29. Yang, J.; Lu, Y.; Guo, A. Platelet-rich plasma protects rat chondrocytes from interleukin-1β-induced apoptosis. *Mol. Med. Rep.* **2016**, *14*, 4075–4082. [CrossRef]
30. Pereira, C.; Scaranari, M.; Benelli, R.; Strada, P.; Reis, R.L.; Cancedda, R.; Gentili, C. Dual Effect of Platelet Lysate on Human Articular Cartilage: A Maintenance of Chondrogenic Potential and a Transient pro-Inflammatory Activity Followed by an Inflammation Resolution. *Tissue Eng. Part A* **2013**, *19*, 1476–1488. [CrossRef] [PubMed]
31. Legendre, F.; Heuze, A.; Boukerrouche, K.; Leclercq, S.; Boumediene, K.; Galera, P.; Domagala, F.; Pujol, J.P.; Ficheux, H. Rhein, the Metabolite of Diacerhein, Reduces the Proliferation of Osteoarthritic Chondrocytes and Synoviocytes without Inducing Apoptosis. *Scand. J. Rheumatol.* **2009**, *38*, 104–111. [CrossRef]
32. Legendre, F.; Bogdanowicz, P.; Martin, G.; Domagala, F.; Leclercq, S.; Pujol, J.P.; Ficheux, H. Rhein, a Diacerhein-Derived Metabolite, Modulates the Expression of Matrix Degrading Enzymes and the Cell Proliferation of Articular Chondrocytes by Inhibiting ERK and JNK-AP-1 Dependent Pathways. *Clin. Exp. Rheumatol.* **2007**, *25*, 546–555. [PubMed]
33. Yang, F.; Hu, H.; Yin, W.; Li, G.; Yuan, T.; Xie, X.; Zhang, C. Autophagy Is Independent of the Chondroprotection Induced by Platelet-Rich Plasma Releasate. *BioMed Res. Int.* **2018**, *2018*, 9726703. [CrossRef]

34. Chen, W.H.; Lo, W.C.; Hsu, W.C.; Wei, H.J.; Liu, H.Y.; Lee, C.H.; Tina Chen, S.Y.; Shieh, Y.H.; Williams, D.F.; Deng, W.P. Synergistic Anabolic Actions of Hyaluronic Acid and Platelet-Rich Plasma on Cartilage Regeneration in Osteoarthritis Therapy. *Biomaterials* **2014**, *35*, 9599–9607. [CrossRef]
35. Anitua, E.; Sánchez, M.; Nurden, A.T.; Zalduendo, M.M.; De la Fuente, M.; Azofra, J.; Andía, I. Platelet-Released Growth Factors Enhance the Secretion of Hyaluronic Acid and Induce Hepatocyte Growth Factor Production by Synovial Fibroblasts from Arthritic Patients. *Rheumatology* **2007**, *46*, 1769–1772. [CrossRef]
36. Van Buul, G.M.; Koevoet, W.L.M.M.; Kops, N.; Bos, P.K.; Verhaar, J.A.N.N.; Weinans, H.; Bernsen, M.R.; Van Osch, G.J.V.M.V.M. Platelet-Rich Plasma Releasate Inhibits Inflammatory Processes in Osteoarthritic Chondrocytes. *Am. J. Sports Med.* **2011**, *39*, 2362–2370. [CrossRef] [PubMed]
37. Woodell-May, J.; Matuska, A.; Oyster, M.; Welch, Z.; O'Shaughnessey, K.; Hoeppner, J. Autologous Protein Solution Inhibits MMP-13 Production by IL-1β and TNFα-Stimulated Human Articular Chondrocytes. *J. Orthop. Res.* **2011**, *29*, 1320–1326. [CrossRef] [PubMed]
38. Wang, C.C.; Lee, C.-H.H.; Peng, Y.J.; Salter, D.M.; Lee, H.S. Platelet-Rich Plasma Attenuates 30-KDa Fibronectin Fragment-Induced Chemokine and Matrix Metalloproteinase Expression by Meniscocytes and Articular Chondrocytes. *Am. J. Sports Med.* **2015**, *43*, 2481–2489. [CrossRef]
39. Wu, C.C.; Chen, W.H.; Zao, B.; Lai, P.L.; Lin, T.C.; Lo, H.Y.; Shieh, Y.H.; Wu, C.H.; Deng, W.P. Regenerative Potentials of Platelet-Rich Plasma Enhanced by Collagen in Retrieving pro-Inflammatory Cytokine-Inhibited Chondrogenesis. *Biomaterials* **2011**, *32*, 5847–5854. [CrossRef]
40. Tamura, T.; Kosaka, N.; Ishiwa, J.; Sato, T.; Nagase, H.; Ito, A. Rhein, an Active Metabolite of Diacerein, down-Regulates the Production of pro-Matrix Metalloproteinases-1, -3, -9 and -13 and up-Regulates the Production of Tissue Inhibitor of Metalloproteinase-1 in Cultured Rabbit Articular Chondrocytes. *Osteoarthr. Cartil.* **2001**, *9*, 257–263. [CrossRef] [PubMed]
41. Roman-Blas, J.A.; Jimenez, S.A. NF-KappaB as a Potential Therapeutic Target in Osteoarthritis and Rheumatoid Arthritis. *Osteoarthr. Cartil.* **2006**, *14*, 839–848. [CrossRef]
42. Zhuo, F.; Li, J.; Wang, Y.H.; Li, M.; Song, F.F.; Liu, Y.L.; Tao, Z.Y. Platelet-Rich Plasma Inhibits Inflammation, Apoptosis, and the NLRP3/Caspase-1 Pathway and Induces Matrix Metalloproteinases and Proliferation of IL-1β-Induced Articular Chondrocytes by Downregulating T-Box Transcription Factor 3. *Eur. J. Inflamm.* **2022**, *20*, 1–10. [CrossRef]
43. Yang, J.; Guo, A.; Li, Q.; Wu, J. Platelet-Rich Plasma Attenuates Interleukin-1β-Induced Apoptosis and Inflammation in Chondrocytes through Targeting Hypoxia-Inducible Factor-2α. *Tissue Cell* **2021**, *73*, 101646. [CrossRef]
44. Moussa, M.; Lajeunesse, D.; Hilal, G.; El Atat, O.; Haykal, G.; Serhal, R.; Chalhoub, A.; Khalil, C.; Alaaeddine, N. Platelet Rich Plasma (PRP) Induces Chondroprotection via Increasing Autophagy, Anti-Inflammatory Markers, and Decreasing Apoptosis in Human Osteoarthritic Cartilage. *Exp. Cell Res.* **2017**, *352*, 146–156. [CrossRef] [PubMed]
45. Yaron, M.; Shirazi, I.; Yaron, I. Anti-Interleukin-1 Effects of Diacerein and Rhein in Human Osteoarthritic Synovial Tissue and Cartilage Cultures. *Osteoarthr. Cartil.* **1999**, *7*, 272–280. [CrossRef]
46. Pelletier, J.P.; Mineau, F.; Fernandes, J.C.; Duval, N.; Martel-Pelletier, J. Diacerhein and Rhein Reduce the Interleukin 1beta Stimulated Inducible Nitric Oxide Synthesis Level and Activity While Stimulating Cyclooxygenase-2 Synthesis in Human Osteoarthritic Chondrocytes. *J. Rheumatol.* **1998**, *25*, 2417–2424. [PubMed]
47. Eitner, A.; Müller, S.; König, C.; Wilharm, A.; Raab, R.; Hofmann, G.O.; Kamradt, T.; Schaible, H.-G. Inhibition of Inducible Nitric Oxide Synthase Prevents IL-1β-Induced Mitochondrial Dysfunction in Human Chondrocytes. *Int. J. Mol. Sci.* **2021**, *22*, 2477. [CrossRef] [PubMed]
48. Abramson, S.B. Osteoarthritis and Nitric Oxide. *Osteoarthr. Cartil.* **2008**, *16*, S15–S20. [CrossRef]
49. Yin, W.; Xu, H.; Sheng, J.; Xu, Z.; Xie, X.; Zhang, C. Comparative Evaluation of the Effects of Platelet-Rich Plasma Formulations on Extracellular Matrix Formation and the NF-KB Signaling Pathway in Human Articular Chondrocytes. *Mol. Med. Rep.* **2017**, *15*, 2940–2948. [CrossRef]
50. Lo, Y.Y.; Conquer, J.A.; Grinstein, S.; Cruz, T.F. Interleukin-1 Beta Induction of c-Fos and Collagenase Expression in Articular Chondrocytes: Involvement of Reactive Oxygen Species. *J. Cell. Biochem.* **1998**, *69*, 19–29. [CrossRef]
51. Gómez-Gaete, C.; Retamal, M.; Chávez, C.; Bustos, P.; Godoy, R.; Torres-Vergara, P. Development, Characterization and in Vitro Evaluation of Biodegradable Rhein-Loaded Microparticles for Treatment of Osteoarthritis. *Eur. J. Pharm. Sci.* **2017**, *96*, 390–397. [CrossRef] [PubMed]
52. Moldovan, F.; Pelletier, J.P.; Jolicoeur, F.C.; Cloutier, J.M.; Martel-Pelletier, J. Diacerhein and Rhein Reduce the ICE-Induced IL-1beta and IL-18 Activation in Human Osteoarthritic Cartilage. *Osteoarthr. Cartil.* **2000**, *8*, 186–196. [CrossRef]
53. Liu, X.; Wang, L.; Ma, C.; Wang, G.; Zhang, Y.; Sun, S. Exosomes Derived from Platelet-Rich Plasma Present a Novel Potential in Alleviating Knee Osteoarthritis by Promoting Proliferation and Inhibiting Apoptosis of Chondrocyte via Wnt/β-Catenin Signaling Pathway. *J. Orthop. Surg. Res.* **2019**, *14*, 470. [CrossRef] [PubMed]
54. Domagala, F.; Martin, G.; Bogdanowicz, P.; Ficheux, H.; Pujol, J.-P. Inhibition of Interleukin-1beta-Induced Activation of MEK/ERK Pathway and DNA Binding of NF-KappaB and AP-1: Potential Mechanism for Diacerein Effects in Osteoarthritis. *Biorheology* **2006**, *43*, 577–587. [PubMed]

55. Cavallo, C.; Filardo, G.; Mariani, E.; Kon, E.; Marcacci, M.; Pereira Ruiz, M.T.; Facchini, A.; Grigolo, B. Comparison of Platelet-Rich Plasma Formulations for Cartilage Healing: An in Vitro Study. *J. Bone Jt. Surg. Am.* **2014**, *96*, 423–429. [CrossRef] [PubMed]
56. Sakata, R.; McNary, S.M.; Miyatake, K.; Lee, C.A.; Van den Bogaerde, J.M.; Marder, R.A.; Reddi, A.H. Stimulation of the Superficial Zone Protein and Lubrication in the Articular Cartilage by Human Platelet-Rich Plasma. *Am. J. Sports Med.* **2015**, *43*, 1467–1473. [CrossRef]

life

MDPI

Article

One-Year Handgrip Strength Change in Kindergarteners Depends upon Physical Activity Status

Akemi Abe [1], Rika Sanui [2], Jeremy P. Loenneke [3] and Takashi Abe [1,4,*]

1 Division of Children's Health and Exercise Research, Institute of Trainology, Fukuoka 814-0001, Japan; amyabe3379@gmail.com
2 Child Health Research Group, Atagohama Kindergarten, Fukuoka 819-0002, Japan; atagohama1@gmail.com
3 Department of Health, Exercise Science, & Recreation Management, Kevser Ermin Applied Physiology Laboratory, The University of Mississippi, Oxford, MS 38677, USA; jploenne@olemiss.edu
4 Institute of Health and Sports Science & Medicine, Graduate School of Health and Sports Science, Juntendo University, Inzai 270-1695, Japan
* Correspondence: t12abe@gmail.com

Abstract: Free play in kindergarten can be roughly divided into fine and gross motor activities, but the effects of these activities on improving handgrip strength are unknown. Therefore, we aimed to compare one-year changes in handgrip strength and forearm flexor muscle size in children separated by preferred play in a kindergarten. One hundred and eleven children were recruited from a local kindergarten. They underwent handgrip strength and forearm muscle thickness measurements, and 95 (49 boys and 46 girls) underwent a second measurement one year after the first measurement. Class teachers assessed the physical activity of everyone in their class after the second measurement. Using three evaluation scores by the class teachers, we divided children into three groups based on the children's preference to play in kindergarten (fine movement vs. gross motor movement). Handgrip strength did not change differently between groups across one year. However, children who liked active playing outside (i.e., gross motor activity) were stronger than others. Furthermore, children who like playing outside observed greater changes than the other groups in the ulna (right hand) and radius muscle thickness (left hand), suggesting that changes in forearm muscle size might be incongruent with changes in handgrip strength among the three activity groups.

Keywords: grip strength; young children; active play; growth and development

Citation: Abe, A.; Sanui, R.; Loenneke, J.P.; Abe, T. One-Year Handgrip Strength Change in Kindergarteners Depends upon Physical Activity Status. *Life* **2023**, *13*, 1665. https://doi.org/10.3390/life13081665

Academic Editor: Clinton T. Rubin

Received: 13 June 2023
Revised: 17 July 2023
Accepted: 29 July 2023
Published: 31 July 2023

1. Introduction

Handgrip strength is a biomarker of current health status and future morbidity/disability in middle-aged and older adults [1]. For example, a study investigated the association between handgrip strength and the incidence of heart disease in 20,829 middle-aged and older adults aged 50 or older [2]. The incidence rate of heart disease was adjusted for covariates such as age, education level, physical activity, body mass index, alcohol, smoking, and medical history. The authors found that those in the highest quartile of handgrip strength had a 35% lower risk of being diagnosed with heart disease compared with those in the lowest quartile in men and 46% in women over 13 years of follow-up. In addition, it is noted that there was a difference of 12 kg for men and 10 kg for women between the highest and lowest quartile cut-off values for handgrip strength in each age group. Similarly, recent large-sized follow-up studies also reported an inverse association between handgrip strength and the incidence rate of type 2 diabetes [3], cancer [4], and dementia [5]. Our article search found over 100 similar articles in the last quarter century (e.g., [6–25]).

Given that handgrip strength can be a biomarker that predicts current and future health status, it seems necessary to discuss how to increase this handgrip strength [26,27].

Recently, we compared differences in handgrip strength among different sports in first-year university male students enrolled in a sports university [28]. We found that handgrip strength was greater in participants who participated in sports with upper-body movements (i.e., kendo and baseball) than those in sports that primarily involve lower-body activities (i.e., soccer). Interestingly, the mean difference between the kendo and soccer groups was approximately 5 kg, but the difference between the two groups has gradually widened over the past 45 years. Similar results were observed in female students [29]. Those results suggest that the type of physical activity performed during the developmental period may affect the handgrip strength acquired by children in the development process.

Although research is limited, previous studies have examined the impact of family- and school-based interventions on handgrip strength in children and adolescents [30–32]. However, the intervention program did not affect handgrip strength in the intervention group compared with the control group. Unfortunately, most studies investigating the effects of school-based physical education classes did not include handgrip strength changes after the exercise intervention [27]. In addition, more recent studies investigating the effects of an exercise training intervention on handgrip strength in preschool-aged children have reported conflicting results; one study found significant improvements in handgrip strength in the intervention group compared to the control group [33], while another did not [34]. However, we could not determine why one study found a benefit and another did not.

In free-play behaviors in kindergarten, some children prefer fine movements (primarily using hands and fingers) and others prefer gross motor activities (primarily using the lower body). It would be meaningful to know the impact of preferred play on changes in handgrip strength during growth. Therefore, this study aimed to compare one-year changes in handgrip strength and forearm muscle size in children separated by preferred play in a kindergarten (fine movement vs. gross motor movement).

2. Materials and Methods

2.1. Study Design

This is a study of kindergarteners conducted in the city of Fukuoka, Japan. This kindergarten has a relatively large (approximately 3100 m^2) lawn garden for children. Data collection took place from October 2021 to November 2022. The measurements were performed in the morning (9:00–10:00 AM, at room temperature of approximately 22 °C) using the same methodological protocols described below. This study received approval from the ethics committee of Seinan Gakuin University (application no SG #2021-2-2) and was conducted according to the Declaration for Helsinki. Children with their parents were fully informed about the purpose of the study and its safety, and written informed consent was obtained from the parents of each child.

2.2. Participants

With the cooperation of the school's staff and parents, 111 young children (56 boys and 55 girls) were recruited from a local kindergarten. Few children used their left hand or mixed hands to eat and write (n = 4). All participants completed the first measurement, but 95 (49 boys and 46 girls) underwent a second measurement one year after the first because some children transferred to other kindergartens due to their parents' jobs (Table 1). Only data from these 95 participants were used for this study.

Table 1. Changes in anthropometric variables, ultrasound-measured forearm muscle thickness, and handgrip strength in boys and girls.

	Boys	Girls
N	49	46
Age (yr)		
Test 1	4.5 ± 0.6	4.6 ± 0.5
Test 2	5.5 ± 0.6	5.6 ± 0.5
Height (cm)		
Test 1	103.9 ± 5.5	103.1 ± 5.0
Test 2	109.9 ± 5.6	109.3 ± 5.4
Change	6.0 ± 0.8	6.2 ± 0.9
Body mass (kg)		
Test 1	17.0 ± 1.9	16.4 ± 2.1
Test 2	18.8 ± 2.4	18.3 ± 2.7
Change	1.8 ± 0.9	1.9 ± 0.9
Muscle thickness ulna, right hand (mm)		
Test 1	21.2 ± 1.7	20.8 ± 2.0
Test 2	23.3 ± 1.7	22.6 ± 2.1
Change	2.0 ± 0.9	1.8 ± 1.3
Muscle thickness radius, right hand (mm)		
Test 1	10.6 ± 1.3	10.1 ± 1.3
Test 2	11.3 ± 1.3	10.8 ± 1.5
Change	0.7 ± 0.8	0.7 ± 0.9
Handgrip strength, right hand (kg)		
Test 1	8.1 ± 2.7	6.6 ± 2.4
Test 2	11.6 ± 2.3	9.8 ± 2.3
Change	3.5 ± 1.6	3.3 ± 2.1

Results are expressed as mean and standard deviation. Statistical differences are noted in the text. The table is meant to be descriptive.

2.3. Handgrip Strength Measurements

Maximum voluntary handgrip strength was measured with the right and left hands using a Smedley handgrip dynamometer (TKK Grip-A, Niigata, Japan) [35,36]. All children were instructed to maintain an upright standing position to keep their arms at their sides. The participants held the dynamometer in their right or left hand with the elbow extended downward without squeezing. The distance of the dynamometer grip bars (grip span) was adjusted to the hand size of the children (the middle phalanx rested on the inner handle) [37]. All children were allowed to perform two maximal trials on each side with a one-minute break. All the participants appeared motivated during the strength tests [38,39]. The highest value on each side was used for data analysis.

2.4. Forearm Muscle Thickness Measurements

Anterior forearm muscle thickness was also measured using B-mode ultrasound (Logiq e; GE, Fairfield, CT, USA) at 30% proximal of forearm length (between the styloid process and the head of the radius) on the right side of the body [40]. A linear scanning head was coated with transmission gel and placed on the skin surface of the measurement site with minimum pressure to achieve a clear image. Two images from the site were stored for offline analysis following data collection. Muscle thickness of the radius (MT-radius) and ulna (MT-ulna) was measured as the perpendicular distance between the adipose tissue–muscle interface and the muscle–bone interface. The average value measured on two images was used for data analysis.

Before ultrasound measurements, standing height and body mass were measured to the nearest 0.1 cm and 0.1 kg, respectively, using a height scale and an electronic weight scale. Forearm length and girth (at 30% proximal of forearm length) were also measured using a flexible tape measure.

2.5. Physical Activity Assessments

Class teachers assessed the physical activity of everyone in their class after the second measurement. The teacher of each class was unaware of any of the study participants' results from the handgrip strength test and ultrasound muscle thickness measurements. We asked the class teachers to evaluate the physical activity level from the following three evaluation points. The first evaluation point concerned whether the children preferred to play indoors or outdoors during free play in kindergarten: (1) Often plays indoors, (2) intermediate, and (3) often plays outdoors. The second evaluation point was whether or not children sweated during free play: (1) Never sweating from play, (2) intermediate, and (3) always sweating from play. The last evaluation point was a question about the type of play. We provided teachers with two different examples of play: One being gross-motor movements (e.g., tag, rope-jumping, dodgeball) and the other being fine movements (e.g., block play, the art of paper folding, drawing pictures). We asked teachers whether or not children were challenged with various play in each preferred play: (1) Often performed the same type of play; (2) intermediate; (3) or performed many different types of challenging play.

From the above three points, we divided them into three groups. For example, children who preferred to sit and play, never sweated from play, and performed relatively similar activities would be rated 1, 1, and 1 and would be assigned to "Group 1". In contrast, children who liked to play outdoors, always sweated from play, and engaged in many types of play would be rated 3, 3, and 3 and would be assigned to "Group 3". Children rated 2 (intermediate) on three evaluation points were assigned to "Group 2." When all three scores were not the same, children were grouped as follows: No children had all different ratings (i.e., 1, 2, and 3) on the three evaluation points. That is, at least two ratings were in agreement. Therefore, we adopted two matching evaluation points to separate the groups. As a result, the number of children in each group was divided as follows: Group 1 (n = 23), Group 2 (n = 34), and Group 3 (n = 38).

2.6. Statistical Analysis

Overall changes in handgrip strength and muscle size were determined using paired sample t-tests. A repeated-measures ANOVA on time with a between-subject factor of sex was used to determine differences in muscle size and strength between boys and girls. To determine the influence of activity level, we used a repeated-measures ANOVA on time with a between-subject factor of activity level. We also included sex as a covariate to determine if that altered the result. Post-hoc comparisons were not adjusted for multiple comparisons. Statistical significance was set at $p < 0.05$. Normality was visually assessed using a Q-Q plot, and Levene's test was used for testing the homogeneity of variance. All statistical analyses were run using Jamovi version 2.3.13.0. Data are presented as mean and 95% confidence intervals unless otherwise stated.

3. Results

3.1. Overall Change in Handgrip Strength and Muscle Size

Handgrip strength increased in both the right (a change of 3.3 (3.0, 3.7) kg) and left (a change of 3.1 (2.7, 3.4) kg) hands. For muscle thickness, there were also increases for MT-ulna (right forearm: 1.9 (1.7, 2.1) mm; left forearm: 1.8 (1.6, 2.1) mm) and MT-radius (right forearm: 0.7 (0.5, 0.8) mm; left forearm: 0.7 (0.5, 0.9) mm) in both the right and left forearms.

3.2. Comparison between Boys and Girls

Handgrip strength did not change differently between boys and girls for either the right hand (time x sex: p = 0.498) or the left hand (time x sex: p = 0.991). Handgrip strength was greater at the second time point compared to the first. However, boys had greater overall strength than girls (when collapsed across time; $p \leq 0.001$). On the right hand, boys were 1.6 (0.7, 2.5) kg stronger, and on the left hand, boys were 1.5 (0.6, 2.4) kg stronger (Table 1).

MT-ulna did not change differently between boys and girls (Table 1) for either the right forearm (time x sex: $p = 0.309$) or the left forearm (time x sex: $p = 0.388$). Muscle thickness was greater at the second time point than the first, but there was no main effect of sex ($p = 0.11$ and $p = 0.1$ for right and left, respectively).

MT-radius did not change differently between boys and girls (Table 1) for either the right forearm (time x sex: $p = 0.91$) or the left forearm (time x sex: $p = 0.388$). Muscle thickness was greater at the second time point than the first, but there was no main effect of sex ($p = 0.06$ and $p = 0.1$ for right and left, respectively).

3.3. Comparison among Three Physical Activity Groups

Handgrip strength did not change differently between activity levels for either the right hand (time x activity level: $p = 0.365$) or the left hand (time x activity level: $p = 0.307$) (Figure 1). Handgrip strength was greater at the second time point compared to the first; however, activity level did influence overall strength when collapsed across time for the right hand ($p = 0.002$) and the left hand ($p = 0.008$). Post-hoc analysis for the right hand found that Group 3 was significantly greater than Group 2 (difference of 1.3 (0.2, 2.3) kg, $p = 0.015$) and Group 1 (difference of 2 (0.9, 3.2) kg, $p = 0.001$). Group 1 was not statistically different from Group 2 ($p = 0.2$). This result held following an adjustment for sex. Post-hoc analysis for the left hand found that Group 3 was significantly greater than Group 1 (difference of 1.8 (0.6, 3.0) kg, $p = 0.002$) but not Group 2 (difference of 0.9 (−0.05, 2.0) kg, $p = 0.06$). Group 2 was also not statistically different from Group 1 ($p = 0.166$). This result held following an adjustment for sex.

MT-ulna changed differently (Figure 2) between activity levels for the right forearm (time x activity level: $p = 0.013$) but not the left forearm (time x activity level: $p = 0.4$). Changes across the year were greatest in Group 3 compared to Group 2 (difference of 0.67 (0.17, 1.1) mm) and Group 1 (difference of 0.68 (0.11, 1.2) mm). There were no differences between Group 2 and Group 1 ($p = 0.986$). The statistical interaction held following an adjustment for sex. When collapsed across time, Group 3 was greater than Group 2 ($p = 0.02$) and Group 1 ($p = 0.03$), but Group 2 was not greater than Group 1 ($p = 0.96$). For MT-ulna of the left forearm, there was a time effect and effect of activity level. MT-ulna was greater at the second time point than the first, and Group 3 was greater than Group 2 (difference of 1.0 (0.26, 1.9) mm, $p = 0.01$). There were no other statistically significant differences. Results remained the same following an adjustment for sex.

MT-radius did not change differently (Figure 3) between activity levels for the right forearm (time x activity level: $p = 0.23$), but it did for the left forearm (time x activity level: $p = 0.033$). Both results held following an adjustment for sex. MT-radius of the right forearm was greater at the second time point than the first. Group 3 had greater MT-radius values than Group 2 (difference of 0.81 (0.23, 1.39) mm; $p = 0.006$) and Group 1 (difference of 0.82 (0.16, 1.47) mm; $p = 0.014$). Group 2 was not different from Group 1 ($p = 0.993$). MT-radius of the left arm changed differently across time between activity levels. Changes across the year in the left forearm were greater in Group 3 and Group 2 compared to Group 1 (Group 3 vs. Group 1: 0.59 (0.1, 1.0) mm; Group 2 vs. Group 1: 0.59 (0.09, 1.0) mm). There was no difference in the differences between Group 3 and Group 2. When collapsed across time, Group 3 was greater than Group 2 ($p = 0.0004$).

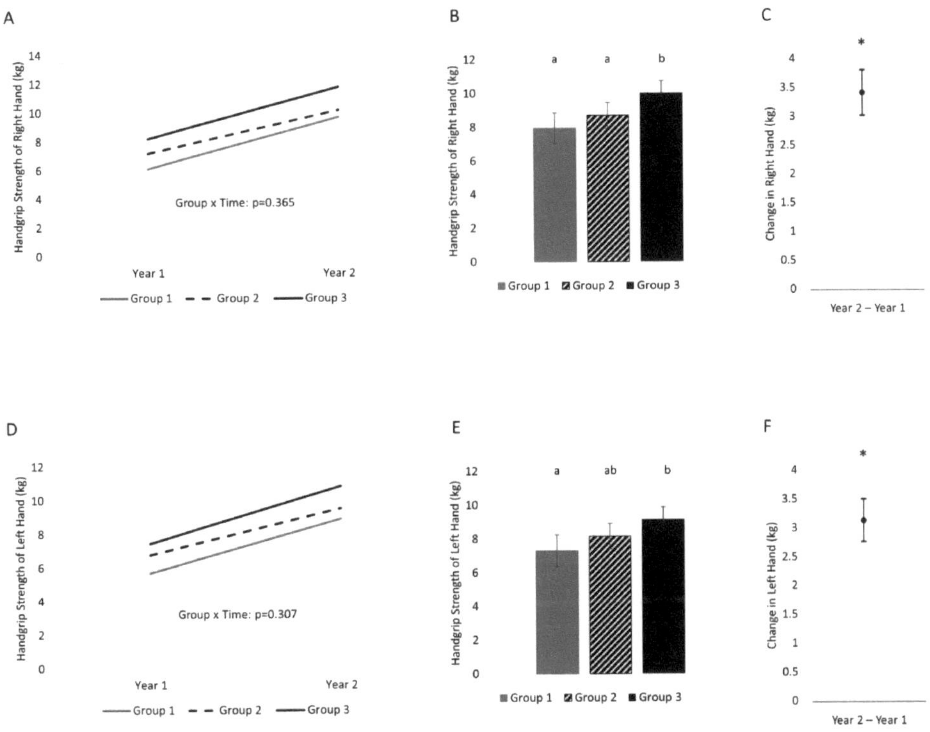

Figure 1. One-year changes in handgrip strength of the right and left hands separated into three groups on the basis of physical activity status. (**A**) Changes across time separated by group (variability of changes are found in Table 2) in the right hand, (**B**) between-subject effect of group (collapsed across time) in the right hand, (**C**) time effect (collapsed across group) in the right hand; (**D**) change across time separated by group (variability of changes are found in Table 2) in the left hand, (**E**) between-subject effect of group (collapsed across time) in the left hand, (**F**) time effect (collapsed across group) in the left hand. Variability is represented by 95% confidence intervals. Conditions that share a letter are not statistically significantly from each other. * indicates a statistically significant time effect.

Table 2. Changes in anthropometric variables, forearm muscle thickness, and handgrip strength in three groups.

	Group 1	Group 2	Group 3
N	23 (9 boys, 14 girls)	34 (15 boys, 19 girls)	38 (25 boys, 13 girls)
Age (yr)			
Test 1	4.4 ± 0.6	4.6 ± 0.5	4.7 ± 0.6
Test 2	5.4 ± 0.6	5.6 ± 0.5	5.7 ± 0.5
Height (cm)			
Test 1	101.9 ± 4.8	103.1 ±5.0	104.9 ± 5.5
Test 2	108.1 ± 5.4	109.1 ± 5.2	110.9 ± 5.5
Body mass (kg)			
Test 1	16.6 ± 2.4	16.1 ± 1.7	17.3 ± 2.0
Test 2	18.4 ± 3.0	17.9 ± 2.2	19.3 ± 2.5
Muscle thickness ulna, right hand (mm)			
Test 1	20.7 ± 2.2	20.7 ± 1.8	21.4 ± 1.6
Test 2	22.4 ± 2.3	22.4 ± 1.7	23.7 ± 1.6
Change	1.7 ± 1.2	1.7 ± 1.1	2.3 ± 1.0

Table 2. *Cont.*

	Group 1	Group 2	Group 3
Muscle thickness ulna, left hand (mm)			
Test 1	20.7 ± 2.2	20.3 ± 1.5	21.2 ± 1.7
Test 2	22.4 ± 2.4	22.1 ± 1.8	23.3 ± 1.7
Change	1.7 ± 1.1	1.8 ± 1.0	2.1 ± 1.4
Muscle thickness radius, right hand (mm)			
Test 1	10.0 ± 1.4	10.1 ± 1.4	10.7 ± 1.0
Test 2	10.7 ± 1.8	10.6 ± 1.4	11.6 ± 1.0
Change	0.7 ± 1.0	0.5 ± 0.7	0.9 ± 0.9
Muscle thickness radius, left hand (mm)			
Test 1	10.4 ± 1.5	9.7 ± 1.5	10.8 ± 1.1
Test 2	10.7 ± 1.6	10.6 ± 1.4	11.7 ± 1.2
Change	0.3 ± 1.0	0.9 ± 0.9	0.9 ± 0.9
Handgrip strength, right hand (kg)			
Test 1	6.1 ± 2.2	7.2 ± 2.8	8.2 ± 2.5
Test 2	9.7 ± 2.6	10.2 ± 2.5	11.8 ± 1.9
Change	3.6 ± 2.0	3.0 ± 1.7	3.6 ± 2.0
Handgrip strength, left hand (kg)			
Test 1	5.7 ± 2.4	6.8 ± 2.6	7.5 ± 2.5
Test 2	8.9 ± 2.8	9.5 ± 2.3	10.8 ± 1.8
Change	3.2 ± 2.0	2.7 ± 1.5	3.4 ± 1.8

Results are expressed as mean and standard deviation. Change = Test 2 − Test 1. Statistical differences are noted in the text. The table is meant to be descriptive.

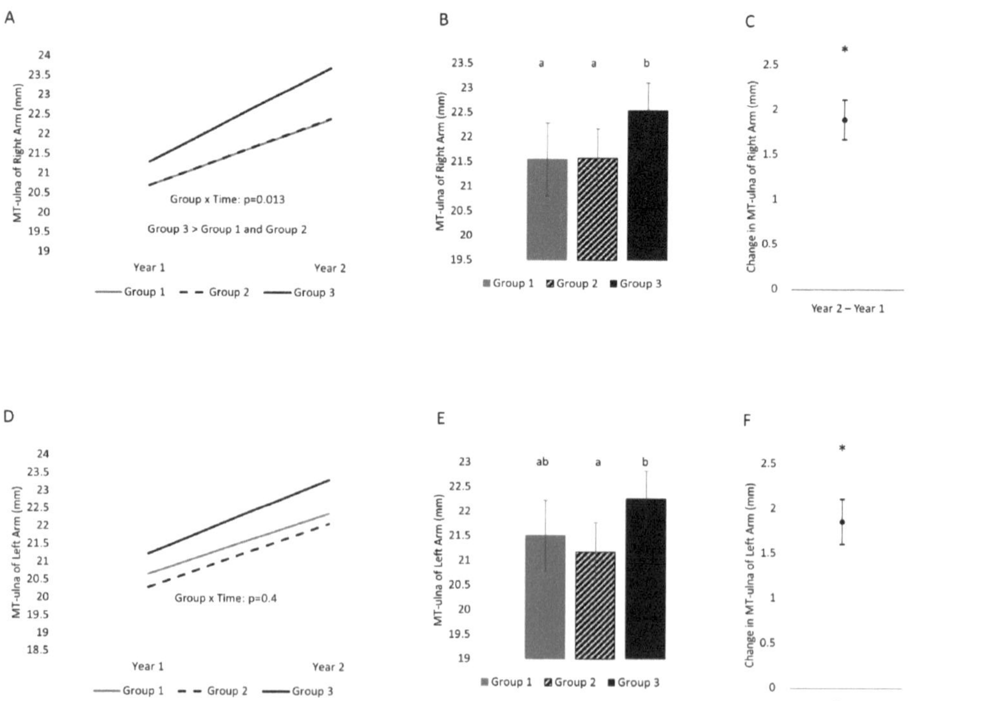

Figure 2. One-year changes in MT-ulna of the right and left hands separated into three groups on the basis of physical activity status. (**A**) Changes across time separated by group (variability of changes are found in Table 2) in the right arm, (**B**) between-subject effect of group (collapsed across time) in the

right arm, (**C**) time effect (collapsed across group) in the right arm; (**D**) change across time separated by group (variability of changes are found in Table 2) in the left arm, (**E**) between-subject effect of group (collapsed across time) in the left arm, (**F**) time effect (collapsed across group) in the left arm. Variability is represented by 95% confidence intervals. Conditions that share a letter are not statistically significantly from each other. * indicates a statistically significant time effect.

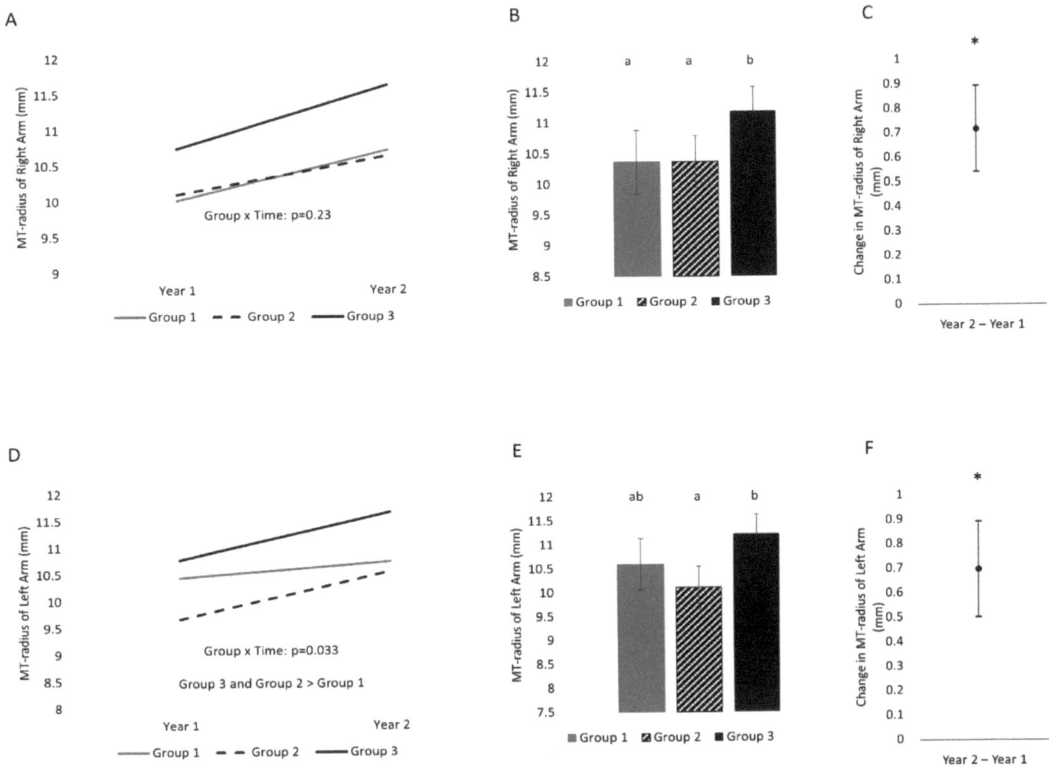

Figure 3. One-year changes in MT-radius of the right and left hands separated into three groups on the basis of physical activity status. (**A**) Changes across time separated by group (variability of changes are found in Table 2) in the right arm, (**B**) between-subject effect of group (collapsed across time) in the right arm, (**C**) time effect (collapsed across group) in the right arm; (**D**) change across time separated by group (variability of changes are found in Table 2) in the left arm, (**E**) between-subject effect of group (collapsed across time) in the left arm, (**F**) time effect (collapsed across group) in the left arm. Variability is represented by 95% confidence intervals. Conditions that share a letter are not statistically significantly from each other. * indicates a statistically significant time effect.

4. Discussion

We investigated whether the change in one-year handgrip strength depended upon the children's physical activity status. Physical activity status was based on the children's preferred play in kindergarten (fine movement vs. gross motor movement). The present study found that a one-year change in handgrip strength was similar among three physical activity groups. However, children who liked active play outside (i.e., gross motor movement) were stronger than children of other groups (i.e., group effect). In contrast, muscle thickness changed differently across groups in MT-ulna of the right hand and MT-radius of the left hand. These results suggest that differences among children already exist as early as kindergarten and that changes in forearm muscle thickness do not always occur in alignment with changes in muscle strength.

4.1. One-Year Change in Handgrip Strength

Active play that children perform outside in kindergarten during free time is an activity that primarily uses the lower body. Previous studies [41,42] observed increased muscle strength of the untrained upper extremities due to resistance training of the lower extremities (called the cross-transfer effect). However, there are no studies on increased handgrip strength with a lower-body exercise intervention, and no such results were found in this study. On the other hand, fine motor activities primarily use the hands and fingers. Therefore, practicing fine motor activities helps children improve their fine motor skills [43].

In the present study, our results showed that a one-year change in handgrip strength was not different among the three active groups, but children who liked active play outside (Group 3) were stronger than other groups. Therefore, children in Group 3 are hypothesized to have been similarly active before the study period, which may have contributed to their greater handgrip strength. Unfortunately, in this study, we could not evaluate the specific play of children, such as types, amount, and intensity before and during this study. Furthermore, we could not investigate what children do with their families after school or on weekends. However, previous studies have reported the possibility that exercise using the upper body during play in children may be involved in improving handgrip strength [27]. For example, one study investigated the effects of upper-body exercise on handgrip strength in an intervention group by comparing it with a control group [44]. The intervention group ($n = 40$, mean age 8.4 years) performed upper-body exercises such as self-supported movements (e.g., wheelbarrow, seal walk, crabwalk) and circuit exercises (e.g., tennis balls for squeezing, strips of rubber tire to pull) three times a week. The control group ($n = 46$, mean age 8.6 years) had a free-play period, which was part of the normal school routine. The changes in handgrip strength were significantly greater ($p < 0.05$) for the intervention group compared to the control group (pre–post change of the right hand: Experimental group = 1.5 kg and control group = 0.3 kg) following a 12-week intervention. More recently, we investigated the effects of the type of sports practiced on handgrip strength in first-year sport university students, as mentioned above [28,29]. The authors selected two types of sporting events with matching physiques (i.e., height and body mass); Soccer ($n = 1127$) targets the lower body, and Kendo ($n = 297$) and Baseball ($n = 698$) use the lower body simultaneously with upper-body movement (including gripping) and report that those in the lower-body-only (Soccer) sports had −3.78 (95% CI: −4.27, −3.29) kg lower handgrip strength than those in the lower + upper body (Kendo and Baseball) sporting events [28]. Comparing each individual sport found that each sport was different from the others with Kendo > Baseball > Soccer (between each sport, $p < 0.001$). In addition, the difference in handgrip strength between Kendo and Soccer was approximately 5 kg in the overall sample. Considering the results of the above-mentioned previous studies and this study, it is expected that grip strength during an object's gripping movements improves handgrip strength during the developmental period. However, further research is needed on the gripping conditions (e.g., intensity and duration) for improving handgrip strength in children and adolescents.

4.2. One-Year Change in Forearm Muscle Thickness

An interesting finding obtained in this study was that changes in handgrip strength and changes in forearm flexor muscle thickness were inconsistent among the three groups with different physical activity preferences. We recently investigated the association between handgrip strength changes and forearm flexor muscle thickness changes in 218 young children different from the sample of this study [45]. The study found that there were significant ($p < 0.001$) within-subject correlations between ulna muscle thickness and handgrip strength (r = 0.50) and radius muscle thickness and handgrip strength (r = 0.59). However, while there was a statistically significant ($p < 0.001$) between-subject relationship between radius muscle thickness and handgrip strength (r = 0.27), there was no significant between-subject correlation between ulna muscle thickness and handgrip strength (r = 0.07). It has been reported that muscle strength and size changes do not always match during resistance training in healthy young adults [46]. Although changes do not necessarily line up, it should be noted that those in Group 3 tended to have the most muscle size and strength.

The reasons for the difference in muscle thickness change in children who liked active playing outside compared with other groups between the left and right arms over one year are unknown. However, considering the ulna muscle thickness includes two major extrinsic flexor muscles of the fingers, whereas the radius muscle thickness involves muscles in the forearm pronation and wrist and elbow joint flexion [47], and differences in how to use the left and right hands may have appeared (e.g., perhaps related to tasks completed with dominant vs. non-dominant hands; most children were right-handed). These are all speculations and future research is needed to clarify this issue.

4.3. *Physical Activity Assessment*

In this study, class teachers assessed their children's physical activity during their free time in a kindergarten, as reported previously [48]. The teachers spend time in kindergarten with the children in their class (approximately between 8:00 AM and 3:00 PM) every weekday. An advantage of the proxy-reported tools over the other measurement tools, such as the accelerometer, is that they could capture the context and type of the behaviors [49]. This study aimed not to quantify children's physical activity (such as intensity and duration) but to understand the kind of play that children prefer. From this point, it is considered that the assessments of physical activity by the teachers were appropriate for measuring the behaviors of interest. Although we view this assessment as appropriate and informative, subjective assessments of physical activity from teachers are imperfect.

5. Conclusions

Free play in kindergarten is roughly divided into fine and gross motor activities. This study observed no difference in one-year changes in handgrip strength between activity groups, but children who liked active playing outside were stronger than other children. These results suggest that there are already differences in strength in young children prior to entering kindergarten. Assuming these children had similar activity levels prior to entering school, these results suggest that children who actively play outdoors may acquire higher handgrip strength than those who prefer indoor play. Regardless of the reason, strength differences between children appear very early in life. Furthermore, changes in forearm muscle thickness might be inconsistent with handgrip strength changes among the three activity groups.

Author Contributions: Conceptualization, A.A., R.S., J.P.L. and T.A.; investigation, A.A., R.S. and T.A.; formal analysis, J.P.L. and T.A.; writing–original draft, A.A. and T.A.; writing—review and editing, J.P.L. All authors have read and agreed to the published version of the manuscript.

Funding: This study was supported by grant support from the Japan Society for the Promotion of Science Grants-in-Aid for Scientific Research (JSPS KAKENHI Grant Number 22K11610).

Institutional Review Board Statement: This study was approved by the ethics committee of Seinan Gakuin University (application no SG #2021-2-2; 9 July 2021).

Informed Consent Statement: Written informed consent was obtained from the parents of each child.

Data Availability Statement: Data are available from the corresponding author upon reasonable request.

Acknowledgments: The authors are grateful to all the children who participated in this study, their caregivers, and all the supporting staff of the kindergarten (Hara, M.; Anai, M.; Ishibashi, A.; Nakahara, S.; Honda, R.; Asai, K.; Murata, S.; Abe, H.).

Conflicts of Interest: The authors have no conflict of interest directly relevant to the content of this article.

References

1. Bohannon, R.W. Grip strength: An indispensable biomarker for older adults. *Clin. Interv. Aging* **2019**, *14*, 1681–1691. [CrossRef] [PubMed]
2. Peralta, M.; Dias, C.M.; Marques, A.; Henriques-Neto, D.; Sousa-Uva, M. Longitudinal association between grip strength and the risk of heart diseases among European middle-aged and older adults. *Exp. Gerontol.* **2023**, *171*, 112014. [CrossRef] [PubMed]
3. Boonpor, J.; Parra-Soto, S.; Petermann-Rocha, F.; Ferrari, G.; Welsh, P.; Pell, J.P.; Sattar, N.; Gill, J.M.R.; Ho, F.K.; Gray, S.R.; et al. Associations between grip strength and incident type 2 diabetes: Findings from the UK Biobank prospective cohort study. *BMJ Open Diabetes Res. Care* **2021**, *9*, e001865. [CrossRef] [PubMed]
4. Parra-Soto, S.; Pell, J.P.; Celis-Morales, C.; Ho, F.K. Absolute and relative grip strength as predictors of cancer: Prospective cohort study of 445552 participants in UK Biobank. *J. Cachexia Sarcopenia Muscle* **2022**, *13*, 325–332. [CrossRef]
5. Esteban-Cornejo, I.; Ho, F.K.; Petermann-Rocha, F.; Lyall, D.M.; Martinez-Gomez, D.; Cabanas-Sanchez, V.; Ortega, F.B.; Hillman, C.H.; Gill, J.M.; Quinn, T.J.; et al. Handgrip strength and all-cause dementia incidence and mortality: Findings from the UK Biobank prospective cohort study. *J. Cachexia Sarcopenia Muscle* **2022**, *13*, 1514–1525. [CrossRef]
6. Laukkanen, P.; Heikkinen, E.; Kauppinen, M. Muscle strength and mobility as predictors of survival in 75-84-year-old people. *Age Ageing* **1995**, *24*, 468–473. [CrossRef]
7. Giampaoli, S.; Ferrucci, L.; Cecchi, F.; Lo Noce, C.; Poce, A.; Dima, F.; Santaquilani, A.; Vescio, M.F.; Menotti, A. Hand-grip strength predicts incident disability in non-disabled older men. *Age Ageing* **1999**, *28*, 283–288. [CrossRef]
8. Metter, E.J.; Talbot, L.A.; Schrager, M.; Conwit, R. Skeletal muscle strength as a predictor of all-cause mortality in healthy men. *J. Gerontol. A Biol. Sci. Med. Sci.* **2002**, *57*, B359–B365. [CrossRef]
9. Al Snih, S.; Markides, K.S.; Ray, L.; Ostir, G.V.; Goodwin, J.S. Handgrip strength and mortality in older Mexican Americans. *J. Am. Geriatr. Soc.* **2002**, *50*, 1250–1256. [CrossRef]
10. Rantanen, T.; Volpato, S.; Ferrucci, L.; Heikkinen, E.; Fried, L.P.; Guralnik, J.M. Handgrip strength and cause-specific and total mortality in older disabled women: Exploring the mechanism. *J. Am. Geriatr. Soc.* **2003**, *51*, 636–641. [CrossRef]
11. Sasaki, H.; Kasagi, F.; Yamada, M.; Fujita, S. Grip strength predicts cause-specific mortality in middle-aged and elderly persons. *Am. J. Med.* **2007**, *120*, 337–342. [CrossRef]
12. Leong, D.P.; Teo, K.K.; Rangarajan, S.; Lopez-Jaramillo, P.; Avezum Jr, A.; Orlandini, A.; Seron, P.; Ahmed, S.H.; Rosengren, A.; Kelishadi, R.; et al. Prognostic value of grip strength: Findings from the prospective urban rural epidemiology (PURE) study. *Lancet* **2015**, *386*, 266–273. [CrossRef]
13. Jeong, W.; Moon, J.Y.; Kim, J.-H. Association of absolute and relative hand grip strength with all-cause mortality among middle-aged and old-aged people. *BMC Geriatr.* **2023**, *23*, 321. [CrossRef] [PubMed]
14. Duchowny, K.A.; Ackley, S.F.; Brenowitz, W.D.; Wang, J.; Zimmerman, S.C.; Caunca, M.R.; Glymour, M.M. Assoaciations between handgrip strength and dementia risk, cognition, and neuroimaging outcomes in UK Biobank cohort study. *JAMA Netw. Open* **2022**, *5*, e2218314. [CrossRef] [PubMed]
15. Lopez-Bueno, R.; Anderson, L.L.; Calatayud, J.; Casana, J.; Grabovac, I.; Oberndorfer, M.; Cruz, B.D.P. Associations of handgrip strength with all-cause and cancer mortality in older adults: A prospective cohort study in 28 countries. *Age Ageing* **2022**, *51*, afac117. [CrossRef]
16. Lopez-Bueno, R.; Anderson, L.L.; Calatayud, J.; Casana, J.; Smith, L.; Jacob, L.; Koyanagi, A.; Lopez-Gil, J.F.; Cruz, B.D.P. Longitudinal association of handgrip strength with all-cause and cardiovascular mortality from a causal framework. *Exp. Gerontol.* **2022**, *168*, 111951. [CrossRef] [PubMed]
17. Li, G.; Qiao, Y.; Lu, Y.; Liu, S.; Ding, Y.; Chen, X.; Ke, C. Role of handgrip strength in predicting new-onset diabetes: Findings from the survey of health, ageing and retirement in Europe. *BMC Geriatr.* **2021**, *21*, 445. [CrossRef] [PubMed]
18. McGrath, R.P.; Vincent, B.M.; Lee, I.-M.; Kraemer, W.J.; Peterson, M.D. Handgrip strength, function, and mortality in older adults: A time-varying approach. *Med. Sci. Sports Exerc.* **2018**, *50*, 2259–2266. [CrossRef]
19. Celis-Morales, C.A.; Welsh, P.; Lyall, D.M.; Steell, L.; Petermann, F.; Anderson, J.; Iliodromiti, S.; Sillars, A.; Graham, N.; Mackay, D.F.; et al. Associations of grip strength with cardiovascular, respiratory, and cancer outcomes and all cause mortality: Prospective cohort study of half a million UK Biobank participants. *BMJ* **2018**, *361*, k1651. [CrossRef]
20. Strand, B.H.; Cooper, R.; Bergland, A.; Jorgensen, L.; Schirmer, H.; Skirbekk, V.; Emaus, N. The association of grip strength from midlife onwards with all- cause and cause-specific mortality over 17 years of follow-up in the Tromsø Study. *J. Epidemiol. Community Health* **2016**, *70*, 1214–1221. [CrossRef]
21. Mainous, A.G., 3rd; Tanner, R.J.; Anton, S.; Jo, A. Grip strength as a marker of hypertension and diabetes in healthy weight adults. *Am. J. Prev. Med.* **2015**, *49*, 850–858. [CrossRef] [PubMed]

22. Kishimoto, H.; Hata, J.; Ninomiya, T.; Nemeth, H.; Hirakawa, Y.; Yoshida, D.; Kumagai, S.; Kitazono, T.; Kiyohara, Y. Midlife and late-life handgrip strength and risk of cause-specific death in a general Japanese population: The Hisayama Study. *J. Epidemiol. Community Health* **2014**, *68*, 663–668. [CrossRef]
23. Newman, A.B.; Kupelian, V.; Visser, M.; Simonsick, E.M.; Goodpaster, B.H.; Kritchevsky, S.B.; Tylavsky, F.A.; Rubin, S.M.; Harris, T.B. Strength, but not muscle mass, is associated with mortality in the health, aging and body composition study cohort. *J. Gerontol. A Biol. Sci. Med. Sci.* **2006**, *61A*, 72–77. [CrossRef]
24. Rantanen, T.; Guraink, J.M.; Foley, D.; Masaki, K.; Leveille, S.; Curb, J.D.; White, L. Midlife hand grip strength as a predictor of old age disability. *JAMA* **1999**, *281*, 558–560. [CrossRef] [PubMed]
25. Fujita, Y.; Nakamura, Y.; Hiraoka, J.; Kobayashi, K.; Sakata, K.; Nagai, M.; Yanagawa, H. Physical-strength tests and mortality among visitors to health-promotion centers in Japan. *J. Clin. Epidemiol.* **1995**, *48*, 1349–1359. [CrossRef] [PubMed]
26. Buckner, S.L.; Dankel, S.J.; Bell, Z.W.; Abe, T.; Loenneke, J.P. The association of handgrip strength and mortality: What does it tell us and what can we do with it? *Rejuvenat. Res.* **2019**, *22*, 230–234. [CrossRef]
27. Abe, T.; Thiebaud, S.R.; Ozaki, H.; Yamasaki, S.; Loenneke, J.P. Children with low handgrip strength: A narrative review of possible exercise strategies to improve its development. *Children* **2022**, *9*, 1616. [CrossRef] [PubMed]
28. Abe, T.; Kohmura, Y.; Suzuki, K.; Someya, Y.; Loenneke, J.P.; Machida, S.; Naito, H. Athletes in sporting events with upper-body gripping movements have greater handgrip strength than those in sporting events that prioritize the lower body. *Am. J. Hum. Biol.* **2023**, *35*, e23891. [CrossRef]
29. Abe, T.; Kohmura, Y.; Suzuki, K.; Someya, Y.; Loenneke, J.P.; Machida, S.; Naito, H. Handgrip strength and Healthspan: Impact of sports during the developmental period on handgrip strength (Juntendo Fitness Plus Study). *Juntendo Med. J.* **2023**, *in press*. [CrossRef]
30. Bogataj, S.; Trajkovic, N.; Cadenas-Sanchez, C.; Sember, V. Effects of school-based exercise and nutrition intervention on body composition and physical fitness in overweight adolescent girls. *Nutrients* **2021**, *13*, 238. [CrossRef]
31. Labayen, I.; Medrano, M.; Arenaza, L.; Maiz, E.; Oses, M.; Martinez-Vizcaino, V.; Ruiz, J.R.; Ortega, F.B. Effects of exercise in addition to a family-based lifestyle intervention program on hepatic fat in children with overweight. *Diabetes Care* **2020**, *43*, 306–313. [CrossRef] [PubMed]
32. Rexen, C.T.; Ersboll, A.K.; Moller, N.C.; Klakk, H.; Wedderkopp, N.; Andersen, L.B. Effects of extra school based physical education on overall physical fitness development—The CHAMPS study DK. Scand. *J. Med. Sci. Sport.* **2015**, *25*, 706–715. [CrossRef]
33. Macak, D.; Popovic, B.; Cadenas-Sanchez, C.; Madic, D.M.; Trajkovic, N. The effects of daily physical activity intervention on physical fitness in preschool children. *J. Sports. Sci.* **2022**, *40*, 146–155. [CrossRef] [PubMed]
34. Wick, K.; Kriemler, S.; Granacher, U. Effects of a strength-dominated exercise program on physical fitness and cognitive performance in preschool children. *J. Strength Cond. Res.* **2021**, *35*, 983–990. [CrossRef]
35. Abe, A.; Yamasaki, S.; Tahara, R.; Loenneke, J.P.; Abe, T. Comparison of handgrip strength values of young children when using two different types of dynamometers. *Am. J. Hum. Biol.* **2022**, *34*, e23771. [CrossRef]
36. Sanchez-Delgado, G.; Cadenas-Sanchez, C.; Mora-Gonzalez, J.; Martinez-Tellez, B.; Chillon, P.; Lof, M.; Ortega, F.B.; Ruiz, J.R. Assessment of Handgrip Strength in Preschool Children Aged 3 to 5 Years. *J. Hand Surg.* **2015**, *40*, 966–972. [CrossRef]
37. Abe, T.; Sanui, R.; Sasaki, A.; Ishibashi, A.; Daikai, N.; Shindo, Y.; Abe, A.; Loenneke, J.P. Optimal grip span for measuring maximum handgrip strength in preschool children. *Int. J. Clin. Med.* **2022**, *13*, 479–488. [CrossRef]
38. Ozaki, H.; Abe, T.; Dankel, S.J.; Loenneke, J.P.; Natsume, T.; Deng, P.; Haito, H. The measurement of handgrip strength in children: Is the peak value truly maximal? *Children* **2020**, *8*, 9. [CrossRef]
39. Abe, A.; Sanui, R.; Loenneke, J.P.; Abe, T. Is the peak value truly maximal when measuring strength in young children? An Updated study. *J. Trainol.* **2022**, *11*, 17–21. [CrossRef]
40. Abe, T.; Ozaki, H.; Abe, A.; Loenneke, J.P. Impact of forearm pronation on ultrasound-measured forearm muscle thickness in children and adolescents. *Imaging* **2022**, *14*, 104–108. [CrossRef]
41. Ben Othman, A.; Behm, D.G.; Chaouachi, A. Evidence of homologous and heterologous effects after unilateral leg training in youth. *Appl. Physiol. Nutr. Metab.* **2018**, *43*, 282–291. [CrossRef] [PubMed]
42. Magdi, H.R.; Maroto-Izquierdo, S.; de Paz, J.A. Ipsilateral lower-to-upper limb cross-transfer effect on muscle strength, mechanical power, and lean tissue mass after accentuated eccentric loading. *Medicina* **2021**, *57*, 445. [CrossRef] [PubMed]
43. Rule, A.C.; Stewart, R.A. Effects of practical life materials on kindergartner's fine motor skills. *Early Child. Educ. J.* **2002**, *30*, 9–13. [CrossRef]
44. Siegel, J.A.; Camaione, D.N.; Manfredi, T.G. The effects of upper body resistance training on prepubescent children. *Pediatr. Exerc. Sci.* **1989**, *1*, 145–154. [CrossRef]
45. Abe, T.; Ozaki, H.; Abe, A.; Machida, S.; Naito, H.; Loenneke, J.P. Longitudinal changes of grip strength and forearm muscle thickness in young children. *Physiol. Int.* 2023, *in press*. [CrossRef]
46. Loenneke, J.P.; Buckner, S.L.; Dankel, S.J.; Abe, T. Exercise-induced changes in muscle size do not contribute to exercise-induced changes in muscle strength. *Sports Med.* **2019**, *49*, 987–991. [CrossRef]
47. Saladin, K.S. Anatomy & Physiology. In *the Unity of Form and Function*, 3rd ed.; McGraw-Hill: New York, NY, USA, 2004; pp. 345–354.

48. Chen, X.; Sekine, M.; Hamanishi, S.; Wang, H.; Hayashikawa, Y.; Yamagami, T.; Kagamimori, S. The validity of nursery teachers' report on the physical activity of young children. *J. Epidemiol.* **2002**, *12*, 367–374. [CrossRef]
49. Phillips, S.M.; Summerbell, C.; Hobbs, M.; Hesketh, K.R.; Saxena, S.; Muir, C.; Hillier-Brown, F.C. A systematic review of the validity, reliability, and feasibility of measurement tools used to assess the physical activity and sedentary behaviour of pre-school aged children. *Int. J. Behav. Nutr. Phys. Act.* **2021**, *18*, 141. [CrossRef]

life

MDPI

Article

Risk Factors and Outcomes of Children with Congenital Heart Disease on Extracorporeal Membrane Oxygenation—A Ten-Year Single-Center Report

Antonio Amodeo [1,2,*,†], Milena Stojanovic [1,2,†], Tugba Erdil [3], Hitendu Dave [1,2], Robert Cesnjevar [1,2], Sebastian Paal [1,2], Oliver Kretschmar [2,4] and Martin Schweiger [1,2]

1 Pediatric Cardiovascular Surgery, Pediatric Heart Center, Department of Surgery, University Children's Hospital Zurich, 8032 Zurich, Switzerland; hitendu.dave@kispi.uzh.ch (H.D.); robert.cesnjevar@kispi.uzh.ch (R.C.)
2 Children's Research Center, University Children's Hospital Zurich, 8032 Zurich, Switzerland
3 Division of General Thoracic Surgery, Inselspital, Bern University Hospital, University of Bern, 3010 Bern, Switzerland
4 Pediatric Cardiology, Pediatric Heart Center, University Children's Hospital Zurich, 8032 Zurich, Switzerland
* Correspondence: antonioamodeo91@gmail.com
† These authors contributed equally to this work.

Abstract: For children born with congenital heart defects (CHDs), extracorporeal life support may be necessary. This retrospective single-center study aimed to investigate the outcomes of children with CHDs on extracorporeal membrane oxygenation (ECMO), focusing on various risk factors. Among the 88 patients, 36 (41%) had a single-ventricle heart defect, while 52 (59%) had a biventricular defect. In total, 25 (28%) survived, with 7 (8%) in the first group and 18 (20%) in the latter. A *p*-value of 0.19 indicated no significant difference in survival rates. Children with biventricular hearts had shorter ECMO durations but longer stays in the intensive care unit. The overall rate of complications on ECMO was higher in children with a single ventricle (odds ratio [OR] 1.57, 95% confidence interval [CI] 0.67–3.7); bleeding was the most common complication in both groups. The occurrence of a second ECMO run was more frequent in patients with a single ventricle (22% vs. 9.6%). ECMO can be effective for children with congenital heart defects, including single-ventricle patients. Bleeding remains a serious complication associated with worse outcomes. Patients requiring a second ECMO run within 30 days have lower survival rates.

Keywords: complications; congenital heart disease; ECMO; extracorporeal life support; mortality; risk factors; single ventricle

Citation: Amodeo, A.; Stojanovic, M.; Erdil, T.; Dave, H.; Cesnjevar, R.; Paal, S.; Kretschmar, O.; Schweiger, M. Risk Factors and Outcomes of Children with Congenital Heart Disease on Extracorporeal Membrane Oxygenation—A Ten-Year Single-Center Report. *Life* **2023**, *13*, 1582. https://doi.org/10.3390/life13071582

Academic Editors: Stefanos Roumeliotis and Giuseppe Minervini

Received: 28 June 2023
Revised: 14 July 2023
Accepted: 17 July 2023
Published: 19 July 2023

1. Introduction

Extracorporeal membrane oxygenation (ECMO) is a well-established therapy utilized in neonates and children. According to the Extracorporeal Life Support Organization (ELSO), the survival rates for patients undergoing ECMO treatment vary depending on the age group and the underlying condition. The survival rate for pediatric patients receiving extracorporeal cardiopulmonary resuscitation (eCPR) is 55%, while the survival rate for neonates receiving ECMO for respiratory problems is 84% [1].

Congenital heart defects (CHDs) are one of many factors that can affect how well children and newborns respond to ECMO. Neonatal children with CHDs have a reported 40% survival rate, compared to 48% for pediatric patients [1]. Patients with single-ventricle physiology within the CHD group are worse than those with biventricular CHDs in terms of outcomes [2]. Studies show that the survival of children in this subgroup is still low, with best-case survival rates being around 40% [3–6].

This study's goal is to give a thorough overview of the particular population of CHD-affected children who need ECMO support. Our analysis aims to determine the risk factors and issues associated with ECMO use in these patients as well as the overall success of ECMO implantation. By examining all of these factors, just as other research groups are doing [7–9], we hope to advance patient care in this population and increase our understanding of CHD management in conjunction with ECMO therapy.

2. Materials and Methods

2.1. Study Design and Patient Population

This study is a retrospective, single-center investigation that aimed to evaluate the outcomes of children diagnosed with CHDs who required ECMO support between the years of 2009 and 2019. The study evaluated children up to the age of 16 and categorized them as either "neonates" if they were up to 30 days old or "pediatric" if they exceeded that age. To ensure the accuracy of the data, exclusion criteria were applied and consisted of excluding patients without a CHD diagnosis and those whose baseline or follow-up data were missing. Notably, patients who underwent a second ECMO run during the same hospital admission were considered separately and labeled as "second ECMO run", with no patient receiving more than two ECMO runs.

2.2. Categorization of Patients Based on CHD Anatomical Classification

The patients were categorized into two groups based on the underlying anatomical classification of their CHD: those with biventricular CHD and those with single-ventricle CHD. The functional single-ventricle heart diagnosis encompassed conditions such as hypoplastic left heart syndrome, tricuspid valve atresia, pulmonary atresia, and borderline left ventricle.

2.3. Factors Leading to ECMO

This study identified five main categories of factors leading to the need for ECMO support: respiratory failure, cardiac failure, sepsis, post-cardiotomy ECMO, and eCPR (Table S1). The failure to wean off cardio-pulmonary bypass (CPB) or the need for ECMO within the first 48 h after a CPB-assisted operation were both referred to as post-cardiotomy ECMO.

Due to the complexity of patient cases, it was often challenging to attribute ECMO support to a single factor, as multiple relevant factors were concurrently present, influencing the decision to initiate ECMO support. In instances where multiple factors were identified, the patient was classified into the categories considered more relevant by two independent senior consultants. Any discrepancies were resolved through discussion until a consensus was reached. Consequently, for the majority of patients, it was established that more than one factor contributed to the need for ECMO support.

2.4. Complications and Criteria for Classifying Complications

A series of complications was defined and encompassed various situations. These included bleeding, reposition of a cannula, disseminated intravascular coagulation (DIC), circuit changes, and cerebrovascular insults (CVIs).

The main criterion for classifying bleeding as a complication was the need to repeat surgery due to bleeding. Any occurrence of bleeding, whether inside or outside the area of the index operation, was taken into account. Bleeding specifically related to ECMO was also considered. Regarding the repositioning of a cannula, such adjustments may be necessary either to improve ECMO flow or to correct unintentional displacement, and they were labeled as complications. The cleaning of cannulas or tubes to address thrombus formation also falls into this category of complications. Disseminated intravascular coagulation was evaluated based on laboratory and clinical assessments, constituting another complication category. This study also accounted for circuit changes, which were defined as changes resulting from the depletion of the oxygenator. In the study, CVI was defined as any thromboembolic event causing a cerebral insult during ECMO, confirmed through magnetic resonance imaging (MRI) or computed tomography (CT). These imaging modalities were interpreted by pediatric radiologists or neuroradiologists, ensuring the accurate identification and confirmation of CVI cases.

2.5. Non-Cardiac Genetic Diseases

In addition to the primary heart defect, some patients also had additional non-cardiac genetic diseases, which were documented separately and listed as "other diagnoses" (Table S2).

2.6. Data Storage and Ethics Approval

All data were safely stored in an Excel sheet protected by a password. The document containing personalized information linked to patient IDs was kept separate from the Excel sheet. The study received ethical approval from the Cantonal Ethics Committee Zurich (BASEC-Nr. 2020-01147).

2.7. Statistical Analysis

Data pertaining to patients and ECMO were gathered from the clinical information system "Phoenix®" provided by CGM Clinical (CompuGroup Medical Schweiz AG, Bern, Switzerland) at the University Children's Hospital Zurich. A comprehensive set of variables was selected for analysis, including date of birth, gender, weight, classification as neonate or pediatric, presence of single-ventricle or biventricular heart, specific congenital heart defect, concomitant diseases, factors leading to ECMO initiation, occurrence of cardiopulmonary resuscitation (CPR) prior to ECMO, previous cardiotomy, last recorded pH and lactate levels before ECMO, type of ECMO implantation, cannulation site, timing of ECMO initiation and removal, occurrence of a second ECMO run, complications experienced while on ECMO, conversion to a ventricular assist device (VAD), length of stay in the intensive care unit (ICU), survival while on ECMO, and survival after a 1-year follow-up. To ensure the accuracy and consistency of the collected data, an Excel sheet was utilized for data collection. Subsequent statistical analysis and evaluation were conducted using the software "R-Studio" [RStudio Team (2020). RStudio: Integrated Development for R. RStudio, PBC, Boston, MA, USA]. Results are given as mean values ± standard deviation or numbers and percentages. Comparisons were performed using Student's *t*-test or the Mann–Whitney *U*-test. Qualitative variables were analyzed using Fisher's exact test. The survival times of the two groups were compared using a log-rank test, with statistical significance assumed at a 2-sided *p*-value of 0.05 or lower.

3. Results

3.1. Study Group

A total of 88 patients received ECMO therapy, including 42 neonates and 43 females. The mean age at ECMO implantation was 1.4 years, with a standard deviation of 3.6 years. The average weight of the patients was 6.9 kg, with a standard deviation of 1.0 kg. Table 1 shows the specific baseline characteristics for both groups.

Table 1. Baseline characteristics.

n	Single Ventricle 36		Biventricular 52	
Age at ECMO implantation in months (mean (±SD))	28	(54.7)	9.9	(31.6)
Male (%)	16	(18)	29	(33)
Female (%)	20	(23)	23	(26)
Neonate (%)	13	(15)	29	(33)
Paediatric (%)	23	(26)	23	(26)
Other diagnosis (%)	5	(6)	16	(18)

Single-ventricle heart defects were found in 36 (41%) of the 88 patients, with hypoplastic left heart syndrome (HLHS) being the most prevalent condition in this cohort, accounting for 23 cases (26%). As shown in Table 2, which displays the distribution of CHD types across the sample, 52 patients (59%) had a congenital heart defect with biventricular physiology.

Table 2. Congenital heart defects.

Cardiac Diagnosis	Total Cases (n = 88)	
	n	%
Single ventricle	36	41
Functional single ventricle (non-HLHS)	13	15
HLHS	23	26
Biventricular	52	59
VSD	24	27
ASD	18	20
AVSD	19	22
TOF	5	6
TGA	14	16
Aortic valve stenosis	11	13
Truncus arteriosus communis	4	5
Pulmonary valve stenosis	3	3
Pulmonary atresia	13	15
IAA	3	3
TAPVD	9	10
Partial anomalous pulmonary venous connection	2	2
DORV	2	2
ALCAPA	3	3
Atrioventricular valve regurgitation	15	17
Myocarditis	1	1
Cardiomyopathy	3	3

In both the single-ventricle and biventricular groups, cardiac failure emerged as the main cause of ECMO. Cardiovascular failure was identified in 33 of the 36 patients with a single-ventricle defect (91%) and 48 patients (92%), respectively, in the biventricular group. Notably, the majority of single-ventricle patients (70%) required ECMO support post-cardiotomy, compared to 55% of the biventricular patients. Respiratory failure was a contributing factor in 44% of single-ventricle cases and in 32% of biventricular cases. Sepsis, on the other hand, was a relatively uncommon cause of ECMO, accounting for 5% of cases in the single-ventricle group and 2% in the biventricular group.

Table 3 provides further information on the ECMO-related data for the two groups.

Table 3. ECMO Data.

	Single Ventricle		Biventricular	
n	36		52	
CPR time in minutes (mean (±SD))	49.44	(40.44)	49.44	(52.78)
Surgery pre-ECMO (%)	33	(37.5)	36	(41)
ECMO pre-surgery (%)	3	(3.4)	11	(12.5)
pH pre-ECMO (mean (±SD))	7.23	(0.15)	7.06	(0.66)
Lactate pre-ECMO (mean (±SD))	6.05	(4.1)	6.93	(5.59)
VA-ECMO (%)	33	(37.5)	48	(54)
VV-ECMO (%)	3	(3.4)	4	(4.5)
Central cannulation (%)	33	(37.5)	44	(50)

3.2. Outcomes

The overall survival rate for children with CHDs receiving ECMO support was found to be poor. Out of the 88 patients included in the study, 54% did not survive while on ECMO support. However, 45% of the patients were successfully weaned off ECMO. Additionally, 6% of the patients required VAD support, and 28% of the patients were discharged from the hospital. Figure 1 presents a schematic representation of the main outcomes in absolute numbers:

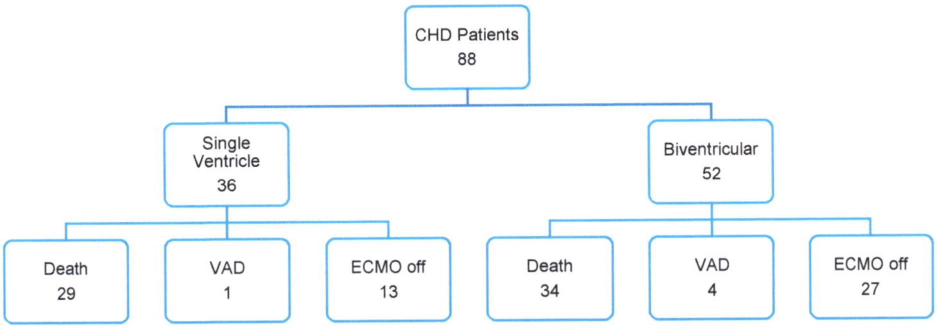

Figure 1. Outcome: this chart shows the number of patients in absolute numbers.

At the time of hospital discharge and one year after, 28% of the patients included in the study were still alive. In total, 7 (28%) of these survivors had a single-ventricular heart, whereas the remaining 18 (72%) had biventricular physiology. Notably, whether univentricular or biventricular, the type of underlying cardiac disease did not show a significant impact on survival outcomes ($p = 0.19$). The survival curve corresponding to these findings is visually represented in Figure 2, providing a graphical representation of the observed survival rates over time.

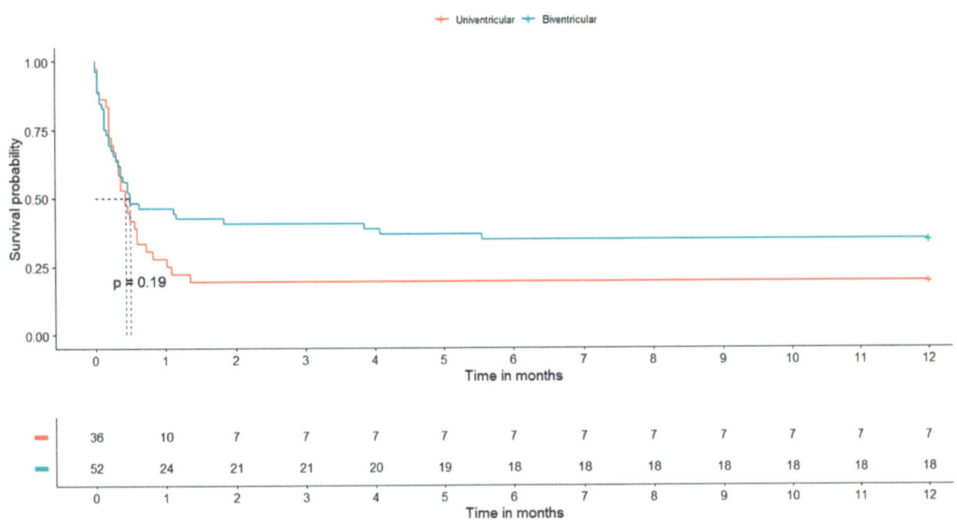

Figure 2. Survival after ECMO. The Kaplan–Meier curve shows the survival time of patients from ECMO implantation to one-year follow-up. The risk table shows survival in absolute numbers.

The average duration of ECMO support was 5.4 days, with a standard deviation of 4.4 days. Compared to children with univentricular hearts, children with biventricular hearts had shorter ECMO support durations while experiencing longer stays in the intensive care unit (ICU). However, the difference in ICU stays between the two groups was not found to be statistically significant (*p*-value: 0.99), as indicated by the analysis. The outcome data are listed in Table 4.

Table 4. Outcome: single ventricle versus biventricular.

n	Single Ventricle 36		Biventricular 52	
ECMO duration in days (mean (±SD))	5.9	(4.7)	5	(4.3)
ICU stay in days (mean (±SD))	16	(14)	23	(34)
Second ECMO run (%)	8	(9)	5	(6)
Change to VAD (%)	1	(1.1)	4	(4.5)

It was found that ECMO-support-related complications were frequent, affecting about 49% of patients. Below and in Table 5 are descriptions of these issues in more detail. Importantly, patients with univentricular hearts showed significantly increased frequency of overall complications (odds ratio: 1.57, 95% confidence interval: 0.67–3.7). The most common complication seen in both groups was bleeding.

Table 5. Complications of ECMO.

n	Single Ventricle 36		Biventricular 52	
Reoperation due to bleeding (%)	9	(10)	15	(17)
Reposition of cannula (%)	8	(9)	11	(12.5)
Cleaning the cannula due to a thrombus (%)	1	(1.1)	0	(-)
DIC (%)	6	(7)	3	(3.4)
Verified CVI (%)	5	(5.6)	2	(2.2)
Circuit change (%)	2	(2.2)	4	(4.5)

Among the 33 patients who underwent eCPR prior to ECMO implantation, 30% survived to hospital discharge and were still alive at one year. Prior to ECMO implantation, CPR lasted an average of 49 min for both groups. The mean time spent performing CPR was notably shorter, at 23 min, among the patients who survived.

3.3. Subgroup Second ECMO Run

An analysis was conducted specifically on the subset of patients who underwent a second ECMO run, which included a total of 13 individuals (15% of the total). Figure 3 illustrates that out of this group, the majority (eight patients) had a single ventricle. With seven cases, hypoplastic left heart syndrome was identified as the most common heart defect.

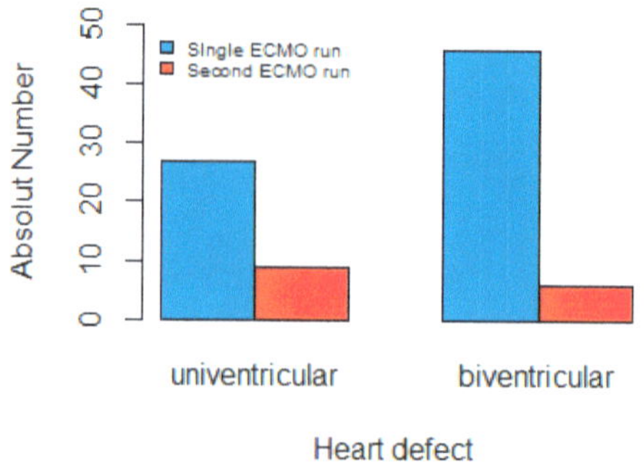

Figure 3. Second ECMO run. The graph shows that 8 children (9%) with univentricular heart defects and 5 children (6%) with biventricular heart defects required a second ECMO run.

Cardiac failure was the main factor leading to ECMO in this group, accounting for 85% of cases, and the second ECMO run was started on average 1.9 days after the first run. The average support duration for the children who needed a second ECMO run was 7.3 days, with a standard variation of 1.2 days. Only 2 of the 13 patients survived through the second ECMO run. These two survivors, who were pediatric patients, both had a single-ventricle heart abnormality.

Complications were observed in 46% of the cases within the subset of patients who underwent a second ECMO run. Among the patients with a univentricular heart defect, complications occurred in four children, representing 50% of this subgroup. Similarly, among the patients with a biventricular heart defect, complications were observed in two individuals, accounting for 40% of this subgroup. Within this cohort, reoperation due to bleeding emerged as the most frequent complication. It is worth highlighting that the two children who survived the second ECMO run did not experience any complications while on ECMO support. Additionally, none of the children in this group required the implantation of a ventricular assist device.

4. Discussion

The use of ECMO in patients with congenital heart disease (CHD) is increasing globally [10–14]. In our study, we found that cardiac failure, not surprisingly, was the most common factor leading to the need for ECMO, followed by post-cardiotomy failure. Almost half of the patients (45%) were successfully weaned from ECMO, while a small but substantial number of patients (n = 6; 7%) required long-term mechanical circulatory support in the form of a ventricular assist device. For those patients who were successfully discharged, the survival rate at one year was consistent with the rate at hospital discharge, with a survival rate of 22% for neonates and 35% for pediatric patients. When we examined the underlying anatomy of the total ECMO cohort, we found that a substantial number (41%) of the patients had single-ventricle hearts. The survival rate for children on ECMO with biventricular heart abnormalities is approximately 40%, and the survival rate for children with single-ventricle hearts is lower [15–17].

The wide range of survival rates reported In the literature is noteworthy and can be attributed to differences in inclusion and exclusion criteria, center size, study dimension (single-center vs. multicenter), and the timing and setting of ECMO deployment (daytime vs. nighttime), even though it has been found that the latter variable was irrelevant in adults [18] and in pediatric patients [19]. Most of the studies found in the literature primarily included children who underwent ECMO after cardiac surgery [12,15,20]. In contrast, our study aimed to include all children who required ECMO, regardless of their correction status or specific heart defect, provided that ECMO was indicated and subsequently implemented. This approach allowed us to avoid selection bias. Our findings are consistent with the survival rate ranges found in the literature [6,15,21] with a survival rate of 35% for biventricular hearts and 19% for single-ventricle hearts. Importantly, we did not observe a significant difference in survival based on the underlying anatomy, whether the patient had a biventricular or univentricular defect. In the literature, there are conflicting reports, with some studies showing no significant difference in outcome as we found [15,22] or showing a better outcome for children with biventricular CHD, when ECMO is needed [16]. It should be noted that dividing patients based on underlying anatomy creates groups (biventricular and single-ventricle CHD) that inherently contain a heterogeneous patient population.

Factors other than anatomy may also impact survival probability. High inotrope scores, pre-ECMO acidosis, elevated pre-ECMO lactate, failure to clear lactate within 24 h, bleeding while on ECMO, fluid overload, peripheral cannulation, renal failure, start of ECMO in the intensive care unit, and length of ECMO support are some of the factors that have been discussed in the literature, although not always with consistent conclusions [23–26]. In terms of pH and lactate levels, we found higher lactate levels and lower mean pH values in the group of children with biventricular hearts (pH 7.06 vs. 7.23, lactate 6.93 vs. 6.05). Even so, this group's likelihood of survival was better than that of children with single-ventricle hearts (35% vs. 19%).

Bleeding during ECMO is identified as a significant risk factor in the literature and is known to reduce the likelihood of survival [12,27,28]. The incidence of bleeding in cardiac patients on ECMO ranges from 25% to 78%, with children who have a structural heart defect being at an increased risk of bleeding [29–32]. Our study also demonstrated a high rate of bleeding complications during ECMO. However, the prevalence of reoperation due to bleeding did not show a significant difference between children with single-ventricle and biventricular hearts (25% vs. 29%). Nonetheless, the mortality rate for children with a single ventricle and this complication was 100%, compared to 80% for children with biventricular CHD.

Given the prevalence of post-cardiotomy cases or failures to wean from cardiopulmonary bypass as reasons for ECMO, the majority of patients in our sample had central cannulation. It is possible that the slightly higher survival rate (27.3% vs. 22.2%) seen in patients with central cannulation can be attributed to the use of larger cannulas and increased flow [33]. The benefits of central cannulation in post-cardiotomy adult patients are being discussed, and contrasting findings have been found in the literature [34,35]. Peripheral ECMO may have the benefit of a lesser risk of bleeding [36] but pose a risk of limb ischemia [37].

Another risk factor can be identified in the presence of genetic abnormalities other than the ones strictly related to CHD. In children with a congenital heart defect, the incidence of non-cardiac and genetic illnesses ranges from 15 to 30% [38,39], which is consistent with the findings in our cohort (24%). According to the abovementioned study by Alsoufi et al., genetic abnormalities are a significant risk factor for mortality. We also observed that children with non-cardiac genetic illnesses had a lower survival rate than those without them (9.5% vs. 26.1%).

Mortality after eCPR is still high, and longer CPR duration correlates with higher mortality [40–42]. In our study population, 38% of children with ECMO received eCPR. Among these, 10 patients (11%) were discharged from hospital and are still alive after one year. It is worth noting that eight patients (9%) had a biventricular circulation, compared to two patients (2.3%) who had a univentricular heart. In our analysis, the mean duration of CPR prior to the implantation of an ECMO device was 49 min; the 10 survivors received CPR for an average of 23 min. We did not look into the neurological outcomes of these patients, but one objective of future studies should be examining the long-term effects of such issues. Several investigations [40,43,44] have shown that neurological complications are frequent in this patient subgroup.

In our analysis, the survival of children who required a second ECMO run was worse compared to those who had only one run (15% vs. 28% survival). Following a second ECMO run, the literature indicates survival rates of about 25% [45–48]. In our cohort, 13 patients (15%) required a second ECMO run, of whom around half (n = 6) were neonates. The outcomes were poor, with only two children surviving the second ECMO run. Both survivors were pediatric patients with hypoplastic left heart syndrome. Although the survival results were lower with the second ECMO run, there were no significant differences in the incidence of complications (45.9% vs. 46.1%).

Limitations

Several limitations should be considered in the interpretation of our findings, given that this study was retrospective and conducted at a single center. The relatively small sample size of 88 patients and the long observation period of 10 years may have implications for the generalizability of the results.

It is important to point out that the decision-making process was frequently influenced by numerous factors rather than a single determinant, and that the indication for ECMO implantation was determined retrospectively based on the data that were available.

We acknowledge that we did not report the ultimate cause of death for the patients in our cohort. While failure of cardiac function recovery could be attributed as a cause of death, it is essential to recognize that there may be other contributing factors, such as sepsis, intracranial hemorrhage, or multi-organ failure, which could have played a significant role. Future studies should aim to provide a more comprehensive analysis of the ultimate causes of mortality in this patient population.

It is important to highlight that our study did not conduct statistical analysis to determine whether there were significant differences between the subgroups of patients who underwent eCPR and those who did not receive CPR, instead choosing to focus on descriptive representation. We were unable to conduct thorough statistical analysis for this particular comparison due to insufficient data (unfortunately, CPR duration data were only available for 18 of the 23 non-survivors). Therefore, our findings regarding the differences between these two variables should be interpreted cautiously. Further research is necessary to identify any appreciable differences in survival or other outcomes between patients who received eCPR and those who did not in order to better understand the features and outcomes of these subgroups.

5. Conclusions

Our findings suggest that neonates and children with congenital heart defects can be successfully treated with ECMO, even in the presence of single-ventricle heart defects. Bleeding, however, continues to be a serious complication linked to worse outcomes. Patients who require a second ECMO run within 30 days continue to have a low survival rate. In order to address the study's limitations and examine options for enhancing results in this patient population, additional research is necessary.

Supplementary Materials: The following supporting information can be downloaded at: https://www.mdpi.com/article/10.3390/life13071582/s1, Table S1: Factors leading to ECMO implantation; Table S2: other diagnosis.

Author Contributions: Conceptualization, M.S. (Martin Schweiger) and A.A.; methodology, M.S. (Martin Schweiger) and A.A.; software, A.A. and M.S. (Milena Stojanovic); validation, M.S. (Martin Schweiger), O.K. and R.C.; formal analysis, A.A., M.S. (Milena Stojanovic) and M.S. (Martin Schweiger); investigation, M.S. (Milena Stojanovic), T.E. and A.A.; resources, H.D., S.P. and M.S. (Martin Schweiger); data curation, M.S. (Milena Stojanovic), T.E. and A.A.; writing—original draft preparation, A.A. and M.S. (Milena Stojanovic); writing—review and editing, A.A., M.S. (Milena Stojanovic), R.C. and M.S. (Martin Schweiger); visualization, A.A. and M.S. (Martin Schweiger); supervision, M.S. (Martin Schweiger) and R.C.; project administration, M.S. (Martin Schweiger) and R.C. All authors have read and agreed to the published version of the manuscript.

Funding: This research received no external funding.

Institutional Review Board Statement: This study was conducted in accordance with the Declaration of Helsinki and approved by the Ethics Committee of "Cantonal Ethic Commission" of Zurich (protocol code 2020-01147; date: 20 May 2020).

Informed Consent Statement: General informed consent was obtained from all of the parents of the subjects involved in this study.

Data Availability Statement: All of the data of this study are in the Hospital Database, available with the software "Phoenix®" of CGM Clinical (CompuGroup Medical Schweiz AG, Bern, Switzerland).

Conflicts of Interest: The authors declare no conflict of interest.

Abbreviations

Abbreviation	Meaning
ALCAPA	anomalous left coronary artery from the pulmonary artery
ASD	atrial septal defect
AVSD	atrioventricular septal defect
CBP	cardiopulmonary bypass
CT	computer tomography
CVI	cerebrovascular insult
CHD	congenital heart disease
DORV	double outlet right ventricle
DIC	disseminated intravascular coagulation
eCPR	extracorporeal cardiopulmonary resuscitation
ECMO	extracorporeal membrane oxygenation
ELSO	extracorporeal life support organization
HLHS	hypoplastic left heart syndrome
IAA	interrupted aortic arch
ICU	intensive care unit
MRI	magnetic resonance imaging
TAPVD	total anomalous pulmonary venous drainage
TGA	transposition of the great arteries
TOF	tetralogy of Fallot
VA	venoarterial
VAD	ventricular assist device
VSD	ventricular septum defect
VV	venovenous

References

1. Thiagarajan, R.R.; Barbaro, R.P.; Rycus, P.T.; McMullan, D.M.; Conrad, S.A.; Fortenberry, J.D.; Paden, M.L.; ELSO member centers. Extracorporeal Life Support Organization Registry International Report 2016. *ASAIO J.* **2017**, *63*, 60–67. [CrossRef] [PubMed]
2. Griselli, M.; Sinha, R.; Jang, S.; Perri, G.; Adachi, I. Mechanical Circulatory Support for Single Ventricle Failure. *Front. Cardiovasc. Med.* **2018**, *5*, 115. [CrossRef]
3. Basgoze, S.; Temur, B.; Aydin, S.; Guzelmeric, F.; Guvenc, O.; Cevik, A.; Iyigun, M.; Erek, E. Outcomes of Extracorporeal Membrane Oxygenation in Patients After Repair of Congenital Heart Defects. *Pediatr. Cardiol.* **2022**, *43*, 1811–1821. [CrossRef] [PubMed]
4. Bacon, M.K.; Gray, S.B.; Schwartz, S.M.; Cooper, D.S. Extracorporeal Membrane Oxygenation (ECMO) Support in Special Patient Populations-The Bidirectional Glenn and Fontan Circulations. *Front. Pediatr.* **2018**, *6*, 299. [CrossRef]
5. Bezerra, R.F.; Pacheco, J.T.; Volpatto, V.H.; Franchi, S.M.; Fitaroni, R.; da Cruz, D.V.; Castro, R.M.; da Silva, L.D.F.; da Silva, J.P. Extracorporeal Membrane Oxygenation After Norwood Surgery in Patients With Hypoplastic Left Heart Syndrome: A Retrospective Single-Center Cohort Study From Brazil. *Front. Pediatr.* **2022**, *10*, 813528. [CrossRef]
6. Mayr, B.; Kido, T.; Holder, S.; Wallner, M.; Vodiskar, J.; Strbad, M.; Ruf, B.; Hager, A.; Ewert, P.; Horer, J.; et al. Single-centre outcome of extracorporeal membrane oxygenation after the neonatal Norwood procedure. *Eur. J. Cardiothorac. Surg.* **2022**, *62*, ezac129. [CrossRef]
7. Raj, S.; Li, S.; Schears, G.J.; Nemergut, M.E.; Gram, K.; Watson, D.; Overman, D.M. Survival-to-Hospital Discharge in Neonates With Congenital Heart Disease Supported With Prolonged Extracorporeal Membrane Oxygenation. *Am. J. Cardiol.* **2023**, *201*, 310–316. [CrossRef]
8. Mahmood, B.; Newton, D.; Pallotto, E.K. Current trends in neonatal ECMO. *Semin. Perinatol.* **2018**, *42*, 80–88. [CrossRef] [PubMed]
9. Zheng, G.; Wang, J.; Chen, P.; Huang, Z.; Zhang, L.; Yang, A.; Wu, J.; Chen, C.; Zhang, J.; Sun, Y.; et al. Epidemiological characteristics and trends in postoperative death in children with congenital heart disease (CHD): A single-center retrospective study from 2005 to 2020. *J. Cardiothorac. Surg.* **2023**, *18*, 165. [CrossRef] [PubMed]
10. Fan, Y.Y.K.; Wong, K.L.; Ho, K.L.C.; Chan, T.L.D.; Lee, O.J.; Yung, C.Y.; Lun, K.S.; Chau, M.C.E.; Chiu, S.W.C.; Cheng, L.C.; et al. Trends in contemporary advanced heart failure management: An in-depth review over 30 years of heart transplant service in Hong Kong. *Korean J. Transplant.* **2022**, *36*, 267–277. [CrossRef] [PubMed]
11. Erdil, T.; Lemme, F.; Konetzka, A.; Cavigelli-Brunner, A.; Niesse, O.; Dave, H.; Hasenclever, P.; Hubler, M.; Schweiger, M. Extracorporeal membrane oxygenation support in pediatrics. *Ann. Cardiothorac. Surg.* **2019**, *8*, 109–115. [CrossRef] [PubMed]
12. Wu, Y.; Zhao, T.; Li, Y.; Wu, S.; Wu, C.; Wei, G. Use of Extracorporeal Membrane Oxygenation After Congenital Heart Disease Repair: A Systematic Review and Meta-Analysis. *Front. Cardiovasc. Med.* **2020**, *7*, 583289. [CrossRef]

13. Bowen, R.E.S.; Graetz, T.J.; Emmert, D.A.; Avidan, M.S. Statistics of heart failure and mechanical circulatory support in 2020. *Ann. Transl. Med.* **2020**, *8*, 827. [CrossRef] [PubMed]
14. Allen, K.Y.; Allan, C.K.; Su, L.; McBride, M.E. Extracorporeal membrane oxygenation in congenital heart disease. *Semin. Perinatol.* **2018**, *42*, 104–110. [CrossRef]
15. ElMahrouk, A.F.; Ismail, M.F.; Hamouda, T.; Shaikh, R.; Mahmoud, A.; Shihata, M.S.; Alradi, O.; Jamjoom, A. Extracorporeal Membrane Oxygenation in Postcardiotomy Pediatric Patients-15 Years of Experience Outside Europe and North America. *Thorac. Cardiovasc. Surg.* **2019**, *67*, 28–36. [CrossRef]
16. Dohain, A.M.; Abdelmohsen, G.; Elassal, A.A.; ElMahrouk, A.F.; Al-Radi, O.O. Factors affecting the outcome of extracorporeal membrane oxygenation following paediatric cardiac surgery. *Cardiol. Young* **2019**, *29*, 1501–1509. [CrossRef]
17. Cho, H.J.; Choi, I.; Kwak, Y.; Kim, D.W.; Habimana, R.; Jeong, I.S. The Outcome of Post-cardiotomy Extracorporeal Membrane Oxygenation in Neonates and Pediatric Patients: A Systematic Review and Meta-Analysis. *Front. Pediatr.* **2022**, *10*, 869283. [CrossRef]
18. Gomez-Sanchez, R.; Garcia-Carreno, J.; Martinez-Solano, J.; Sousa-Casasnovas, I.; Juarez-Fernandez, M.; Devesa-Cordero, C.; Sanz-Ruiz, R.; Gutierrez-Ibanes, E.; Elizaga, J.; Fernandez-Aviles, F.; et al. Off-Hours versus Regular-Hours Implantation of Peripheral Venoarterial Extracorporeal Membrane Oxygenation in Patients with Cardiogenic Shock. *J. Clin. Med.* **2023**, *12*, 1875. [CrossRef]
19. AbuHassan, H.R.; Arafat, A.A.; Albabtain, M.A.; Alwadai, A.H.; AlArwan, K.M.; Ali, A.A.; Rasheed, S.; Babikr, N.B.; Shaikh, S.F. Postcardiotomy extracorporeal membrane oxygenation in patients with congenital heart disease; the effect of place of initiation. *Perfusion* **2023**. [CrossRef]
20. Joo, S.; Cho, S.; Lee, J.H.; Min, J.; Kwon, H.W.; Kwak, J.G.; Kim, W.H. Postcardiotomy Extracorporeal Membrane Oxygenation Support in Patients with Congenital Heart Disease. *J. Chest Surg.* **2022**, *55*, 158–167. [CrossRef]
21. Luna, A.O.; Kuhnell, P.; Wooton, S.; Handler, S.S.; Wright, G.; Hammel, J.; Tweddell, J.S.; Chan, T. Factors Associated with Inability to Discharge After Stage 1 Palliation for Single Ventricle Heart Disease: An Analysis of the National Pediatric Cardiology Quality Improvement Collaborative Database. *Pediatr. Cardiol.* **2022**, *43*, 1298–1310. [CrossRef]
22. Melvan, J.N.; Davis, J.; Heard, M.; Trivedi, J.R.; Wolf, M.; Kanter, K.R.; Deshpande, S.R.; Alsoufi, B. Factors Associated With Survival Following Extracorporeal Cardiopulmonary Resuscitation in Children. *World J. Pediatr. Congenit. Heart Surg.* **2020**, *11*, 265–274. [CrossRef]
23. Roeleveld, P.P.; Mendonca, M. Neonatal Cardiac ECMO in 2019 and Beyond. *Front. Pediatr.* **2019**, *7*, 327. [CrossRef]
24. Amodeo, A.; Erdil, T.; Vanetta, C.; Steigmiller, K.; Schmiady, M.; Schweiger, M.; Pretre, R.; Dave, H. Serum lactate at 24 hours is associated with outcome in children requiring extracorporeal membrane oxygenation for pulmonary causes—A retrospective, observational study. *Swiss Med. Wkly.* **2020**, *150*, w20358. [CrossRef]
25. Ren, Y.Q.; Zhang, Y.C.; Shi, J.Y.; Shan, Y.J.; Sun, T.; Zhou, Y.P.; Cui, Y. Analysis of risk factors of central nervous system complications supported on extracorporeal membrane oxygenation. *Zhonghua Er Ke Za Zhi* **2022**, *60*, 1059–1065. [CrossRef]
26. Edes, I.F.; Nemeth, B.T.; Hartyanszky, I.; Szilveszter, B.; Kulyassa, P.; Fazekas, L.; Polos, M.; Nemeth, E.; Becker, D.; Merkely, B. Predictors of mortality following extracorporeal membrane oxygenation support in an unselected, critically ill patient population. *Postep. Kardiol. Interwencyjnej* **2021**, *17*, 290–297. [CrossRef]
27. Carmona, C.; Nellis, M.E.; Karam, O. Anticoagulation and hemostasis on extracorporeal membrane oxygenation. *Curr. Opin. Pediatr.* **2023**, *35*, 297–302. [CrossRef]
28. Saini, A.; Spinella, P.C. Management of anticoagulation and hemostasis for pediatric extracorporeal membrane oxygenation. *Clin. Lab. Med.* **2014**, *34*, 655–673. [CrossRef]
29. Dalton, H.J.; Reeder, R.; Garcia-Filion, P.; Holubkov, R.; Berg, R.A.; Zuppa, A.; Moler, F.W.; Shanley, T.; Pollack, M.M.; Newth, C.; et al. Factors Associated with Bleeding and Thrombosis in Children Receiving Extracorporeal Membrane Oxygenation. *Am. J. Respir. Crit. Care Med.* **2017**, *196*, 762–771. [CrossRef]
30. Drop, J.G.; Erdem, O.; Wildschut, E.D.; van Rosmalen, J.; de Maat, M.P.M.; Kuiper, J.W.; Houmes, R.J.M.; van Ommen, C.H. Use of rotational thromboelastometry to predict hemostatic complications in pediatric patients undergoing extracorporeal membrane oxygenation: A retrospective cohort study. *Res. Pract. Thromb. Haemost.* **2021**, *5*, e12553. [CrossRef]
31. Werho, D.K.; Pasquali, S.K.; Yu, S.; Donohue, J.; Annich, G.M.; Thiagarajan, R.R.; Hirsch-Romano, J.C.; Gaies, M.G.; Extracorporeal Life Support Organization Member, C. Hemorrhagic complications in pediatric cardiac patients on extracorporeal membrane oxygenation: An analysis of the Extracorporeal Life Support Organization Registry. *Pediatr. Crit. Care Med.* **2015**, *16*, 276–288. [CrossRef]
32. Ankola, A.A.; Bailly, D.K.; Reeder, R.W.; Cashen, K.; Dalton, H.J.; Dolgner, S.J.; Federman, M.; Ghassemzadeh, R.; Himebauch, A.S.; Kamerkar, A.; et al. Risk Factors Associated With Bleeding in Children With Cardiac Disease Receiving Extracorporeal Membrane Oxygenation: A Multi-Center Data Linkage Analysis. *Front. Cardiovasc. Med.* **2021**, *8*, 812881. [CrossRef]
33. Harvey, C. Cannulation for Neonatal and Pediatric Extracorporeal Membrane Oxygenation for Cardiac Support. *Front. Pediatr.* **2018**, *6*, 17. [CrossRef]
34. Radakovic, D.; Hamouda, K.; Penov, K.; Bening, C.; Sayed, S.; Gietzen, C.; Leyh, R.G.; Aleksic, I. Central Versus Peripheral Arterial Cannulation for Veno-Arterial Extracorporeal Membrane Oxygenation in Post-Cardiotomy Patients. *ASAIO J.* **2021**, *67*, 67–73. [CrossRef]

35. Biancari, F.; Kaserer, A.; Perrotti, A.; Ruggieri, V.G.; Cho, S.M.; Kang, J.K.; Dalen, M.; Welp, H.; Jonsson, K.; Ragnarsson, S.; et al. Central versus Peripheral Postcardiotomy Veno-Arterial Extracorporeal Membrane Oxygenation: Systematic Review and Individual Patient Data Meta-Analysis. *J. Clin. Med.* **2022**, *11*, 7406. [CrossRef]
36. Kanji, H.D.; Schulze, C.J.; Oreopoulos, A.; Lehr, E.J.; Wang, W.; MacArthur, R.M. Peripheral versus central cannulation for extracorporeal membrane oxygenation: A comparison of limb ischemia and transfusion requirements. *Thorac. Cardiovasc. Surg.* **2010**, *58*, 459–462. [CrossRef]
37. Alhijab, F.A.; Tantawy, T.M.; Ismail, H.H.; AlBarrak, M.; Adam, A.I.; Belghith, M.; Hassan, E.; Pragliola, C.; Albabtain, M.A.; Arafat, A.A. Venoarterial extracorporeal membrane oxygenation for postcardiotomy cardiogenic shock: The impact of cannulation strategy on survival. *Perfusion* **2022**. [CrossRef]
38. Alsoufi, B.; Gillespie, S.; Mahle, W.T.; Deshpande, S.; Kogon, B.; Maher, K.; Kanter, K. The Effect of Noncardiac and Genetic Abnormalities on Outcomes Following Neonatal Congenital Heart Surgery. *Semin. Thorac. Cardiovasc. Surg.* **2016**, *28*, 105–114. [CrossRef]
39. Furlong-Dillard, J.; Bailly, D.; Amula, V.; Wilkes, J.; Bratton, S. Resource Use and Morbidities in Pediatric Cardiac Surgery Patients with Genetic Conditions. *J. Pediatr.* **2018**, *193*, 139–146. [CrossRef]
40. Sperotto, F.; Gearhart, A.; Hoskote, A.; Alexander, P.M.A.; Barreto, J.A.; Habet, V.; Valencia, E.; Thiagarajan, R.R. Cardiac arrest and cardiopulmonary resuscitation in pediatric patients with cardiac disease: A narrative review. *Eur. J. Pediatr.* **2023**. [CrossRef]
41. De Mul, A.; Nguyen, D.A.; Doell, C.; Perez, M.H.; Cannizzaro, V.; Karam, O. Prognostic Evaluation of Mortality after Pediatric Resuscitation Assisted by Extracorporeal Life Support. *J. Pediatr. Intensive Care* **2019**, *8*, 57–63. [CrossRef]
42. Wengenmayer, T.; Rombach, S.; Ramshorn, F.; Biever, P.; Bode, C.; Duerschmied, D.; Staudacher, D.L. Influence of low-flow time on survival after extracorporeal cardiopulmonary resuscitation (eCPR). *Crit. Care* **2017**, *21*, 157. [CrossRef]
43. Speth, M.; Munch, F.; Purbojo, A.; Glockler, M.; Toka, O.; Cesnjevar, R.A.; Ruffer, A. Pediatric Extracorporeal Life Support Using a Third Generation Diagonal Pump. *ASAIO J.* **2016**, *62*, 482–490. [CrossRef]
44. Marino, B.S.; Tabbutt, S.; MacLaren, G.; Hazinski, M.F.; Adatia, I.; Atkins, D.L.; Checchia, P.A.; DeCaen, A.; Fink, E.L.; Hoffman, G.M.; et al. Cardiopulmonary Resuscitation in Infants and Children With Cardiac Disease: A Scientific Statement From the American Heart Association. *Circulation* **2018**, *137*, e691–e782. [CrossRef]
45. Brown, G.; Moynihan, K.M.; Deatrick, K.B.; Hoskote, A.; Sandhu, H.S.; Aganga, D.; Deshpande, S.R.; Menon, A.P.; Rozen, T.; Raman, L.; et al. Extracorporeal Life Support Organization (ELSO): Guidelines for Pediatric Cardiac Failure. *ASAIO J.* **2021**, *67*, 463–475. [CrossRef]
46. Shuhaiber, J.; Thiagarajan, R.R.; Laussen, P.C.; Fynn-Thompson, F.; del Nido, P.; Pigula, F. Survival of children requiring repeat extracorporeal membrane oxygenation after congenital heart surgery. *Ann. Thorac. Surg.* **2011**, *91*, 1949–1955. [CrossRef]
47. Bohuta, L.; d'Udekem, Y.; Best, D.; Alexander, P.; Barozzi, L.; Butt, W. Outcomes of second-run extracorporeal life support in children: A single-institution experience. *Ann. Thorac. Surg.* **2011**, *92*, 993–996. [CrossRef]
48. d'Udekem, Y.; Shime, N.; Lou, S.; MacLaren, G. Recurrent or prolonged mechanical circulatory support: Bridge to recovery or road to nowhere? *Pediatr. Crit. Care Med.* **2013**, *14*, S69–S72. [CrossRef]

life

Systematic Review

The Role of Blood Oxygen Level Dependent Signal Variability in Pediatric Neuroscience: A Systematic Review

Michael F. Dinatolo [1,*], Daiana Roxana Pur [1], Roy Eagleson [2,3] and Sandrine de Ribaupierre [2,4]

1 Schulich School of Medicine and Dentistry, Western University, London, ON N6A 5C1, Canada; dpur2024@meds.uwo.ca
2 Brain and Mind Institute, Western University, London, ON N6A 5B7, Canada; eagleson@uwo.ca (R.E.); sderibau@uwo.ca (S.d.R.)
3 Department of Electrical and Computer Engineering, Western University, London, ON N6A 3K7, Canada
4 Department of Clinical Neurological Sciences, Schulich School of Medicine and Dentistry, Western University, London, ON N6A 5C1, Canada
* Correspondence: mdinatol@uwo.ca

Abstract: Background: As pediatric BOLD Signal Variability (SV) analysis is relatively novel, there is a need to provide a foundational framework that gives researchers an entry point into engaging with the topic. This begins with clarifying the definition of BOLD signal variability by identifying and categorizing the various metrics utilized to measure BOLD SV. Methods: A systematic review of the literature was conducted. Inclusion criteria were restricted to studies utilizing any metric of BOLD SV and with individuals younger than 18 in the study population. The definition of BOLD SV was any measure of intra-individual variability in the BOLD signal. Five databases were searched: Psychinfo, Healthstar, MEDLINE, Embase, and Scopus. Results: A total of 17 observational studies, including male (n = 1796) and female (n = 1324) pediatric participants were included. Eight studies quantified variability as the amount of deviation from the average BOLD signal, seven used complexity-based metrics, three used correlation measures of variability, and one used the structure of the hemodynamic response function. In this study, 10 methods of quantifying signal variability were identified. Associations and trends in BOLD SV were commonly found with age, factors specific to mental and/or neurological disorders such as attention deficit disorder, epilepsy, psychotic symptoms, and performance on psychological and behavioral tasks. Conclusions: BOLD SV is a potential biomarker of neurodevelopmental and neurological conditions and symptom severity in mental disorders for defined pediatric populations. Studies that establish clinical trends and identify the mechanisms underlying BOLD SV with a low risk of bias are needed before clinical applications can be utilized by physicians.

Keywords: BOLD signal variability; pediatrics; biomarker; fMRI; neurodevelopment

check for updates

Citation: Dinatolo, M.F.; Pur, D.R.; Eagleson, R.; de Ribaupierre, S. The Role of Blood Oxygen Level Dependent Signal Variability in Pediatric Neuroscience: A Systematic Review. *Life* **2023**, *13*, 1587. https://doi.org/10.3390/life13071587

Academic Editor: Wenceslao Peñate

Received: 9 May 2023
Revised: 27 June 2023
Accepted: 10 July 2023
Published: 19 July 2023

1. Introduction

Variability in the blood-oxygen-level-dependent (BOLD) signal has emerged as a metric with potential clinical relevance. It is no longer viewed as simply "noise" from confounding events during functional magnetic resonance imaging (fMRI) [1–3] at its most inclusive, BOLD signal variability, hereafter referred to as BOLD SV, is a measure of the intraindividual change of the measured BOLD signal, a proxy for neural activity. BOLD SV has been associated with age and cognitive function over the lifespan [1], as well as clinical symptoms in eating disorders [2], attention deficit hyperactivity disorder (ADHD) [3], or 22q11.2 deletion syndrome [4]. Although it is true that other physiological pulsations can confound the true neural activation found in the BOLD signal, the predictability of these associations should decrease after regression of these confounding post-analysis techniques such as independent component analysis (ICA) denoising and RETROspective Image CORrection (RETROICOR) [1,5]. This allows for the isolation of neural activation effects from other external and physiological contributions that confound the association and improve the signal-to-noise ratio [1].

Overall, younger individuals are reported to be more variable in neural processing than older populations. Older populations report reduced BOLD SV during aging, primarily in subcortical regions. In addition, correlations have been made between poorer performance and reduced BOLD SD in these regions [6]. Although BOLD SV of individual brain regions presents differing trends across the lifespan, an inverted U-shaped trend of cognitive performance and whole brain variability level is observed over the lifespan. Specific trends in the pediatric period have yet to be investigated [6–10].

Despite the growth of BOLD SV being utilized in pediatric research, there remains inconsistency around its definition and the metrics used to characterize variability. Which metrics exist and which should be used is unclear, rendering BOLD SV challenging to apply or interpret in a standardized manner, especially in a clinical setting. For example, cortical morphology metrics such as cortical thickness confound BOLD SV measurements, but this is not consistently demonstrated or accounted for across all metrics [11].

Understanding pediatric BOLD SV may provide insight into critical neuro-developmental processes including maturation of neurotransmitter systems, pruning and neuroplasticity, myelination and white matter integrity, and functional network changes [7,8,10,12]. For example, higher BOLD SV in medial prefrontal areas comprising the default mode network (DMN) has been shown to positively correlate with ADHD symptom severity [3]. Importantly, infancy and adolescence are unique periods of brain development in which early screening and surveillance can mitigate neurodevelopmental issues. Diagnosing neurological and developmental disorders early on in a child's life can result in earlier identification, and therefore, improved chances for intervention [2]. BOLD SV has the potential to be established as a neurodevelopmental biomarker and contribute to the diagnosis, prognosis, and treatment of neurological disorders in pediatric development [1].

As pediatric BOLD SV is relatively novel, there is a need to provide a foundational framework that gives researchers an entry point into engaging with the topic. BOLD SV is not yet clearly defined, nor is it measured using a single metric of variability deemed more effective in clinical and research environments. This systematic review attempts to clarify the definition of BOLD SV by identifying and categorizing the various metrics used to measure BOLD SV, and how each metric has been utilized in the literature.

2. Materials and Methods

2.1. Operational Definitions

BOLD SV, in this review, was defined as any measure of intra-individual variance in the BOLD signal. The BOLD signal was acquired signal correlated with changes to blood flow and blood oxygenation to localized regions of the brain [13]. The signal also had to characterize the flow of oxygenated hemoglobin being used to support neuronal activity [13]. This definition was chosen to ensure a comprehensive set of all definitions, which are presently not well defined in the BOLD SV literature.

2.2. Article Search Strategy

The preferred reporting items for a systematic review and meta-analysis (PRISMA) guidelines were used to conduct the systematic review [14]. The electronic literature search was conducted in November 2021 by using MEDLINE (2003 to 2021), Ovid Healthstar (2003–2021), Psychinfo (2003–2021), and Embase (2003 to 2021) through the Ovid platform, as well as the Scopus (2003 to 2021) database. Google Scholar was also searched, although no additional citations were captured. The same strategy was used for each database to search for controlled vocabulary and keywords. These key terms were: BOLD Signal AND (Variability OR standard deviation OR Mean Successive Difference) AND (Paediatric OR Adolescent OR Youth OR Infant). Forward and backward citation tracing was conducted to search for articles that may not have been captured in electronic databases or Google Scholar.

2.3. Study Inclusion and Exclusion

Articles included used BOLD SV to measure intra-individual variability, or variability changes across the lifespan. Measures of BOLD SV used to adjust for signal noise and other confounders were excluded. All studies possessed participants in their final study sample that were under the age of 18, even if individuals over the age of 18 were included in the study. The inclusion criteria permitted both studies that used an observational or experimental design. Only results relevant to pediatric samples were included in the final extraction. Review papers, conference abstracts and letters to editor case reports and case studies, non-peer-reviewed studies, populations over 18, non-human studies, non-English papers, editorials, and any study without enough data (i.e., did not identify age) were all excluded.

2.4. Study Selection and Quality Assessment

A two-stage screening process was conducted to identify relevant articles. All articles were first identified through electronic database searches and imported into the systematic review management system known as Covidence. Duplicates of captured articles were then removed. Abstract and Title screening was completed by two authors (MD, DRP) who screened inclusively to avoid the removal of potentially relevant articles. Then, a full-text review was independently conducted by two authors (MD, DRP). The review team collaboratively reviewed full-text articles and resolved conflicts. Risk of bias (ROB) and quality assessment was then conducted using the Downs and Black checklist [15].

2.5. Data Synthesis

Mean and standard deviations (SD) described the study population's age and the number of control and diseased patients. In addition, the number and percentage of analysis conducted in studies, and the total number of male and female participants were also calculated from all studies included. Given the heterogeneity of the identified BOLD SV definition subgroups, and of the pediatric populations studied, a meta-analysis was not performed. A data extraction spreadsheet was developed to capture information pertaining to the definitions, study characteristics, sample characteristics, patient characteristics, variability metrics, scales, independent variables, and results of each article. Tables were constructed to summarize study characteristics, BOLD SV metrics and associated findings, and study objectives. Figures were constructed to summarize the results of the search via the PRISMA flowchart, summarize overall findings of Metric type and prevalence, and summarize significant findings in the literature.

3. Results

3.1. Study Sample

Of the five databases searched, Psychinfo contained 20 results, Healthstar had 41, Medline had 46, Embase had 96, and Scopus had A total of 185 unique studies were identified, and 17 studies were included. The PRISMA flowchart depicts how many studies were included or excluded at each screening step (Figure 1). This study included 10 different metrics of BOLD SV, a total of 3258 participants, and 2869 total pediatrics (1796 M/1324 F). Of the 17 studies, 8 used deviation from the average BOLD signal [4,10,16–20], 4 used correlational measures of BOLD SV [7,21–23], 7 used signal complexity [17,19,20,24–27], and 1 used the structure of the HRF [28] (Table 1). Metrics classification and associated findings can be found in Table 2.

Table 1. BOLD Signal Variability Study Characteristics.

Title	Author and Year	Location (Region, Country)	Study Design	Age of Subjects	Sex	Sample Size	Case Definition
Age-Associated Patterns in Gray Matter Volume, Cerebral Perfusion and BOLD Oscillations in Children and Adolescents	Bray et al., 2017 [26]	Calgary, Alberta, Canada	Cross-Sectional	Mean = 13.8, SD = 3.12 Range = 7–18	Typically developing females = 34 Typically developing males = 25	Typically developing = 59	All participants healthy (No cases)
BOLD SV and complexity in children and adolescents with and without autism spectrum disorder	Easson, et al., 2019 [17]	Toronto, Ontario, Canada	Cross-Sectional	ASD Group Mean = 13.25, SD = 2.87 ASD Group Range = [9.6–17.80] Typically Developing Mean = 13.42 SD = 3.21 Typically Developing Range [8.10–17.60]	ASD Males = 20 Typically Developing Males = 17	ASD = 20 Typically Developing = 17 Total Sample Size = 37	Autism spectrum disorder was defined by the Autism Brain Imaging Data Exchange (ABIDE) II database (Where cases ascertained from)
Changes in BOLD variability are linked to the development of variable response inhibition: BOLD variability and variable response inhibition	Thompson et al., 2020 [7]	London, UK	Cross-Sectional	Children Range = [10–12] Children Mean = 11.56, SD = 0.83 Adult Range = [18–26] Adult Mean = 21.55, SD = 2.31	Females = 10 Males = 9	Children 10–12 = 19 Adults 18–26 = 26 Total = 45	All participants healthy (No cases)
Creative internally directed cognition is associated with reduced BOLD variability	Roberts, et al., 2020 [18]	Auckland, New Zealand	Cross-Sectional	Range = [17–25] Mean = 21 years, SD = 4 years	8 Males and 16 Females	24 typically developing	All participants healthy (No cases)
Disentangling resting-state BOLD variability and PCC functional connectivity in 22q11.2 deletion syndrome	Zöller et al., 2017 [4]	Geneva, Switzerland	Case Control	22q11.2 Gene Age Range = [9.0–24.8] Mean 22q11.2 Gene Age = 16.53 ± 4.25 Control Group Age Range = [9.5–24.9] Mean Control Group Age = 16.44 ± 4.20	Males = 21 Females = 29	Healthy Controls = 50 (22/28) 2q11.2DS = 50 (21/29) Total = 100	50 patients with 22q11.2DS, which is a specific type of microdeletion in chromosome 22
Individual Differences in Reading Skill Are Related to Tiral-by-Trial Neural Activation Variability in the Reading Network	Malins et al., 2017 [21]	United States	Cross-Sectional	Discovery Sample Range = [7.8–11.3] Discovery Sample Mean = 9.3, SD = 0.6 Confirmation Sample Range = [7.5–11.3] Confirmation Sample Mean = 9.4, SD = 1.1	Sample 1 females: 18 female Sample 1 males: 26 male Sample 2 females: 14 female Sample 2 males: 18 males	Sample 1 = 44 Sample 2 = 32 Total = 76	All participants healthy (No cases)
Moment-to-Moment BOLD Signal Variability Reflects Regional Changes in Neural Flexibility across the Lifespan	Nomi et al., 2017 [16]	Miami, Florida USA	Cross-Sectional	Slow repetition time Range = [6–85] Slow repetition time Mean = 42.26, SD = 23.60 Fast repetition time Range = [6–85] Fast repetition time Mean = 42.46, SD = 23.30	191 participants, 132 Female, 59 male	191 Participants	All participants healthy (No cases)
Neural correlates of inhibitory control and functional genetic variation in the dopamine D4 receptor gene	Mulligan et al., 2014 [23]	Alberta, Canada	Cross-Sectional	All Participants are 18	Female population = 33 Male population = 29	7R+ = 23 7R − control = 39 Total = 62	(R7+) group (dopamine D4 receptor gene (DRD4) with 7 repeats in the Variable Number of Tandem Repeats section (VNTR) of DRD4)
Neural, electrophysiological and anatomical basis of brain-network variability and its characteristic changes in mental disorders	Zhang et al., 2016 [22]	Nanjing, PR, China	Case Control	Total Study Age Range = [8–25] UM Sample Controls = 15.1 +/− 3.7 Autism = 3.6 +/− 2.4 Peking University-PKU Sample Controls = (11.4 +/− 1.9) ADHD = (12.1 +/− 2.0) New York University-NYU Controls = (12.2 +/− 3.1) ADHD = (12.2 +/− 13.1)	Autism UM dataset controls = (48/16) Autism UM dataset Autism = (31/7) ADHD PKU dataset controls = (84/59) ADHD PKU dataset ADHD = (89/10) ADHD NYU dataset controls = (54/54) ADHD NYU dataset ADHD = (106/34)	Autism MU dataset controls = 64 Autism MU dataset Autism = 38 ADHD PKU dataset controls = 143 ADHD PKU dataset ADHD = 99 ADHD NYU dataset controls = 108 ADHD NYU dataset ADHD = 140 Total = 592 (we only use a subset of 1180 total in this study due to age exclusions)	Schizophrenia case definition as defined in the Taiwan Dataset 1 (Guo et al., 2014); and the COBRE Dataset 2. Autism case definition as defined by the definition as defined in the New York University-NYU Dataset 3 and University of Melbourne-UM Dataset 4 (which are from ABIDE Consortium) ADHD case definition was defined by the Peking University-PKU Dataset 5; and New York University-NYU Dataset 6 which are included from 1000 participants derived from the Functional Connectome Project
Psychotic symptoms influence the development of anterior cingulate BOLD variability in 22q11.2 deletion syndrome	Zöller et al., 2018 [29]	Geneva Switzerland	Case-Control	Between 10 and 30 years old	PS+ = 28 (12/16) PS− = 29 (14/15) Healthy controls = 69 (30/39)	22q11.2 gene = 57 Healthy Controls = 69 Total = 126	Chromosome 22q11.2 deletion syndrome (22q11DS) is defined as a neurodevelopmental disorder associated with "a broad phenotype of clinical, cognitive, and psychiatric features". It is a specific type of microdeletion in chromosome 22

Table 1. *Cont.*

Title	Author and Year	Location (Region, Country)	Study Design	Age of Subjects	Sex	Sample Size	Case Definition
Temporal fractal analysis of the rs-BOLD signal identifies brain abnormalities in autism spectrum disorder	Dona et al., 2017 [24]	Austin, Texas, United States	Case-Control	ASD (12.7 ± 2.4 y/o) 55 age-matched (14.1 ± 3.1 y/o) healthy controls	ASD = 46 male and 9 females, Healthy controls = 38 male and 9 females.	ASD = 55 Healthy Control = 55 Total = 110	ASD and age-matched controls. Definition of ASD defined by NITRC database and the ABIDE project
Variability of the hemodynamic response as a function of age and frequency of epileptic discharge in children with epilepsy	Jacobs et al., 2007 [28]	Germany and Montreal Canada	Cross-Sectional	Range = [5 months-18 years] (Mean and SD not calculated)	12 Female, 25 Male	37	Epilepsy, case definition of epilepsy not explicit but EEG-fMRI data were ascertained in children who met the following criteria: (1) An indication for an anatomical scan on the basis of the necessity to investigate a lesion seen on a prior anatomical MRI scan or to diagnose them with epilepsy syndrome and exclude pathological changes. (2) Participants had frequent spikes (N 10 in 20 min) identified on EEG outside the scanner, without occurrence in bursts.
Evaluation of spontaneous regional brain activity in weight-recovered anorexia nervosa	Seidel et al., 2020 [19]	Germany	Case Control Study	Total Study Range = 15.5–29.7 recAN Mean = 22.06, SD = 3.38 HC Mean = 22.05, SD = 3.34	Healthy Control = 65 Female recAN = 65 female	Healthy Control = 65 recAN = 65 Total = 130	Recovered Anorexia Nervosa (Weight Recovered). Defined as recAN subjects had to (1) maintain a body mass index (BMI) (kg/m^2) > 18.5 (if older than 18 years) or above the 10th age percentile (if younger than 18 years); (2) menstruate; and (3) have not binged, purged, or engaged in restrictive eating patterns during at least 6 months before the study.
Complexity of low-frequency blood oxygen level-dependent fluctuations covaries with local connectivity	Anderson et al., 2013 [20]	N/A	Cross-Sectional	Range = [7–30] Mean = 8.3, SD = 5.6	Male = 590 Female = 429	1019	Not Specified
Fractal Analysis of Brain Blood Oxygenation Level Dependent (BOLD) Signals from Children with Mild Traumatic Brain Injury (mTBI)	Dona et al., 2017 [25]	N/A	Cross-Sectional	mTBI Subjects = 13.4 ± 2.3 Age-matched Healthy Controls = 13.5 ± 2.34	N/A	mTBI = 15 Healthy Control = 56 Total = 71	Case Control
The longitudinal relationship between BOLD signal variability changes and white matter maturation during early childhood	Wang et al., 2021 [10]	Canada and Australia	Cross-Sectional	Range = 1.97–8.0 years Mean age at intake = 4.42 ± 1.27	Females = 43 Males = 40	83	None
Frequency-specific alterations of the resting-state BOLD signals in nocturnal enuresis: an fMRI Study	Zheng et al., 2021 [27]	China	Case Control	Range approx. = [7–12] NE Patients 9.27(± 1.760) Control 9.68(± 1.601)	NE males = 57 NE Females = 14 Control Males = 19 Control Females = 16	Children with nocturnal enuresis (NE) = 129 Healthy controls = 37	Case Control

Abbreviations: BOLD, Blood oxygen level dependent; SV, signal variability; $BOLD_{SD}$, blood oxygen level dependent standard deviation, GMV, gray matter volume; fALLF fractional amplitude of low-frequency fluctuations; ASD, autism spectrum disorder; DRD4, Dopamine Receptor D4; VNTR, Variable Number of Tandem Repeats; VNTR 7-repeats present, 7R+; No VNTR 7-repeats present, 7R−; ADHD, attention deficit hyperactive disorder; recAN weight-recovered anorexia; acAN, acute anorexia; fMRI, functional magnetic resonance imaging; resting state, rs; recovered anorexia, recAN; MSSD, mean square successive difference; mTBI, mild traumatic brain injury, NE, nocturnal enuresis.

Table 2. Classification of BOLD Signal Variability Metrics.

Metric Type	Authors	Variability Metric	Description	Findings and Associations
Deviation from Average BOLD Signal	(Roberts et al., 2020 [18], Zöller et al., 2017 [4], Zöller et al., 2018 [30], Wang et al., 2021 [10], Anderson et al. 2013 [20])	$BOLD_{SD}$	Quantified the deviation of average BOLD signal from the mean signal.	BOLD Signal variability globally increased with age in all metrics (some regions decrease) BOLD SV in dACC did not change over age in PS+ patients and increased in PS−. Variability increased with age in the DMN. Positively correlated with GE in structural networks and negatively correlated with performance in ASD behavioral severity (SRS). Negative associations with indexes of creativity
	(Nomi et al., 2017a [16], Seidel et al., 2020 [19], Amanda K. Easson and McIntosh 2019 [17])	sMSSD	Calculated by subtracting the amplitude of the signal at time point t from time point t + 1, squaring, and then averaging the resulting values from the entire voxel time course.	
Correlational Measures of BOLD Signal Variance	(Zhang et al., 2016 [22])	Temporal Variance	The BOLD time series were segmented into non-overlapping windows, a whole brain signal measure is obtained using Pearson correlation, and a region's variability is compared to others.	Lower variability of DMN in schizophrenia, and increased variability in Autism/ADHD. Changes in variability were closely related to symptom scores and in the 10% most variable regions. Variability increases with age in the inhibition network. More variability in the network was associated with less variability in behavioral performance. Low variability in the DMN was correlated with high FC. Lower variability in 7R+ when compared to 7R− when participants successfully inhibited a prepotent motor response. Primarily seen in the prefrontal cortex, occipital lobe, and cerebellum.
	(Malins et al., 2018 [21], and Mulligan et al., 2014 [23])	GLM Derived Variance	GLM produced trial β series estimates of the signal which was used to estimate a variance.	
	(Thompson et al., 2021 [7])	Differences of Residuals	The difference in the variability between the two residual models.	
Signal Complexity	(Amanda K. Easson and McIntosh 2019 [17])	Sample Entropy	SE was used in identifying repetitive patterns in a time series. The degree of regularity of these patterns of activation was also observed, with fewer complex signals being more random.	Positive correlations were identified between entropy, GE, and age. Negative correlations with SRS severity scores and FD in social and non-social tasks, ADIR and ADOS. Grey matter rs-BOLD FD in mTBI patients had reduced FD. Power law exponents remained unchanged or decreased with age and are linearly related to ReHo, which covaried across subjects and gray matter regions. Grey matter rs-BOLD FD in mTBI patients had reduced FD. The fALFF increased with age, distinguishing posterior, and anterior regions. Higher fALFF values in recAN patient's cerebellum and the inferior temporal gyrus compared to controls. The fALFF decreased in the right insula in children with NE.
	(Dona et al., 2017a [24] and Dona et al., 2017b [25])	Fractal Dimension	Measure of the structural complexity of a signal derived from hurst exponents and quantified structural complexity across different predefined time windows.	
	(Anderson et al., 2013 [20])	Power Law Exponents	Power-based index of sinusoidal amplitudes in the BOLD signal. Signal that follows fractal characteristics that were self-similar within and across frequencies over a time series were measured.	
	(Seidal et al., 2020 [19], Zheng et al., 2021 [27], Bray 2017 [26])	Fractional amplitude of low-frequency fluctuations (fALFF)	The ratio of the low-frequency power spectrum, specifically in the range of 0.01–0.08 Hz, to the entire signal frequency range.	
Structure of Hemodynamic Response Function	(Jacobs et al., 2008 [28])	HRF Structure	Using the structure of the HRF, like peak time, amplitude or other signal characteristics not mentioned above.	Could not identify an age-specific HRF. Longer peak times of the HRF 0 to 2 yrs.

Abbreviations: BOLD, Blood oxygen level dependent; $BOLD_{SD}$, blood oxygen level dependent standard deviation; fALLF fractional amplitude of low-frequency fluctuations; ASD, autism spectrum disorder; ADHD, attention deficit hyperactive disorder; FD, fractal dimension; HRF, hemodynamic response function; HRF, hemodynamic response function; recAN weight-recovered anorexia; acAN, acute anorexia; ReHo, regional homogeneity fMRI, functional magnetic resonance imaging; resting state, rs; recovered anorexia, recAN; MSSD, mean square successive difference; mTBI, mild traumatic brain injury. A total of eight studies measured variability as a deviation from the mean BOLD signal time series [4,10,16–20,30]. Of these, five studies utilized $BOLD_{SD}$ as a measure of variability [4,10,18,20,30], and three used mean sample standard deviation (MSSD) [16,17,19] of the BOLD signal. In addition, four studies utilized correlational metrics to quantify the variability in the BOLD Signal [7,21–23]. This included two articles producing a beta series derived from linear modeling or regression to quantify variability [21,23], and one with a difference of residuals-based calculation [7]. Seven studies were identified that used a complexity-based metric of BOLD SV [17,19,20,24–27]. Of these, three used Fractional amplitude of low-frequency fluctuation (fALFF) as a metric of variability [19,26,27], two used fractal density (FD) [24,25], one used sample entropy (SE) [17], and one used power law exponents [20]. Finally, only one study used changes in key features of the hemodynamic response as a measure of variability [28]. Figure 2 is a graphical representation of the four categories of variability metrics.

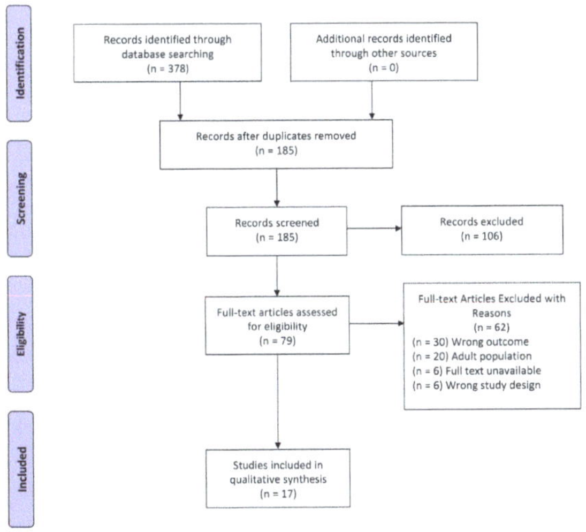

Figure 1. The Preferred Reporting Items for Systematic Reviews and Meta-Analyses (PRISMA) Diagram.

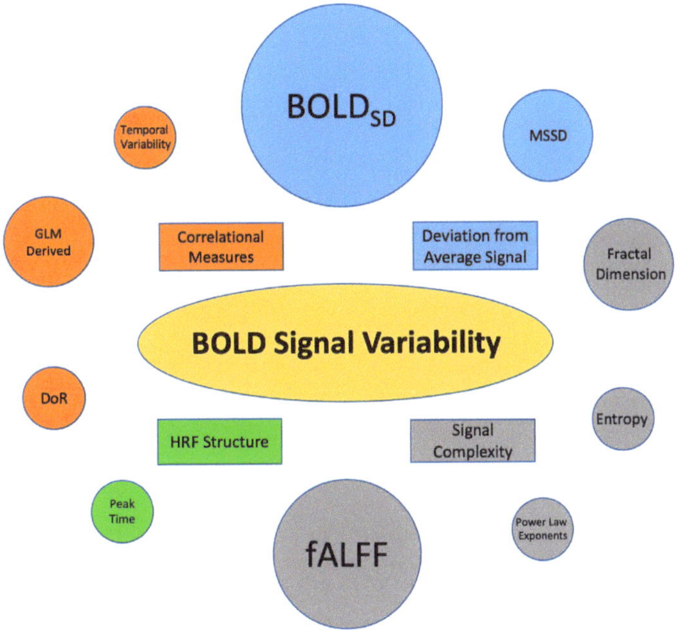

Figure 2. Summary of BOLD SV Metric Prevalence in the Pediatric Literature. Circles of the same color belong to a common metric subtype. The area of each circle is proportionate to the number of papers published that utilized the metric. BOLDSD appeared in six papers, making the largest circle. Colors were used to indicate metrics belonging to a common subtype of variability (i.e., Deviation from Average BOLD Signal). Abbreviations: $BOLD_{SD}$, Blood Oxygen Level Dependent Signal Standard Deviation; MSSD, Mean Successive Square Difference; fALFF, Fractional amplitude of low-frequency fluctuation; HRF, Hemodynamic Response Function; DoR, Difference of Residuals; GLM, General linear Model.

3.2. Study Characteristics

As presented in Table 1, all studies were observational. Of these 11/17, (65%) are cross-sectional studies and 6/17 (35%) are case control. Here, 11/17 of the studies exclusively included children (those under the age of 18) and 6/17 included a mixed population that included more than one child in their study population.

The statistical analyses performed in the included studies were heterogenous, with the most common being partial least squares analysis (n = 4, 24%) [10,17,18,30], followed by temporal fractal analysis (n = 2, 12%) [24,25] and principle component analysis (PCA) (n = 1, 5.9%) [26]. Age-based variability trends (n = 5, 29.4%) [4,16,26,28,30], behavioral and psychological task performance (n = 2, 12%) [18,21], and mental disorders (n = 5, 29%) [17,19,22,24,30], neurological disorders (e.g., Autism, ADHD, schizophrenia/psychotic symptoms, and anorexia) (n = 3, 18%) [25,27,28], and genetic conditions (n = 3, 18%) [4,23,30], were examined in relation to BOLD SV. Table A1 indicates the various objectives of the included articles.

3.3. BOLD SV Metrics

Variability metrics were grouped into four categories: BOLD signal deviation from the mean, measures of BOLD SV derived through a correlational analysis of the signal, measures of BOLD signal complexity, and measures that utilize characteristics of the hemodynamic response function (HRF). Table 2 presents the descriptions of each variability metric identified in the review.

3.4. Findings Associated with Deviation from the Average BOLD Signal

3.4.1. Standard Deviation of the BOLD Signal ($BOLD_{SD}$)

Five studies utilized $BOLD_{SD}$ (n = 5, 72.5%) [4,10,18,20,30] quantifying an average amount of deviation from the typical BOLD signal (Table 2). Most studies had the objective of characterizing variability differences between healthy or typically developing controls and those with a mental disorder, neurological issue, or genetic condition (n = 2, 40%) [4,30]. The next most common objective was identifying lifespan and age-based patterns in variability (n = 2, 40%) [4,30]. Only one of these studies looked at structural changes across the lifespan (n = 1, 20%) [8], while the rest looked at network-based changes (n = 4, 80%) [4,10,20,30].

A longitudinal study of white matter structure in healthy children, and a cross-sectional study on 22q11.2 deletion syndrome, assessed aging and its effect on $BOLD_{SD}$ of the brain and age-related variability patterns, respectively. A global association of increasing $BOLD_{SD}$ with age, particularly in the frontal gyrus, supramarginal gyrus, middle temporal gyrus, and superior parietal lobule was reported [10]. BOLD SV and white matter micro and macro structure metrics such as white matter volume, mean fractional anisotropy (FA), and mean diffusivity (MD) measured at younger ages were predictive of BOLD SV at older ages [10]. $BOLD_{SD}$ associations with these macro and micro structural alterations changed over the lifespan and across various regions throughout the brain.

Two studies focused on 22q11.2 deletion syndrome, a genetic disorder commonly associated with schizophrenia, and its relationship to $BOLD_{SD}$ [4,30]. Strong positive psychotic symptoms (PS+) were associated with aberrant age relationships and concurrently saw BOLD SV increase in visual regions and decrease in the cortices of the prefrontal and orbitofrontal regions of the brain [4]. Both of the studies identified elevated and reduced $BOLD_{SD}$ across different brain regions, often being lower in regions of the DMN (medial prefrontal cortex, posterior cingulate cortex (PCC), and lateral parietal cortex) [4,30]. Notably, the lack of association between age and $BOLD_{SD}$ was identified in the dACC or DMN of patients with high psychotic symptom scores (PS+) [30] or schizophrenia, which was typical of healthy controls [4,30] and populations with less severe psychotic symptoms (PS-) and the 22q11.2 deletion [30]. This resulted in globally reduced variability in the dACC region of children with PS+ when compared to children with PS- [30].

A task-based study measured internally directed creative cognition using a future simulation task, and an alternate uses task (AUT) also has correlations with $BOLD_{SD}$.

Performance, which acts as an index of creativity, was negatively correlated with the $BOLD_{SD}$ [18].

3.4.2. Mean Successive Squared Difference (MSSD)

MSSD is another way deviation from the average signal is measured (Table 1). Three studies utilized MSSD as a metric of BOLD SV [16,17,19] (n = 3, 27.5%). Although heterogeneous, studies in this section focused on diseased-based findings, one study assessed BOLD SV's relationship to autism spectrum disorder (ASD) [17] and another assessed lifespan-related trends in various networks across the brain [16]. The third study looked at recovered anorexia patients but found no significant findings using the metric [19].

A cross-sectional study of ASD and typically developing individuals used MSSD as a metric to quantify BOLD SV. Variability increased linearly in the SN nodes (anterior insula) and the ventral temporal cortex and decrease across subcortical, visual, sensorimotor, DMN, and central executive network (CEN) regions [16,17]. When MSSD was used in a population of children with ASD, positive associations between MSSD of the BOLD time series and GE in structural networks are present. Brain regions that had positive correlations with GE also had a negative correlation with behavioral severity scores such as the social responsiveness scale (SRS) [17].

3.5. *Findings Associated with Correlational Measures of BOLD SV*

The following section includes all metrics that attained variability measures through correlation-based methods (n = 4, 24%). This includes temporal variability, GLM-derived measures of variability, and the BOLD% signal change. Appendix A Table A2 includes the definitions of these metrics.

3.5.1. Temporal Variability

Temporal variability was assessed in one study, which included subjects with mental disorders and healthy controls (n = 1, 25%) [22]. In typically developing children, age-related trends demonstrated significant increases in temporal variability across the inhibition network, from childhood to adulthood [22]. When characterizing relationships in mental disorders, children with schizophrenia had decreased BOLD SV in DMN regions associated with higher activity and connectivity compared to typically developing patients. This decreased variability was also associated with neurocognitive symptoms characteristic of schizophrenia [22]. Increased variability was seen in subcortical regions (thalamus, putamen, and pallidum) in these patients, while children with ADHD, saw increased BOLD SV in regions of the DSN and decreased BOLD SV in subcortical regions. Variability levels were not the same in the DMN regions of typically developing children with autism and ADHD, with the medial frontal areas mainly affected in ASD, and the posterior cingulate in ADHD [22]. Importantly, regions with the highest variability in controls, (i.e., trans modal areas) have lower levels of variability in disorders [22]. Those areas in controls with the lowest variability, such as primary sensory regions, are more prevalent in mental disorders [22].

According to a study, 50% of regions with significant changes in BOLD SV in the three disorders are in the top 10% of regions with the highest or lowest variability in controls [22]. Negative correlations between the variability of the signal in a brain region and its level of activity were found. Low DMN variability was consistently identified alongside strong functional connectivity (FC) within the DMN during resting state fMRI [22].

3.5.2. Multilinear and General Linear Model (GLM)-Derived Variance Measurement

Two studies used multilinear models or GLM-derived variance measures (n = 2, 50%) [21,23]. A reading skill task was used to investigate deviations from the mean BOLD signal by measuring the standard deviation of a beta series representing mean activation. In the left inferior frontal gyrus pars triangularis, the SD of the series appears to account for additional variance in reading skill, measured as task performance [21].

Only one study measured BOLD SV as the % change in signal. This study was task-based, studying a "Go/No-Go" behavioral task in children and assessed neural factors associated with inhibitory control and genetic variation in the Dopamine (DA) receptor gene, having seven repeats in the variable number of tandem repeats (VNTR) of the DA receptor gene DRD4 (7R+). The presence of seven repeats in the VNTR region of DRD4 (7R+) is associated with psychiatric disorders that present self-regulation issues such as ADHD [23]. Lower variability was found in those with 7R+ when compared to 7R− groups during successfully inhibited prepotent motor response. This was observed in two regions located in the prefrontal cortex, one in the cerebellum and one in the occipital lobe [23]. There were no differences in behavioral performance of the "Go/No-Go" task and correlations between task-related BOLD responses were not observed during the task [23].

3.5.3. Difference of Residuals

One cross-sectional study used the difference of residuals metric (n = 1, 25%) [7]. This variability metric compares the difference in variability between the two residual models of observed and expected BOLD response. BOLD SV in the inhibition network was reported as lower in children than adults during a successful stopping task [7].

3.6. *Findings Associated with Signal Complexity*

Signal complexity (as defined in Table 2) was also used to measure the variability in the BOLD signal. Signal complexity is also described as the unpredictability of a signal over its time series [31]. Seven studies were identified that utilized this metric (n = 7, 41%) [17,19,20,24–27].

3.6.1. Entropy/Sample Entropy

Another way BOLD SV is estimated is by using an entropy metric such as sample entropy (SE). SE is used to identify repetitive patterns in a time series, and the degree of regularity of patterns of activation observed [31].

Only one study used an entropy-based metric of BOLD SV in populations of children with and without autism spectrum disorder (n = 1, 14%) [17]. Distributed brain regions showed increases in MSSD and entropy from childhood through adolescence and positive correlations between entropy, general efficiency (GE), and age in both ASD and typically developing groups [17]. Negative correlations with SRS scores and entropy [17]. Lower levels of sample entropy are seen in ASD individuals during social and non-social tasks [17].

3.6.2. Fractal Dimensionality

Two studies used fractal dimension, obtained by fractal analysis, as a measure of the complexity derived from hurst exponents (n = 2, 29%) [24,25]. FD is a statistical measure of how completely a fractal appears to fill the space in the geometric sense. When used for signals, it can become a metric of structural complexity across a given time domain [32].

Reduced signal complexity was seen in ASD participants with respect to controls in the amygdala, the vermis, the basal ganglia, and the hippocampus. Decreases were correlated with autism diagnostic interview-revised (ADI-R) and autism diagnostic observation schedule (ADOS) scores [24]. The nucleus accumbens and the caudate head showed significantly reduced fractal dimension. Regions of the cerebellum in the ASD cohort showed significantly reduced FD, particularly in the vermis with mild correlations with the Autism Diagnostic Interview restricted and repetitive behaviors (ADIRRB) and Autism Diagnostic Observation Schedule Restricted and Repetitive Behaviors (ADOSRRB) metrics [24].

A cross-sectional study of children with mTBI utilized FD as a metric of BOLD SV. There were 11 brain regions where FD significantly decreased for mTBI patients, including the caudate nucleus and nucleus accumbens [25]. The FD also decreased for mTBI patients when compared with the uninjured control group in both these areas [11].

3.6.3. Power-Based Metrics

Power or spectral density-based variability metrics are an index of the signal amplitude of sinusoidal oscillations within and across frequencies over a time series [8]. This signal, which demonstrates scale-free behavior, requires fractal-like self-similarity in a spatial or temporal scale to use a power law measure of complexity [20].

Only one study used this metric to quantify complexity in healthy participants (n = 1, 14%) [20]. Increases in complexity were found throughout the whole brain during adolescence and early adulthood, excluding the DMN and attention control networks. Complexity did not change with age in a subset of gray matter regions and dorsal attention networks [20]. Decreases in complexity were observed in other regions of the brain, but the largest reductions occurred in the subcortical gray nuclei [20]. A strong positive correlation between local connectivity (ReHo) and complexity in endogenous brain activity fluctuations was also identified [20]. White matter and areas of gray matter with lower local connectivity exhibited more randomness in their BOLD fluctuations. In the basal ganglia, thalami, and spinocerebellum. relatively lower complexity than would be predicted from ReHo [20] was observed.

3.6.4. Fractional Amplitude of Low-Frequency Fluctuation (fALFF)

Three studies utilized fALFF as a metric of complexity (n = 3, 43%) [19,26,27]. One cross-sectional study found that fALFF metrics were associated with age, with 5.2% of the variability in age attributed to complexity. They distinguished areas of the DMN and salience network in occipital, temporal, superior parietal, and pre- and post-central gyral regions. The age-associated fALFF component was also distinguishable from the posterior from anterior cortical regions. Anterior regions of the DMN had a more evident decline compared to posterior regions not a part of the DMN [26].

Two studies identified used fALFF in populations with mental disorders or neurological conditions [19,27]. It was found that in children with nocturnal enuresis (NE), fALFF was higher in the right insula and in the typical spectral band. Regional Homogeneity (ReHo) rose in the left insula and the right thalamus in children with NE, and the right insula saw increased fALFF in NE patients [27]. In the slow-5 frequency band, fALFF increased in the superior cerebellum and superior temporal gyrus in those with NE. The fALFF in slow-2 was primarily seen in white matter and was observed to be negative in other bands [27]. In anorexia nervosa patients and healthy controls, values indicated alterations in the temporal gyrus and cerebellum of recovered anorexic patients. Between-group differences in fALFF were also observed in the cerebellum, specifically in the vermis [19].

3.7. Findings Associated with Characteristics of the Hemodynamic Response Function (HRF)

The hemodynamic response function (HRF) describes the behavior of the BOLD response over time by measuring the change in the HRF with respect to time. A single cross-sectional study uses the "time to peak" in the function, as well as the overall shape, as a metric of variability.

A study of pediatric epilepsy patients discovered that the shape of the HRF changes in children, specifically, the amplitude decreases significantly with greater EEG spike frequency in epileptic patients. When looking at age-related trends in these patients, the intrasubject variability of the amplitude of the HRF does not vary significantly across the age groups of epileptic children [28]. In epilepsy cases, authors reported differences in age could not be distinguished using time-to-peak or amplitude-based metrics of the HRF [28].

4. Discussion

4.1. Summary of Evidence

4.1.1. Metric Utilization

A total of 17 studies and 10 unique metrics of BOLD SV were included in this review. These metrics were categorized into four types of variability measures: Eight used deviation from average BOLD signal, four used correlational measures of BOLD SV, seven used signal complexity, and one used the structure of the HRF. In addition, only seven studies included healthy controls (HCs) exclusively, while 10 included patients with neurological, psychiatric, or genetic disorders.

Presently, deviation-based and complexity-based metrics appear to be the most viable for clinical application and utilization in pediatric BOLD SV research, as the majority of studies included that used these metrics, produced significant results. In addition, complexity and deviation-based methods of quantifying signal variability have been previously established in other neuroscientific contexts that use biomedical signal analysis such as brain variability, heart rate variability, and variability in respiratory rates [33,34]. This attests to these metrics' promise as future biomarkers of BOLD SV. These metrics have been associated with neurophysiological, psychological, genetic, and developmental findings and have been presented in these studies. The pediatric BOLD SV literature specifically includes global and regional changes or associations of variability and neurostructural alterations, factors relating to mental and neurological disorders, genetic markers of disease, and psychological performance and aging (Table 2).

Deviation-based metrics can be used in the BOLD SV literature to describe how much the magnitude of the BOLD signal changes in the *y*-axis compared to the baseline level of activation over the course of the time series. Deviation-based metrics appear to be more versatile, as they are used to assess pathological or non-pathologically related trends in neuropsychological development [4,18]. This includes developmental, pathological, and psychologically relevant findings in the BOLD SV literature (Table 2). Complexity metrics best describe the degree of structure and information of signals and how associated they are with other functional networks [35]. Signals can have equal amounts of deviation from the average but still differ in complexity. Studies included in this review report on only developmental or age-related trends, neurological pathologies, and mental disorders (Table 2) since aging and pathologies of the nervous system result in signal degradation over time [35–37]. Typically, the more complex a signal is, the less it is impacted by unhealthy pathologies or age-related complexity degradation, and the metric should be utilized with this in mind.

Non-deviation or non-complexity-based subgroups include HRF metrics and correlational BOLD SV metrics. HRF-based variation currently is not well established or justified as an effective BOLD SV metric, given the single study using the HRF variability metric did not show significant results [28]. Correlational metrics are highly specific to statistical models utilized in the study, and it is unclear how useful they will be unless they can be applied to clinical settings in a standardized manner. Unlike the HRF, however, they have produced significant results that have established pediatric BOLD SV trends [21,22].

4.1.2. The Inverted U Trend and BOLD SV

Global increases in whole brain BOLD SV were associated with aging in three of the four metric types in pediatric populations. The literature has competing perspectives on age-based variability trends. Typically, an inverted U-like pattern of variability is reported over the lifespan, suggesting that variability is functionally related to cognitive performance, and increases through childhood to adulthood and decreases in older age [8]. Multiple studies included in this review demonstrate that in both resting state and task-based protocols, whole brain variability increased from 0–18 years of age [4,17,24,30]. This inverted U may relate to the development of cognitive capacity, dynamic range, and therefore, efficiency that increases in childhood, peaks in young adulthood, and declines in older age [8]. One cross-sectional study that was identified proposed that lifespan-based trends in BOLD SV are better characterized by networks that simultaneously increase and decrease in variance over the lifespan. They report resting state fMRI data, which indicates regions of the SN nodes (anterior insula) and the ventral temporal cortex increase while there are decreases across subcortical, visual, sensorimotor, DMN, and CEN regions [16].

Though not established yet in pediatrics, the inverted U trends of cognitive performance and variability over the lifespan also follow dopamine signaling strength [38].

Cognition appears to change as DA signaling strength becomes too low or too high, and may play a role in the change in variability throughout the lifespan [38,39]. It should be noted that higher levels of BOLD SV have been specifically associated with elevated levels of cognitive flexibility [8]. In younger and older adults, suboptimal dopamine synthesis capacity is also associated with reduced cognitive flexibility, in addition to reduced BOLD SV [38,40].

4.1.3. BOLD SV Trends in Mental and Neurological Conditions

BOLD SV trends were identified in individuals with ASD, ADHD, schizophrenia, epilepsy, NE, recovered anorexia mTBI, and VNTR 7R deletion syndrome. In all disorders, atypical variability trends were uniquely observed across a variety of brain regions and compared to health controls. Regions associated with mental disorders, brain injury, and higher symptom severity were also associated with changes in variability.

Interestingly, lower variability of DMN specifically was seen in those with schizophrenia, while increased DMN variability in Autism/ADHD was identified, reporting opposite relationships [22]. Schizophrenia and ASD/ADHD's opposite variability trends in similar regions may be a result of their differing function in the social development patterns associated with the two diseases [3,29,41]. In the identified mental disorders, variability trends were inconsistent across regions, with some showing increases, aligning with the global variability trend, while others showed decreases or no change, breaking the trend. Elevated and reduced variability levels compared to healthy controls were consistent across all studies with a focus on mental disorders and neurological conditions, often in affected regions (Figure 3).

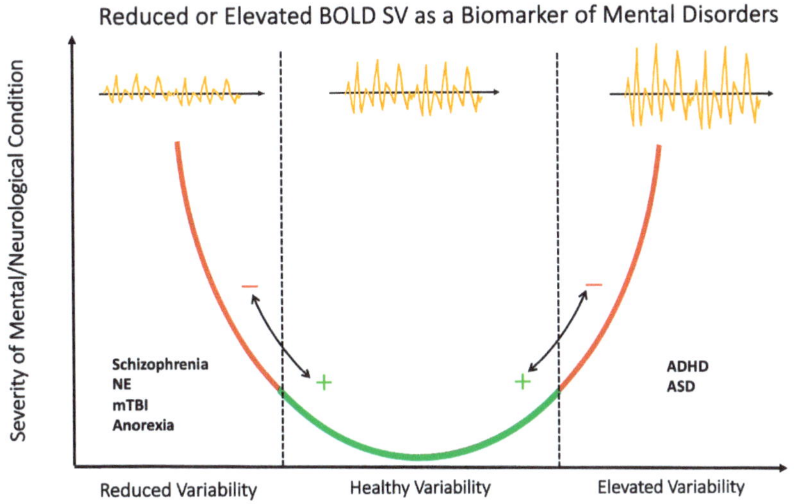

Figure 3. Reduced or Elevated BOLD SV as a Biomarker of Mental Disorders. When symptom severity scores and other markers of mental and neurological condition severity are present, BOLD SV is often reported as elevated or reduced in regions associated with the condition. Though it has promise as a biomarker, this model is only a representation of trends in the present literature. Abbreviations: NE, nocturnal enuresis; mTBI, mild traumatic brain injury, ADHD, Attention Deficit Hyperactive Disorder; ASD, autism spectrum disorder.

4.2. Recommendations for Clinical Applications

Though it is likely that deviation-based or complexity-based metrics have the potential to be used as a clinical biomarker in the future, not enough information is known at this time to make specific assessments on which metrics if any should be used and applied to clinical environments at this stage. More studies conducted using these metrics will allow for a more comprehensive appraisal of BOLD SV metrics. For instance, each metric's ability to be used in combination with signal processing and statistical techniques to mitigate confounding from non-neuronal sources of BOLD SV should be considered before clinical utilization.

Although the variability in neuronal activity is a key component of BOLD SV, there are other significant contributing sources to variability before processing, filtering, and statistical modeling, and ICA techniques are applied to the signal. Non-neuronal physiological sources of BOLD SV include brain hemodynamics influenced by heartbeat, respiration, and low-frequency oscillations (LFOs). LFOs in and of themselves are derived from a multitude of sources, potentially including Mayer waves, vasomotion from oscillations in vascular tone, CO_2 vasodilation, variations in heart rate or respiratory volumes, gastric oscillations seen using electrogastrograms, and aliased signals of cardiac and respiration due to long signal repetition times (TRs) [42].

These three categories of physiological factors contribute to BOLD SV due to their ability to impact fluctuations in oxygenated hemoglobin concentration in various regions of the brain. Heart rate, vasodilation vasoconstriction, respiratory rate, and respiratory depth over the course of the signal can all cause oxygenated hemoglobin concentration to change independent of brain region activation. This can result in the true associations or effects of BOLD SV being confounded by non-neuronal sources [43]. For instance, age or disease-related correlations with decreased BOLD SV could truly be a result of a decrease in resting cerebral blood flow, cerebral metabolic rate of O_2 consumption, and vascular reactivity from aging or disease-related causes. If this variability is not removed or controlled for in the analysis inferences from study conclusions cannot be validly applied to clinical practice [43,44].

These non-neuronal sources of signal can contribute between 20% and 70% of total BOLD SV prior to filtering, component analysis, or other correction steps [42]. Non-neuronal LFO variability is a particularly important target for controlling confounding. The LFO frequency range is where the neuronally related contributions to the BOLD signal can be found and is generally within the range of the low-frequency band (0–0.15 Hz) [45,46]. This is a consequence of the speed at which neuronal activation occurs relative to confounding physiological sources of BOLD SV [45,46]. Caution should be exercised when preparing raw signal for analysis. Approximately 30% of BOLD SV in grey matter is non-neuronal BOLD SV in the same 0–15 Hz frequency range that neuronal BOLD SV is found [42,45,46]. Each contributor to non-neuronal BOLD SV must be mitigated or removed from the signal through statistical modeling to control for these sources of variability. This should be carried out post spectral filtering of the BOLD signal, which already removes 10–15% of the variability in the BOLD signal derived from respiration and cardiac factors [43,47]. If certain metrics are better equipped to isolate neuronal BOLD SV in this frequency range, they should be favored in clinical and non-clinical practice.

Future areas of investigation into BOLD SV should continue to focus on developing BOLD SV into a biomarker of neurodevelopment and a risk factor for neurological issues and mental disorders such as schizophrenia would be a critical advancement of the pediatric BOLD SV literature. Reduced or elevated levels of BOLD SV in particular may identify the need for early intervention or treatment in pediatric populations [48]. In addition, given global variability's associations with age in childhood development, there are benefits to producing standardized thresholds of BOLD SV in a typical healthy patient across the different neurodevelopmental milestones in different populations (healthy, diseased, injured, etc.). This can be for associated brain regions, networks, or across the whole brain. This would allow for the establishment of BOLD SV as a biomarker of neurodevelopment and neurological conditions. To achieve this, consistent use of BOLD SV metrics in the literature and the recruitment of larger pediatric cohorts with a low risk of bias is vital. For BOLD SV to be a useful clinical biomarker, researchers must produce normative and non-normative distributions of BOLD SV for various regions of the brain in healthy populations and those affected by different neurodevelopmental disorders, respectively.

4.3. Future Directions and Limitations

Given the plethora of metrics identified, future studies should seek to implement multiple variability metrics into their analysis to validate that their findings are consistent, while simultaneously ensuring high-quality evidence is procured. Although it appears deviation-based and complexity-based metrics are most utilized, complexity-based metrics were primarily utilized in assessing associations between BOLD SV and either aging or developmental trends, or neurological pathologies or mental disorders. To verify if these metrics are more effective at characterizing variability in these populations, more work must be done to logically standardize these metrics in a way that highlights the strengths and weaknesses of each from a signal-processing perspective. Each metric should be utilized across diverse populations of patients so that findings may contribute to a future common framework for BOLD SV metric utilization.

A complimentary risk of bias analysis was conducted (Table A2), identifying that included articles displayed a risk of bias for external and internal validity overall. Using the Modified Downs and Black checklist identified total scores of 64% for reporting bias, 37% for external validity, 42% for internal validity bias, 37% for internal validity confounding, and an 11% score for power (Table A2). An overall score of 47% was obtained from all articles (Table A2). Criteria that were not included in studies were given a score of 0 unless otherwise indicated. In addition, seven studies included healthy controls while the rest were cross-sectional and included none. Of the 17 studies, 10 (n = 10, 59%) studies included patients with neurological, psychiatric, or genetic disorders. Many of the findings identified come from cross-sectional and case-control studies with a risk of bias. These studies are both observational and non-randomized, making it difficult to make etiologic or casual statements regarding risk factors' effect on variability. Higher quality evidence with a lower risk of bias will be important to the future of this promising and developing field in order to validate present trends in the literature [38,39]. Once studies on BOLD SV present higher-quality results in terms of typical and atypical pediatric populations, BOLD SV can be used as an important biomarker for neurodevelopment.

Author Contributions: Conceptualization, M.F.D., D.R.P., S.d.R., R.E.; writing—original manuscript preparation, M.F.D.; writing—review and editing, M.F.D., D.R.P., S.d.R., R.E.; visualization, M.F.D.; supervision, S.d.R., R.E. All authors have read and agreed to the published version of the manuscript.

Funding: Senior authors have research funding from NSERC (S.dR, R.E.), Epic Games MegaGrant Recipients (S.d.R R.E) and London Health Science Center (Paediatric Neurosurgery and Neuroscience Chair, S.d.R).

Institutional Review Board Statement: Not applicable.

Informed Consent Statement: Not applicable.

Data Availability Statement: No new data were created or analyzed in this study. Data sharing is not applicable to this article.

Conflicts of Interest: The authors declare no conflict of interest.

Appendix A

Table A1. Objectives of Included Studies.

Author and Year	Title	Objectives of Included Articles	Application
Bray et al., 2017 [26]	Age-Associated Patterns in Gray Matter Volume, Cerebral Perfusion and BOLD Oscillations in Children and Adolescents	Characterize patterns in GMV, CBF, fALFF, age, and their relation to structural and functional connectivity.	Identification of structural and functional relationships in pediatric brain development
Easson, et al., 2019 [17]	BOLD Signal Variability and complexity in children and adolescents with and without autism spectrum disorder	Assess both BOLD variability and BOLD complexity in children and adolescents with ASD and age-matched typically developing participants.	Identification of pathophysiology of ASD
Thompson et al., 2021 [7]	Changes in BOLD variability are linked to the development of variable response inhibition: BOLD variability and variable response inhibition	Effect on intra-individual variability in a response inhibition task and behavioral variability across the lifespan.	Identification of response inhibition trends during development
Roberts et al., 2020 [18]	Creative internally directed cognition is associated with reduced BOLD variability	Identify the relationship between BOLD variability, mean BOLD Signal, and creativity tasks that required flexible thinking in various fMRI tasks.	Identify trends of BOLD SV and creativity/flexibility
Zöller et al., 2017 [4]	Disentangling resting-state BOLD variability and PCC functional connectivity in 22q11.2 deletion syndrome	Investigate relationships between 22q11.2 deletion syndrome associated alterations in BOLD SV and age-relationship throughout the cortex of children and adolescents.	Clinical: identify pathophysiology and symptom severity of 22q11.2 deletion and schizophrenia
Malins et al., 2018 [21]	Individual Differences in Reading Skill Are Related to Tiral-by-Trial Neural Activation Variability in the Reading Network	Determine whether trial-by-trial neural activation variability accounts for variance in reading skill and in what direction.	Identify trends of BOLD SV and variance in reading skill
Nomi et al., 2017 [16]	Moment-to-Moment BOLD Signal Variability Reflects Regional Changes in Neural Flexibility across the Lifespan	Determine regional variability trends across the lifespan using rs-fMRI data across ages 6–85.	Identify brain variability trends in healthy brain development
Mulligan et al., 2014 [23]	Neural correlates of inhibitory control and functional genetic variation in the dopamine D4 receptor gene	Demonstrate carriers of DRD4 (7R+) have reduced prefrontal inhibitory control than non-carriers (7R−) confirmed by locally reduced BOLD % signal change and Go/No-Go task performance.	Clinical: identify pathophysiology of genetic alterations (addition of 7 tandem repeats) of the DRD4 receptor gene

Table A1. *Cont.*

Author and Year	Title	Objectives of Included Articles	Application
Zhang et al., 2016 [22]	Neural, electrophysiological, and anatomical basis of brain-network variability and its characteristic changes in mental disorders	Characterize temporal variability of the functional architecture of pediatrics with mental disorders in associated regions and networks and establish functional-structural relationships.	Clinical: identify pathophysiology and symptom severity of ADHD, ASD, and schizophrenia and identify SV trends in typically developing patients
Zöller et al., 2017 [29]	Psychotic symptoms influence the development of anterior cingulate BOLD variability in 22q11.2 deletion syndrome	Use the BOLD signal and $BOLD_{SD}$ to assess brain dynamics in patients with psychotic symptoms seen in schizophrenia.	Clinical: identify pathophysiology and symptom severity of schizophrenia
Dona et al., 2017 [24]	Temporal fractal analysis of the rs-BOLD signal identifies brain abnormalities in autism spectrum disorder	Utilize a model-free complexity analysis based on the fractal dimension of the rs-BOLD signal to identify BOLD SV trends in children with ASD.	Identify pathophysiology and symptom severity ASD
Jacobs et al., 2008 [28]	Variability of the hemodynamic response as a function of age and frequency of epileptic discharge in children with epilepsy	Identify age-related changes in the HRF after interictal epileptic discharge and identify the relationship between the number of spikes and a change in the HRF.	Clinical: Identify Pathophysiology of Epilepsy/interictal epileptic discharge in development
Seidel et al., 2020 [19]	Evaluation of spontaneous regional brain activity in weight-recovered anorexia nervosa	Investigate intrinsic regional brain activity differences between recAN, acAN, and healthy controls using resting-state measures of fALFF, ReHo (as reported in acAN, MSSD, DC, and VHMC (as new measures of spontaneous regional brain activity).	Clinical: Identify long-term effects and pathophysiology of recAN and patients
Anderson et al., 2013 [20]	Complexity of low-frequency blood oxygen level-dependent fluctuations covaries with local connectivity	Determine if BOLD fluctuations exhibit temporal complexity associated with local connectivity (ReHo), across gray matter regions utilizing power law behavior.	Identify associations between grey matter ReHo and temporal complexity
Dona et al., 2017 [25]	Fractal Analysis of Brain Blood Oxygenation Level Dependent (BOLD) Signals from Children with Mild Traumatic Brain Injury (mTBI)	Utilize FD to quantify local neural activity in the brain as a metric of functional changes in mTBI patients.	Clinical: Identification of pathophysiology of mTBIs.

Table A1. *Cont.*

Author and Year	Title	Objectives of Included Articles	Application
Wang et al., 2021 [10]	The longitudinal relationship between BOLD signal variability changes and white matter maturation during early childhood	Investigate longitudinal relationships between BOLD SV, age, and white matter structure in early childhood.	Identify variability trends between brain region SV, structure, and age.
Zheng et al., 2021 [27]	Frequency-specific alterations of the resting-state BOLD signals in nocturnal enuresis: an fMRI Study	Use associations of spontaneous brain activity and scores on urinary intention-related wakefulness in 5 frequency bands to detect abnormalities of activity in local brain regions of children with nocturnal enuresis.	Identify pathophysiology of NE

Note on Abbreviations: BOLD, Blood oxygen level dependent; SV, signal variability; $BOLD_{SD}$, blood oxygen level dependent standard deviation, GMV, gray matter volume; CBF, cerebral blood flow; fALLF fractional amplitude of low-frequency fluctuations; ASD, autism spectrum disorder; DRD4, Dopamine Receptor D4; ADHD, attention deficit hyperactive disorder; FD, fractal dimension; HRF, hemodynamic response function; recAN weight-recovered anorexia; acAN, acute anorexia; ReHo, regional homogeneity fMRI, functional magnetic resonance imaging; resting state, rs; recovered anorexia, recAN; MSSD, mean square successive difference; DC, degree centrality; VHMC, inter-hemispheric synchronicity; mTBI, mild traumatic brain injury, NE, nocturnal enuresis.

Table A2. Scores from the Downs and Black Checklist for Quality Assessment.

	Scoring						
	Reporting	**External Validity**	**Bias**	**Confounding**	**Power**	**Total**	**%**
Author(s) (Year)	Items 1–10	Items 11–13	Items 14–20	Items 21–26	Item 27 *	Total/28	Percentage
Bray et al., 2017 [26]	6	2	3	2	0	13	46.4%
Easson et al., 2019 [17]	7	1	3	3	0	14	50%
Thompson et al., 2021 [7]	7	0	2	2	1	12	42.9%
Roberts et al., 2020 [18]	7	0	3	2	0	12	42.9%
Zöller et al., 2017 [4]	8	1	3	3	0	15	53.6%
Malins et al., 2018 [21]	7	1	4	1	0	13	46.4%

Table A2. *Cont.*

	Scoring						
	Reporting	**External Validity**	**Bias**	**Confounding**	**Power**	**Total**	**%**
Nomi et al., 2017 [16]	7	1	2	2	0	12	42.9%
Mulligan et al., 2014 [23]	7	1	3	3	0	14	50%
Zhang et al., 2016 [22]	8	1	3	2	0	14	50%
Zöller et al., 2018 [30]	7	1	3	2	0	13	46.4%
Dona et al., 2017 [24]	7	1	3	2	1	14	50%
Jacobs et al., 2008 [28]	7	1	3	1	0	12	42.9%
Seidel et al., 2020 [19]	8	0	3	3	1	15	53.6%
Anderson et al., 2013 [20]	6	2	3	1	0	12	42.9%
Dona et al., 2017 [25]	7	2	3	3	0	15	53.6%
Wang et al., 2021 [10]	7	2	3	3	0	15	53.6%
Zheng et al., 2021 [27]	7	2	3	3	0	15	53.6%
Total	120/187	19/51	50/119	38/102	3/27	230/486	47.3%
%	64.2%	37.3%	42.0%	37.3%	11.1%	47.3%	X

* Note: Modified Downs and Blacks checklist, 27 questions were used to score the risk of bias for each article, in each section, and to estimate an overall risk of bias. Item 27 was given no points if the study's power was not reported. This table uses an "X" to identify a cell that cannot be filled with valid information.

References

1. Garrett, D.D.; Kovacevic, N.; McIntosh, A.R.; Grady, C.L. Blood Oxygen Level-Dependent Signal Variability Is More than Just Noise. *J. Neurosci.* **2010**, *30*, 4914–4921. [CrossRef] [PubMed]
2. Spalatro, A.V.; Amianto, F.; Huang, Z.; D'Agata, F.; Bergui, M.; Abbate Daga, G.; Fassino, S.; Northoff, G. Neuronal Variability of Resting State Activity in Eating Disorders: Increase and Decoupling in Ventral Attention Network and Relation with Clinical Symptoms. *Eur. Psychiatry* **2019**, *55*, 10–17. [CrossRef]
3. Nomi, J.S.; Schettini, E.; Voorhies, W.; Bolt, T.S.; Heller, A.S.; Uddin, L.Q. Resting-State Brain Signal Variability in Prefrontal Cortex Is Associated with ADHD Symptom Severity in Children. *Front. Hum. Neurosci.* **2018**, *12*, 90. [CrossRef] [PubMed]
4. Zöller, D.; Schaer, M.; Scariati, E.; Padula, M.C.; Eliez, S.; Van De Ville, D. Disentangling Resting-State BOLD Variability and PCC Functional Connectivity in 22q11.2 Deletion Syndrome. *Neuroimage* **2017**, *149*, 85–97. [CrossRef]
5. Jones, T.B.; Bandettini, P.A.; Birn, R.M. Integration of Motion Correction and Physiological Noise Regression in FMRI. *NeuroImage* **2008**, *42*, 582–590. [CrossRef] [PubMed]
6. Grady, C.L.; Garrett, D.D. Understanding Variability in the BOLD Signal and Why It Matters for Aging. *Brain Imaging Behav.* **2014**, *8*, 274–283. [CrossRef]
7. Thompson, A.; Schel, M.A.; Steinbeis, N. Changes in BOLD Variability Are Linked to the Development of Variable Response Inhibition. *Neuroimage* **2021**, *228*, 117691. [CrossRef]
8. Garrett, D.D.; Samanez-Larkin, G.R.; MacDonald, S.W.S.; Lindenberger, U.; McIntosh, A.R.; Grady, C.L. Moment-to-Moment Brain Signal Variability: A next Frontier in Human Brain Mapping? *Neurosci. Biobehav. Rev.* **2013**, *37*, 610–624. [CrossRef] [PubMed]
9. Mella, N.; de Ribaupierre, S.; Eagleson, R.; de Ribaupierre, A. Cognitive Intraindividual Variability and White Matter Integrity in Aging. *Sci. World J.* **2013**, *2013*, 350623. [CrossRef]
10. Wang, H.; Ghaderi, A.; Long, X.; Reynolds, J.E.; Lebel, C.; Protzner, A.B. The Longitudinal Relationship between BOLD Signal Variability Changes and White Matter Maturation during Early Childhood. *NeuroImage* **2021**, *242*, 118448. [CrossRef]
11. Pur, D.R.; Eagleson, R.A.; de Ribaupierre, A.; Mella, N.; de Ribaupierre, S. Moderating Effect of Cortical Thickness on BOLD Signal Variability Age-Related Changes. *Front. Aging Neurosci.* **2019**, *11*, 46. [CrossRef]
12. Pur, D.; Eagleson, R.; Ribaupierre, S. de C.4 Distinct BOLD Signal Variability Changes in Temporal and Occipital Cortices in Pediatric Epilepsy. *Can. J. Neurol. Sci.* **2022**, *49*, S7. [CrossRef]
13. Zou, Q.-H.; Zhu, C.-Z.; Yang, Y.; Zuo, X.-N.; Long, X.-Y.; Cao, Q.-J.; Wang, Y.-F.; Zang, Y.-F. An Improved Approach to Detection of Amplitude of Low-Frequency Fluctuation (ALFF) for Resting-State FMRI: Fractional ALFF. *J. Neurosci. Methods* **2008**, *172*, 137–141. [CrossRef]
14. Page, M.J.; McKenzie, J.E.; Bossuyt, P.M.; Boutron, I.; Hoffmann, T.C.; Mulrow, C.D.; Shamseer, L.; Tetzlaff, J.M.; Akl, E.A.; Brennan, S.E.; et al. The PRISMA 2020 Statement: An Updated Guideline for Reporting Systematic Reviews. *BMJ* **2021**, *372*, n71. [CrossRef]
15. Downs, S.H.; Black, N. The Feasibility of Creating a Checklist for the Assessment of the Methodological Quality Both of Randomised and Non-Randomised Studies of Health Care Interventions. *J. Epidemiol. Community Health* **1998**, *52*, 377–384. [CrossRef] [PubMed]
16. Nomi, J.S.; Bolt, T.S.; Ezie, C.E.C.; Uddin, L.Q.; Heller, A.S. Moment-to-Moment BOLD Signal Variability Reflects Regional Changes in Neural Flexibility across the Lifespan. *J. Neurosci.* **2017**, *37*, 5539–5548. [CrossRef] [PubMed]
17. Easson, A.K.; McIntosh, A.R. BOLD Signal Variability and Complexity in Children and Adolescents with and without Autism Spectrum Disorder. *Dev. Cogn. Neurosci.* **2019**, *36*, 100630. [CrossRef]
18. Roberts, R.P.; Grady, C.L.; Addis, D.R. Creative, Internally-Directed Cognition Is Associated with Reduced BOLD Variability. *NeuroImage* **2020**, *219*, 116758. [CrossRef] [PubMed]
19. Seidel, M.; Geisler, D.; Borchardt, V.; King, J.A.; Bernardoni, F.; Jaite, C.; Roessner, V.; Calhoun, V.; Walter, M.; Ehrlich, S. Evaluation of Spontaneous Regional Brain Activity in Weight-Recovered Anorexia Nervosa. *Transl. Psychiatry* **2020**, *10*, 395. [CrossRef]
20. Anderson, J.S.; Zielinski, B.A.; Nielsen, J.A.; Ferguson, M.A. Complexity of Low-frequency Blood Oxygen Level-dependent Fluctuations Covaries with Local Connectivity. *Hum. Brain Mapp.* **2013**, *35*, 1273–1283. [CrossRef]
21. Malins, J.G.; Pugh, K.R.; Buis, B.; Frost, S.J.; Hoeft, F.; Landi, N.; Mencl, W.E.; Kurian, A.; Staples, R.; Molfese, P.J.; et al. Individual Differences in Reading Skill Are Related to Trial-by-Trial Neural Activation Variability in the Reading Network. *J. Neurosci.* **2018**, *38*, 2981–2989. [CrossRef]
22. Zhang, J.; Cheng, W.; Liu, Z.; Zhang, K.; Lei, X.; Yao, Y.; Becker, B.; Liu, Y.; Kendrick, K.M.; Lu, G.; et al. Neural, Electrophysiological and Anatomical Basis of Brain-Network Variability and Its Characteristic Changes in Mental Disorders. *Brain* **2016**, *139*, 2307–2321. [CrossRef] [PubMed]
23. Mulligan, R.C.; Kristjansson, S.D.; Reiersen, A.M.; Parra, A.S.; Anokhin, A.P. Neural Correlates of Inhibitory Control and Functional Genetic Variation in the Dopamine D4 Receptor Gene. *Neuropsychologia* **2014**, *62*, 306–318. [CrossRef] [PubMed]
24. Dona, O.; Hall, G.B.; Noseworthy, M.D. Temporal Fractal Analysis of the Rs-BOLD Signal Identifies Brain Abnormalities in Autism Spectrum Disorder. *PLoS ONE* **2017**, *12*, e0190081. [CrossRef]
25. Dona, O.; Noseworthy, M.D.; DeMatteo, C.; Connolly, J.F. Fractal Analysis of Brain Blood Oxygenation Level Dependent (BOLD) Signals from Children with Mild Traumatic Brain Injury (MTBI). *PLoS ONE* **2017**, *12*, e0169647. [CrossRef] [PubMed]
26. Bray, S. Age-associated Patterns in Gray Matter Volume, Cerebral Perfusion and BOLD Oscillations in Children and Adolescents. *Hum. Brain Mapp.* **2017**, *38*, 2398–2407. [CrossRef] [PubMed]

27. Zheng, X.; Sun, J.; Lv, Y.; Wang, M.; Du, X.; Jia, X.; Ma, J. Frequency-Specific Alterations of the Resting-State BOLD Signals in Nocturnal Enuresis: An FMRI Study. *Sci. Rep.* **2021**, *11*, 12042. [CrossRef]
28. Jacobs, J.; Hawco, C.; Kobayashi, E.; Boor, R.; LeVan, P.; Stephani, U.; Siniatchkin, M.; Gotman, J. Variability of the Hemodynamic Response as a Function of Age and Frequency of Epileptic Discharge in Children with Epilepsy. *Neuroimage* **2008**, *40*, 601–614. [CrossRef] [PubMed]
29. Zöller, D.; Padula, M.C.; Sandini, C.; Schneider, M.; Scariati, E.; Van De Ville, D.; Schaer, M.; Eliez, S. Psychotic Symptoms Influence the Development of Anterior Cingulate BOLD Variability in 22q11.2 Deletion Syndrome. *Schizophr. Res.* **2018**, *193*, 319–328. [CrossRef] [PubMed]
30. Richman, J.S.; Lake, D.E.; Moorman, J.R. Sample Entropy. In *Methods in Enzymology*; Numerical Computer Methods, Part E.; Academic Press: Cambridge, MA, USA, 2004; Volume 384, pp. 172–184.
31. Raghavendra, B.S.; Dutt, D.N. Computing Fractal Dimension of Signals Using Multiresolution Box-Counting Method. *Int. J. Inf. Math. Sci.* **2010**, *6*, 50–65. [CrossRef]
32. Castiglioni, P.; Faes, L.; Valenza, G. Assessing Complexity in Physiological Systems through Biomedical Signals Analysis. *Entropy* **2020**, *22*, 1005. [CrossRef]
33. Garrett, D.D.; Kovacevic, N.; McIntosh, A.R.; Grady, C.L. The Importance of Being Variable. *J. Neurosci.* **2011**, *31*, 4496–4503. [CrossRef]
34. Glass, L.; Mackey, M.C. *From Clocks to Chaos: The Rhythms of Life*; Princeton University Press: Princeton, NJ, USA, 1988; ISBN 978-0-691-08496-1.
35. Amaral, L.A.N.; Díaz-Guilera, A.; Moreira, A.A.; Goldberger, A.L.; Lipsitz, L.A. Emergence of Complex Dynamics in a Simple Model of Signaling Networks. *Proc. Natl. Acad. Sci. USA* **2004**, *101*, 15551–15555. [CrossRef] [PubMed]
36. Goldberger, A.L.; Amaral, L.A.N.; Hausdorff, J.M.; Ivanov, P.C.; Peng, C.-K.; Stanley, H.E. Fractal Dynamics in Physiology: Alterations with Disease and Aging. *Proc. Natl. Acad. Sci. USA* **2002**, *99*, 2466–2472. [CrossRef]
37. Li, S.-C.; Lindenberger, U.; Bäckman, L. Dopaminergic Modulation of Cognition across the Life Span. *Neurosci. Biobehav. Rev.* **2010**, *34*, 625–630. [CrossRef]
38. Guitart-Masip, M.; Salami, A.; Garrett, D.; Rieckmann, A.; Lindenberger, U.; Bäckman, L. BOLD Variability Is Related to Dopaminergic Neurotransmission and Cognitive Aging. *Cereb. Cortex* **2016**, *26*, 2074–2083. [CrossRef] [PubMed]
39. Berry, A.S.; Shah, V.D.; Baker, S.L.; Vogel, J.W.; O'Neil, J.P.; Janabi, M.; Schwimmer, H.D.; Marks, S.M.; Jagust, W.J. Aging Affects Dopaminergic Neural Mechanisms of Cognitive Flexibility. *J. Neurosci.* **2016**, *36*, 12559–12569. [CrossRef]
40. Crespi, B.; Badcock, C. Psychosis and Autism as Diametrical Disorders of the Social Brain. *Behav. Brain Sci.* **2008**, *31*, 241–261, discussion 261-320. [CrossRef] [PubMed]
41. Tong, Y.; Hocke, L.M.; Frederick, B.B. Low Frequency Systemic Hemodynamic "Noise" in Resting State BOLD FMRI: Characteristics, Causes, Implications, Mitigation Strategies, and Applications. *Front. Neurosci.* **2019**, *13*, 787. [CrossRef]
42. Chang, C.; Cunningham, J.P.; Glover, G.H. Influence of Heart Rate on the BOLD Signal: The Cardiac Response Function. *NeuroImage* **2009**, *44*, 857–869. [CrossRef]
43. D'Esposito, M.; Deouell, L.Y.; Gazzaley, A. Alterations in the BOLD FMRI Signal with Ageing and Disease: A Challenge for Neuroimaging. *Nat. Rev. Neurosci.* **2003**, *4*, 863–872. [CrossRef]
44. Howseman, A.; Zeki, S.; Josephs, O.; Henson, R.N.A. Event-Related Functional Magnetic Resonance Imaging: Modelling, Inference and Optimization. *Philos. Trans. R. Soc. London. Ser. B Biol. Sci.* **1999**, *354*, 1215–1228. [CrossRef]
45. Logothetis, N.K.; Pauls, J.; Augath, M.; Trinath, T.; Oeltermann, A. Neurophysiological Investigation of the Basis of the FMRI Signal. *Nature* **2001**, *412*, 150–157. [CrossRef]
46. Tong, Y.; Hocke, L.M.; Fan, X.; Janes, A.C.; deB Frederick, B. Can Apparent Resting State Connectivity Arise from Systemic Fluctuations? *Front. Hum. Neurosci.* **2015**, *9*, 285. [CrossRef]
47. Hadders-Algra, M. Early Diagnostics and Early Intervention in Neurodevelopmental Disorders—Age-Dependent Challenges and Opportunities. *J. Clin. Med.* **2021**, *10*, 861. [CrossRef] [PubMed]
48. Alavash, M.; Lim, S.-J.; Thiel, C.; Sehm, B.; Deserno, L.; Obleser, J. Dopaminergic Modulation of Hemodynamic Signal Variability and the Functional Connectome during Cognitive Performance. *NeuroImage* **2018**, *172*, 341–356. [CrossRef] [PubMed]

life

Article

Lessons from Polyomavirus Immunofluorescence Staining of Urinary Decoy Cells

Sahra Pajenda [1], Zsofia Hevesi [2], Michael Eder [1], Daniela Gerges [1,*], Monika Aiad [1], Oliver Koldyka [3], Wolfgang Winnicki [1], Ludwig Wagner [1], Farsad Eskandary [1] and Alice Schmidt [1]

1 Division of Nephrology and Dialysis, Department of Internal Medicine III, Medical University of Vienna, 1090 Vienna, Austria; sahra.pajenda@meduniwien.ac.at (S.P.); michael.eder@meduniwien.ac.at (M.E.); monika.aiad@students.boku.ac.at (M.A.); farsad.eskandary@meduniwien.ac.at (F.E.); alice.schmidt@meduniwien.ac.at (A.S.)

2 Center for Brain Research, Medical University of Vienna, 1090 Vienna, Austria; szofia.hevesi@meduniwien.ac.at

3 Division of Endocrinology and Metabolism, Department of Internal Medicine III, Medical University of Vienna, 1090 Vienna, Austria; oliver.koldyka@meduniwien.ac.at

* Correspondence: daniela.gerges@meduniwien.ac.at

Abstract: Decoy cells that can be detected in the urine sediment of immunosuppressed patients are often caused by the uncontrolled replication of polyomaviruses, such as BK-Virus (BKV) and John Cunningham (JC)-Virus (JCV), within the upper urinary tract. Due to the wide availability of highly sensitive BKV and JCV PCR, the diagnostic utility of screening for decoy cells in urine as an indicator of polyomavirus-associated nephropathy (PyVAN) has been questioned by some institutions. We hypothesize that specific staining of different infection time-dependent BKV-specific antigens in urine sediment could allow cell-specific mapping of antigen expression during decoy cell development. Urine sediment cells from six kidney transplant recipients (five males, one female) were stained for the presence of the early BKV gene transcript lTag and the major viral capsid protein VP1 using monospecific antibodies, monoclonal antibodies and confocal microscopy. For this purpose, cyto-preparations were prepared and the BK polyoma genotype was determined by sequencing the PCR-amplified coding region of the VP1 protein. lTag staining began at specific sites in the nucleus and spread across the nucleus in a cobweb-like pattern as the size of the nucleus increased. It spread into the cytosol as soon as the nuclear membrane was fragmented or dissolved, as in apoptosis or in the metaphase of the cell cycle. In comparison, we observed that VP1 staining started in the nuclear region and accumulated at the nuclear edge in 6–32% of VP1$^+$ cells. The staining traveled through the cytosol of the proximal tubule cell and reached high intensities at the cytosol before spreading to the surrounding area in the form of exosome-like particles. The spreading virus-containing particles adhered to surrounding cells, including erythrocytes. VP1-positive proximal tubule cells contain apoptotic bodies, with 68–94% of them losing parts of their DNA and exhibiting membrane damage, appearing as "ghost cells" but still VP1$^+$. Specific polyoma staining of urine sediment cells can help determine and enumerate exfoliation of BKV-positive cells based on VP1 staining, which exceeds single-face decoy staining in terms of accuracy. Furthermore, our staining approaches might serve as an early readout in primary diagnostics and for the evaluation of treatment responses in the setting of reduced immunosuppression.

Keywords: BK-polyomavirus; decoy cell; polyoma nephropathy; large T antigen; VP1

check for updates

Citation: Pajenda, S.; Hevesi, Z.; Eder, M.; Gerges, D.; Aiad, M.; Koldyka, O.; Winnicki, W.; Wagner, L.; Eskandary, F.; Schmidt, A. Lessons from Polyomavirus Immunofluorescence Staining of Urinary Decoy Cells. *Life* **2023**, *13*, 1526. https://doi.org/10.3390/life13071526

Academic Editor: Won Kim

Received: 22 May 2023
Revised: 28 June 2023
Accepted: 6 July 2023
Published: 7 July 2023

1. Introduction

Among kidney transplant recipients under immunosuppressive therapy, uncontrolled reactivation or primary infection with the human polyomaviruses 1 (BK-Virus, BKV) and less often 2 (John Cunningham, JC-Virus, JCV) can turn into a common complication that is mostly observed within the early phase after transplantation [1]. Patients may develop increasing viremia that can result—if not timely reversed by lowering immunosuppression—into functional decline of the kidney transplant and ultimately lead to polyomavirus-associated nephropathy (PyVAN), with a substantial degree of advanced early graft loss [2]. The routine screening for BKV/JCV via PCR in blood is currently thought to represent the gold standard and has become a mainstay of post-transplant surveillance in most centers [3]. To date, the primary response to a sustained increase in viral replication is the concerted reduction of immunosuppression that, in the majority of cases, will lead to resolving viremia. In refractory cases, as some small interventional studies have shown, the administration of foscarnet, cidofovir, leflunomide and/or intravenous immunoglobulins (IVIG) can be used, although the overall level of evidence for these approaches is quite low [4]. Experimental approaches such as adaptive virus-specific T-cell therapy exist; however, no other therapeutic solutions are yet known in routine clinical practice [5].

Polyomavirus transmission occurs via the fecal-oral route in childhood, but normally healthy individuals show no symptoms during BKV/JCV primary infection. Overall, 83 to 90% of adults in Europe show a robust humoral immune response against these polyomaviruses as a sign of prior exposition to this pathogen [6]. However, in a low percentage of healthy individuals (0–6%), intermittent viruria without viremia can be observed, which has not been shown to be associated with any pathologic process [7,8]. On the contrary, immunocompromised patients are more likely to show symptomatic infection and viremia. Thereby, kidney transplant recipients tend to develop BK-viremia and less often JC-viremia, although rare cases of JCPyVAN have been described, which are thought to follow a more latent disease course compared to BKPyVAN [7,9]. In those patients, BK/JC-viremia typically follows an antecedental constant rise of viruria. The test for polyomavirus copy number in plasma therefore has a high sensitivity for identifying patients at risk of developing PyVAN [10–12].

BK virus-transformed decoy cells appear in urine, which can be identified via cytology and quantified as a percentage of total urine cells [4,13]. These so-called decoy cells in urine can serve as a specific surrogate for BKV/JC viremia and PyVAN, but show an overall low sensitivity in panoptic staining, which increases moderately with the amount of decoy cells in urine. However, infected cells identified by double immunostaining allow a more specific diagnosis of BKPyVAN [14]. In this case, decoy cells are former renal epithelial cells that have been infected and have undergone a process that has allowed BKV/JCV to replicate, and thus the cell moves from the resting phase to the S phase of the cell cycle. This is achieved by inhibiting the retinoblastoma tumor suppressor via binding to the large tumor antigen (lTag) and the associated effects on host-cell DNA and virus genome replication [15–17] by using the host's replisome [18]. As a result, the nucleus develops a disproportionate nuclear/cytoplasmic ratio during the transition from the G_0 to the S phase of the cell cycle, which has also been incorporated into the current pathologic hallmarks of cytopathic changes often seen in kidney transplant biopsies with PyVAN [19–21]. Further morphological changes are nuclear inclusions and shiny staining [22]. The major site of BK replication is the proximal tubule epithelial cell, but as shown by in vitro experiments, BK infection can cause marked changes in gene transcript and protein expression by two days after infection [23]. This affects proteins involved in energy metabolism, detoxification, tumor necrosis factor signaling and protein translation. However, it has also been shown that infection can occur in uroepithelial cells further distal from the renal tubular cells, such as the urinary bladder [14,22].

The double-stranded 5000 bp genome of the BKV or JCV encodes early transcribed genes, such as the lTag, and late-transcribed genes, of which VP1 is the major capsid protein that forms the outer layer of the viral capsid [24,25]. The lTag protein is translated in the nucleus shortly after infection of the cell and forms hexameric structures that bind to the viral genome ORI with their origin-binding domain [26,27], initiating replication of the BK- or JC viral genome. Transcription of the VP1 gene is initiated later, and virus particle formation may be initiated soon thereafter.

We hypothesized that staining various time-dependent polyomavirus-specific proteins in the urine sediment of patients with known viremia and assessing their localization in cellular compartments during different phases of the cell cycle could enable us to identify a tool to assist clinicians in making treatment decisions, such as reduction of immunosuppression or as yet unknown antiviral treatments. In this pilot project, we focused on lTag as the most important member of the early transcriptional part of the BKV genome, and especially on the VP1 protein as the most important part of the late transcriptional part. VP1 staining was used to follow virus particle synthesis and its passage through the cell and its environment. We evaluated the expression and distribution pattern of lTag and VP1 by immunostaining and confocal microscopy in urine sediment cells of patients with PyVAN.

2. Patients and Methods

2.1. Patients

Five male and one female kidney transplant patients aged 51–61 years, diagnosed with BK viremia, had undergone allograft biopsy because of an acute increase of sCr combined with BK viremia and urinary decoy cells.

Morning urine sediment was obtained and separated into two portions. One part was used for cytopreparations as described below. The other part was lysed in TRIzol and frozen at −20 °C for further analysis.

2.2. Virus Genotype Definition

The total RNA was isolated by phase separation by adding 200 µL chloroform to the TRIzol lysate and spinning at 12,000× *g* for 10 min. The aqueous phase was taken off and mixed with 650 µL of isopropanol, out of which the RNA was precipitated by pelleting at 12,000× *g* for 10 min. Following a wash with 75% ethanol, the semidry RNA pellet was redissolved in nuclease-free water and used for cDNA transcription. In brief, 800 ng of total RNA was mixed with random primers in a volume of 12 µL and heated for 3 min at 65 °C, followed by chilling in ice water. The dNTP, reaction buffer, Ribolock and RNA Aid were then added and 5 min annealing at 25 °C was followed by cDNA synthesis at 42 °C for 60 min. The process was stopped by heating the sample at 80 °C for 10 min.

As primers for the VP1 PCR reaction, the forward primer ATGGCCCCAACCAAAAG and reverse primer TTAAAGCATTTTGGTTGCAATTG were used. The cycling conditions were initially 5 min denaturing at 94 °C followed by 30 cycles at 94 °C for 30 s denaturing, 55 °C for annealing and 68 °C for 60 s for synthesis. The resultant PCR product was then submitted for Sanger sequencing.

2.3. Cytopreparations

Morning urine was collected in a sterile container and aliquots of 7 mL were centrifuged at 2000× *g* for 10 min. The supernatant was discarded and the cell pellet was resuspended in 1 mL of culture medium (RPMI supplemented with 10% calf serum). Next, 70 µL of the resulting cell suspension was added to the funnel of the cytocentrifuge and spun at 1200 rpm for 3 min. The cytopreparation was air-dried and subsequently fixed in acetone for 5 min. The slide was then wrapped in aluminum and frozen at −25 °C. For immunostaining, the frozen slides were thawed under air flow, maintaining the aluminum wrapping until ambient temperature was reached to prevent water condensation and protein denaturation.

2.4. Immunofluorescence

After thawing the cytoslides, a hydrophobic circle was drawn around the cell-containing area and 30 µL of PBS was applied to this area to rehydrate the preparation. After rehydration, approximately 60 µL of the antibody solution was applied to the cytopreparation, which was incubated overnight in a humidified chamber at 4 °C on a shaking platform. For detecting the large T-antigen, the affinity purified anti-SV40 large T-antigen-specific antibody (diluted 1:100) PAS 112036 was used (Invitrogen, Waltham, MA, USA), and for staining BK polyoma virus VP1, the monoclonal (diluted 1:30) MAB:33242 clone 4942 (Invitrogen) was used. The next morning, the cytopreparation was washed in PBS with constant agitation of the wash liquid. Then, the secondary antibody solution Alexa-Fluor 488 goat anti rabbit IgG (A11008) or Alexa-Fluor 594 goat anti mouse IgG (H+L) (A11032, Invitrogen) was applied to the labeled areas containing the cells. After 60 min incubation in the moist chamber, the slides were washed in PBS for 10 min with constant stirring. For nuclear DNA staining, a three-minute staining with DAPI was performed before washing. Finally, an embedding solution and a glass coverslip were applied before images were recorded using an Axiovert confocal microscope.

3. Results

We used reverse transcription of RNA from the urine sediment of six BKPyVAN patients (Table 1), and VP1 transcripts from the late coding region of BK polyomavirus were amplified by PCR and sequenced. Thereby, BK virus genotype 1 was identified in all six patients. Confocal microscopy of these urine sediment cells was used to localize the product of the early coding region lTag and the late coding portion VP1. For this purpose, cytopreparations were stained by immunofluorescence.

Table 1. Demographic data of the six kidney transplant patients. ADPKD: autosomal dominant polycystic kidney disease, BK PCR: BK polyomavirus PCR, eGFR: estimated glomerular filtration rate, KTX: kidney transplantation, NP: nephropathy, * 95% granulocytes. BK PCR data are given in copy numbers per ml blood plasma.

	Case 1	Case 2	Case 3	Case 4	Case 5	Case 6
Age	61	58	52	60	51	60
Gender	m	m	m	m	m	f
Underlying disease	ADPKD	ADPKD	Reflux NP	Diabetic NP.	Undefined	Undefined
eGFR (MDRD) mL/min	15	32	12	42	24.51	24.51
BK PCR (Plasma)	5.2×10^4	4.1×10^5	1×10^2	2.3×10^4	4×10^3	3×10^8
Decoy cells in urine (%)	50	20	30	40	90	5 *
Months after KTX	6	2	96	27	4	14

3.1. LTag Distribution

LTag staining was performed on urine sediment when about 20% of urine sediment cells resembled decoy cells. The distribution of lTag took place within the nucleus (Figure 1). It began at specific locations within the nucleus when the nucleus still maintained its normal size (Figures 1 and 2). The distribution spread over the nucleus in a 'spiderweb' fashion (Figure 1). During the phase when nuclear staining was most intense, little staining was found in the cytoplasm (Figures 2 and 3). When the nuclear membrane dissolved in the mitotic cycle (Figures 2 and 3A,C) or was destroyed in apoptosis (Figure 1C, insert), lTag staining distributed into the cytoplasm. This redistribution of the protein was typically observed in the green monkey kidney cell line COS. The nuclear lTag in its variable staining intensity was distributed in a reticular pattern, but was seen in the cytoplasm when the metaphase chromosome plate was formed (Figure 3).

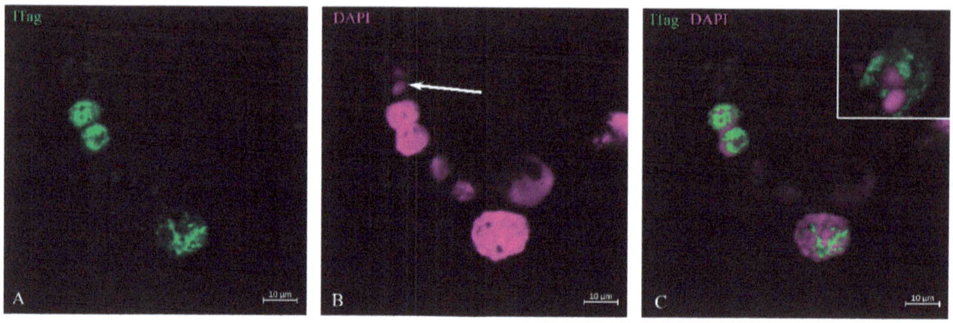

Figure 1. Cytopreparation of urine sediment and lTag immunofluorescence staining. Out of eight tubular epithelial cells, six presented morphological disparities: three presented with disproportionately enlarged nuclei, two with moderately enlarged nuclei and one with apoptotic bodies. Two cells with moderately enlarged nuclei and the decoy cell in the lower part of the figure showed distinct lTag nuclear staining (**A**). In the upper part of the image, the cell shows apoptotic bodies (long-tailed arrow, (**B**)). This part of the image is shown as an insert at higher magnification in (**C**). In this cell, the lTag staining has spread from the apoptotic bodies into the cytosol. Cells with normal-sized nuclei are weakly lTag-positive at specific sites of the nucleus (**C**).

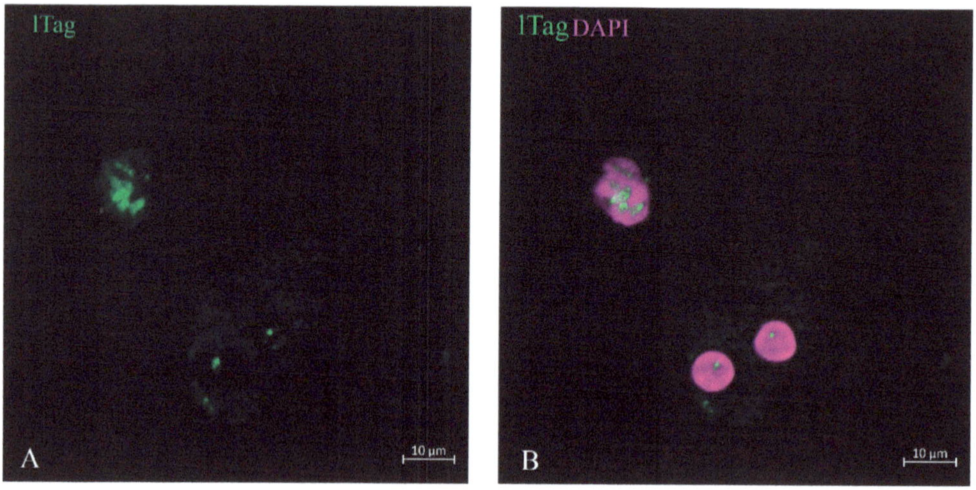

Figure 2. Ltag-positive tubular cells at different stages of the cell cycle. The cell in late telophase, or representing an endocycling cell with absence of cell division but with already separated nuclei, still had cytosolic staining and incipient nuclear spot staining at a specific location (**A**). The cell in the upper part showed nuclear spiderweb-like staining, but its nuclear chromatin did not show a clear border and shaded out into the cytosol (**B**).

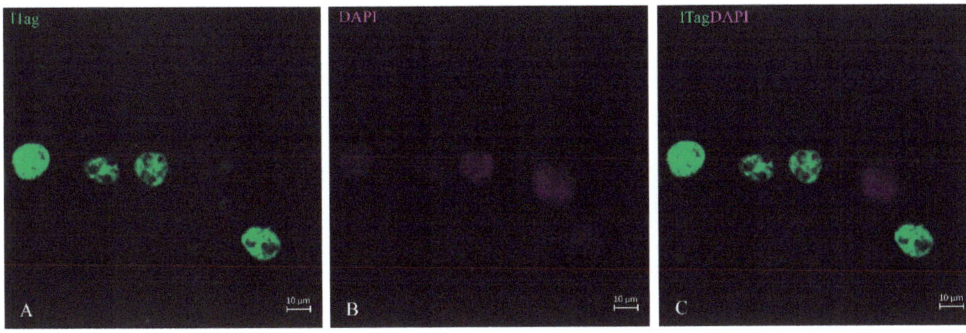

Figure 3. Green monkey kidney cell line ltag staining. Cos cells, known to be positive for the SV40 lTag, showed the typical strict nuclear staining pattern in variable intensity, but this staining spread into the cytosol (**A**,**C**) when the nuclear membrane was dissolved, such as at the metaphase stage of the cell cycle shown by DAPI stain (**B**).

3.2. *VP1 Translation and Distribution*

After lTag transcription and translation was deployed, further steps represent the production of virus capsid proteins. The outer layer of the capsid is the VP1, which is supplemented by VP2 and VP3 in the inner compartment of the virion. Its transcription and translation is achieved by host-cell enzymes in a strictly concerted mode. As already demonstrated, in the case of viruses, this can happen within the nucleus of the host cell [28], or the proteins are shuttled back into the nucleus from the cytosol due to the nuclear localization signal. We were able to show that in decoy cells of human BKPyVAN patients, the VP1 staining in cells with intact morphology could be restricted to the nucleus and its outer rim where it is concentrated (Figure 4A,C). As shown in the cell (Figure 4), the outer rim of the nucleus underwent some sort of demarcation and it was not entirely clear whether the virus particles had already passed the nuclear membrane. About 16–20% of VP1-positive cells were found at this stage of virus infection depending on the patient and specimen (Table 2). In contrast to these cells were decoy cells with a disintegrated nucleus and reduced DNA staining by DAPI, such as in Figure 5, or in an apoptotic nucleus (Figures 6 and 7), where VP1 staining was distributed all over the cytoplasm (Figure 5) and seemed to represent a late stage of infection. In general, these cells were characterized by much stronger VP1 staining and represented the dominant version of the positive cells (80–84%, see Table 2). The staining intensity and thereby virus particle content showed remarkably different extent and differed from cell to cell. On rare occasions, these cells even appeared in clusters (Figure 7) and were positive for AQP1 as a marker of proximal tubular origin. In most of them, the cytoplasmic membrane appeared to be destroyed or had lesions.

Table 2. Percentage of VP1 staining cells at different stage of virus production. Faint nuclear staining with intact morphology was much less frequent than cells with nuclear fragmentation and membrane damage resembling ghost cells.

	Start of Virus Production at Nucleus (%)	Ghost Cells Membrane Damage (%)
Case 1	6	94
Case 2	18	82
Case 3	20	80
Case 4	16	84
Case 5	21	79
Case 6	32	68

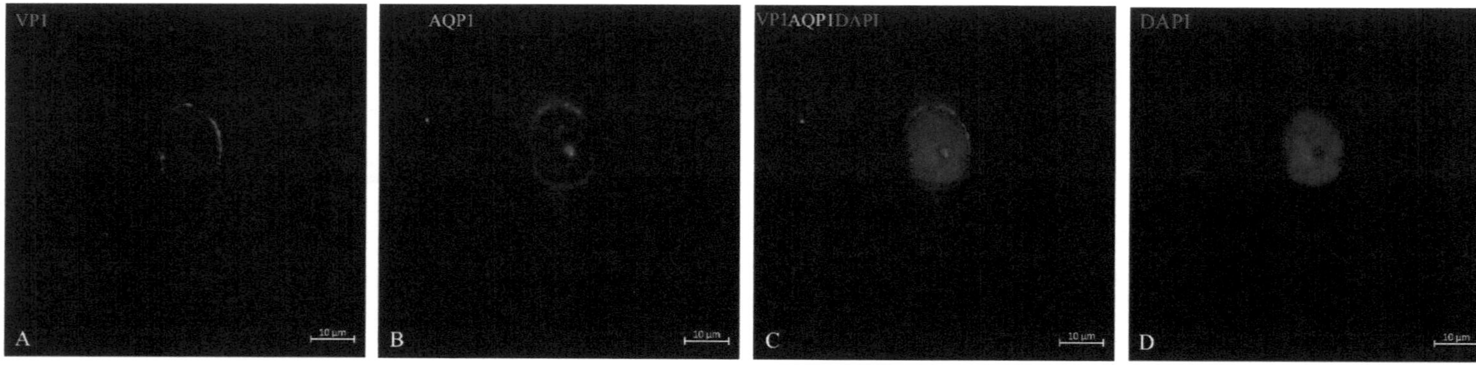

Figure 4. Encapsulation and production of the virus in the nucleus based on VP1 staining. Proximal tubule epithelial cell showed weak, homogeneous VP1 staining throughout the nuclear region, but with higher intensity at the nuclear margin (**A**); the cell was further defined by AQP1 staining (**B**). It is not clear whether the virus had passed through the nuclear pores or was concentrated in the outer region of the nucleus (**C**). This represented an early stage of infection, which was representative for 16–20% of VP1-positive cells in these patients. This is a representative picture, which was observed in such a status of virus replication from these patients. DAPI staining is shown in (**D**).

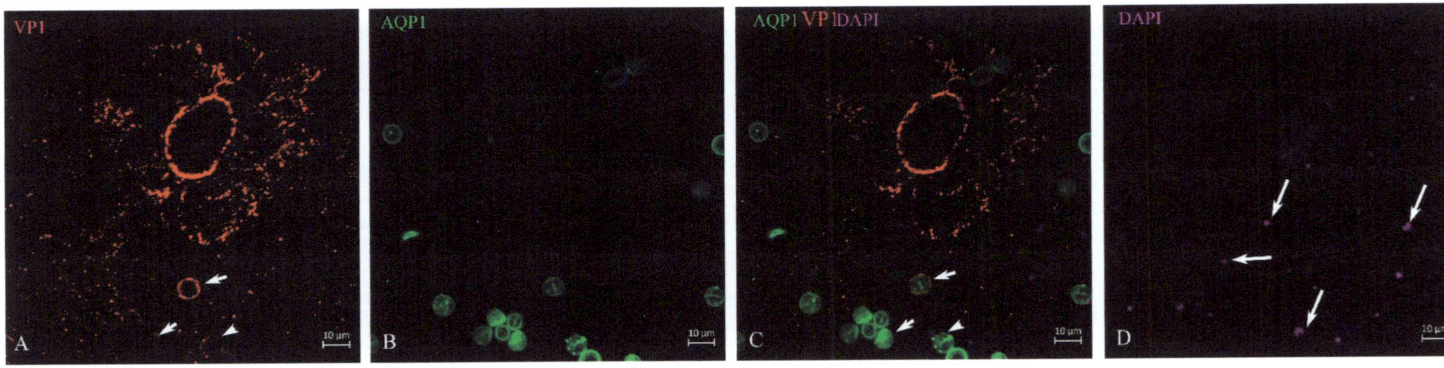

Figure 5. BK virus distribution within the cell and surroundings. Proximal tubular epithelial cell with AQP1 staining (**B**) over the nucleus. VP1 staining at the outer edge of the nucleus was retained, whose cytosol might have partly disintegrated and VP1-positive virus particles were distributed in a web-like fashion in exosome size inside of the cell and the area around it (**A**). This nucleus exhibited reduced DNA staining by DAPI (**D**). Erythrocytes known to be positive for AQP1 (**B**,**C**) were marked by VP1 (short-tailed arrows (**A**)) because of membrane binding of the BK virus. Apoptotic bodies floating around in the urine at the time of decoy cell collection (DAPI long-tailed arrows (**D**).

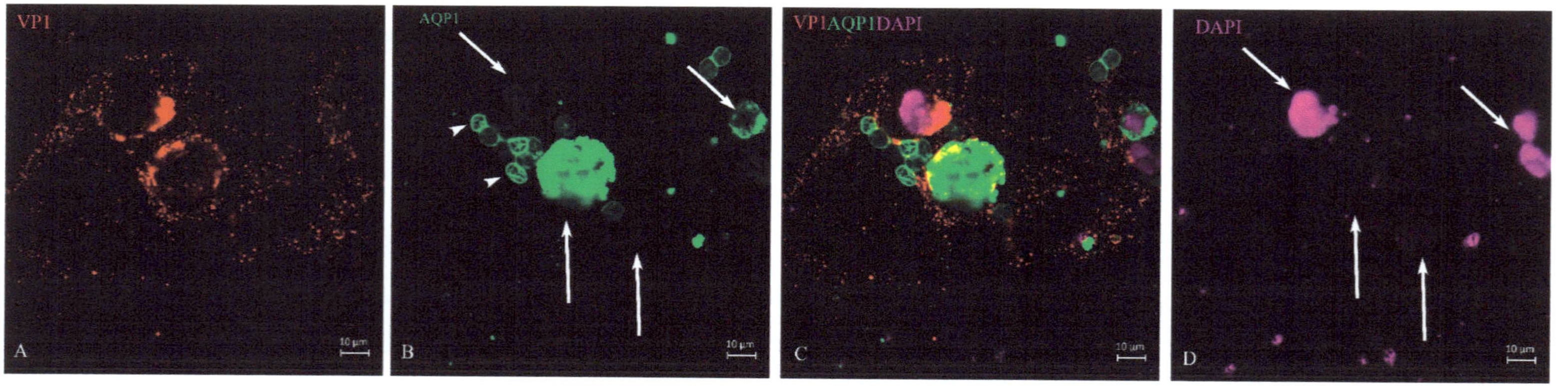

Figure 6. BK virus spreading in the surroundings of ghost cells. Partially disrupted proximal tubule epithelial cells and VP1-positive viral particles spreading around the cells in an exosome-like size (**A**). The ghost cells showed different intensities of AQP1 staining (green, long-tailed arrows (**B**,**C**)) and erythrocytes (short-tailed arrows (**B**)). DNA staining by DAPI (**D**) showed separated apoptotic bodies and the greatly reduced nuclear staining in the ghost cells (long-tailed arrows (**B**,**D**) and the fragmented nucleus in the upper part of the image (**D**).

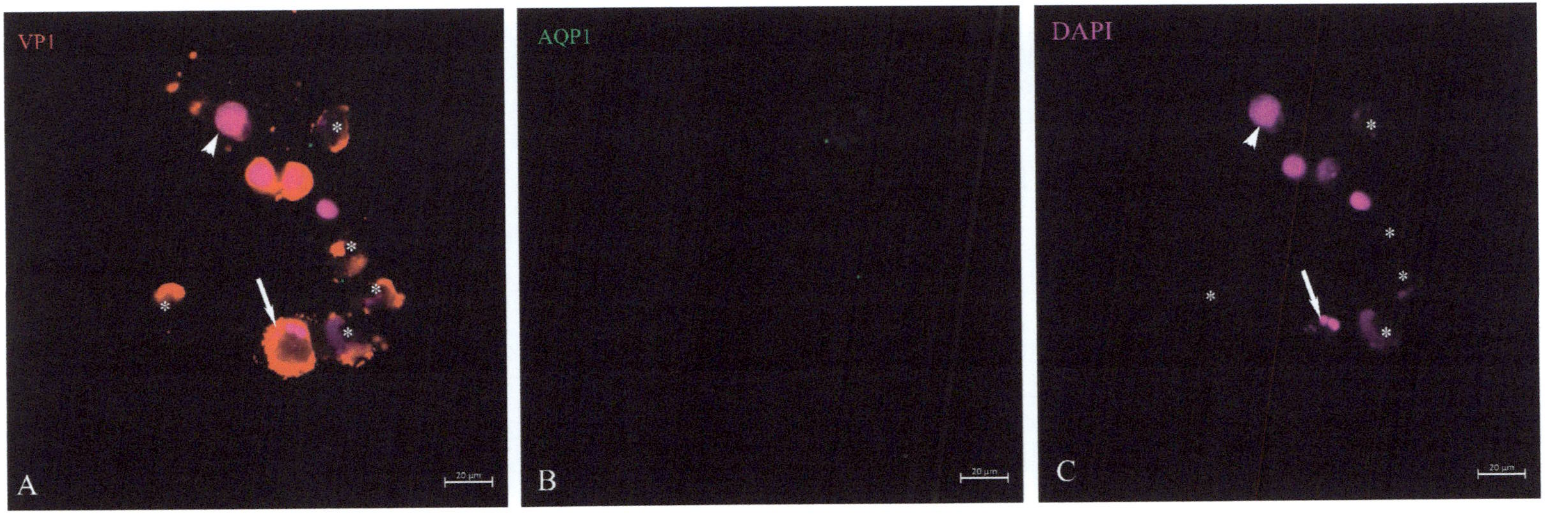

Figure 7. VP1 and AQP1 immunostaining of urine sediment decoy cells in asynchronous stage of infection. A cluster of VP1-positive staining cells (**A**). AQP1 as marker for proximal tubular cells (**B**). Small green particles represent cell fragments (**B**). One of the VP1-positive staining cells (**A**) showed apoptotic bodies indicated by a long-tailed arrow (**C**) and reduced DNA staining of the entire nuclear area. This is a cell in the late stage of infection. The cell with enlarged nucleus (short-tailed arrow (**C**)) in the upper part showed low VP1 stain (**A**) and might therefore be in the early phase of infection and virus replication (**A**). Six ghost cells with reduced nuclear DNA staining (**C**) still showed positive VP1 staining (**A**) and are marked with an asterisk (*).

When the cytoplasmic membrane was ruptured, the virus particles dispersed in the environment, probably encapsulated in exosomes (Figure 6). When also present in urine, we found that some of these exosome-like particles attached to erythrocyte membranes (Figure 5, short-tail arrows) and stained the membrane edge to very different degrees. This is consistent with the fact that in earlier experiments, the erythrocyte agglutination test has been used in human polyomavirus research [29]. The VP1 staining of tubular epithelial cells was highly variable (Figure 7), indicating the asynchronous infection stage of these urinary sediment cells. Some of them could not be identified as decoy cells by simple H/E staining. The disproportionately enlarged nucleus did not go along with high VP1 expression (Figure 7). DAPI staining of the nuclear DNA was frequently reduced and nuclear borders were not clearly demarcated in up to 40% of decoy cells, and apoptotic bodies (arrow in Figure 7) were seen in up to 10% of decoy cells which stained for VP1. Fragments of cells were found all over the cyto-preparation which contained less than 10% VP1 staining (Figure 6).

3.3. *VP1 and lTag-Positive Decoy Cells in Process of Apoptosis*

Apoptosis, programmed cell death, is a specific process that can either be induced by certain types of immune cells, e.g., when the expression of danger signals or microbial/viral proteins on target cells is recognized by them (extrinsic), or under circumstances when distinct intracellular signals shift the overall cellular response towards the apoptosis pathways (intrinsic). In the case of polyomavirus-infected renal epithelial cells, they will often become targets of specific cytolytic T cells and NK cells upon recognition by an adequate immune response [30–32]. The number of late-stage apoptotic cells with highly condensed chromatin and nuclear DNA distributed in apoptotic bodies varies from day to day. However, it must be assumed that these cells received the hit while intact and subsequently exfoliated from the basement membrane and shed. Such cells are still positive for lTag, but apoptotic bodies are negative; rather, the protein is distributed throughout the cytosol (Figure 1C insert). As expected, these apoptotic cells were positive for VP1 to varying degrees (Figures 6 and 7). In addition, apoptotic bodies floated in the urine (Figure 6), which entered the urine sediment through centrifugation conditions, as indicated in the Methods section, but these were negative for VP1 staining. Such a scenario was caused by VP1-positive cell ghosts that have spread their entire nucleus except for a minimal DNA residue, and from which VP1-positive small microsomes were released (Figure 6). Such mode of virus release was observed in all six patients, but the percentage of decoy cells with such virus-spreading conditions was not more than 3–4%.

4. Discussion

In this work, we focused on urinary sediment cell morphology and its relationship to early gene expression in terms of lTag, and the late gene product VP1 as an indicator for BK polyomavirus production and particle formation. This question was investigated by using lTag and virus capsid specific antibodies and observing the lTag protein distribution and the VP1 protein that forms the outer layer of the virion by confocal microscopy.

Firstly, we focused on the lTag as the early transcribed gene of the polyoma virus, incorporating a nuclear localization sequence similar to that of the SV40 virus [33], and therefore detected within the nucleus starting shortly after nuclear separation in the telophase. It spread in a 'spider web' fashion all over the nucleus in resting cells at specific stages of infection. We could show that it was redistributed into the cytosol when the nuclear membrane was dissolved, such as in the cell cycle, or destroyed, as in apoptosis. Whether lTag staining in apoptotic or mitotic cells detected the intact lTag protein or only a fragmented form or a specific splice variant [34] must be left open for this method.

In a second step, regarding gene translation from the late coding region [24] and virion assembly, it was clearly demonstrated, confirming the work of previous authors [35], that virus production is initiated and accomplished mainly in the nucleus. Subsequently, the virus particles spread through the cytosol and were distributed in the environment in exosome-sized vesicles. Earlier work has associated the promyelocytic leukemia nuclear bodies with JCV production sites and have termed these "virus factories" [36]. This morphology of viral spread, as shown by this work, has not yet been demonstrated, but previous authors have suggested that the BK polyoma virus hides in extracellular vesicles [37], so-called exosomes, to evade immune defense. This could help explain why the virus can still spread even when patients are positive for BK antibodies. Embedding of JC polyomavirus in extracellular vesicles has been shown by earlier authors [38], and our morphologic work supports this theory.

The third important observation of this work is that erythrocyte membranes are susceptible to BK virus binding, which could serve as a vehicle for transport of virions, which then leads to randomly distributed foci of BKPyVAN in kidney transplant recipients. If this erythrocyte binding is also true for the JC virus, this could help explain the transmission of virions from the kidney to the brain.

Previous authors have used dual immunocytochemistry to identify the origin of decoy cells and whether they originate from the ureterorenal region or urinary bladder [14]. We used AQP1 as a marker for proximal tubular cells [39,40].

Testing urine sediment for decoy cells has, without debate, gained importance, and various methods, such as Sternberg–Malbin staining, have improved availability and show excellent discriminative potential from other cells of the urinary tract [41,42]. Combined confocal immunostaining for proteins specific to the early and late stages of infection will extend the specificity for counting polyomavirus-infected cells beyond simple decoy staining. Various stages of apoptotic cells and ghost cells can be detected as virus carriers. These would be overlooked in panoptic decoy cell staining. However, it must remain open whether the extremely high viral replication in them, where the virus completely takes over the transcription and translation machinery, has led to intrinsic apoptosis. Nevertheless, extrinsic apoptosis caused by cytolytic immune cells remains another option. In particular, this could occur after modification of immunosuppression.

According to our data, the combination of a high number of decoy cells, especially when identified by immunostaining with BK-virus-specific antibodies, in conjunction with the BK virus copy number in the plasma, seems to be a strong indication of an ongoing infection of the allograft with BK virus. This is true, especially when the copy number reaches 10,000 copies per mL [43]. It is not yet decided whether this can replace the allograft biopsy and serve as a liquid biopsy in the future. Because the BK virus infection sites in the allograft are unevenly and patchily distributed, BK immunostaining in fine-needle biopsies can miss the infection in up to 10–30% of cases [10].

Another important question is whether the timing of a biopsy and decision-making is significantly facilitated by these two non-invasive testing methods. This question cannot be answered clearly in this study. However, follow-up of patients with proven BKPyVAN undergoing modified immunosuppression shows a decreasing number of decoy cells in the urine and, with some delay, a decrease in viral copies in the plasma. Consequently, the two methods combined, plasma copy numbers and immunostained decoy cells in urine, should be able to assess the status of viral replication in the allograft. However, we noted decoy cells in low percentages (1–4%) for several months while allograft function was stable. The cells in which the BK virus replicates could also originate from a site distal to the nephron. But still, this is important as the virus exhibits oncogenic potential and BK-positive urothelial carcinomas are frequent among transplant patients [44], or an already ongoing BK-virus-induced malignant process might be the origin of exfoliation [31].

This work stresses that monitoring decoy cells by urine cytology and virus-specific immunostaining is important information for the care of kidney transplant patients. Routine hematoxylin/eosin examination of decoy cells misses some of the infected cells, especially when large amounts of inflammatory cells are present, which is observed in about 20% of kidney transplant patients for various reasons, e.g., concurrent asymptomatic urinary tract infections.

5. Limitations of This Work

Immunostaining with mAbs is complicated by the specificity of the antibodies, which may result in missing BK mutants with rare genotypes. In addition, the virus replication rate in the cells must reach a certain level for the staining intensity to reach the detection limit. Although the antibody used works excellently in patients positive for the BK polyomavirus genotype 1, it is not clear whether this will be the case in other genotypes.

6. Conclusions

Diagnostics need to become more specific, as much more has been learned in recent years about the twelve characterized members of the human polyomavirus and the specific association with human disease. Therefore, immunostaining of decoy cells in the urine sediment for routine diagnostics needs to be further explored and improved. This might become of significant value for clinical application.

Author Contributions: S.P., Z.H., D.G., M.E., W.W., A.S., F.E. and L.W. designed experiments; Z.H., S.P., M.E., O.K., M.A., F.E. and L.W. performed experiments and analyzed data; A.S., D.G. and F.E. procured funding; and D.G., W.W., F.E. and L.W. wrote the manuscript. All authors have read and agreed to the published version of the manuscript.

Funding: This research was funded by the Medical Scientific Fund of the Mayor of the City of Vienna, grant numbers 22100 and 22099.

Institutional Review Board Statement: This study was approved by the Ethics committee of the Medical University of Vienna (EK 1065/2021).

Informed Consent Statement: Written informed consent was obtained from all study participants.

Data Availability Statement: All data ae provided within this publication.

Conflicts of Interest: The authors declare no conflict of interest.

References

1. Hariharan, S.; Israni, A.K.; Danovitch, G. Long-Term Survival after Kidney Transplantation. *N. Engl. J. Med.* **2021**, *385*, 729–743. [CrossRef] [PubMed]
2. Mohamed, M.; Parajuli, S.; Muth, B.; Astor, B.C.; Panzer, S.E.; Mandelbrot, D.; Zhong, W.; Djamali, A. In kidney transplant recipients with BK polyomavirus infection, early BK nephropathy, microvascular inflammation, and serum creatinine are risk factors for graft loss. *Transpl. Infect. Dis.* **2016**, *18*, 361–371. [CrossRef]
3. Nickeleit, V.; Singh, H.K.; Dadhania, D.; Cornea, V.; El-Husseini, A.; Castellanos, A.; Davis, V.G.; Waid, T.; Seshan, S.V. The 2018 Banff Working Group classification of definitive polyomavirus nephropathy: A multicenter validation study in the modern era. *Am. J. Transplant.* **2021**, *21*, 669–680. [CrossRef] [PubMed]
4. Hirsch, H.H.; Randhawa, P.S.; AST Infectious Diseases Community of Practice. BK polyomavirus in solid organ transplantation—Guidelines from the American Society of Transplantation Infectious Diseases Community of Practice. *Clin. Transplant.* **2019**, *33*, e13528. [CrossRef] [PubMed]
5. Nelson, A.S.; Heyenbruch, D.; Rubinstein, J.D.; Sabulski, A.; Jodele, S.; Thomas, S.; Lutzko, C.; Zhu, X.; Leemhuis, T.; Cancelas, J.A.; et al. Virus-specific T-cell therapy to treat BK polyomavirus infection in bone marrow and solid organ transplant recipients. *Blood Adv.* **2020**, *4*, 5745–5754. [CrossRef]
6. Egli, A.; Infanti, L.; Dumoulin, A.; Buser, A.; Samaridis, J.; Stebler, C.; Gosert, R.; Hirsch, H.H. Prevalence of polyomavirus BK and JC infection and replication in 400 healthy blood donors. *J. Infect. Dis.* **2009**, *199*, 837–846. [CrossRef]
7. Drachenberg, C.B.; Hirsch, H.H.; Papadimitriou, J.C.; Gosert, R.; Wali, R.K.; Munivenkatappa, R.; Nogueira, J.; Cangro, C.B.; Haririan, A.; Mendley, S.; et al. Polyomavirus BK versus JC replication and nephropathy in renal transplant recipients: A prospective evaluation. *Transplantation* **2007**, *84*, 323–330. [CrossRef]
8. Coleman, D.V.; Wolfendale, M.R.; Daniel, R.A.; Dhanjal, N.K.; Gardner, S.D.; Gibson, P.E.; Field, A.M. A prospective study of human polyomavirus infection in pregnancy. *J. Infect. Dis.* **1980**, *142*, 1–8. [CrossRef]
9. Wiegley, N.; Walavalkar, V.; Aujla, H.; Chen, L.X.; Huang, Y.; Lee, B.K.; Jen, K.Y. Clinicopathologic Characteristics of JC Virus Nephropathy in Kidney Transplant Recipients. *Transplantation* **2021**, *105*, 1069–1076. [CrossRef]
10. Hirsch, H.H.; Vincenti, F.; Friman, S.; Tuncer, M.; Citterio, F.; Wiecek, A.; Scheuermann, E.H.; Klinger, M.; Russ, G.; Pescovitz, M.D.; et al. Polyomavirus BK replication in de novo kidney transplant patients receiving tacrolimus or cyclosporine: A prospective, randomized, multicenter study. *Am. J. Transplant.* **2013**, *13*, 136–145. [CrossRef]

11. Schaub, S.; Hirsch, H.H.; Dickenmann, M.; Steiger, J.; Mihatsch, M.J.; Hopfer, H.; Mayr, M. Reducing immunosuppression preserves allograft function in presumptive and definitive polyomavirus-associated nephropathy. *Am. J. Transplant.* **2010**, *10*, 2615–2623. [CrossRef] [PubMed]
12. Petrov, R.; Elbahloul, O.; Gallichio, M.H.; Stellrecht, K.; Conti, D.J. Monthly screening for polyoma virus eliminates BK nephropathy and preserves renal function. *Surg. Infect.* **2009**, *10*, 85–90. [CrossRef]
13. Hirsch, H.H.; Knowles, W.; Dickenmann, M.; Passweg, J.; Klimkait, T.; Mihatsch, M.J.; Steiger, J. Prospective study of polyomavirus type BK replication and nephropathy in renal-transplant recipients. *N. Engl. J. Med.* **2002**, *347*, 488–496. [CrossRef] [PubMed]
14. Chen, X.-T.; Chen, W.-F.; Hou, X.-T.; Yang, S.-C.; Yang, H.-F.; Li, J.; Deng, R.-H.; Huang, Y.; Nuertai, Y.; Wang, C.-X.; et al. Non-invasive urinary sediment double-immunostaining predicts BK polyomavirus associated-nephropathy in kidney transplant recipients. *Ann. Transl. Med.* **2020**, *8*, 235. [CrossRef] [PubMed]
15. Kim, H.Y.; Ahn, B.Y.; Cho, Y. Structural basis for the inactivation of retinoblastoma tumor suppressor by SV40 large T antigen. *Embo J.* **2001**, *20*, 295–304. [CrossRef]
16. DeCaprio, J.A.; Garcea, R.L. A cornucopia of human polyomaviruses. *Nat. Rev. Microbiol.* **2013**, *11*, 264–276. [CrossRef]
17. Harris, K.F.; Christensen, J.B.; Imperiale, M.J. BK virus large T antigen: Interactions with the retinoblastoma family of tumor suppressor proteins and effects on cellular growth control. *J. Virol.* **1996**, *70*, 2378–2386. [CrossRef]
18. Sowd, G.A.; Fanning, E. A wolf in sheep's clothing: SV40 co-opts host genome maintenance proteins to replicate viral DNA. *PLoS Pathog.* **2012**, *8*, e1002994. [CrossRef]
19. Gai, M.; Lanfranco, G.; Segoloni, G.P. "Decoy cells" in urine. *Transplant. Proc.* **2005**, *37*, 4309–4310. [CrossRef]
20. Maia, T.M.; Silva, S.F.; Silva, S.L.; Holanda, M.C.; Nascimento, J.M.; Ferreira, M.V. Polyomavirus-infected decoy cells in cytocentrifuged urine cytology specimens from renal transplant recipients. *Acta Cytol.* **2011**, *55*, 445–448. [CrossRef]
21. Drachenberg, C.B.; Beskow, C.O.; Cangro, C.B.; Bourquin, P.M.; Simsir, A.; Fink, J.; Weir, M.R.; Klassen, D.K.; Bartlett, S.T.; Papadimitriou, J.C. Human polyoma virus in renal allograft biopsies: Morphological findings and correlation with urine cytology. *Hum. Pathol.* **1999**, *30*, 970–977. [CrossRef]
22. Nickeleit, V.; Hirsch, H.H.; Binet, I.F.; Gudat, F.; Prince, O.; Dalquen, P.; Thiel, G.; Mihatsch, M.J. Polyomavirus infection of renal allograft recipients: From latent infection to manifest disease. *J. Am. Soc. Nephrol.* **1999**, *10*, 1080–1089. [CrossRef]
23. An, P.; Cantalupo, P.G.; Zheng, W.; Saenz-Robles, M.T.; Duray, A.M.; Weitz, D.; Pipas, J.M. Single-Cell Transcriptomics Reveals a Heterogeneous Cellular Response to BK Virus Infection. *J. Virol.* **2021**, *95*, 10–1128. [CrossRef]
24. White, M.K.; Safak, M.; Khalili, K. Regulation of gene expression in primate polyomaviruses. *J. Virol.* **2009**, *83*, 10846–10856. [CrossRef]
25. Hurdiss, D.L.; Morgan, E.L.; Thompson, R.F.; Prescott, E.L.; Panou, M.M.; Macdonald, A.; Ranson, N.A. New Structural Insights into the Genome and Minor Capsid Proteins of BK Polyomavirus using Cryo-Electron Microscopy. *Structure* **2016**, *24*, 528–536. [CrossRef] [PubMed]
26. Meinke, G.; Phelan, P.J.; Kalekar, R.; Shin, J.; Archambault, J.; Bohm, A.; Bullock, P.A. Insights into the initiation of JC virus DNA replication derived from the crystal structure of the T-antigen origin binding domain. *PLoS Pathog.* **2014**, *10*, e1003966. [CrossRef] [PubMed]
27. Chang, Y.P.; Xu, M.; Machado, A.C.D.; Yu, X.J.; Rohs, R.; Chen, X.S. Mechanism of Origin DNA Recognition and Assembly of an Initiator-Helicase Complex by SV40 Large Tumor Antigen. *Cell Rep.* **2013**, *3*, 1117–1127. [CrossRef] [PubMed]
28. David, A.; Dolan, B.P.; Hickman, H.D.; Knowlton, J.J.; Clavarino, G.; Pierre, P.; Bennink, J.R.; Yewdell, J.W. Nuclear translation visualized by ribosome-bound nascent chain puromycylation. *J. Cell Biol.* **2012**, *197*, 45–57. [CrossRef]
29. Ou, W.C.; Wang, M.; Fung, C.Y.; Tsai, R.T.; Chao, P.C.; Hseu, T.H.; Chang, D. The major capsid protein, VP1, of human JC virus expressed in Escherichia coli is able to self-assemble into a capsid-like particle and deliver exogenous DNA into human kidney cells. *J. Gen. Virol.* **1999**, *80 Pt 1*, 39–46. [CrossRef]
30. Cioni, M.; Leboeuf, C.; Comoli, P.; Ginevri, F.; Hirsch, H.H. Characterization of Immunodominant BK Polyomavirus 9mer Epitope T Cell Responses. *Am. J. Transplant.* **2016**, *16*, 1193–1206. [CrossRef]
31. Meier, R.P.H.; Muller, Y.D.; Dietrich, P.Y.; Tille, J.C.; Nikolaev, S.; Sartori, A.; Labidi-Galy, I.; Ernandez, T.; Kaur, A.; Hirsch, H.H.; et al. Immunologic Clearance of a BK Virus-associated Metastatic Renal Allograft Carcinoma. *Transplantation* **2021**, *105*, 423–429. [CrossRef] [PubMed]
32. Comoli, P.; Basso, S.; Azzi, A.; Moretta, A.; De Santis, R.; Del Galdo, F.; De Palma, R.; Valente, U.; Nocera, A.; Perfumo, F.; et al. Dendritic Cells Pulsed with Polyomavirus BK Antigen Induce Ex Vivo Polyoma BK Virus–Specific Cytotoxic T-Cell Lines in Seropositive Healthy Individuals and Renal Transplant Recipients. *J. Am. Soc. Nephrol.* **2003**, *14*, 3197–3204. [CrossRef] [PubMed]
33. Lanford, R.E.; Butel, J.S. Construction and characterization of an SV40 mutant defective in nuclear transport of T antigen. *Cell* **1984**, *37*, 801–813. [CrossRef] [PubMed]
34. Abend, J.R.; Joseph, A.E.; Das, D.; Campbell-Cecen, D.B.; Imperiale, M.J. A truncated T antigen expressed from an alternatively spliced BK virus early mRNA. *J. Gen. Virol.* **2009**, *90*, 1238–1245. [CrossRef] [PubMed]
35. Erickson, K.D.; Bouchet-Marquis, C.; Heiser, K.; Szomolanyi-Tsuda, E.; Mishra, R.; Lamothe, B.; Hoenger, A.; Garcea, R.L. Virion Assembly Factories in the Nucleus of Polyomavirus-Infected Cells. *PLoS Pathog.* **2012**, *8*, e1002630. [CrossRef]
36. Maul, G.G.; Negorev, D.; Bell, P.; Ishov, A.M. Review: Properties and assembly mechanisms of ND10, PML bodies, or PODs. *J. Struct. Biol.* **2000**, *129*, 278–287. [CrossRef]

37. Giannecchini, S. Evidence of the Mechanism by Which Polyomaviruses Exploit the Extracellular Vesicle Delivery System during Infection. *Viruses* **2020**, *12*, 585. [CrossRef]
38. Morris-Love, J.; O'Hara, B.A.; Gee, G.V.; Dugan, A.S.; O'Rourke, R.S.; Armstead, B.E.; Assetta, B.; Haley, S.A.; Atwood, W.J. Biogenesis of JC polyomavirus associated extracellular vesicles. *J. Extracell. Biol.* **2022**, *1*, e43. [CrossRef]
39. Gerges, D.; Hevesi, Z.; Schmidt, S.H.; Kapps, S.; Pajenda, S.; Geist, B.; Schmidt, A.; Wagner, L.; Winnicki, W. Tubular epithelial progenitors are excreted in urine during recovery from severe acute kidney injury and are able to expand and differentiate in vitro. *PeerJ* **2022**, *10*, e14110. [CrossRef]
40. Schnermann, J.; Chou, C.L.; Ma, T.; Traynor, T.; Knepper, M.A.; Verkman, A.S. Defective proximal tubular fluid reabsorption in transgenic aquaporin-1 null mice. *Proc. Natl. Acad. Sci. USA* **1998**, *95*, 9660–9664. [CrossRef]
41. Yan, L.; Guo, H.; Han, L.; Huang, H.; Shen, Y.; He, J.; Liu, J. Sternheimer-Malbin Staining to Detect Decoy Cells in Urine of 213 Kidney Transplant Patients. *Transplant. Proc.* **2020**, *52*, 823–828. [CrossRef] [PubMed]
42. Sekito, T.; Araki, M.; Yoshinaga, K.; Maruyama, Y.; Sadahira, T.; Nishimura, S.; Wada, K.; Watanabe, M.; Watanabe, T.; Tanabe, K.; et al. Presence of decoy cells for 6 months on urine cytology efficiently predicts BK virus nephropathy in renal transplant recipients. *Int. J. Urol.* **2021**, *28*, 1240–1246. [CrossRef] [PubMed]
43. Nickeleit, V.; Singh, H.K.; Randhawa, P.; Drachenberg, C.B.; Bhatnagar, R.; Bracamonte, E.; Chang, A.; Chon, W.J.; Dadhania, D.; Davis, V.G.; et al. The Banff Working Group Classification of Definitive Polyomavirus Nephropathy: Morphologic Definitions and Clinical Correlations. *J. Am. Soc. Nephrol.* **2018**, *29*, 680–693. [CrossRef] [PubMed]
44. Müller, D.C.; Rämö, M.; Naegele, K.; Ribi, S.; Wetterauer, C.; Perrina, V.; Quagliata, L.; Vlajnic, T.; Ruiz, C.; Balitzki, B.; et al. Donor-derived, metastatic urothelial cancer after kidney transplantation associated with a potentially oncogenic BK polyomavirus. *J. Pathol.* **2018**, *244*, 265–270. [CrossRef] [PubMed]

life

MDPI

Systematic Review

Critical Overview of Serous Endometrial Intraepithelial Cancer Treatment: Systematic Review of Adjuvant Options

Carlo Ronsini [1], Antonella Reino [1], Rossella Molitierno [1], Maria Giovanna Vastarella [1], Elvira La Mantia [2] and Pasquale De Franciscis [1,*]

1 Department of Woman, Child and General and Specialized Surgery, University of Campania "Luigi Vanvitelli", Largo Madonna Delle Grazie, 1, 80138 Naples, Italy; carlo.ronsini@unicampania.it (C.R.); mariagiovanna.vastarella@studenti.unicampania.it (M.G.V.)
2 Pathology Unit, University of Campania "L. Vanvitelli", Via Luciano Armanni, 80138 Naples, Italy
* Correspondence: pasquale.defranciscis@unicampania.it

Abstract: SEIC is a non-invasive lesion of the endometrial epithelium considered to be the precursor to uterine serous carcinoma (USC) and is just as aggressive as USC. Currently, there are no reliable data about the behavior and prognosis of SEIC; therefore, the therapeutic management approach is not clear. **Method**: A systematic search of the Pubmed, Scopus and Embase databases was conducted, following the recommendations in the Preferred Reporting Items for Systematic Reviews and Meta-Analyses (PRISMA). **Results**: Of the 296 studies that matched the search criteria, only 9 met the inclusion criteria, covering a total of 81 patients. The main disease-presenting pattern was AUB (abnormal uterine bleeding). In 31 cases, SEIC was associated with extrauterine disease. All patients underwent hysterectomy and salpingo-oophorectomy, while only 15 of the 81 patients received adjuvant treatments. In the patients receiving adjuvant therapy, the RR was 42.67%, the DFS was 35.71% and the OS was 57.13%. In patients subjected to follow-up alone, the RR was only 28.78%, the DFS was 59.1% and the OS was 66.6%. **Conclusions**: The presence of an extrauterine disease significantly worsens outcomes, regardless of adjuvant treatment. In cases of disease confined to the uterine mucosa alone, the prognosis is good and follow-up allows a good control of the disease; however, adjuvant therapy could further increase survival rates and reduce relapse rates.

Keywords: serous endometrial intraepithelial carcinoma; SEIC; MUSC; adjuvant therapy; relapse

check for updates

Citation: Ronsini, C.; Reino, A.; Molitierno, R.; Vastarella, M.G.; La Mantia, E.; De Franciscis, P. Critical Overview of Serous Endometrial Intraepithelial Cancer Treatment: Systematic Review of Adjuvant Options. *Life* **2023**, *13*, 1429. https://doi.org/10.3390/life13071429

Academic Editor: Nihar R. Nayak, Stefanos Roumeliotis and Giuseppe Minervini

Received: 31 March 2023
Revised: 22 May 2023
Accepted: 13 June 2023
Published: 22 June 2023

1. Introduction

Serous endometrial intraepithelial carcinoma (SEIC) is also described in the literature as 'minimal uterine serous carcinoma' (MUSC), 'serous endometrial intraepithelial neoplasia', 'endometrial carcinoma in situ', 'non-invasive endometrial serous carcinoma' and 'superficial serous carcinoma'. It represents a non-invasive lesion of the endometrial epithelium [1]. As with invasive serous carcinoma of the uterus (USC), it constitutes an aggressive histological form of type II endometrial cancer. Although previously considered a pre-cursor of USC, recent evidence demonstrates its aggressive behavior and its ability to extensively metastasize extrauterine, despite the absence of myometrial invasion and lymph-vascular involvement [2,3]. Several studies suggest that superficial intraepithelial carcinoma may spread through the tubes or lymphatic vessels within the peritoneal cavity. However, its behavior is currently unpredictable [4]. Although there are no International guidelines, the WHO recommends surgical staging of the disease (hysterectomy, bilateral salpingo-oophorectomy, omentectomy, lymph node removal, or peritoneal dissection and biopsy). The scarcity with which it occurs and the variable prognosis reported in the literature mean that there is no non-ambiguous adjuvant therapy. Data are available in the literature on the use of chemotherapy and on follow-up models [4–6]. The purpose of this review is to investigate the effects of adjuvant treatments on the prognosis of the disease.

2. Materials and Methods

The selected registrations complied with the PRISMA (Preferred Reporting Items for Systematic Reviews and Meta-Analysis) guidelines [7]. We registered this systematic review on the PROSPERO site with protocol number 403507.

2.1. Search Methods

A systematic search of the Pubmed, EMBASE and Scopus databases was carried out in February 2023. Studies were considered if they had been included in published material since their first release. No country restrictions were carried out. The search criteria adopted to identify studies applicable to the subject of the review were: "intraepithelial serum endometrial carcinoma" OR "minimal serous uterine carcinoma" OR "SEIC".

2.2. Studies Selection

Study selection was made independently by AR and RM. In disputed cases, CR decided to include or exclude. The inclusion criteria were: (1) studies including patients with the diagnosis of serous intraepithelial uterine carcinoma; (2) studies including patients who underwent surgical staging; (3) studies reporting at least one outcome of interest (recurrence rate; recurrence type; surgical staging; type of adjuvant treatment; survival report); and (4) peer-reviewed articles, published originally. Nonoriginal studies, preclinical trials, animal trials, abstract-only publications and articles in languages other than English were excluded. Wherever possible, the authors of studies that were only published as congress abstracts were contacted via email and asked to provide their data. The primary outcome of interest was the recurrence of the disease. The studies selected and all reasons for exclusion are given in the Preferred Reporting Items for Systematic Reviews and Meta-Analyses (PRISMA) flowchart (Figure 1). All included studies were assessed regarding potential conflicts of interest.

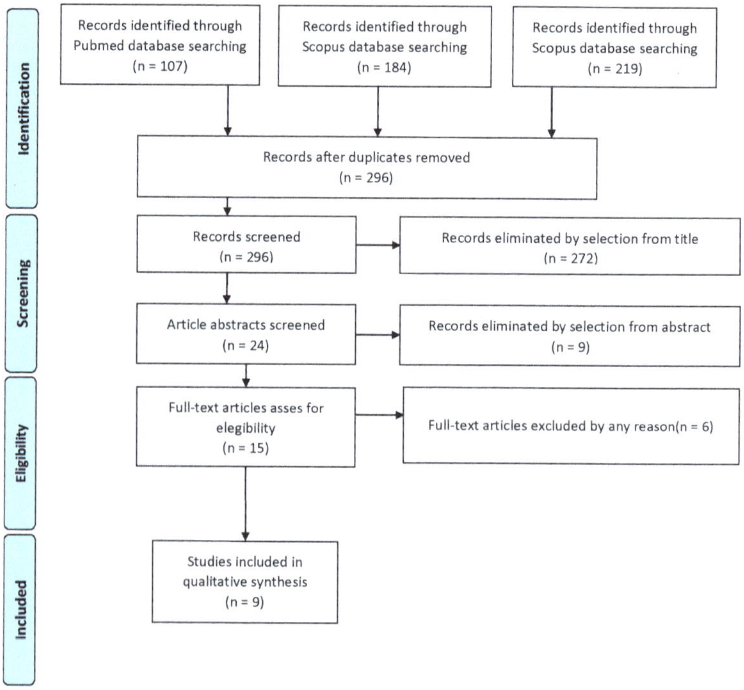

Figure 1. PRISMA Flow-chart.

2.3. Data Extraction

AR and RM extracted data for all relevant series and case reports. We extracted data on tumor characteristics (stage, histological subtype, LVSI status, grading), surgical approach, morbidity and oncological issues such as recurrences, deaths and recurrence rate (RR). We also collected data on adjuvant therapy (Number of cycles, type of drugs). In addition, data on follow-up and survival status reported as "not evident disease (NED", "alive with disease (AWD)", "death of disease (DOD)" and "death of other causes (DOC)" were also extracted. We also evaluated disease-free survival (DFS) as the time in months from the surgery to the recurrence or the last follow-up and overall survival (OS) as the time in months from the diagnosis to the recurrence or the last follow-up.

2.4. Quality Assessment

We assessed the quality of the included studies using the Newcastle–Ottawa scale (NOS) [8]. This assessment scale uses three broad factors (selection, comparability and outcome), with the scores ranging from 0 (lowest quality) to 8 (best quality). Two authors (CR and PDF) independently rated the study's quality. Any disagreement was subsequently resolved by discussion or consultation with AR. We report the NOS Scale scores in Appendix A.

3. Results

3.1. Studies' Characteristics

After the database search, 296 articles matched the search criteria. After removing records with no full text, duplicates and wrong study design (e.g., reviews), 15 were eligible. Of those, nine matched the inclusion criteria and were included in the systematic review. All nine studies were non-comparative, single-armed, or case-report studies evaluating the therapeutic management of SEICs. The countries where the studies were conducted, the publication year range, the study design, the type of surgery and adjuvant therapy, the mean follow-up and the number of participants are summarized in Table 1. Overall, the publication years ranged from 2000 to 2021 while the follow-up period ranged from 9 to 84 months.

3.2. Patients' Characteristics

The clinical characteristics of the patients are summarized in Table 2. A total of 81 patients were analyzed. The mean patient age was 66.24 (range 42–83 y). The main presenting patterns were AUB (41 of 81 patients), a cervical smear positive for endometrial malignant cells (17 of 81 patients) and abdominal distension/discomfort (6 of 81 patients). In one case, an irregular endometrial thickening was found using TV-US. The mode of presentation was unknown in four patients. In 79 of 81 patients, the final diagnosis was SEIC/SSC, in 2 patients, it was grade 1 endometroid adenocarcinoma and in 5 cases, the SEIC was associated with intraepithelial carcinoma or serous carcinoma of the ovary. In these cases, the presence of serous ovarian carcinoma was considered as an extrauterine disease of the SEIC and it was not possible to define whether the origin of the disease was adnexal or uterine. In 31 cases, extrauterine disease, including fallopian-tube, omental, ovarian, peritoneal, bowel and lymph node metastases, focal tubal intraepithelial carcinoma and intraepithelial or serous ovarian cancer was found. All patients underwent total or radical hysterectomy, salpingo-oophorectomy and complete or partial surgical staging. A total of 66 of 81 patients did not receive any adjuvant treatment, while 12 patients underwent adjuvant chemotherapy alone, 2 patients received radiotherapy and chemotherapy and 1 patient underwent whole abdomen and pelvic radiotherapy only. In eight of the nine studies, patients with stage IA disease did not receive adjuvant therapy. In just one case, a 42-year-old patient diagnosed with SEIC stage IA received adjuvant chemotherapy [12].

Table 1. Studies' characteristics.

Name Year	Country	Study Design	N of Participants	Surgery	Adjuvant Therapy	F/UP (months)
Wheeler 2000 [2]	USA	Retrospective cohort-study monocentric	21	H ± BSO± Partial/complete surgical staging	None (12 pt) Platinum-based CHT (8 pt) WAPRT (1 pt)	27
Hui 2005 [9]	USA	Retrospective cohort-study monocentric	40	H + BSO + pelvic lymph node dissection ± omentum sampling	None	25.8
Abushahin 2011 [10]	USA	Case series	5	TAH+BSO± partial/complete surgical staging	None (2 pt) CHT (2 pt) RT+CHT (1 pt)	54
Kawano 2011 [3]	Japan	Case report	1	TAH + BSO+ EILN biopsy	6 cycles CHT (cisplatin + doxorubicin) +RT of left supraclavicolar region	37
Pathiraja 2013 [6]	UK	Case series	5	Complete surgical staging (3 pt), incomplete surgical staging (2pt)	None	16.6
Ono 2014 [11]	Japan	Prospective, cohort-study monocentric	6	RH + BSO + LN (3 pt) TAH + BSO (2 pt) TAH + BSO + OMT (1 pt)	None	36
Kawata 2017 [12]	Japan	Case report	1	TAH + BSO + Partial OMT+ pelvic and paraaortic LN	6 cycles CHT (paclitaxel+doxorubicin+carboplatin)	9
Han 2020 [13]	South Korea	Case report	1	TAH + BSO + Pelvic LN	None	84
Shimizu 2021 [14]	Japan	Case report	1	TAH + BSO + Partial OMT+ pelvic and paraaortic LN	6 cycles CHT (carboplatin, paclitaxel, bevacizumab)	9

BSO: bilateral salpingo-oophorectomy; EILN: external iliac lymph node; H: hysterectomy; LN: lymphadenectomy; OMT: omentectomy; RH: radical hysterectomy; TAH: total abdominal hysterectomy; WAPRT: whole abdomen and pelvic radiotherapy.

Table 2. Clinical characteristics of patients.

Name, Year	Age/ Mean Age	Presentation	Stage	Final Diagnosis	Extrauterine Disease	Follow-Up
Wheeler, 2000 [2]	65 y	PMB (14 pt), cervical smear positive for malignant cells (6 pt), ABD (1 pt)	IA-IVB	SEIC/SSC SEIC + IC-ovary (3 pt)	IC-ovary (3 pt), fallopian tube metastases (1 pt), omentum metastases (2 pt), bowel metastases (1 pt), none (14 pt)	NED (2 pt) AWD (2 pt) DOD (3 pt) DOC (1 pt)
Hui, 2005 [9]	66.5 y	PMB (20 pt), Cervical HPV (1 pt), pap smear positive (7 pt), ABD (8 pt), unknown (4 pt)	IA-IVB	SEIC/SSC	Omentum (14 pt) Ovary (12 pt) Fallopian tube (7 pt) Pelvic peritoneum (7 pt) Abdomen organ surface (6 pt) LN (5 pt)	NED (20 pt) DOD (9 pt) AWD (4 pt) DOC (1 pt)
Abushahin, 2011 [10]	63.4 y	Abdominal discomfort (2 pt), PMB (1 pt), abnormal cervical smear (2 pt)	IA-IIIA	SEIC (4 pt) SEIC + OSC (1 pt)	Focal TIC (1 pt), omental implants (2 pt),	AWD (2 pt) DOD (2 pt) AWOD (1 pt)
Kawano, 2011 [3]	61 y	PMB	IIIC	Grade 1 endometrioid adenocarcinoma	Metastatic lymph node	NED
Pathiraja, 2013 [6]	72 y	PMB	IA	SEIC	None	NED (2 pt) DOD (2 pt) AWD (1 pt)
Ono, 2014 [11]	74.5 y	PMB (3 pt); ABD (1 pt); abnormal cervical smear (1 pt); unknown (1 pt)	IA-IIIB	SEIC (2 pt) SSC (3 pt) SEIC-SSC (1 pt)	Omentum and ovaries micrometastases (1 pt); None (5 pt)	NED (3 pt) DOD (2 pt) AWD (1 pt)

Table 2. *Cont.*

Name, Year	Age/ Mean Age	Presentation	Stage	Final Diagnosis	Extrauterine Disease	Follow-Up
Kawata, 2017 [12]	42 y	AUB	IA	SEIC	None	NED
Han, 2020 [13]	61 y	Irregular endometrial thickening observed by TV-US	IA	Grade 1 endometrioid carcinoma	None	Metastatic recurrence
Shimizu, 2021 [14]	57 y	Abdominal pain	IIIA1 with SEIC	OSC + SEIC	Ovarian cancer, metastatic paraaortic lymph-lode	NED

ABD: abdominal distension; IC: intraepithelial carcinoma; OSC: ovarian serous cancer; PMB: postmenopausal bleeding; SSC: superficial serous carcinoma; TIC: tubal intraepithelial carcinoma; NED: no evidence of disease; AWD: alive with disease; DOD: dead of disease; DOC: dead of other causes; AWOD: alive without disease.

3.3. Outcomes

All nine of the selected studies presented RR, OS, or DFS data. These results are summarized in Tables 3 and 4. In 46 of 81 patients, there was no evidence of disease at the end of follow-up, 12 patients were alive with the disease, 18 patients died from the disease and 2 patients died from other causes. In two studies, 62.5% and 33.3% of patients receiving adjuvant chemotherapy, respectively, relapsed [2,10], while, in three studies, none of the patients relapsed [3,12,14]. Among patients not receiving any adjuvant treatment, only in one study were no relapses reported [13], and the average recurrence rate was 28.78%, ranging from 16.6% to 100%, and the DFS was 59.1%. In the patients receiving adjuvant chemotherapy, the average recurrence rate was 42.67%, ranging from 25% to 100%, and the DFS was 35.71%. In the case report by Han et al. [13], the patient developed multifocal abdominopelvic peritoneal metastases 7 years after surgery, while none of the 12 patients showed signs of disease during the average 33.1 months of follow-up. In the other studies, DFS ranged from 40% to 52.2%. The OS of the patients who underwent adjuvant chemotherapy was 57.13%, while the OS of the follow-up-only group was 66.6%.

Table 3. Oncological Outcome.

Nome	3Y DFS * (%)	3Y OS ° (%)	4.5Y DFS * (%)	4.5Y OS ° (%)
Wheeler 2000 [2]	33.3	42.8	9.5	9.5
Hui 2005 [9]	17.5	17.5	10	10
Abushahin 2011 [10]	20	80	20	40
Kawano 2011 [3]	100	100	-	-
Pathiraja 2013 [6]	-	-	-	-
Ono 2014 [11]	33.3	33.3	-	-
Kawata 2017 [12]	-	-	-	-
Han 2020 [13]	100	100	100	100
Shimizu 2021 [14]	-	-	-	-

* Disease-Free Survival. ° Overall Survival.

Table 4. Recurrence Rate.

	ADJCHT			FUP		
Name	**RR ′ (%)**	**DFS * (%)**	**OS ° (%)**	**RR ′ (%)**	**DFS * (%)**	**OS ° (%)**
Wheeler 2000 [2]	62.5	25	50	0	100	91.6
Hui 2005 [9]	-	-	-	32.5	52.5	62.5
Abushahin 2011 [10]	33.3	0	33.3	50	50	100
Kawano 2011 [3]	0	100	100	-	-	-
Pathiraja 2013 [6]	-	-	-	60	40	60
Ono 2014 [11]	-	-	-	16.6	50	66.6
Kawata 2017 [12]	0	100	100	-	-	-
Han 2020 [13]	-	-	-	100	0	-
Shimizu 2021 [14]	0	100	100	-	-	-

′ Recurrence Rate * Disease-Free Survival ° Overall Survival.

4. Discussion

The scarcity of data in the literature demonstrates that SEIC is an infrequent diagnosis in clinical practice. Furthermore, from this review, it appears that 38% of cases are associated with extrauterine disease, detected at diagnosis, in contrast to the typical behavior of carcinoma in situ of the other organs. Dunton et al. detected metastases in 30–60% of SEIC cases [15]. Beyond its rarity, the understanding of this disease is also hindered by its histological characteristics. As reported in the data, it is often associated with ovarian serous carcinoma. Parallel to this other tumor, it presents a particular tropism of the peritoneal surface, even without visible locoregional infiltration. For these reasons, a diagnosis of SEIC is unlikely to be reflected in recommendations for surgical staging of endometrial carcinomas.

Two studies have described simultaneous SEIC and ovarian carcinoma. It was impossible to determine whether these were two independent neoplasms or if the SEIC had developed previously [2,14]. Serous endometrial and ovarian tumors may have similar characteristics under the microscope and may be difficult to distinguish because of their structure alone. Molecular profiling of the tumor can be helpful. This could discriminate between the presence of synchronous or metastatic tumors. Similarly, with synchronous endometrioid tumors of the endometrium and ovary, several molecular markers have been identified for differential diagnosis [16,17]. Another in-depth study that could help is the study of the tumor microenvironment, which could show differences in the genesis of both tumors [18]. Therefore, the best therapeutic management for patients with SEIC is unclear. If the tumor is clinically confined to the mucosa of the endometrium (stage IA), the most common treatment is total hysterectomy [19]. In some cases, pelvic and para-aortic lymph node removal may also be performed to assess whether the tumor has spread.

SEIC typically presents with postmenopausal bleeding, and, although the data available in the literature are numerically scarce, there is no evidence of a close correlation with risk factors such as nulliparity, late menopause, obesity and hormone replacement therapy [6]. Analysis of the literature shows that the prognosis is poor if even a minimal microscopic extrauterine disease is found, independent of the adjuvant treatment. In a study conducted by Wheeler et al., seven patients with extrauterine disease underwent chemotherapy, of which four died despite adjuvant therapy; the remaining three relapsed [2]. Conversely, the lack of extrauterine disease may be associated with a 94% chance of survival [9]. Complete surgical staging, followed by extensive sampling, is essential to define the most appropriate prognosis and therapy management. The absence of myometrial or lymphovascular space invasion was insufficient to predict the absence of extrauterine disease [20]. Due to its nature, the disease is particularly aggressive. However, in the absence of incontrovertible objective evidence of the benefit of adjuvant therapy, there is a risk of worsening iatrogenic morbidity without affecting the prognosis. Therefore, although the benefits of adjuvant treatments are not yet clear [21,22], it appears necessary to opt for additional treatments or close follow-up in patients who have undergone incomplete surgical staging. Adjuvant treatments were adopted in most cases in patients with advanced stages of the disease, except for one study in which the more aggressive approach could be justified by the young age of the patient examined, albeit with stage IA disease [12]. The patients who were followed had promising results. Of these, 19 had an extrauterine disease at diagnosis and 47 did not. However, despite being patients with stage IA disease, about one-third of patients relapsed or did not survive. A total of 66 of 81 patients had no adjuvant treatment. In particular, 20 patients died, 18 due to the disease and 2 due to other causes, while 12 patients showed signs of disease at subsequent check-ups. In most studies, it was not specified whether the disease was persistent or a recurrence.

Analyzing the data relating only to patients who did not present extrauterine disease at diagnosis, it emerged that 83% of patients subjected to FUP alone survived without evidence of disease, 6.4% developed recurrence and only approximately 1/10 of the sample died. These findings change significantly in patients with extra-uterine disease at the time of diagnosis. In fact, about half (47%) of patients undergoing follow-up alone died, 26% relapsed and the remaining percentage showed no signs of disease at subsequent follow-ups. Han described a recurrence 7 years after surgery in a woman with stage I SEIC who received an annual outpatient follow-up [13]. It is, therefore, possible to infer that follow-up is a very valid option only in patients who do not have extrauterine disease at the time of diagnosis. An additional consideration should be made regarding the incidental diagnosis of SEIC. Indeed, in clinical practice, it is more common to have a diagnosis of an intramucosal tumor following demolitive surgery. It is not always associated with adequate surgical staging. In the absence of data on the impact on the prognosis of complete staging, and given the high risk of distant microscopic involvement, this view might justify the view that adopting adjuvant therapies, even in patients with early-stage disease, could improve patient outcomes. It should be pointed out, however, that major international guidelines currently cover a limited follow-up approach [23]. However, these recommendations are based on trials that have not presented any cancer cases other than endometrioid limited to the mucosa, making their applicability questionable [24,25]. Indeed, the comparison between adjuvant and follow-up-only patients showed that adjuvant therapy could actually bring benefits in terms of overall survival and a reduction in relapses. However, if the comparison is made between patients with extrauterine disease and patients with disease confined to the uterus, examining the outcomes of patients undergoing adjuvant therapy or only follow-up in each respective group, the results partly conflict with the preliminary analysis. In particular, in patients with extrauterine disease, adjuvant therapy does not seem to have brought the expected benefits. In fact, regardless of the adjuvant therapy, about half of the patients died. That said, adjuvant treatments compared to follow-up alone have reduced rates of recurrence in patients with extrauterine disease (33.3% vs. 26.3%). In patients with disease confined to the uterus, among those subjected to only follow-up, the percentage of deaths was 10.6% while none of the patients undergoing adjuvant therapies died. However, in the latter case, the sample examined is too small from which to draw conclusions with high statistical value. Our review is severely limited by the scarcity of literature data, mainly represented by case reports. However, by reporting what has been systematically published on the topic, our review can provide a basis for further clinical knowledge concerning SEIC. In our opinion, the most important future step will be the molecular characterization of the tumor [26]. Indeed, the histological division into serous and endometroid may be limiting and unrepresentative of the molecular mechanisms underlying the curious behavior of SEIC. In particular, the most common molecular alterations in serous carcinoma of the uterus are: mutations of p53, p16 FBXW7 and PPP2R1A, HER2 overexpression, PIK3CA mutation or amplification, Cyclin E1 amplification and variable ER/PR expression [27,28]. Multiple targeted therapies have been evaluated to treat endometrial cancer in recent years. For example, dual HER2 inhibition by Trastuzumab and Pertuzumab showed antitumor activity in USC cell lines [29]. The PIK3CA inhibitor Copanlisib caused a decrease in tumor volume in five cases [30]; another preclinical result suggests that combination regimens using C-ERB/PIK3CA/AKT/mTOR inhibitors may improve responses and induce long-lasting clinical responses in patients with USC [31]; and in pre-clinical models of Cyclin E1 overexpression, the CDK2/9 inhibition has been suggested to have efficacy [32]. The routine use of the BRCA analysis was only introduced in 2014. Therefore, since the studies in question predate that date, there is a lack of data in this regard. Further studies may also consider this important prognostic factor in the therapeutic management of these patients.

In conclusion, it can be said that if the presence of SEIC is suspected, (1) it is useful to proceed to an adequate staging of the disease, in view of the high probability of extrauterine disease; (2) that the presence of an extrauterine disease significantly worsens outcomes, regardless of adjuvant treatment and that instead; and (3) in cases of disease confined to the uterine mucosa alone, the prognosis is good and follow-up allows a good control of the disease. We can, therefore, say that adjuvant therapy could further increase survival rates and reduce relapse rates in patients with uterine-confined disease and that future work, aimed at deepening the molecular signature of SEIC, will be needed to expand knowledge on this topic.

Author Contributions: Conceptualization C.R.; methodology, C.R. and A.R.; validation, P.D.F. and C.R.; formal analysis, R.M.; data curation, A.R. and R.M.; writing—original draft preparation, A.R.; writing—review and editing, C.R. and M.G.V.; visualization, P.D.F. and E.L.M.; supervision C.R. All authors have read and agreed to the published version of the manuscript.

Funding: This research received no external funding.

Institutional Review Board Statement: Not applicable.

Informed Consent Statement: Not applicable.

Conflicts of Interest: The authors declare no conflict of interest.

Appendix A

Table A1. Newcastle–Ottawa Scale.

	Selection				Comparability	Outcome			
Single-Arm Study	*Representativeness of Exposed Cohort*	*Selection of Non-Exposed Cohort*	*Ascertainment of Exposure*	*Outcome of Interest Was Not Present at Start of Study*	*Comparability of Cohorts*	*Assessment Outcome*	*Follow-Up Long Enough for Outcome to Occur?*	*Adequacy of Follow-Up*	**Quality Score**
Wheeler 2000	+	+	+	+	+	+	-	-	6
Hui 2005	-	+	+	+	-	-	-	-	3
Abushahin 2011	+	+	+	+	-	+	-	-	5
Kawano 2011	-	-	+	+	-	+	+	+	5
Pathiraja 2013	-	+	+	+	-	+	-	-	4
Ono 2014	-	+	+	+	-	+	+	+	6
Kawata 2017	-	-	+	+	-	+	-	-	3
Han 2020	-	-	+	+	-	+	+	+	5
Shimizu 2021	-	-	+	+	-	+	-	-	3

References

1. IARC. *World Health Organization Classification of Tumours: Female Genital Tumours*, 5th ed.; IARC: Lyon, France, 2020.
2. Wheeler, D.T.; Bell, K.A.; Kurman, R.J.; Sherman, M.E. Minimal uterine serous carcinoma: Diagnosis and clinicopathologic correlation. *Am. J. Surg. Pathol.* **2000**, *24*, 797–806. [CrossRef] [PubMed]
3. Kawano, K.; Ushijima, K.; Yokomine, M.; Fukui, A.; Ijichi, M.; Kamura, T. A case of minimal uterine serous carcinoma with distant lymph node metastasis without peritoneal dissemination. *J. Gynecol. Oncol.* **2011**, *22*, 53. [CrossRef] [PubMed]
4. Slaager, C.; Hofhuis, W.; Hoogduin, K.; Ewing-Graham, P.; van Beekhuizen, H. Serous endometrial intraepithelial carcinoma (SEIC): Current clinical practice in The Netherlands. *Eur. J. Obs. Gynecol. Reprod. Biol.* **2021**, *265*, 25–29. [CrossRef] [PubMed]
5. Giuntoli, R.L., 2nd; Gerardi, M.A.; Yemelyanova, A.V.; Ueda, S.M.; Fleury, A.C.; Diaz-Montes, T.P.; Bristow, R.E. Stage I noninvasive and minimally invasive uterine serous carcinoma: Comprehensive staging associated with improved survival. *Int. J. Gynecol. Cancer* **2012**, *22*, 273–279. [CrossRef]
6. Pathiraja, P.; Dhar, S.; Haldar, K. Serous endometrial intraepithelial carcinoma: A case series and literature review. *Cancer Manag. Res.* **2013**, *5*, 117–122. [CrossRef]
7. Moher, D. Preferred reporting items for systematic reviews and meta-analyses: The PRISMA statement. *PLoS Med.* **2009**, *6*, 7. [CrossRef]
8. Wells, G.; Shea, B.; O'Connell, D.; Peterson, J.; Welch, V.; Losos, M.; Tugwell, P. The Newcastle-Ottawa Scale (NOS) for Assessing the Quality of Nonrandomised Studies in Meta-Analyses. 2013. Available online: http://www.ohri.ca/programs/clinical_epidemiology/oxford.asp (accessed on 22 May 2023).
9. Hui, P.; Kelly, M.; O'Malley, D.M.; Tavassoli, F.; Schwartz, P.E. Minimal uterine serous carcinoma: A clinicopathological study of 40 cases. *Mod. Pathol.* **2005**, *18*, 75–82. [CrossRef]
10. Abushahin, N.; Zhang, T.; Chiang, S.; Zhang, X.; Hatch, K.; Zheng, W. Serous endometrial intraepithelial carcinoma arising in adenomyosis: A report of 5 cases. *Int. J. Gynecol. Pathol.* **2011**, *30*, 271–281. [CrossRef]
11. Ono, K.; Hayashi, H.; Tateno, M.; Tanaka, R.; Suzuki, R.; Maruyama, Y.; Miyagi, Y.; Furuya, M. Uterine superficial serous carcinomas and extensive serous endometrial intraepithelial carcinomas: Clinicopathological analysis of 6 patients. *Int. J. Clin Exp. Pathol.* **2014**, *7*, 7979–7988.
12. Kawata, M.; Miyoshi, A. Serous Endometrial Intraepithelial Carcinoma: Case Report and Literature Review. *J. Clin.* Gynecol. Obstet. **2017**, *6*, 49–52. [CrossRef]
13. Han, J.; Kim, H.S. Abdominopelvic Metastasis of Endometrial Serous Carcinoma Initially Misdiagnosed as Early-Stage Low-Grade Endometrioid Carcinoma: The Importance of Recognizing Minimal Uterine Serous Carcinoma. *Case Rep. Oncol.* **2020**, *13*, 1537–1544. [CrossRef] [PubMed]
14. Shimizu, M.; Yamanaka, K.; Azumi, M.; Tomimoto, M.; Washio, K.; Takahashi, R.; Nagamata, S.; Murata, Y.; Yamasaki, Y.; Terai, Y. A case of synchronous serous ovarian cancer and uterine serous endometrial intraepithelial carcinoma. *J. Ovarian Res.* **2021**, *14*, 87. [CrossRef] [PubMed]
15. Dunton, C.J.; Balsara, G.; McFarland, M.; Hernandez, E. Uterine papillary serous carcinoma: A review. *Obs. Gynecol. Surv.* **1991**, *46*, 97–102. [CrossRef] [PubMed]
16. Connell, P.P.; Rotmensch, J.; Waggoner, S.; Mundt, A.J. The significance of adnexal involvement in endometrial carcinoma. *Gynecol. Oncol.* **1999**, *74*, 74–79. [CrossRef] [PubMed]
17. Soliman, P.T.; Slomovitz, B.M.; Broaddus, R.R.; Sun, C.C.; Oh, J.C.; Eifel, P.J.; Gershenson, D.M.; Lu, K.H. Synchronous primary cancers of the endometrium and ovary: A single institution review of 84 cases. *Gynecol. Oncol.* **2004**, *94*, 456–462. [CrossRef] [PubMed]
18. Lucidi, A.; Buca, D.; Ronsini, C.; Tinari, S.; Bologna, G.; Buca, D.; Leombroni, M.; Liberati, M.; D'Antonio, F.; Scambia, G.; et al. Role of Extracellular Vesicles in Epithelial Ovarian Cancer: A Systematic Review. *Int. J. Mol. Sci.* **2020**, *21*, 8762. [CrossRef]
19. Gueli Alletti, S.; Restaino, S.; Finelli, A.; Ronsini, C.; Lucidi, A.; Scambia, G.; Fanfani, F. Step by Step Total Laparoscopic Hysterectomy with Uterine Arteries Ligation at the Origin. *J. Minim. Invasive Gynecol.* **2020**, *27*, 22–23. [CrossRef]
20. Goff, B.A.; Kato, D.; Schmidt, R.A.; Ek, M.; Ferry, J.A.; Muntz, H.G.; Cain, J.M.; Tamimi, H.K.; Figge, D.C.; Greer, B.E. Uterine papillary serous carcinoma: Patterns of metastatic spread. *Gynecol. Oncol.* **1994**, *54*, 264–268. [CrossRef]
21. Kelly, M.G.; O'Malley, D.M.; Hui, P.; McAlpine, J.; Yu, H.; Rutherford, T.J.; Azodi, M.; Schwartz, P.E. Improved survival in surgical stage I patients with uterine papillary serous carcinoma (UPSC) treated with adjuvant platinum-based chemotherapy. *Gynecol. Oncol.* **2005**, *98*, 353–359. [CrossRef]
22. Thomas, M.B.; Mariani, A.; Cliby, W.A.; Keeney, G.A.; Podratz, K.C.; Dowdy, S.C. Role of systematic lymphadenectomy and adjuvant therapy in stage I uterine papillary serous carcinoma. *Gynecol. Oncol.* **2007**, *107*, 186–189. [CrossRef]
23. Concin, N.; Matias-Guiu, X.; Vergote, I.; Cibula, D.; Mirza, M.R.; Marnitz, S.; Ledermann, J.; Bosse, T.; Chargari, C.; Fagotti, A.; et al. ESGO/ESTRO/ESP guidelines for the management of patients with endometrial carcinoma. *Int. J. Gynecol. Cancer* **2021**, *31*, 12–39. [CrossRef] [PubMed]
24. Barney, B.M.; Petersen, I.A.; Mariani, A.; Dowdy, S.C.; Bakkum-Gamez, J.N.; Haddock, M.G. The role of vaginal brachytherapy in the treatment of surgical stage I papillary serous or clear cell endometrial cancer. *Int. J. Radiat. Oncol. Biol. Phys.* **2013**, *85*, 109–115. [CrossRef] [PubMed]

25. Wortman, B.G.; Creutzberg, C.L.; Putter, H.; Jürgenliemk-Schulz, I.M.; Jobsen, J.J.; Lutgens, L.C.H.W.; van der Steen-Banasik, E.M.; Mens, J.W.M.; Slot, A.; Stenfert Kroese, M.C.; et al. Ten-year results of the PORTEC-2 trial for high-intermediate risk endometrial carcinoma: Improving patient selection for adjuvant therapy. *Br. J. Cancer* **2018**, *119*, 1067–1074. [CrossRef] [PubMed]
26. Perrone, E.; De Felice, F.; Capasso, I.; Distefano, E.; Lorusso, D.; Nero, C.; Arciuolo, D.; Zannoni, G.F.; Scambia, G.; Fanfani, F. The immunohistochemical molecular risk classification in endometrial cancer: A pragmatic and high-reproducibility method. *Gynecol. Oncol.* **2022**, *165*, 585–593. [CrossRef]
27. Lee, E.K.; Fader, A.N.; Santin, A.D.; Liu, J.F. Uterine serous carcinoma: Molecular features, clinical management, and new and future therapies. *Gynecol. Oncol.* **2021**, *160*, 322–332. [CrossRef] [PubMed]
28. Yen, T.T.; Wang, T.L.; Fader, A.N.; Shih, I.M.; Gaillard, S. Molecular Classification and Emerging Targeted Therapy in Endometrial Cancer. *Int. J. Gynecol. Pathol.* **2020**, *39*, 26–35. [CrossRef]
29. El-Sahwi, K.; Bellone, S.; Cocco, E.; Cargnelutti, M.; Casagrande, F.; Bellone, M.; AbuKhalaf, M.; Buza, N.; Tavassoli, F.A.; Hui, P.; et al. In vitro activity of pertuzumab in combination with trastuzumab in uterine serous papillary adenocarcinoma. *Br. J. Cancer* **2010**, *102*, 134–143. [CrossRef]
30. Santin, A.D.; Filiaci, V.; Bellone, S.; Ratner, E.S.; Mathews, C.A.; Cantuaria, G.; Gunderson, C.C.; Rutledge, T.; Buttin, B.M.; Lankes, H.A.; et al. Phase II evaluation of copanlisib, a selective inhibitor of Pi3kca, in patients with persistent or recurrent endometrial carcinoma harboring PIK3CA hotspot mutations: An NRG Oncology study (NRG-GY008). *Gynecol. Oncol. Rep.* **2020**, *31*, 100532. [CrossRef]
31. Lopez, S.; Cocco, E.; Black, J.; Bellone, S.; Bonazzoli, E.; Predolini, F.; Ferrari, F.; Schwab, C.L.; English, D.P.; Ratner, E.; et al. Dual HER2/PIK3CA targeting overcomes single-agent acquired resistance in HER2-amplified uterine serous carcinoma cell lines in vitro and in vivo. *Mol. Cancer Ther.* **2015**, *14*, 2519–2526. [CrossRef]
32. Cocco, E.; Lopez, S.; Black, J.; Bellone, S.; Bonazzoli, E.; Predolini, F.; Ferrari, F.; Schwab, C.L.; Menderes, G.; Zammataro, L.; et al. Dual CCNE1/ PIK3CA Targeting Is Synergistic in CCNE1-Amplified/PIK3CA-mutated Uterine Serous Carcinomas In Vitro and In Vivo. *Br. J. Cancer* **2016**, *115*, 303–311. [CrossRef]

life

MDPI

Article

Neonicotinoid Imidacloprid Affects the Social Behavior of Adult Zebrafish by Damaging Telencephalon Neurons through Oxidation Stress, Inflammation, and Apoptosis

Kou-Toung Chung [1], Li-Wen Chen [2], Hung-Wei Tseng [2] and Chung-Hsin Wu [3,*]

[1] Department of Chemical Engineering, Army Academy of ROC, Taoyuan City 320, Taiwan; chungkoutoung@gmail.com

[2] Department of Science Education and Application, National Taichung University of Education, Taichung City 403, Taiwan; liwenchen@mail.ntcu.edu.tw (L.-W.C.); ives0208@hotmail.com (H.-W.T.)

[3] School of Life Science, National Taiwan Normal University, Taipei 106, Taiwan

* Correspondence: megawu@ntnu.edu.tw; Tel.: +886-2-77496363

Abstract: The neonicotinoid imidacloprid is a widely used insecticide worldwide. We assessed the effects of acute and chronic imidacloprid exposure on the social behavior of adult zebrafish. We assembled simple apparatus to detect 2D locomotion: a single camera capture system and two specially designed water tanks. We then used the tracking and heat maps of the behavior trajectories of zebrafish subjected to sham and imidacloprid exposure and compared their social behavior. Furthermore, histomorphology and immunohistochemistry of their brain tissue sections were performed to clarify possible neurotoxicity due to imidacloprid exposure in our adult zebrafish. Our results showed that imidacloprid exposure significantly reduced the zebrafish's swimming speed, distance traveled, acceleration, and deceleration. The longer the imidacloprid exposure, the more severe the locomotor behavior disability. Furthermore, imidacloprid exposure significantly reduced heterosexual attractive behavior between the different sexes, as well as defensive alert behavior among males. Our histomorphology and immunohistochemistry evidence showed imidacloprid exposure may lead to neuronal oxidative stress, inflammation, apoptosis, and damage in the telencephalon of adult zebrafish. Thus, we suggested that neonicotinoid imidacloprid exposure can damage the telencephalon neurons of adult zebrafish through oxidative stress, inflammation, and apoptosis and then affect the social behavior of adult zebrafish.

Keywords: imidacloprid; oxidative stress; inflammation; apoptosis; telencephalon; zebrafish

Citation: Chung, K.-T.; Chen, L.-W.; Tseng, H.-W.; Wu, C.-H. Neonicotinoid Imidacloprid Affects the Social Behavior of Adult Zebrafish by Damaging Telencephalon Neurons through Oxidation Stress, Inflammation, and Apoptosis. *Life* **2023**, *13*, 1418. https://doi.org/10.3390/life13061418

Academic Editors: Stefanos Roumeliotis, Giuseppe Minervini and Anca Oana Docea

Received: 31 May 2023
Revised: 12 June 2023
Accepted: 15 June 2023
Published: 20 June 2023

1. Introduction

The neonicotinoid imidacloprid has been widely used as a pesticide because it negatively affects the nervous system of insects. It has an adequate insecticidal effect at a small dose. Consequently, imidacloprid has become an emerging pesticide for the control of agricultural pests. When insects ingest imidacloprid, the nicotinic acetylcholine receptors (nAChRs) in their nerve synapses become disturbed; this hinders the normal transmission of nerve messages, which negatively influences the insects' behavior [1]. Although imidacloprid is an extremely potent neurotoxic insecticide, it can also act as an nAChR activator [2]. Pharmacologic studies have shown that the blocking of acetylcholine receptors (AChRs) impairs memory formation, whereas acetylcholine promotes memory and learning functions. When AChRs in the hippocampus are damaged, severe deficits occur in spatial recognition and working memory [3]. However, in agriculture, pesticides such as imidacloprid are typically applied by spraying an entire area. As such, organisms other than insects may ingest them. In recent years, many studies have focused on the damage caused by neonicotinoid pesticides to nonpests such as honeybees. For instance, in honeybees, the ingestion of nectar containing imidacloprid and thiamethoxam may result in a major drop in honey production [4]. Moreover, excessive use of imidacloprid may reduce the number of wild honeybees because long-term exposure to imidacloprid has been noted to hamper the memory and learning functions of honeybees [5]. Furthermore, imidacloprid exposure may cause olfactory and visual dysfunction in honeybees in their larval stages [6]. As such, the use of neonicotinoid neurotoxic pesticides, such as imidacloprid, severely threatens the survival of pollinating insects such as honeybees, butterflies, and flower flies. For example, exposure to a small amount of imidacloprid can affect the flight path recognition ability of honeybees such that both the efficiency of their nectar collection as well as the number of bees returning to the hive decrease [7].

Many recent studies have reported the effects of imidacloprid exposure in vertebrates such as amphibians, fish, and mammals. Stacey et al. [8] observed that in the wood frog (*Lithobates sylvaticus*), exposure to neonicotinoid imidacloprid at 1, 10, and 100 μg/L during tadpole development may affect the ability of young frogs to sense or respond to predators. Vignet et al. [9] studied the effects of neonicotinoid pesticides on medaka and zebrafish development and behavior and observed that imidacloprid exposed for 5–14 days from 0.2 to 2000 μg/L had a sublethal effect on both types of fish. Burke et al. [10] found that in mice, exposure to imidacloprid (0.5 mg/kg/day) during pregnancy tended to result in lower fertility and body weight during adulthood, whereas exposure during developmental years negatively affected behavior and brain function during adulthood. Sriapha et al. [11] performed a case study on imidacloprid poisoning and found that imidacloprid with estimated doses of ingestion ranging from 2 to 35 g may increase the hepatic injury risk in humans. These results imply that imidacloprid-related injury during the embryo and infant stages may affect performance through adulthood and that even adult individuals can develop varying degrees of injury, including nonimmediate injury, after ingesting imidacloprid. Nerve repair is generally more difficult than muscle repair. For instance, damage to the cranial nerves during development can affect cognitive development to varying degrees. Tomizawa [12] reported that long-term exposure to imidacloprid (1 mg/kg/BW/day) may cause nAChR overexpression in the brain tissue of mammals, resulting in brain damage. In addition, Duzguner and Erdogan [13,14] reported that long-term exposure to 10 μM imidacloprid may induce inflammation and increase oxidative stress in the central nervous system of rats, eventually leading to neuronal apoptosis.

Insecticides can pose a serious threat to the survival of many animals in the wild. Neonicotinoid insecticides such as imidacloprid are widely used in agricultural production because they are easy to use, cheap, and effective. However, the excessive or incorrect use of pesticides may eventually result in water pollution. Therefore, in recent years, studies have increasingly used zebrafish as a model animal in experiments for detecting agricultural pesticides in the environment. In studies on the effects of pollution on water ecology, fish behavior patterns and the underlying neural transmission mechanisms have been employed to monitor water pollution and its potential impact on organisms. Zebrafish is one of the fish species recommended for aquatic acute toxicity testing by the OECD (Organization of Economic Cooperation and Development) not only because its developmental changes are easy to observe but also because it grows rapidly, is easy and inexpensive to raise, and has strong fecundity. In addition, the mechanism underlying its embryonic development is similar to that underlying mammalian embryonic development; it has various organ systems that are similar to those in humans, and its complete genetic database has been established [15]. As such, the zebrafish has become a major indicator organism in aquatic ecotoxicology, which can sensitively detect the toxicity of trace environmental pollutants. When the zebrafish is affected by environmental pollutants, its sensory system receives vital information, which passes through the central nervous system [16]. Systematic regulation of various physiological systems means that it exhibits behaviors such as swarming, aggression, fear, and vigilance [17]. Therefore, the behavior of zebrafish can be used as a crucial indicator in behavioral research. Several studies on imidacloprid have focused on embryonic development [18], but few studies have assessed adult individuals of vertebrates such as fish and mammals. In the present study, we determined the possible effects of imidacloprid exposure on the social behavior of adult zebrafish.

2. Materials and Methods

2.1. Animal Preparation

Adult wild-type zebrafish (*Danio rerio*) were obtained from Academia Sinica (Taipei, Taiwan). They were reared in circulating tap water at room temperature and were fed twice a day. Zebrafish, fish food, and other supplies were purchased from local pet shops (Taipei, Taiwan) for these studies. Zebrafish were kept in 10-gallon holding tanks and were fed live brine shrimp, microworms, and Tetramin staple food ad libitum. Experiments were conducted on 16-week-old adult zebrafish that were a useful animal model to study the effects of acute and chronic imidacloprid exposure on social behavior because it is a gregarious fish that can express behaviors such as swarming, aggression, fear, and vigilance. The behavioral performance of zebrafish was studied in the current experiments, which complied with guidelines of the IACUC and were approved by the IACUC of our university (protocol no.: No. 103018).

2.2. Imidacloprid Preparation and Treatment

Imidacloprid was purchased from Sigma-Aldrich (St. Louis, MO, USA; PESTANAL, analytical standard; concentration $\leq$ 100%; empirical formula (Hill Notation): $C_9H_{10}ClN_5O_2$; molecular weight: 255.66; CAS number: 138261-41-3). Imidacloprid is a neonicotinoid insecticide in the chloronicotinyl nitroguanidine chemical family. The International Union of Pure and Applied Chemistry (IUPAC) name is 1-(6-chloro-3-pyridylmethyl)-N-nitroimidazolidin-2-ylideneamine and the Chemical Abstracts Service (CAS) registry number is 138261-41-3. The molecular structure of imidacloprid is listed in Table 1. Imidacloprid powder was dissolved in 0.5% dimethyl sulfoxide (Sigma-Aldrich) as a cosolvent that was diluted with tap water to concentrations of 0.1, 0.5, and 1.0 ppm. During the observation experiment, which lasted 5 consecutive days, the solution was refreshed daily. The excrement in the fish tank was cleaned daily, and imidacloprid consumed during the experiment was supplemented, as required. Based on the fact that imidacloprid has an impact on the movement trajectory of zebrafish and does not cause fish death, we selected the initial concentrations of imidacloprid to be 0.1, 0.5, and 1.0 ppm; in order to avoid premature death of zebrafish in the 5-day experiment, a concentration of 0.1 ppm was chosen for the 5-day experiment. All the stock solutions were used at a room temperature of 25 °C.

Table 1. Molecular structure, molecular formula, and molecular weight of imidacloprid.

Molecular structure	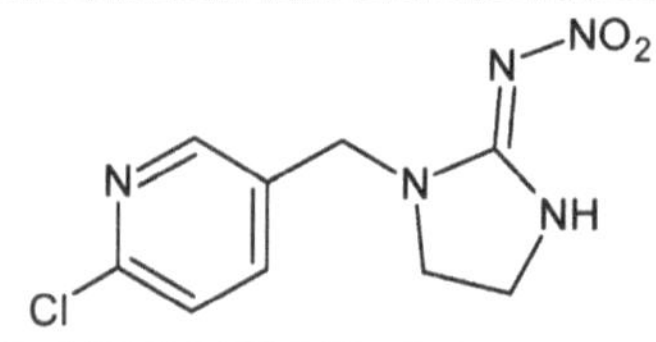
Molecular formula	$C_9H_{10}ClN_5O_2$
Molecular weight	255.662 g/mol

2.3. Locomotor Behavior Assay of the Zebrafish

The zebrafish were exposed to imidacloprid at different concentrations (0.1, 0.5, and 1.0 ppm) at different time points (0, 24, 48, 72, 96, and 120 h) for locomotion testing. Locomotor behavior of zebrafish was examined and tracked daily using a high-speed camera (Mikrotron-GmbH, Unterschleißheim, Germany) and were then analyzed using EthoVision-X (Noldus, Wageningen, The Netherlands). The behavioral performance of zebrafish in the current experiments was recorded and tracked daily for 20 min. Locomotor behavior assays of the zebrafish such as the swimming velocity and distance were examined using a high-speed camera.

2.4. Social Interaction Assay of the Zebrafish

We placed a female and a male zebrafish in two adjacent fish tanks. We recorded the movement trajectories of the female or male zebrafish in the separate fish tanks when a baffle plate was placed between the fish tanks to prevent the zebrafish from seeing each other. When the baffle plate was removed and the zebrafish saw each other in adjacent tanks, the movement trajectories of the female and male zebrafish were recorded again. In addition to recording the movement distance and speed and maximum acceleration and deceleration of the female and male zebrafish, we analyzed the relative distance between the female and male zebrafish, which was named the heterosexual attraction distance. Changes in this distance were considered to denote effects on the heterosexual attraction of the fish.

We placed one male zebrafish each into two adjacent fish tanks. We recorded the movement trajectories of the zebrafish in the separate fish tanks when a baffle plate was placed between the fish tanks. When the baffle plate was removed, the movement trajectories of the zebrafish were recorded again. In addition to recording the movement distance and speed and maximum acceleration and deceleration of both the zebrafish, we analyzed the relative distance between the two male zebrafish, which was named the vigilant confrontation distance. Changes in this distance were considered to denote effects on the defensive alert behavior of the fish.

2.5. Hematoxylin and Eosin Staining and Immunohistochemical Staining of Zebrafish Brain Tissue

Male zebrafish were anesthetized and perfused with PBS containing 4% formaldehyde (EM grade glutaraldehyde solution, Sigma-Aldrich). Brain tissue samples from male zebrafish were fixed with 4% formaldehyde (Sigma-Aldrich) and embedded in paraffin. Brain tissue specimens were cut into 5 μm thick sections using a tissue microtome, and then, sections were mounted on glass slides. Some brain tissue sections were stained with hematoxylin and eosin (H&E) (Sigma-Aldrich) to assess tissue integrity. Other myocardial tissue sections were subjected to immunohistochemical (IHC) staining with SOD2 (Cat. numbers ab110300; Abcam, Cambridge, UK), tumor necrosis factor (TNF)-α (Cat. numbers #3707; Cell Signaling Technology, Danvers, MA, USA), and caspase-3 (Cat. numbers #9662; Cell Signaling Technology) for 1 h at a room temperature of 25 °C. By incubating with biotinylated secondary antibody (NovolinkTM Polymer Detection System l, Leica Biosystems Newcastle Ltd., Newcastle, UK) for 30 min and avidin–biotin–horseradish peroxidase (HRP) complex (Novolink™ Polymer Detection System l, Leica Biosystems Newcastle Ltd.) for an additional 30 min. IHC was visualized using DAB Chromogen (NovolinkTM Polymer Detection System 1, Leica Biosystems Newcastle Ltd.), and slides were counterstained with hematoxylin (NovolinkTM Polymer Detection System 1, Leica Biosystems Newcastle Ltd.).

2.6. Statistical Analysis

In this study, SigmaPlot 12.5 (Systat Software Inc., San Jose, CA, USA) was used for data analysis and chart production. All data are shown as mean ± standard error of the mean (SEM). Differences among different groups of zebrafish were assessed using one-way or two-way analysis of variance (ANOVA). Student–Newman–Keuls multiple comparisons post hoc test was performed if a significant F-value was obtained. Significance was defined as $p < 0.05$.

3. Results

3.1. Effects of Imidacloprid Exposure on Optic Tectum of Adult Zebrafish

Through H&E staining, we assessed neuronal injury in the optic tectum sections of the adult male zebrafish after 5 days of sham and imidacloprid exposure at various concentrations (Figure 1). We observed that the neuron number in the optic tectum sections was significantly higher in the adult zebrafish exposed to the sham treatment than in those exposed to imidacloprid (Figure 1A). Moreover, neuron density in these sections was significantly lower in adult zebrafish exposed to imidacloprid than in those that received the sham treatment (Figure 1B). Furthermore, as the imidacloprid concentration was increased, the neuron density decreased gradually and significantly (Figure 1B).

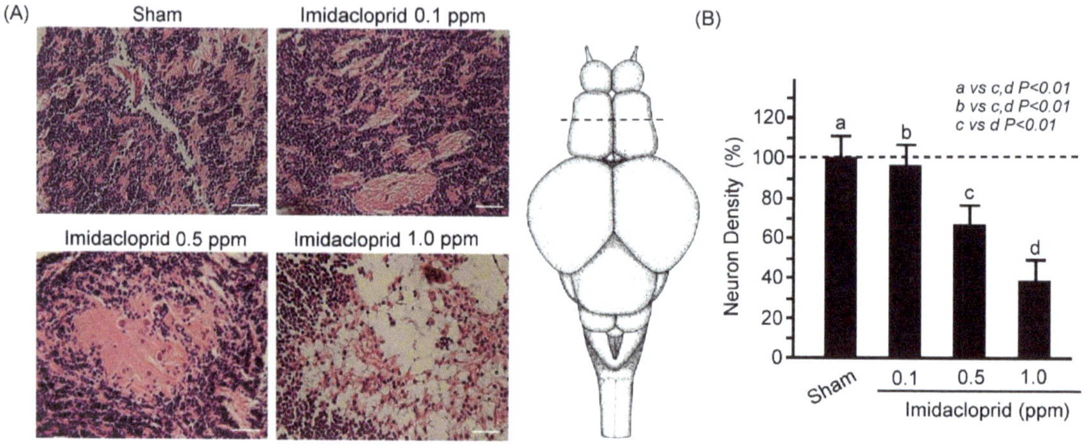

Figure 1. (**A**) H&E staining showing neuronal injury in telencephalon sections of an adult male zebrafish after 5 days of sham treatment and imidacloprid treatment at various concentrations. Scale bar = 25 μm. The dotted line shows transverse sections across a zebrafish adult brain in the telencephalon. (**B**) Neuron density in telencephalon sections of adult male zebrafish without (a: sham) and with imidacloprid (b: 0.1, c: 0.5, and d: 1.0 ppm) treatment after 5 days of exposure. Data are presented as mean ± SEM and were obtained from 10 independent experiments. One-way ANOVA followed by the Student–Newman–Keuls multiple comparison post-test. The differences in the median values among the treatment groups were greater than would be expected by chance; there is a statistically significant difference (*p* (Factor A) = 0.01).

Anti-oxidative stress SOD2 expressions were examined in the brain tissue of an adult male zebrafish using IHC staining and are shown in Figure 2A. SOD2 is a crucial antioxidant enzyme associated with oxidative stress. We observed that SOD2 protein expression in the brain tissue was weaker in the adult male zebrafish subjected to imidacloprid treatment than in those subjected to the sham treatment. Moreover, as the imidacloprid was concentration increased, SOD2 expression in the brain tissue of the adult male zebrafish exhibited a gradual decrease (Figure 2A).

TNF-α expression, an inflammation marker, in the brain tissue of an adult male zebrafish was examined and is shown in Figure 2B. We observed that TNF-α expression in the brain tissue of the adult male zebrafish subjected to imidacloprid treatment was higher than in those subject to the sham treatment. As the imidacloprid concentration was increased, TNF-α expression gradually increased in the brain tissue of the adult male zebrafish (Figure 2B).

Finally, caspase-3 expression, an apoptosis marker, in the brain tissue of an adult male zebrafish was examined, as shown in Figure 2C. We observed that caspase-3 expression in the brain tissue of the adult male zebrafish subjected to imidacloprid treatment was higher than in those subjected to the sham treatment. As the imidacloprid concentration increased, caspase-3 expression gradually increased in the brain tissue of the adult male zebrafish (Figure 2C). Taken together, these results confirmed that imidacloprid may cause neurotoxicity through oxidative stress, inflammation, and apoptosis in the brain tissue of the adult male zebrafish.

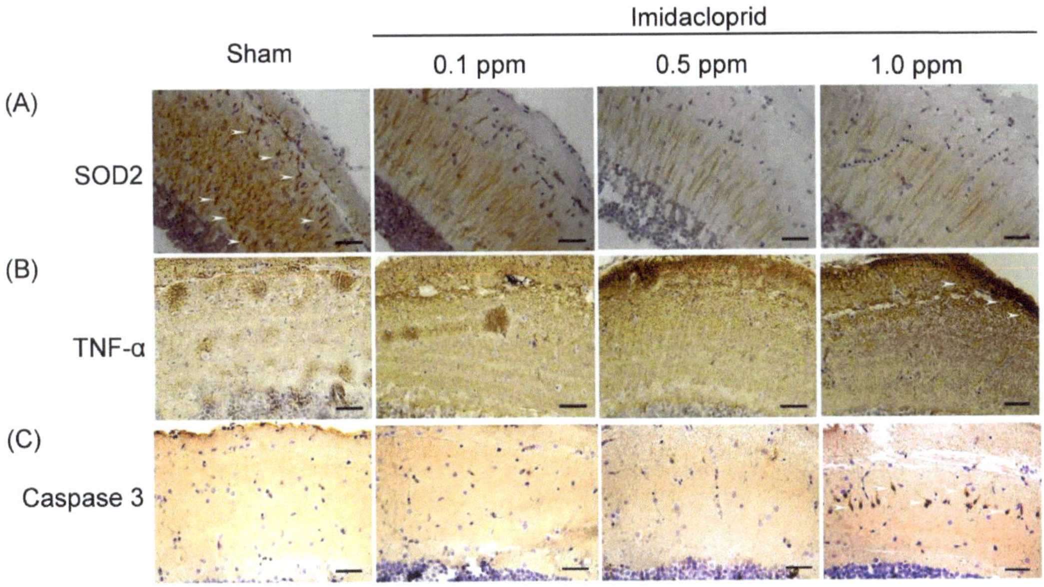

Figure 2. IHC staining showing neuronal (**A**) oxidative stress, (**B**) inflammation, and (**C**) apoptosis in telencephalon sections of adult male zebrafish without (sham) and with imidacloprid (0.1, 0.5, and 1.0 ppm) treatment after 5 days of exposure. The arrows denote positive expression of proteins related to neuronal antioxidative stress (SOD2), inflammation (TNF-α), and apoptosis (caspase-3). Scale bar = 100 μm.

3.2. Effects of Acute and Chronic Imidacloprid Exposure on Locomotor Behavior of Adult Zebrafish

Using a Noldus Ethovision-XT animal behavior trajectory tracking analysis system, we analyzed the locomotor behavior of a single adult male zebrafish after they had spent 12 h in clean water and water environments containing different concentrations of imidacloprid. The movement trajectory map and movement trajectory heat map of the zebrafish were recorded for 10 min. According to the results shown in Figure 3A, compared with the zebrafish not exposed to imidacloprid, those exposed to different concentrations of imidacloprid moved more slowly and a shorter distance and had lower maximum acceleration and deceleration after 12 h; the nonimidacloprid group exhibited the best locomotor behavior, whereas the group with the highest imidacloprid exposure exhibited the worst locomotor behavior. These results are corroborated by the bar charts shown in Figure 3B ($p < 0.01$ or 0.05).

We next explored the changes in locomotor behavior of adult male zebrafish immersed in a fixed concentration (0.1 ppm) of imidacloprid for different exposure durations (1, 2, 3, 4, or 5 days). As shown in Figure 4A, the locomotor behavior of the male zebrafish after exposure to 0.1 ppm imidacloprid for 5 consecutive days was recorded using our tracking analysis system. We observed that the longer the exposure time, the more significant the decrease in the average movement distance and speed as well as maximum acceleration and deceleration. These results are corroborated by the bar charts shown in Figure 4B ($p < 0.01$ or 0.05).

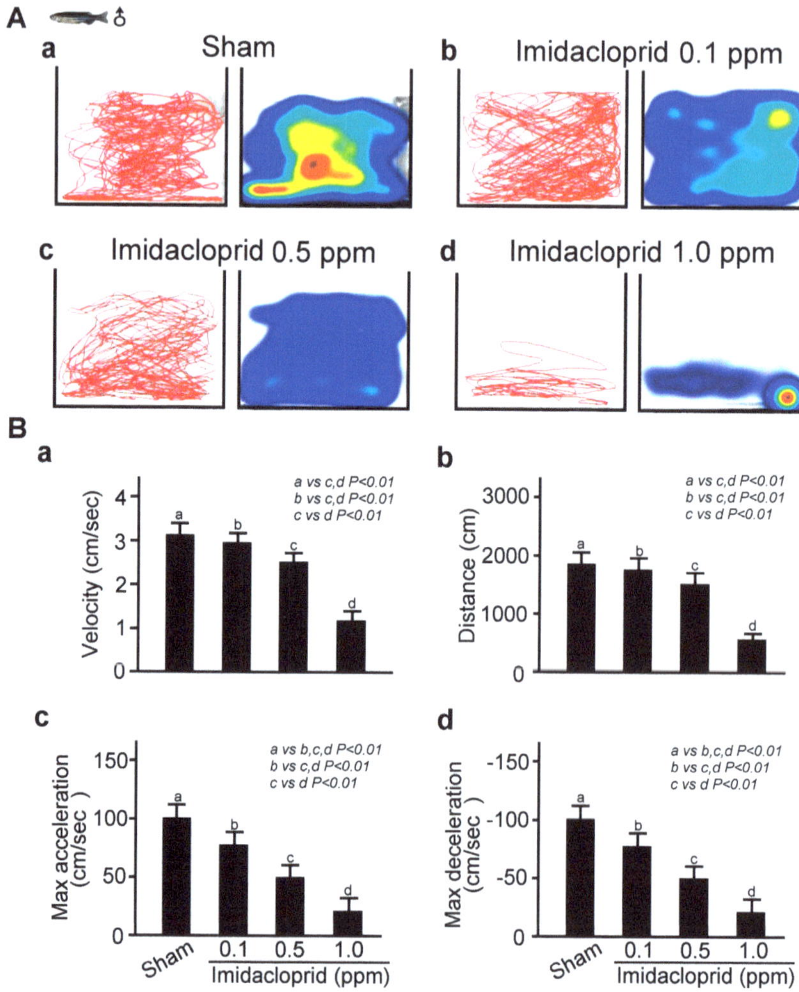

Figure 3. Locomotor behavior disability in adult male zebrafish exposed to imidacloprid for 24 h at various concentrations in a novel tank diving test. (**A**) Tracking and heat maps of the behavior trajectory of a male zebrafish without imidacloprid treatment (sham) and with imidacloprid treatment at various concentrations (0, 0.1, 0.5, and 1.0 ppm) after 24 h of exposure. (**B**) Bar charts showing swimming ability in quantified movement speed (**a**), movement distance (**b**), maximum acceleration (**c**), and maximum deceleration (**d**) in adult male zebrafish without imidacloprid treatment (sham) and with imidacloprid treatment at various concentrations (a: 0, b: 0.1, c: 0.5, and d: 1.0 ppm) after 12 h of exposure. Data are presented as mean ± SEM and were obtained from 10 independent experiments. The differences in the median values among the treatment groups were greater than would be expected by chance; there is a statistically significant difference (p (Factor A) = 0.01).

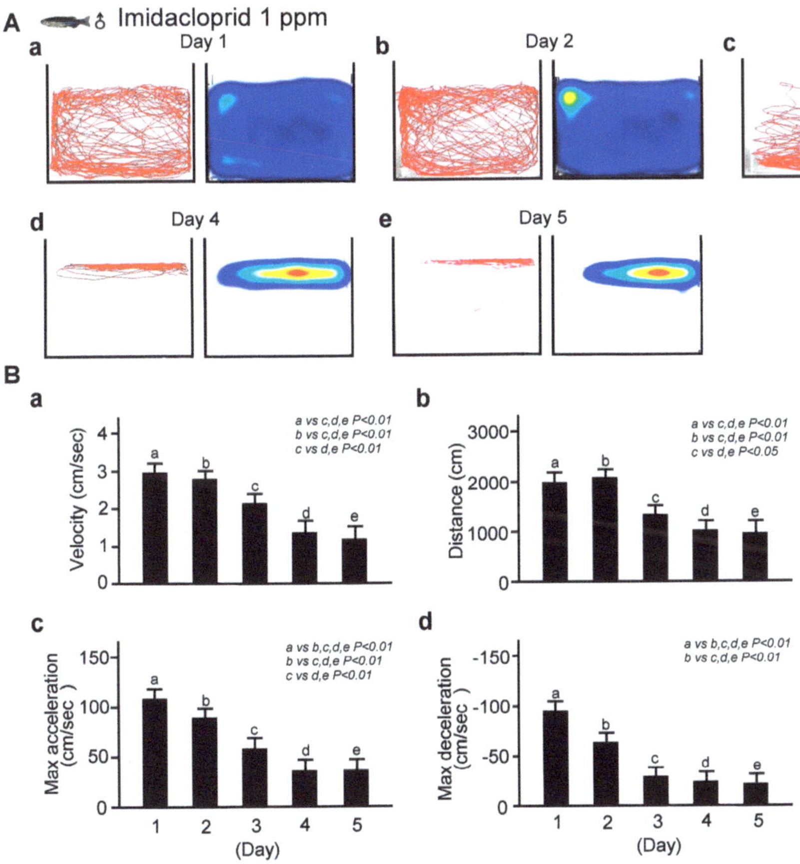

Figure 4. Locomotor behavior disability in adult male zebrafish exposed to 0.1 ppm imidacloprid for various exposure times in a novel tank diving test. (**A**) Tracking and heat maps of the behavior trajectory of male zebrafish without imidacloprid treatment (sham) and with 0.1 ppm imidacloprid treatment after various exposure times (1, 2, 3, 4, and 5 days). (**B**) Bar charts showing swimming ability in quantified movement speed (**a**), movement distance (**b**), maximum acceleration (**c**), and maximum deceleration (**d**)—in adult male zebrafish without imidacloprid treatment (sham) and with 0.1 ppm imidacloprid treatment after various exposure times (a: 1, b: 2, c: 3, d: 4, and e: 5 days). Data are presented as mean ± SEM and were obtained from 10 independent experiments. The differences in the median values among the treatment groups were greater than would be expected by chance; there is a statistically significant difference (p (Factor A) = 0.01).

3.3. Effects of Imidacloprid Exposure on Social Interaction of Adult Zebrafish

We further examined the effects of imidacloprid exposure on social interaction in adult zebrafish by analyzing the movement trajectories of zebrafish in two adjacent fish tanks. As shown in Figure 5A, we found that in a clean water environment, the movement distance and speed and maximum acceleration and deceleration were similar for the male and female zebrafish in separate tanks when the baffle plate was present; however, they then decreased when the baffle plates were removed, indicating heterosexual attraction. However, after exposure to 0.1 ppm imidacloprid, the heterosexual attraction between the female and male fish was significantly weaker (Figure 5B, $p < 0.01$ or 0.05).

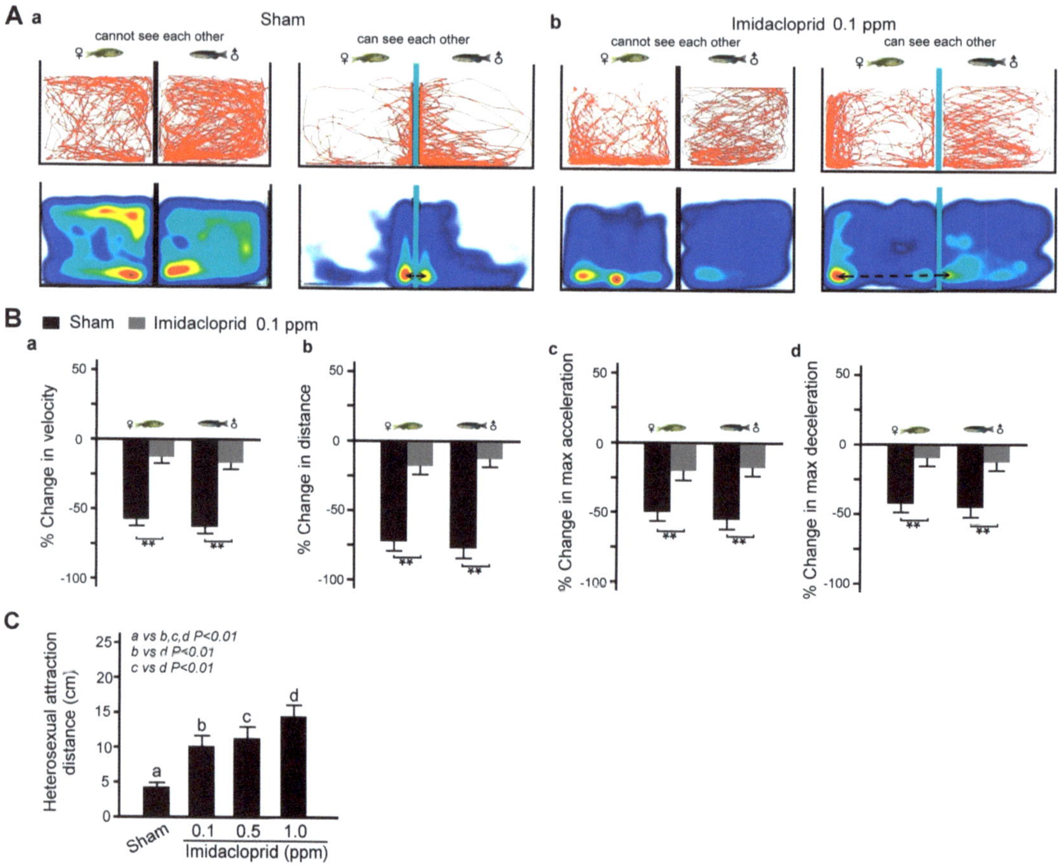

Figure 5. Heterosexual attraction disability in adult male and female zebrafish after 5 days of imidacloprid exposure in a novel tank diving test. (**A**) Tracking and heat maps of the behavior trajectory of a male and a female zebrafish without imidacloprid treatment (sham) and with 0.1 ppm imidacloprid treatment for 5 days. The dotted lines denote the heterosexual attraction distance. (**B**) Bar charts showing swimming ability in quantified movement speed (**a**), movement distance (**b**), maximum acceleration (**c**), and maximum deceleration (**d**) in adult male and female zebrafish without imidacloprid treatment (sham) and with 0.1 ppm imidacloprid treatment for 5 days. (**C**) Bar chart showing quantified heterosexual attraction distance without imidacloprid treatment (sham) and with imidacloprid treatment (a: 0, b: 0.1, c: 0.5, and d: 1.0 ppm) for 5 days. Data are presented as mean ± SEM (n = 10 for each group, ** $p < 0.01$).

Two male zebrafish were placed one each in adjacent fish tanks, and the zebrafish could not see each other due to a baffle plate between the tanks. As shown in Figure 6A, we found that in a clean water environment, the movement distance and speed as well as maximum acceleration and deceleration of two male zebrafish in separate tanks were similar when the baffle plate was employed; additionally, they decreased when the baffle plate was removed, indicating defensive alert behavior because the behavior of male zebrafish in the two tanks is compared to a defensive alert. However, after exposure to imidacloprid, this behavior was significantly decreased (Figure 6B).

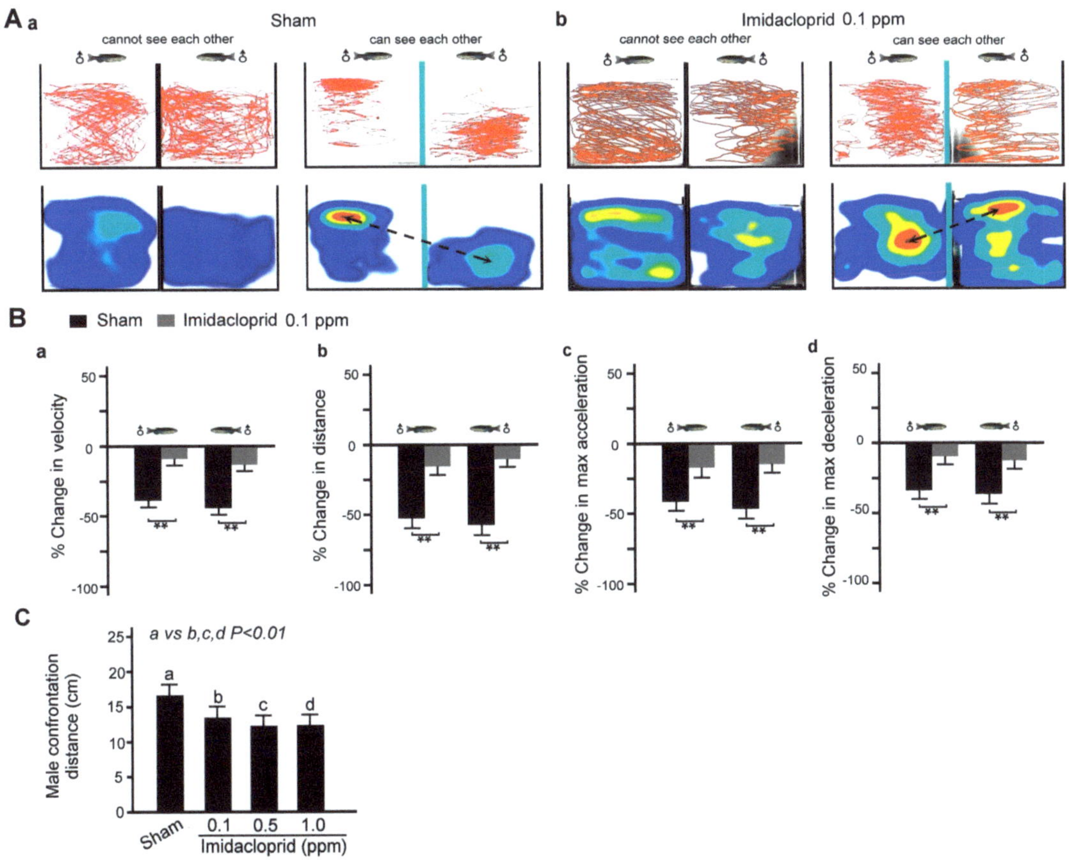

Figure 6. Defensive alert behavior disability in two adult male zebrafish after 5 days of imidacloprid exposure in a novel tank diving test. (**A**) Tracking and heat maps of the behavior trajectory of two male zebrafish without imidacloprid treatment (sham) and with 0.1 ppm imidacloprid treatment for 5 days. The dotted lines denote the vigilant confrontation distance. (**B**) Bar charts showing swimming ability in quantified movement speed (**a**), movement distance (**b**), maximum acceleration (**c**), and maximum deceleration (**d**) in two adult male zebrafish without imidacloprid treatment (sham) and with 0.1 ppm imidacloprid treatment for 5 days. (**C**) Bar chart showing quantified confrontation distance without imidacloprid treatment (sham) and with imidacloprid treatment (a: 0, b: 0.1, c: 0.5, and d: 1.0 ppm) for 5 days. Data are presented as mean ± SEM (n = 10 for each group; ** $p < 0.01$).

4. Discussion

To adapt to their environment and survival needs, fish require skills such as spatial learning and predator evasion so as to identify and avoid predators as well as find suitable breeding grounds. We found that regardless of their sex, the movement distance and speed as well as maximum movement acceleration and deceleration of adult zebrafish were significantly altered by imidacloprid exposure; the longer the imidacloprid exposure, the more severe the locomotor behavior disability. Moreover, imidacloprid significantly reduced the heterosexual attraction between an adult male and an adult female zebrafish and significantly affected defensive alert behavior between two adult male zebrafish. Because the zebrafish is a gregarious fish, it displays behaviors such as grouping, aggression, fear, and vigilance; different nuclei in the brain dominate these social behaviors. Our results demonstrated that imidacloprid exposure significantly negatively affected the performance of social behaviors such as mutual attraction and mutual alertness in zebrafish, indicating that exposure to a systemic pesticide such as imidacloprid may damage the neural nuclei in the brain related to emotion or courtship behavior.

The forebrain of the goldfish develops into the telencephalon, a brain area responsible for cognitive learning and emotional regulation. Moreover, in goldfish, damage to the outer telencephalon causes disturbance in spatial memory [19], whereas that to the inner telencephalon leads to disturbance in emotional memory [20]. The goldfish telencephalon is equivalent to the limbic system of mammals in that the function of the medial telencephalic pallium is equivalent to that of the amygdala in the limbic system—the nucleus that controls emotional memory. If the medial telencephalic pallium is damaged, goldfish lose memory of their past experiences of fear [20]. Furthermore, the function of the lateral telencephalic pallium in goldfish is similar to that of the hippocampus, which controls spatial cognition and emotional expression [21]. The zebrafish has gradually been developed as an animal model for exploring cognitive functions, and some studies have indicated that it has the ability to learn and remember fear experiences [22]. In addition, the administration of nicotine receptor agonists to zebrafish can improve cognitive learning [23,24].

The ADME (absorption, distribution, metabolism, and elimination) of imidacloprid exposure has been reported in many studies. Imidacloprid is rapidly and completely absorbed and distributed after oral administration in rats; after exposure, the peak plasma level of imidacloprid is reached within 2 h, whereas the peaks in liver, kidney, lung, and skin levels occur after 48 h in rats [25]. Imidacloprid is mainly metabolized in the liver and then excreted through urine. Imidacloprid can be oxidatively cleaved into 6-chloronicotinic acid, which is further metabolized through glutathione binding to form mercaptonicotinic acid and hippuric acid. In addition, imidacloprid can be metabolized through imidazolidine ring hydroxylation, thus generating 5-hydroxyl and alkene derivatives [26]. Approximately 90% of imidacloprid is eliminated within 24 h of exposure: 75–80% through urine and 10–15% through feces via biliary excretion [27]. The differences between species are believed to be due to differences in metabolic rates and associated cumulative oxidative damage. Therefore, different species demonstrate differing changes in the pharmacokinetics of ADME and other aspects of susceptibility to hazards associated with a toxicant such as imidacloprid.

Imidacloprid is a highly potent neurotoxic insecticide; it blocks AChRs in hippocampal neurons and impairs memory formation [3]. Long-term exposure to imidacloprid may damage neurons in the brain and impair the memory and learning functions of honeybees [5]. We previously reported that in bats, imidacloprid exposure can cause neuronal apoptosis in the CA1 area of the hippocampus and the medial entorhinal cortex related to memory learning in the brain, which in turn triggers spatial memory impairment [28]. In addition, we previously revealed that inflammation and mitochondrial-dysfunction-related apoptosis in the hippocampal CA1 and medial entorhinal cortex areas may induce orientation disorder and spatial memory dysfunction [29]. In the current study, the results of our histomorphology and IHC staining using brain tissue sections indicated that imidacloprid exposure causes neuronal oxidative stress, inflammation, apoptosis, and damage in the telencephalon of adult zebrafish. Extremely high imidacloprid concentrations have been reported to induce a considerable increase in reactive oxygen species (ROS) levels in the zebrafish liver and enhance the activities of SOD, CAT, and GST, which scavenge excess ROS. ROS attack cell membranes, leading to an increase in MDA, which causes DNA damage and increases GST scavenging activity [30].

5. Conclusions

The neonicotinoid imidacloprid is considered to be one of the most commonly detected neonicotinoid insecticides in surface waters. Imidacloprid concentrations in surface waters range from 0.001 to 320 ppb, while some estimates of accidental spills can even be as high as 1.8 to 7.3 ppm, which can adversely affect aquatic organisms [31,32]. Our behavioral and histological experiments showed that adult zebrafish exposure to the 0.1–1.0 ppm neonicotinoid imidacloprid can affect the performance of zebrafish social behavior, which we believe is partly due to imidacloprid damaging neurons in the telencephalon of zebrafish through oxidative stress, inflammation, and apoptosis. (Figure 7). From the results of this experiment, we believe that the behavioral responses of zebrafish can be used as a biomarker for assessing environmental toxicological risks.

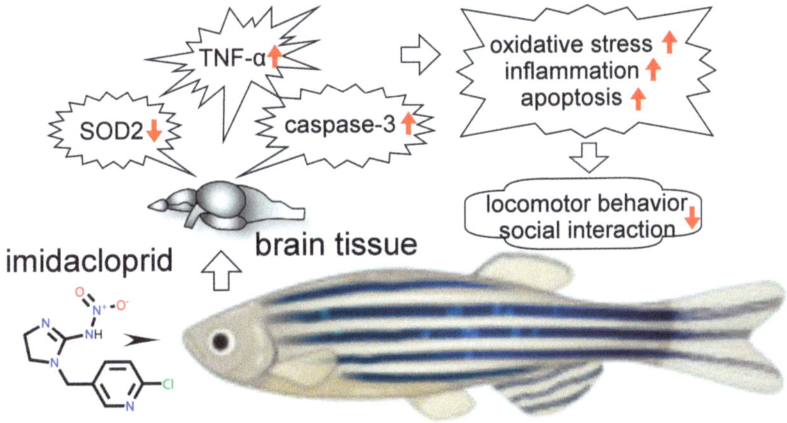

Figure 7. Possible pathological mechanism underlying brain damage induced by imidacloprid in zebrafish. Our behavioral and histological experiments showed that adult zebrafish exposure to the neonicotinoid imidacloprid may affect the performance of zebrafish social behavior because imidacloprid may damage neurons in the telencephalon of zebrafish.

Author Contributions: Conceptualization and methodology, K.-T.C. and H.-W.T.; investigation, L.-W.C.; writing—original draft preparation, K.-T.C. and H.-W.T.; writing—review and editing, C.-H.W. All authors have read and agreed to the published version of the manuscript.

Funding: This research received no external funding.

Institutional Review Board Statement: The study of the behavioral performance of zebrafish in the current experiments complied with the guidelines of the IACUC and was approved by the IACUC of our university (protocol no.: No. 103018).

Informed Consent Statement: Not applicable.

Data Availability Statement: Not applicable.

Acknowledgments: We are grateful to Wallace Academic Editing for editing and revising this paper.

Conflicts of Interest: The authors declare no conflict of interest.

References

1. Chao, S.L.; Casida, J.E. Interaction of Imidacloprid Metabolites and Analogs with the Nicotinic Acetylcholine Receptor of Mouse Brain in Relation to Toxicity. *Pestic. Biochem. Physiol.* **1997**, *58*, 77–88. [CrossRef]
2. Matsuda, K.; Shimomura, M.; Ihara, M.; Akamatsu, M.; Sattelle, D.B. Neonicotinoids Show Selective and Diverse Actions on Their Nicotinic Receptor Targets: Electrophysiology, Molecular Biology, and Receptor Modeling Studies. *Biosci. Biotechnol. Biochem.* **2005**, *69*, 1442–1452. [CrossRef] [PubMed]
3. Tang, Y.; Mishkin, M.; Aigner, T.G. Effects of muscarinic blockade in perirhinal cortex during visual recognition. *Proc. Natl. Acad. Sci. USA* **1997**, *94*, 12667–12669. [CrossRef] [PubMed]
4. Chambers, R.G.; Chatzimichael, K.; Tzouvelekas, V. Sub-lethal concentrations of neonicotinoid insecticides at the field level affect negatively honey yield: Evidence from a 6-year survey of Greek apiaries. *PLoS ONE* **2019**, *14*, e0215363. [CrossRef]
5. Decourtye, A.; Armengaud, C.; Renou, M.; Devillers, J.; Cluzeau, S.; Gauthier, M.; Pham-Delègue, M.-H. Imidacloprid impairs memory and brain metabolism in the honeybee (*Apis mellifera* L.). *Pestic. Biochem. Physiol.* **2004**, *78*, 83–92. [CrossRef]
6. Dively, G.P.; Embrey, M.S.; Kamel, A.; Hawthorne, D.J.; Pettis, J.S. Assessment of chronic sublethal effects of imidacloprid on honey bee colony health. *PLoS ONE* **2015**, *10*, e0118748.

7. Kenna, D.; Cooley, H.; Pretelli, I.; Ramos Rodrigues, A.; Gill, S.D.; Gill, R.J. Pesticide exposure affects flight dynamics and reduces flight endurance in bumblebees. *Ecol. Evol.* **2019**, *9*, 5637–5650. [CrossRef]
8. Stacey, S.Y.; Lee, J.; Stacey, A.R. Effects of neonicotinoids on putative escape behavior of juvenile wood frogs (*Lithobates sylvaticus*) chronically exposed as tadpoles. *Environ. Toxicol. Chem.* **2018**, *37*, 3115–3123.
9. Vignet, C.; Cappello, T.; Fu, Q.; Lajoie, K.; De Marco, G.; Clérandeau, C.; Mottaz, H.; Maisano, M.; Hollender, J.; Schirmer, K.; et al. Imidacloprid induces adverse effects on fish early life stages that are more severe in Japanese medaka (*Oryzias latipes*) than in zebrafish (*Danio rerio*). *Chemosphere* **2019**, *225*, 470–478. [CrossRef]
10. Burke, A.P.; Niibori, Y.; Terayama, H.; Ito, M.; Pidgeon, C.; Arsenault, J.; Camarero, P.R.; Cummins, C.L.; Mateo, R.; Sakabe, K.; et al. Mammalian Susceptibility to a Neonicotinoid Insecticide after Fetal and Early Postnatal Exposure. *Sci. Rep.* **2018**, *8*, 16639. [CrossRef]
11. Sriapha, C.; Trakulsrichai, S.; Intaraprasong, P.; Wongvisawakorn, S.; Tongpoo, A.; Schimmel, J.; Wananukul, W. Imidaclo-prid poisoning case series: Potential for liver injury. *Clin. Toxicol.* **2020**, *58*, 136–138. [CrossRef]
12. Tomizawa, M.; Cowan, A.; Casida, J.E. Analgesic and Toxic Effects of Neonicotinoid Insecticides in Mice. *Toxicol. Appl. Pharmacol.* **2001**, *177*, 77–83. [CrossRef] [PubMed]
13. Duzguner, V.; Erdogan, S. Acute oxidant and inflammatory effects of imidacloprid on the mammalian central nervous sys-tem and liver in rats. *Pestic. Biochem. Physiol.* **2010**, *97*, 13–18. [CrossRef]
14. Duzguner, V.; Erdogan, S. Chronic exposure to imidacloprid induces inflammation and oxidative stress in the liver & central nervous system of rats. *Pestic. Biochem. Physiol.* **2012**, *104*, 58–64. [CrossRef]
15. Hill, A.J.; Teraoka, H.; Heideman, W.; Peterson, R.E. Zebrafish as a model vertebrate for investigating chemical toxicity. *Toxicol. Sci.* **2005**, *86*, 6–19. [PubMed]
16. Lin, W.; Huang, Z.; Zhang, W.; Ren, Y. Investigating the neurotoxicity of environmental pollutants using zebrafish as a model organism: A review and recommendations for future work. *Neurotoxicology* **2023**, *94*, 235–244. [CrossRef]
17. Lai, K.P.; Gong, Z.; Tse, W.K.F. Zebrafish as the toxicant screening model: Transgenic and omics approaches. *Aquat. Toxicol.* **2021**, *234*, 105813. [CrossRef]
18. Zhang, B.; Yang, X.; Zhao, J.; Xu, T.; Yin, D. Studying Neurobehavioral Effects of Environmental Pollutants on Zebrafish Larvae. *J. Vis. Exp.* **2020**, *156*, e60818. [CrossRef]
19. Rodríguez, F.; Durán, E.; Gómez, A.; Ocaña, F.M.; Alvarez, E.; Jiménez-Moya, F.; Broglio, C.; Salas, C. Cognitive and emo-tional functions of the teleost fish cerebellum. *Brain Res. Bull.* **2005**, *66*, 365–370. [CrossRef]
20. Portavella, M.; Vargas, J.P. Emotional and spatial learning in goldfish is dependent on different telencephalic pallial systems. *Eur. J. Neurosci.* **2005**, *21*, 2800–2806. [CrossRef]
21. Portavella, M.; Torres, B.; Salas, C. Avoidance Response in Goldfish: Emotional and Temporal Involvement of Medial and Lateral Telencephalic Pallium. *J. Neurosci.* **2004**, *24*, 2335–2342. [CrossRef]
22. Xu, X.; Scott-Scheiern, T.; Kempker, L.; Simons, K. Active avoidance conditioning in zebrafish (*Danio rerio*). *Neurobiol. Learn. Mem.* **2007**, *87*, 72–77. [CrossRef]
23. Levin, E.D.; Chen, E. Nicotinic involvement in memory function in zebrafish. *Neurotoxicol. Teratol.* **2004**, *26*, 731–735. [CrossRef]
24. Levin, E.D.; Limpuangthip, J.; Rachakonda, T.; Peterson, M. Timing of nicotine effects on learning in zebrafish. *Psychopharmacology* **2006**, *184*, 547–552. [CrossRef]
25. Gupta, R.C.; Milatovic, D. Insecticides. In *Biomarkers in Toxicology*; Gupta, R.C., Ed.; Academic Pres: Amsterdam, The Netherlands; Elsevier: Amsterdam, The Netherlands, 2014; pp. 389–407.
26. Wang, X.; Anadón, A.; Wu, Q.; Qiao, F.; Ares, I.; Martínez-Larrañaga, M.R.; Yuan, Z.; Martínez, M.A. Mechanism of Neon-icotinoid Toxicity: Impact on Oxidative Stress and Metabolism. *Annu. Rev. Pharmacol. Toxicol.* **2018**, *58*, 471–507. [CrossRef] [PubMed]
27. Ensley, S.M. Neonicotinoids. In *Veterinary Toxicology: Basic and Clinical Principles*; Gupta, R.C., Ed.; Academic Pres: Amsterdam, The Netherlands; Elsevier: Amsterdam, The Netherlands, 2012; pp. 596–598.
28. Hsiao, C.-J.; Lin, C.-L.; Lin, T.-Y.; Wang, S.-E.; Wu, C.-H. Imidacloprid toxicity impairs spatial memory of echolocation bats through neural apoptosis in hippocampal CA1 and medial entorhinal cortex areas. *Neuroreport* **2016**, *27*, 462–468. [CrossRef] [PubMed]
29. Wu, C.-H.; Lin, C.-L.; Wang, S.-E.; Lu, C.-W. Effects of imidacloprid, a neonicotinoid insecticide, on the echolocation system of insectivorous bats. *Pestic. Biochem. Physiol.* **2020**, *163*, 94–101. [CrossRef] [PubMed]
30. Ge, W.; Yan, S.; Wang, J.; Zhu, L.; Chen, A.; Wang, J. Oxidative Stress and DNA Damage Induced by Imidacloprid in Zebrafish (*Danio rerio*). *J. Agric. Food Chem.* **2015**, *63*, 1856–1862. [CrossRef]
31. Morrissey, C.A.; Mineau, P.; Devries, J.H.; Sanchez-Bayo, F.; Liess, M.; Cavallaro, M.C.; Liber, K. Neonicotinoid contamination of global surface waters and associated risk to aquatic invertebrates: A review. *Environ. Int.* **2015**, *74*, 291–303. [CrossRef]
32. Thunnissen, N.; Lautz, L.; van Schaik, T.; Hendriks, A. Ecological risks of imidacloprid to aquatic species in the Netherlands: Measured and estimated concentrations compared to species sensitivity distributions. *Chemosphere* **2020**, *254*, 126604. [CrossRef]

life

Review

Shedding Light on the Cell Biology of Platelet-Derived Extracellular Vesicles and Their Biomedical Applications

Preeti Kumari Chaudhary †, Sanggu Kim † and Soochong Kim *

Laboratory of Veterinary Pathology and Platelet Signaling, College of Veterinary Medicine, Chungbuk National University, Cheongju 28644, Republic of Korea; chaudharypreety11@gmail.com (P.K.C.); tkdrnfld@naver.com (S.K.)
* Correspondence: skim0026@cbu.ac.kr; Tel.: +82-43-249-1846
† These authors contributed equally to this work.

Abstract: EVs are membranous subcellular structures originating from various cells, including platelets which consist of biomolecules that can modify the target cell's pathophysiological functions including inflammation, cell communication, coagulation, and metastasis. EVs, which are known to allow the transmission of a wide range of molecules between cells, are gaining popularity in the fields of subcellular treatment, regenerative medicine, and drug delivery. PEVs are the most abundant EVs in circulation, being produced by platelet activation, and are considered to have a significant role in coagulation. PEV cargo is extremely diverse, containing lipids, proteins, nucleic acids, and organelles depending on the condition that induced their release and can regulate a wide range of biological activities. PEVs, unlike platelets, can overcome tissue barriers, allowing platelet-derived contents to be transferred to target cells and organs that platelets cannot reach. Their isolation, characterization, and therapeutic efficacy, on the other hand, are poorly understood. This review summarizes the technical elements of PEV isolation and characterization methods as well as the pathophysiological role of PEVs, including therapeutic potential and translational possibility in diverse disciplines.

Keywords: platelets; PEVs; hemostasis; inflammation; angiogenesis; wound healing; carcinogenesis; therapy

check for updates

Citation: Chaudhary, P.K.; Kim, S.; Kim, S. Shedding Light on the Cell Biology of Platelet-Derived Extracellular Vesicles and Their Biomedical Applications. *Life* **2023**, *13*, 1403. https://doi.org/10.3390/life13061403

Academic Editor: Yong Weon Yi, Stefanos Roumeliotis and Giuseppe Minervini

Received: 5 May 2023
Revised: 1 June 2023
Accepted: 15 June 2023
Published: 16 June 2023

1. Introduction

EVs are membranous subcellular structures originating from various cells, including platelets through a wide range of biomechanism [1]. EVs are divided into subpopulations based on morphology, size, content, cellular origin, and the functions they perform [2]. The EVs can bundle active cargo such as proteins, nucleic acids, and lipids and convey it to a recipient cell, whether close or far away, and thus, they can modify the destination cell's pathophysiological functions including inflammation, cell communication, coagulation, and metastasis in the process [3]. EVs have enormous promise for the advancement of innovative biological treatments. Recently, EVs are being engineered as a disease-modifying biotherapy for age-related degeneration and as medication delivery vehicles for cancer, immunological, and inflammatory illnesses.

The most common type of EVs in circulation are PEVs, which are released upon activation of platelets by various factors [4]. PEVs have capabilities comparable to platelets and are thus thought to have an impact on a variety of biological processes such as coagulation, wound healing, and inflammation. PEVs have been shown to stimulate cellular differentiation, hence improving musculoskeletal or neurological regeneration. Unlike platelets, PEVs can pass across tissue barriers, extending their capabilities outside of the blood [5]. PEVs do not have legal and safety issues, can be obtained as a byproduct from whole-blood donations, bring no concerns regarding contamination or immunological reactions, and are unable to multiply because they lack a functioning nucleus. Therefore, using PEVs instead can have the desirable advantage of boosting the benefits of their clinical application. However, PEVs are poorly understood in terms of standardization, heterogeneity, repeatability, and storage conditions. It is unknown how PEVs package their machinery, transport it to other cells, and communicate between the cells in order to alter the pathophysiology of the target cells.

In this review, we summarize the technical features of PEV isolation and characterization approaches including the pathophysiological role of PEVs. In addition, this review will also look at the advantages and limitations of therapeutic applications of PEVs to grasp the fundamental needs for their clinical translation.

2. Extracellular Vesicles

EVs are lipid bilayer-delimited particles that are generated by nearly all types of cells in a normal manner but are unable to proliferate like cells. EVs are a tool for intercellular communication, facilitating the interchange of a wide variety of chemicals between nearby or far-away cells. EVs usually contain lipids, nucleic acids, and proteins, particularly those connected to the cell membrane, the cytosol, and those involved in lipid metabolism [6,7]. The diversity of cell types and functional states, as well as the various biogenetic pathways, all contribute to the variability of EVs. Exosomes, microvesicles, and apoptotic bodies are the three primary subtypes of EVs, distinguished by their biogenesis, release mechanisms, size, composition, and function [8]. As a brief explanation, exosomes are encased in a single outer membrane, typically ranging from 30 to 150 nm, released by all types of the cell through the endosomal pathway, and present in various kinds of body fluids [6,7]. Exosomal vesicles specifically originate by inward budding of early endosomes' limiting membranes, which develop into multivesicular bodies (MVBs) in the process [9]. Exosomes are engaged in the cell's endocytic and material trafficking processes, playing a part in protein sorting, recycling, storage, transport, and release, specifically [10]. Alix, TSG101, HSC70, and HSP90 are expected to be expressed by exosomes and can be used as "exosomal marker proteins" [11,12]. Exosomes frequently contain the tetraspanin proteins including CD63, CD9, and CD81. Exosomes have a role in cell-to-cell communication, cell maintenance, tumor progression, and cellular waste management, and they behave as antigen-presenting vesicles and promote immunological responses [13].

Microvesicles are EVs that develop from the cell membrane by directly outward budding, or pinching, and typically have diameters between 100 nm and 1000 nm. Microvesicles mostly contain cytosolic and cell membrane-associated proteins, such as tetraspanins. Integrins, heat shock proteins, cytoskeletal proteins, and proteins with post-translational modifications including glycosylation and phosphorylation are other proteins that are frequently found in microvesicles [14]. Initially, it was believed that microvesicles were a cellular dumping or maintenance process, similarly to exosomes, by which the cell would get rid of waste [9]. However, microvesicles are now recognized to play a role in cell–cell communication between nearby and distant cells. Likewise, dying cells discharge apoptotic bodies into the extracellular environment. According to reports, they can be as little as 50 nm or as large as 5000 nm in diameter, with most apoptotic bodies being on the larger side [15]. During cell contraction, increasing hydrostatic pressure causes the cell membrane to separate from the cytoskeleton, resulting in the generation of these apoptotic bodies [16]. Apoptotic bodies, as opposed to exosomes and microvesicles, include intact organelles, chromatin, and modest levels of glycosylated proteins [16]. So, it makes sense to anticipate seeing larger quantities of proteins associated with the nucleus, mitochondria, Golgi apparatus, and endoplasmic reticulum (such as histones), among other structures.

3. Origin of PEVs

Platelets are anucleated, discoid cells that originate from megakaryocytes in the bone marrow and circulate in the bloodstream with a physiological count of 150,000 to 450,000 platelets/μL of blood and a lifespan of 8–10 days. The resting platelet consists of alpha granules, dense granules, lysosomal granules, and glycogen granules, which contain various kinds of proteins, growth factors, angiogenic factors, chemokines, immune mediators, etc. that are involved in various pathophysiological activities of the platelet (Table 1) [17]. The activation of platelets leads to the development of hemostasis and thrombosis. Upon vascular injury, von Willebrand Factor (vWF) and collagen become exposed to the extracellular matrix which binds with their respective receptors present in the platelet and activates the platelet. The activated platelet releases adenosine diphosphate (ADP) and generates thromboxane A_2, which further recruits the circulating platelet in the bloodstream, activates them, and forms the hemostatic plug by converting fibrinogen to fibrin in the presence of thrombin.

Under normal circumstances, the circulating microvesicles found in the plasma come mostly from megakaryocytes. However, in pathological conditions, microvesicles are produced by activated platelets. Upon activation of platelets by a variety of agonists, platelets readily generate EVs as well (cellular plasma membrane (microvesicles) or endosomal compartment (exosomes)) that remain circulating in the bloodstream. Chargaff and West initially documented PEVs as coagulant lipoproteins that were separated from platelets by differential centrifugation [18]. Shortly after, electron microscopic analyses of α-granule release from platelets also imaged small vesicles being released, which were referred to as exosomes [19,20]. Data from various electron microscopy demonstrated that depending on the type of agonist stimulation, there are two types of PEVs released: small vesicles (exosomes) with a diameter of ~40 to 100 nm that expose CD63 and are undetectable by flow cytometry, and larger vesicles (microvesicles) with a diameter of 100 to 1000 nm that expose annexin-V and express αIIb-β3 and β1, GP1bα, and P-selectin, which enables Factor X and prothrombin [14,21]. It is widely acknowledged that megakaryocytes and platelets are the main sources of EVs in blood circulation [22,23]. Another research demonstrated the first proof that PEVs may have both pro- and anti-coagulatory effects, even though PEVs had previously only been linked to procoagulant activity [24]. Now, PEV cargo is considered to be highly diverse consisting of proteins, growth factors, nucleic acids, and organelles that are present in the platelet itself (as shown in Table 1) and are engaged in diverse biological activities in different cell types. PEVs can infiltrate into various organs and tissues where they contribute to more distant cellular communication. This makes it possible to deliver platelet-derived material to cells and organs that platelets cannot reach.

Table 1. Various chemical modulators present in platelets.

Location	Type	Chemical Modulators	References
	Adhesive proteins	P-selectin Fibrinogen Von Willebrand factor Fibronectin Thrombospondin-1 Thrombospondin-2 Laminin-8 Vitronectin	[25–31]
	Growth factors	EGF IGF-1 HGF TGF-β PDGF	[32–36]
	Angiogenic factors	VEGF PDGF FGF	[37–39]
α-granules	Chemokines	CXCL1/2/5/6/7/8/12 CCL2/3/5/7 (RANTES) IL1β CD40L Proteases	[40–50]

Table 1. *Cont.*

Location	Type	Chemical Modulators	References
	Coagulation factors	Factor V Protein S Factor XI Factor XIII Kininogens Plasminogen	[51–56]
	Integral membrane proteins	Integrin αIIbβ3 GPIba-IX-V GPVI TLT-1 P-selectin	[25,57–60]
	Immune mediators	Complement C3/C4 precursor Factor D/H C1 inhibitor Immunoglobulins	[61–65]
	Protease inhibitors	α2-antiplasmin PAI-1 α2-antitrypsin α2-macroglobulin TFPI C1-inhibitor	[64,66–70]
	Proteoglycans	MMP2, MMP9	[71]
Dense granules	Amines	Serotonin Histamine	[72,73]
	Bivalent cations	Ca^{2+} Mg^{2+}	
	Nucleotides Polyphosphates	ATP ADP GTP GDP	

EGF: epidermal growth factor; IGF-1: insulin-like growth factor 1; HGF: hepatocyte growth factor; TGF-β: transforming growth factor-β; PDGF: platelet-derived growth factor; VEGF: vascular-endothelial growth factor; FGF: fibroblast growth factor; PAI-1: plasminogen activator inhibitor-1; TFPI: tissue factor inhibitor; MMP: matrix metalloprotease.

4. Isolation and Detection of Platelet-Derived Extracellular Vesicles

While there are several PEV isolation techniques that have been invented, the lack of consistent and optimum techniques is a significant barrier to introducing exosomes in the clinical and experimental field. Most of the PEV isolation methods are divided into platelet isolation and PEV isolation. Platelets must be very pure at this time, so not only simple centrifugation methods but also a 10–17% iodixanol gradient or leukocyte reduction filtration by PVC-citrate storage bag are used to isolate completely pure platelets [23,74]. Additionally, PEVs can be isolated from platelet lysate [75,76], platelet derivatives, and plasma [77]. After that, platelets can be completely activated not only with platelet agonists including collagen, thrombin, collagen-related peptide (CRP), ADP, and thrombin receptor-activating peptide (TRAP)-6, but also with lipopolysaccharide (LPS), Ca^{2+} ionophore, and LPS-binding protein [23]. The most commonly known method is the centrifugation technique, which obtains PEVs from the supernatant from which platelets and cell debris have been removed through centrifugation. This technique can also separate various types of EVs such as microvesicles and exosomes by adding more steps of centrifugation. However, it has been known that high-speed centrifugation should be used with precaution because it can affect the concentration of EVs, their size, or their biochemical composition via the generation of EV aggregates [78]. In addition, gel-filtration via size-exclusion chromatography, immunoaffinity chromatography using disk with anti-human CD61 antibody [77], and/or anti-CD-41, CD63, CD9, and CD81 antibody-covered beads can be applied to further separate the desired PEVs [74,75,79,80]. Although it is not currently applied to PEV isolation, precipitation is known to be used as a technique for EV isolation and purification in several other cells [81]. Detailed PEV preparation conditions that can be applied are mentioned in Table 2.

Table 2. Various PEV preparation conditions used to date [23,75–77,80,82–84].

Method of Isolation	Approaches	Advantages	Disadvantages
Platelet activation	**Activation for 30 min** - Thrombin 1 U/mL - Collagen 10 μg/mL - CRP-XL 1 μg/mL - ADP 60 μM - TRAP-6 10 μM - Thrombin 1 U/mL + collagen 10 μg/mL - Ca^{2+} ionophore 10 μM **Activation for 3 h** - LPS 100 ng/mL - LBP 100 ng/mL - CD14 100 ng/mL **Activation by $CaCl_2$**	- Characteristically different types of PEVs can be produced - Enhances PEVs release	- Lower procoagulant activity - Expensive
Centrifugation	**PEV preparation** - 800–5000× *g* for 5 min–30 min **Purification** - 20,000× *g* for 60 min **Microvesicle pellet preparation** - 2500–12,000× *g* for 15 min–60 min **Exosome pellet preparation** - 20,000–120,000× *g* 40 min–18 h	- Cost efficient - Pure preparation	- Low reproducibility - Possibility of exosomes damage
Membrane filtration	**PEV preparation** - 0.2 μm pore membrane filtration **PEV purification** - 0.8 μm pore membrane filtration	- Simple procedure - Process many samples at the same time - Pure preparation	- Deformation of vesicles (less exosomal proteins)
Gel filtration (size exclusion chromatography)	**Further isolation** - Isolating 0.5 mL of 26 fraction, harvest fraction 9–12 - Isolating 24–30 fraction	- High reproducibility - Pure preparation - Preserves vesicle integrity - Prevent PEV aggregation	- Need specialized equipment - Expensive
Immunoaffinity chromatography	**Further isolation** - Filtering sample with the disk with anti-human CD61 antibody at a flow rate of 0.5 mL/min repeated five times.	- Fast and easy - Enrichment of hundred to thousand-fold	- Expensive
Iodixanol density gradient	**Further isolation** - Collect the band from the 30% and 10% interface	- Pure preparations without viral particles	- Sample loss - Unable to separate large particles with similar sedimentation rates
Immuno-bead capturing	**Further isolation** - Incubate sample with Anti-CD63, CD9, and CD81 antibody covered beads	- High reproducibility - Pure preparation	- Not suitable for large-volume samples

5. Analysis and Detection of Platelet Extracellular Vesicles

After the preparation of the PEVs, several analyses are applied for confirmation and characterization of them. One of the most commonly used methods is nanoparticle tracking analysis (NTA). This method gives the position, vesicle concentration, and size of particles suspended in a fluid by detecting the light they scatter [85]. It can detect nanoparticles ranging from 10 nm to 2000 nm. However, particles smaller than 50 nm are not well identified, and contaminants in the sample such as protein aggregates and cell fragments can be detected. In this case, utilizing 0.02 μm filtration or immuno-labeling the particle can specify the target particles [86]. Dynamic light scattering (DLS), a method similar to NTA, estimates scattering intensity from bulk samples, unlike NTA. The main advantage of DLS is that it can measure particles ranging from 1 nm to 6 μm. However, purification is still required because the data can only be trusted if just there is the presence of one sort of particle [87]. Flow cytometry, a method of detecting, counting, and sorting single-file passage targets using a laser beam, is another approach often employed in EV analysis [88]. This approach has the advantage of determining the absolute number of particles, although it only detects particles over 200 nm and frequently detects many vesicles as one when concentrations are high (swarming effect) [89]. Furthermore, electron microscopes are utilized for PEV detection, and not only the size of the vesicle but also its exact form can be viewed through direct measurement, but structural damage may be occurred through high surface tension during evaporation of water [90]. There are many additional approaches, such as tunable resistive pulse sensing, atomic force microscopy, and mass spectrometry, but it is important to evaluate based on the purpose and size of the target.

6. PEVs in Health and Diseases

PEVs have been associated with both noninfectious chronic inflammatory diseases (e.g., atherosclerosis, diabetes, coronary artery disease, and hypertension) and infectious diseases (e.g., influenza and COVID-19) as well as other pathophysiology. The diverse roles of PEVs in various fields are shown in Figure 1 and are summarized below:

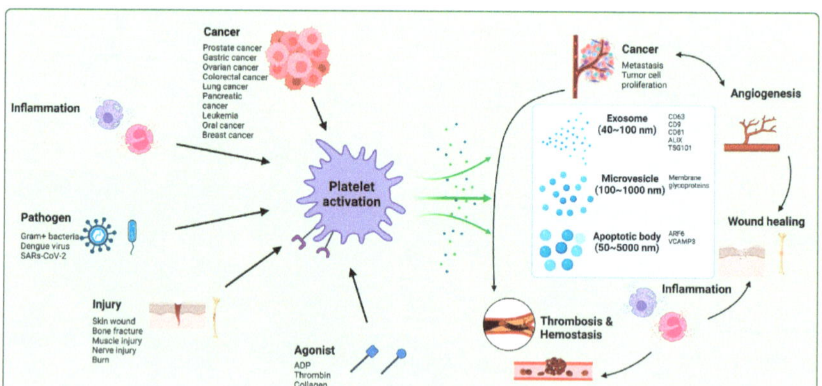

Figure 1. The effect of PEVs in diverse pathophysiological processes. Activation of platelet by various stimuli including cancer, inflammation, pathogens, and injury leads to the release of EVs: exosomes, microvesicles, and apoptotic body The EVs can bundle active cargo such as proteins, nucleic acids, and lipids and convey it to a recipient cell, whether close or far away; thus, they can modify the destination cell's pathophysiological functions including inflammation, cell communication, angiogenesis, coagulation, and metastasis in the process. "Created with BioRender.com".

6.1. *PEVs in Hemostasis, Coagulation, and Hemorrhagic Shock*

Worldwide, trauma is responsible for more than 500,000 deaths each year, and severe hemorrhage leading to trauma-induced coagulopathy (TIC) characterizes the majority of these cases [91]. Platelet and plasma therapy have been shown to decrease hemorrhage-associated mortality in TIC patients [92]. One of the known primary activities assigned to platelet EVs is coagulation [4,18]. The surface of circulating PEVs has been shown to be 50–100-fold more procoagulant than activated platelets [93]. Negatively charged phosphatidylserine and tissue factor (TF) exposed to the surface of PEVs have been substantially attributed to their pro-coagulant activities. PEVs express binding sites for coagulation factors such as activated factor V and factor VIII as well as thrombin [93–95]. EV clearance was recently demonstrated to be aided by coating PS with lactadherin, which reduced coagulopathy and improved survival in a traumatic brain injury mouse model [96]. PEVs produce activated protein C, which is known to be involved coagulation process [24]. Following severe trauma, treatment with PEVs has been shown to enhance hemostasis, stop blood loss, and slow the development of hemorrhagic shock [85]. Since platelets cannot be kept and must be utilized within five days of withdrawal, PEV preparation clearly outperforms platelet transfusion in terms of storage. Investigating plasma proteins, blood cells, and the endothelium is important to have a thorough grasp of the hemodynamic physiology of PEVs. Taken together, although platelets and PEVs have numerous functional similarities, including a strong procoagulant capacity, PEVs may be a better option for hemostasis. However, before these encouraging results can be applied to clinical practice, more study is required to characterize the PEV isolates in greater detail. Investigating the interaction between proteins and cells present in the blood, and the endothelium is important to have a thorough grasp of hemodynamic physiology. By doing so, we can explore the dynamics of the biomarkers and have the opportunity to gauge the treatment's immediate impact on coagulation.

6.2. PEVs in Immune Response and Inflammation

PEVs have a significant effect on the pathophysiology of the immune system by increasing in quantity or changing granule contents. PEV is released by platelet activation mediated by platelet agonists in a physiologic state and inflammation and/or infection in a pathologic state [97,98]. Various viruses trigger the release of PEV, of which dengue virus induces PEV release through c-type lectin (CLEC)-2 of the platelet [99]. Additionally, COVID-19 has recently been found to induce PEV release through CLEC-2 [100] and elevate $PF4^+$ and $HMGF1^+$ PEVs, which are elevated in sepsis [101,102]. It is known that several Gram-positive bacteria increase the release of EVs, but this has not been elucidated in PEVs [103]. Generated PEVs are involved in a variety of immune-related pathways, and they interact with mononuclear cells more than other inflammatory cells. PEVs can deposit inflammatory mediators such as CCL5 onto the endothelium surface, resulting in the recruitment of mononuclear cells during rolling [104]. Additionally, PEVs increased the adhesion of monocytes to endothelial cells by arachidonic acid and protein kinase C activation in a time- and dose-dependent manner [105]. In addition, PEVs bind to monocytes via p-selectin-p-selectin glycoprotein ligands-1, and this is sustained by phosphatidylserine binding, at which GPIbα transfers to the monocyte, which is recruited into the blood vessel and stimulate angiogenesis [106]. Additionally, PEVs have the ability to change the distribution of monocyte subsets towards intermediate $CD14^+$ $CD16^+$ monocytes with inflammatory properties [107]. PEVs also can significantly increase the expression of MMP 9, hydrogen peroxide, and pro-inflammatory factors, including C5a and tumor necrosis factor (TNF) [108]. PEV is also known to interact with several other inflammatory cells. Recently, PEVs have been known to interact with T-lymphocyte [109]. PEVs induced the differentiation of naive $CD4^+$ T Cells into $Foxp3^+$ regulatory T cells by TGF-β, and they induced immunosuppressive response by decreasing the release of IFNr, TNFα, and IL-6 [110]. Furthermore, unlike platelets, PEVs circulate in lymph and express MHC-1 to perform co-activation with lymphocytes via CD40L and OX40L [111]. However, the role of PEVs in T-lymphocyte, including proliferation, differentiation, and cytokine production, needs further research [109]. Additionally, it is known that PEVs can enhance inflammatory response by capturing and activating neutrophils and endothelial cells to promote interaction [112]. In particular, PEVs worsen the symptoms by activating neutrophils through heterocomplexes of TLR2 and CLEC5a [99], and they increase the activity of EV-TF [113]. PEVs eventually induce a number of diseases, including rheumatoid arthritis (RA) and systemic lupus erythematosus (SLE). PEVs in RA enter the lymphatic system and influence joint vascular leakage via the fibrinogen receptor αIIbβ3 and serotonin [114]. A high number of influxed microvesicles, the majority of which carried the platelet marker CD41a, were found in synovial fluid from an RA patient and stimulated monocyte adhesion to the endothelium, thus increasing the ICAM-1 in monocytes [115,116]. In addition, presence of intra-vesicular arachidonic acid in PEVs increases monocyte adhesion to endothelial cells, which further transfers the lipids and lipid metabolism in cells, eventually inducing atherosclerosis and inflammation [117]. Furthermore, PEVs promote inflammation through serotonin and IL-1 in SLE an autoimmune disease, as well as RA [118,119]. PEVs also can spread infection by delivering functional viral RNA from cell to cell in several viral infections [120,121]. As a result, PEVs are intimately linked to immunity, including release by immune-mediated disease, interaction with inflammatory cells, and expression of immune-mediated disease symptoms.

6.3. PEVs in Angiogenesis and Wound Healing

PEVs can indirectly increase angiogenesis in the inflammatory induction and the subsequent hypoxic condition in the vascular injury [122]. However, PEVs further induce angiogenesis through various mechanisms. PEVs are known to secrete various angiogenic growth factors including lipid growth factors (sphingosine-1-phosphate) [123] RANTES [124] and several growth factors (VEGF, FGF-2, bFBF, PDGF, TFG-beta, EGF, hybridoma growth factor, MMP-2, MMP-9) [123,125–128]. Increased VEGF, FGF-2, and lipid growth factors induce endothelial progenitor cells differentiation, endothelial proliferation, chemotaxis, tube formation, and stimulating resident mature endothelial cells via PTX-sensitive G protein, extracellular signal-regulated kinase, phosphoinositide 3-kinases, AKT, and Src kinase activation [123,125–127,129]. Furthermore, PEVs amplify the vaso-regenerative potential of endothelial progenitor cells (EPCs) and support the maintenance of vascular integrity after arterial injury through recruitment, migration, and differentiation via CXCR4 sensitization and by providing CD31, vWF, and lectin phenotype of EPCs [129,130]. PEVs also contain angiogenic microRNAs (miRNAs), including miR-320, miR-25, and miR-126. Among these, miR-126 has the ability to down-regulate vascular cell adhesion molecule-1 upon the VEGF, thereby contributing to endothelial migration and proliferation [131]. The angiogenic effect of PEV changes in several disease conditions. PEVs in patients with pulmonary arterial hypertension induced more transcription and translation of VEGF-A, and FGF, further promoting endothelial cell activation through escape lysosomal degradation [132]. In addition, the PEVs improve the process of revascularization in ischemic myocardium [125]. On the other hand, Nitric oxide (NO) and bacterial elements can trigger the PEV release and further induce caspase-3 activation and apoptosis of target endothelial cells through active ROS/RNS generation by NADPH oxidase and NO synthase via redox-signaling pathway type II in sepsis [133,134]. In addition, PEVs secreted from PM2.5 (fine dust)-exposed platelets significantly reduced the proliferation of vascular endothelium by changing miRNAs level, decreasing the effective angiogenic factors and increasing proinflammatory factors (ICAM-1, IL-6, and TNF-a), ROS level, and apoptosis (up-regulation of cytochrome-C, BAX, and cleaved caspase-3, and down-regulation of Bcl-2) [135]. As a result, PEVs can be an effective therapeutic target in a certain disease state, and they can also be a candidate for investigating delayed or augmented angiogenesis in numerous diseases with unknown angiogenesis mechanisms.

6.4. PEVs in Carcinogenesis

PEVs are influenced by tumor cells and, in turn, influence tumor cells by various mechanisms in different tumor cell types. It is known that PEVs are increased by several types of tumors including tumor including prostate cancer [136,137], gastric cancer [138], ovarian cancer [139], colorectal cancer [140–142], lung cancer [143], pancreatic cancer [141], acute lymphoblastic leukemia, oral squamous cell carcinoma [144], and breast cancer [145]. Increased PEVs raise the level of factors, such as VEGF, IL-6, RANTET, fibrinogen, and TNF-α, which increases metastasis and cancer grade [138,144], and eventually, this significantly reduces median survival time [136]. This increase in PEVs is especially pronounced in the presence of a large tumor, distant metastases, or invasiveness [145]. In addition, the increase in D-dimer may have come from an increase in PEVs, which promotes thrombosis [137,139,140]. All of these tumor-induced PEV alterations are also seen in proteomics. Increased HLA and PSMD2 levels in PEVs derived from colorectal cancer patients promote immune response, and an increase in HLA elevates platelet activity, resulting in accelerated carcinogenesis [142]. However, further research is needed to determine whether the increase in PEVs number is the result of chemotherapy [136,143,146,147].

On the other hand, PEVs also affect tumor cells. PEVs enhance tumor cell invasion by stimulating MMP-2 synthesis and secretion [148]. PEVs transfer CD41 to lung cancer and induce the phosphorylation of mitogen-activated protein kinase (MAPK) p42/44, serine/threonine kinases, and membrane type 1-matrix metalloproteinase (MT1-MMP), which stimulate proliferation, upregulate cyclin D2 expression, and increase trans-Matrigel chemo-invasion [149]. Furthermore, PEVs stimulate mRNA expression of angiogenic factors, including MMP-9, VEGF, IL-8, and HGF, which promote lung cancer metastasis. Additionally, miR-939 in PEVs increases the migration, proliferation, and expression of molecules associated with epithelial–mesenchymal transition in epithelial ovarian cancer mediated by sPLA$_2$-IIa [150]. Tropomyosin 3 (TPM3) mRNA, which has been associated with metastasis in breast cancer, significantly increases the platelet of breast cancer patients, which transmit TPM3 mRNA to breast cancer through PEVs, giving breast cancer a migrative phenotype [151]. Moreover, PEVs aggregate breast cancer cells, bind and internalize to the breast cancer cell, and stimulate migration and invasion via phosphorylating p38 MAPK and myosin light chain [152]. PEVs from colorectal cancer patients accelerate metastasis by increasing EMT markers TWIST1 and VIM in the colorectal cancer cell line, as well as enhancing COX2 and TxA2 generation to promote cancer development [142]. In addition, colorectal cancer cell line acquired the capacity to produce 12-HETE from PEVs generated from platelet type 12-LOX, which is detected in adenoma or adenocarcinoma patients [153]. Furthermore, EMT genes expression are suppressed by 12-LOX inhibitors, suggesting that they can be utilized as a treatment for cancer. However, PEVs can suppress the growth of lung and colon carcinomas by miR-24 by inhibiting mitochondrial noncoding small nucleolar RNA mt-Nd2 and Snora75 [154]. PEVs also inhibit the expression of the EMT marker CDH1 [142]. Not only the characteristics of each tumor by PEVs but also the contradictory findings of PEVs on tumor growth should be thoroughly investigated in order to identify the mechanisms and efficient treatment of the tumor in the future.

7. Therapeutic Applications and Future Perspectives of PEVs

PEVs are bioproduct that have recently been used in regenerative medicine through their functions including inflammation, hemostasis, angiogenesis, and cell proliferation, and it is gaining attention dues to their efficiency more than platelets [155]. In addition, the research has not been thoroughly conducted, and thus, possibilities in various fields are expected. In breast cancer cell lines (MDA-MB-231, SKBR3, and BT474 but not MCF-7 cells), PEVs efficiently interact with all except MCF-7 [156]. Similarly, in rheumatic arthritis, platelet exosome displays antigens that are detected by rheumatic arthritis-specific autoantibodies [157]. In the case of a COVID-19 patient, proteins linked to cardiovascular disease and pro-thrombotic/endothelial damage factors were elevated in EVs from severe cases. However, in moderate cases, levels of TF, CD163, and EN-RAGE were lower compared to severe cases [157]. Thus, if proteomic and genomic profiling of PEVs is completed, it can serve as a biomarker. Furthermore, PEVs can bind with integrin and membrane glycoproteins such as GPIIbIIIa (CD41/CD61 or integrin αIIbβ3), GPIaIIa (CD49b/CD29), GPIba (CD42b), P-selectin (CD62P), platelet endothelial cell adhesion molecule-1 (CD31), and GP53, allowing us to employ it in drug delivery. Additionally, since cells inhibit apoptosis by exporting their intracellular caspase-3 through EVs to perform waste management, platelet homeostasis research can be undertaken by controlling PEV release [158]. Moreover, it has been known that cells secrete viral DNA and RNA via EV in a viral infection state, and thus, it will be available as an identifying mechanism for spreading and as a new virucidal target [159,160]. In addition, PEVs are taken up by cancer cells, causing them to produce corresponding substances by transferring molecules (as discussed earlier) [153]. Beyond just drug delivery, this mechanism can provide a new approach to preventing or improving various pathological conditions. However, there are many hurdles to using these PEVs in clinical practice. PEVs derived from optimized preparation from blood without blood-related infectious diseases should be treated with appropriate treatment methods and should be kept for a long time without degradation. Additionally, we should know exactly in which diseases PEVs should not be utilized.

Author Contributions: Conceptualization, S.K. (Soochong Kim), P.K.C. and S.K. (Sanggu Kim); validation, S.K. (Soochong Kim); investigation, P.K.C. and S.K. (Sanggu Kim); writing—original draft, P.K.C. and S.K. (Sanggu Kim); writing—review and editing, S.K. (Soochong Kim); supervision, S.K. (Soochong Kim). All authors have read and agreed to the published version of the manuscript.

Funding: This research was funded by National Research Foundation of Korea (NRF-2022R1A2C1003638), the Basic Research Lab Program (2022R1A4A1025557) through the NRF of Korea funded by the Ministry of Science and ICT, the Korea Institute of Planning and Evaluation for Technology in Food, Agriculture, Forestry and Fisheries (IPET) through Agriculture, Food and Rural Affairs Convergence Technologies Program for Educating Creative Global Leader, funded by Ministry of Agriculture, Food and Rural Affairs (MAFRA; 320005-4), and the National IT Industry Promotion Agency (NIPA) of Korea grant funded by the Korea government (MSIT) (S2005-22-1031).

Institutional Review Board Statement: Not applicable.

Informed Consent Statement: Not applicable.

Data Availability Statement: Data is contained within the article.

Conflicts of Interest: The authors declare no conflict of interest.

Abbreviations

EV	Extracellular vesicle
PEV	Platelet-derived extracellular vesicle
vWF	Von Willebrand factor
ADP	Adenosine diphosphate
EGF	Epidermal growth factor
IGF-1	Insulin-like growth factor-1
HGF	Hepatocyte growth factor
TGF-β	Transforming growth factor-β
PDGF	Platelet-derived growth factor
VEGF	Vascular-endothelium growth factor
FGF	Fibroblast growth factor
PAI-1	Plasminogen activator inhibitor-1
TFPI	Tissue factor inhibitor
MMP	Matrix metalloprotease
CRP	Collagen-related protein
TRAP	Thrombin receptor-activating protein
LPS	Lipopolysaccharide
NTA	Nanoparticle Tracking Analysis
TIC	Trauma-induced coagulopathy
TF	Tissue factor
CLEC	C-type lectin
RA	Rheumatoid arthritis
SLE	Systematic lupus erythematosus
EPC	Endothelial progenitor cell

miRNAs	Micro RNAs
NO	Nitric Oxide
MAPK	Mitogen-activated kinase

References

1. Buzas, E.I.; György, B.; Nagy, G.; Falus, A.; Gay, S. Emerging role of extracellular vesicles in inflammatory diseases. *Nat. Rev. Rheumatol.* **2014**, *10*, 356–364. [CrossRef] [PubMed]
2. Théry, C.; Witwer, K.W.; Aikawa, E.; Alcaraz, M.J.; Anderson, J.D.; Andriantsitohaina, R.; Antoniou, A.; Arab, T.; Archer, F.; Atkin-Smith, G.K. Minimal information for studies of extracellular vesicles 2018 (MISEV2018): A position statement of the International Society for Extracellular Vesicles and update of the MISEV2014 guidelines. *J. Extracell. Vesicles* **2018**, *7*, 1535750. [CrossRef] [PubMed]
3. Boilard, E.; Duchez, A.-C.; Brisson, A. The diversity of platelet microparticles. *Curr. Opin. Hematol.* **2015**, *22*, 437–444. [CrossRef] [PubMed]
4. Berckmans, R.J.; Nieuwland, R.; Böing, A.N.; Romijn, F.P.; Hack, C.E.; Sturk, A. Cell-derived microparticles circulate in healthy humans and support low grade thrombin generation. *Thromb. Haemost.* **2001**, *85*, 639–649.
5. Puhm, F.; Boilard, E.; Machlus, K.R. Platelet extracellular vesicles: Beyond the blood. *Atertio. Thromb. Vasc. Biol.* **2021**, *41*, 87–96. [CrossRef]
6. Zaborowski, M.P.; Balaj, L.; Breakefield, X.O.; Lai, C.P. Extracellular vesicles: Composition, biological relevance, and methods of study. *Bioscience* **2015**, *65*, 783–797. [CrossRef]
7. Bebelman, M.P.; Smit, M.J.; Pegtel, D.M.; Baglio, S.R. Biogenesis and function of extracellular vesicles in cancer. *Pharmacol. Ther.* **2018**, *188*, 1–11. [CrossRef]
8. Veziroglu, E.M.; Mias, G.I. Characterizing extracellular vesicles and their diverse RNA contents. *Front. Genet.* **2020**, *11*, 700. [CrossRef]
9. Yáñez-Mó, M.; Siljander, P.R.-M.; Andreu, Z.; Bedina Zavec, A.; Borràs, F.E.; Buzas, E.I.; Buzas, K.; Casal, E.; Cappello, F.; Carvalho, J. Biological properties of extracellular vesicles and their physiological functions. *J. Extracell. Vesicles* **2015**, *4*, 27066. [CrossRef]
10. Guerra, K.; Ventura, M. Bioética, imigração e assistência à saúde: Tensões e convergências sobre o direito humano à saúde no Brasil na integração regional dos países. *Cad. Saúde Colet.* **2017**, *25*, 123–129. [CrossRef]
11. Morita, E.; Sandrin, V.; Chung, H.Y.; Morham, S.G.; Gygi, S.P.; Rodesch, C.K.; Sundquist, W.I. Human ESCRT and ALIX proteins interact with proteins of the midbody and function in cytokinesis. *EMBO J.* **2007**, *26*, 4215–4227. [CrossRef]
12. Géminard, C.; De Gassart, A.; Blanc, L.; Vidal, M. Degradation of AP2 during reticulocyte maturation enhances binding of hsc70 and Alix to a common site on TFR for sorting into exosomes. *Traffic* **2004**, *5*, 181–193. [CrossRef]
13. Chaput, N.; Théry, C. Exosomes: Immune properties and potential clinical implementations. *Semin Immunopathol.* **2011**, *33*, 419–440. [CrossRef]
14. Heijnen, H.F.; Schiel, A.E.; Fijnheer, R.; Geuze, H.J.; Sixma, J.J. Activated Platelets Release Two Types of Membrane Vesicles: Microvesicles by Surface Shedding and Exosomes Derived from Exocytosis of Multivesicular Bodies and α-Granules. *Blood J. Am. Soc. Hematol.* **1999**, *94*, 3791–3799.
15. Borges, F.T.; Reis, L.; Schor, N. Extracellular vesicles: Structure, function, and potential clinical uses in renal diseases. *Braz. J. Med. Biol. Res.* **2013**, *46*, 824–830. [CrossRef]
16. Wickman, G.; Julian, L.; Olson, M. How apoptotic cells aid in the removal of their own cold dead bodies. *Cell Death Differ.* **2012**, *19*, 735–742. [CrossRef]
17. Senzel, L.; Gnatenko, D.V.; Bahou, W.F. The platelet proteome. *Curr. Opin. Hematol.* **2009**, *16*, 329–333. [CrossRef]
18. Chargaff, E.; West, R. The biological significance of the thromboplastic protein of Wood. *J. Biol. Chem.* **1946**, *166*, 189–197. [CrossRef]
19. Webber, A.J.; Johnson, S.A. Platelet participation in blood coagulation aspects of hemostasis. *Am. J. Pathol.* **1970**, *60*, 19.
20. Crawford, N. The presence of contractile proteins in platelet microparticles isolated from human and animal platelet-free plasma. *Br. J. Haematol.* **1971**, *21*, 53–69. [CrossRef]
21. Sandberg, H.; Bode, A.P.; Dombrose, F.A.; Hoechli, M.; Lentz, B.R. Expression of coagulant activity in human platelets: Release of membranous vesicles providing platelet factor 1 and platelet factor 3. *Thromb. Res.* **1985**, *39*, 63–79. [CrossRef] [PubMed]
22. Flaumenhaft, R.; Dilks, J.R.; Richardson, J.; Alden, E.; Patel-Hett, S.R.; Battinelli, E.; Klement, G.L.; Sola-Visner, M.; Italiano, J.E., Jr. Megakaryocyte-derived microparticles: Direct visualization and distinction from platelet-derived microparticles. *J. Am. So. Hematol.* **2009**, *113*, 1112–1121. [CrossRef] [PubMed]
23. Aatonen, M.T.; Öhman, T.; Nyman, T.A.; Laitinen, S.; Grönholm, M.; Siljander, P.R.-M. Isolation and characterization of platelet-derived extracellular vesicles. *J. Extracell. Vesicles* **2014**, *3*, 24692. [CrossRef] [PubMed]
24. Tans, G.; Rosing, J.; Thomassen, M.C.; Heeb, M.J.; Zwaal, R.; Griffin, J.H. Comparison of anticoagulant and procoagulant activities of stimulated platelets and platelet-derived microparticles. *Blood* **1991**, *77*, 2641–2648. [CrossRef] [PubMed]
25. Hayashi, S.-i.; Watanabe, N.; Nakazawa, K.; Suzuki, J.; Tsushima, K.; Tamatani, T.; Sakamoto, S.; Isobe, M. Roles of P-selectin in inflammation, neointimal formation, and vascular remodeling in balloon-injured rat carotid arteries. *Circ. J.* **2000**, *102*, 1710–1717. [CrossRef]

26. Sørensen, B.; Tang, M.; Larsen, O.H.; Laursen, P.N.; Fenger-Eriksen, C.; Rea, C.J. The role of fibrinogen: A new paradigm in the treatment of coagulopathic bleeding. *Thromb. Res.* **2011**, *128*, S13–S16. [CrossRef]
27. Peyvandi, F.; Garagiola, I.; Baronciani, L. Role of von Willebrand factor in the haemostasis. *Blood Transfus.* **2011**, *9*, s3–s8.
28. Huveneers, S.; Truong, H.; Fässler, R.; Sonnenberg, A.; Danen, E.H. Binding of soluble fibronectin to integrin α5β1–link to focal adhesion redistribution and contractile shape. *J. Cell Sci.* **2008**, *121*, 2452–2462. [CrossRef]
29. Zhang, K.; Li, M.; Yin, L.; Fu, G.; Liu, Z. Role of thrombospondin-1 and thrombospondin-2 in cardiovascular diseases. *Int. J. Mol. Med.* **2020**, *45*, 1275–1293. [CrossRef]
30. Fujiwara, H.; Kikkawa, Y.; Sanzen, N.; Sekiguchi, K. Purification and Characterization of Human Laminin-8: Laminin-8 Stimulates Cell Adhesion and Migration through A3β1 and A6β1integrins. *J. Biol. Chem.* **2001**, *276*, 17550–17558. [CrossRef]
31. Madsen, C.D.; Ferraris, G.M.S.; Andolfo, A.; Cunningham, O.; Sidenius, N. uPAR-induced cell adhesion and migration: Vitronectin provides the key. *J. Cell Biol.* **2007**, *177*, 927–939. [CrossRef]
32. Wong, R.W.C.; Guillaud, L. The role of epidermal growth factor and its receptors in mammalian CNS. *Cytokine Growth Factor Rev.* **2004**, *15*, 147–156. [CrossRef]
33. Clemmons, D.R.; Snyder, P.; Martin, K. Physiology of Insulin-Like Growth Factor 1. Up to Date Website. 2014. Available online: https://www.uptodate.com/contents/physiology-of-insulin-like-growth-factor-1 (accessed on 21 April 2023).
34. Oliveira, A.G.; Araújo, T.G.; Carvalho, B.d.M.; Rocha, G.Z.; Santos, A.; Saad, M.J. The role of hepatocyte growth factor (HGF) in insulin resistance and diabetes. *Front. Endocrinol.* **2018**, *9*, 503. [CrossRef]
35. Nagaraj, N.S.; Datta, P.K. Targeting the transforming growth factor-β signaling pathway in human cancer. *Expert Opin. Investig. Drugs* **2010**, *19*, 77–91. [CrossRef]
36. Kardas, G.; Daszyńska-Kardas, A.; Marynowski, M.; Brząkalska, O.; Kuna, P.; Panek, M. Role of platelet-derived growth factor (PDGF) in asthma as an immunoregulatory factor mediating airway remodeling and possible pharmacological target. *Front. Pharmacol.* **2020**, *11*, 47. [CrossRef]
37. Niu, G.; Chen, X. Vascular endothelial growth factor as an anti-angiogenic target for cancer therapy. *Curr. Drug Targets* **2010**, *11*, 1000–1017. [CrossRef]
38. Raica, M.; Cimpean, A.M. Platelet-derived growth factor (PDGF)/PDGF receptors (PDGFR) axis as target for antitumor and antiangiogenic therapy. *Pharmaceuticals* **2010**, *3*, 572–599. [CrossRef]
39. Jia, T.; Jacquet, T.; Dalonneau, F.; Coudert, P.; Vaganay, E.; Exbrayat-Héritier, C.; Vollaire, J.; Josserand, V.; Ruggiero, F.; Coll, J.-L. FGF-2 promotes angiogenesis through a SRSF1/SRSF3/SRPK1-dependent axis that controls VEGFR1 splicing in endothelial cells. *BMC Biol.* **2021**, *19*, 173. [CrossRef]
40. Bernhard, S.; Hug, S.; Stratmann, A.E.P.; Erber, M.; Vidoni, L.; Knapp, C.L.; Thomaß, B.D.; Fauler, M.; Nilsson, B.; Ekdahl, K.N. Interleukin 8 elicits rapid physiological changes in neutrophils that are altered by inflammatory conditions. *J. Innate. Immun.* **2021**, *13*, 225–241. [CrossRef]
41. Brown, A.J.; Sepuru, K.M.; Sawant, K.V.; Rajarathnam, K. Platelet-derived chemokine CXCL7 dimer preferentially exists in the glycosaminoglycan-bound form: Implications for neutrophil–platelet crosstalk. *Front. Immunol.* **2017**, *8*, 1248. [CrossRef]
42. Sawant, K.V.; Poluri, K.M.; Dutta, A.K.; Sepuru, K.M.; Troshkina, A.; Garofalo, R.P.; Rajarathnam, K. Chemokine CXCL1 mediated neutrophil recruitment: Role of glycosaminoglycan interactions. *Sci. Rep.* **2016**, *6*, 33123. [CrossRef] [PubMed]
43. Disteldorf, E.M.; Krebs, C.F.; Paust, H.-J.; Turner, J.-E.; Nouailles, G.; Tittel, A.; Meyer-Schwesinger, C.; Stege, G.; Brix, S.; Velden, J. CXCL5 drives neutrophil recruitment in TH17-mediated GN. *Clin. J. Am. Soc. Nephrol.* **2015**, *26*, 55–66. [CrossRef] [PubMed]
44. Wang, G.; Huang, W.; Wang, S.; Wang, J.; Cui, W.; Zhang, W.; Lou, A.; Geng, S.; Li, X. Macrophagic Extracellular Vesicle CXCL2 Recruits and Activates the Neutrophil CXCR2/PKC/NOX4 Axis in Sepsis. *J. Immunol. Res.* **2021**, *207*, 2118–2128. [CrossRef] [PubMed]
45. Jovic, S.; Linge, H.; Shikhagaie, M.; Olin, A.; Lannefors, L.; Erjefält, J.; Mörgelin, M.; Egesten, A. The neutrophil-recruiting chemokine GCP-2/CXCL6 is expressed in cystic fibrosis airways and retains its functional properties after binding to extracellular DNA. *Mucosal Immunol.* **2016**, *9*, 112–123. [CrossRef] [PubMed]
46. Isles, H.M.; Herman, K.D.; Robertson, A.L.; Loynes, C.A.; Prince, L.R.; Elks, P.M.; Renshaw, S.A. The CXCL12/CXCR4 signaling axis retains neutrophils at inflammatory sites in zebrafish. *Front. Immunol.* **2019**, *10*, 1784. [CrossRef]
47. Aldinucci, D.; Colombatti, A. The inflammatory chemokine CCL5 and cancer progression. *Mediators Inflamm.* **2014**, *2014*, 292376. [CrossRef]
48. Xue, M.L.; Thakur, A.; Cole, N.; Lloyd, A.; Stapleton, F.; Wakefield, D.; Willcox, M.D. A critical role for CCL2 and CCL3 chemokines in the regulation of polymorphonuclear neutrophils recruitment during corneal infection in mice. *Immunol. Cell Biol.* **2007**, *85*, 525–531. [CrossRef]
49. Ford, J.; Hughson, A.; Lim, K.; Bardina, S.V.; Lu, W.; Charo, I.F.; Lim, J.K.; Fowell, D.J. CCL7 is a negative regulator of cutaneous inflammation following Leishmania major infection. *Front. Immunol.* **2019**, *9*, 3063. [CrossRef]
50. Kaneko, N.; Kurata, M.; Yamamoto, T.; Morikawa, S.; Masumoto, J. The role of interleukin-1 in general pathology. *Inflamm. Regen.* **2019**, *39*, 1–16. [CrossRef]
51. Lam, W.; Moosavi, L. *Physiology, Factor V*; StatPearls Publishing: Treasure Island, FL, USA, 2019.
52. Pilli, V.; Plautz, W.; Majumder, R. The journey of protein S from an anticoagulant to a signaling molecule. *JSM Biochem. Mol. Biol.* **2016**, *3*, 1014.
53. Emsley, J.; McEwan, P.A.; Gailani, D. Structure and function of factor XI. *Blood J. Am. Soc. Hematol.* **2010**, *115*, 2569–2577. [CrossRef]

54. Shaz, B.H.; Hillyer, C.D. *Transfusion Medicine and Hemostasis: Clinical and Laboratory Aspects*; Newnes: Oxford, UK, 2013.
55. Wu, Y. Contact pathway of coagulation and inflammation. *Thromb. J.* **2015**, *13*, 17. [CrossRef]
56. Baker, S.K.; Strickland, S. A critical role for plasminogen in inflammation. *J. Exp.* **2020**, *217*, e20191865. [CrossRef]
57. Albert, F.; Christopher, N.F. The platelet fibrinogen receptor: From megakaryocyte to the mortuary. *JRSM Cardiovasc. Dis.* **2012**, *1*, cvd-2012. [CrossRef]
58. Andrews, R.K.; Gardiner, E.E.; Shen, Y.; Whisstock, J.C.; Berndt, M.C. Glycoprotein Ib–IX–V. *Int. J. Biochem. Cell Biol.* **2003**, *35*, 1170–1174. [CrossRef]
59. Moroi, M.; Jung, S.M. Platelet glycoprotein VI: Its structure and function. *Thromb. Res.* **2004**, *114*, 221–233. [CrossRef]
60. Schmoker, A.M.; Pearson, L.M.P.; Cruz, C.; Flores, L.G.C.; Branfeild, S.; Torres, F.D.P.; Fonseca, K.; Cantres, Y.M.; Ramirez, C.A.S.; Melendez, L.M. Defining the TLT-1 interactome from resting and activated human platelets. *J. Proteom.* **2020**, *215*, 103638. [CrossRef]
61. Girardi, G.; Lingo, J.J.; Fleming, S.D.; Regal, J.F. Essential role of complement in pregnancy: From implantation to parturition and beyond. *Front. Immunol.* **2020**, *11*, 1681. [CrossRef]
62. Biesma, D.H.; Hannema, A.J.; van Velzen-Blad, H.; Mulder, L.; van Zwieten, R.; Kluijt, I.; Roos, D. A family with complement factor D deficiency. *J. Clin. Investig.* **2001**, *108*, 233–240. [CrossRef]
63. Ferreira, V.P.; Pangburn, M.K.; Cortés, C. Complement control protein factor H: The good, the bad, and the inadequate. *Mol. Immunol.* **2010**, *47*, 2187–2197. [CrossRef]
64. Schmaier, A.H.; Smith, P.M.; Colman, R.W. Platelet C1-inhibitor. A secreted alpha-granule protein. *J. Clin. Investig.* **1985**, *75*, 242–250. [CrossRef] [PubMed]
65. Schroeder Jr, H.W.; Cavacini, L. Structure and function of immunoglobulins. *J. Allergy Clin. Immunol.* **2010**, *125*, S41–S52. [CrossRef] [PubMed]
66. Maron, B.A.; Loscalzo, J. The role of platelets in fibrinolysis. In *Platelets*; Elsevier: Amsterdam, The Netherlands, 2007; pp. 415–430.
67. Damare, J.; Brandal, S.; Fortenberry, Y.M. Inhibition of PAI-1 antiproteolytic activity against tPA by RNA aptamers. *Nucleic Acid Ther.* **2014**, *24*, 239–249. [CrossRef] [PubMed]
68. Bergin, D.A.; Hurley, K.; McElvaney, N.G.; Reeves, E.P. Alpha-1 antitrypsin: A potent anti-inflammatory and potential novel therapeutic agent. *Arch. Immunol. Ther. Exp.* **2012**, *60*, 81–97. [CrossRef] [PubMed]
69. Borth, W. α2 "Macroglobulin, a multifunctional binding protein with targeting characteristics. *FASEB J.* **1992**, *6*, 3345–3353. [CrossRef]
70. Kato, H. Tissue factor pathway inhibitor; its structure, function and clinical significance. *Pol. J. Pharmacol.* **1996**, *48*, 67–72.
71. Cancemi, P.; Aiello, A.; Accardi, G.; Caldarella, R.; Candore, G.; Caruso, C.; Ciaccio, M.; Cristaldi, L.; Di Gaudio, F.; Siino, V. The role of matrix metalloproteinases (MMP-2 and MMP-9) in ageing and longevity: Focus on sicilian long-living individuals (LLIs). *Mediat. Inflamm.* **2020**, *2020*, 8635158. [CrossRef]
72. Duerschmied, D.; Bode, C. The role of serotonin in haemostasis. *Hämostaseologie* **2009**, *29*, 356–359.
73. Mannaioni, P.; Di Bello, M.; Raspanti, S.; Gambassi, F.; Mugnai, L.; Masini, E. Platelet histamine: Characterization of the proaggregatory effect of histamine in human platelets. *Int. Arch. Allergy. Immunol.* **1992**, *99*, 394–396. [CrossRef]
74. Boing, A.N.; van der Pol, E.; Grootemaat, A.E.; Coumans, F.A.; Sturk, A.; Nieuwland, R. Single-step isolation of extracellular vesicles by size-exclusion chromatography. *J. Extracell. Vesicles* **2014**, *3*, 23430. [CrossRef]
75. Nyam-Erdene, A.; Nebie, O.; Delila, L.; Buee, L.; Devos, D.; Chou, S.Y.; Blum, D.; Burnouf, T. Characterization and Chromatographic Isolation of Platelet Extracellular Vesicles from Human Platelet Lysates for Applications in Neuroregenerative Medicine. *ACS Biomater. Sci. Eng.* **2021**, *7*, 5823–5835. [CrossRef]
76. Antich-Rossello, M.; Forteza-Genestra, M.A.; Calvo, J.; Gaya, A.; Monjo, M.; Ramis, J.M. Platelet-derived extracellular vesicles promote osteoinduction of mesenchymal stromal cells. *Bone Joint Res.* **2020**, *9*, 667–674. [CrossRef]
77. Multia, E.; Tear, C.J.Y.; Palviainen, M.; Siljander, P.; Riekkola, M.L. Fast isolation of highly specific population of platelet-derived extracellular vesicles from blood plasma by affinity monolithic column, immobilized with anti-human CD61 antibody. *Anal. Chim. Acta* **2019**, *1091*, 160–168. [CrossRef]
78. Linares, R.; Tan, S.; Gounou, C.; Arraud, N.; Brisson, A.R. High-speed centrifugation induces aggregation of extracellular vesicles. *J. Extracell. Vesicles* **2015**, *4*, 29509. [CrossRef]
79. Aatonen, M.; Valkonen, S.; Boing, A.; Yuana, Y.; Nieuwland, R.; Siljander, P. Isolation of Platelet-Derived Extracellular Vesicles. *Methods Mol. Biol.* **2017**, *1545*, 177–188.
80. Vajen, T.; Benedikter, B.J.; Heinzmann, A.C.A.; Vasina, E.M.; Henskens, Y.; Parsons, M.; Maguire, P.B.; Stassen, F.R.; Heemskerk, J.W.M.; Schurgers, L.J.; et al. Platelet extracellular vesicles induce a pro-inflammatory smooth muscle cell phenotype. *J. Extracell. Vesicles* **2017**, *6*, 1322454. [CrossRef]
81. Van Deun, J.; Mestdagh, P.; Sormunen, R.; Cocquyt, V.; Vermaelen, K.; Vandesompele, J.; Bracke, M.; De Wever, O.; Hendrix, A. The impact of disparate isolation methods for extracellular vesicles on downstream RNA profiling. *J. Extracell. Vesicles* **2014**, *3*, 24858. [CrossRef]
82. Karimi, N.; Dalirfardouei, R.; Dias, T.; Lotvall, J.; Lasser, C. Tetraspanins distinguish separate extracellular vesicle subpopulations in human serum and plasma—Contributions of platelet extracellular vesicles in plasma samples. *J. Extracell. Vesicles* **2022**, *11*, e12213. [CrossRef]

83. Preusser, C.; Hung, L.H.; Schneider, T.; Schreiner, S.; Hardt, M.; Moebus, A.; Santoso, S.; Bindereif, A. Selective release of circRNAs in platelet-derived extracellular vesicles. *J. Extracell. Vesicles* **2018**, *7*, 1424473. [CrossRef]
84. Lopez, E.; Srivastava, A.K.; Burchfield, J.; Wang, Y.W.; Cardenas, J.C.; Togarrati, P.P.; Miyazawa, B.; Gonzalez, E.; Holcomb, J.B.; Pati, S.; et al. Platelet-derived- Extracellular Vesicles Promote Hemostasis and Prevent the Development of Hemorrhagic Shock. *Sci. Rep.* **2019**, *9*, 17676. [CrossRef]
85. Boyd, R.D.; Pichaimuthu, S.K.; Cuenat, A. New approach to inter-technique comparisons for nanoparticle size measurements; using atomic force microscopy, nanoparticle tracking analysis and dynamic light scattering. *Colloids Surf. A. Physicochem.* **2011**, *387*, 35–42. [CrossRef]
86. Comfort, N.; Cai, K.; Bloomquist, T.R.; Strait, M.D.; Ferrante, A.W., Jr.; Baccarelli, A.A. Nanoparticle Tracking Analysis for the Quantification and Size Determination of Extracellular Vesicles. *J. Vis. Exp.* **2021**, *169*, e62447.
87. Szatanek, R.; Baj-Krzyworzeka, M.; Zimoch, J.; Lekka, M.; Siedlar, M.; Baran, J. The Methods of Choice for Extracellular Vesicles (EVs) Characterization. *Int. J. Mol. Sci.* **2017**, *18*, 1153. [CrossRef] [PubMed]
88. Van der Pol, E.; Coumans, F.A.; Grootemaat, A.E.; Gardiner, C.; Sargent, I.L.; Harrison, P.; Sturk, A.; van Leeuwen, T.G.; Nieuwland, R. Particle size distribution of exosomes and microvesicles determined by transmission electron microscopy, flow cytometry, nanoparticle tracking analysis, and resistive pulse sensing. *J. Thromb. Haemost.* **2014**, *12*, 1182–1192. [CrossRef] [PubMed]
89. Van Der Pol, E.; Van Gemert, M.; Sturk, A.; Nieuwland, R.; Van Leeuwen, T. Single vs. swarm detection of microparticles and exosomes by flow cytometry. *J. Thromb. Haemost.* **2012**, *10*, 919–930. [CrossRef]
90. Malenica, M.; Vukomanovic, M.; Kurtjak, M.; Masciotti, V.; Dal Zilio, S.; Greco, S.; Lazzarino, M.; Krusic, V.; Percic, M.; Jelovica Badovinac, I.; et al. Perspectives of Microscopy Methods for Morphology Characterisation of Extracellular Vesicles from Human Biofluids. *Biomedicines* **2021**, *9*, 603. [CrossRef]
91. Thetford, C.; Myers, L. Establishing a Regional Trauma Preventable/Potentially Preventable Death Rate. *Ann. Surg.* **2018**, 1–8.
92. Holcomb, J.B.; Tilley, B.C.; Baraniuk, S.; Fox, E.E.; Wade, C.E.; Podbielski, J.M.; del Junco, D.J.; Brasel, K.J.; Bulger, E.M.; Callcut, R.A. Transfusion of plasma, platelets, and red blood cells in a 1: 1: 1 vs a 1: 1: 2 ratio and mortality in patients with severe trauma: The PROPPR randomized clinical trial. *Jama* **2015**, *313*, 471–482. [CrossRef]
93. Sinauridze, E.I.; Kireev, D.A.; Popenko, N.Y.; Pichugin, A.V.; Panteleev, M.A.; Krymskaya, O.V.; Ataullakhanov, F.I. Platelet microparticle membranes have 50-to 100-fold higher specific procoagulant activity than activated platelets. *J. Thromb. Haemost.* **2007**, *97*, 425–434.
94. Kerris, E.W.; Hoptay, C.; Calderon, T.; Freishtat, R.J. Platelets and platelet extracellular vesicles in hemostasis and sepsis. *J. Investig. Med.* **2020**, *68*, 813–820. [CrossRef]
95. Gardiner, C.; Harrison, P.; Belting, M.; Böing, A.; Campello, E.; Carter, B.S.; Collier, M.E.; Coumans, F.; Ettelaie, C.; van Es, N. Extracellular vesicles, tissue factor, cancer and thrombosis–discussion themes of the ISEV 2014 Educational Day. *J. Extracell. Vesicles* **2015**, *4*, 26901. [CrossRef]
96. Zhou, Y.; Cai, W.; Zhao, Z.; Hilton, T.; Wang, M.; Yeon, J.; Liu, W.; Zhang, F.; Shi, F.-D.; Wu, X. Lactadherin promotes microvesicle clearance to prevent coagulopathy and improves survival of severe TBI mice. *J. Am. Soc. Hematol.* **2018**, *131*, 563–572. [CrossRef]
97. Raeven, P.; Zipperle, J.; Drechsler, S. Extracellular vesicles as markers and mediators in sepsis. *Theranostics* **2018**, *8*, 3348–3365. [CrossRef]
98. Cappellano, G.; Raineri, D.; Rolla, R.; Giordano, M.; Puricelli, C.; Vilardo, B.; Manfredi, M.; Cantaluppi, V.; Sainaghi, P.P.; Castello, L.; et al. Circulating Platelet-Derived Extracellular Vesicles Are a Hallmark of SARS-CoV-2 Infection. *Cells* **2021**, *10*, 85. [CrossRef]
99. Sung, P.S.; Huang, T.F.; Hsieh, S.L. Extracellular vesicles from CLEC2-activated platelets enhance dengue virus-induced lethality via CLEC5A/TLR2. *Nat. Commun.* **2019**, *10*, 2402. [CrossRef]
100. Sung, P.S.; Hsieh, S.L. C-type lectins and extracellular vesicles in virus-induced NETosis. *J. Biomed. Sci.* **2021**, *28*, 46. [CrossRef]
101. Sartori, M.T.; Zurlo, C.; Bon, M.; Bertomoro, A.; Bendo, R.; Bertozzi, I.; Radu, C.M.; Campello, E.; Simioni, P.; Fabris, F. Platelet-Derived Microparticles Bearing PF4 and Anti-GAGS Immunoglobulins in Patients with Sepsis. *Diagnostics* **2020**, *10*, 627. [CrossRef]
102. Maugeri, N.; De Lorenzo, R.; Clementi, N.; Antonia Diotti, R.; Criscuolo, E.; Godino, C.; Tresoldi, C.; Angels for COVID-Bio, B.S.G.B.; Bonini, C.; Clementi, M.; et al. Unconventional CD147-dependent platelet activation elicited by SARS-CoV-2 in COVID-19. *J. Thromb. Haemost.* **2022**, *20*, 434–448. [CrossRef]
103. Bose, S.; Aggarwal, S.; Singh, D.V.; Acharya, N. Extracellular vesicles: An emerging platform in gram-positive bacteria. *Microb. Cell* **2020**, *7*, 312–322. [CrossRef]
104. Mause, S.F.; von Hundelshausen, P.; Zernecke, A.; Koenen, R.R.; Weber, C. Platelet microparticles: A transcellular delivery system for RANTES promoting monocyte recruitment on endothelium. *Arterioscler. Thromb. Vasc. Biol.* **2005**, *25*, 1512–1518. [CrossRef]
105. Barry, O.P.; Pratico, D.; Savani, R.C.; FitzGerald, G.A. Modulation of monocyte-endothelial cell interactions by platelet microparticles. *J. Clin. Investig.* **1998**, *102*, 136–144. [CrossRef] [PubMed]
106. Chimen, M.; Evryviadou, A.; Box, C.L.; Harrison, M.J.; Hazeldine, J.; Dib, L.H.; Kuravi, S.J.; Payne, H.; Price, J.M.J.; Kavanagh, D.; et al. Appropriation of GPIbalpha from platelet-derived extracellular vesicles supports monocyte recruitment in systemic inflammation. *Haematologica* **2020**, *105*, 1248–1261. [CrossRef] [PubMed]

107. Lee, S.J.; Yoon, B.R.; Kim, H.Y.; Yoo, S.J.; Kang, S.W.; Lee, W.W. Activated Platelets Convert CD14(+)CD16(-) Into CD14(+)CD16(+) Monocytes with Enhanced FcgammaR-Mediated Phagocytosis and Skewed M2 Polarization. *Front. Immunol.* **2020**, *11*, 611133. [CrossRef] [PubMed]
108. Vasina, E.M.; Cauwenberghs, S.; Feijge, M.A.; Heemskerk, J.W.; Weber, C.; Koenen, R.R. Microparticles from apoptotic platelets promote resident macrophage differentiation. *Cell Death Dis.* **2011**, *2*, e211. [CrossRef]
109. Zmigrodzka, M.; Witkowska-Pilaszewicz, O.; Pingwara, R.; Winnicka, A. Platelet Extracellular Vesicles Are Taken up by Canine T Lymphocytes but Do Not Play a Role in Their Proliferation, Differentiation and Cytokine Production In Vitro. *Int. J. Mol. Sci.* **2022**, *23*, 5504. [CrossRef]
110. Sadallah, S.; Amicarella, F.; Eken, C.; Iezzi, G.; Schifferli, J.A. Ectosomes released by platelets induce differentiation of CD4+T cells into T regulatory cells. *Thromb. Haemost.* **2014**, *112*, 1219–1229.
111. Marcoux, G.; Laroche, A.; Hasse, S.; Tamagne, M.; Tessandier, N.; Becker, Y.L.C.; Zufferey, A.; Levesque, T.; Allaeys, I.; Karakeussian-Rimbaud, A.; et al. Platelet-Derived Extracellular Vesicles Actively Process Proteins and Present Antigen via MHC Class I [abstract]. *Res. Pract. Thromb. Haemost.* **2020**, *4*, 3011–3023.
112. Kuravi, S.J.; Harrison, P.; Rainger, G.E.; Nash, G.B. Ability of Platelet-Derived Extracellular Vesicles to Promote Neutrophil-Endothelial Cell Interactions. *Inflammation* **2019**, *42*, 290–305. [CrossRef]
113. Hottz, E.D.; Azevedo-Quintanilha, I.G.; Palhinha, L.; Teixeira, L.; Barreto, E.A.; Pao, C.R.R.; Righy, C.; Franco, S.; Souza, T.M.L.; Kurtz, P.; et al. Platelet activation and platelet-monocyte aggregate formation trigger tissue factor expression in patients with severe COVID-19. *Blood* **2020**, *136*, 1330–1341. [CrossRef]
114. Tessandier, N.; Melki, I.; Cloutier, N.; Allaeys, I.; Miszta, A.; Tan, S.; Milasan, A.; Michel, S.; Benmoussa, A.; Levesque, T.; et al. Platelets Disseminate Extracellular Vesicles in Lymph in Rheumatoid Arthritis. *Arterioscler. Thromb. Vasc. Biol.* **2020**, *40*, 929–942. [CrossRef]
115. Boilard, E.; Nigrovic, P.A.; Larabee, K.; Watts, G.F.; Coblyn, J.S.; Weinblatt, M.E.; Massarotti, E.M.; Remold-O'Donnell, E.; Farndale, R.W.; Ware, J.; et al. Platelets amplify inflammation in arthritis via collagen-dependent microparticle production. *Science* **2010**, *327*, 580–583. [CrossRef]
116. Rautou, P.E.; Leroyer, A.S.; Ramkhelawon, B.; Devue, C.; Duflaut, D.; Vion, A.C.; Nalbone, G.; Castier, Y.; Leseche, G.; Lehoux, S.; et al. Microparticles from human atherosclerotic plaques promote endothelial ICAM-1-dependent monocyte adhesion and transendothelial migration. *Circ. Res.* **2011**, *108*, 335–343. [CrossRef]
117. Bui, K.L.; Nyberg, A.; Maltais, F.; Saey, D. Functional Tests in Chronic Obstructive Pulmonary Disease, Part 1: Clinical Relevance and Links to the International Classification of Functioning, Disability, and Health. *Ann. Am. Thorac. Soc.* **2017**, *14*, 778–784. [CrossRef]
118. Knijff-Dutmer, E.A.; Koerts, J.; Nieuwland, R.; Kalsbeek-Batenburg, E.M.; van de Laar, M.A. Elevated levels of platelet microparticles are associated with disease activity in rheumatoid arthritis. *Arthritis Rheum.* **2002**, *46*, 1498–1503. [CrossRef]
119. Burbano, C.; Villar-Vesga, J.; Orejuela, J.; Munoz, C.; Vanegas, A.; Vasquez, G.; Rojas, M.; Castano, D. Potential Involvement of Platelet-Derived Microparticles and Microparticles Forming Immune Complexes during Monocyte Activation in Patients with Systemic Lupus Erythematosus. *Front. Immunol.* **2018**, *9*, 322. [CrossRef]
120. Valadi, H.; Ekstrom, K.; Bossios, A.; Sjostrand, M.; Lee, J.J.; Lotvall, J.O. Exosome-mediated transfer of mRNAs and microRNAs is a novel mechanism of genetic exchange between cells. *Nat. Cell Biol.* **2007**, *9*, 654–659. [CrossRef]
121. Bello-Morales, R.; Ripa, I.; Lopez-Guerrero, J.A. Extracellular Vesicles in Viral Spread and Antiviral Response. *Viruses* **2020**, *12*, 623. [CrossRef]
122. Angelo, L.S.; Kurzrock, R. Vascular endothelial growth factor and its relationship to inflammatory mediators. *Clin. Cancer Res.* **2007**, *13*, 2825–2830. [CrossRef]
123. Kim, H.K.; Song, K.S.; Chung, J.H.; Lee, K.R.; Lee, S.N. Platelet microparticles induce angiogenesis in vitro. *Br. J. Haematol.* **2004**, *124*, 376–384. [CrossRef]
124. Ohtsuka, M.; Sasaki, K.; Ueno, T.; Seki, R.; Nakayoshi, T.; Koiwaya, H.; Toyama, Y.; Yokoyama, S.; Mitsutake, Y.; Chibana, H.; et al. Platelet-derived microparticles augment the adhesion and neovascularization capacities of circulating angiogenic cells obtained from atherosclerotic patients. *Atherosclerosis* **2013**, *227*, 275–282. [CrossRef]
125. Brill, A.; Dashevsky, O.; Rivo, J.; Gozal, Y.; Varon, D. Platelet-derived microparticles induce angiogenesis and stimulate post-ischemic revascularization. *Cardiovasc. Res.* **2005**, *67*, 30–38. [CrossRef] [PubMed]
126. Guo, S.C.; Tao, S.C.; Yin, W.J.; Qi, X.; Yuan, T.; Zhang, C.Q. Exosomes derived from platelet-rich plasma promote the re-epithelization of chronic cutaneous wounds via activation of YAP in a diabetic rat model. *Theranostics* **2017**, *7*, 81–96. [CrossRef] [PubMed]
127. Tao, S.C.; Yuan, T.; Rui, B.Y.; Zhu, Z.Z.; Guo, S.C.; Zhang, C.Q. Exosomes derived from human platelet-rich plasma prevent apoptosis induced by glucocorticoid-associated endoplasmic reticulum stress in rat osteonecrosis of the femoral head via the Akt/Bad/Bcl-2 signal pathway. *Theranostics* **2017**, *7*, 733–750. [CrossRef] [PubMed]
128. Sun, C.; Feng, S.B.; Cao, Z.W.; Bei, J.J.; Chen, Q.; Zhao, W.B.; Xu, X.J.; Zhou, Z.; Yu, Z.P.; Hu, H.Y. Up-Regulated Expression of Matrix Metalloproteinases in Endothelial Cells Mediates Platelet Microvesicle-Induced Angiogenesis. *Cell Physiol. Biochem.* **2017**, *41*, 2319–2332. [CrossRef] [PubMed]

129. Mause, S.F.; Ritzel, E.; Liehn, E.A.; Hristov, M.; Bidzhekov, K.; Muller-Newen, G.; Soehnlein, O.; Weber, C. Platelet microparticles enhance the vasoregenerative potential of angiogenic early outgrowth cells after vascular injury. *Circulation* **2010**, *122*, 495–506. [CrossRef] [PubMed]
130. Prokopi, M.; Pula, G.; Mayr, U.; Devue, C.; Gallagher, J.; Xiao, Q.; Boulanger, C.M.; Westwood, N.; Urbich, C.; Willeit, J.; et al. Proteomic analysis reveals presence of platelet microparticles in endothelial progenitor cell cultures. *Blood* **2009**, *114*, 723–732. [CrossRef]
131. Bordin, A.; Chirivi, M.; Pagano, F.; Milan, M.; Iuliano, M.; Scaccia, E.; Fortunato, O.; Mangino, G.; Dhori, X.; De Marinis, E.; et al. Human platelet lysate-derived extracellular vesicles enhance angiogenesis through miR-126. *Cell Prolif.* **2022**, *55*, e13312. [CrossRef]
132. Khandagale, A.; Aberg, M.; Wikstrom, G.; Bergstrom Lind, S.; Shevchenko, G.; Bjorklund, E.; Siegbahn, A.; Christersson, C. Role of Extracellular Vesicles in Pulmonary Arterial Hypertension: Modulation of Pulmonary Endothelial Function and Angiogenesis. *Arterioscler. Thromb. Vasc. Biol.* **2020**, *40*, 2293–2309. [CrossRef]
133. Janiszewski, M.; Do Carmo, A.O.; Pedro, M.A.; Silva, E.; Knobel, E.; Laurindo, F.R. Platelet-derived exosomes of septic individuals possess proapoptotic NAD(P)H oxidase activity: A novel vascular redox pathway. *Crit. Care Med.* **2004**, *32*, 818–825. [CrossRef]
134. Gambim, M.H.; do Carmo Ade, O.; Marti, L.; Verissimo-Filho, S.; Lopes, L.R.; Janiszewski, M. Platelet-derived exosomes induce endothelial cell apoptosis through peroxynitrite generation: Experimental evidence for a novel mechanism of septic vascular dysfunction. *Crit. Care* **2007**, *11*, R107. [CrossRef]
135. Kong, L.; Li, K.; Gao, L.; Yin, A.; Zhou, L.; Teng, G.; Huang, P. Mediating effects of platelet-derived extracellular vesicles on PM(2.5)-induced vascular endothelial injury. *Ecotoxicol. Environ. Saf.* **2020**, *198*, 110652. [CrossRef]
136. Helley, D.; Banu, E.; Bouziane, A.; Banu, A.; Scotte, F.; Fischer, A.M.; Oudard, S. Platelet microparticles: A potential predictive factor of survival in hormone-refractory prostate cancer patients treated with docetaxel-based chemotherapy. *Eur. Urol.* **2009**, *56*, 479–484. [CrossRef]
137. Haubold, K.; Rink, M.; Spath, B.; Friedrich, M.; Chun, F.K.; Marx, G.; Amirkhosravi, A.; Francis, J.L.; Bokemeyer, C.; Eifrig, B.; et al. Tissue factor procoagulant activity of plasma microparticles is increased in patients with early-stage prostate cancer. *Thromb. Haemost.* **2009**, *101*, 1147–1155.
138. Kim, H.K.; Song, K.S.; Park, Y.S.; Kang, Y.H.; Lee, Y.J.; Lee, K.R.; Kim, H.K.; Ryu, K.W.; Bae, J.M.; Kim, S. Elevated levels of circulating platelet microparticles, VEGF, IL-6 and RANTES in patients with gastric cancer: Possible role of a metastasis predictor. *Eur. J. Cancer* **2003**, *39*, 184–191. [CrossRef]
139. Rank, A.; Liebhardt, S.; Zwirner, J.; Burges, A.; Nieuwland, R.; Toth, B. Circulating microparticles in patients with benign and malignant ovarian tumors. *Anticancer Res.* **2012**, *32*, 2009–2014.
140. Hron, G.; Kollars, M.; Weber, H.; Sagaster, V.; Quehenberger, P.; Eichinger, S.; Kyrle, P.A.; Weltermann, A. Tissue factor-positive microparticles: Cellular origin and association with coagulation activation in patients with colorectal cancer. *Thromb. Haemost.* **2007**, *97*, 119–123. [CrossRef]
141. Mege, D.; Panicot-Dubois, L.; Ouaissi, M.; Robert, S.; Sielezneff, I.; Sastre, B.; Dignat-George, F.; Dubois, C. The origin and concentration of circulating microparticles differ according to cancer type and evolution: A prospective single-center study. *Int. J. Cancer* **2016**, *138*, 939–948. [CrossRef]
142. Contursi, A.; Fullone, R.; Szklanna-Koszalinska, P.; Marcone, S.; Lanuti, P.; Taus, F.; Meneguzzi, A.; Turri, G.; Dovizio, M.; Bruno, A. Tumor-Educated Platelet Extracellular Vesicles: Proteomic Profiling and Crosstalk with Colorectal Cancer Cells. *Cancers* **2023**, *15*, 350. [CrossRef]
143. Nomura, S.; Yasunaga, K. Influence of platelet-derived microparticles on coagulation in a lung cancer patient receiving chemotherapy. *Chest* **1993**, *103*, 979–980. [CrossRef]
144. Ren, J.G.; Man, Q.W.; Zhang, W.; Li, C.; Xiong, X.P.; Zhu, J.Y.; Wang, W.M.; Sun, Z.J.; Jia, J.; Zhang, W.F.; et al. Elevated Level of Circulating Platelet-derived Microparticles in Oral Cancer. *J. Dent. Res.* **2016**, *95*, 87–93. [CrossRef]
145. Toth, B.; Liebhardt, S.; Steinig, K.; Ditsch, N.; Rank, A.; Bauerfeind, I.; Spannagl, M.; Friese, K.; Reininger, A.J. Platelet-derived microparticles and coagulation activation in breast cancer patients. *Thromb. Haemost.* **2008**, *100*, 663–669. [CrossRef] [PubMed]
146. Trappenburg, M.C.; van Schilfgaarde, M.; Bredewold, E.O.; van Aalderen, M.C.; Spronk, H.M.; Ten Cate, H.; Leyte, A.; Terpstra, W.E. Elevated numbers and altered subsets of procoagulant microparticles in breast cancer patients using endocrine therapy. *Thromb. Res.* **2011**, *127*, 363–369. [CrossRef] [PubMed]
147. Yenigurbuz, F.D.; Kizmazoglu, D.; Ates, H.; Erdem, M.; Tufekci, O.; Yilmaz, S.; Oren, H. Analysis of apoptotic, platelet-derived, endothelial-derived, and tissue factor-positive microparticles of children with acute lymphoblastic leukemia during induction therapy. *Blood Coagul. Fibrinolysis* **2019**, *30*, 149–155. [CrossRef] [PubMed]
148. Dashevsky, O.; Varon, D.; Brill, A. Platelet-derived microparticles promote invasiveness of prostate cancer cells via upregulation of MMP-2 production. *Int. J. Cancer* **2009**, *124*, 1773–1777. [CrossRef]
149. Janowska-Wieczorek, A.; Wysoczynski, M.; Kijowski, J.; Marquez-Curtis, L.; Machalinski, B.; Ratajczak, J.; Ratajczak, M.Z. Microvesicles derived from activated platelets induce metastasis and angiogenesis in lung cancer. *Int. J. Cancer* **2005**, *113*, 752–760. [CrossRef]
150. Tang, M.; Jiang, L.; Lin, Y.; Wu, X.; Wang, K.; He, Q.; Wang, X.; Li, W. Platelet microparticle-mediated transfer of miR-939 to epithelial ovarian cancer cells promotes epithelial to mesenchymal transition. *Oncotarget* **2017**, *8*, 97464–97475. [CrossRef]

151. Yao, B.; Qu, S.; Hu, R.; Gao, W.; Jin, S.; Ju, J.; Zhao, Q. Delivery of platelet TPM3 mRNA into breast cancer cells via microvesicles enhances metastasis. *FEBS Open Bio* **2019**, *9*, 2159–2169. [CrossRef]
152. Zara, M.; Guidetti, G.F.; Boselli, D.; Villa, C.; Canobbio, I.; Seppi, C.; Visconte, C.; Canino, J.; Torti, M. Release of Prometastatic Platelet-Derived Microparticles Induced by Breast Cancer Cells: A Novel Positive Feedback Mechanism for Metastasis. *TH Open* **2017**, *1*, e155–e163. [CrossRef]
153. Contursi, A.; Schiavone, S.; Dovizio, M.; Hinz, C.; Fullone, R.; Tacconelli, S.; Tyrrell, V.J.; Grande, R.; Lanuti, P.; Marchisio, M. Platelets induce free and phospholipid-esterified 12-hydroxyeicosatetraenoic acid generation in colon cancer cells by delivering 12-lipoxygenase. *J. Lipid Res.* **2021**, *62*, 100109. [CrossRef]
154. Michael, J.V.; Wurtzel, J.G.T.; Mao, G.F.; Rao, A.K.; Kolpakov, M.A.; Sabri, A.; Hoffman, N.E.; Rajan, S.; Tomar, D.; Madesh, M.; et al. Platelet microparticles infiltrating solid tumors transfer miRNAs that suppress tumor growth. *Blood* **2017**, *130*, 567–580. [CrossRef]
155. Widyaningrum, R.; Wu, Y.W.; Delila, L.; Lee, D.Y.; Wang, T.J.; Burnouf, T. In vitro evaluation of platelet extracellular vesicles (PEVs) for corneal endothelial regeneration. *Platelets* **2022**, *33*, 1237–1250. [CrossRef]
156. Vismara, M.; Zara, M.; Negri, S.; Canino, J.; Canobbio, I.; Barbieri, S.S.; Moccia, F.; Torti, M.; Guidetti, G.F. Platelet-derived extracellular vesicles regulate cell cycle progression and cell migration in breast cancer cells. *Biochim. Biophys. Acta Mol. Cell Res.* **2021**, *1868*, 118886. [CrossRef]
157. Cloutier, N.; Tan, S.; Boudreau, L.H.; Cramb, C.; Subbaiah, R.; Lahey, L.; Albert, A.; Shnayder, R.; Gobezie, R.; Nigrovic, P.A.; et al. The exposure of autoantigens by microparticles underlies the formation of potent inflammatory components: The microparticle-associated immune complexes. *EMBO Mol. Med.* **2013**, *5*, 235–249. [CrossRef]
158. Szabo-Taylor, K.; Ryan, B.; Osteikoetxea, X.; Szabo, T.G.; Sodar, B.; Holub, M.; Nemeth, A.; Paloczi, K.; Pallinger, E.; Winyard, P.; et al. Oxidative and other posttranslational modifications in extracellular vesicle biology. *Semin. Cell Dev. Biol.* **2015**, *40*, 8–16. [CrossRef]
159. Takahashi, A.; Okada, R.; Nagao, K.; Kawamata, Y.; Hanyu, A.; Yoshimoto, S.; Takasugi, M.; Watanabe, S.; Kanemaki, M.T.; Obuse, C.; et al. Exosomes maintain cellular homeostasis by excreting harmful DNA from cells. *Nat. Commun.* **2017**, *8*, 15287. [CrossRef]
160. Baglio, S.R.; van Eijndhoven, M.A.; Koppers-Lalic, D.; Berenguer, J.; Lougheed, S.M.; Gibbs, S.; Leveille, N.; Rinkel, R.N.; Hopmans, E.S.; Swaminathan, S.; et al. Sensing of latent EBV infection through exosomal transfer of 5′pppRNA. *Proc. Natl. Acad. Sci. USA* **2016**, *113*, E587–E596. [CrossRef]

life

Article

Geranylgeraniol Application in Human Osteoblasts and Osteoclasts for Reversal of the Effect of Bisphosphonates

Junho Jung [1,*], Jung Soo Park [2], Jeewan Chun [3], Bilal Al-Nawas [4], Thomas Ziebart [5] and Yong-Dae Kwon [1,*]

1 Department of Oral & Maxillofacial Surgery, School of Dentistry, Kyung Hee University, Seoul 02447, Republic of Korea
2 Department of Periodontology, Korea University Anam Hospital, Seoul 02841, Republic of Korea
3 Department of Dentistry, Graduate School, Kyung Hee University, Seoul 02447, Republic of Korea
4 Department of Oral and Maxillofacial Surgery, University Medical Center of the Johannes Gutenberg University Mainz, 55131 Mainz, Germany
5 Department of Oral and Maxillofacial Surgery, University Hospital Giessen and Marburg of the Philipps University of Marburg, 35043 Marburg, Germany
* Correspondence: ssa204@khu.ac.kr (J.J.); yongdae.kwon@gmail.com (Y.-D.K.)

Abstract: Nitrogen-containing bisphosphonates lead to the depletion of geranylgeranyl pyrophosphate involved in the mevalonate pathway. The effect of geranylgeraniol (GGOH) on human osteoblast and osteoclast activities suppressed by zoledronate was investigated in this study. The effect of GGOH on human osteoblasts and osteoclasts subjected to treatment with zoledronate was analyzed by assessing cell viability, osteoclast differentiation, resorption ability, gene expression, and protein synthesis. Cell viability suppressed by bisphosphonates in osteoblasts and osteoprogenitor cells was restored with GGOH. Osteoclast differentiation was analyzed by vitronectin receptor immunofluorescence staining, and the addition of GGOH to zoledronate significantly increased osteoclast differentiation compared with zoledronate alone. A trend of reversal of osteoclast resorption by GGOH was observed; however, it was not significant in all groups. The expression of ALP, type 1 collagen, and RUNX2 in osteoblasts was recovered by the addition of GGOH. Only CALCR expression in osteoclasts was significantly recovered by GGOH addition in the zoledronate group. Although the activities of osteoblasts and osteoclasts were not entirely restored, the possibility that the topical application of GGOH in MRONJ patients or patients with dental problems and bisphosphonates might lessen the risk of development and recurrence of MRONJ is shown.

Keywords: geranylgeraniol; GGOH; bisphosphonates; medication-related osteonecrosis of the jaw; MRONJ; mevalonate pathway

check for updates

Citation: Jung, J.; Park, J.S.; Chun, J.; Al-Nawas, B.; Ziebart, T.; Kwon, Y.-D. Geranylgeraniol Application in Human Osteoblasts and Osteoclasts for Reversal of the Effect of Bisphosphonates. *Life* **2023**, *13*, 1353. https://doi.org/10.3390/life13061353

Academic Editor: Peter Zioupos

Received: 8 May 2023
Revised: 1 June 2023
Accepted: 6 June 2023
Published: 8 June 2023

1. Introduction

Bisphosphonates are pharmacological agents that have been used for over 40 years for the treatment of bone diseases, such as osteoporosis, Paget's disease, osteogenesis imperfecta, multiple myeloma, fibrous dysplasia, and bone metastasis mainly caused by prostate and breast cancer [1–7]. However, medication-related osteonecrosis of the jaw (MRONJ) was first described in 2003, and several cases of osteonecrosis with a history of administration of bisphosphonates have been reported [8,9]. Considering their efficacy and cost-effectiveness, it is not surprising that bisphosphonates continue to be broadly used for the prevention and treatment of such diseases, despite the exhibition and development of various complications [10–12]. As the number of elderly individuals increases, the prevalence of bone diseases also increases, and the prescription of bisphosphonates and the complications resulting from their use are expected to remain high [13].

Nitrogen-containing bisphosphonates inhibit the actions of farnesyl pyrophosphate synthase, an enzyme involved in the mevalonate pathway, leading to the depletion of geranylgeranyl pyrophosphate (GGPP), an intermediate in the mevalonate pathway [14,15].

GGPP is an essential substrate for post-translational prenylation of small GTP-binding proteins, such as Rab and Rho family proteins [16,17]. Since geranylgeraniol (GGOH) serves as a substrate for GGPP formation, supplementation of GGOH may help resume prenylation of small GTP-binding proteins that play a key role in cell survival, despite the presence of bisphosphonates [18,19]. Therefore, several studies have noticed and focused on the possibility of rescuing cells by using this strategy [18–22].

Although clear standards for treatment of MRONJ have not been determined thus far, early surgical interventions are gaining preference among oral and maxillofacial surgeons, as higher success rates for the management of MRONJ have been reported [23]. However, there is a possibility that surgical treatment may act as a trigger for MRONJ development. Therefore, adjunctive therapies, including the administration of teriparatide, pentoxifylline, and tocopherol to reduce surgical morbidity, have been suggested [24,25]. As described above, if GGOH can aid the recovery of the cellular damage caused by bisphosphonates, it may emerge as a potential candidate for the treatment of MRONJ. Additionally, the use of GGOH as a preventive measure can also be considered. The effectiveness of GGOH in rescuing and preventing cellular damage has been recently presented [26,27],

Thus, this study aimed to investigate the effect of GGOH on human osteoblast and osteoclast activities, including cell proliferation, osteoclastogenesis, resorption ability, gene expression, and protein synthesis, in the presence of various bisphosphonates.

2. Materials and Methods

2.1. Cell Culture

Commercially available human osteoblast cells (PromoCell) and human osteoclast precursors (Lonza) were cultured in their respective culture media (PromoCell and Lonza) at 37 °C with 5% CO_2, and the media were replaced with fresh media every three days. The osteoblasts were passaged when they reached 70–80% confluence in a 75 cm^2 culture flask (Corning, New York, NY, USA) using Accutase solution (Sigma-Aldrich, St. Louis, MO, USA). Osteoblasts from passages 4 to 7 were used in the experiments and seeded onto appropriate plates at a density of 2×10^4 cells/cm^2. The osteoclast precursors were seeded onto appropriate plates for each experiment at a density of 4×10^4 cells/cm^2, and human receptor activators of nuclear factor kappa-B ligand (RANKL; 40 ng/mL, Sigma-Aldrich) and human macrophage colony stimulating factor (M-CSF; 25 ng/mL, Sigma-Aldrich) were added to induce osteoclast differentiation.

2.2. Bisphosphonates and Geranylgeraniol

Nitrogen-containing bisphosphonates, namely, Zometa (zoledronate, Novartis Pharma, Basel, Switzerland) and Alendron (alendronate, Hexal AG; Novartis group, Holzkirchen, Germany), and a non-nitrogen-containing bisphosphonate, Bonefos (clodronate, Bayer, Leverkusen, Germany), were used for the experiments, and geranylgeraniol (GGOH) purchased from Sigma-Aldrich was supplemented along with bisphosphonate treatment. The alendronate tablet was pulverized and dissolved in phosphate-buffered saline (PBS). Subsequently, the pH of the solution was adjusted, and the solution was sterilized by filtration.

2.3. Cell Viability

The viability of human osteoblasts and human osteoclast precursors was determined using the MTT colorimetric assay (Sigma-Aldrich). Osteoblasts and osteoclast precursor cells were seeded onto 24-well plates at a density of 2×10^4 cells/cm^2 and incubated for 24 h. Bisphosphonates, namely, zoledronate (Zol), alendronate (Aln), and clodronate (Clod), were added to the wells (0, 10, and 50 μM) with or without GGOH (10 μM). The above-mentioned range of concentrations was selected, because in vivo concentrations in plasma shortly after zoledronate infusion are approximately 5 μM, and these doses roughly correspond to the standard oncology dose regimens of 1 year and 4 years (32, 33). The assay was conducted in triplicate, with three replicates for each experiment. After incubation for a duration of 72 h, MTT solution was added to the wells and the plates were incubated for

4 h. Cells were subjected to lysis for 30 min using a lysis buffer (isopropanol and 2 N HCl, 49:1), and the optical density (OD) was measured at 570 nm using a spectrophotometric microplate reader (Synergy HT; BioTek, Winooski, VT, USA).

2.4. Vitronectin Receptor Staining and Cell Count

To analyze osteoclast differentiation, vitronectin receptor (VNR) immunofluorescence staining was performed. VNR-positive multinucleated cells (cells with more than 2 nuclei) were considered osteoclasts. The osteoclast precursors were seeded onto 96-well plates at a density of 4×10^4 cells/cm^2, and human receptor activators of nuclear factor kappa-B ligand (RANKL; 40 ng/mL, Sigma-Aldrich) and human macrophage colony stimulating factor (M-CSF; 25 ng/mL, Sigma-Aldrich) were added. The assay was conducted in triplicate. After incubation for a duration of 24 h, bisphosphonates (50 μM) with or without GGOH (10 μM) were added and the plates were incubated for 72 h. Subsequently, the cells were subjected to fixation in 3.7% paraformaldehyde for 20 min at 25 °C and blocked with goat serum (Thermo Fisher Scientific, Waltham, MA, USA) for 30 min at 25 °C. The cells were then incubated with anti-human CD51/61 antibody (MAB1976Z, 1:200; EMD Millipore, Temecula, CA, USA) for 1 h at 25 °C and with a secondary fluorescent antibody (ab150113, 1:500; Abcam, Cambridge, United Kingdom) for 1 h at 25 °C. Images were obtained using a fluorescence microscope (BZ-9000; Keyence, Osaka, Japan) and subsequently merged with the DAPI images for nuclei staining. For each group, fifteen different areas, each measuring 0.01 cm^2, were selected, and a cell count was performed using ImageJ software. The proportion of cells with more than two nuclei among the total cell population was calculated.

2.5. Bone Resorption Pit Assay

After incubation of osteoclast precursor cells with M-CSF and RANKL for 72 h as per the methods described above, the cells were counted and seeded onto 24-well hydroxyapatite-coated plates (Corning) at a density of 2×10^4 cells/cm^2. The assay was conducted in quadruplicate with two replicates for each experiment. After incubation for a duration of 24 h, bisphosphonates (10 and 50 μM) with or without GGOH (10 μM) were added. Following incubation for 72 h, resorption pits were observed using an inverted phase-contrast microscope and analyzed by measuring the resorbed area using ImageJ software.

2.6. Messenger RNA Extraction and Quantitative Real-Time Polymerase Chain Reaction

Osteoblasts were seeded onto 6-well plates and incubated with Aln and Zol (50 μM) with or without GGOH (10 μM) for 72 h. Osteoclast precursors were also seeded onto 6-well plates and differentiated into osteoclasts by RANKL and M-CSF stimulation. Thereafter, Aln and Zol, with or without GGOH, were added for the conduction of treatment for 72 h. Subsequently, the cells were harvested using Accutase solution, and mRNA extraction was performed. The amount of extracted mRNA was measured spectrophotometrically at 260 nm. Complementary DNA synthesis was performed using a cDNA synthesis kit (iScrip; Bio-Rad, Hilden, Germany) and a thermal cycler (peqSTAR 96 Universal Gradient; PeqLab, Erlangen, Germany). The sequences of primers used in the experiment are listed in Table 1. iQ SYBR Green Supermix (Bio-Rad) was used to conduct polymerase chain reactions (PCRs). The PCR cycling conditions used in the present study were as follows: initial denaturation at 95 °C for 5 min, 40 cycles of denaturation at 95 °C for 30 s, annealing at 56 °C for 30 s, and elongation at 71 °C for 20 s, with final elongation at 65 °C for 0.5 s and then at 95 °C for 5 s (CFX Connect; Bio-Rad). Amplification of PCR products was confirmed by performing a melting curve analysis. The expression levels of target genes were normalized using glyceraldehyde 3-phosphate dehydrogenase (GAPDH) and were quantified using the ΔΔCT method [28]. The assay was conducted in triplicate, with three replicates for each experiment.

Table 1. Primer sequences used for RT-PCR.

Gene	Forward (5′-3′)	Reverse (5′-3′)
ALP	CCGTGGCAACTCT ATCTTTGG	GCCATACAGGAT GGCAGTGA
OC	AAGAGACCCAGG CGCTACCT	AACTCGTCACAG TCCGGATTG
M-CSF	CTCCAGAGAGAG GAGCCTGA	AGTATAGACACT CGTCACTGGTG
RANKL	ATACCCTGATGAAAGGAGGA	GGGGCTCAATCTATATCTCG
COL1	CCCTGGAAAGAATGGAGATGAT	ACTGAAACCTCTGTGTCCCTTCA
RUNX2	AGCAAGGTTCAACGATCTGAGAT	TTTGTGAAGACGGTTATGGTCAA
RANK	TGTGGCACTGGATCAATGAG	GTCTTGCTGACCAATGAGAG
TRAP	GATCCTGGGTGCAGACTTCA	GCGCTTGGAGATCTTAGAGT
CALCR	GACAACTGCTGGCTGAGTG	GAAGCAGTAGATGGTCGCAA
CSF1R	GGCTCCTGGGCCTTCATACC	CAAAGGCTCCAGCTCCGAGG
c-Fos	TGTCTGTGGCTTCCCTTGAT	ATCAAAGGGCTCGGTCTTCA
OSCAR	GAGTAGCTGAAAGGAAGACGCGAT	CAGAGCGCTGATTGGTCCATCTTA

2.7. Western Blot Analysis

Osteoblasts were incubated with zoledronate (50 μM) for 72 h. Subsequently, the cells were subjected to lysis with RIPA buffer (Sigma-Aldrich) containing a phosphatase inhibitor cocktail (Sigma-Aldrich). Protein concentration was determined using a BCA protein assay kit. Sodium dodecyl sulfate-polyacrylamide gel electrophoresis (SDS-PAGE) was used to separate proteins, which were then transferred onto a PVDF membrane, followed by blocking for 1 h. The membrane was then incubated for 24 h at 4 °C with primary antibodies against the following molecules: alkaline phosphatase (ALP), macrophage colony-stimulating factor (M-CSF), receptor activator of nuclear factor kappa-B ligand (RANKL), and type 1 collagen (cat. nos. ab108337, ab52864, ab9957, and ab138492, respectively; dilutions of 1:10,000, 1:50,000, 1 μg/mL, and 1:1000, respectively; Abcam), RUNX2 (cat no. 12556, dilution 1:1000, Cell Signaling Technology, Danvers, MA, USA), β-actin (cat. no. sc-47778, dilution 1:3000, Santa Cruz Biotechnology, Dallas, TX, USA). Subsequently, they were incubated with anti-mouse and anti-rabbit secondary horseradish peroxidase-conjugated antibodies (cat. nos. 111-035-003 and 115-035-003, both with dilutions of 1:5000; Jackson ImmunoResearch Laboratories, West Grove, PA, USA) for 1 h at room temperature. The immunoreactive proteins were determined using enhanced ECL chemiluminescence and a detection device (Fusion Solo S; Vilber, Marne-la-Vallée, France).

2.8. Statistical Analysis

The Kruskal–Wallis test and the Mann–Whitney *U* test with Bonferroni correction were used to perform statistical analyses. Two-way ANOVA with Dunnett's T3 test was used to analyze the osteoclast differentiation count, as the normality of data was proven. All statistical analyses were performed using SPSS (version 25.0; IBM Corp). Statistical significance was set at $p < 0.05$.

3. Results

3.1. Cell Viability

Based on the statistical analysis results, a significant difference was observed between the groups in osteoblasts (Figure 1). Bisphosphonate treatment decreased cell viability compared to that observed in the control group ($p < 0.001$). The Zol 50 μM group showed the most considerable decrease among the bisphosphonate-treated groups. The addition of GGOH demonstrated a statistically significant improvement in cell viability in the Aln and Zol groups ($p = 0.038$ and 0.002, respectively).

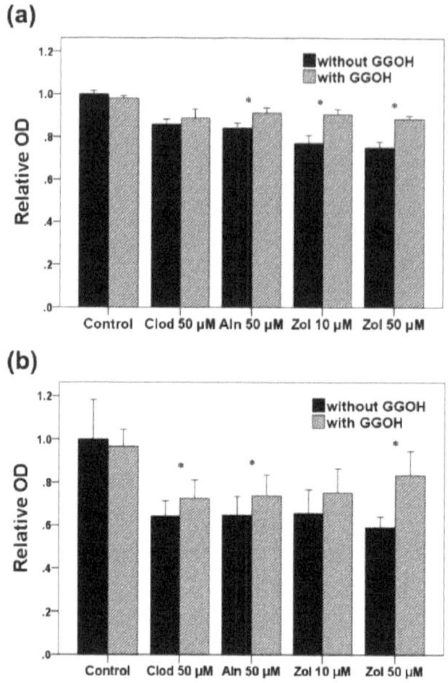

Figure 1. Cell viability assessed in osteoblasts (**a**) and osteoclast precursors (**b**). The values have been normalized relative to the control. Asterisks (*) represent statistical significance for comparisons of the groups with GGOH and without GGOH addition ($p < 0.05$), and the error bars indicate standard deviations. Clod, clodronate; Aln, alendronate; Zol, zoledronate; GGOH, geranylgeraniol.

Regarding osteoclast progenitors, a significant difference was observed between the groups ($p < 0.001$). Zol 50 μM was determined as the most potent inhibitor of cell viability. Cell viability was significantly improved by GGOH supplementation ($p < 0.001$), except in the Zol 10 μM group ($p = 0.089$).

3.2. Osteoclast Differentiation

Osteoclast differentiation was evaluated by counting the number of cells with more than two nuclei, showing positive results for VNR, and by calculating the proportion of such cells among the total cell population (Figures 2 and 3). A statistically significant difference was observed between the groups ($p = 0.019$). The number of osteoclasts decreased with bisphosphonate treatment, and Zol showed the most considerable potency among bisphosphonates, followed by Aln and Clod. The addition of GGOH to Zol significantly increased osteoclast differentiation compared to that observed with Zol alone ($p = 0.027$). In the Clod and Aln groups, although the differentiation increased with GGOH, the increase was not found to be statistically significant.

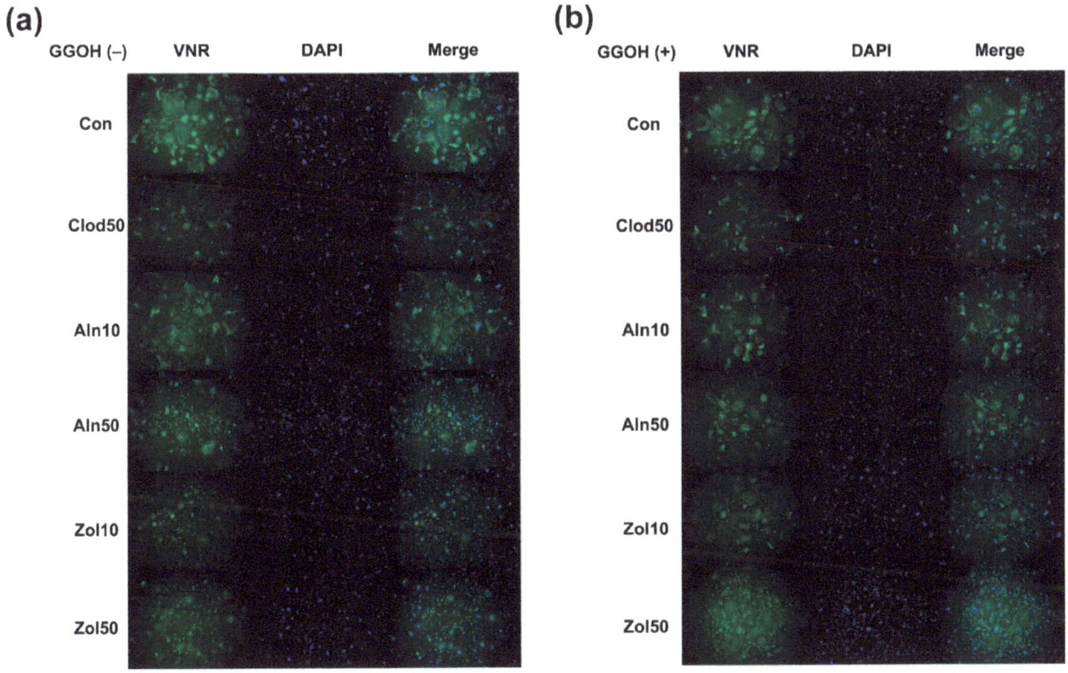

Figure 2. Vitronectin receptor (VNR) immunofluorescence staining conducted for cells with GGOH (**a**) and without GGOH addition (**b**). VNR-positive multinucleated cells (cells with more than two nuclei) were considered osteoclasts. Clod, clodronate; Aln, alendronate; Zol, zoledronate; GGOH, geranylgeraniol.

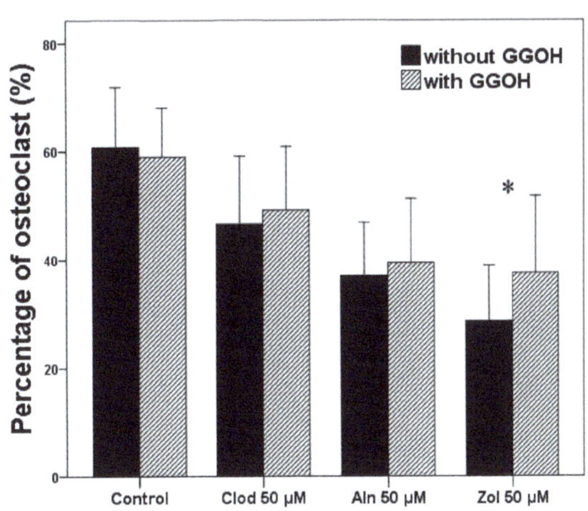

Figure 3. VNR-positive multinucleated cell counts. The percentage of multinucleated cell (cells with more than two nuclei) was determined with respect to the total cell number. Asterisks (*) represent statistical significance for comparisons of the groups with GGOH and without GGOH addition ($p < 0.05$), and the error bars indicate standard deviations. Clod, clodronate; Aln, alendronate; Zol, zoledronate; GGOH, geranylgeraniol.

3.3. Resorption Area Analysis

To analyze the resorption ability of osteoclasts and the extent of osteoclast differentiation, a resorption pit assay was conducted (Figure 4). A significant difference in resorption area was observed between the groups. The resorption area decreased with the addition of bisphosphonates. The most considerable decrease in resorption was observed in the Zol 50 μM group ($p < 0.001$). Although a trend of reversal of the resorption of osteoclasts by GGOH was observed, it was not statistically significant in all groups (Control, Clod, Aln, and Zol groups; $p = 0.094$, $p = 0.574$, $p = 0.645$, and $p = 0.072$, respectively).

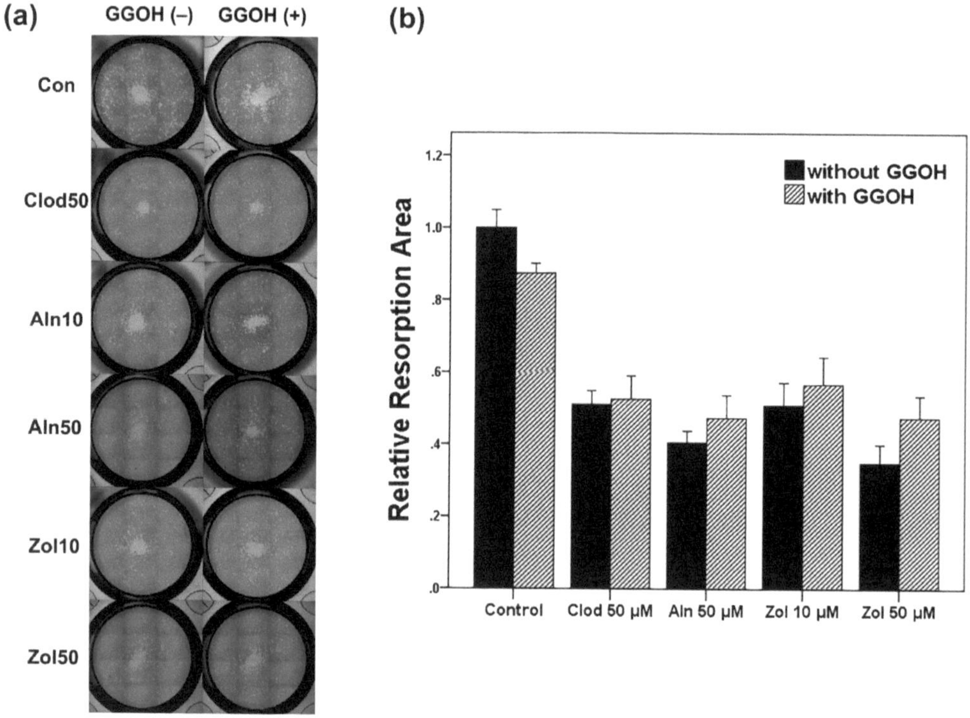

Figure 4. (**a**) Resorption pit assay conducted to analyze the resorption ability of osteoclast and osteoclast differentiation. (**b**) The resorbed area measured was normalized relative to the control. Asterisks (*) represent statistical significance for comparisons of the groups with GGOH and without GGOH addition ($p < 0.05$), and the error bars indicate standard deviations. Clod, clodronate; Aln, alendronate; Zol, zoledronate; GGOH, geranylgeraniol.

3.4. Gene Expression and Protein Synthesis

3.4.1. Osteoblasts

qRT-PCR was performed to analyze the gene expression of the osteogenic markers and osteoclastogenesis-stimulating genes, including ALP, RUNX2, type 1 collagen, osteocalcin, M-CSF, and RANKL (Figure 5).

The gene expression of ALP, type 1 collagen, and RUNX2 in osteoblasts significantly decreased as bisphosphonates were administered compared to the control group ($p < 0.001$). The addition of GGOH reversed the effects of bisphosphonates on the expression of the above-mentioned genes ($p < 0.001$). Although no statistical significance was observed in the gene expression of M-CSF, bisphosphonates decreased the expression and GGOH reversed the action of Zol ($p = 0.836$). RANKL and osteocalcin gene expression levels increased with bisphosphonate treatment, and GGOH significantly enhanced the expression ($p = 0.001$).

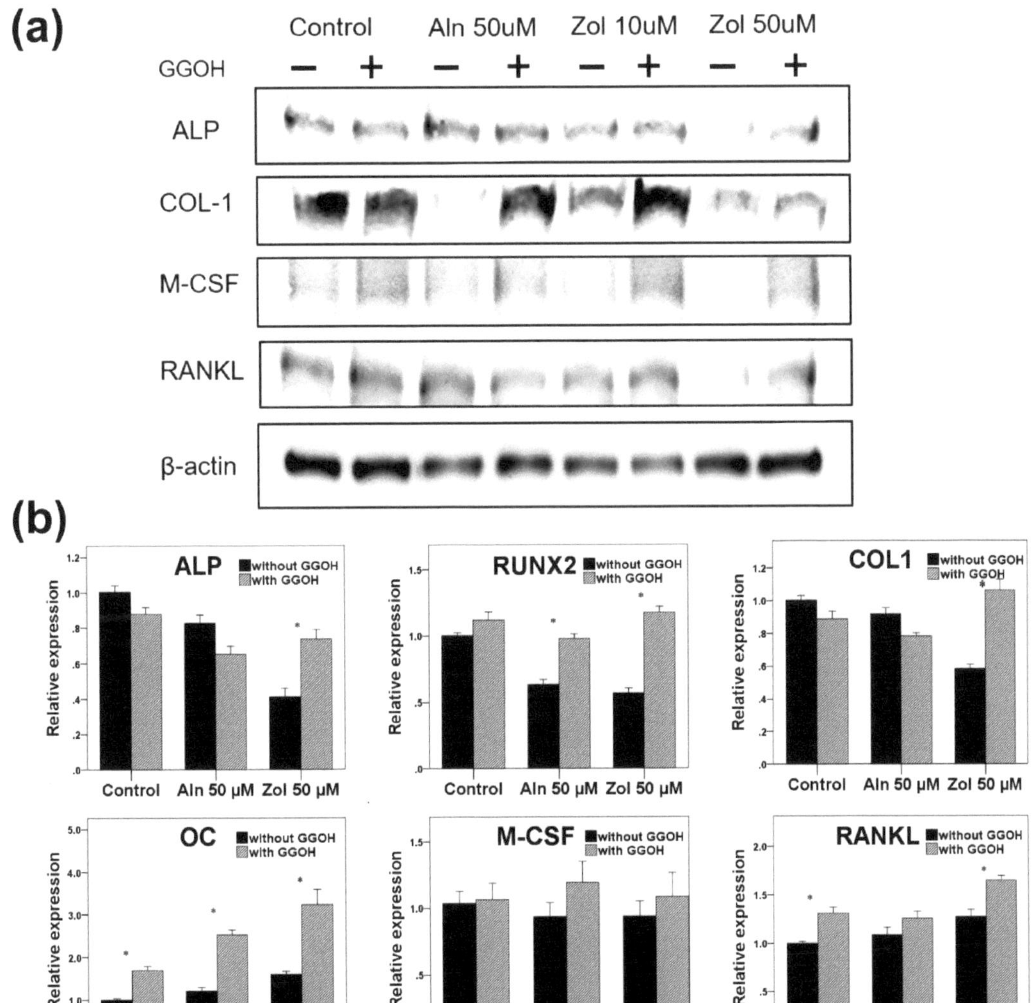

Figure 5. (**a**) Western blot analysis and (**b**) qRT-PCR conducted for osteoblasts. The gene expression levels have been normalized relative to the control. Asterisks (*) represent statistical significance for comparisons of the groups with GGOH and without GGOH addition ($p < 0.05$), and the error bars indicate standard deviations. ALP, alkaline phosphatase; COL1, type 1 collagen; OC, osteocalcin; M-CSF, macrophage colony stimulating factor; RANKL, receptor activator of nuclear factor kappa-B ligand; Aln, alendronate; Zol, zoledronate; GGOH, geranylgeraniol.

Western blot analysis (Figure 5) showed that incubation with Zol (50 μM) reduced the expression of ALP, type 1 collagen, M-CSF, and RANKL compared to the control. ALP, M-CSF, and RANKL expression demonstrated recovery with the addition of GGOH to the osteoblasts.

3.4.2. Osteoclasts

qRT-PCR was performed to analyze the expression of genes related to osteoclast differentiation and activity, including receptor activator of nuclear factor kappa-B (RANK), TRAP, calcitonin receptor (CALCR), colony stimulating factor 1 receptor (CSF1R), c-Fos, and osteoclast-associated receptor (OSCAR) (Figure 6).

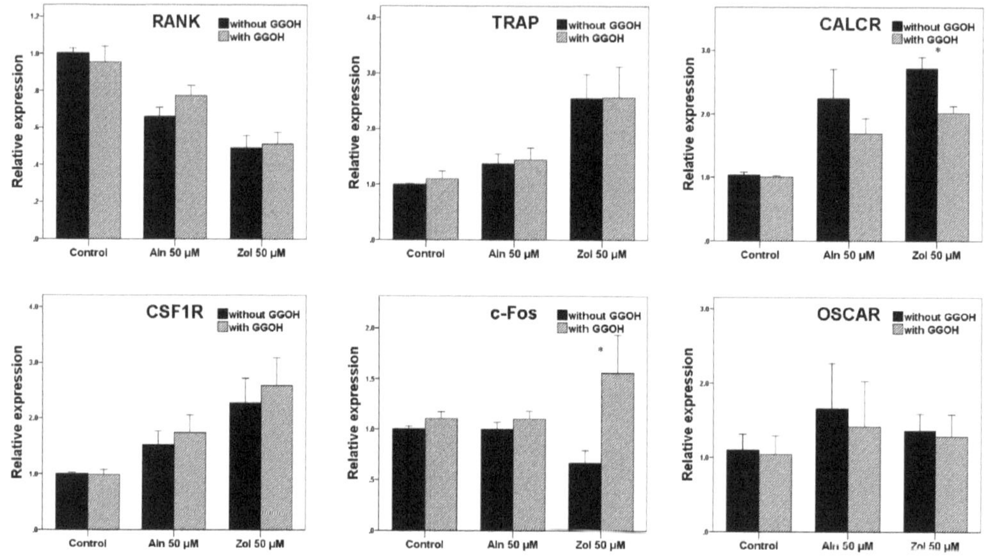

Figure 6. qRT-PCR analysis conducted for osteoclasts. The gene expression levels have been normalized relative to the control. Asterisks (*) represent statistical significance for comparisons of the groups with GGOH and without GGOH addition ($p < 0.05$), and the error bars indicate standard deviations. RANK, receptor activator of nuclear factor kappa-B; TRAP, tartrate-resistant acid phosphatase; CALCR, calcitonin receptor; CSF1R, colony stimulating factor 1 receptor; c-Fos, OSCAR, osteoclast-associated receptor; Aln, alendronate; Zol, zoledronate; GGOH, geranylgeraniol.

Bisphosphonate treatment significantly increased the gene expression of TRAP, CALCR, CSF1R, and OSCAR compared to the control group. However, only CALCR expression was significantly recovered by GGOH in the Zol group ($p = 0.011$). In the case of TRAP and CSF1R, GGOH treatment did not cause a significant difference in expression ($p = 0.730$ and $p = 0.258$, respectively). The gene expression of RANK and c-Fos in the bisphosphonate-treated group was significantly decreased compared to that observed in the control. The effect of GGOH increased the gene expression of RANK; however, the difference was not statistically significant ($p = 0.895$). GGOH had a significant effect on c-Fos expression after Zol treatment ($p = 0.030$).

4. Discussion

Almost 20 years have elapsed since the first documentation of MRONJ, and it has emerged as a disease well recognized by clinicians [29]. Several attempts to unearth the nature of the disease have been reported; however, an established pathophysiology or treatment regimen remain unavailable. Several hypotheses regarding the cause of the disease have been suggested. Impaired bone turnover, exertion of cell toxicity against various cell types, bacterial infection, and inflammation occurring due to dental problems and microtrauma have been considered as contributing factors. MRONJ is therefore considered a multifactorial disease [30]. Among these possible causes, impaired bone turnover occurring due to downregulated osteoclast and osteoblast activities plays a critical role in the development of MRONJ.

MRONJ was first reported in patients subjected to treatments using nitrogen-containing bisphosphonates, and such bisphosphonates are broadly prescribed as antiresorptive agents for the treatment of various bone diseases. Nitrogen-containing bisphosphonates inhibit the actions of farnesyl pyrophosphate synthase (FPPS), an enzyme involved in the mevalonate pathway, leading to the depletion of geranylgeranyl pyrophosphate (GGPP), an essential substrate for the post-translational prenylation of small GTP-binding proteins, such as those belonging to Rab and Rho subfamilies [14,15]. The prenylated small GTP-binding proteins act as molecular switches during signal transduction and help regulate cellular processes and functions, including cell growth and survival, differentiation and proliferation, gene expression, and energy metabolism [31,32]. Thus, undermining of the function and viability of osteoclasts and osteoblasts by nitrogen-containing bisphosphonates leads to a reduction in the extent of bone remodeling, and the use of nitrogen-containing bisphosphonates has been ascertained as the main cause of MRONJ.

Certain researchers have focused on the application of geranylgeraniol (GGOH) as a potential therapeutic approach, as it serves as a substrate for GGPP and undergoes conversion to GGPP [18]. A study conducted by Ziebart et al. reported that the addition of GGOH reversed the effect of nitrogen-containing bisphosphonates, resulting in increased cell viability and migration and decreased cell apoptosis [18]. Another study also reported that the cytotoxic effect of Zol on osteoblasts was reversed by GGOH addition [33]. Furthermore, the prenylation of Rap1A, a GTP-binding protein, was restored by GGOH addition in the presence of bisphosphonates exerting effects on human osteoclasts [27].

Decreased osteoclasts and their suppressed resorption ability under bisphosphonates have a critical effect on the occurrence of MRONJ due to impaired bone turnover. However, they have not been investigated in human osteoclasts, despite the importance of doing so. The present study focused on analyzing human osteoclast differentiation and activities, and the results showed positive effects of GGOH exerted on human osteoblasts and osteoclasts subjected to treatment with Zol. Notably, osteoclast differentiation compromised by Zol treatment was restored to a certain extent, although this level was not sufficient to reach values demonstrated by the control. Given that the expression levels of M-CSF and RANKL reduced by BPS in osteoblasts were also recovered by GGOH, it is assumed that it has the potential to not only promote increased bone formation but also enhance osteoclastogenesis. The addition of GGOH also tends to improve hydroxyapatite resorption. Given that the expression levels of M-CSF and RANKL reduced by BPS in osteoblasts were also recovered by GGOH, it is assumed that it has the potential to not only promote increased bone formation but also enhance osteoclastogenesis and bone resorption in vivo. Gene expression, such as ALP, collagen 1, RANKL, and RUNX2 expression in osteoblasts and C-Fos and CALCR expression in osteoclasts, was significantly recovered with the addition of GGOH. Interestingly, not all genes and proteins were affected. Since protein prenylation is mediated not only by the action of geranylgeranyl transferase, but also by the action of farnesyltransferase for farnesylation of proteins [32,34], the sole addition of GGOH may be insufficient to fully restore cellular function, and as a result the gene expression and protein expression were not correlated accordingly.

Aln and Clod also exhibited suppressive effects on cell survival, osteoclastogenesis, resorption, and gene expression. As Clod is not a nitrogen-containing BP that acts via the mevalonate pathway, it is not surprising that GGOH has no impact on cells treated with Clod. However, in the case of Aln, the effect of GGOH was also not profound. Although 10 μM of GGOH increased the viability of osteoclast precursors treated with Aln, similar to Zol, there was no statistically significant impact on osteoclast differentiation. Considering that the drug potency of Aln is lower than that of Zol, resulting in a lesser effect on bone turnover, higher concentrations of Aln could be comparable to Zol, and supplementation with varying amounts of GGOH might lead to improved results.

As demonstrated by the present study, GGOH addition antagonized the effect of Zol and, as a result, the activities of osteoblasts and osteoclasts were restored. However, the effect of GGOH was exerted on a limited number of genes. The Ras superfamily, influenced by FPPS, comprises various subfamilies, including Ras, Rho, Rab, Ran, and Arf [35], and the prenylation of the proteins is mediated by three enzymes, namely, farnesyltransferase, geranylgeranyltransferase-I, and geranylgeranyltransferase-II [27,30]; therefore, another type of isoprenoid, farnesol, may play an important role in the rescue of cellular functions. Additionally, the effect of GGOH was not sufficient to reach values demonstrated by the control. Different concentrations of GGOH may lead to the obtainment of better results, although the cytotoxic effect of GGOH was also observed at an extremely high concentration (80 μM) [27]. Furthermore, considering the well-established role of osteoblasts in regulating osteoclastogenesis, conducting a co-culture experiment involving osteoblasts and osteoclast progenitors under the influence of BPs and GGOH treatment, followed by the assessment of gene and protein expression, would provide valuable insights into the molecular mechanisms underlying the effects of BPs and GGOH on the interplay between osteoblasts and osteoclasts.

To manage the conditions associated with MRONJ, various adjuvant therapies, including hyperbaric oxygen (HBO) therapy, parathyroid hormone analog teriparatide treatment, and laser treatment, have been reported [30]. However, a fundamental approach at the cellular level has not been applied in clinical settings thus far. The results show a possibility that the topical application of GGOH in MRONJ patients along with surgical treatment, or, for preventive purposes, during dentoalveolar surgery in patients with bisphosphonates, might lessen the risk of development and recurrence of medication-related osteonecrosis of the jaw (MRONJ), since GGOH aids the recovery of cell viability and functions, resulting in improved bone turnover. Moreover, the anti-inflammatory and neuroprotective effects of GGOH have also been reported, in addition to antagonization of the effect of bisphosphonates [36]. However, preclinical and clinical studies are essential to verify the results and its possible use in clinical settings. Systemic administration may not be recommended because of the possible risk of compromising the purpose of bisphosphonate therapy.

Author Contributions: Conceptualization, B.A.-N. and Y.-D.K.; Methodology, T.Z.; Validation, B.A.-N. and T.Z.; Formal Analysis, J.S.P.; Investigation, J.J., J.S.P. and J.C.; Writing—Original Draft Preparation, J.J.; Writing—Review and Editing, J.J. and Y.-D.K.; Visualization, J.J.; Supervision, Y.-D.K.; Funding Acquisition, J.J. All authors have read and agreed to the published version of the manuscript.

Funding: This study was supported by the International Team for Implantology (ITI) (grant no. 1171_2016).

Institutional Review Board Statement: Not applicable.

Informed Consent Statement: Not applicable.

Data Availability Statement: Data supporting the reported results can be provided upon reasonable request.

Conflicts of Interest: The authors declare no conflict of interest.

References

1. Walsh, J.P.; Ward, L.C.; Stewart, G.O.; Will, R.K.; Criddle, R.A.; Prince, R.L.; Stuckey, B.G.; Dhaliwal, S.S.; Bhagat, C.I.; Retallack, R.W.; et al. A randomized clinical trial comparing oral alendronate and intravenous pamidronate for the treatment of Paget's disease of bone. *Bone* **2004**, *34*, 747–754. [CrossRef] [PubMed]
2. Majoor, B.C.; Appelman-Dijkstra, N.M.; Fiocco, M.; van de Sande, M.A.; Dijkstra, P.S.; Hamdy, N.A. Outcome of Long-Term Bisphosphonate Therapy in McCune-Albright Syndrome and Polyostotic Fibrous Dysplasia. *J. Bone Miner. Res.* **2017**, *32*, 264–276. [CrossRef] [PubMed]
3. Parisi, M.S.; Oliveri, M.B.; Mautalen, C.A. Bone mineral density response to long-term bisphosphonate therapy in fibrous dysplasia. *J. Clin. Densitom.* **2001**, *4*, 167–172. [CrossRef] [PubMed]
4. McKeage, K.; Plosker, G.L. Zoledronic acid: A pharmacoeconomic review of its use in the management of bone metastases. *Pharmacoeconomics* **2008**, *26*, 251–268. [CrossRef]
5. Smith, M.R. Zoledronic acid to prevent skeletal complications in cancer: Corroborating the evidence. *Cancer Treat. Rev.* **2005**, *31* (Suppl. 3), 19–25. [CrossRef]

6. Hosaka, S.; Katagiri, H.; Niwakawa, M.; Harada, H.; Wasa, J.; Murata, H.; Takahashi, M. Radiotherapy combined with zoledronate can reduce skeletal-related events in renal cell carcinoma patients with bone metastasis. *Int. J. Clin. Oncol.* **2018**, *23*, 1127–1133. [CrossRef]
7. Russell, R.G. Bisphosphonates: The first 40 years. *Bone* **2011**, *49*, 2–19. [CrossRef]
8. McGowan, K.; McGowan, T.; Ivanovski, S. Risk factors for medication-related osteonecrosis of the jaws: A systematic review. *Oral Dis.* **2018**, *24*, 527–536. [CrossRef]
9. Yamada, S.I.; Kurita, H.; Kondo, E.; Suzuki, S.; Nishimaki, F.; Yoshimura, N.; Morioka, M.; Ishii, S.; Kamata, T. Treatment outcomes and prognostic factors of medication-related osteonecrosis of the jaw: A case- and literature-based review. *Clin. Oral Investig.* **2019**, *23*, 3203–3211. [CrossRef]
10. Hernlund, E.; Svedbom, A.; Ivergard, M.; Compston, J.; Cooper, C.; Stenmark, J.; McCloskey, E.V.; Jonsson, B.; Kanis, J.A. Osteoporosis in the European Union: Medical management, epidemiology and economic burden. A report prepared in collaboration with the International Osteoporosis Foundation (IOF) and the European Federation of Pharmaceutical Industry Associations (EFPIA). *Arch. Osteoporos.* **2013**, *8*, 136. [CrossRef]
11. Saad, F. Clinical benefit of zoledronic acid for the prevention of skeletal complications in advanced prostate cancer. *Clin. Prostate Cancer* **2005**, *4*, 31–37. [CrossRef]
12. Abrahamsen, B. Adverse effects of bisphosphonates. *Calcif. Tissue Int.* **2010**, *86*, 421–435. [CrossRef]
13. Reid, I.R. Osteonecrosis of the jaw: Who gets it, and why? *Bone* **2009**, *44*, 4–10. [CrossRef]
14. Luckman, S.P.; Hughes, D.E.; Coxon, F.P.; Graham, R.; Russell, G.; Rogers, M.J. Nitrogen-containing bisphosphonates inhibit the mevalonate pathway and prevent post-translational prenylation of GTP-binding proteins, including Ras. *J. Bone Miner. Res.* **1998**, *13*, 581–589. [CrossRef]
15. Rogers, M.J.; Crockett, J.C.; Coxon, F.P.; Monkkonen, J. Biochemical and molecular mechanisms of action of bisphosphonates. *Bone* **2011**, *49*, 34–41. [CrossRef]
16. Sinensky, M.; Lutz, R.J. The prenylation of proteins. *Bioessays* **1992**, *14*, 25–31. [CrossRef]
17. Palsuledesai, C.C.; Distefano, M.D. Protein prenylation: Enzymes, therapeutics, and biotechnology applications. *ACS Chem. Biol.* **2015**, *10*, 51–62. [CrossRef]
18. Ziebart, T.; Koch, F.; Klein, M.O.; Guth, J.; Adler, J.; Pabst, A.; Al-Nawas, B.; Walter, C. Geranylgeraniol—A new potential therapeutic approach to bisphosphonate associated osteonecrosis of the jaw. *Oral Oncol.* **2011**, *47*, 195–201. [CrossRef]
19. Zafar, S.; Coates, D.E.; Cullinan, M.P.; Drummond, B.K.; Milne, T.; Seymour, G.J. Zoledronic acid and geranylgeraniol regulate cellular behaviour and angiogenic gene expression in human gingival fibroblasts. *J. Oral Pathol. Med.* **2014**, *43*, 711–721. [CrossRef]
20. Koneski, F.; Popovic-Monevska, D.; Gjorgoski, I.; Krajoska, J.; Popovska, M.; Muratovska, I.; Velickovski, B.; Petrushevska, G.; Popovski, V. In vivo effects of geranylgeraniol on the development of bisphosphonate-related osteonecrosis of the jaws. *J. Craniomaxillofac. Surg.* **2018**, *46*, 230–236. [CrossRef]
21. Pabst, A.M.; Kruger, M.; Ziebart, T.; Jacobs, C.; Sagheb, K.; Walter, C. The influence of geranylgeraniol on human oral keratinocytes after bisphosphonate treatment: An in vitro study. *J. Craniomaxillofac. Surg.* **2015**, *43*, 688–695. [CrossRef] [PubMed]
22. Pabst, A.M.; Kruger, M.; Sagheb, K.; Ziebart, T.; Jacobs, C.; Blatt, S.; Goetze, E.; Walter, C. The influence of geranylgeraniol on microvessel sprouting after bisphosphonate substitution in an in vitro 3D-angiogenesis assay. *Clin. Oral Investig.* **2017**, *21*, 771–778. [CrossRef] [PubMed]
23. Favia, G.; Tempesta, A.; Limongelli, L.; Crincoli, V.; Maiorano, E. Medication-related osteonecrosis of the jaw: Surgical or non-surgical treatment? *Oral Dis.* **2018**, *24*, 238–242. [CrossRef]
24. Jung, J.; Yoo, H.Y.; Kim, G.T.; Lee, J.W.; Lee, Y.A.; Kim, D.Y.; Kwon, Y.D. Short-Term Teriparatide and Recombinant Human Bone Morphogenetic Protein-2 for Regenerative Approach to Medication-Related Osteonecrosis of the Jaw: A Preliminary Study. *J. Bone Miner. Res.* **2017**, *32*, 2445–2452. [CrossRef] [PubMed]
25. Owosho, A.A.; Estilo, C.L.; Huryn, J.M.; Yom, S.K. Pentoxifylline and tocopherol in the management of cancer patients with medication-related osteonecrosis of the jaw: An observational retrospective study of initial case series. *Oral Surg. Oral Med. Oral Pathol. Oral Radiol.* **2016**, *122*, 455–459. [CrossRef]
26. Zafar, S.; Cullinan, M.P.; Drummond, B.K.; Seymour, G.J.; Coates, D.E. Effects of zoledronic acid and geranylgeraniol on angiogenic gene expression in primary human osteoclasts. *J. Oral Sci.* **2020**, *62*, 79–83. [CrossRef]
27. Fliefel, R.M.; Entekhabi, S.A.; Ehrenfeld, M.; Otto, S. Geranylgeraniol (GGOH) as a Mevalonate Pathway Activator in the Rescue of Bone Cells Treated with Zoledronic Acid: An In Vitro Study. *Stem Cells Int.* **2019**, *2019*, 4351327. [CrossRef]
28. Livak, K.J.; Schmittgen, T.D. Analysis of relative gene expression data using real-time quantitative PCR and the 2(-Delta Delta C(T)) Method. *Methods* **2001**, *25*, 402–408. [CrossRef]
29. Marx, R.E. Pamidronate (Aredia) and zoledronate (Zometa) induced avascular necrosis of the jaws: A growing epidemic. *J. Oral Maxillofac. Surg.* **2003**, *61*, 1115–1117. [CrossRef]
30. Ruggiero, S.L.; Dodson, T.B.; Fantasia, J.; Goodday, R.; Aghaloo, T.; Mehrotra, B.; O'Ryan, F. American Association of Oral and Maxillofacial Surgeons position paper on medication-related osteonecrosis of the jaw—2014 update. *J. Oral Maxillofac. Surg.* **2014**, *72*, 1938–1956. [CrossRef]
31. Wennerberg, K.; Rossman, K.L.; Der, C.J. The Ras superfamily at a glance. *J. Cell Sci.* **2005**, *118*, 843–846. [CrossRef]
32. Jeong, A.; Suazo, K.F.; Wood, W.G.; Distefano, M.D.; Li, L. Isoprenoids and protein prenylation: Implications in the pathogenesis and therapeutic intervention of Alzheimer's disease. *Crit. Rev. Biochem. Mol. Biol.* **2018**, *53*, 279–310. [CrossRef]

33. Zafar, S.; Coates, D.E.; Cullinan, M.P.; Drummond, B.K.; Milne, T.; Seymour, G.J. Effects of zoledronic acid and geranylgeraniol on the cellular behaviour and gene expression of primary human alveolar osteoblasts. *Clin. Oral Investig.* **2016**, *20*, 2023–2035. [CrossRef]
34. Casey, P.J.; Solski, P.A.; Der, C.J.; Buss, J.E. p21ras is modified by a farnesyl isoprenoid. *Proc. Natl. Acad. Sci. USA* **1989**, *86*, 8323–8327. [CrossRef]
35. Colicelli, J. Human RAS superfamily proteins and related GTPases. *Sci. STKE* **2004**, *2004*, RE13. [CrossRef]
36. Ho, H.J.; Shirakawa, H.; Giriwono, P.E.; Ito, A.; Komai, M. A novel function of geranylgeraniol in regulating testosterone production. *Biosci. Biotechnol. Biochem.* **2018**, *82*, 956–962. [CrossRef]

life

MDPI

Brief Report

Gender-Related Differences in the Levels of Ambulatory BP and Intensity of Antihypertensive Treatment in Patients Undergoing Peritoneal Dialysis

Ioannis Kontogiorgos [1], Panagiotis I. Georgianos [1], Vasilios Vaios [1], Georgia Vareta [1], Eleni Georgianou [1], Apostolos Karligkiotis [1], Vasiliki Sgouropoulou [1], Konstantia Kantartzi [2], Pantelis E. Zebekakis [3,*] and Vassilios Liakopoulos [1]

[1] 2nd Department of Nephrology, AHEPA Hospital, Aristotle University of Thessaloniki, 54636 Thessaloniki, Greece
[2] Department of Nephrology, Democritus University of Thrace, 68100 Alexandroupolis, Greece
[3] Section of Hypertension, 1st Department of Medicine, AHEPA Hospital, Aristotle University of Thessaloniki, 54636 Thessaloniki, Greece
* Correspondence: pzempeka@auth.gr; Tel./Fax: +30-2310-994620

Abstract: Prior studies have shown that among patients with chronic kidney disease not yet on dialysis, the faster progression of kidney injury in men than in women is, at least partly, explained by sex differences in ambulatory blood pressure (BP) control. The present study aimed to investigate potential differences in the levels of ambulatory BP and intensity of antihypertensive treatment between men and women with end-stage kidney disease undergoing long-term peritoneal dialysis (PD). In a case-control design, 48 male PD patients were matched for age and heart failure status with 48 female patients in a 1:1 ratio. Ambulatory BP monitoring was performed with an oscillometric device, the Mobil-O-Graph (IEM, Stolberg, Germany). The BP-lowering medications actually taken by the patients were prospectively recorded. No gender-related differences were observed in 24 h systolic BP (129.0 ± 17.9 vs. 128.5 ± 17.6 mmHg, p = 0.890). In contrast, 24 h diastolic BP was higher in men than in women (81.5 ± 12.1 vs. 76.8 ± 10.3 mmHg, p = 0.042). As compared with women, men were being treated with a higher average number of antihypertensive medications daily (2.4 ± 1.1 vs. 1.9 ± 1.1, p = 0.019) and were more commonly receiving calcium-channel-blockers (70.8% vs. 43.8%, p = 0.007) and β-blockers (85.4% vs. 66.7%, p = 0.031). In conclusion, the present study shows that among PD patients, the levels of ambulatory BP and intensity of antihypertensive treatment are higher in men than in women. Longitudinal studies are needed to explore whether these gender-related differences in the severity of hypertension are associated with worse cardiovascular outcomes for male patients undergoing PD.

Keywords: ambulatory blood pressure; antihypertensive therapy; peritoneal dialysis; sex differences

Citation: Kontogiorgos, I.; Georgianos, P.I.; Vaios, V.; Vareta, G.; Georgianou, E.; Karligkiotis, A.; Sgouropoulou, V.; Kantartzi, K.; Zebekakis, P.E.; Liakopoulos, V. Gender-Related Differences in the Levels of Ambulatory BP and Intensity of Antihypertensive Treatment in Patients Undergoing Peritoneal Dialysis. *Life* **2023**, *13*, 1140. https://doi.org/10.3390/life13051140

Academic Editor: Alexey V. Polonikov

Received: 10 April 2023
Revised: 2 May 2023
Accepted: 7 May 2023
Published: 8 May 2023

1. Introduction

Hypertension is an important cause of cardiovascular morbidity and mortality in both the general population and in patients with end-stage kidney disease (ESKD) undergoing long-term peritoneal dialysis (PD) [1,2]. In the general population, the trajectories for blood pressure (BP) with ageing differ between men and women [3]. Hypertension is less frequent in young women than in men of the same age. Thereafter, there is a progressive elevation in the levels of BP in women. At approximately the fourth decade of life, the prevalence of hypertension does not substantially differ between the two genders. However, in the elderly, the severity of hypertension is greater in women than in men [3]. Furthermore, evidence from clinical studies suggests that there are sex differences in the severity of hypertension-mediated target-organ damage. As compared with men, women have been shown to carry a greater risk of developing left ventricular hypertrophy, concentric cardiac remodeling, and subclinical left ventricular diastolic dysfunction [4,5].

Prior studies have shown that there are gender-related differences in the severity of hypertension in patients with chronic kidney disease who are not yet on dialysis [6,7]. For example, in a prospective observational study that enrolled 906 hypertensive patients with predialysis CKD, the worse ambulatory BP control in men than in women at baseline was associated with a higher risk of incident ESKD and all-cause mortality in men over a median follow-up of 10.7 years [8]. It remains unclear whether such gender-related differences in ambulatory BP control exist in patients with ESKD who have even more severe hypertension. Accordingly, the present study aimed to provide a comparison of ambulatory BP levels and intensity of antihypertensive treatment between men and women with ESKD receiving long-term PD.

2. Materials and Methods

This was a secondary analysis incorporating data from a cross-sectional study that was conducted in 4 PD centers in Northern Greece aiming to investigate the epidemiology of hypertension in the PD population [2]. Patients were enrolled in the study if they met the following inclusion criteria: (i) ESKD patients who had been treated with continuous ambulatory or automated PD for at least 3 months, and (ii) patients who had signed informed written consents. Patients were excluded from this study in the case of: (i) chronic atrial fibrillation or other arrhythmia; (ii) adjustments to the PD regimen and/or changes in the prescribed antihypertensive medications during the last 2 weeks; (iii) acute peritonitis or other infectious/bleeding complications during the past 1 month; (iv) a body mass index of $\geq$40 kg/m^2; (v) the presence of nonfunctioning arteriovenous fistula in both arms that limited the possibility of accurate assessment of BP; and (vi) recent hospitalization for acute coronary syndrome or stroke. All clinical procedures were carried out in accordance with the Declaration of Helsinki and its latest amendments. The study protocol was approved by the Ethics Committee of the School of Medicine, Aristotle University of Thessaloniki (code of approval: 448/18-07-18), and it was registered in http://www.clinicaltrials.gov (accessed on 18 July 2018) (unique identifier: NCT03607747).

For the aims of the present analysis, a member of the investigative team (I.K.), who did not participate in the enrollment process and was unaware of the BP readings, matched at a 1:1 rate 48 male PD patients with 48 female PD patients for age and history of heart failure. All participants visited their PD unit to complete the prespecified protocol procedures. Data on demographic characteristics, medical history, laboratory parameters, antihypertensive treatment, and the prescribed PD regimen were prospectively collected.

Office BP measurements were taken by a nurse trained in this technique, according to the 2018 European Society of Hypertension/European Society of Cardiology (ESC/ESH) guidelines [9]. In all 4 PD centers, office BP was recorded with a validated automated device, the HEM–705 CP (Omron, Healthcare). More specifically, after a 5 min seated rest period, a cuff of appropriate size was fitted to the non-dominant (or non-fistula) arm and 3 BP measurements were performed 1 min apart. These 3 consecutive BP recordings were averaged to provide a standardized office BP measurement.

Ambulatory BP monitoring was performed for 24 h with an oscillometric device, the Mobil-O-Graph (IEM, Stolberg, Germany). Office and ambulatory BP readings were taken from the same arm to avoid inter-arm differences between these 2 techniques. The device was programmed to record ambulatory BP at 20 min intervals in the daytime period (07:00–23:00) and at 30 min intervals in the nighttime period (23:00–07:00). The ambulatory BP monitoring was judged as accurate if >80% of the readings were valid with no more than 2 non-consecutive daytime hours with <2 valid recordings and no more than 1 nighttime hour without a valid BP recording [10].

Hypertension was diagnosed based on at least one of the three following criteria: (i) standardized office BP of $\geq$140/90 mmHg; (ii) average 24-h ambulatory BP of $\geq$130/80 mmHg; and (iii) the use of at least 1 antihypertensive agent of any category.

The continuous variables are presented as means $\pm$ standard deviations (SDs) or medians and interquartile ranges (IQRs). The categorical variables are reported as frequencies (n) and percentages (%). The Kolmogorov–Smirnov test was used to examine if each variable was normally distributed. Comparisons of the continuous data between males and females were performed with an independent *t*-test or a Mann–Whitney U test, as appropriate. Between-group comparisons of the categorical variables were performed with a Chi-squared test or a Fisher's exact test. All tests were two-tailed, and a *p*-value of <0.05 was considered statistically significant. The analysis was conducted using the Statistical Package for Social Sciences (SPSS) version 27.0 (SPSS, Chicago, IL, USA).

3. Results

The study enrollment procedure is depicted in Figure 1. A total of 225 patients were assessed for eligibility. Of these, 145 patients fulfilled the inclusion/exclusion criteria and provided informed written consent. After the exclusion of 5 patients because of invalid or incomplete ambulatory BP monitoring, a total of 140 patients with complete datasets were finally included in the study. The overall population consisted of 54 female and 86 male PD patients. After the matching procedure for age and heart failure status, 48 pairs of women and men were created. Their basic demographic, clinical, and laboratory characteristics are presented in Table 1. As expected, due to the case-control design of this study, age and history of heart failure did not differ between the female and male participants. As compared with the men, the women had lower body weights (70.5 ± 15.2 vs. 77.9 ± 12.9 kg, $p = 0.012$) and lower levels of serum creatinine (5.9 (4.8–7.6) vs. 8.0 (5.5–13.9), $p = 0.008$). With respect to the mode of PD, the proportion of patients receiving continuous ambulatory PD was higher in the group of women than in the group of men (54.2% vs. 29.2%, $p = 0.013$). There were no statistically significant differences between the two genders in the prevalence of cardiovascular comorbidities, in the smoking status, or in other basic hematological or biochemical parameters (Table 1).

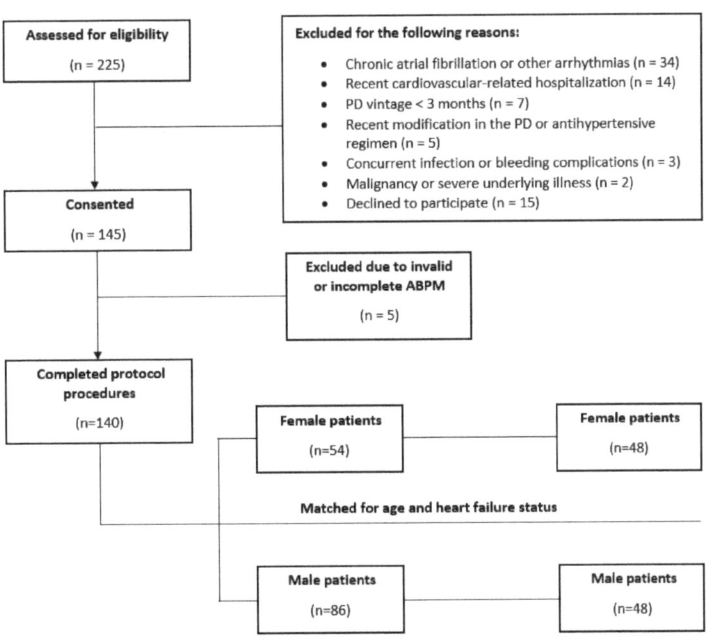

Figure 1. Flow diagram of the patient enrollment process of the study.

Table 1. Demographic, clinical, and laboratory characteristics of the male and female PD patients.

Parameter	Men (n = 48)	Women (n = 48)	*p*-Value
Age (years)	62.5 (54.0–70.5)	62 (53.3–70.8)	0.956
Weight (kg)	77.9 ± 12.9	70.5 ± 15.2	0.012
BMI (kg/m^2)	26.6 ± 4.0	27.5 ± 5.9	0.356
Time on PD (months)	21.0 (6.0–39.0)	21.5 (7.0–44.8)	0.867
Continuous ambulatory PD (n, %)	14 (29.2%)	26 (54.2%)	0.013
Peritoneal ultrafiltration (L)	0.6 (0.4–1.0)	0.8 (0.5–1.0)	0.412
Dialysate-to-plasma creatinine ratio	0.69 ± 0.10	0.67 ± 0.11	0.232
Peritoneal transport status (n, %)			
Low	3 (6.3%)	6 (12.5%)	
Low-average	13 (27.1%)	13 (27.1%)	
High-average	27 (56.3%)	23 (47.9%)	
High	5 (10.4%)	6 (12.5%)	
Residual diuresis ≥ 0.5 L/day (n, %)	35 (72.9%)	33 (68.8%)	0.653
Comorbidities (n, %)			
Diabetes mellitus	20 (41.7%)	18 (37.5%)	0.676
Dyslipidemia	33 (68.8%)	33 (68.8%)	1.000
Coronary artery disease	16 (33.3%)	11 (22.9%)	0.256
Peripheral vascular disease	8 (16.7%)	3 (6.3%)	0.109
Heart failure	9 (18.8%)	9 (18.8%)	1.000
Current smokers (n, %)	11 (22.9%)	7 (14.6%)	0.296
Laboratory parameters			
Hemoglobin (g/dL)	11.5 (10.9–12.6)	11.2 (10.3–11.9)	0.065
Serum urea (mg/dL)	123.9 ± 34.8	112.7 ± 32.4	0.106
Serum creatinine (mg/dL)	8.0 (5.5–13.9)	5.9 (4.8–7.6)	0.008
Serum albumin (g/dL)	3.9 (3.5–4.0)	3.7 (3.6–4.0)	0.371
Serum sodium (mEq/L)	138 (137–140)	138 (136–140)	0.474
Serum potassium (mEq/L)	4.5 ± 0.6	4.4 ± 0.6	0.516

Abbreviations: BMI = body mass index; PD = peritoneal dialysis. The continuous data are presented as means ± SDs or medians (IQRs).

As shown in Table 2, no significant differences between men and women were detected in the office systolic BP and office diastolic BP. The average 24 h ambulatory systolic BPs were similar in both groups (129.0 ± 17.9 vs. 128.5 ± 17.6 mmHg, p = 0.890). In contrast, the average 24 h ambulatory diastolic BP was significantly higher in men than in women (81.5 ± 12.1 vs. 76.8 ± 10.3, p = 0.042). These gender-related differences were consistent during both the daytime and nighttime periods. In detail, the daytime ambulatory diastolic BP (82.5 ± 11.8 vs. 78.1 ± 10.4, p = 0.052) and nighttime ambulatory diastolic BP (78.8 ± 14.0 vs. 73.8 ± 11.1 vs. p = 0.056) were higher in men than in women. The office and ambulatory heart rates were similar for the two groups. In addition, volume status, as assessed with the method of bioimpedance spectroscopy, did not significantly differ between the men and the women (Table 2).

There were no significant gender-related differences in the prevalence of hypertension either with the use of office recordings (93.8% vs. 89.6%, p = 0.460) or the use of the reference-standard method of ambulatory BP monitoring (93.8% vs. 91.7%, p = 0.695) for the diagnosis of hypertension. However, the men were being treated with a higher average number of antihypertensive medications daily (2.4 ± 1.1 vs. 1.9 ± 1.1, p = 0.019). Furthermore, as compared with the women, the men were more commonly being treated with calcium channel blockers (70.8% vs. 43.8%, p = 0.007) and β-blockers (85.4% vs. 66.7%, p = 0.031). In contrast, the male patients were less frequently receiving treatment with mineralocorticoid receptor antagonists than the women (4.2% vs. 20.8%, p = 0.014).

Table 2. Blood pressure measurements, volume statuses, and antihypertensive agents used in treating the male and female PD patients.

Parameter	Men (n = 48)	Women (n = 48)	*p*-Value
Office BP			
Systolic (mmHg)	135.5 ± 21.0	134.4 ± 18.2	0.768
Diastolic (mmHg)	79.6 ± 11.6	80.1 ± 14.1	0.856
Ambulatory 24 h BP			
Systolic (mmHg)	129.0 ± 17.9	128.5 ± 17.6	0.890
Diastolic (mmHg)	81.5 ± 12.1	76.8 ± 10.3	0.042
Ambulatory daytime BP			
Systolic (mmHg)	129.6 ± 17.6	129.7 ± 17.5	0.991
Diastolic (mmHg)	82.5 ± 11.8	78,1 ± 10.4	0.052
Ambulatory nighttime BP			
Systolic (mmHg)	127.0 ± 19.8	125.9 ± 18.8	0.776
Diastolic (mmHg)	78.8 ± 14.0	73.8 ± 11.1	0.056
HR (bpm)			
Office HR	73.7 ± 9.8	74.9 ± 11.7	0.573
Ambulatory 24 h HR	72.4 ± 8.1	72.3 ± 9.9	0.964
Ambulatory daytime HR	73.5 ± 0.3	73.6 ± 10.7	0.949
Ambulatory nighttime HR	69.6 ± 8.6	69.0 ± 9.1	0.730
Prevalence of hypertension			
Ambulatory BP ≥ 130/80 mmHg or antihypertensive drug use (n, %)	45 (93.8%)	44 (91.7%)	0.695
Office BP ≥ 140/90 mmHg or antihypertensive drug use (n, %)	45 (93.8%)	43 (89.6%)	0.460
Volume status			
BIS-derived overhydration index (L)	1.7 (0.1–3.3)	0.8 (−0.3–1.9)	0.071
Overhydration index > 2.5 L (n, %)	16 (33.3%)	8 (16.7%)	0.059
Patients treated with antihypertensives (n, %)	45 (93.8%)	42 (87.5%)	0.294
Number of antihypertensive medications (n, %)	2.4 ± 1.1	1.9 ± 1.1	0.019
Antihypertensive agent classes			
ACEIs/ARBs	25 (52.1%)	22 (45.8%)	0.540
CCBs	34 (70.8%)	21 (43.8%)	0.007
β-blockers	41 (85.4%)	32 (66.7%)	0.031
α-blockers	6 (12.5%)	1 (2.1%)	0.111
MRAs	2 (4.2%)	10 (20.8%)	0.014
Central acting agents	7 (14.6%)	3 (6.3%)	0.181

Abbreviations: BIS = bioimpendence spectroscopy; bpm = beats per minute; ACEI = angiotensin-converting enzyme inhibitor; ARB = angiotensin receptor blocker; BP = blood pressure; CCB = calcium channel blocker; HR = heart rate; MRA = mineralocorticoid receptor antagonist.

4. Discussion

The present study showed that among patients undergoing long-term PD, the levels of ambulatory BP were higher in men than in women. In addition, the intensity of antihypertensive treatment, such as the average number of prescribed BP-lowering medications as well as the use of calcium channel blockers and β-blockers, was greater in the male PD patients than in the female PD patients. The findings of the present study are accordant with the results of a prior cross-sectional analysis that compared the rates of ambulatory BP control between 129 male and 91 female patients receiving maintenance hemodialysis [11]. In this study, the 48 h ambulatory systolic BPs (137.2 ± 17.4 vs. 132.2 ± 19.2 mmHg, $p = 0.045$) and 48 h ambulatory diastolic BPs (81.9 ± 12.1 vs. 75.9 ± 11.7 mmHg, $p < 0.001$) were higher in men than in women [11]. Although the prevalence of hypertension did not differ between the two genders, the rates of 48 h ambulatory BP control were significantly lower in the male hemodialysis patients than in the female hemodialysis patients [11]. Similarly, another prior cross-sectional study showed that among kidney transplant recipients, the rates of 24 h ambulatory BP control were significantly lower in the female patients as compared with the male patients (16.9 vs. 30.3%, $p = 0.029$), despite the more intensive use of antihypertensive drug therapy in the men [12]. Taken together, the results of the present study and prior studies show that for the whole spectrum of ESKD, the severity of hypertension is greater in male patients than in female patients.

These sex-related differences in BP levels have biological plausibility. Mechanistic studies have provided evidence that the differences between the two genders in the activation of the renin-angiotensin system (RAS) and the sympathetic nervous system, nitric oxide metabolism as well as the release of sex hormones may mediate the greater severity of hypertension in men than in women [6,13]. Animal studies have shown that there is a higher activation in the AngII–AT1–ACE axis and a faster response to AngII infusion in male hypertensive rats than in female hypertensive rats [14,15]. Additionally, female hormones play a pivotal role in BP regulation. Postmenopausal women have been shown to have higher BP levels whereas the initiation of estrogen replacement therapy is accompanied by improvements in BP profiles [16,17]. Pro-inflammatory T-cells may also explain the sex differences in BP levels, with hypertensive women having more protective immune profiles and lower interleukin-17 levels, resulting in better BP control as compared with men [13,18].

The strength of the present study lies in its careful evaluation of hypertension with the concomitant use of standardized office and ambulatory BP measurements. Unlike the cross-sectional design of prior studies [9,10], an important advantage of the present work was the fact that our study followed a blinded matching procedure in group formation, mitigating the confounding effects of age and history of heart failure on the severity of hypertension. However, there are also some weaknesses that need to be acknowledged. First, the sample size of our study was relatively small; therefore, our analysis may not have been adequately powered to detect statistical significance in the small differences in the office and ambulatory BP levels between the males and females. Second, our study did not follow a longitudinal design and did not explore potential associations between ambulatory BP levels and the risk for adverse cardiovascular events for the two genders. Third, the measurements of the office and ambulatory BP were performed in a single time-point at baseline. Therefore, this study could not evaluate longitudinal changes in the severity of hypertension for the males and females.

Larger and longer-term observational studies are needed to confirm or refute the results of our analysis. If such gender-related differences in the severity of hypertension truly exist, then the worse ambulatory BP measurements in men might be a plausible mechanistic explanation for the sex differences in cardiovascular outcomes among patients receiving kidney replacement therapy.

Author Contributions: Investigation, V.V., G.V. and P.I.G.; data curation, I.K., P.I.G., E.G., A.K. and V.S.; writing—original draft preparation, I.K. and P.I.G.; writing—review and editing, E.G., A.K., V.S., K.K., P.E.Z. and V.L.; supervision, V.L. and P.E.Z. All authors have read and agreed to the published version of the manuscript.

Funding: This research received no external funding.

Institutional Review Board Statement: The study was conducted in accordance with the Declaration of Helsinki, and it was approved by the Ethics Committee of the School of Medicine, Aristotle University of Thessaloniki (code of approval: 448, 18 July 2018).

Informed Consent Statement: Informed consent was obtained from all subjects involved in the study.

Data Availability Statement: The data used in this study are not publicly available due to privacy and ethical concerns. These data may be shareable after contacting the corresponding author.

Conflicts of Interest: The authors declare no conflict of interest.

References

1. Georgianos, P.I.; Vaios, V.; Sgouropoulou, V.; Eleftheriadis, T.; Tsalikakis, D.G.; Liakopoulos, V. Hypertension in Dialysis Patients: Diagnostic Approaches and Evaluation of Epidemiology. *Diagnostics* **2022**, *12*, 2961. [CrossRef] [PubMed]
2. Vareta, G.; Georgianos, P.I.; Vaios, V.; Sgouropoulou, V.; Roumeliotis, S.; Georgoulidou, A.; Dounousi, E.; Eleftheriadis, T.; Papagianni, A.; Balaskas, E.V.; et al. Epidemiology of Hypertension among Patients on Peritoneal Dialysis Using Standardized Office and Ambulatory Blood Pressure Recordings. *Am. J. Nephrol.* **2022**, *53*, 139–147. [CrossRef] [PubMed]
3. Ji, H.; Kim, A.; Ebinger, J.E.; Niiranen, T.J.; Claggett, B.L.; Bairey Merz, C.N.; Cheng, S. Sex Differences in Blood Pressure Trajectories Over the Life Course. *JAMA Cardiol.* **2020**, *5*, 255. [CrossRef] [PubMed]
4. Cuspidi, C.; Gherbesi, E.; Sala, C.; Tadic, M. Sex, Gender, and Subclinical Hypertensiveorgan Damage—Heart. *J. Hum. Hypertens* **2022**. [CrossRef] [PubMed]
5. Cuspidi, C.; Faggiano, A.; Tadic, M. Hypertensive Organ Damage: The Vulnerable Heart of Women. *J. Hum. Hypertens* **2023**. [CrossRef] [PubMed]
6. Carrero, J.J.; Hecking, M.; Chesnaye, N.C.; Jager, K.J. Sex and Gender Disparities in the Epidemiology and Outcomes of Chronic Kidney Disease. *Nat. Rev. Nephrol.* **2018**, *14*, 151–164. [CrossRef] [PubMed]
7. Ricardo, A.C.; Yang, W.; Sha, D.; Appel, L.J.; Chen, J.; Krousel-Wood, M.; Manoharan, A.; Steigerwalt, S.; Wright, J.; Rahman, M.; et al. Sex-Related Disparities in CKD Progression. *JASN* **2019**, *30*, 137–146. [CrossRef] [PubMed]
8. Minutolo, R.; Gabbai, F.B.; Agarwal, R.; Garofalo, C.; Borrelli, S.; Chiodini, P.; Signoriello, S.; Paoletti, E.; Ravera, M.; Bellizzi, V.; et al. Sex Difference in Ambulatory Blood Pressure Control Associates with Risk of ESKD and Death in CKD Patients Receiving Stable Nephrology Care. *Nephrol. Dial. Transplant.* **2021**, *36*, 2000–2007. [CrossRef] [PubMed]
9. Williams, B.; Mancia, G.; Spiering, W.; Agabiti Rosei, E.; Azizi, M.; Burnier, M.; Clement, D.L.; Coca, A.; de Simone, G.; Dominiczak, A.; et al. 2018 ESC/ESH Guidelines for the Management of Arterial Hypertension: The Task Force for the Management of Arterial Hypertension of the European Society of Cardiology and the European Society of Hypertension. *J. Hypertens.* **2018**, *36*, 1953–2041. [CrossRef] [PubMed]
10. Parati, G.; Stergiou, G.; O'Brien, E.; Asmar, R.; Beilin, L.; Bilo, G.; Clement, D.; de la Sierra, A.; de Leeuw, P.; Dolan, E.; et al. European Society of Hypertension Practice Guidelines for Ambulatory Blood Pressure Monitoring. *J. Hypertens.* **2014**, *32*, 1359–1366. [CrossRef] [PubMed]
11. Theodorakopoulou, M.P.; Karagiannidis, A.G.; Alexandrou, M.-E.; Polychronidou, G.; Karpetas, A.; Giannakoulas, G.; Papagianni, A.; Sarafidis, P.A. Sex Differences in Ambulatory Blood Pressure Levels, Control and Phenotypes of Hypertension in Hemodialysis Patients. *J. Hypertens.* **2022**, *40*, 1735–1743. [CrossRef] [PubMed]
12. Korogiannou, M.; Sarafidis, P.; Theodorakopoulou, M.P.; Alexandrou, M.E.; Xagas, E.; Argyris, A.; Protogerou, A.; Ferro, C.J.; Boletis, I.N.; Marinaki, S. Sex Differences in Ambulatory Blood Pressure Levels, Control, and Phenotypes of Hypertension in Kidney Transplant Recipients. *J. Hypertens.* **2022**, *40*, 356–363. [CrossRef] [PubMed]
13. Song, J.-J.; Ma, Z.; Wang, J.; Chen, L.-X.; Zhong, J.-C. Gender Differences in Hypertension. *J. Cardiovasc. Trans. Res.* **2020**, *13*, 47–54. [CrossRef] [PubMed]
14. Hilliard, L.M.; Nematbakhsh, M.; Kett, M.M.; Teichman, E.; Sampson, A.K.; Widdop, R.E.; Evans, R.G.; Denton, K.M. Gender Differences in Pressure-Natriuresis and Renal Autoregulation: Role of the Angiotensin Type 2 Receptor. *Hypertension* **2011**, *57*, 275–282. [CrossRef] [PubMed]
15. Brown, R.D.; Hilliard, L.M.; Head, G.A.; Jones, E.S.; Widdop, R.E.; Denton, K.M. Sex Differences in the Pressor and Tubuloglomerular Feedback Response to Angiotensin II. *Hypertension* **2012**, *59*, 129–135. [CrossRef] [PubMed]
16. Fardoun, M.; Dehaini, H.; Shaito, A.; Mesmar, J.; El-Yazbi, A.; Badran, A.; Beydoun, E.; Eid, A.H. The Hypertensive Potential of Estrogen: An Untold Story. *Vasc. Pharmacol.* **2020**, *124*, 106600. [CrossRef] [PubMed]
17. Reckelhoff, J.F. Gender Differences in the Regulation of Blood Pressure. *Hypertension* **2001**, *37*, 1199–1208. [CrossRef] [PubMed]
18. Gillis, E.E.; Sullivan, J.C. Sex Differences in Hypertension: Recent Advances. *Hypertension* **2016**, *68*, 1322–1327. [CrossRef] [PubMed]

life

MDPI

Opinion

Central Centrifugal Cicatricial Alopecia in the Adolescent Population: An Overview of Available Literature

Victoria Palmer [1,*,†] and Manuel Valdebran [2,3,†]

1 King's Medical Center, St. Catherine, Portmore JM00000, Jamaica
2 Department of Dermatology and Dermatologic Surgery, Medical University of South Carolina, Charleston, SC 29425, USA
3 Department of Pediatrics, Medical University of South Carolina, Charleston, SC 29425, USA
* Correspondence: vpalmer@kingsmedcentre.com; Tel.: +1-(929)-268-0638
† These authors contributed equally to this work.

Abstract: Central centrifugal cicatricial alopecia (CCCA) is a lymphocytic scarring alopecia that predominantly affects women of African descent. Recent studies have demonstrated prevalence in children and adolescents, as well as Asian populations. A thorough search of Pubmed, Cochrane Database of Systematic Reviews, OVID Medline and Google Scholar was conducted using keywords such as "central centrifugal cicatricial alopecia", "scarring hair loss", "scarring alopecia", "hot comb alopecia", "pediatric" and "adolescent". The results yielded few articles in the literature that directly addressed CCCA in the adolescent population, with three articles providing details of the presentation in the form of case series and retrospective reviews. The presentation in the adolescent population was found to be varied, ranging from asymptomatic to symptomatic and involving diffuse to patchy hair loss in only the vertex and/or frontal and parietal scalp. Genetic and environmental etiologies were found to be statistically significant, and markers of metabolic dysregulation predisposing patients to diabetes mellitus and breast cancer were also uncovered. The differential diagnosis of patients who present with hair loss in the adolescent population should therefore be broad, and a low threshold for biopsies should be adopted to confirm CCCA in suspected patients. This will have future implications for reduced morbidity and public health.

Keywords: central centrifugal cicatricial alopecia; scarring alopecia; pediatric; scarring hair loss; skin of colour; public health

check for updates

Citation: Palmer, V.; Valdebran, M. Central Centrifugal Cicatricial Alopecia in the Adolescent Population: An Overview of Available Literature. *Life* **2023**, *13*, 1022. https://doi.org/10.3390/life13041022

Academic Editor: Enzo Berardesca

Received: 3 March 2023
Revised: 8 April 2023
Accepted: 14 April 2023
Published: 15 April 2023

1. Introduction

Central Centrifugal Cicatricial Alopecia (CCCA) is a lymphocytic scarring alopecia seen more commonly in adult women of African descent, with emerging literature also suggesting a prevalence in adolescent Black and Asian populations [1–3]. The aetiology of CCCA is multifactorial, ranging from genetic predisposition to traumatic hairstyling practices [2]. The association with metabolic syndrome and breast cancer also promotes inquiry into relevant genetic markers and potential public health implications [3–7]. Therefore, a high index of suspicion in the adolescent population should be maintained as there is wide variability in the presentation of CCCA. This review aims to classify the aetiology, presentation, histopathology, diagnosis and significance of treatment of CCCA in the adolescent population.

2. Epidemiology

The documented incidence of scarring hair loss at the vertex, predominantly presumed to be CCCA, is 5.6% in the US [4]. Women of African descent have a higher predilection for the condition, with a female: male ratio of 3:1 [8]. Adolescent patients tend to have a late presentation, like their adult counterparts [9]. Six patients with biopsy-proven cases of CCCA had an average of 32.4 months from symptom onset to presentation [10]. This differs from a study by Imhof et al., which reports that the average time from symptom onset to the diagnosis of scarring alopecia in the pediatric population was 17.1 months [11]. However, cases of CCCA were not included in this cohort, and it should be noted that the primary target population was White or Multiracial. Epidemiological data regarding the age of symptom onset is limited; however, studies have demonstrated an average age of 14 years, ranging from 11–15 years old [10,12,13]. This is in keeping with other average ages of primary cicatricial alopecias [11]. Concurrent psychiatric co-morbidities included anxiety (22.2%) and depression (22.2%) [9,11].

3. Aetiology

A genetic component of CCCA has been observed: inheritance is noted to be in an autosomal dominant pattern with partial/variable penetrance in familial cases [9,10,14–16]. Additionally, the role of anticipation is also being studied: in a study by Eginli et al., four of five adolescent patients with CCCA had a first-degree relative, their mothers, with the condition [10]. The same finding was documented in an asymptomatic South African 11-year-old girl who had biopsy-proven CCCA, diagnosed after she was screened because of her mother's CCCA diagnosis [12]. Scalp biopsies of CCCA have also demonstrated an upregulation of genes involved in fibroblast proliferation, collagen formation, and wound healing [9]. People of colour, i.e., Fitzpatrick phototypes IV–VI, have an increased proportion of fibroblasts relative to their White counterparts [1]. This finding may provide insight into the disparate incidence in the former population, as fibroblasts are a core component of wound healing and abnormalities with this process, manifesting in conditions such as keloids, which also prevails in People of Colour (POC) [17]. Therefore, the finding by Eginli et al. that two pediatric patients with biopsy-confirmed CCCA had previous scalp surgery may be linked to this pathogenesis [10]. Additionally, peptidyl arginine deiminase type III (PADI3), a gene involved in lipid metabolism and hair shaft formation, may be downregulated in patients with CCCA [9,15]. This decrease in expression, as well as concomitant missense and splice mutations, ultimately leads to decreased follicular development and abnormalities of the hair shaft resulting in increased hair fragility and breakage [9,15]. A disruption of pro-inflammatory and anti-inflammatory factors has also been noted to contribute to the pathogenesis. For example, matrix metalloproteinase 9 (MMP9) is a biomarker associated with dysregulated pathways of fibrosis and is upregulated in severe cases of CCCA [18]. This dysregulation is translated clinically by the low-grade inflammation seen on dermoscopy and histopathology with the subsequent progression to fibrosis [15].

Ethnic hair practices are the most debated aetiology for CCCA. While the majority of patients with CCCA have reported traumatic hairstyling practices (chemical relaxers/braids/hotcombs/weaves) at least once in their lifetime, these findings may not be causative [13,14]. Chemical relaxers have not consistently been associated with statistically significant findings [4,19,20]. Rather, bacterial scalp infections and tension-inducing hairstyles such as weaves/extensions and braids/cornrows have the most statistically significant correlation with clinically diagnosed CCCA, although this still remains a matter of debate [21–23]. The hypothesis that alopecia may result from tension-inducing hairstyles is consistent with the dysregulated pro-inflammatory and anti-inflammatory signals involved in the pathogenesis of CCCA; Further histopathological studies comparing the extent of inflammation between tension-inducing hairstyles and chemical relaxers would be useful in delineating a clearer association. Tension hairstyles are applied relatively frequently and involve consistent traction and subsequent inflammation for days to weeks at a time, while chemical relaxers are briefly applied to the scalp and are most frequently reapplied at 4-to-8-week intervals. The level of inflammation in tension hairstyles, though presumably milder, may therefore have a more profound cumulative effect. This is of cultural significance as hair grooming practices involving the use of heavy beads, cornrows and tight ponytails start at an early age in the African American community, highlighting the necessity of parent education.

4. Clinical Associations

Evidence demonstrates that CCCA may be a marker of metabolic dysregulation [7,11,15]. Roche et al. demonstrated that nonobese women with biopsy-proven CCCA had over a 3× risk of developing diabetes mellitus type 2 than their age, race and sex-matched controls ((OR (95% CI)): 3.26 (1.33–8.04); p-value < 0.05)) [7]. A 4.68× increase in the odds of having uterine leiomyomas compared with race-, age-, and sex-matched controls was also observed in a retrospective study at Johns Hopkins Hospital ($p < 0.001$) [24]. Additionally, Brown et al. demonstrated that in patients with biopsy-proven CCCA (159 of 742), 4.4% had a history of breast cancer compared with the 4079 controls (1.8%) (odds ratio 2.49; 95% confidence interval 1.06–4.92; $p = 0.02$) [25]. Both latter conditions are associated with an abnormal proliferation of fibrous tissue and once again demonstrate a crossover of the pathogenesis to different organ systems. The average age of diagnosis of breast cancer was 62.9 years [25]. While the types of breast cancer were not delineated in the study, an association between dysregulated PADI3, upregulated MMP9, triple-negative inflammatory breast cancer (TNIBC), and triple-negative non-inflammatory breast cancer (TN-NIBC) has been documented in the literature [5,6,23]. Triple-negative breast cancer appears more frequently in women aged 40 and younger than in older women. Black and Latina women are more predisposed to develop TNBC than white women. Women who have the gene change BRCA1 are also more likely to develop TNBC than other women [26]. Further investigation is therefore needed into the types of breast cancer diagnosed in the retrospective cross-sectional study by Brown et al., as it may help to broaden the scope of associated genetic markers to screen in the younger population [25].

5. Presentation

Eginli et al. analysed the scalp symptoms of six patients aged 14–19 who had symptom onset of biopsy-proven CCCA at 11–17 years old [10]. The primary clinical manifestation of the disease was scalp pruritus, scaling and tender papules and pustules (n: 5/6 = 83%). However, one patient was asymptomatic (n: 1/6 = 17%). The distribution of alopecia and associated signs were diverse: areas involved ranged from patchy hair loss confined to the vertex (n: 4/6 = 67%) or also involving the parietal area (n: 1/6 = 17%) or frontal scalp (n: 2/6 = 33%), diffuse thinning by the temples (n: 1/6 = 17%), diffuse erythema without scale (n: 1/6 = 17%) or diffuse scaling (n: 2/6 = 33%) (Figure 1).

These broad presentations are in keeping with Dlova et al.'s findings of an asymptomatic 11-year-old girl with small areas of scarring on her vertex and frontal scalp, as well as Shah et al.'s findings of an 18-year-old male with pruritus, scaling/crusting, bleeding and pustules/papules for 3 years [12,13]. Of note, the majority of these patients had no history of chemical or traumatic exposure to their hair. This reinforces the importance of genetic predisposition in the pathophysiology and the importance of maintaining a wide differential diagnosis, as seen in Table 1 below.

Although long-standing tinea capitis is a known precipitator of secondary scarring alopecia, further studies are needed to delineate the complete association between fungal/bacterial infections and CCCA. *Trichophyton tonsurans* tinea capitis infections have a predilection for Afro-American and Afro-Caribbean children in both North America and Europe, with a study in London demonstrating that 91% of *T. tonsurans* tinea capitis occurred in Afro-Caribbean children [27]. Potential causes for this finding include the practice of tight braiding, which expose the scalp's stratum corneum to fungal spores, as well as the application of oils, which may adhere to and retain spores [27]. The tight braiding hypothesis would subsequently increase the risk of developing CCCA in those who are genetically acceptable. Therefore, it would be reasonable to screen for CCCA in Afro-American or Afro-Caribbean children who present with pruritus, scaling, hair loss and black dots on dermoscopy, especially if they have a history of tension-inducing hairstyles and a maternal family history of CCCA, as all of these findings overlap with the presentation of CCCA. In addition, *T. tonsurans* can also exist as a carrier state in asymptomatic children, so these authors propose that asymptomatic children with clinical features suggestive of CCCA also have laboratory tests done to assess for concurrent infection [27].

Table 1. Differential diagnoses of primary and secondary scarring alopecias in the pediatric population [11].

Type of Scarring Alopecia	Symptoms	Distribution of Scalp Alopecia
Central Centrifugal Cicatricial Alopecia	Scalp pruritus, scaling, tender papules or pustules, asymptomatic	Vertex, frontal, parietal or patchy distribution
Folliculitis Decalvans	Follicular hyperkeratosis, tufting, pustules, scalp induration and atrophy, mild pain or discomfort	Vertex or patchy distribution
Lichen Planopilaris (LPP)	Single or multiple plaques with itching, stinging or burning	Classic LPP: Confluent random plaques FFA: Primarily frontotemporal involvement Lasseur-Graham-Little-Picardi: Patchy distribution
Aplasia Cutis Congenita	Asymptomatic; characterised by absence of skin	Primarily vertex involvement
Tina Capitis	Scalp pruritus, scaling, tender papules or pustules, asymptomatic	Patchy distribution
Morphea (Localised Scleroderma)	Erythematous patches or plaques with itching, tenderness or asymptomatic	Variable
Discoid Lupus Erythematosus	Scaling, erythematous annular plaques, asymptomatic	Variable
Dissecting Cellulitis	Painful nodules and abscesses, scaling	Variable
Keratosis Follicularis Spinulosa Decalvans	Keratotic follicular papules, atrophic depression	Variable

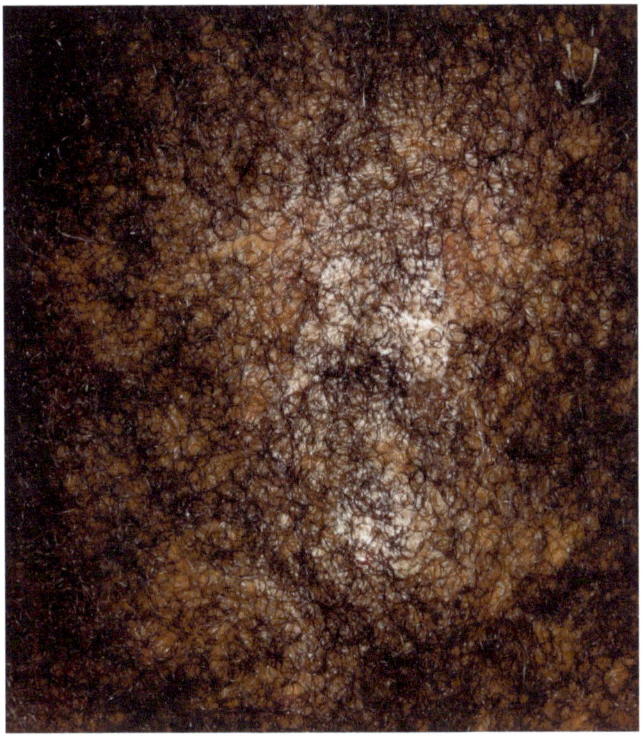

Figure 1. Patchy scarring alopecia with underlying erythema and erosions in male patient with biopsy-proven CCCA.

6. Histopathology and Dermoscopy

The histopathologic features of CCCA are consistent across age groups [12]. Table 2 describes the histopathological findings of CCCA in pediatric populations from studies currently available in the literature.

Table 2. Histopathological findings of CCCA in various pediatric populations.

Study	Age at Time of Biopsy (Age at Onset of Symptoms)	Histopathologic Findings of Biopsy-Proven-CCCA
Dlova et al. [12]	11 (No Data)	Perifollicular and perivascular lymphoid cell infiltrate with eccentric thinning of the follicular epithelium with concentric lamellar fibroplasia
Eginli et al. [10]	14 (11) 15 (13) 16 (12) 17 (15) 19 (16) 19 (17)	Concentric perifollicular fibrosis and lymphocytes at the level of the infundibulum and isthmus
Shah et al. [13]	18 (15–16)	Scarring, perifollicular fibrosis, fibrotic tracts, inflammatory infiltrate, few follicles

In the active stages of CCCA, there is follicular lichenoid inflammation; in the later stages, follicular fibrosis prevails [16]. The main diagnostic features of histopathology for CCCA are:

1. Reduced follicular density with altered architecture because of absent or reduced and miniaturised sebaceous glands [16];
2. Premature desquamation of the inner root sheath (very sensitive for CCCA, even in the absence of other findings) [16];
3. Perifollicular fibrosis and mild inflammatory infiltrate; CD3 and CD4 t-lymphocyte involvement in affected and unaffected follicles, with CD4 predominance in affected follicles and an increased CD1a:CD3 ratio [9,16] (Figures 2 and 3);
4. Lamellar hyperkeratosis or parakeratosis [16];
5. Naked hair shafts in the dermis [16];
6. Follicular miniaturisation [16];
7. Increased distance between affected follicles and small blood vessel clusters (BVCs; i.e., the perifollicular mucinous fibroplasia from chronic inflammation results in diminished blood supply [9].

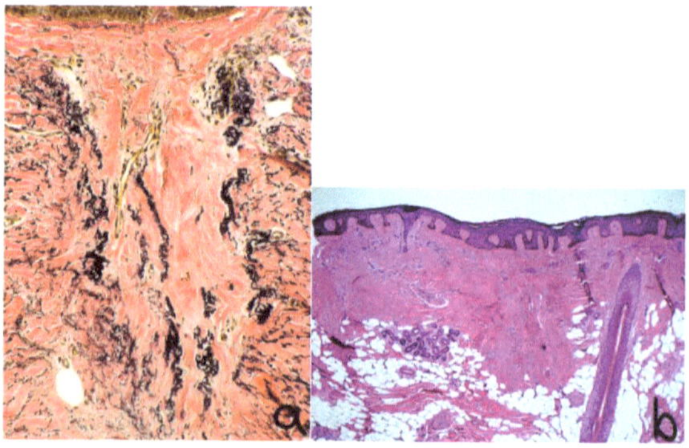

Figure 2. Histology: ×40 vertical sections showing (**a**) preservation and duplication of elastic sheath, (**b**) condensation of dermal collagen, broad fibrous tract with hair granuloma. Stained with hematoxylin.

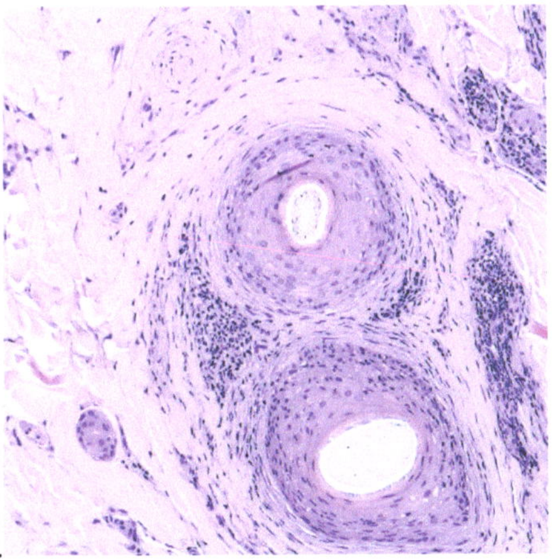

Figure 3. Histology ×40 horizontal section showing concentric lamellar fibroplasia and perifollicular inflammation. Stained with hematoxylin.

Dermoscopic findings include perihilar white/grey halos, loss of follicular ostia, perifollicular hyperpigmentation/erythema, polytrichia and hair shaft variability, pin-point white macules, and broken hairs resembling black dots [14,15]. Currently, there are no data correlating dermoscopy and pathology findings with disease evolution.

7. Management

Treatment of CCCA is notoriously challenging, and multiple therapies are often deployed, particularly in patients with advanced stages of hair loss. Early intervention is paramount to delay and/or prevent follicular burnout [21]. History includes documentation of hair and scalp symptoms, with the physician maintaining a high index suspicion as hair loss may present only as hair breakage at the vertex. The physician should also aim to confirm the diagnosis of CCCA with a biopsy to rule out other inflammatory disorders, such as lichen planopilaris (LPP) or folliculitis decalvans, which would influence subsequent management. Furthermore, documentation of hair grooming practices, gynaecological history, surgical history, medication use and dietary intake should also be obtained [9].

Treatments focus on decreasing potential triggers leading to fibrosis [9,10]. One of the first-line therapies is, therefore, behavioural modification: Although no consensus for hair styling recommendations has been reached, based on the conflicting data in the literature, it is advisable to refrain from tension-inducing hairstyles and chemical relaxers. The authors also suggest education about "protective hairstyles". "Protective hairstyles" have been advertised by hair stylists on social media with the goal of reducing daily manipulation of the hair as well as harsh environmental exposures [28]. These hairstyles range from cornrows and bantu knots to braided lace wigs and crotchet styling [28]. However, the use of hair extensions and tugging on the hair for braiding may inadvertently apply excess tension to the scalp and exacerbate the underlying inflammation [9,10,15,28]. Parents should therefore be acutely aware of signs that their child's hairstyle is too tight. Symptoms of excessive traction include discomfort and pruritus, and signs include visible tenting and folliculitis of the scalp [29]. If any of these signs or symptoms are observed, parents are advised to remove the hairstyle immediately [29]. In general, a braid is considered loose enough if a pencil can slip underneath the braid easily.

Additional anti-inflammatory therapies involve the application of daily high-potency topical corticosteroids, monthly intralesional corticosteroids +/− oral anti-inflammatory antibiotics such as tetracyclines, topical minoxidil and as-needed anti-dandruff shampoos [9,10]. Topical 10% metformin and oral metformin formulations have also been prescribed based on the association of CCCA with metabolic syndrome [23,29]. A six-month trial of these first-line therapies may be utilised before considering re-evaluating the diagnosis and/or considering alternate second-line therapies (Figure 4).

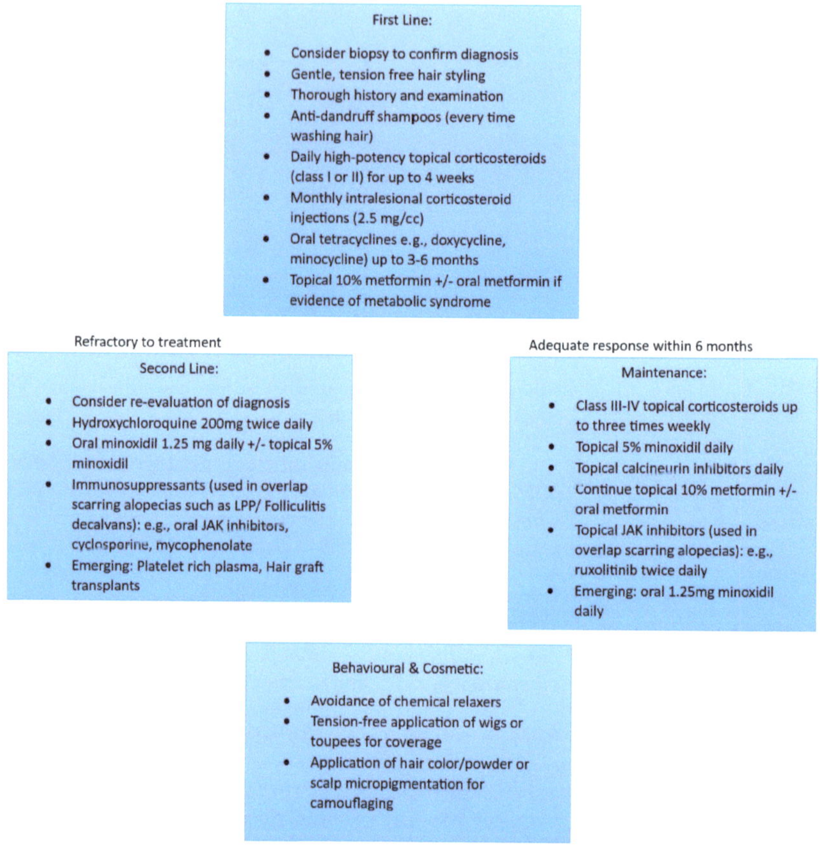

Figure 4. Illustrating the recommended management of CCCA. Adapted from George EA et al. [9].

For responders, results are maintained with mild–moderate potency topical corticosteroids, topical calcineurin inhibitors and topical/oral minoxidil. For refractory cases, if there was a significant infiltrate on initial biopsy, consider another type of cicatricial alopecia, such as LPP or folliculitis decalvans, in the differential diagnosis. Other strategies also include re-biopsy, reviewing the initial biopsy or seeking a second opinion. Second-line therapies include hydroxychloroquine, oral immunomodulators and oral/topical minoxidil. Immunosuppressants such as cyclosporine, mycophenolate and oral/topical JAK inhibitors are generally reserved for overlapping cases of scarring alopecia such as the aforementioned LPP or folliculitis decalvans. Surgery may be directed at end-stage biopsy-proven CCCA, in which there is no active inflammation for at least 9 to 12 months. Emerging therapies such as platelet-rich plasma injections and hair graft transplants have been described [9,14].

8. Recommendations

The postulated genetic anticipation promotes the recommendation that entire families should be screened if anyone presents with CCCA. This could be a method of decreasing the morbidity, such as concomitant anxiety and depression, associated with the disease [11]. The association between breast cancer and diabetes mellitus type II are also additional reasons to implement screening in these populations. Further studies should demonstrate the type of breast cancer associated with CCCA, as triple-negative breast cancer is associated with dysregulated PADI3 and MMP9 [5]. Women with the BRCA1 mutation are more likely to develop TNIBC; therefore, screening of this genetic marker in adolescent women with CCCA could potentially be of clinical utility [26].

9. Conclusions

Few studies are available in the literature outlining the presentation, management and prognosis of adolescent patients with CCCA. Awareness of CCCA in this population is paramount as the clinical presentation largely overlaps with tinea capitis scalp infections, which similarly prevail in Afro-American and Afro-Caribbean populations. A low threshold for screening and obtaining a biopsy in areas with follicular dropout should be used, particularly if first-degree relatives have concurrent hair loss. The public health implications of screening for BRCA1 mutations and diabetes mellitus type 2 should also be further researched.

Author Contributions: Conceptualisation, V.P. and M.V.; methodology, V.P and MV.; formal analysis, V.P. and M.V; data curation, V.P and M.V.; writing—original draft preparation, V.P.; writing—review and editing: M.V and V.P; supervision: M.V. All authors have read and agreed to the published version of the manuscript.

Funding: This research received no external funding.

Institutional Review Board Statement: Not applicable.

Informed Consent Statement: Informed consent was obtained for all clinical photographs included in this review.

Data Availability Statement: Data sharing is not applicable to this article as no datasets were generated or analysed during the current study.

Acknowledgments: Special thanks to Dirk Elston, who offered his expertise and clinical and histopathological photographs for this review.

Conflicts of Interest: The authors declare no conflict of interest.

References

1. Taylor, S.C.; Kelly, A.P.; Lim, H.; Serrano, A.M. *Taylor and Kelly's Dermatology for Skin of Color 2/E*; McGraw Hill Professional: New York, NY, USA, 2016.
2. Mitchell, K.N.; Tay, Y.K.; Heath, C.R.; Trachtman, R.; Silverberg, N.B. Emerging issues in pediatric skin of color, part 1. *Pediatr. Dermatol.* **2021**, *38*, 20–29. [CrossRef] [PubMed]
3. Goldberg, L.J.; Castelo-Soccio, L.A. Alopecia: Kids are not just little people. *Clin. Dermatol.* **2015**, *33*, 622–630. [CrossRef] [PubMed]
4. Olsen, E.A.; Callender, V.; McMichael, A.; Sperling, L.; Anstrom, K.J.; Shapiro, J.; Roberts, J.; Durden, F.; Whiting, D.; Bergfeld, W. Central hair loss in African American women: Incidence and potential risk factors. *J. Am. Acad. Dermatol.* **2011**, *64*, 245–252. [CrossRef] [PubMed]
5. Funakoshi, Y.; Wang, Y.; Semba, T.; Masuda, H.; Hout, D.; Ueno, N.T.; Wang, X. Comparison of molecular profile in triple-negative inflammatory and non-inflammatory breast cancer not of mesenchymal stem-like subtype. *PLoS ONE* **2019**, *14*, e0222336. [CrossRef] [PubMed]
6. Cheng, T.; Chen, P.; Chen, J.; Deng, Y.; Huang, C. Landscape analysis of matrix metalloproteinases unveils key prognostic markers for patients with breast cancer. *Front. Genet.* **2022**, *12*, 2769. [CrossRef]
7. Roche, F.C.; Harris, J.; Ogunleye, T.; Taylor, S.C. Association of type 2 diabetes with central centrifugal cicatricial alopecia: A follow-up study. *J. Am. Acad. Dermatol.* **2022**, *86*, 661–662. [CrossRef] [PubMed]
8. Sperling, L.C.; Cowper, S.E. The histopathology of primary cicatricial alopecia. *Semin. Cutan. Med. Surg.* **2006**, *25*, 41–50. [CrossRef]
9. George, E.A.; Matthews, C.; Roche, F.C.; Taylor, S.C. Beyond the Hot Comb: Updates in Epidemiology, Pathogenesis, and Treatment of Central Centrifugal Cicatricial Alopecia from 2011 to 2021. *Am. J. Clin. Dermatol.* **2023**, *24*, 81–88. [CrossRef]
10. Eginli, A.N.; Dlova, N.C.; McMichael, A. Central Centrifugal Cicatricial Alopecia in Children: A Case Series and Review of the Literature. *Pediatr. Dermatol.* **2017**, *34*, 133–137. [CrossRef] [PubMed]
11. Imhof, R.L.; Cantwell, H.M.; Proffer, S.L.; Tolkachjov, S.N.; Torgerson, R.R.; Tollefson, M.M. The spectrum of pediatric scarring alopecia: A retrospective review of 27 patients seen at Mayo Clinic. *Pediatr. Dermatol.* **2021**, *38*, 580–584. [CrossRef]

12. Dlova, N.C.; Forder, M. Central centrifugal cicatricial alopecia: Possible familial aetiology in two African families from South Africa. *Int. J. Dermatol.* **2012**, *51* (Suppl. S1), 17–20. [CrossRef]
13. Shah, S.K.; Alexis, A.F. Central centrifugal cicatricial alopecia: Retrospective chart review. *J. Cutan. Med. Surg.* **2010**, *14*, 212–222. [CrossRef] [PubMed]
14. Taylor, S.C.; Gathers, R.C.; Callender, V.D.; Rodriguez, D.A.; Badreshia-Bansal, S. *Treatments for Skin of Color E-Book*; Elsevier Health Sciences: Amsterdam, The Netherlands, 2011.
15. Lawson, C.N.; Bakayoko, A.; Callender, V.D. Central Centrifugal Cicatricial Alopecia: Challenges and Treatments. *Dermatol. Clin.* **2021**, *39*, 389–405. [CrossRef] [PubMed]
16. Herskovitz, I.; Miteva, M. Central centrifugal cicatricial alopecia: Challenges and solutions. *Clin. Cosmet. Investig. Dermatol.* **2016**, *9*, 175–181. [CrossRef]
17. Huang, C.; Wu, Z.; Du, Y.; Ogawa, R. The Epidemiology of Keloids. In *Textbook on Scar Management*; Téot, L., Mustoe, T.A., Middelkoop, E., Gauglitz, G.G., Eds.; Springer: Cham, Switzerland, 2020. [CrossRef]
18. Jamerson, T.A.; Conover Talbot, C., Jr.; Dina, Y.; Kwatra, S.G.; Garza, L.A.; Aguh, C. Gene expression profiling suggests severe, extensive central centrifugal cicatricial alopecia may be both clinically and biologically distinct from limited disease subtypes. *Exp. Dermatol.* **2022**, *31*, 789–793. [CrossRef]
19. Gathers, R.C.; Jankowski, M.; Eide, M.; Lim, H.W. Hair grooming practices and central centrifugal cicatricial alopecia. *J. Am. Acad. Dermatol.* **2009**, *60*, 574–578. [CrossRef] [PubMed]
20. Khumalo, N.P.; Gumedze, F. Traction: Risk factor or coincidence in central centrifugal cicatricial alopecia? *Br. J. Dermatol.* **2012**, *167*, 1191–1193. [CrossRef] [PubMed]
21. Whiting, D.A.; Olsen, E.A. Central centrifugal cicatricial alopecia. *Dermatol. Ther.* **2008**, *21*, 268–278. [CrossRef]
22. Suchonwanit, P.; Hector, C.E.; Bin Saif, G.A.; McMichael, A.J. Factors afecting the severity of central centrifugal cicatricial alopecia. *Int. J. Dermatol.* **2016**, *55*, e338–e343. [CrossRef]
23. Kyei, A.; Bergfeld, W.F.; Piliang, M.; Summers, P. Medical and environmental risk factors for the development of central centrifugal cicatricial alopecia: A population study. *Arch. Dermatol.* **2011**, *147*, 909–914. [CrossRef]
24. Dina, Y.; Okoye, G.A.; Aguh, C. Association of Uterine Leiomyomas With Central Centrifugal Cicatricial Alopecia. *JAMA Dermatol.* **2018**, *154*, 213–214. [CrossRef] [PubMed]
25. Brown-Korsah, J.B.; Roche, F.C.; Taylor, S.C. Association of breast and colorectal cancer in patients with central centrifugal cicatricial alopecia: A retrospective, cross-sectional pilot study. *J. Am. Acad. Dermatol.* **2021**, *84*, 859–860. [CrossRef] [PubMed]
26. National Cancer Institute. *Surveillance, Epidemiology, and End Results Program (SEER) Database*; National Cancer Institute: Bethesda, MD, USA, 2018.
27. Ameen, M. Epidemiology of superficial fungal infections. *Clin. Dermatol.* **2010**, *28*, 197–201. [CrossRef] [PubMed]
28. Afifi, L.; Oparaugo, N.C.; Hogeling, M. Review of traction alopecia in the pediatric patient: Diagnosis, prevention, and management. *Pediatr. Dermatol.* **2021**, *38*, 42–48. [CrossRef] [PubMed]
29. Ayandibu, G.; Bergfeld, W. Retrospective cohort study to assess the prevalence of different factors of metabolic syndrome in central centrifugal cicatricial alopecia patients. *J. Am. Acad. Dermatol.* **2018**, *79*, AB246.

life

MDPI

Article

Bone-Marrow-Derived Mesenchymal Stem Cells Attenuate Behavioral and Cognitive Dysfunction after Subarachnoid Hemorrhage via HMGB1–RAGE Axis Mediation

Harry Jung [1,†], Dong Hyuk Youn [1,†], Jeong Jin Park [2,3,*] and Jin Pyeong Jeon [4,*]

1 Institute of New Frontier Research Team, Hallym University College of Medicine, Chuncheon 24252, Republic of Korea
2 Department of Neurology, Konkuk University Medical Center, Seoul 05030, Republic of Korea
3 Department of Neurosurgery, Kangwon National University College of Medicine, Chuncheon 24341, Republic of Korea
4 Department of Neurosurgery, Hallym University College of Medicine, Chuncheon 24253, Republic of Korea
* Correspondence: medicalstory@gmail.com (J.J.P.); jjs6553@daum.net (J.P.J.)
† These authors contributed equally to this work.

Abstract: We evaluated the therapeutic effects of bone-marrow-derived mesenchymal stem cells (BMSCs) on behavioral and cognitive function in a mouse model of mild subarachnoid hemorrhage (SAH) and explored the underlying mechanisms in conjunction with the HMGB1–RAGE axis. The SAH models were generated in a total of 126 male C57BL/6J mice via endovascular perforation and evaluated 24 h and 72 h after the intravenous administration of BMSCs (3×10^5 cells). The BMSCs were administered once, at 3 h, or twice, at 3 h and 48 h after the model induction. The therapeutic effects of the BMSCs were compared to those of the saline administration. Compared to saline-treated SAH-model mice, at 3 h, the mice with mild SAH treated with the BMSCs showed significant improvements in their neurological scores and cerebral edema. The administration of the BMSCs decreased the mRNA expression of HMGB1, RAGE, TLR4, and MyD88, as well as the protein expression of HMGB1 and phosphorylated NF-kB p65. Furthermore, the numbers of slips per walking time, impairments in short-term memory, and the recognition of novel objects were improved. There was some improvement in inflammatory-marker levels and cognitive function according to the BMSCs' administration times, but no large differences were seen. The administration of BMSCs improved behavioral and cognitive dysfunction by ameliorating HMGB1–RAGE axis-mediated neuroinflammation after SAH.

Keywords: subarachnoid hemorrhage; bone-marrow mesenchymal stem cells; cognitive impairment; high-mobility group box 1

Citation: Jung, H.; Youn, D.H.; Park, J.J.; Jeon, J.P. Bone-Marrow-Derived Mesenchymal Stem Cells Attenuate Behavioral and Cognitive Dysfunction after Subarachnoid Hemorrhage via HMGB1–RAGE Axis Mediation. *Life* **2023**, *13*, 881. https://doi.org/10.3390/life13040881

Academic Editors: Giuseppe Minervini and Stefanos Roumeliotis

Received: 6 March 2023
Revised: 21 March 2023
Accepted: 25 March 2023
Published: 26 March 2023

1. Introduction

Subarachnoid hemorrhage (SAH) is a neurological disease with a high rate of in-hospital mortality, which ranges from 20 to 30%. The pooled incidence of SAH was reported to be 21.4 per 100,000 person-years [1,2]. The main focus of research on SAH is on improving patient survival by effectively preventing rebleeding (clipping vs. coiling) and minimizing neurological complications, such as delayed cerebral ischemia (DCI) and hydrocephalus. However, although favorable neurological outcomes are achieved by the use of appropriate treatments, a significant number of SAH survivors complain of behavioral deficits or changes such as motor weakness, sensory changes, and balance problems, and exhibit cognitive dysfunction in various domains of visual and verbal memory, as well as a decline in executive functions [3]. Hunt–Hess grades greater than 2, a thick SAH, and DCI are well-known risk factors for behavioral and cognitive dysfunction [4,5]. Subarachnoid hemorrhage can result in behavioral and cognitive dysfunction by altering functional connectivity [6]. Despite good neurological outcomes, persistent behavioral and cognitive dysfunction impairs quality of life. Nevertheless, the research on therapeutics for SAH patients is limited compared to the research on therapies for those with neurodegenerative diseases or ischemic stroke.

Stem-cell treatments have been investigated for use in treating some brain diseases, especially degenerative brain diseases, in anticipation of replacing injured neuronal cells and reconstructing damaged neural circuits using stem cells [7–9]. Among various types of stem cell, mesenchymal stem cells (MSCs) are advantageous in terms of immune tolerance because they express fewer major histocompatibility complex class I molecules and are easily obtained and handled [10]. Previous studies on MSC treatments for SAH have focused on ameliorating neuroinflammation in the early phase after the ictus of SAH [11,12]. Khalili et al. [11] first reported that MSC treatment 24 h after SAH significantly improved functional recovery and reduced apoptosis. Liu et al. [12] reported that bone-marrow-derived stem-cell (BMSC) treatment 1 h after SAH contributed to decreased brain water content and blood–brain barrier (BBB) permeability by inhibiting Notch1-dependent neuroinflammation. However, few studies have examined whether MSC treatment is linked to the attenuation of behavioral and cognitive dysfunction. Neuroinflammation itself is widely recognized as a potential mediator of behavioral and cognitive dysfunction [13]. In particular, high-mobility-group box protein 1 (HMGB1) has received attention in the study of various disease conditions, since it is released by glial cells and neurons after brain damage [14]. The HMGB1 continuously binds to toll-like receptors (TLRs) and the receptor for advanced glycation end products (RAGE), activating inflammatory responses [14]. The anti-HMGB1 antibody improved behavioral performance and reduced oxidative stress in injured brains after hemorrhage [15]. The suppression of HMGB1, TLR, and RAGE was shown to halt the progression of amyloid-beta (Aß) loading in Alzheimer's disease (AD) and diabetes-related dementia [16,17]. Thus, we investigated the therapeutic effects of BMSCs on behavioral and cognitive dysfunction after SAH and explored the underlying mechanisms in conjunction with HMGB1-mediated neuroinflammation in an experimental mouse model of mild SAH.

2. Materials and Methods

2.1. Experimental SAH Model

The C57BL/6J male mice, 8–10 weeks of age and weighing 20–25 g, were obtained from the Laboratory Animal Resources Center of Hallym University. The animals were provided with regular food and water ad libitum under a 12-h dark/light cycle at 24 °C and 55 ± 10% humidity. The SAH model was generated using the endovascular perforation technique, as described previously [4,18]. The mice were anesthetized with 2.5% isoflurane in oxygen. Next, a vertical incision was made on the midline of the neck, and the external and common carotid arteries were exposed. Subsequently, sharpened 5-0 Prolene suture material was inserted in the external carotid artery and advanced, ultimately perforating the distal internal carotid artery (ICA), which is divided into the anterior and middle cerebral arteries. Mice in the sham-operated group underwent the same procedure, except for arterial perforation [19]. In this study, we used only mild-SAH-model mice evaluated at 24 h based on modified Garcia neurological scale scores of 16 and 17 [19,20]. At the end of the study, mice were hyperanesthetized with 3.5% isoflurane in oxygen for 5 min. After confirming that each mouse's heart had stopped, the brain was isolated. For histology analysis, mice were anesthetized with 2.5% isoflurane in oxygen followed by cardiac perfusion before their brains were collected. After separating the mouse brains, brain-tissue samples, from which the olfactory bulb and cerebellum were removed using a microblade, were used for analysis. Next, the isolated tissues were homogenized using Omni Bead mill homogenizer (Omni International, Kennesaw, GA, USA). All animal experiments were approved by the Institutional Animal Care and Use Committee (IACUC) of Hallym University (no: HallymR1 2021-50).

2.2. BMSC Culture

The BMSCs isolated from normal human bone marrow without disease were purchased from ATCC (PCS-500-012, Manassas, VA, USA). We confirmed BMSCs with pluripotent marker expression of SOX2, OCT4, and Nanog for at least 5 passages. We cultured BMSCs by referring to previous papers [21,22]. Cells were plated at a density of 1×10^6 cells in a 100-mm culture dish in high-glucose Dulbecco's modified Eagle medium (DMEM), 10% fetal bovine serum (FBS), and 100 U/mL penicillin/streptomycin (Gibco, Grand Island, NY, USA). After 48 h, nonadherent cells contained in the medium were removed, and fresh culture medium was added to the adherent mononuclear cells, which represented BMSCs. All BMSCs used in this experiment were from passage 5. The BMSCs (3×10^5 cells) were administrated intravenously to the mice.

2.3. BMSC Administration

A total of 126 male C57BL/6J mice were randomly divided into 6 groups (Supplemental Figure S1). After SAH induction, BMSCs were administered to the mice once, at 3 h, or twice, at 3 h and 48 h, and the treatment effects were evaluated at 24 h and 72 h, respectively. In detail, the analysis groups were: (1) normal controls (Normal); (2) SAH mice treated with saline at 3 h and evaluated at 24 h (24 h-S-3 h); (3) SAH mice treated with BMSCs at 3 h and evaluated at 24 h (24 h-B-3 h); (4) SAH mice treated with saline at 3 h and evaluated at 72 h (72 h-S-3 h); (5) SAH mice treated with BMSCs at 3 h and evaluated at 72 h (72 h-B-3 h); (6) SAH mice administered saline twice, at 3 h and 48 h, and evaluated at 72 h (72 h-S-3 h/48 h); and (7) SAH mice treated with administered BMSCs twice, at 3 h and 48 h, and evaluated at 72 h (72 h-B-3 h/48 h). The results were compared to those of mice administered saline.

2.4. RNA Isolation and Quantitative RT-PCR

Total RNA in the brain tissues was extracted using easy-BLUE Total RNA Extraction Kit and reverse-transcribed into cDNA using Maxime RT PreMix Kits (iNtRON Biotechology, Inc., Santa Cruz, MA, USA). The mRNA purity was measured using an Eppendorf BioSpectrometer Basic (Eppendorf, Hamburg, Germany). The A260/A280 ratio was used in this study to indicate the mRNA purity, which ranged from 1.9 to 2.0. Quantitative real-time polymerase chain reaction (qRT-PCR) analysis was performed in triplicate for each sample using SYBR Green PCR Kits (Applied Biosystems, Foster City, CA, USA) for 60 cycles with a 3-step program of 15 s of denaturation at 94 °C, 30 s of annealing at 55 °C, and 30 s of extension at 70 °C. Amplification specificity was assessed by melting-curve analysis. The sequences of the qRT-PCR primers are presented in Supplemental Table S1. Glyeraldehyde-3-phosphate dehydrogenase (GAPDH) was used as the endogenous control. The qRT-PCR results were analyzed using the $2^{-\Delta\Delta ct}$ method.

2.5. Western Blots

After lysing brain tissues in radio-immunoprecipitation assay buffer supplemented with a proteinase-inhibitor cocktail, the protein concentrations were measured using the Pierce BCA Protein Assay Kit (Thermo Fisher Scientific Inc., Waltham, MA, USA). Proteins (15 ug) were separated by 10–15% sodium dodecyl sulfate–polyacrylamide-gel electrophoresis (SDS PAGE) and transferred onto polyvinylidene-fluoride membranes. The membranes were blocked in 1% bovine serum albumin (BSA) for 1 h at room temperature and incubated with primary antibodies overnight at 4 °C. The following primary antibodies were used: interleukin (IL)-6 (1:500, Santa Cruz Biotechnology, Dallas, TX, USA), tumor necrosis factor (TNF)-α (1:500, Santa Cruz Biotechnology), COX-2 (1:1000, Abcam, Waltham, MA, USA), HMGB1 (1:1000, Cell Signaling Technology, Danvers, MA, USA), nuclear factor (NF)-kB p65 (1:1000, Cell Signaling Technology), and phosphor-NF-kB p65 (1:1000, Cell Signaling Technology). The membranes were washed three times for 15 min in tris-buffered saline with 0.1% Tween 20 and then incubated with HRP-linked secondary antibody. The bots were exposed to X-ray film for 1–5 min and analyzed by ImageJ software (Image J 1.49v,

National Institutes of Health). Rationales for investigating various markers used in this study are presented in the Supplemental Method Section.

2.6. Brain Water Content

The wet weights of the mouse brains were obtained and the brains were dried in the oven at 100 °C for 3 h to obtain the dry weights, as in a previous report [23]. Cerebral edema was measured by the following formula: brain water content percentage = [(wet weight − dry weight)/wet weight] × 100% [23].

2.7. Behavioral and Cognitive Dysfunction

Behavioral assessments were conducted using modified Garcia neurological scale scores and the beam-walking test, according to previous studies [4,24]. The beams were located horizontally and 50 cm above the table. Briefly, in the beam-walking test, mice were trained to cross an illuminated alley (10 cm wide and 33 cm long) and move straight to the opposite side, located at the end of the alley. Their hindlimbs were then coated with non-toxic ink, and the mice were allowed to walk through a small tunnel on a sheet of white paper. This results of 1–2 trials were recorded until 10 clearly visible footprints per animal were obtained. Mice were trained to traverse a beam 2 cm in diameter and then a beam 1 cm in diameter. The latency time to traverse each beam and latency time to fall were recorded. Cognitive dysfunction was assessed using Y-maze and novel object recognition (NOR) tests. The Y-maze test was used to assess short-term spatial memory. Each mouse was placed in a white Y-maze with three arms, which were designated A, B, and C. Each arm was 40 cm long, 12 cm high, and 10 cm wide. Each mouse was placed at the end of the starting arm and allowed to move freely through the maze for 5 min. Alternation behavior was defined as consecutive entries into three arms. The major outcome was spontaneous alternation (alternation index = alternation/maximum alternation × 100). The NOR test was performed according to our previous report (Supplemental Data) [23]. The mice were habituated for 10 min for two days in an open square field (65 × 45 × 30 cm) and then trained with two identical objects (A1 and A2) in opposite quadrants in the arena. After 24 h, the mice were exposed to a familiar object (A1) and a novel object (B1) for 10 min. Twenty-four h and seventy-tow h after the SAH, mouse activity was evaluated by changing the distance between A1 and the novel object (C1) in the 10-min open-field test. Object preference was measured once, at s distance between the mouse's nose and the object of less than 2 cm. All mouse-behavior tests were recorded by a video tracking system and described using heatmap image tracking (NoldusEthoVision XT, Leesburg, VA, USA) [23].

2.8. Statistical Analysis

All data are presented as the means with standard errors of the mean (SEM). One-way analysis of variance (ANOVA) with post hoc Bonferroni correction was conducted for all possible pairwise comparisons [25]. Any p-values of less than 0.05, 0.01, and 0.001 are represented by *, **, and *** in the figures, respectively [26]. All statistical analyses were conducted using GraphPad Prism software (v.8.0; GraphPad Software Inc., San Diego, CA, USA).

3. Results

3.1. Effect of BMSC on the In Vivo SAH Model

We explored the therapeutic effects of the BMSCs on neurological deficits and cerebral edema after the SAH induction in the mice (Figure 1 and Figure S1). Compared to the control group, the mice with mild SAH administered saline at 3 h exhibited definite blood clots in the basal cistern and decreased neurological scores with increased cerebral edema at 24 h and 72 h. In particular, although the amount of clotted blood decreased visually at 72 h, the neurologic scores and edema continued to deteriorate. The mice with mild SAH and BMSC administration at 3 h showed significantly improved neurological scores with decreased cerebral edema compared to the mice with mild SAH and saline administration

(17.3 ± 0.6 in the BMSC treatment group vs. 15.7 ± 0.6 in the saline treatment group; $p < 0.005$). When measured at 72 h, the neurologic scores and cerebral edema showed no significant improvements compared to the measurements at 24 h. To examine the differences in the therapeutic effects at 72 h according to the number of administrations, the BMSCs were administered twice, 3 h and 48 h after the model induction. Contrary to our expectations, similar effects on the neurological scores and brain water content were seen in the mice with mild SAH treated with BMSCs twice compared to a single administration of BMSCs.

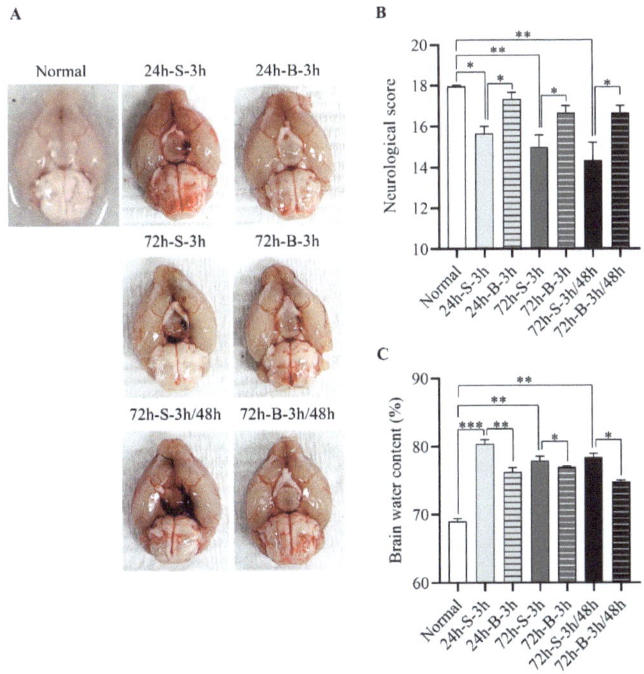

Figure 1. Therapeutic effects of BMSC on the in vivo SAH model. (**A**) Representative brain images of the normal control and in vivo SAH model mice treated with saline or BMSCs observed at 24 h or 72 h after model induction. (**B**,**C**) Comparison of neurological scores (n = 6) and brain water content (n = 6) according to the treatment method. * $p < 0.05$, ** $p < 0.01$, and *** $p < 0.001$. The data represent the mean ± standard error of the mean (SEM).

3.2. Histological Examination, Neuronal Apoptosis, and Inflammation

The H&E staining performed 24 h after SAH induction showed that the mice with mild SAH and saline administration had decreased luminal areas in the distal ICA, with increased wall thickness compared to those administered the BMSCs (Figure 2A). More pronounced thick blood in the subarachnoid space and thick subarachnoid layers over the convexities were observed at 24 h after the SAH in the saline-treated group compared to the BMSC-treated group. The H & E staining at 72 h showed thin layers on the convexities and decreased numbers of invading cells under the pia mater after the administration of the BMSCs. The lumen diameter of the distal ICA was 576.4 ± 75.1 μm for the normal mice. It was decreased to 269.8 ± 10.9 μm at 24 h after the SAH induction. The wall thickness of the distal ICA was 36.8 ± 3.8 μm for the normal mice. It increased to 72.5 ± 7.0 μm at 24 h after the SAH induction. Anatomically, the lumen area and the thickness of distal ICA were similar to those of the normal-mice group after the administration of the BMSCs at 3 h and 48 h after the SAH induction. At 72 h after the SAH induction, the wall thickness was 46.3 ± 1.6 μm for the single-BMSC-administration group and 62.3 ± 4.8 μm for the saline-administration group (Figure 2B,C).

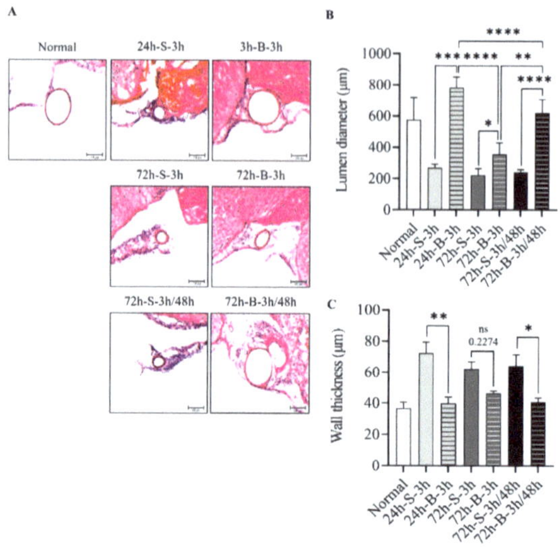

Figure 2. Change in histological examination, lumen size, and wall thickness for BMSC in the in vivo SAH model. (**A–C**) Representative hematoxylin and eosin-stained coronal sectioned images of the distal internal carotid artery according to treatment method, such as saline or BMSC, observed at 24 h or 72 h after SAH induction (n = 6). Error bars, mean SEM, ns: not significant, * $p < 0.05$, ** $p < 0.01$, *** $p < 0.005$, and **** $p < 0.001$.

The mRNA- and protein-expression levels of IL-6, TNF-α, and COX-2 were significantly decreased after the BMSC administration at both 24 h and 72 h after the SAH induction compared to the control group (Figure 3A–F). In particular, the IL-6 and COX-2 proteins decreased more after two BMSC administrations than after one.

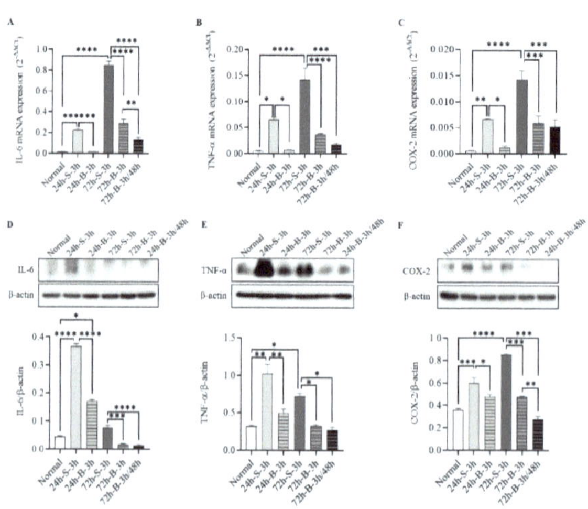

Figure 3. Comparisons of mRNAs (**A–C**) and proteins (**D–F**) of IL-6, TNF-α, and COX-2 in in vivo SAH model mice according to the treatment method (n = 6). Error bars, mean SEM, * $p < 0.05$, ** $p < 0.01$, *** $p < 0.005$, and **** $p < 0.001$.

3.3. Changes in HMGB1–RAGE Axis Inflammation

To determine inflammatory changes in the HMGB1–RAGE axis after the BMSC administration, we measured the mRNA-expression levels of HMGB1, RAGE, TLR4, and MyD88 using qRT-PCR, and the protein-expression levels of HMGB1, total NF-kB p65, and phospho-NF-kB p65 by Western blotting. The BMSC administration decreased the mRNA expression of HMGB1, RAGE, TLR4, and MyD88 after the SAH induction (Figure 4A–D). Reductions in TLR4 and MyD88 mRNA expression were seen at 72 h. The protein expressions of HMGB1 and phosphorylated NF-kB p65 decreased after the BMSC administration (Figure 4E,F). In particular, NF-kB p65 decreased more when the BMSCs were administered twice compared to once.

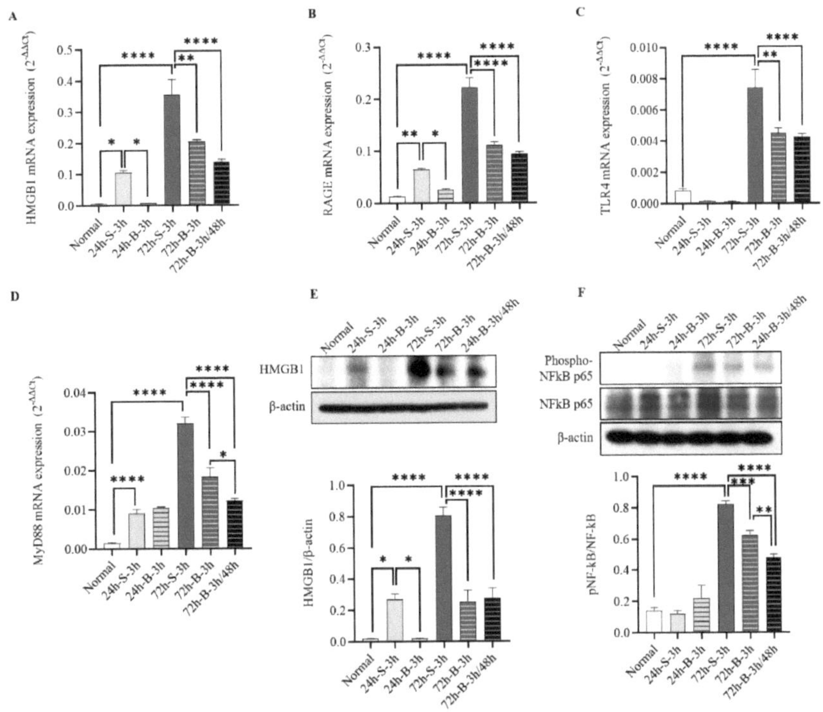

Figure 4. Changes in HMGB1–RAGE axis inflammation. (**A–D**) The mRNA expression of HMGB1–RAGE inflammation by HMGB1, RAGE, TLR4, and MyD88 using qRT-PCR in in vivo SAH-model mice based on treatment. (**E,F**) Comparison of HMGB1, total NF-kB p65, and phospho-NF-kB p65 according to the treatment method (n = 6). Error bars, mean SEM, * $p < 0.05$, ** $p < 0.01$, *** $p < 0.005$, and **** $p < 0.001$.

3.4. Behavior and Cognition

The BMSC administration improved the motor activity and balance (Figure 5 and Figure S2). The slip number/sec for walking in the normal mice was 0.013 ± 0.003 n/sec. It increased to 4.667 ± 1.258 n/sec at 24 h after the SAH induction in the saline-administered mice (Figure 5A,B). The alteration/maximum alteration rate in the normal mice was 74.4 ± 4.6%. It decreased to 48.6 ± 0.9% at 24 h after the SAH induction in the saline-administered mice. In particular, more improvements were seen after administering the BMSCs twice, at 3 h and 48 h, compared to once (Figure 5C,D). On the NOR test, the percentage of identical object (A1 and A2) recognition after the training phase and the percentage of familiar object (A1) and novel object (B1) recognition did not significantly differ between the groups (Supplemental Figure S2). After the SAH induction, the recognition index of a novel object (C1) by the SAH-model mice treated with the BMSCs at 3 h was significantly higher than in those treated with the saline at 24 h. The novel recognition rate was higher when the BMSCs were administered twice, at 3 h and 48 h, compared to the saline-administered group, but there was no significant difference compared to the group administered BMSCs once, at 3 h (Figure 5E,F).

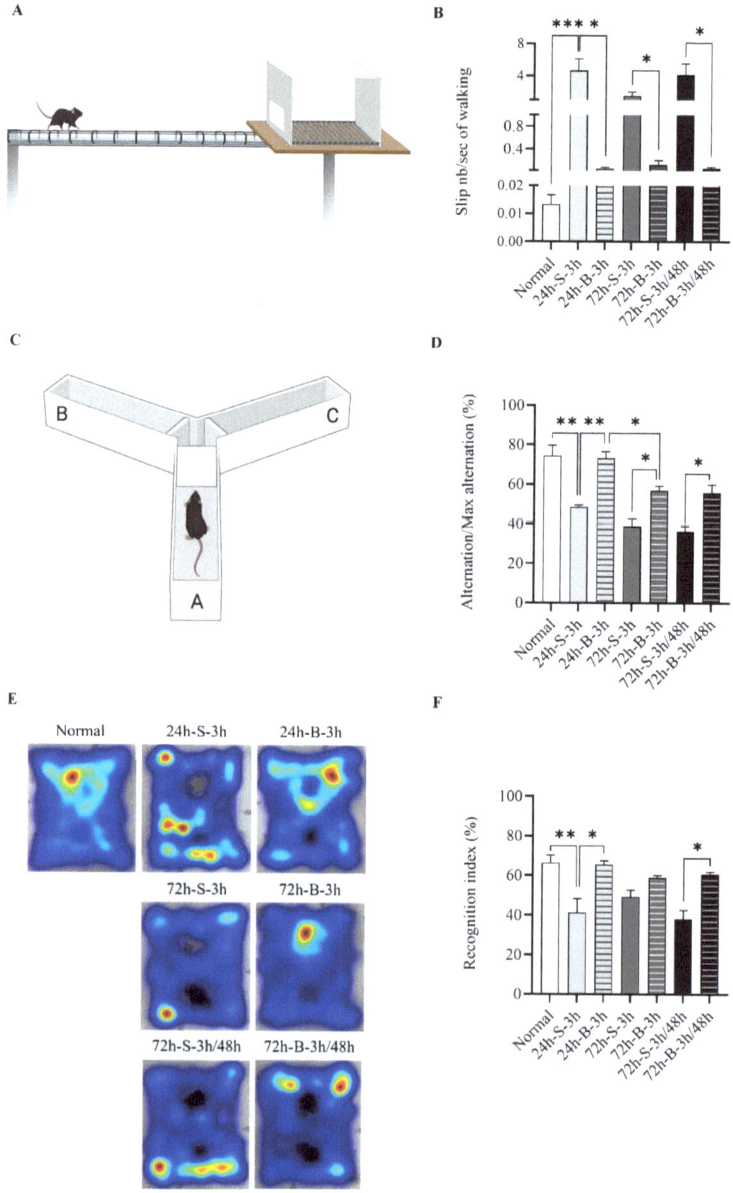

Figure 5. Effect of BMSC on behavior and cognitive dysfunction in in vivo SAH-model mice analyzed by beam-walking (**A**,**B**), the Y-maze (**C**,**D**), and NOR tests (**E**,**F**) (n = 9). Error bars, mean SEM, * $p < 0.05$, ** $p < 0.01$, and *** $p < 0.005$. The data represent the mean ± SEM.

4. Discussion

Despite favorable outcomes in patients after SAH, behavioral and cognitive dysfunction can persist, limiting daily activities [3,27]. Nevertheless, few studies have focused on the effect of stem cells on the recovery from these dysfunctions. Unlike SAH, the treatment of various neurological disorders with MSCs has been widely investigated [28–30]. Lee et al. [31] reported that patients with multiple-system atrophy treated with MSCs showed improvements in cerebellar dysfunction. Additionally, BMSC administration facilitated reductions in Aß and increased the expression of microRNA-146a in the hippocampus, reducing cognitive impairment [29,32]. Since neuroinflammation plays an important role in neurological disorders, we focused on the HMGB1–RAGE axis. Our findings showed that the expression of HMGB1 increased 6 h after the SAH induction. A single administration of BMSCs at 3 h reduced cognitive impairment while maintaining reductions in apoptosis and inflammatory cytokines within 24 h. However, these increased again after 72 h. Although the mild-SAH-model mice without BMSC administration showed some recovery after 72 h, the therapeutic effects were small. There was no difference on the NOR test between the saline- and BMSC-treated groups at 72 h. However, there was a difference at 72 h between multiple BMSC treatments and the saline treatment. Early brain injury (EBI) occurs immediately after SAH. Delayed cerebral ischemia (DCI) starts from 48 to 72 h after SAH ictus. It typically appears on day 4–10, unlike other forms of intracerebral hemorrhage. This characteristically causes inflammation and DCI, not immediately after SAH, but after some time [33]. Accordingly, additional BMSC treatment may be necessary to prevent secondary brain damage due to DCI, as well as to alleviate the inflammation caused by the initial brain damage in SAH to improve clinical symptoms, including cognitive impairment. Thus, administering BMSCs at different times could be more effective in restoring behavioral and cognitive dysfunction via persistent reductions in HMGB1–RAGE-mediated neuroinflammation. To confirm our hypothesis, we administered the BMSCs twice, at 3 h and 48 h after SAH induction, and compared the therapeutic effects to those of a single BMSC administration. Although the overall differences were not large, some improvements in inflammation and cognitive function were seen in the mild SAH. It is likely that the treatment effect would have been higher in cases of severe SAH. Therefore, it is thought that multiple BMSC treatments might be needed to prevent both EBI and DCI, rather than a single BMSC treatment, in order to improve neurological outcomes for SAH patients in actual clinical practice.

The optimal delivery method and therapeutic dose of BMSCs for SAH have not been determined. In this study, we selected an intravenous approach for BMSC transplantation, out of several delivery routes. Subarachnoid hemorrhage refers to bleeding that suddenly occurs in the subarachnoid space, which causes brain damage due to increased intracranial pressure. Thus, damage to the brain parenchyma is often not localized in patients with SAH compared to those with intracranial hemorrhage or traumatic brain injury. In addition, continuous cerebrospinal-fluid drainage (e.g., extraventricular drainage and lumbar drain) to relieve increased intracranial pressure is frequently performed after surgery. Overall, intravenous administration is more clinically useful and noninvasive than intraventricular or intraparenchymal approaches to BMSC transplantation following SAH. However, the trapping of BMSCs in the peripheral organs, particularly the lungs, is a concern after the administration of BMSCs [30]. Jung et al. [34] reported serial cases of pulmonary embolisms after multiple intravenous administrations of human-adipose-tissue-derived stem cells (AMSCs) for treating cervical herniated intervertebral discs. Although BMSCs with a molecular size of 7 μm exhibited a higher passage rate through the lungs than 18-μm AMSCs, it is necessary to design a delivery method that increases the number of BMSCs that reach the target brain region without being trapped in peripheral organs and that produces small-sized stem cells that pass through the BBB to increase the utility of BMSCs in patients with SAH in the future.

The optimal cell dosage of BMSCs for administration also remains undecided. However, it can be determined by the type of lesion and the purpose of the treatment. Zhang et al. [35] reported that a single administration of 3 to 4 $\times$ 10^5 ADSCs improved neurological function by maintaining BBB stability after cerebral hemorrhage. Referring to the results of this study, we administered 3 $\times$ 10^5 BMSCs to a mouse model of SAH. Nevertheless, varying doses should be tested to identify the therapeutic effects of stem cells in different species, as well as the optimal stem-cell type and delivery route. In addition, higher doses may be needed to identify stem cells' effects in humans. An 80-year-old SAH patient experienced neurological improvement after receiving 1 $\times$ 10^7 allogenic MSCs three days after ictus [36]. Therefore, it is necessary to study optimal doses according to the purpose and species, including human patients, in the future.

Administered MSCs were observed in damaged brains in a SAH model [11]. This finding suggests that MSCs migrated to an injured brain may be responsible for treatment efficacy and neuronal differentiation. The MSCs exhibited neuroplastic effects after injury by differentiating into glial cells, neurons, and endothelial cells after intravenous administration [11]. However, the main protective influence of BMSCs is thought to occur through their paracrine effects, particularly those of exosomes [7]. Xiong et al. [7] reported that the administration of exosomes derived from BMSCs improved neurological functions and reduced brain swelling via the anti-inflammatory effects of miRNA129-5p. In addition, exosomes secreted from BMSCs were taken up into astrocytes, which are involved in synapse formation [29]. Accordingly, investigations of the therapeutic effect of BMSC-derived exosomes in cognition improvement in SAH, particularly focusing on astrocytes, are required.

This study has some limitations. First, we only enrolled mice with mild SAH and evaluated the therapeutic efficacy of the BMSCs based on neurological scores, not CT scans. When a severe-SAH model was generated, it was difficult to properly identify cognition changes due to the severe neurological damage. In addition, since CTs were not taken, varying amounts of SAH could have exerted similar effects on neurologic functioning. Accordingly, the results of this study were limited in that the cognitive-function-recovery effect was only seen in mice with mild SAH and a relatively good prognosis. Second, we focused on the EBI and analyzed the cognitive-function effects of BMSCs with a focus on reducing neuroinflammation via the HMGB-RAGE axis. Delayed cerebral ischemia, which mostly occurs between days 4 and 10 after ictus, can cause neurologic deterioration and aggravate neuroinflammation [33]. Eagles et al. [4] reported that DCI was a risk factor for behavioral and cognitive dysfunctions after SAH. Although DCI is more common in severe SAH, with a larger amount of initial bleeding than in mild SAH, further stem-cell studies are needed to reduce DCI in patients with mild SAH. Third, we did not compare the BMSC treatment to other treatments, but only found that the HMGB1–RAGE axis-mediated neuroinflammation was reduced by the administration of the BMSCs. Haruma et al. [37] reported that an anti-MGB1 antibody attenuated the activation of cerebrocortical microglia due to brain injury. Thus, a comparative analysis of the combined therapeutic efficacy of BMSCs and HMGB1 inhibition using small interfering RNA (siRNA) or monoclonal antibodies is needed in the future. Fourth, we did not evaluate how the BMSC administration affected the HMGB1/RAGE axis, and no significant effect on TLR4 was seen in the mice with mild SAH (Figure 6). In general, HMGB1 released from neuronal cells or glia cells activates RAGE and TLR4, resulting in neuroinflammation [14]. Zhang et al. [38] reported that siRNA-HMGB1 treatment decreased the expression of the RAGE protein, but not that of TLR4, in stress-induced microglial-mediated neuroinflammation. Accordingly, it is necessary to study the mechanism of how the administration of BMSCs contributes to decreasing neuroinflammation via the HMGB1–RAGE axis. Fifth, we harvested the brains using a standardized method for dissecting brain tissues while confirming the anatomical structure to ensure that the same brain regions were dissected from each mouse. Nevertheless, the brain-harvesting process can be imperfect, and these differences might have affected the results. Finally, we did not perform immunohistochemical staining to confirm the specific cellular localization of the increased mRNAs and proteins. While qRT-PCR and Western blotting are useful for quantifying gene- and protein-expression levels, they cannot provide information on the spatial distribution of these molecules within cells or tissues. Accordingly, future studies should investigate the use of immunohistochemical staining to localize the expression of mRNAs and proteins to determine the cellular and subcellular localizations of these molecules in cerebral arteries or brain tissues.

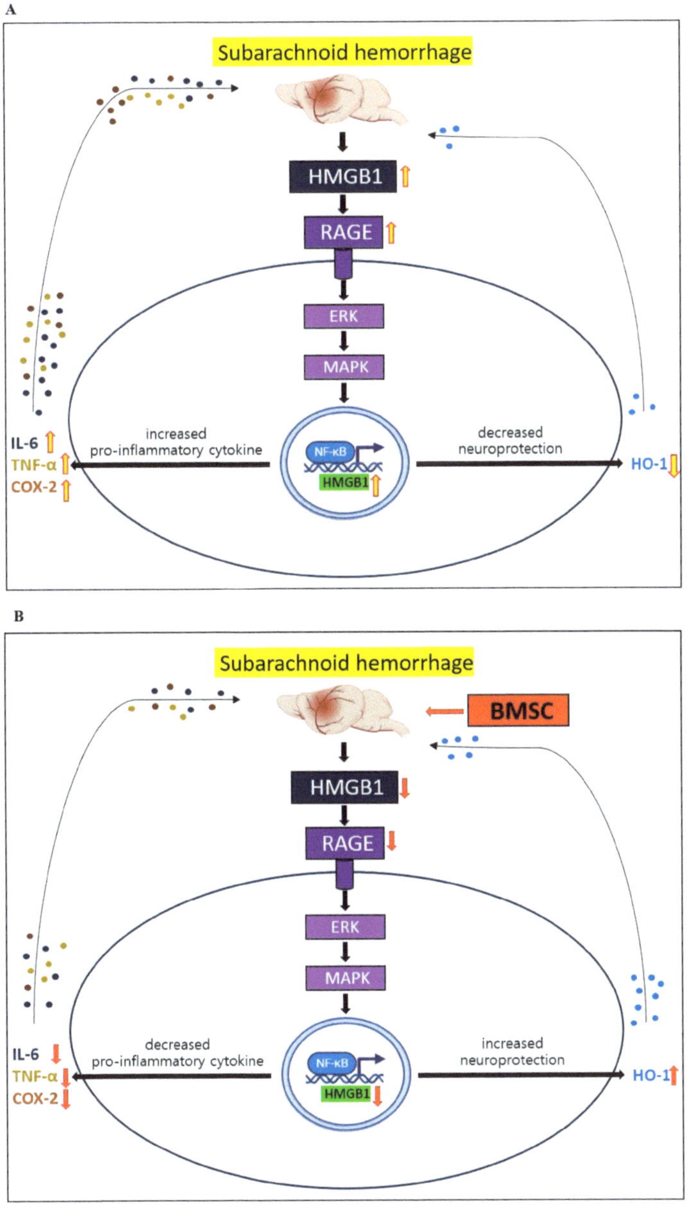

Figure 6. Schema showing therapeutic effects of saline administration (**A**) and BMSC administration (**B**) on SAH model mice in vivo. The administration of BMSCs may contribute to improvements in behavioral and cognitive dysfunction, mainly by relieving HMGB1–RAGE axis-mediated neuroinflammation.

5. Conclusions

The administration of BMSCs reduced behavioral and cognitive dysfunction by ameliorating HMGB1–RAGE axis-mediated neuroinflammation after mild SAH in mice.

Supplementary Materials: The following supporting information can be downloaded at: https://www.mdpi.com/article/10.3390/life13040881/s1, Figure S1: Experimental design of the study; Figure S2: Representative tracing images of NOR tests including training and memory tasks before SAH induction (A) and quantification of recognition in percentages (B,C); Table S1: Sequence of all primers used for qRT-PCR analysis; Figure S3: Raw data of Western blotting. References [39–45] are cited in Supplementary Materials.

Author Contributions: Conceptualization, J.P.J.; methodology, H.J. and D.H.Y.; investigation, H.J. and D.H.Y.; writing—original draft preparation, H.J. and D.H.Y.; writing—review and editing, J.P.J. and J.J.P.; funding acquisition, J.P.J. All authors have read and agreed to the published version of the manuscript.

Funding: This work was supported by the National Research Foundation of Korea (NRF) grant funded by the Korea government (MSIT) (no. 2022R1A5A8019303) and the Hallym University Research Fund.

Institutional Review Board Statement: All animal experiments were approved by the Institutional Animal Care and Use Committee (IACUC) of Hallym University (no: HallymR1 2021-50).

Informed Consent Statement: Patient consent was waived as this was an animal study.

Data Availability Statement: Not applicable.

Acknowledgments: Harry Jung and Dong Hyuk Youn contributed equally to this work and should both be considered first authors. Jin Pyeong Jeon and Jeong Jin Park are co-corresponding authors of this work.

Conflicts of Interest: The authors declare no conflict of interest.

References

1. Linn, F.H.; Rinkel, G.J.; Algra, A.; van Gijn, J. Incidence of subarachnoid hemorrhage: Role of region, year, and rate of computed tomography: A meta-analysis. *Stroke* **1996**, *27*, 625–629. [CrossRef]
2. Mourelo-Farina, M.; Pertega, S.; Galeiras, R. A Model for Prediction of In-Hospital Mortality in Patients with Subarachnoid Hemorrhage. *Neurocrit. Care* **2021**, *34*, 508–518. [CrossRef]
3. Ravnik, J.; Starovasnik, B.; Sesok, S.; Pirtosek, Z.; Svigelj, V.; Bunc, G.; Bosnjak, R. Long-term cognitive deficits in patients with good outcomes after aneurysmal subarachnoid hemorrhage from anterior communicating artery. *Croat. Med. J.* **2006**, *47*, 253–263.
4. Eagles, M.E.; Tso, M.K.; Macdonald, R.L. Cognitive Impairment, Functional Outcome, and Delayed Cerebral Ischemia After Aneurysmal Subarachnoid Hemorrhage. *World Neurosurg.* **2019**, *124*, e558–e562. [CrossRef]
5. Haug Nordenmark, T.; Karic, T.; Sorteberg, W.; Sorteberg, A. Predictors of cognitive function in the acute phase after aneurysmal subarachnoid hemorrhage. *Acta Neurochir.* **2019**, *161*, 177–184. [CrossRef]
6. Chung, D.Y.; Oka, F.; Jin, G.; Harriott, A.; Kura, S.; Aykan, S.A.; Qin, T.; Edmiston, W.J.; Lee, H.; Yassen, M.A.; et al. Subarachnoid hemorrhage leads to early and persistent functional connectivity and behavioral changes in mice. *J. Cereb. Blood Flow Metab.* **2021**, *41*, 975–985. [CrossRef]
7. Xiong, L.; Sun, L.; Zhang, Y.; Peng, J.; Yan, J.; Liu, X. Exosomes from Bone Marrow Mesenchymal Stem Cells Can Alleviate Early Brain Injury After Subarachnoid Hemorrhage Through miRNA129-5p-HMGB1 Pathway. *Stem. Cells Dev.* **2020**, *29*, 212–221. [CrossRef]
8. Shichinohe, H.; Kuroda, S.; Sugiyama, T.; Ito, M.; Kawabori, M. Bone marrow stromal cell transplantation attenuates cognitive dysfunction due to chronic cerebral ischemia in rats. *Dement. Geriatr. Cogn. Disord.* **2010**, *30*, 293–301. [CrossRef]
9. Kim, J.T.; Youn, D.H.; Kim, B.J.; Rhim, J.K.; Jeon, J.P. Recent Stem Cell Research on Hemorrhagic Stroke: An Update. *J. Korean Neurosurg. Soc.* **2022**, *65*, 161–172. [CrossRef]
10. Skok, M. Mesenchymal stem cells as a potential therapeutic tool to cure cognitive impairment caused by neuroinflammation. *World J. Stem. Cells.* **2021**, *13*, 1072–1083. [CrossRef]
11. Khalili, M.A.; Anvari, M.; Hekmati-Moghadam, S.H.; Sadeghian-Nodoushan, F.; Fesahat, F.; Miresmaeili, S.M. Therapeutic benefit of intravenous transplantation of mesenchymal stem cells after experimental subarachnoid hemorrhage in rats. *J. Stroke Cerebrovasc. Dis.* **2012**, *21*, 445–451. [CrossRef]

12. Liu, W.; Li, R.; Yin, J.; Guo, S.; Chen, Y.; Fan, H.; Li, G.; Li, Z.; Li, X.; Zhang, X.; et al. Mesenchymal stem cells alleviate the early brain injury of subarachnoid hemorrhage partly by suppression of Notch1-dependent neuroinflammation: Involvement of Botch. *J. Neuroinflamm.* **2019**, *16*, 8. [CrossRef]
13. Kumar, A. Editorial: Neuroinflammation and Cognition. *Front. Aging Neurosci.* **2018**, *10*, 413. [CrossRef]
14. Paudel, Y.N.; Shaikh, M.F.; Chakraborti, A.; Kumari, Y.; Aledo-Serrano, A.; Aleksovska, K.; Alvim, M.K.M.; Othman, I. HMGB1: A Common Biomarker and Potential Target for TBI, Neuroinflammation, Epilepsy, and Cognitive Dysfunction. *Front. Neurosci.* **2018**, *12*, 628. [CrossRef]
15. Wang, D.; Liu, K.; Wake, H.; Teshigawara, K.; Mori, S.; Nishibori, M. Anti-high mobility group box-1 (HMGB1) antibody inhibits hemorrhage-induced brain injury and improved neurological deficits in rats. *Sci. Rep.* **2017**, *7*, 46243. [CrossRef]
16. Paudel, Y.N.; Angelopoulou, E.; Piperi, C.; Othman, I.; Aamir, K.; Shaikh, M.F. Impact of HMGB1, RAGE, and TLR4 in Alzheimer's Disease (AD): From Risk Factors to Therapeutic Targeting. *Cells* **2020**, *9*, 383. [CrossRef]
17. Jeong, J.H.; Lee, D.H.; Song, J. HMGB1 signaling pathway in diabetes-related dementia: Blood-brain barrier breakdown, brain insulin resistance, and Abeta accumulation. *Biomed. Pharmacother.* **2022**, *150*, 112933. [CrossRef]
18. Schuller, K.; Buhler, D.; Plesnila, N. A murine model of subarachnoid hemorrhage. *J. Vis. Exp.* **2013**, *81*, e50845.
19. Sugawara, T.; Ayer, R.; Jadhav, V.; Zhang, J.H. A new grading system evaluating bleeding scale in filament perforation subarachnoid hemorrhage rat model. *J. Neurosci. Methods* **2008**, *167*, 327–334. [CrossRef]
20. Garcia, J.H.; Wagner, S.; Liu, K.F.; Hu, X.J. Neurological deficit and extent of neuronal necrosis attributable to middle cerebral artery occlusion in rats. Statistical validation. *Stroke* **1995**, *26*, 627–634. [CrossRef]
21. Chu, D.T.; Phuong, T.N.T.; Tien, N.L.B.; Tran, D.K.; Thanh, V.V.; Quang, T.L.; Truong, D.T.; Pham, V.H.; Ngoc, V.T.N.; Chu-Dinh, T.; et al. An Update on the Progress of Isolation, Culture, Storage, and Clinical Application of Human Bone Marrow Mesenchymal Stem/Stromal Cells. *Int. J. Mol. Sci.* **2020**, *21*, 708. [CrossRef]
22. Delorme, B.; Charbord, P. Culture and characterization of human bone marrow mesenchymal stem cells. *Methods Mol. Med.* **2007**, *140*, 67–81.
23. Youn, D.H.; Tran, N.M.; Kim, B.J.; Kim, Y.; Jeon, J.P.; Yoo, H. Shape effect of cerium oxide nanoparticles on mild traumatic brain injury. *Sci. Rep.* **2021**, *11*, 15571. [CrossRef]
24. Pedard, M.; El Amki, M.; Lefevre-Scelles, A.; Compere, V.; Castel, H. Double Direct Injection of Blood into the Cisterna Magna as a Model of Subarachnoid Hemorrhage. *J. Vis. Exp.* **2020**, *162*, 975–985. [CrossRef]
25. Kim, C.K.; Kim, T.; Choi, I.Y.; Soh, M.; Kim, D.; Kim, Y.J.; Park, H.; Park, S.P.; Park, S.; Yu, T.; et al. Ceria nanoparticles that can protect against ischemic stroke. *Angew. Chem. Int. Ed. Engl.* **2012**, *51*, 11039–11043. [CrossRef]
26. Bae, Y.H.; Joo, H.; Bae, J.; Hyeon, S.J.; Her, S.; Ko, E.; Choi, H.G.; Ryu, H.; Hur, E.; Lee, B.D. Brain injury induces HIF-1alpha-dependent transcriptional activation of LRRK2 that exacerbates brain damage. *Cell Death Dis.* **2018**, *9*, 1125. [CrossRef]
27. Han, S.W.; Kim, B.J.; Kim, T.Y.; Lim, S.H.; Youn, D.H.; Hong, E.P.; Rhim, J.K.; Park, J.J.; Lee, J.J.; Cho, Y.J.; et al. Association of Haptoglobin Phenotype With Neurological and Cognitive Outcomes in Patients With Subarachnoid Hemorrhage. *Front. Aging Neurosci.* **2022**, *14*, 819628. [CrossRef]
28. Andrzejewska, A.; Dabrowska, S.; Lukomska, B.; Janowski, M. Mesenchymal Stem Cells for Neurological Disorders. *Adv. Sci.* **2021**, *8*, 2002944. [CrossRef]
29. Nakano, M.; Kubota, K.; Kobayashi, E.; Chikenji, T.S.; Saito, Y.; Konari, N.; Fujimiya, M. Bone Marrow-Derived Mesenchymal Stem Cells Improve Cognitive Impairment in an Alzheimer's Disease Model by Increasing the Expression of *microRNA*-146a in hippocampus. *Sci. Rep.* **2020**, *10*, 10772. [CrossRef]
30. Zhang, S.; Lachance, B.B.; Moiz, B.; Jia, X. Optimizing Stem Cell Therapy after Ischemic Brain Injury. *J. Stroke* **2020**, *22*, 286–305. [CrossRef]
31. Lee, P.H.; Kim, J.W.; Bang, O.Y.; Ahn, Y.H.; Joo, I.S.; Huh, K. Autologous mesenchymal stem cell therapy delays the progression of neurological deficits in patients with multiple system atrophy. *Clin. Pharmacol. Ther.* **2008**, *83*, 723–730. [CrossRef]
32. Lee, J.K.; Jin, H.K.; Endo, S.; Schuchman, E.H.; Carter, J.E.; Bae, J.S. Intracerebral transplantation of bone marrow-derived mesenchymal stem cells reduces amyloid-beta deposition and rescues memory deficits in Alzheimer's disease mice by modulation of immune responses. *Stem Cells* **2010**, *28*, 329–343. [CrossRef]
33. Al-Mufti, F.; Amuluru, K.; Smith, B.; Damodara, N.; El-Ghanem, M.; Singh, I.P.; Dangayach, N.; Gandhi, C.D. Emerging Markers of Early Brain Injury and Delayed Cerebral Ischemia in Aneurysmal Subarachnoid Hemorrhage. *World Neurosurg.* **2017**, *107*, 148–159. [CrossRef]
34. Jung, J.W.; Kwon, M.; Choi, J.C.; Shin, J.W.; Park, I.W.; Choi, B.W.; Kim, J.Y. Familial occurrence of pulmonary embolism after intravenous, adipose tissue-derived stem cell therapy. *Yonsei Med. J.* **2013**, *54*, 1293–1296. [CrossRef]
35. Zhang, Y.; Deng, H.; Hu, Y.; Pan, C.; Wu, G.; Li, Q.; Tang, Z. Adipose-derived mesenchymal stem cells stereotactic transplantation alleviate brain edema from intracerebral hemorrhage. *J. Cell Biochem.* **2019**, *120*, 14372–14382. [CrossRef]
36. Brunet, M.C.; Chen, S.H.; Khandelwal, P.; Hare, J.M.; Starke, R.M.; Peterson, E.C.; Yavagal, D.R. Intravenous Stem Cell Therapy for High-Grade Aneurysmal Subarachnoid Hemorrhage: Case Report and Literature Review. *World Neurosurg.* **2019**, *128*, 573–575. [CrossRef]
37. Haruma, J.; Teshigawara, K.; Hishikawa, T.; Wang, D.; Liu, K.; Wake, H.; Mori, S.; Takahashi, H.K.; Sugiu, K.; Date, I.; et al. Anti-high mobility group box-1 (HMGB1) antibody attenuates delayed cerebral vasospasm and brain injury after subarachnoid hemorrhage in rats. *Sci. Rep.* **2016**, *6*, 37755. [CrossRef]

38. Zhang, S.; Hu, L.; Jiang, J.; Li, H.; Wu, Q.; Ooi, K.; Wang, J.; Feng, Y.; Zhu, D.; Xia, C. HMGB1/RAGE axis mediates stress-induced RVLM neuroinflammation in mice via impairing mitophagy flux in microglia. *J. Neuroinflamm.* **2020**, *17*, 15. [CrossRef]
39. Gallyas, F., Jr. Acute changes of pro-inflammatory markers and corticosterone in experimental subarachnoid haemorrhage: A prerequisite for severity assessment. *PLoS ONE* **2019**, *14*, e0220467.
40. Muhammad, S.; Grote, A. Interleukin 6 and Aneurysmal Subarachnoid Hemorrhage. A Narrative Review. *Int. J. Mol. Sci.* **2021**, *22*, 4133.
41. Ayer, R.; Hadhav, V.; Sugawara, T.; Zhang, J.H. The neuroprotective effects of cyclooxygenase-2 inhibition in a mouse model of aneurysmal subarachnoid hemorrhage. *Acta Neurochir. Suppl.* **2011**, *111*, 145–149.
42. Paudel, Y.N.; Angelopoulou, E.; Piperi, C.; Othman, I.; Shaikh, M.F. HMGB1-Mediated Neuroinflammatory Responses in Brain injuries: Potential Mechanisms and Therapeutic Opportunities. *Int. J. Mol. Sci.* **2020**, *21*, 4609. [CrossRef]
43. Wang, L.; Geng, G.; Zhu, T.; Chen, W.; Li, X.; Gu, J.; Jiang, E. Progress in Research on TLR4-Mediated Inflammatory Response Mechanisms in Brain Injury after Subarachnoid Hemorrhage. *Cells* **2022**, *23*, 3781. [CrossRef]
44. Ahmed, H.; Khan, M.A.; Kahlert, U.D.; Niemelä, M.; Hänggi, D.; Chaudhry, S.R.; Muhammad, S. Role of Adaptor Protein Myeloid Differentiation 88 (MyD88) in Post-Subarachnoid Hemorrhage: A Systematic Review. *Int. J. Mol. Sci.* **2021**, *22*, 4185. [CrossRef]
45. Shao, A.; Wu, H.; Hong, Y.; Tu, S.; Sun, X.; Wu, Q.; Zhao, Q.; Zhang, J.; Sheng, J. Hydrogen-Rich Saline Attenuated Subarachnoid Hemorrhage-Induced Early Brain Injury in Rats by Suppressing Inflammatory Response: Possible Involvement of NF-kB Pathway and NLRP3 Inflammasome. *Mol. Neurobiol.* **2016**, *53*, 3462–3467. [CrossRef]

life

MDPI

Communication

WNT16 Regulation of the Articular Chondrocyte Phenotype in Mice

Subburaman Mohan [1,2,3], Shelia Pourteymoor [1] and Chandrasekhar Kesavan [1,2,*]

1 Musculoskeletal Disease Center, VA Loma Linda Healthcare System, Loma Linda, CA 92357, USA
2 Department of Medicine, Loma Linda University, Loma Linda, CA 92354, USA
3 Orthopedic Surgery, Loma Linda University, Loma Linda, CA 92354, USA
* Correspondence: chandrasekhar.kesavan@va.gov; Tel.: +1-909-825-7084 (ext. 1553); Fax: +1-909-796-1680

Abstract: The anabolic effects of WNT16 on osteoblasts are well established, however, little is known regarding the role of WNT16 in chondrocytes. In this study, we evaluated *Wnt16* expression and its biological effects on mouse articular chondrocytes (ACs), since these cells are key to the development of osteoarthritis. While ACs derived from the long bone epiphysis of 7-day old C57BL/6J mice express multiple *Wnts*, *Wnt5b and Wnt16* represent the two most highly expressed *Wnts* (expressed at several-fold higher levels than other *Wnts*). Treatment of serum-free AC cultures, with 100 ng/mL of recombinant human (rh) WNT16 for 24 h (hrs), increased proliferation (20%, $p < 0.05$) and expression levels of makers (*Sox9 and Col2*) of immature chondrocytes at both 24 h and 72 h, while *Acan* increased at 72 h. Expression of *Mmp9*, a marker of mature chondrocytes was decreased at 24 h. Additionally, WNT16 treatment regulated expression levels of *Wnt* ligands in a biphasic manner, inhibiting its expression at 24 h, while stimulating expression at 72 h. To determine whether WNT16 exerted anabolic effects on the AC phenotype, ex vivo cultures of tibial epiphyses were treated with rhWNT16 or vehicle for 9 days, and the articular cartilage phenotype was evaluated by safranin O cartilage staining and expression of articular cartilage marker genes. Both articular cartilage area and expression levels of AC markers were increased after rhWNT16 treatment. Our data suggest that Wnt16 expressed in ACs may play a role in regulating joint cartilage homeostasis via its direct effect, as well as through modulating the expression of other *Wnt* ligands.

Keywords: WNT16; osteoarthritis; chondrocytes; mice; chondrogenesis; cell culture

check for updates

Citation: Mohan, S.; Pourteymoor, S.; Kesavan, C. WNT16 Regulation of the Articular Chondrocyte Phenotype in Mice. *Life* **2023**, *13*, 878. https://doi.org/10.3390/life13040878

Academic Editors: Stefanos Roumeliotis, Sanda M. Cretoiu and Giuseppe Minervini

Received: 28 January 2023
Revised: 7 March 2023
Accepted: 21 March 2023
Published: 25 March 2023

1. Introduction

The cartilage around the joints acts as a cushion between bones in healthy individuals, by absorbing shock during physical activity. In response to acute joint trauma, obesity, aging and bone fracture, cartilage tends to deteriorate because of the activation of sequential events, including inflammation, apoptosis and matrix degradation, which triggers a chronic remodeling process in the joint cartilage over time [1,2]. This remodeling leads to a clinical condition known as osteoarthritis (OA), a progressive degenerative joint cartilage disease affecting over 240 million people globally (10% men and 18% women), especially in our aging population, leading to disability, a poor quality of life and an increased mortality rate [3–5]. Presently, there are no available effective therapies for OA [6,7]. Therefore, understanding the biology of articular cartilage development and identifying signaling mechanisms that are perturbed during OA is important for developing future strategies to treat joint disease.

In terms of regulatory molecules important for articular cartilage development, recent clinical studies have reported increased Wingless-related Integration site (*Wnt*) *16* expression in injured joints, in the temporomandibular junction after blocking canonical WNT signaling, and in lumbar facet joint OA. However, it was unclear if this increased expression initiated anabolic or catabolic effects [8–12]. In response to injury, transgenic animal studies have reported that mice deficient in *Wnt16* expression exhibited a severe OA phenotype compared with wild-type mice. [13]. While these studies have implicated a role for *Wnt16* in the articular cartilage phenotype, the issue of whether *Wnt16* is expressed in articular chondrocytes and exerts significant biological effects on articular chondrocytes remains to be established. The findings of this study demonstrate that articular chondrocytes expressed *Wnt16*, and that exogenous treatment with recombinant WNT16 promoted the articular chondrocyte phenotype, as evidenced by increased chondrocyte proliferation and expression of articular cartilage marker genes.

2. Materials and Methods

2.1. Chondrocyte Culture

Cells from the epiphyseal region of long bones were collected from euthanized 7-day old C57BL/6J mice ($n = 6$), as described [14]. The cells were cultured in alpha-minimal essential medium (αMEM) containing 10% fetal bovine serum (FBS) with antibiotics (penicillin 100 units/mL and streptomycin 100 μg/mL), for 3 days. The cells were passaged once, and the first-passage cells were used for experiments.

2.2. Gene Expression

Approximately 200,000 cells were platted per well in 6-well plates, and cultured in αMEM containing 10% FBS with antibiotics for 48 h (hrs), followed by another 24 h in αMEM containing 0.1% bone serum albumin (BSA) and antibiotics. Thereafter, the cells were treated with or without 100 ng/mL of recombinant human (rh) WNT16 (R&D Systems, Minneapolis, MN, USA) or vehicle (1X phosphate buffered saline), and were cultured in αMEM containing 0.1% BSA and antibiotics. The experiments were terminated 24 or 72 h after WNT16 treatment. Total ribonucleic acid (RNA) was isolated from cells treated with vehicle and WNT16 using a Qiagen isolation kit protocol, per the manufacturer's instructions. Two hundred nanograms of purified total RNA was used to synthesize the first strand complementary deoxyribose nuclei acid (cDNA) by reverse transcription, as per the manufacturer's instructions (Bio-Rad, Irvine, CA, USA). The first strand of DNA was subjected to real-time PCR amplification, using a SYBR green master mix and gene-specific primers (IDT DNA Technology, San Diego, CA, USA) on a ViiA7 real-time PCR system (Applied Biosystems, Waltham, MA, USA). The endogenous control (*18S*) was used to normalize the data [15,16], and the normalized values were subjected to the $2^{\Delta\Delta}$Ct (where C+ is contraction threshold) formula, to calculate the fold change between the vehicle and experimental groups [17].

2.3. Proliferation Assay

The first-passage chondrocytes (4000 cells/well) were plated in a 96-well plate and cultured in αMEM containing 10% FBS with antibiotics for 48 h, followed by another 24 h in αMEM containing 0.1% BSA with antibiotics. The cells were then treated with vehicle (1X PBS) or 100 ng/mL of rhWNT16 (R&D System, Minneapolis, MN, USA) in αMEM containing 0.1% BSA and antibiotics. Proliferation was assessed 48 h after WNT16 treatment using a Cy-Quant Dye kit (Life Technologies, Carlsbad, CA, USA), according to the manufacturer's instructions.

2.4. Ex Vivo Joint Culture and Histology

We collected right and left intact femoral head bones that were connected to the hip, from euthanized 6-month-old male C57BL/6J mice. Briefly, the whole intact femoral head was isolated by cutting at the junction of the femoral neck. The femoral head width was approximately 0.95–1 mm, and the length from the head to the neck junction was 1 mm. The femoral head was cultured in αMEM with 0.1% BSA and antibiotics in 96-well plates. A 100 μL medium was added to each well so that the femoral head was completely immersed in the media. The media was replaced every day. The right femoral head joint was treated with 100 ng of rhWNT16 once/day for 9 days, while the corresponding left femoral head joint was treated with vehicle (1X PBS). Nine days after WNT16 or vehicle treatment, the femoral heads were fixed in 10% formalin for 24 h, and then washed and stored in 1X PBS. Six-micron paraffin-embedded sections were prepared from these samples, processed, and stained with safranin O [14]. The stained area was outlined in both the rhWNT16- and vehicle-treated groups, using the Image J software. The difference in the staining area was calculated as a percentage using this formula: (treated value − vehicle value)/vehicle value ∗ 100).

2.5. Ex Vivo Joint Culture and Gene Expression

Right and left proximal tibial epiphyses, with attached articular cartilage, were collected from euthanized 6-month and 10-month-old male C57BL/6J mice under sterile conditions, and cultured in αMEM with 0.1% BSA and antibiotics. The right tibial articular cartilage was treated with 100 ng/mL of rhWNT16 once/day for 7 days, while the corresponding left tibia articular cartilage was treated with vehicle (1X PBS). The media was changed every day for both groups. Seven days after WNT16 treatment, the tibia epiphyses with articular cartilage from 6-month and 10-month-old mice were used for total RNA isolation (Qiagen, MD, USA). Purified total RNA was used to synthesize the first strand of cDNA by reverse transcription, according to the manufacturer's instructions (Bio-Rad, CA, USA). Quantitative real-time PCR was used to determine the expression levels of genes using the SYBR green dye approach, as described above. Gene-specific primers were designed with the Vector NTI software and ordered from IDT DNA technologies. Data normalization was accomplished using an endogenous control (*18s*) to correct for variations in the RNA quality among samples. The normalized CT values were used to calculate the fold change using the $2^{-\Delta\Delta}$Ct formula [17].

2.6. Statistical Analysis

The Student *t*-test was used to compare the difference between the treatment vs. non-treatment groups. A *p*-value of <0.05 was considered statistically significant. Values are presented as the mean ± standard error mean (SEM).

3. Results and Discussion

Clinical and animal model studies have reported increased *Wnt16* expression in OA knees compared to control knees. Furthermore, it has been shown that Wnt16 treatment of human cartilage explants via a peptide-based nanoplatform to deliver *Wnt16* mRNA was effective in maintaining cartilage homeostasis, and that over-expression of *Wnt16* using an adenovirus reduced the progression of OA in an animal model [18,19]. While these findings suggest a role for WNT16 in the pathogenesis of OA, the issue of whether *Wnt16* is expressed in articular chondrocytes and exerts significant biological effects remains to be examined. We, therefore, evaluated the expression levels of *Wnt* ligands by real-time PCR in the RNA samples isolated from articular chondrocytes of 7-day old C57BL/J mice. We used the *18s* gene as an endogenous control to normalize our expression data. Of the *Wnt*s examined, *Wnt5b* showed the lowest expression, and was therefore used as a baseline to compare the expression of the other *Wnt* ligands. We found that, except for *Wnt10a* (below detectable limit), all other *Wnt*s examined were expressed in articular chondrocytes, but at different levels (Figure 1A). *Wnt5a* and *Wnt16* were found to be expressed at much higher levels than other *Wnt*s in articular chondrocytes. Both canonical (*Wnts 2a, 3a* and *10b*) and non-canonical (*Wnts 4, 5a, 6a and 16*) *Wnt*s were expressed by articular chondrocytes, suggesting that both signaling pathways may be involved in the development and maintenance of the articular cartilage phenotype.

To determine the WNT16 biological effects on chondrocytes, we tested if rhWNT16 modulates proliferation of articular chondrocytes. We chose a 100 ng/mL dosage based on a dose-response study that revealed a maximum biological effect at this dose in MC3T3-E1 mouse osteoblasts [20]. Furthermore, we chose human rhWNT16 protein for the study, because the WNT16 protein is 92% conserved between mouse and human, and the long-term goal of research is to determine if we could use human rhWNT16 protein as a therapy to promote joint cartilage homeostasis. We found that cells treated with rhWNT16 showed a 20% increase in proliferation 48 h after WNT16 treatment. Terminal differentiation of articular chondrocytes into hypertrophic chondrocytes is a known cause for the pathogenesis of osteoarthritis [21]. We, therefore, determined the effects of WNT16 on expression levels of markers of the transition of immature to mature chondrocytes [22]. We found that the markers that reflect the transition of stem cells to chondrocytes *Sox5* ($p = 0.06$), *Sox9* ($p = 0.04$) and type-2 collagen (*Col2*) ($p < 0.01$)) (Figure 1B) increased in response to WNT16 treatment. By contrast, a marker that is highly expressed in hypertrophic chondrocytes that undergoes apoptosis, *Mmp9*, was reduced ($p < 0.01$) 24 h post WNT16 treatment. After 72 h treatment with rhWNT16, expression levels of the articular cartilage markers, *Sox5* ($p < 0.05$), *Col2* ($p < 0.05$) and aggrecan (*Acan* ($p = 0.06$)) remained increased, showing a sustained anabolic effect (Figure 1B). Importantly, the decrease in *Mmp9* and increase in expression of transcription factors (*Sox5, 9*) upon WNT16 treatment suggests that the WNT16 treatment acts to maintain the articular chondrocyte fate. In our study, we chose a serum-free medium (0.1% BSA) to test the effects of exogenously added Wnt16, since sera contain a number of growth factors that could interact with Wnt16 effects and make the data difficult to interpret. In future studies, we will determine if serum growth factors modify Wnt16 biological effects in chondrocytes.

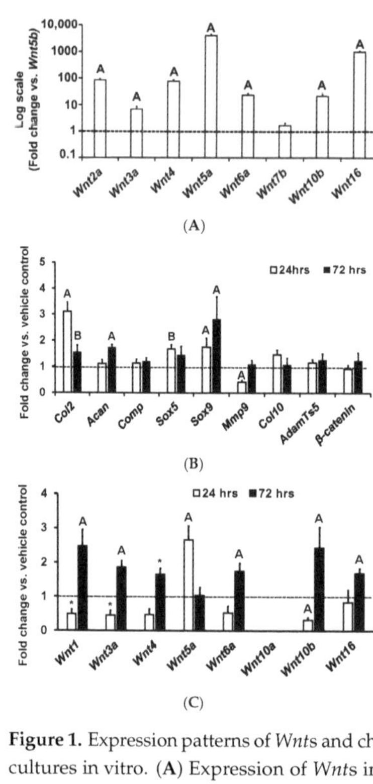

Figure 1. Expression patterns of *Wnts* and chondrocyte marker genes in primary articular chondrocyte cultures in vitro. (**A**) Expression of *Wnts* in cultured articular chondrocytes isolated from 1-week-old C57BL/6J mice (fold-change data vs. *Wnt5b* is expressed in the log scale). (**B**) Quantitation of expression of genes 24 ($n = 5$) and 72 h post rhWNT*16* treatment ($n = 5$) in chondrocytes derived from epiphyses of 1-week-old C57BL/6J mice. (**C**) Quantitation of expression of *Wnt* ligands 24 and 72 h post rhWNT16 treatment in chondrocytes isolated from the epiphyses of 1-week-old C57BL/6J mice ($n = 3$). Values are the mean ± SEM. ^{A} $p < 0.05$ and ^{B} $p = 0.06$ vs. vehicle, * $p = 0.08$ vs. vehicle. The *x*-axis represents the genes studied and *y*-axis reflects fold-change in expression.

To determine if the WNT16 effects were mediated in part by modulating the expression of other Wnt ligands, we evaluated expression levels of *Wnt*s known to influence chondrogenesis 24 or 72 h after rhWNT16 treatment in articular chondrocytes (Figure 1C). We found that WNT16 affects the expression of multiple *Wnt*s in articular chondrocytes. Twenty-four-hour WNT16 treatment suppressed the expression of *Wnt1*, *Wnt3a* and *Wnt10b*, and increased the expression of *Wnt5a*, which has been reported to have an anabolic effect on cartilage (Figure 1C). However, at 72 h WNT16 treatment increased expression of *Wnt1, Wnt3a, Wnt4, Wnt6A, Wnt10b and Wnt16*. Overall, the expression data suggest that WNT16 modulates expression of other *Wnt*s, in both a positive and negative manner.

In humans, joint cartilage damage is very common in young adults and middle-aged adults. To determine if WNT16 could produce anabolic effects in the articular cartilage of adult mice, we isolated the femoral head up to the neck junction with intact articular surfaces from 6-month-old male (corresponds to adult humans) C57BL/6J mice, and cultured them for 9 days with and without rhWNT16. Staining of the histological femoral head sections with safranin O revealed an increased articular cartilage staining area in femoral heads treated with WNT16, compared to joints treated with the vehicle (Figure 2A,B). Consistent with the histology data showing the anabolic effects of rhWNT16, we found that a 7-day treatment with rhWNT16 increased the expression levels of markers of chondrogenesis (*Col2, Sox5, Acan, β-catenin* and *Comp*) in cultured tibia epiphyseal articular cartilage regions from 6-month-old, as well as from 10-month-old (corresponds to middle-aged humans) C57BL/6J mice, compared to the vehicle-treated cultures (Figure 2C).

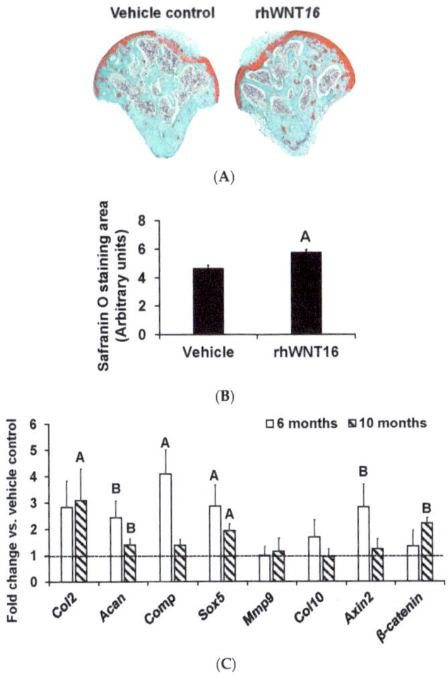

Figure 2. Illustration of the femoral head safranin O staining and expression patterns of chondrocyte marker genes in ex vivo cultures of tibia epiphysis regions which contain articular cartilage. (**A**) Histology image of safranin O stained areas and (**B**) quantitation of safranin-O-stained areas in 6-month-old male femoral heads cultured ex vivo and treated with rhWNT16 vs. vehicle. (**C**) Quantitation of expression levels of genes from epiphyseal regions of the tibia with articular cartilage, isolated from 6- and 10-month-old male C57BL/6J mice and cultured ex vivo with 100 ng rhWNT16 vs. vehicle for 7 days in vitro. $n = 5$/group, values are the mean ± SEM, ^{A} $p < 0.05$ vs. vehicle and ^{B} $p = 0.08$ vs. vehicle.

The limitations of this study include a lack of confirmation of gene expression data by corresponding changes in protein levels, and the failure to establish a causal role for Wnt16 expressed in articular chondrocytes in regulating the articular cartilage phenotype. Our future investigations will focus on the in vivo role of Wnt16 in regulating the articular cartilage phenotype.

4. Conclusions

Articular chondrocytes express WNT16, and exogenous treatment with WNT16 stimulates mRNA levels of the genes involved in regulating joint cartilage homeostasis directly, as well as through modulating expression of other *Wnt* ligands.

Author Contributions: Conceptualization, S.M. and C.K.; methodology, S.M. and C.K.; validation, S.M. and C.K.; formal analysis, C.K.; data curation, C.K. and S.P.; writing—original draft preparation, S.M. and C.K.; writing—review and editing, S.M. and C.K.; funding acquisition, S.M. All authors have read and agreed to the published version of the manuscript.

Funding: The work was supported by funding from the Veteran's Administration (101 BX001396 and 1K6 BX005381) and National Institutes of Arthritis and Musculoskeletal and Skin Diseases (R01 AR048139) awarded to Subburaman Mohan. All work was performed in facilities provided by the VA.

Institutional Review Board Statement: The study was conducted according to the guidelines of the National Institutes of Health (USA) and approved by the Institutional Animal Care and Use Committee of the Jerry L. Pettis Memorial Veterans Affairs Medical Center (ACORP number: 0029/204 and approval date 4.20.2017).

Informed Consent Statement: Not applicable.

Data Availability Statement: Raw data are available upon request.

Acknowledgments: The authors thank Donna Strong for proofreading the manuscript.

Conflicts of Interest: The authors declare no conflict of interest.

References

1. Zichella, L.; Gramolini, R. Autotransfusion during cesarean section. *Am. J. Obstet. Gynecol.* **1990**, *162*, 295. [CrossRef] [PubMed]
2. Buckwalter, J.A.; Brown, T.D. Joint injury, repair, and remodeling: Roles in post-traumatic osteoarthritis. *Clin. Orthop. Relat. Res.* **2004**, *426*, 7–16. [CrossRef]
3. Chen, D.; Shen, J.; Zhao, W.; Wang, T.; Han, L.; Hamilton, J.L.; Im, H.J. Osteoarthritis: Toward a comprehensive understanding of pathological mechanism. *Bone Res.* **2017**, *5*, 16044. [CrossRef] [PubMed]
4. Nelson, A.E. Osteoarthritis year in review 2017: Clinical. *Osteoarthr. Cartil.* **2018**, *26*, 319–325. [CrossRef] [PubMed]
5. Xing, D.; Xu, Y.; Liu, Q.; Ke, Y.; Wang, B.; Li, Z.; Lin, J. Osteoarthritis and all-cause mortality in worldwide populations: Grading the evidence from a meta-analysis. *Sci. Rep.* **2016**, *6*, 24393. [CrossRef]
6. Grassel, S.; Muschter, D. Recent advances in the treatment of osteoarthritis. *F1000Research* **2020**, *9*, 1–17. [CrossRef]
7. Liu, Y.; Shah, K.M.; Luo, J. Strategies for Articular Cartilage Repair and Regeneration. *Front. Bioeng. Biotechnol.* **2021**, *9*, 770655. [CrossRef]
8. Blom, A.B.; Brockbank, S.M.; van Lent, P.L.; van Beuningen, H.M.; Geurts, J.; Takahashi, N.; van der Kraan, P.M.; van de Loo, F.A.; Schreurs, B.W.; Clements, K.; et al. Involvement of the Wnt signaling pathway in experimental and human osteoarthritis: Prominent role of Wnt-induced signaling protein 1. *Arthritis Rheum.* **2009**, *60*, 501–512. [CrossRef]
9. Dell'accio, F.; De Bari, C.; Eltawil, N.M.; Vanhummelen, P.; Pitzalis, C. Identification of the molecular response of articular cartilage to injury, by microarray screening: Wnt-16 expression and signaling after injury and in osteoarthritis. *Arthritis Rheum.* **2008**, *58*, 1410–1421. [CrossRef]
10. Tornqvist, A.E.; Nilsson, K.H.; Li, L.; Ohlsson, C.; Moverare-Skrtic, S. Induced inactivation of Wnt16 in young adult mice has no impact on osteoarthritis development. *PLoS ONE* **2022**, *17*, e0277495. [CrossRef]
11. Hua, B.; Qiu, J.; Ye, X.; Liu, X. Intra-articular injection of a novel Wnt pathway inhibitor, SM04690, upregulates Wnt16 expression and reduces disease progression in temporomandibular joint osteoarthritis. *Bone* **2022**, *158*, 116372. [CrossRef] [PubMed]
12. Wu, C.; Yu, J.; Xu, G.; Bao, G.; Zhang, J.; Xue, P.; Jiang, J.; Chen, J.; Chen, C.; Hong, H.; et al. Wnt16 protects chondrocytes from lumbar facet joint osteoarthritis through the Wnt/beta-catenin pathway in low back pain patients. *Somatosens. Mot. Res.* **2021**, *38*, 339–346. [CrossRef]
13. Nalesso, G.; Thomas, B.L.; Sherwood, J.C.; Yu, J.; Addimanda, O.; Eldridge, S.E.; Thorup, A.S.; Dale, L.; Schett, G.; Zwerina, J.; et al. WNT16 antagonises excessive canonical WNT activation and protects cartilage in osteoarthritis. *Ann. Rheum. Dis.* **2017**, *76*, 218–226. [CrossRef]

14. Cheng, S.; Pourteymoor, S.; Alarcon, C.; Mohan, S. Conditional Deletion of the Phd2 Gene in Articular Chondrocytes Accelerates Differentiation and Reduces Articular Cartilage Thickness. *Sci. Rep.* **2017**, *7*, 45408. [CrossRef] [PubMed]
15. Al-Sabah, A.; Stadnik, P.; Gilbert, S.J.; Duance, V.C.; Blain, E.J. Importance of reference gene selection for articular cartilage mechanobiology studies. *Osteoarthr. Cartil.* **2016**, *24*, 719–730. [CrossRef] [PubMed]
16. Peng, X.X.; Zhao, R.L.; Song, W.; Chu, H.R.; Li, M.; Song, S.Y.; Li, G.Z.; Liang, D.C. Selection of suitable reference genes for normalization of quantitative real-time PCR in cartilage tissue injury and repair in rabbits. *Int. J. Mol. Sci.* **2012**, *13*, 14344–14355. [CrossRef]
17. Mohan, S.; Wergedal, J.E.; Das, S.; Kesavan, C. Conditional disruption of miR17-92 cluster in collagen type I-producing osteoblasts results in reduced periosteal bone formation and bone anabolic response to exercise. *Physiol. Genom.* **2015**, *47*, 33–43. [CrossRef]
18. Tong, W.; Zeng, Y.; Chow, D.H.K.; Yeung, W.; Xu, J.; Deng, Y.; Chen, S.; Zhao, H.; Zhang, X.; Ho, K.K.; et al. Wnt16 attenuates osteoarthritis progression through a PCP/JNK-mTORC1-PTHrP cascade. *Ann. Rheum. Dis.* **2019**, *78*, 551–561. [CrossRef]
19. Yan, H.; Hu, Y.; Akk, A.; Rai, M.F.; Pan, H.; Wickline, S.A.; Pham, C.T.N. Induction of WNT16 via Peptide-mRNA Nanoparticle-Based Delivery Maintains Cartilage Homeostasis. *Pharmaceutics* **2020**, *12*, 73. [CrossRef]
20. Ozeki, N.; Mogi, M.; Hase, N.; Hiyama, T.; Yamaguchi, H.; Kawai, R.; Kondo, A.; Nakata, K. Wnt16 Signaling Is Required for IL-1beta-Induced Matrix Metalloproteinase-13-Regulated Proliferation of Human Stem Cell-Derived Osteoblastic Cells. *Int. J. Mol. Sci.* **2016**, *17*, 221. [CrossRef]
21. Dreier, R. Hypertrophic differentiation of chondrocytes in osteoarthritis: The developmental aspect of degenerative joint disorders. *Arthritis Res. Ther.* **2010**, *12*, 216. [CrossRef] [PubMed]
22. Li, J.; Dong, S. The Signaling Pathways Involved in Chondrocyte Differentiation and Hypertrophic Differentiation. *Stem Cells Int.* **2016**, *2016*, 2470351. [CrossRef] [PubMed]

life

MDPI

Case Report

Immunoglobulin G4-Related Disease-Associated Dermatitis with Pruritus: A Positive Response to Dupilumab

Tyler C. Beck [1,*,†], John Plante [1,†], India Robinson [1], Katsiaryna Khatskevich [2], Jessica A. Forcucci [1,2] and Manuel Valdebran [1,3]

1 Department of Dermatology and Dermatologic Surgery, Medical University of South Carolina, Charleston, SC 29425, USA
2 Department of Pathology and Laboratory Medicine, Medical University of South Carolina, Charleston, SC 29425, USA
3 Department of Pediatrics, Medical University of South Carolina, Charleston, SC 29425, USA
* Correspondence: beckt@musc.edu
† These authors contributed equally to this work.

Abstract: Immunoglobulin G4-related disease (IgG4-RD) is a rare fibro-inflammatory condition characterized by IgG4-expressing plasma cell infiltration of the skin and other organs, leading to profound itchiness. Oral corticosteroids are the first-line therapy for IgG4-RD but relapses and potential side effects are common. In this case, we discuss a patient with a hyperpigmented, scaling dermatitis on his arms, back, and chest with lichen amyloidosis (LA) that incompletely responded to corticosteroids. He had reduced quality of life secondary to chronic pruritus. Dupilumab, an IL-4 and IL-13 inhibitor, was initiated. He experienced a transient worsening, followed by complete resolution of his itch with remission of his rash. While the pathogenesis of IgG4-RD is not entirely understood, a T-helper 2 (Th2) immune response has been implicated, with interleukins (IL) 4, 5, 10, and 13 playing a role in IgG4 class switch, resulting in eosinophilia and elevated IgE. The strong response of dupilumab in this case may provide evidence in favor of the involvement of IL-4 and IL-13 in the pathogenesis of cutaneous IgG4-RD. Future clinical studies involving larger patient populations may be warranted.

Keywords: dupilumab; biologic; dermatitis; lichen amyloidosis; primary cutaneous amyloidosis; primary localized cutaneous amyloidosis; IgG4-related disease; IgG4-related skin disease; immunoglobulin G4-related disease; immunoglobulin G4-related skin disease

check for updates

Citation: Beck, T.C.; Plante, J.; Robinson, I.; Khatskevich, K.; Forcucci, J.A.; Valdebran, M. Immunoglobulin G4-Related Disease-Associated Dermatitis with Pruritus: A Positive Response to Dupilumab. *Life* **2023**, *13*, 833. https://doi.org/10.3390/life13030833

Academic Editors: Ron Kohen and Enzo Berardesca

Received: 17 November 2022
Revised: 1 January 2023
Accepted: 17 March 2023
Published: 20 March 2023

1. Introduction

Immunoglobulin G4-related disease (IgG4-RD) is a rare fibro-inflammatory condition characterized by IgG4-expressing plasma cell infiltration of the skin and other organs [1]. IgG4-RD typically affects middle-aged or elderly males and can present with widespread cutaneous and systemic manifestations [2–5]. Cutaneous IgG4-RD exhibits a heterogenous clinical picture but commonly presents alongside internal organ involvement as erythematous and pruritic papules, nodules, or plaques on the head and neck or trunk. Oral corticosteroids are first-line therapy for IgG4-RD. However, relapses are common and potential side effects are multiple [6]. Here we present the unique case of IgG4-related disease associated dermatitis and pruritus (IgG4-ADP) with lichen amyloidosis (LA); a condition that is often secondary to chronic pruritus [7–11]. The patient did not tolerate rituximab and had a variable response to corticosteroids but demonstrated a complete response to dupilumab.

2. Case Report

Our patient is a Middle Eastern male with a past medical history of asthma and allergic rhinitis. In 1989, he presented at 36 years of age to an outside institution with sclerosing cholangitis and pancreatitis. He was diagnosed with IgG4-RD after serologic evaluation and a strong response to steroids. Over the next several decades, he experienced intermittent disease flaring on low–moderate dose prednisone. Of note, in 2016, he was diagnosed with stage IV chronic kidney disease secondary to systemic IgG4-RD; however, his renal function remained unchanged over the course of this case report (Table A1 in Appendix A).

He first presented to our institution in 2016 with fatigue and elevated blood urea nitrogen (BUN) (68 mg/dL) (normal range (NR): 5–25 mg/dL) and serum creatinine (2.8) (NR: 0.6–1.3 mg/dL), as well as a low estimated glomerular filtration rate (eGFR) of 23. His liver function tests (LFTs) were within normal reference ranges. A renal biopsy demonstrating severe interstitial nephritis with fibrosis was suspected by nephrology to be IgG4-related tubulointerstitial nephritis. At that time, he was diagnosed with stage IV chronic kidney disease (CKD). He quickly responded to high-dose steroids and was discharged on 20 mg/day of prednisone.

During a rheumatology appointment in late 2016, the patient reported fatigue and severe, progressive pruritus over the past several months, interfering greatly with his quality of life. A diffuse, erythematous, confluent papular rash was observed on his back and arms. Dry eyes and mouth were also present, and his serum IgG was 506 mg/dL (normal range (NR): 1–123 mg/dL). During this visit, the patient reported that a rash and severe, diffuse pruritus had started on his back and arms several years ago and was refractory to hydroxyzine, famotidine, moisturizing creams, dapsone cream, and topical corticosteroids. A prior biopsy showed interface dermatitis and perivascular inflammation with eosinophils.

Steroid-sparing therapy with rituximab was initiated at the end of 2016. His rash and pruritus quickly improved, and his symptoms remained well-controlled after a steroid taper until November of 2019. His IgG4 level at that time was within the normal range (10 mg/dL). His pruritus later returned, and a hyperpigmented, scaling rash on his arms, back, and chest was identified. Rheumatology then placed a dermatology referral. Rituximab was continued through the middle of 2020 until he was hospitalized for suspected rituximab-induced neutropenia. He was discharged on 10 mg/day of prednisone without rituximab. His pruritus worsened over the next several months despite the addition of topical corticosteroids, and he presented to our dermatology clinic toward the end of 2020. His exam was remarkable for ill-defined, erythematous plaques on his abdomen (Figure 1A) and dark tan papules on bilateral forearms and left leg (Figure 1B,C).

Lab work was significant for peripheral eosinophilia, and a workup resulted in the following: a positive antinuclear antibodies test (1:80 nucleolar pattern); elevated absolute eosinophil count (AEC) (2820 cells/mcL) (NR: 30–350 cells/mcL); elevated IgE (281 IU/mL) (NR:1.5–144 IU/mL); normal adrenocorticotropic hormone, cortisol, and tryptase levels; and negative strongyloides and toxocara antibodies. A tangential biopsy of his abdomen demonstrated spongiotic dermatitis with mixed superficial and perivascular infiltrates with eosinophils (Figure 2A). An incisional biopsy of his right forearm showed small deposits of amyloid in the superficial papillary dermis, and the diagnosis of LA was made (Figure 2B,C). Subepidermal deposition of amyloid correlates to keratinocyte-derived amyloid rather than a systemic origin.

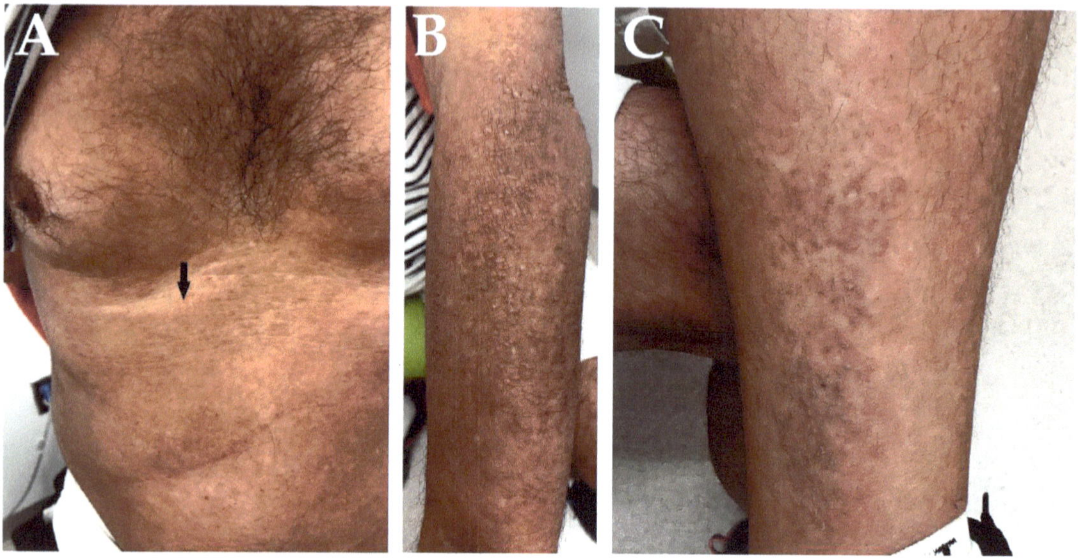

Figure 1. (**A**) Immunoglobulin G4-related disease-associated dermatitis involving the abdomen (arrow). Lichen amyloidosis involving the left forearm (**B**) and left leg (**C**) prior to initiating dupilumab therapy.

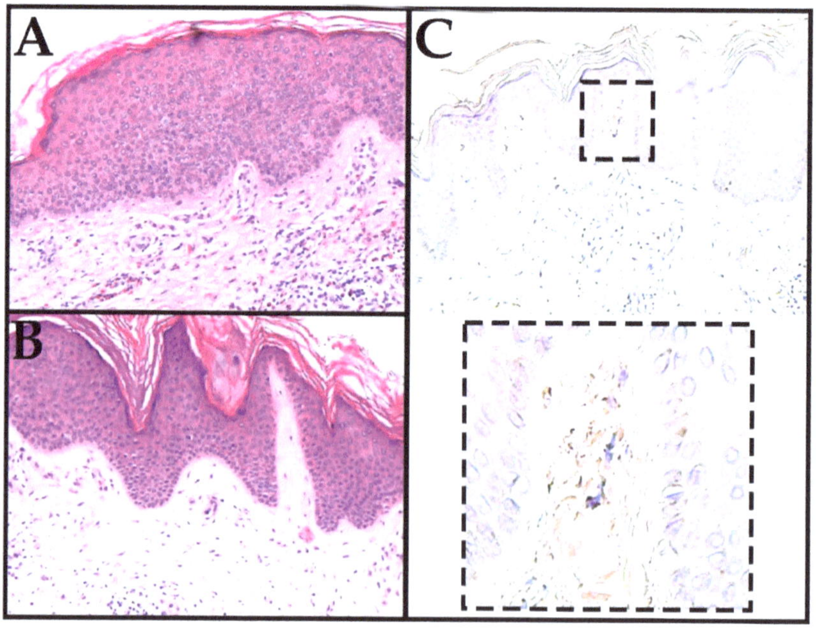

Figure 2. (**A**) A shave biopsy from the patient's forearm showed spongiotic dermatitis with mixed superficial perivascular inflammation with notable eosinophils (H&E 200×). (**B**) The biopsy revealed lichen amyloidosis (H&E 200×). (**C**) Congo Red staining highlighted small amyloid deposits in the superficial papillary dermis (200× with digital zoom).

Given the constellation of conditions contributing to his pruritus, such as IgG4-RD, LA, and atopy, a course of dupilumab therapy was initiated at 600 mg as a loading dose followed by 300 mg biweekly injections. Worsening pruritus and erythema were reported after one month, and his AEC increased to 3610 cells/mcL. During this time, no changes in liver or renal function were observed and no new medications were initiated. One month later, his pruritus had significantly improved spontaneously, and his AEC was 580 cells/mcL. Three months after starting dupilumab, he noted further improvement in his pruritus, and his prednisone was tapered to 5 mg/day. His AEC was 220 cells/mcL, and his IgG was 382 mg/dL.

At his 4-month follow-up appointment in early 2021, he reported a remarkable improvement in his quality of life. His LA demonstrated significant improvement (Figure 3), and his AEC had further decreased to 90. His pruritus is still well-controlled on dupilumab after two years of treatment. His most recent labs revealed an AEC of 160 cells/mcL, IgE of 141 IU/mL, and C3 of 85 mg/dL (NR: 88–201). At his most recent follow-up in the spring of 2022 his eosinophil and neutrophil counts remained normalized, and he remained in remission from his dermatitis and pruritus.

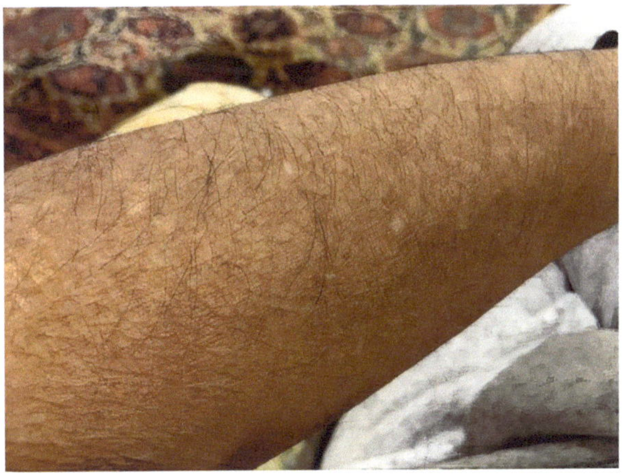

Figure 3. Left forearm demonstrating resolution of hyperpigmented papules after 4 months of dupilumab therapy.

3. Discussion

Given our patient's clinicopathologic features and lab results, including peripheral eosinophilia and elevated IgE, we concluded his cutaneous findings and pruritus were compatible with a cutaneous manifestation of IgG4-RD that we termed IgG4-ADP [2,12]. Attempts to control his IgG4-RD, LA, and atopy with corticosteroids and anti-histamines were unsuccessful. As such, novel approaches to treat his disease were initiated.

While the pathogenesis of IgG4-RD is not entirely understood, a T-helper 2 (Th2) immune response has been implicated, with interleukins (IL) 4, 5, 10, and 13 playing a role in IgG4 class switch, resulting in eosinophilia and elevated IgE. Dupilumab is an IL-4 and IL-13 antagonist that potentially inhibits Th2 IL production. In addition, dupilumab may inhibit IL-31 production, a cytokine implicated in pruritus [10]. This is a plausible explanation for the strong response of our patient's pruritic cutaneous disease to dupilumab.

We report a case where dermatitis, itch, and peripheral eosinophilia were resolved with dupilumab treatment, with a significant improvement in quality of life sustained two years post-treatment initiation. This report provides additional insight into the pathogenesis of these diseases and further supports the efficacy of dupilumab in itch-related processes. Our patient experienced dramatically improved quality of life with initiation of therapy.

Awareness of cytokines activated by IgG4 and how they manifest clinically and in ancillary studies is important for targeted therapy. Future clinical study of dupilumab and its use in the treatment of both systemic and cutaneous IgG4-RD in larger patient populations should be considered.

4. Limitations

This case report was not without limitations. Although skin biopsies cannot directly prove lesions are connected, the constellation of findings such as elevated eosinophils leading to pruritus and spongiotic dermatitis, as well as response to treatment, demonstrate evidence of a connection to IgG4-RD.

Author Contributions: Conceptualization, M.V., J.P., T.C.B. and I.R.; writing—original draft preparation, T.C.B., J.P., K.K. and J.A.F.; writing—review and editing, M.V., J.P., T.C.B., I.R., K.K. and J.A.F. All authors have read and agreed to the published version of the manuscript.

Funding: This research received no external funding.

Institutional Review Board Statement: Ethical review and approval were waived for this study as the case report does not include any identifying information.

Informed Consent Statement: Informed consent was obtained from the patient involved in the case report.

Data Availability Statement: No new data were generated in the creation of this case report.

Conflicts of Interest: The authors declare no conflict of interest.

Appendix A

Table A1. Lab Values Assessing Renal and Liver Function.

	4/16	1/17	11/19	6/20	8/20	11/20	1/21	3/21	9/21	2/22	Units
BUN	68	61	51	45	79	45	48	41	43	47	mg/dL
CR	2.8	3.1	2.4	2.1	3.1	2.7	2.6	2.7	2.8	2.7	mg/dL
eGFR	23.0	20.0	27.0	32.0	20.0	23.5	24.6	23.5	22.3	23.3	mL/min/1.73 sqm
Bili (Total)	0.5	0.6	0.8	0.8	0.6	0.7	0.8	0.8	0.9	1.1	mg/dL
AST	24	23	27	19	31	21	14	20	21	21	U/L
ALT	35	31	25	24	42	24	17	20	20	20	U/L
ALP	88	84	86	82	69	84	93	81	116	119	U/L

Lab values remained relatively unchanged over the course of the case report. The patient demonstrated poor renal function at baseline, which remained consistent over the course of his treatment. Abbreviations: BUN (blood urea nitrogen); CR (creatinine); eGFR (estimated glomerular filtration rate); Bili (Total) (total bilirubin); AST (aspartate transaminase); ALT (alanine transaminase); ALP (alkaline phosphatase). Normal ranges: BUN (5–25 mg/dL); CR (0.6–1.3 mg/dL); eGFR (>60 mL/min/1.73 sqm); Bili (Total) (0.0–1.0 mg/dL); AST (14–50 U/L); ALT (10–40 U/L); ALP (50–136 U/L).

References

1. Wisniowski-Yáñez, A.; Zavala-García, G.; Hernández-Molina, G.; González-Duarte, A.; la Mora, J.D.-D.; Ángeles-Ángeles, A.; Martín-Nares, E. Amyloid A amyloidosis secondary to immunoglobulin G4–related disease. *Rheumatology* **2020**, *60*, e97–e98. [CrossRef] [PubMed]
2. Takayama, R.; Ueno, T.; Saeki, H. Immunoglobulin G4-related disease and its skin manifestations. *J. Dermatol.* **2017**, *44*, 288–296. [CrossRef] [PubMed]
3. Charrow, A.; Imadojemu, S.; Stephen, S.; Ogunleye, T.; Takeshita, J.; Lipoff, J.B. Cutaneous manifestations of IgG4-related disease (RD): A systematic review. *J. Am. Acad. Dermatol.* **2016**, *75*, 197–202. [CrossRef] [PubMed]
4. Shenoy, A.; Mohandas, N.; Gottlieb, A. Cutaneous and systemic IgG4-related disease: A review for dermatologists. *Dermatol. Online J.* **2019**, *25*, 1. [CrossRef]
5. Bennett, A.E.; Fenske, N.A.; Rodriguez-Waitkus, P.; Messina, J.L. IgG4-related skin disease may have distinct systemic manifestations: A systematic review. *Int. J. Dermatol.* **2016**, *55*, 1184–1195. [CrossRef] [PubMed]

6. Shirakashi, M.; Yoshifuji, H.; Kodama, Y.; Chiba, T.; Yamamoto, M.; Takahashi, H.; Uchida, K.; Okazaki, K.; Ito, T.; Kawa, S.; et al. Factors in glucocorticoid regimens associated with treatment response and relapses of IgG4-related disease: A multicentre study. *Sci. Rep.* **2018**, *8*, 10262. [CrossRef] [PubMed]
7. Weidner, T.; Illing, T.; Elsner, P. Primary Localized Cutaneous Amyloidosis: A Systematic Treatment Review. *Am. J. Clin. Dermatol.* **2017**, *18*, 629–642. [CrossRef] [PubMed]
8. Kaltoft, B.; Schmidt, G.; Lauritzen, A.F.; Gimsing, P. Primary localised cutaneous amyloidosis–a systematic review. *Dan. Med. J.* **2013**, *60*, A4727. [PubMed]
9. Mehrotra, K. Primary Cutaneous Amyloidosis: A Clinical, Histopathological and Immunofluorescence Study. *J. Clin. Diagn. Res.* **2017**, *11*, WC01–WC05. [CrossRef] [PubMed]
10. Humeda, Y.; Beasley, J.; Calder, K. Clinical resolution of generalized lichen amyloidosis with dupilumab: A new alternative therapy. *Dermatol. Online J.* **2020**, *26*, 18. [CrossRef]
11. Ladizinski, B.; Lee, K.C. Lichen amyloidosis. *Can. Med. Assoc. J.* **2013**, *186*, 532. [CrossRef] [PubMed]
12. Della Torre, E.; Mattoo, H.; Mahajan, V.; Carruthers, M.; Pillai, S.; Stone, J.H. Prevalence of atopy, eosinophilia, and IgE elevation in IgG4-related disease. *Allergy* **2013**, *69*, 269–272. [CrossRef] [PubMed]

life

Review

The Protective Role of Ozone Therapy in Kidney Disease: A Review

Luis Fernando Delgadillo-Valero [1,2], Estefani Yaquelin Hernández-Cruz [2,3] and José Pedraza-Chaverri [2,*]

1 Faculty of Medicine, National Autonomous University of Mexico, Mexico City 04360, Mexico
2 Laboratory F-315, Department of Biology, Faculty of Chemistry, National Autonomous University of Mexico, Mexico City 04510, Mexico
3 Postgraduate in Biological Sciences, National Autonomous University of Mexico, Ciudad Universitaria, Mexico City 04510, Mexico
* Correspondence: pedraza@unam.mx

Abstract: Ozone (O_3) is a reactive oxygen species (ROS) that can interact with cellular components and cause oxidative stress. Following said logic, if O_3 induces such a stressful milieu, how does it exert antioxidant functions? This is mediated by controlled toxicity produced by low concentrations of O_3, which enhance the cell's suppliance of antioxidant properties without causing any further damage. Therapeutic concentrations vary extensively, although 50 μg/mL is commonly used in experimental and clinical procedures, given that augmented concentrations might work as germicides or cause endogenous damage. O_3 therapy has been shown to be effective when applied before or after traumatic renal procedures, whether caused by ischemia, xenobiotics, chronic damage, or other models. In this review, we focus on discussing the role of O_3 therapy in different models of kidney damage associated with fibrosis, apoptosis, oxidative stress, and inflammation. We integrate and report knowledge about O_3 in renal therapy, debunking skepticism towards unconventional medicine, explaining its proven therapeutic properties, and thus providing background for its use in further research as well as in clinical settings.

Keywords: ozone; ozone therapy; kidney disease; oxidative stress; antioxidants defense; inflammation

Citation: Delgadillo-Valero, L.F.; Hernández-Cruz, E.Y.; Pedraza-Chaverri, J. The Protective Role of Ozone Therapy in Kidney Disease: A Review. *Life* **2023**, *13*, 752. https://doi.org/10.3390/life13030752

Academic Editors: Stefanos Roumeliotis and Giuseppe Minervini

Received: 15 February 2023
Revised: 5 March 2023
Accepted: 7 March 2023
Published: 10 March 2023

1. Introduction

Kidneys are organs of great biological importance. They receive approximately 25% of the cardiac output, and their main functions are filtrating blood, keeping a homeostatic plasma volume, and regulating vascular pH and ion concentration in circulation, amongst many others. They achieve this by reabsorbing necessary biological metabolites and depurating toxic or unhelpful ones through a complex tubular system formed by nephrons [1]. Kidney diseases are described as a group of multicausal syndromes and impaired diagnostic markers (oliguria, albuminuria, or proteinuria, rise of creatinine excretion, or diminished filtration rate, all of which measure renal function) that can be categorized according to their evolution time in acute kidney injury (AKI), before 7 days; acute kidney disease (AKD), up to 3 months; and chronic kidney disease (CKD), after 3 months. They are highly prevalent and represent a global health issue. For instance, AKI is experienced by 1 in 5 hospitalized patients worldwide [2] and has a high mortality rate of approximately 21%. However, more severe stages, such as patients needing kidney replacement therapy, are associated with higher mortality (46%) and unaffordable costs. In 2012, 864,226 deaths were attributable for CKD and predictions suggest mortality will increase, even when CKD is currently the fourteenth cause of death worldwide, with 12 deaths per 100,000 individuals [3].

Conventional therapeutics as the disease progresses are often targeted only towards reducing risk factors, such as diabetes, hypertension, and dyslipidaemia, which might aggravate the disease and favor its progression by causing glomerulosclerosis, endothelial damage, salt retention, volume overload, and tubular atrophy [3,4]. Such treatments are also intended to compensate diminished renal function. For example, recommendations from the National Institute of Health include diuretics and renin- angiotensin aldosterone system (RAAS) inhibitors, which are not only useful as treatment for hypertension, but might also compensate for lost electrolyte excretion and diminish albuminuria, respectively [5]. Reducing blood pressure is important given the high prevalence of this disease, which is present in about half of the American population [6] and is one of the main causes of CKD along with diabetes, furtherly discussed in the text. Other international treatment guidelines, e.g., the Mexican Clinical Practice Guide, suggest treatment with SGLT-2 inhibitors to reduce CKD progression in diabetic patients, as well as the use of statins to reduce cardiovascular events [7]. Chronic and end stage renal conditions often need kidney replacement therapy, which includes renal transplant, hemodialysis, and peritoneal dialysis treatment [8]. The survival rate in dialyzed patients is approximately 55% after five years, less than expected for the general population [9]. Besides reported oxidative damage observed in CKD and dialyzed patients [10], the Kidney Disease Improving Global Outcomes (KDIGO) 2012 Clinical Practice Guideline for the Evaluation and Management of CKD does not include any antioxidant treatment in its recommendations [11].

Medical costs associated only to free for service Medicare beneficiaries with CKD can sum up to 49 billion dollars each year [12], even when prevention of kidney disease is promoted with strategies, such as weight control, patient education, diet, exercise, and identifying additional risk factors, e.g., dehydration, anemia, cancer, hypovolaemia, hypoxia, use of nephrotoxic drugs, heart failure, sepsis, hepatorenal syndrome, amongst others [13]. Therefore, finding alternative therapies for patients with kidney diseases, including CKD, AKI, or those needing a transplant, is vital. Ozone (O_3) is a molecule consisting of three unstably bound oxygen atoms that has been used as a novel therapy in many diseases. It is formed naturally when a di-oxygen molecule (O_2) binds to atomic oxygen, formed by ultraviolet (UV) radiation. Moreover, it is artificially created, using O_3 concentrators, which work through the electrical discharge of gas, creating an airtight barrier that prevents O_2 from passing through, forcing it to dissociate and form O_3 instead [14]. O_3 is considered a reactive oxygen species (ROS). In other words, it is more reactive than O_2. However, since it does not have unpaired electrons, it is considered a non-radical one that can react with biological cell structures, such as lipids, proteins, and nucleic acids. O_3 can also promote reactions that form reactive species, such as hydroxyl radicals; such toxic characteristics have also been described as possible antimicrobial mechanisms [15].

Considering the above factors, the purpose of this review is to integrate and present knowledge about O_3 in renal therapy, debunking skepticism towards non-conventional medicine, explaining its proven therapeutic properties, and thus providing background for its use in further research as in clinical settings.

2. O_3 Mechanism of Action

To understand O_3 mechanism of action and chemical properties, O_3 must be identified as a ROS, a molecule with a great oxidizing capacity. ROS are classified as non-radicals and free radicals (with one or more uncoupled electrons). However, O_3 is among the non-radicals [16]. O_3 can react by itself with biological structures, such as amino acids (especially aromatic), enzymes, deoxyribonucleic acid (DNA), as well as membrane glycoproteins and lipids. However, due to its instability in the gaseous phase, water solution, or in combination with other extracellular substances, it can dissolve in a chain reaction to form a variety of free radicals, such as hydroxyl radical ($^{\bullet}OH$) and superoxide radicals ($O_2^{\bullet-}$), which acquire missing electrons by oxidizing biological components. Eventually, when the breakdown of ozone is inhibited, the chain reaction ends. This is because organic and inorganic substances, such as stable carbonate ions (CO_3^{2-}) and bicarbonate (HCO_3), react with OH radicals to form secondary radicals that do not generate superoxide radicals. Another example of termination is the reaction of two free radicals ($^{\bullet}OH + HO_2^{\bullet} \rightarrow O_2 + H_2O$) [17].

The ROS created from the interactions of O_3 and O_3 itself oxidize the cysteinyl thiols of Kelch-like ECH-associated protein 1 (KEAP1), a protein that keeps nuclear erythroid factor 2 (Nrf2) ubiquitinated and, therefore, destroyed by the proteasome. Such an event leads Nrf2, a transcription factor, to translocate to the nucleus, where it regulates oxidative damage by inducing antioxidant response elements (ARE) [18], including antioxidant enzymes that serve as protective responses that delay, prevent, or remove oxidative damage, via catalytic or scavenger activity of free radicals. Examples of upregulated antioxidant proteins include catalase (CAT), superoxide dismutase (SOD), glutathione peroxidase (GSH-Px), glutathione s-transferase (GSTr), heme oxygenase-1 (HO-1), NADPH quinone oxidoreductase 1 (NQO1), and heat shock protein-70 (HSP70) [19]. O_3 therapy also works by inducing controlled oxidation of polyunsaturated fatty acids (PUFAs) found in cell membranes. This creates ozonated lipid products (LOPs), which are important signal transducers and regulators of inflammation [20]. LOPs (specifically hydroxy-hydroperoxides) exacerbate Nrf2 nuclear translocation by oxidizing cysteine residues, promoting KEAP1-Nrf2 dissociation and activation of Nrf2-ARE pathways [21,22]. Furthermore, they increase the phosphorylation of Nrf2 by casein kinase 2 (CK2) [21]. In addition, LOPs have a hormetic response since, at low concentrations, they downregulate activation of nuclear factor kappa B (NF-κB) and inflammatory cytokines and increase antioxidant and anti-inflammatory compounds. High concentrations stimulate potential antimicrobial and chemotactic responses by activating phospholipase A2 and phospholipase C, which via intracellular cascades, including that of the arachidonic acid, stimulate the synthesis of NF-κB and, therefore, pro-inflammatory cytokines, e.g., interleukins (IL) 1 and 6 and tumor necrosis factor-alpha (TNF-α), transforming growth factor beta (TGF-β), as well as the cyclooxygenase (COX) [23]. This explains how controlled and nontoxic oxidation by O_3 mediates the upregulation of antioxidant and anti-inflammatory defenses (Figure 1).

O_3 is applied in situ due to its short life, as it can only be stored for about 40 min at 20 degrees Celsius. Routes of O_3 dosing vary depending on the goals and location of therapy and include rectal insufflation and autohemotherapy (for systematic effects), as well as topic and infiltrative therapy (for localized effects, such as musculoskeletal and germicide) [19]. On the contrary, administration through the respiratory pathway is contraindicated due to the insufficient antioxidant capacity of this system and the narrowing effects caused by O_3 on the airway [20]. The therapeutic window range is proposed to be between 20 and 80 μg/mL of O_3 per gram of blood [24].

Therapeutic effects commonly observed in the kidney after the administration of O_3 administration include amelioration of renal function, measured through plasma clearance of endogenous metabolites, blood urea nitrogen (BUN), and serum creatinine (SCr). Hence, those molecules filtrated and depurated by the kidney [25] at lesser levels after O_3 treatment infer protection [26–31]. In addition, O_3 therapy has been reported to decrease morphological damage mainly evidenced under photon microscopy, including medullary hemorrhage, tubular necrosis, glomerular damage, collagen deposition, and fibrosis markers, such as α-smooth muscle actin (α-SMA) and TGF [26–33], besides increasing the suppressor of mothers against decapentaplegic-7 (SMAD-7) [33]. Furthermore, O_3 therapy reduces inflammation, as evidenced by a diminished expression of cytokines, such as IL, TNF-α, monocyte chemoattractant protein-1 (MCP-1), and intercellular adhesion molecule-1 (ICAM-1), as well as the toll Like receptor 4 (TLR 4)-NFkB pathway [26,34]. Another therapeutic effect is the diminishment of lipid peroxidation, which represents the oxidative stress induced by polyunsaturated fatty acids. A useful marker to quantify this is via malondialdehyde (MDA) [35], which diminishes its renal expression when treated with O_3 [28,29,31,33].

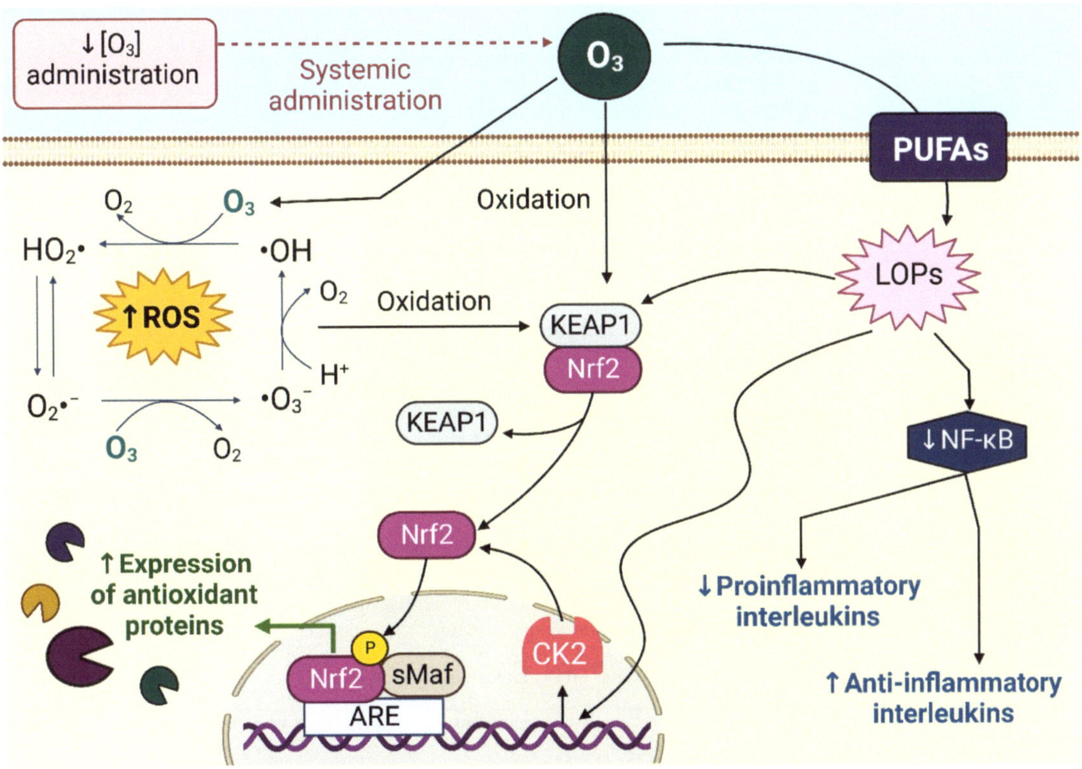

Figure 1. Mechanism of action of the administration of low concentrations of ozone (O_3). O_3 forms free radicals, such as the hydroxyl radical (•OH) and superoxide radicals ($O_2^{\bullet-}$), due to different chain reactions. The free radicals formed, and O_3 oxidized Kelch-like ECH-associated protein 1 (KEAP1), promoting nuclear translocation of nuclear erythroid factor 2 (Nrf2). Nrf2 in the nucleus binds to the antioxidant response element (ARE) and induces the transcription of antioxidant enzymes. Nrf2 nuclear translocation is exacerbated by the action of ozonated lipid products (LOPs) formed by the oxidation of polyunsaturated fatty acids (PUFAs). LOPs act by oxidizing KEAP1 and increasing casein kinase 2 (CK2) synthesis, increasing Nrf2 phosphorylation. In addition, LOPs decreases the expression of nuclear factor kappa B (NF-κB), promising the decrease of proinflammatory cytokines and increasing the concentration of anti-inflammatory cytokines. P: phosphorylation, ROS: reactive oxygen species, sMaf: small musculoaponeurotic fibrosarcoma. Created with Biorender.com, accessed on 10 February 2023.

3. Damage Models and O_3 Effect

3.1. O_3 Therapy Protects the Kidney against Ischemic Damage

Ischemic damage in renal tissue occurs when kidneys experiment periods of diminished or restricted blood supply. In contrast, oxidative damage occurs when tissue is re-oxygenated, which might happen during experimental procedures in rats, such as clamping and unclamping renal pedicle, or during renal transplantation [36]. This kind of damage is proposedly produced through xanthine oxidase (XO). This enzyme degrades nucleotides upon cell ischemia. However, after O_2 reperfusion, XO forms uric acid and high quantities of superoxide radical, which further produces oxidative stress [37]. This explains why treatment with XO inhibitors, such as tungsten [37], allopurinol [38], or even XO knockout models [14], ameliorates ischemia-reperfusion injury (IRI) and oxidative stress after short periods of ischemia. Finding auxiliary treatments for oxidative damage is clinically important since ischemic-producing scenarios are highly prevalent. Just in 2010, for instance, more than 2 million patients received renal transplants [39].

O_3 therapy has previously been used before IRI (preconditioning) [26–28,33,40,41] or after IRI (postconditioning) [29–32,42] and has been described as a potential treatment (Table 1). O_3 therapy is demonstrated to act with similar efficacy, but not synergic, to that achieved when IRI preconditioning is made with other protective strategies, such as inducing short, repeated periods of ischemia before the main IRI. This prepares the renal tissue against the IRI via similar controlled mechanisms as that of the O_3 and is called ischemic (pre)conditioning [43]. Interestingly, when administered after the main IRI, ischemic postconditioning in conjunction with O_3 therapy upregulate beneficial effects and even diminishes cell death [44]. After transplantation, rats also show a protective effect against the oxidative state when treated with O_3 [45,46]. Antioxidant enzymes are also upregulated in cultured kidney cells after they were submitted to hypoxia and reoxygenation [47].

Nitric oxide (NO) and NO synthase (endothelial, eNOS, and inducible, iNOS) have been proposed as oxidants that damage renal tubules through highly reactive peroxynitrite [48]. However, NO was found to be a protective mechanism favored by O_3 therapy against IRI inflammation and vasoconstriction caused by Endothelin-1 [27,28]. In fact, nitrate-derived NO, when applied topically, is an effective therapy against IRI damage [49].

In summary, O_3 therapy, either before or after IRI, improves kidney damage by decreasing markers of kidney damage, inflammation, and fibrosis. Therefore, it is a good treatment for ischemic injuries such as kidney transplantation, iatrogenic trauma, partial nephrectomy, heart failure, and hypovolemia, among other prevalent clinical conditions that reduce renal blood flow, such as those that produce AKI.

Table 1. Ozone (O_3) effects on ischemic damage models.

Damage Model	Induced Procedure	O_3 Administration	Effects in O_3 Treated Rats	Ref.
O_3 oxidative preconditioning Therapy				
Kidney transplantation	Right Nephrectomy and left transplant	15 (1 daily) preconditioning rectal insufflations 1 mg/kg at [50 μg/mL] to the donor rat	↑ SOD, GSH Px ↓ SCr, BUN, MDA ↓ Morphologic damage ↓ IL-6, IL-18, COX2 ↓ NF-κB, HMGB1	[45]
Kidney transplantation	Right nephrectomy and left transplant	15 (1 daily) preconditioning rectal insufflations 1 mg/kg at [50 μg/mL] to the donor rat	↑ SOD, GSH, CAT ↑ Nrf2, HO-1 ↓ SCr, BUN, MDA ↓ Morphologic damage	[46]
Right nephrectomy and left pedicle clamping	45 min ischemia 24 h reperfusion	Preconditioning therapy 15 previous rectal insufflations, 1 mg/kg at [50 μg/mL]	↓ BUN, SCr ↓ Medullar Hemorrhage ↓ TNF-α, IL-1β, IL-6, ICAM-1, ↓ MCP-1, TLR4, NF-kB	[26]
Right nephrectomy and left pedicle clamping	60 min ischemia 60 min reperfusion	Preconditioning therapy OA, 1 mL of blood added with 5 mL of O_3 [50 μg/mL] before and after IR	↑ iNOS ↑ β NADPH diaphorase ↓ BUN, SCr ↓ Medullar damage	[27]
Right nephrectomy and left pedicle clamping	45 min ischemia 24, 48, 72 h reperfusion	Preconditioning therapy 15 previous rectal insufflations, 1 mg/kg at [50 μg/mL]	↑ GSH, GSH-Px, SOD ↑ NO, iNOS, eNOS ↓ BUN, SCr ↓ Morphologic damage ↓ MDA ↓ ET-1	[28]
Right nephrectomy and left pedicle clamping	45 min ischemia 8-week reperfusion	Preconditioning therapy rectal pathway, 1 mg/kg at [50 μg/dL]	↑ SMAD-7 ↓ α- SMA, TGF-β BUN, SCr not significant	[33]
Right nephrectomy and left pedicle clamping	45 min ischemia and reperfusion	Preconditioning 15 (1 daily) doses by rectal insufflation, 1 mg/kg at [50 μg/mL]	↓ SCr, BUN, MDA ↓ Morphologic damage ↓ICAM-1, IL-1β, TNF-α, Caspase 3	[40]
Bilateral pedicle clamping	30 min ischemia and 3 h reperfusion	Preconditioning 15 (1 daily) 2.5–2.6 mL at [50 mg/mL] at a dose of 0.5 mg/kg by rectal insufflation	↑ RPF, GFR (inulin) ↑ SOD ↓ Morphologic damage	[41]

Table 1. *Cont.*

Damage Model	Induced Procedure	O_3 Administration	Effects in O_3 Treated Rats	Ref.
O_3 oxidative postconditioning therapy				
Bilateral Renal Artery Occlusion	60 min ischemia 6 h reperfusion	Postconditioning therapy single 0.7 μg/kg i.p. immediately after reperfusion	↑ SOD, GSH-Px, ↓ SCr, BUN ↓ AST, Neopterin ↓ MDA, PCC, NOx ↓ Morphologic damage	[31]
Left nephrectomy and right pedicle clamping	45 min ischemia 24 h reperfusion	Postconditioning therapy 1 and 2 mg/kg; 15 (1 daily) doses after IRI at [50 μg/mL] by rectal insufflation	↑ SOD ↓ SCr, BUN, MDA ↓ Morphologic damage ↓ BAX, PARP, CREB, c-Fos	[30]
Right Nephrectomy and Left pedicle clamping	45 min ischemia 10 days reperfusion	Postconditioning therapy 10 daily rectal insufflations after IRI, a 2.5 mL volume at 0.5 mg/kg/min [50 μg/mL]	↑ SOD ↓ SCr, BUN ↓ MDA, MPO ↓ Morphologic damage ↓ α-SMA, TGF-β, p-SMAD-2	[29]
Renal vascular bundles clamping	60 min ischemia 10 days reperfusion	Postconditioning therapy Daily 10 days after IRI At 0.5 mg/kg/min via rectal insufflation	↓ Proteinuria ↑ RPF, Glomerular Filtration Rate ↓ Morphologic Damage	[32]
Bilateral Renal Artery Occlusion	60 min ischemia and 10-day reperfusion	10 (1 daily) 2.5–2.6 mL at [50 mg/mL], representing a dose of 0.5 mg/kg weight rectal insufflations	↑ CAT, SOD ↓ SCr, Fructosamine ↓ Phospholipase A2	[42]
Right nephrectomy and left pedicle clamping	45 min ischemia and 24 h reperfusion	Ischemic Preconditioning vs. O_3 Preconditioning, 15 rectal insufflations at [50 μg/mL])	↑ NO ↑ GSH, GSP-Px, SOD ↓ BUN, SCr, MDA	[43]
Right nephrectomy and left pedicle clamping	45 min ischemia and 24 h reperfusion	Comparison Ischemic Post conditioning vs. O_3 post conditioning, 2 mg/kg	↓ IL 1, IL 18, Caspase 1 ↓ SCr, BUN, MDA ↓ Morphologic Damage	[44]

Abbreviatures: ↑: significant increase, ↓: significant decrease, α-SMA: α-smooth muscle actin, AST: aspartate aminotransferase, BAX: bcl-2-associated X, BUN: blood urea nitrogen, CAT: catalase, COX2: cyclooxygenase 2, CREB: cAMP response element-binding, eNOS: endothelial nitric oxide synthase, ET-1: endothelin-1, FF: filtration fraction, GFR: glomerular filtration rate, GSH-Px: glutathione peroxidase, GSH: glutathione, HMGB1: high mobility group Box 1, HO-1: heme oxygenase-1, ICAM-1: intercellular adhesion molecule-1, IL-1β: interleukin-1β, IL-6: interleukin-6, iNOS: inducible nitric oxide synthase, IRI: ischemia/reperfusion injury, MCP-1: monocyte chemoattractant protein 1, MDA: malondialdehyde, NF-kB: nuclear factor kappa B, NO: nitric oxide, O_3: ozone, OA: ozonated autohemotherapy, PARP: polymerase 1, PCC: protein carbonyl content, RPF: renal plasma fraction, SCr: serum creatinine, SMAD-7 and -2: suppressor of mothers against decapentaplegic family members 7 and 2, SOD: superoxide dismutase, β NADPH diaphorase: β-nicotinamide adenine dinucleotide phosphate diaphorase, TGF-β: transforming growth factor β, TLR 4: Toll-Like receptor 4, TNF-α: tumor necrosis factor α.

3.2. O_3 Therapy Protects the Kidney against Xenobiotic-Induced Damage

Xenobiotics are exogenous chemicals not synthesized by a certain organism; therefore, they are not essential for its physiological functions and processes. That way, synthetical drugs, metals, and environmental factors, amongst others, are considered as such [50]. In this section, the mechanisms through which some of these xenobiotics cause nephrotoxicity will be discussed; along with the described protective effects of O_3 therapy against it, looking forward to discovering the usage of new therapeutic alternatives against damaging products we are constantly in contact with (Table 2).

Acetaminophen (APAP), a common anti-inflammatory drug, has been demonstrated to produce severe nephrotoxicity [51]. Proposed mechanisms include APAP's hepatic degradation and further enzymatic formation of a highly toxic and reactive metabolite, N-acetyl-p-benzoquinone (NAPQI), which glutathione (GSH) normally neutralizes. However, in APAP overdose, NAPQI is formed in major quantities, proving uncontainable by antioxidant enzymes, and therefore producing oxidative damage, especially in proximal tubules [52]. O_3 therapy has proven to be an effective antioxidant therapy by enhancing antioxidant enzymes and diminishing oxidation [51]. Interestingly, the administration of O_3 therapy in APAP induced nephrotoxicity, when combined with another antioxidant therapy, N-acetylcysteine (NAC), produced no significant changes in the kidney's function (creatinine, urea) and inflammation (IL-6, IL-10) but did produce significant changes against oxidative stress, showing lower levels of MDA, as well as a reduction of histopathologic glomerular, tubular, and interstitial damage [53].

Cadmium (Cd) is a heavy non-essential metal that is accumulated in body tissues progressively [54] and to which humans are exposed through air particles [55], occupational exposure [56] and seafood such as mollusks, crustaceans, or fish [57]. Cd can produce nephrotoxicity by many mechanisms, including DNA damage, altered gene expression, and, most importantly, oxidative damage by depleting cells' antioxidant defenses, such as selenium, which binds to Cd to neutralize it [58]. Other proteins, e.g., metallothionein (MT), bind Cd in others to diminish its toxicity in organs such as kidneys and testis [59,60]. O_3 therapy can diminish Cd accumulation, augment MT levels, and reduce morphologic damage, serving as an effective protective mechanism against Cd^{2+} renal damage [59]. It also reduces N-acetyl-β-D-glucosaminidase (NAG) [61], a lysosomal enzyme found mainly in proximal convoluted tubules, its function is the digestion of cell's glycoconjugates [62]. The NAG increase is mediated by loss of the tubular brush border, thus liberating the enzyme into the urine [63]; such an increase is associated with pathologic processes such as Cd intoxication and malignancies of the kidney, liver, pancreas, lung, and breast, amongst many others [61,64], as well as an increased risk of requiring dialysis treatment and lethality in hospitalized patients [63]. Even when stimulating lipid peroxidation, as a result, O_3 was also demonstrated to induce antioxidant enzymes in Cd-treated rats [65].

Some antineoplastics are proven to cause nephrotoxicity. For instance, doxorubicin, often known as Adriamycin, binds to cell membranes and inhibits nucleotide replication. However, it can be oxidized into forming reactive species like hydroxyl radicals [66]. It is demonstrated to cause severe progressive damage, fibrosis, and proteinuria [67]. O_3 therapy, in certain doses, has proven to mediate protective effects against this morphologic damage, and arterial pressure, as well as proteinuria, have been ameliorated in rats receiving this treatment [68].

Another example is cisplatin (CDDP), an FDA (American Food and Drug Administration) approved treatment for advanced solid cancers such as that of the testis, ovary, and bladder [69]. CDDP is a molecule composed of a single platinum atom bound to chloride and ammonium; due to its small size, it filtrates freely into the glomerular barrier without tubular reabsorption [70]. It then enters tubular cells and dissociates into its toxic components, which damage DNA, membrane transporters, and mitochondrial function, thus producing oxidative stress, inflammation, and apoptosis [70,71]. O_3 has been used as a therapy against CDDP induced damage, improving function and augmenting antioxidant defenses. Thiobarbituric acid reactive substances (TBARS, an assay used to measure lipid peroxidation; [72]), as well as NAG and morphologic damage, displayed decreased values when treated with O_3 [73–75]. Protective effects, however, varied according to the administered O_3 concentration, given that the administration of 0.36 mg/kg might be therapeutic [60] or might not [75]. On the other hand, 1.1 mg/kg always shows protective tendencies in CDDP-induced damage [73–75]. Higher concentrations, e.g., 1.8 mg/kg, might be protective [62]. However, due to the high formation rate of hydrogen peroxide and oxidative stress mediated by O_3, toxic effects might be produced [73]. Very similar protective morphologic, anti-inflammatory, and antioxidant effects have been found against the damage induced by methotrexate, another cancer drug, in the kidneys, as well as the intestines and liver [76].

Radiographic contrast media (CM) is constantly used in clinical procedures which require the observation of vascular compartments. Mechanisms through which CM might cause renal dysfunction include direct oxygen-free radical damage, modified hemodynamics, and hypoxic renal medullary injury mediated by shortness of blood flow and an increase in tubular O_2 supply. Therefore, the employment of CM produces high toxicity [77], which can be treated with O_3. Neutrophil gelatinase-associated lipocalin (NGAL) is a damage marker observed in contrast-induced nephropathy (CIN) which augmented its expression when treated with O_3; no further discussion was provided, although the initial oxidation by O_3 might have produced it [78,79].

In the medical field, the use of xenobiotics as drugs to treat and diagnose diseases is an irreplaceable factor. However, during their metabolism and excretion, some might become nephrotoxic by accumulation, directing damage, the formation of free radicals, and depletion of antioxidant substances. This represents a risk for patients with neoplasia or other conditions which require constant chemical induction or those in contact with environmental components such as Cd, which is also demonstrated to cause similar renal damage. However, O_3 is an effective treatment against this damage, at least experimentally, and thus the importance of further research in clinical environments.

Table 2. Ozone (O_3) effects on chemical-induced damage models.

Damage Model	Induced Procedure	O_3 Administration	Effects in O_3 Treated Rats	Ref.
APAP toxicity	A 1.0 g/kg dose suspended in H_2O, 3 mL: orally	Single i.p. 0.7 mg/kg dose at [60 mg/mL] Immediately after APAP induction	↑ SOD, GSH-Px ↓ SCr, BUN ↓ MDA ↓ Morphologic damage	[51]
APAP toxicity	A 1.0 g/kg dose suspended in H_2O, 3 mL: gastric tube	5 daily 0.7 mg/kg doses i.p. at [60 mg/mL] Immediately after APAP induction	↑ GSH-Px, IL-10 ↓ Morphologic damage ↓ MDA ↓TNF-α	[53]
Experimental toxic adriamycin-induced glomerulonephritis	Adriamycin single 7.5 mg/kg dose through a jugular vein; 10-week evolution	After 10 weeks, daily for 15 days at 0.3 mg/kg or 0.5 mg/kg or 0.7 mg/kg, or 1.1 mg/kg	(0.3 mg/kg) ↓ Arterial pressure ↓ Proteinuria (0.5 mg/kg) ↓ Morphologic damage (0.7 and 1.1 mg/kg) No significant changes	[68]
Cd intoxication	Drinking water with Cd^{2+} (50 mg/L) in the form of Cadmium Acetate for 12 weeks	10 (1 daily) 1 mL i.p. doses at [40 μg/mL]	↓ Morphologic damage ↓ Glomerulonephritis ↓ NAG	[61]
Cd Intoxication	Drinking water with Cd^{2+} (50 mg/L) in the form of Cadmium Acetate for 12 weeks	10 (1 daily) 1 mL i.p. doses at [40 μg/mL]	↑ MT ↓ Morphologic damage	[59]
CDDP induced nephrotoxicity	Single 6 mg/kg CDDP injection	Preconditioning 15 (1 daily) doses by rectal insufflation, 9 mL at concentrations of [0.36, 0.72, 1.1, 1.8, 2.5 mg/kg]	↑ GSH, SOD, CAT, GSH-Px ↓ SCr ↓ TBARS	[73]
CDDP induced nephrotoxicity	Single 6 mg/kg CDDP injection	Postconditioning 6 (1 daily) rectal insufflations, 9 mL volume with concentrations of: 10 mg at [0.36 mg/kg] or 30 mg at [1.10 mg/kg] or 50 mg at [1.80 mg/kg]	↑ GSH, SOD, CAT, GSH-Px ↓ SCr ↓ TBARS	[75]
CDDP induced nephrotoxicity	Single 6 mg/kg CDDP injection	Daily; 5 days before and 5 days after CDDP injection. i.p.at 1.1 mg/kg	↑ CAT, SOD ↑ NAG, TGF-β1, IL-6 ↓ Morphologic damage ↓Urea, creatinine, uric acid, phosphorus, calcium, sNGAL, albumin ↓ NF-a, IL-1B,	[74]
CIN	10 mg/kg injected through the tail vein	1. 6 h before and 6 h after OR 2. For 5 days after; contrast agent introduction. O_3 at 1 mg/kg, 95% i.p.	1. ↑ NGAL ↓Hemorrhage 2. ↑TAC, similar SCr ↓Renal tubular injury	[79]
CIN	6 mL/kg of meglumine/sodium diatrizoate through the tail vein	Five 0.7 mg/kg/d doses i.p. [70 μg/mL] For 5 days before CIN	↑ NO ↑ TAS ↓ SCr, BUN ↓ MDA ↓ Tubular necrosis	[78]

Abbreviatures: ↑: significant increase, ↓: significant decrease, APAP: acetaminophen, BUN: blood urea nitrogen, CAT: catalase, Cd: cadmium, CDDP: cisplatin, CIN: contrast-induced nephropathy, GSH: glutathione, GSH-Px: glutathione peroxidase, IL-10: interleukin 10, i.p.: intraperitoneal route, MDA: malondialdehyde, MT: metallothionine, NAG: N-acetyl-β-D-glucosaminidase, NGAL: neutrophil gelatinase-associated lipocalin, NO: nitric oxide, O_3: ozone, SCr: serum creatinine, SOD: superoxide dismutase, TAC: total antioxidant capacity, TAS: total antioxidant system, TBARS: thiobarbituric acid reactive substances, TGF-β1: transforming growth factor β1, TNF-α: tumor necrosis factor-alpha.

3.3. O_3 Therapy Protects the Kidney against CKD

CKD is a major global health issue due to its high worldwide prevalence. In 2010, an analysis showed that about 500 million adults over 20 years old suffered from this disease [80]. As its name suggests, CKD is a progressive condition in which kidney function diminishes progressively, as indicated by a lesser glomerular filtration rate (GFR) (<60 mL/min per 1.73 m^2) or the presence of pathologic markers, such as albuminuria, hematuria, glucosuria, or other abnormalities detected by imaging, for at least three months [3]. Many factors are involved in its development, such as hypertension, pollution, glomerulonephritis, and, most importantly, type 2 diabetes mellitus [81]. In this section, the effects of O_3 therapy against CKD will be discussed, hoping to decipher the use of new therapeutic alternatives to delay or prevent this pathology (Table 3).

Several procedures are induced in rats to simulate CKD, such as subtotal (5/6) nephrectomy, which exposes remaining renal tissue to high pressure and perfusion, eventually diminishing renal function and hence great inflammation. O_3 can ameliorate this condition, enhancing kidney function and antioxidant status. TBARS showed higher levels, possibly due to O_3 mediated oxidative stress [82,83]. Adenine administration also simulates CKD through its enzymatic degradation by xanthine dehydrogenase and further accumulation of the product 2,8-dihydroxyadenine (DHA) in the renal tubules, leading to inflammation and oxidative stress [84]. O_3 ameliorated this damaging condition mainly by stimulating the expression of antioxidant enzymes and reducing inflammation [85,86].

Diabetic kidney disease (DKD) is the main cause of CKD. It is a chronic condition caused by diabetes (whether type 1 or 2) via apoptosis, formation of free radicals, advanced glycation end-products (AGES), inflammatory cytokines, and other growth molecules. [87]. Diagnosis is made essentially through diminished GFR and proteinuria in humans. Risk factors include smoking habits and high arterial pressure. The discussion of this disease becomes important since its prevalence, and therefore that of CKD, is augmenting [88]. In experimental DKD studies that use streptozotocin (STZ) as a toxic component to β-cells, O_3 has shown beneficial anti-apoptotic and antioxidative effects in response [89,90].

Table 3. Ozone (O_3) effects on chronic kidney damage models.

Damage Model	Induced Procedure	O_3 Administration	Effects in O_3 Treated Rats	Ref.
Adenine Induced CKD	0.75% adenine diet for 4 weeks	1.1 mg/kg at [50 μg/mL] Via rectal insufflation	↓ SCr, BUN, K, Ca ↓ Morphologic damage ↓ MCP-1, TNFα, IL-1b, IL-6 ↓TLR 4, NFkB, p65	[85]
Subtotal Nephrectomy CKD	Right nephrectomy and left subtotal ablation. 10-week evolution	1.1 mg/kg at [50 μg/mL] Via rectal insufflation Once a day for 2 weeks	↓ TNFα, IL-1β, IL-6, ↓ SCr, BUN, K, Ca ↓ Morphologic damage ↓NLRP3, NFkB, ASC, Caspase 1	[82]
Subtotal Nephrectomy CKD	Right nephrectomy and left subtotal ablation. 10-week evolution	2.5 mL at [50 μg/mL] Dose of 0.5 mg/kg Once a day for 15 days	↑ RPF, GFR ↑ SOD, CAT, GSH, TBARS ↓ Systolic arterial pressure ↓ SCr, BUN ↓ Morphologic damage	[83]
Diabetic Nephropathy	Streptozotocin induced Diabetes 6-week evolution	1.1 mg/kg [50 μg/mL] i.p.	↑ SOD, GPx, CAT ↓ BP, Hb A_{1c} % ↓ BUN, SCr, AR, MDA	[89]
Diabetic Nephropathy	Streptozotocin induced Diabetes 6-week evolution	1.1 mg/kg [50 μg/mL] once a day for 6 weeks	↓ Caspases 1, 3, 9; HIF-1α, TNF-α, Glc, morphologic damage	[90]

Abbreviatures: ↑: significant increase, ↓: significant decrease, AR: aldose reductase, ASC: apoptosis-associated speck-like protein containing a CARD, BP: blood pressure, BUN: blood urea nitrogen, Ca: calcium, CAT: catalase, CKD: chronic kidney disease, GFR: glomerular filtration rate, Glc: glucose, GPx: glutathione peroxidase, GSH: glutathione, Hb A_{1c} %: glycosylated hemoglobin, HIF-1α: hypoxia inducible factor 1α, IL: Interleukins, i.p.: intraperitoneal route, K: potassium, MDA: malondialdehyde, MCP-1: monocyte chemoattractant protein-1, NFkB: nuclear factor kappa B, NLRP3: NLR family pyrin domain containing 3, O_3: ozone, p65: 5 kDa polypeptide, RPF: renal plasma flow, SCr: serum creatinine, SOD: superoxide dismutase, TBARS: thiobarbituric acid reactive substances, TLR 4: Toll-Like receptor 4, TNF-α: tumor necrosis factor-alpha.

CKD usually reaches an advanced terminal stage, which require therapy for replacing renal function, or dialysis, as the indicated treatment [91]. O_3 has been shown as a coadjutant therapy to dialysis, as demonstrated by case reports in which conventional treatment did not work. For example, Biedunkiewicz and collaborators [92] described the case of a dialyzed patient with calciphylaxis-induced ulcerations who did not respond to antibiotics and surgical treatment. Ozonated autohemotherapy in concentrations of 50 μg/mL, as well as O_3 topic administration, allowed a successful skin transplant. Authors propose that effects are mediated through O_3 induced the synthesis of platelet-derived growth factor (PDGF), TGF-β1, and IL-8. Paolo and collaborators [93] described the case of a hemodialyzed patient who presented necrotizing fasciitis and a fatal prognosis. However, after extracorporeal blood oxygenation and ozonization (EBOO) and O_3 topic administration, drastic wellness, including diminished hyperpyrexia and restoration of skin lesions, was reported. EBOO might be a more comfortable and practical alternative to O_3 administration to patients over i.p. or rectal insufflation pathways, and its safety has also been proven experimentally [94]. A clinical trial in hemodialyzed patients conducted by Tylicki and collaborators [82] showed diminished GSH levels after nine weeks of O_3 treatment, possibly caused by an augmented antioxidant system that consumes GSH. The same authors found no difference in NK cell activity after O_3 therapy, indicating it as a safe treatment in hemodialyzed patients [95]. Interestingly, another case report concluded that this therapy might cause heart failure in complex patients, such as those with CKD, diabetes, and hypertension. This association resulted from the speculation that O_3 therapy augmented K^+ serum levels, which, along the diminished excretion, produced sinus arrest [96]. Contrasting effects were found by Gu and collaborators [97], who treated patients suffering from chronic hepatitis with O_3 and, while measuring kidney function, found diminished renal damage, augmented renal blood flow, and even a significant association with lesser fatalities.

To sum up, CKD is usually caused by diabetes. Both are highly prevalent, and dialysis is the standard treatment in advanced stages. O_3 treatment is useful against these chronic diseases by reducing inflammation and oxidative stress. On top of that, O_3 works as a coadjutant therapy for dialyzed patients to ameliorate not only kidney function, but aggravated topical microbial infections, which are common. Figure 2 shows the effects of ozone on ischemia/reperfusion, renal damage by xenobiotics, and chronic kidney disease.

3.4. *Otherapeutic Uses of O_3 in Kidney*

Extracorporeal shock wave lithotripsy is the first-line treatment for patients with renal calculi of under 2.0 cm; therapy fragments such stones and is highly efficient. Nevertheless, adverse effects such as hematuria might be present after the procedure [98]. Experimentally, O_3 treatment has been proven as effective against the morphological and oxidative damage caused by shock wave therapy [99]. The novel therapy, due to its antimicrobial capacity, has also ameliorated oxidative damage caused by microorganisms in kidney infection (pyelonephritis) [88] and septic shock in kidneys [100], as well as in other organs [101].

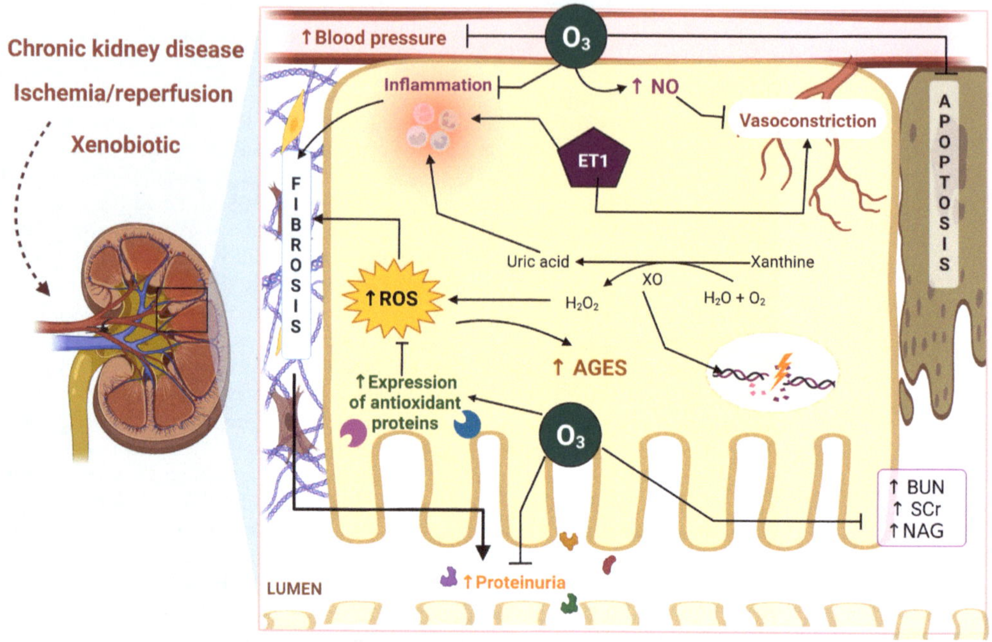

Figure 2. Effects of ozone therapy (O_3) against xenobiotics, ischemia-reperfusion (IRI) and chronic kidney disease (CKD). O_3 inhibits inflammation and ROS production by increasing the expression of antioxidant enzymes in all models. Additionally, during IRI, xanthine oxidase (XO) degrades nucleotides and forms uric acid, generating large amounts of reactive oxygen species (ROS) and inflammation. Endothelin-1 (ET-1) causes vasoconstriction and exacerbates inflammation leading to fibrosis. O_3 therapy increases nitric oxide (NO), which inhibits vasoconstriction. While O_3, by inhibiting ROS, causes a decrease in advanced glycation end products (AGES) and apoptosis, preventing CKD. H_2O: water, H_2O_2: hydrogen peroxide, O_2: oxygen molecule, NAG: N-acetyl-β-D-glucosaminidase. Created with Biorender.com, accessed on 10 February 2023.

4. Concluding Remarks and Future Directions

Renal pathologies are currently a public global health issue, which is highly prevalent and diminishes life quality and quantity, besides being expensive for the governments and patients. After presenting this work, the conclusion that O_3 therapy is an effective treatment against kidney injury can be stated, mainly against oxidative damage and inflammation caused by renal diseases, whether experimentally produced or in less reported clinical environments.

More research is needed to determine therapeutic regimes. The need to standardize the treatment into one most effective application comes from observing the incredible variety of doses, concentrations, and administration times amongst publications. The determination of its specific security and efficacy in humans also needs to be conducted, although adverse effects are not commonly reported when therapy is administered in the right doses; the reason why it is becoming more accepted, not only experimentally for a variety of models, but clinically as an auxiliary treatment for renal pathologies *per se*, or even other pathologies in patients on kidney support. Therefore, an exhortation to researchers to publish their O_3 experimental results is intended; as well as an address to clinicians to publish their therapeutic O_3 cases and, in such cases, evaluate renal markers in renal disease high-risk patients before and after the therapy, even when kidney injury is not their main therapeutic goal, since O_3 treatment is commonly used in other clinical contexts.

Author Contributions: L.F.D.-V. designed the work, coordinated and carried out the bibliographic search, and wrote the manuscript. E.Y.H.-C. reviewed and supported graphics. J.P.-C. reviewed and supervised the manuscript. All authors have read and agreed to the published version of the manuscript.

Funding: This research was funded by Consejo Nacional de Ciencia y Tecnología (CONACYT) México, Grants Numbers A1-S-7495, by Programa de Apoyo a Proyectos de Investigación e Innovación Tecnológica (PAPIIT), Grant Numbers IN202219 and IN200922 of the Universidad Nacional Autónoma de México (UNAM), and by Programa de Apoyo a la Investigación y el Posgrado (PAIP), Grant Number 5000-9105.

Institutional Review Board Statement: Not applicable.

Informed Consent Statement: Not applicable.

Data Availability Statement: Not applicable.

Acknowledgments: Estefani Yaquelin Hernández-Cruz wants to thank CONACYT for providing the doctoral study scholarship she is receiving (779741).

Conflicts of Interest: The authors declare no conflict of interest.

References

1. Pawlina, W.; Ross, M. *Histology: A Text and Atlas: With Correlated Cell and Molecular Biology*, 8th ed.; Wolters Kluwer Health: Philadelphia, PA, USA, 2018.
2. Susantitaphong, P.; Cruz, D.N.; Cerda, J.; Abulfaraj, M.; Alqahtani, F.; Koulouridis, I.; Jaber, B.L. World Incidence of AKI: A Meta-Analysis. *Clin. J. Am. Soc. Nephrol.* **2013**, *8*, 1482–1493. [CrossRef] [PubMed]
3. Webster, A.C.; Nagler, E.V.; Morton, R.L.; Masson, P. Chronic Kidney Disease. *Lancet* **2017**, *389*, 1238–1252. [CrossRef] [PubMed]
4. Ku, E.; Lee, B.J.; Wei, J.; Weir, M.R. Hypertension in CKD: Core Curriculum 2019. *Am. J. Kidney Dis.* **2019**, *74*, 120–131. [CrossRef] [PubMed]
5. National Kidney Disease Education Program. *Making Sense of CKD—A Concise Guide for Managing Chronic Kidney Disease in the Primary Care Setting*; NIH Publication: Bethesda, MD, USA, 2014; No. 14-7989.
6. Centers for Disease Control and Prevention (CDC). *Estimated Hypertension Prevalence, Treatment, and Control among U.S. Adults*; US Department of Health and Human Services: Atlanta, GA, USA, 2021.
7. CENETEC. *Prevención, Diagnóstico y Tratamiento de La Enfermedad Renal Crónica*; Guía de Referencia Rápida, Guía de Práctica Clínica; CENETEC: Cuauhtémoc, Mexico, 2012.
8. Kellum, J.A.; Romagnani, P.; Ashuntantang, G.; Ronco, C.; Zarbock, A.; Anders, H.-J. Acute kidney injury. *Nat. Rev. Dis. Prim.* **2021**, *7*, 52. [CrossRef] [PubMed]
9. Nordio, M.; Limido, A.; Maggiore, U.; Nichelatti, M.; Postorino, M.; Quintaliani, G. Survival in Patients Treated by Long-term Dialysis Compared with the General Population. *Am. J. Kidney Dis.* **2012**, *59*, 819–828. [CrossRef]
10. De Vecchi, A.F.; Bamonti, F.; Novembrino, C.; Ippolito, S.; Guerra, L.; Lonati, S.; Salini, S.; Aman, C.S.; Scurati-Manzoni, E.; Cighetti, G.M. Free and total plasma malondialdehyde in chronic renal insufficiency and in dialysis patients. *Nephrol. Dial. Transplant.* **2009**, *24*, 2524–2529. [CrossRef]
11. KDIGO Guidelines. Chapter 3: Management of progression and complications of CKD. *Kidney Int. Suppl.* **2013**, *3*, 73–90. [CrossRef]
12. Honeycutt, A.A.; Segel, J.E.; Zhuo, X.; Hoerger, T.J.; Imai, K.; Williams, D. Medical Costs of CKD in the Medicare Population. *J. Am. Soc. Nephrol.* **2013**, *24*, 1478–1483. [CrossRef]
13. Mehta, R.L.; Cerdá, J.; Burdmann, E.A.; Tonelli, M.; García-García, G.; Jha, V.; Susantitaphong, P.; Rocco, M.; Vanholder, R.; Sever, M.S.; et al. International Society of Nephrology's 0by25 initiative for acute kidney injury (zero preventable deaths by 2025): A human rights case for nephrology. *Lancet* **2015**, *385*, 2616–2643. [CrossRef]
14. Heim, C.; Glas, K. Ozone I: Characteristics/Generation/Possible Applications. *Brew. Sci.* **2011**, *64*, 8–12.
15. Nogales, C.G.; Ferreira, M.B.; Lage-Marques, J.L. Comparison of the Antimicrobial Activity of Three Different Concentrations of Aqueous Ozone on Pseudomonas Aeruginosa, Staphylococcus Aureus, and Entero-Coccus Faecalis—In Vitro Study. *Rev. Española Ozonoterapia* **2014**, *4*, 9–15.
16. Halliwell, B.; Gutteridge, J.M.C. *Free Radicals in Biology and Medicine*; Oxford University Press: Oxford, UK, 2015; ISBN 9780198717478.
17. Greene, A.K.; Güzel-Seydim, Z.B.; Seydim, A.C. Chemical and Physical Properties of Ozone. In *Ozone in Food Processing*; Wiley-Blackwell: Oxford, UK, 2012; pp. 19–32.
18. Ma, Q. Role of Nrf2 in Oxidative Stress and Toxicity. *Annu. Rev. Pharmacol. Toxicol.* **2013**, *53*, 401–426. [CrossRef] [PubMed]
19. Hidalgo-Tallón, F.J.; Torres-Morera, L.M.; Baeza-Noci, J.; Carrillo-Izquierdo, M.D.; Pinto-Bonilla, R. Updated Review on Ozone Therapy in Pain Medicine. *Front. Physiol.* **2022**, *13*, 840623. [CrossRef] [PubMed]

20. Khan, S.A.; Smith, N.L.; Wilson, A.L.; Gandhi, J.; Vatsia, S. Ozone therapy: An overview of pharmacodynamics, current research, and clinical utility. *Med. Gas Res.* **2017**, *7*, 212. [CrossRef]
21. Delgado-Roche, L.; Riera-Romo, M.; Mesta, F.; Hernández-Matos, Y.; Barrios, J.M.; Martínez-Sánchez, G.; Al-Dalaien, S.M. Medical ozone promotes Nrf2 phosphorylation reducing oxidative stress and pro-inflammatory cytokines in multiple sclerosis patients. *Eur. J. Pharmacol.* **2017**, *811*, 148–154. [CrossRef]
22. Viebahn-Hänsler, R.; Fernández, O.S.L.; Fahmy, Z. Ozone in Medicine: The Low-Dose Ozone Concept—Guidelines and Treatment Strategies. *Ozone Sci. Eng.* **2012**, *34*, 408–424. [CrossRef]
23. Cenci, A.; Macchia, I.; La Sorsa, V.; Sbarigia, C.; Di Donna, V.; Pietraforte, D. Mechanisms of Action of Ozone Therapy in Emerging Viral Diseases: Immunomodulatory Effects and Therapeutic Advantages With Reference to SARS-CoV-2. *Front. Microbiol.* **2022**, *13*, 871645. [CrossRef]
24. Bocci, V. Biological and Clinical Effects of Ozone. Has Ozone Therapy a Future in Medicine? *Br. J. Biomed. Sci.* **1999**, *56*, 270–279.
25. Huidobro, E.J.; Tagle, R.; Guzmán, A.M. Creatinina y Su Uso Para La Estimación de La Velocidad de Filtración Glomerular. *Rev. Med. Chil.* **2018**, *146*, 344–350. [CrossRef]
26. Xing, B.; Chen, H.; Wang, L.; Weng, X.; Chen, Z.; Li, X. Ozone oxidative preconditioning protects the rat kidney from reperfusion injury via modulation of the TLR4-NF-κB pathway. *Acta Cir. Bras.* **2015**, *30*, 60–66. [CrossRef]
27. Foglieni, C.; Fulgenzi, A.; Belloni, D.; Sciorati, C.; Ferrero, E.; Ferrero, M.E. Ozonated autohemotherapy: Protection of kidneys from ischemia in rats subjected to unilateral nephrectomy. *BMC Nephrol.* **2011**, *12*, 61. [CrossRef]
28. Chen, H.; Xing, B.; Liu, X.; Zhan, B.; Zhou, J.; Zhu, H.; Chen, Z. Ozone Oxidative Preconditioning Protects the Rat Kidney from Reperfusion Injury: The Role of Nitric Oxide. *J. Surg. Res.* **2008**, *149*, 287–295. [CrossRef] [PubMed]
29. Jiang, B.; Su, Y.; Chen, Q.; Dong, L.; Zhou, W.; Li, H.; Wang, Y. Protective Effects of Ozone Oxidative Postconditioning on Long-term Injury after Renal Ischemia/Reperfusion in Rat. *Transplant. Proc.* **2020**, *52*, 365–372. [CrossRef] [PubMed]
30. Wang, L.; Chen, Z.; Liu, Y.; Du, Y.; Liu, X. Ozone oxidative postconditioning inhibits oxidative stress and apoptosis in renal ischemia and reperfusion injury through inhibition of MAPK signaling pathway. *Drug Des. Dev. Ther.* **2018**, *12*, 1293–1301. [CrossRef] [PubMed]
31. Oztosun, M.; Akgul, E.O.; Cakir, E.; Cayci, T.; Uysal, B.; Ogur, R.; Ozcan, A.; Ozgurtas, T.; Guven, A.; Korkmaz, A. The Effects of Medical Ozone Therapy on Renal Ischemia/Reperfusion Injury. *Ren. Fail.* **2012**, *34*, 921–925. [CrossRef]
32. Fernández, A.; González, L.; Calunga, J.L.; Rodríguez, S.; Santos, E. Ozone Postconditioning in Renal Ischaemia-Reperfusion Model. Functional and Morphological Evidences. *Soc. Española Nefrol.* **2011**, *31*, 379–504.
33. Wang, L.; Chen, H.; Liu, X.-H.; Chen, Z.-Y.; Weng, X.-D.; Qiu, T.; Liu, L.; Zhu, H.-C. Ozone oxidative preconditioning inhibits renal fibrosis induced by ischemia and reperfusion injury in rats. *Exp. Ther. Med.* **2014**, *8*, 1764–1768. [CrossRef]
34. Abbas, A.; Lichtman, A.; Pillai, S. *Cellular and Molecular Immunology*, 10th ed.; Elsevier: Edinburgh, UK, 2021.
35. Repetto, M.; Semprine, J.; Boveris, A. Lipid Peroxidation: Chemical Mechanism, Biological Implications and Analytical Determination. In *Lipid Peroxidation*; IntechOpen: London, UK, 2012. [CrossRef]
36. Pérez Fernandez, R.; Martín Mateo, M.C.; De Vega, L.; Bustamante Bustamante, J.; Herrero, M.; Bustamante Munguira, E. Antioxidant enzyme determination and a study of lipid peroxidation in renal transplantation. *Ren. Fail.* **2002**, *24*, 353–359. [CrossRef]
37. Linas, S.L.; Whittenburg, D.; Repine, J.E. Role of xanthine oxidase in ischemia/reperfusion injury. *Am. J. Physiol. Physiol.* **1990**, *258*, F711–F716. [CrossRef]
38. Zhou, J.-Q.; Qiu, T.; Zhang, L.; Chen, Z.-B.; Wang, Z.-S.; Ma, X.-X.; Li, D. Allopurinol preconditioning attenuates renal ischemia/reperfusion injury by inhibiting HMGB1 expression in a rat model. *Acta Cir. Bras.* **2016**, *31*, 176–182. [CrossRef]
39. Liyanage, T.; Ninomiya, T.; Jha, V.; Neal, B.; Patrice, H.M.; Okpechi, I.; Zhao, M.-h.; Lv, J.; Garg, A.X.; Knight, J.; et al. World-wide access to treatment for end-stage kidney disease: A systematic review. *Lancet* **2015**, *385*, 1975–1982. [CrossRef] [PubMed]
40. Chen, H.; Xing, B.; Liu, X.; Zhan, B.; Zhou, J.; Zhu, H.; Chen, Z. Ozone oxidative preconditioning inhibits inflammation and apoptosis in a rat model of renal ischemia/reperfusion injury. *Eur. J. Pharmacol.* **2008**, *581*, 306–314. [CrossRef] [PubMed]
41. Barber, E.; Menéndez, S.; León, O.S.; Barber, M.O.; Merino, N.; Calunga, J.L.; Cruz, E.; Bocci, V. Prevention of renal injury after induction of ozone tolerance in rats submitted to warm ischaemia. *Mediat. Inflamm.* **1999**, *8*, 37–41. [CrossRef] [PubMed]
42. Calunga, J.L.; Trujillo, Y.; Zamora, Z.; Alonso, Y.; Merino, N.; Montero, T.; Menéndez, S. Ozone oxidative post-conditioning in acute renal failure. *J. Pharm. Pharmacol.* **2009**, *61*, 221–227. [CrossRef]
43. Chen, H.; Xing, B.; Liu, X.; Zhan, B.; Zhou, J.; Zhu, H.; Chen, Z. Similarities Between Ozone Oxidative Preconditioning and Ischemic Preconditioning in Renal Ischemia/Reperfusion Injury. *Arch. Med. Res.* **2008**, *39*, 169–178. [CrossRef]
44. Wang, L.; Chen, Z.; Weng, X.; Wang, M.; Du, Y.; Liu, X. Combined Ischemic Postconditioning and Ozone Postconditioning Provides Synergistic Protection Against Renal Ischemia and Reperfusion Injury Through Inhibiting Pyroptosis. *Urology* **2019**, *123*, 296.e1–296.e8. [CrossRef]
45. Wang, Z.; Han, Q.; Guo, Y.-L.; Liu, X.-H.; Qiu, T. Effect of ozone oxidative preconditioning on inflammation and oxidative stress injury in rat model of renal transplantation. *Acta Cir. Bras.* **2018**, *33*, 238–249. [CrossRef]
46. Qiu, T.; Wang, Z.-S.; Liu, X.-H.; Chen, H.; Zhou, J.-Q.; Chen, Z.-Y.; Wang, M.; Jiang, G.-J.; Wang, L.; Yu, G.; et al. Effect of ozone oxidative preconditioning on oxidative stress injury in a rat model of kidney transplantation. *Exp. Ther. Med.* **2017**, *13*, 1948–1955. [CrossRef]

47. Wang, L.; Chen, H.; Liu, X.-H.; Chen, Z.-Y.; Weng, X.-D.; Qiu, T.; Liu, L. The protective effect of ozone oxidative preconditioning against hypoxia/reoxygenation injury in rat kidney cells. *Ren. Fail.* **2014**, *36*, 1449–1454. [CrossRef]
48. Yu, L.; Gengaro, P.; Niederberger, M.; Burke, T.J.; Schrier, R.W. Nitric oxide: A mediator in rat tubularhypoxia/reoxygenation injury. *Proc. Natl. Acad. Sci. USA* **1994**, *91*, 1691–1695. [CrossRef]
49. Tripatara, P.; Patel, N.S.; Webb, A.; Rathod, K.; Lecomte, F.M.; Mazzon, E.; Cuzzocrea, S.; Yaqoob, M.M.; Ahluwalia, A.; Thiemermann, C. Nitrite-Derived Nitric Oxide Protects the Rat Kidney against Ischemia/Reperfusion Injury In Vivo: Role for Xanthine Oxidoreductase. *J. Am. Soc. Nephrol.* **2007**, *18*, 570–580. [CrossRef] [PubMed]
50. Juchau, M.R.; Chen, H. Developmental Enzymology. In *Handbook of Developmental Neurotoxicology*; Elsevier: Humana Totowa, NJ, USA, 1998; pp. 321–337.
51. Demirbag, S.; Uysal, B.; Guven, A.; Cayci, T.; Ozler, M.; Ozcan, A.; Kaldirim, U.; Surer, I.; Korkmaz, A. Effects of medical ozone therapy on acetaminophen-induced nephrotoxicity in rats. *Ren. Fail.* **2010**, *32*, 493–497. [CrossRef]
52. Reshi, M.S.; Yadav, D.; Uthra, C.; Shrivastava, S.; Shukla, S. Acetaminophen-induced renal toxicity: Preventive effect of silver nanoparticles. *Toxicol. Res.* **2020**, *9*, 406–412. [CrossRef] [PubMed]
53. Ucar, F.; Taslipinar, M.Y.; Alp, B.F.; Aydin, I.; Aydin, F.N.; Agilli, M.; Toygar, M.; Ozkan, E.; Macit, E.; Oztosun, M.; et al. The Effects of N-Acetylcysteine and Ozone Therapy on Oxidative Stress and Inflammation in Acetaminophen-Induced Nephrotoxicity Model. *Ren. Fail.* **2013**, *35*, 640–647. [CrossRef]
54. Lewis, G.; Coughlin, L.; Jusko, W.; Hartz, S. Contribution of cigarette smoking to cadmium accumulation in man. *Lancet* **1972**, *299*, 291–292. [CrossRef] [PubMed]
55. Vijayakumar, V.; Abern, M.; Jagai, J.; Kajdacsy-Balla, A. Observational Study of the Association between Air Cadmium Exposure and Prostate Cancer Aggressiveness at Diagnosis among a Nationwide Retrospective Cohort of 230,540 Patients in the United States. *Int. J. Environ. Res. Public Health* **2021**, *18*, 8333. [CrossRef]
56. Singh, P.; Mitra, P.; Goyal, T.; Sharma, S.; Sharma, P. Blood lead and cadmium levels in occupationally exposed workers and their effect on markers of DNA damage and repair. *Environ. Geochem. Health* **2020**, *43*, 185–193. [CrossRef]
57. Ramon, D.; Morick, D.; Croot, P.; Berzak, R.; Scheinin, A.; Tchernov, D.; Davidovich, N.; Britzi, M. A survey of arsenic, mercury, cadmium, and lead residues in seafood (fish, crustaceans, and cephalopods) from the south-eastern Mediterranean Sea. *J. Food Sci.* **2021**, *86*, 1153–1161. [CrossRef]
58. Rani, A.; Kumar, A.; Lal, A.; Pant, M. Cellular mechanisms of cadmium-induced toxicity: A review. *Int. J. Environ. Health Res.* **2013**, *24*, 378–399. [CrossRef]
59. Milnerowicz, H.; Śliwińska-Mossoń, M.; Sobiech, K.A. The effect of ozone on the expression of metallothionein in tissues of rats chronically exposed to cadmium. *Environ. Toxicol. Pharmacol.* **2017**, *52*, 27–37. [CrossRef]
60. Ohta, H.; Qi, Y.; Ohba, K.; Toyooka, T.; Wang, R.-S. Role of metallothionein-like cadmium-binding protein (MTLCdBP) in the protective mechanism against cadmium toxicity in the testis. *Ind. Health* **2019**, *57*, 570–579. [CrossRef] [PubMed]
61. Śliwińska-Mossoń, M.; Sobiech, K.; Dolezych, B.; Madej, P.; Milnerowicz, H. N-acetyl-beta-D-Glucosaminidase in Tissues of Rats Chronically Exposed to Cadmium and Treated with Ozone. *Ann. Clin. Lab. Sci.* **2019**, *49*, 193–203. [PubMed]
62. Le Hir, M.; Dubach, U.C.; Schmidt, U. Quantitative distribution of lysosomal hydrolases in the rat nephron. *Histochem.* **1979**, *63*, 245–251. [CrossRef] [PubMed]
63. Liangos, O.; Perianayagam, M.C.; Vaidya, V.S.; Han, W.K.; Wald, R.; Tighiouart, H.; MacKinnon, R.W.; Li, L.; Balakrishnan, V.S.; Pereira, B.J.; et al. Urinary N-Acetyl-β-(D)-Glucosaminidase Activity and Kidney Injury Molecule-1 Level Are Associated with Adverse Outcomes in Acute Renal Failure. *J. Am. Soc. Nephrol.* **2007**, *18*, 904–912. [CrossRef]
64. Boyer, M.J.; Tannock, I.F. Lysosomes, Lysosomal Enzymes, and Cancer. *Adv. Cancer Res.* **1992**, *60*, 269–291.
65. Łaszczyca, P.; Kawka-Serwecińska, E.; Witas, I.; Dolezych, B.; Falkus, B.; Mekail, A.; Ziółkowska, B.; Madej, P.; Migula, P. Lipid peroxidation and activity of antioxidative enzymes in the rat model of ozone therapy. *Mater. Med. Pol.* **1996**, *28*, 155–160.
66. U.S. Food and Drug Administration (FDA). *ADRIAMYCIN (DOXOrubicin HCl) for Injection*; FDA: Silver Spring, MD, USA, 2020.
67. Okuda, S.; Oh, Y.; Tsuruda, H.; Onoyama, K.; Fujimi, S.; Fujishima, M. Adriamycin-induced nephropathy as a model of chronic progressive glomerular disease. *Kidney Int.* **1986**, *29*, 502–510. [CrossRef]
68. Calunga, J.; Bello, M.; Chaple, M.; Barber, E.; Menéndez, S.; Merino, N. Ozonoterapia en la glomerulonefritis tóxica experimental por adriamicina. *Rev. Cuba. Invest. Biomed.* **2004**, *23*, 139–143.
69. U.S. Food and Drug Administration (FDA). Cisplatin Injection. Available online: https://www.accessdata.fda.gov/drugsatfda_docs/label/2019/018057s089lbl.pdf (accessed on 19 October 2022).
70. Sánchez-González, P.D.; López-Hernández, F.J.; Lopez-Novoa, J.M.; Morales, A.I. An integrative view of the pathophysiological events leading to cisplatin nephrotoxicity. *Crit. Rev. Toxicol.* **2011**, *41*, 803–821. [CrossRef]
71. Jo, S.-K.; Cho, W.Y.; Sung, S.A.; Kim, H.K.; Won, N.H. MEK inhibitor, U0126, attenuates cisplatin-induced renal injury by decreasing inflammation and apoptosis. *Kidney Int.* **2005**, *67*, 458–466. [CrossRef]
72. Ghani, M.A.; Barril, C.; Bedgood, D.R., Jr.; Prenzler, P.D. Measurement of antioxidant activity with the thiobarbituric acid reactive substances assay. *Food Chem.* **2017**, *230*, 195–207. [CrossRef] [PubMed]
73. Borrego, A.; Zamora, Z.B.; González, R.; Romay, C.; Menéndez, S.; Hernández, F.; Montero, T.; Rojas, E. Protection by ozone preconditioning is mediated by the antioxidant system in cisplatin-induced nephrotoxicity in rats. *Mediat. Inflamm.* **2004**, *13*, 13–19. [CrossRef]

74. Mohamed, A.A.-R.; Khater, S.I.; Metwally, M.M.; Bin Emran, T.; Nassan, M.A.; El-Emam, M.M.A.; Mostafa-Hedeab, G.; El-Shetry, E.S. TGF-β1, NAG-1, and antioxidant enzymes expression alterations in Cisplatin-induced nephrotoxicity in a rat model: Comparative modulating role of Melatonin, Vit. E and Ozone. *Gene* **2022**, *820*, 146293. [CrossRef]
75. González, R.; Borrego, A.; Zamora, Z.; Romay, C.; Hernández, F.; Menéndez, S.; Montero, T.; Rojas, E. Reversion by ozone treatment of acute nephrotoxicity induced by cisplatin in rats. *Mediat. Inflamm.* **2004**, *13*, 307–312. [CrossRef] [PubMed]
76. Kesik, V.; Uysal, B.; Kurt, B.; Kismet, E.; Koseoglu, V. Ozone ameliorates methotrexate-induced intestinal injury in rats. *Cancer Biol. Ther.* **2009**, *8*, 1623–1628. [CrossRef]
77. Heyman, S.N.; Rosenberger, C.; Rosen, S. Regional alterations in renal haemodynamics and oxygenation: A role in contrast medium-induced nephropathy. *Nephrol. Dial. Transplant.* **2005**, *20*, i6–i11. [CrossRef]
78. Kurtoglu, T.; Durmaz, S.; Akgullu, C.; Gungor, H.; Eryilmaz, U.; Meteoglu, I.; Karul, A.; Boga, M. Ozone preconditioning attenuates contrast-induced nephropathy in rats. *J. Surg. Res.* **2015**, *195*, 604–611. [CrossRef] [PubMed]
79. Ozturk, O.; Eroglu, H.A.; Ustebay, S.; Kuzucu, M.; Adali, Y. An experimental study on the preventive effects of N-acetyl cysteine and ozone treatment against contrast-induced nephropathy. *Acta Cir. Bras.* **2018**, *33*, 508–517. [CrossRef]
80. Mills, K.T.; Xu, Y.; Zhang, W.; Bundy, J.D.; Chen, C.-S.; Kelly, T.N.; Chen, J.; He, J. A systematic analysis of worldwide population-based data on the global burden of chronic kidney disease in 2010. *Kidney Int.* **2015**, *88*, 950–957. [CrossRef]
81. Kalantar-Zadeh, K.; Jafar, T.H.; Nitsch, D.; Neuen, B.L.; Perkovic, V. Chronic kidney disease. *Lancet* **2021**, *398*, 786–802. [CrossRef]
82. Yu, G.; Bai, Z.; Chen, Z.; Chen, H.; Wang, G.; Wang, G.; Liu, Z. The NLRP3 inflammasome is a potential target of ozone therapy aiming to ease chronic renal inflammation in chronic kidney disease. *Int. Immunopharmacol.* **2017**, *43*, 203–209. [CrossRef] [PubMed]
83. Calunga, J.L.; Zamora, Z.B.; Borrego, A.; Del Río, S.; Barber, E.; Menéndez, S.; Hernández, F.; Montero, T.; Taboada, D. Ozone Therapy on Rats Submitted to Subtotal Nephrectomy: Role of Antioxidant System. *Mediat. Inflamm.* **2005**, *2005*, 221–227. [CrossRef] [PubMed]
84. Zhao, Y.-Y.; Feng, Y.-L.; Bai, X.; Tan, X.-J.; Lin, R.-C.; Mei, Q. Ultra Performance Liquid Chromatography-Based Metabonomic Study of Therapeutic Effect of the Surface Layer of Poria cocos on Adenine-Induced Chronic Kidney Disease Provides New Insight into Anti-Fibrosis Mechanism. *PLoS ONE* **2013**, *8*, e59617. [CrossRef] [PubMed]
85. Chen, Z.; Liu, X.; Yu, G.; Chen, H.; Wang, L.; Wang, Z.; Qiu, T.; Weng, X. Ozone therapy ameliorates tubulointerstitial inflammation by regulating TLR4 in adenine-induced CKD rats. *Ren. Fail.* **2016**, *38*, 822–830. [CrossRef]
86. Yu, G.; Liu, X.; Chen, Z.; Chen, H.; Wang, L.; Wang, Z.; Qiu, T.; Weng, X. Ozone Therapy Could Attenuate Tubulointerstitial Injury in Adenine-Induced CKD Rats by Mediating Nrf2 and NF-KB. *Iran J. Basic Med. Sci.* **2016**, *19*, 1136–1143.
87. Umanath, K.; Lewis, J.B. Update on Diabetic Nephropathy: Core Curriculum 2018. *Am. J. Kidney Dis.* **2018**, *71*, 884–895. [CrossRef]
88. Tuttle, K.R.; Bakris, G.L.; Bilous, R.W.; Chiang, J.L.; de Boer, I.H.; Goldstein-Fuchs, J.; Hirsch, I.B.; Kalantar-Zadeh, K.; Narva, A.S.; Navaneethan, S.D.; et al. Diabetic Kidney Disease: A Report from an ADA Consensus Conference. *Diabetes Care* **2014**, *37*, 2864–2883. [CrossRef]
89. Morsy, M.D.; Hassan, W.N.; Zalat, S. Improvement of renal oxidative stress markers after ozone administration in diabetic nephropathy in rats. *Diabetol. Metab. Syndr.* **2010**, *2*, 29. [CrossRef]
90. Güçlü, A.; Erken, H.A.; Erken, G.; Dodurga, Y.; Yay, A.; Özçoban, Ö.; Şimşek, H.; Akçılar, A.; Kocak, F.E. The effects of ozone therapy on caspase pathways, TNF-α, and HIF-1α in diabetic nephropathy. *Int. Urol. Nephrol.* **2015**, *48*, 441–450. [CrossRef]
91. Varghese, R.T.; Jialal, I. Diabetic Nephropathy. Available online: https://www.ncbi.nlm.nih.gov/books/NBK534200/ (accessed on 9 November 2022).
92. Biedunkiewicz, B.; Tylicki, L.; Lichodziejewska-Niemierko, M.; Liberek, T.; Rutkowski, B. Ozonetherapy in a dialyzed patient with calcific uremic arteriolopathy. *Kidney Int.* **2003**, *64*, 367–368. [CrossRef]
93. Di Paolo, N.; Bocci, V.; Cappelletti, F.; Petrini, G.; Gaggiotti, E. Necrotizing Fasciitis Successfully Treated with Extracorporeal Blood Oxygenation and Ozonization (EBOO). *Int. J. Artif. Organs* **2002**, *25*, 1194–1198. [CrossRef] [PubMed]
94. Sancak, E.B.; Turkön, H.; Çukur, S.; Erimsah, S.; Akbas, A.; Gulpinar, M.T.; Toman, H.; Sahin, H.; Uzun, M. Major Ozonated Autohemotherapy Preconditioning Ameliorates Kidney Ischemia-Reperfusion Injury. *Inflammation* **2016**, *39*, 209–217. [CrossRef] [PubMed]
95. Biedunkiewicz, B.; Tylicki, L.; Rachon, D.; Hak, L.; Nieweglowski, T.; Chamienia, A.; Debska-Slizien, A.; Mysliwska, J.; Rutkowski, B. Natural Killer Cell Activity Unaffected by Ozonated Autohemotherapy in Patients with End-Stage Renal Disease on Maintenance Renal Replacement Therapy. *Int. J. Artif. Organs* **2004**, *27*, 766–771. [CrossRef] [PubMed]
96. Tang, W.-J.; Jiang, L.; Wang, Y.; Kuang, Z.-M. Ozone therapy induced sinus arrest in a hypertensive patient with chronic kidney disease. *Medicine* **2017**, *96*, e9265. [CrossRef]
97. Gu, X.-B.; Yang, X.-J.; Zhu, H.-Y.; Xu, Y.-Q.; Liu, X.-Y. Effect of medical ozone therapy on renal blood flow and renal function of patients with chronic severe hepatitis. *Chin. Med. J.* **2010**, *123*, 2510–2513.
98. Torricelli, F.C.M.; Danilovic, A.; Vicentini, F.; Marchini, G.S.; Srougi, M.; Mazzucchi, E. Extracorporeal shock wave lithotripsy in the treatment of renal and ureteral stones. *Rev. Assoc. Med. Bras.* **2015**, *61*, 65–71. [CrossRef]
99. Uğuz, S.; Demirer, Z.; Uysal, B.; Alp, B.F.; Malkoc, E.; Guragac, A.; Turker, T.; Ateş, F.; Karademir, K.; Ozcan, A.; et al. Medical ozone therapy reduces shock wave therapy-induced renal injury. *Ren. Fail.* **2016**, *38*, 974–981. [CrossRef]

100. Madej, P.; Plewka, A.; Madej, J.A.; Nowak, M.; Plewka, D.; Franik, G.; Golka, D. Ozonotherapy in an Induced Septic Shock. I. Effect of Ozonotherapy on Rat Organs in Evaluation of Free Radical Reactions and Selected Enzymatic Systems. *Inflammation* **2007**, *30*, 52–58. [CrossRef]
101. Madej, P.; Plewka, A.; Madej, J.A.; Plewka, D.; Mroczka, W.; Wilk, K.; Dobrosz, Z. Ozone Therapy in Induced Endotoxemic Shock. II. The Effect of Ozone Therapy Upon Selected Histochemical Reactions in Organs of Rats in Endotoxemic Shock. *Inflammation* **2007**, *30*, 69–86. [CrossRef]

life

Essay

Theoretical Framework for the Study of Genetic Diseases Caused by Dominant Alleles

Michael F. Roberts [1,*] and Stephen E. Bricher [2]

1 Department of Biology, Linfield University, McMinnville, OR 97128, USA
2 Department of Mathematics and Computer Science, Linfield University, McMinnville, OR 97128, USA
* Correspondence: mrobert@linfield.edu

Abstract: We propose a theoretical basis for analyzing several features of genetic diseases caused by dominant alleles, including: disease prevalence, genotype penetrance, and the relationship between causal genotype frequency and disease frequency. In addition, we provide a theoretical framework for accurate diagnosis and clinical approaches for disease study, including two examples in which inaccurate and incomplete diagnoses affect the estimates of disease prevalence: First, the disease iceberg effect shows that disease prevalence is often underestimated due to errors introduced by inaccurate diagnosis; second, because lifetime risk of disease is cumulative, and therefore an increasing function of age, measurements of prevalence are inaccurate if people of all ages are not included. Finally, we discuss the aggregation of genetic diseases. We identify theoretical and computational deficiencies associated with using the sibling recurrence-risk ratio as a measure of familial aggregation. We develop an alternative concept of aggregation and propose an associated measure that does not experience the deficiencies. Throughout, we provide clinicians and researchers practical implications of our theoretical framework.

Keywords: genetic disease; prevalence; penetrance; accurate diagnosis; disease iceberg effect; cumulative lifetime risk; familial aggregation

check for updates

Citation: Roberts, M.F.; Bricher, S.E. Theoretical Framework for the Study of Genetic Diseases Caused by Dominant Alleles. *Life* **2023**, *13*, 733. https://doi.org/10.3390/life13030733

Academic Editors: Giuseppe Minervini and Stefanos Roumeliotis

Received: 18 January 2023
Revised: 8 February 2023
Accepted: 13 February 2023
Published: 8 March 2023

1. Introduction

Determining the genetic basis for diseases is an important part of population genetics and epidemiology, as disorders can be caused both by a person's genetic predisposition and by environmental influences. The accurate allocation of the cause between genes and the environment allows a better understanding of disease mechanisms and promotes techniques for diagnosing and combating disease [1,2].

The analysis of genetic diseases has a long history. Garrod [3] first drew attention to the relation between inheritance of recessive alleles and the appearance of alkaptonuria in human families. This work ultimately led to the understanding that body characteristics (phenotype) are primarily determined by cellular proteins and that genes (genotype) specify these proteins (e.g., enzymes). Genetic diseases are phenotypes; thus, a genetic disease is similar to any phenotype specified by a genotype [4]. Though different genetic diseases may have different biochemical bases, their transmission processes are identical, and each can be characterized as being caused by recessive or dominant alleles. We focus on single-gene disorders caused by dominant alleles and assume an autosomal "two-allele" model for the genotype-phenotype relationship; consequently, we will not discuss multi-gene or sex-linked diseases.

Our purpose is to clarify the relationship between disease-causing genotypes and the presence of the disease, as well as to clarify the role of accurate diagnosis. We identify theoretical and computational deficiencies associated with the current measure of familial aggregation and propose an alternative concept of aggregation and its measure. Our intention is therefore to describe the theoretical issues clearly, to show why accurate diagnosis is lacking in some cases, as well as to provide replacements for commonly used approaches that experience theoretical and computational deficiencies. Throughout, we provide clinicians and researchers practical implications of our theoretical framework.

In developing our theoretical framework, we will use: probability as a relative frequency; a set theoretic approach to probability; partitions and the law of total probability; conditional probabilities and their properties; population parameters and their estimators; and large-sample-size confidence intervals. As the background for the underlying probability and statistical concepts used, we recommend References [5,6].

Unbiased clinical studies can provide accurate estimates of population parameters (e.g., allele frequency, genotype penetrance, or disease prevalence), which are required for meaningful inferences about disease characteristics. Readers interested in specific protocols for obtaining unbiased clinical studies may see [7] for an in-depth discussion of clinical study design—including strategies for minimizing biases, the statistical analysis of the data, and ethical issues. In addition, we suggest two clinically oriented works that give additional perspectives on specific genetic diseases [1,2].

2. Disease-Causing Genotypes and Prevalence

We discuss disease-causing genotypes and their relationship to the presence of the associated disease caused by a dominant allele, including their role in determining the disease's frequency in the population.

Traits (phenotypes) are divided into categories determined by genotypes written for convenience as if they consisted of only two alleles [8]. Indeed, most treatments of population genetics [9] focus on a two-allele model, while acknowledging a more complete treatment recognizes that genes have multiple alleles. Nonetheless, even genotype models describing more than two alleles [9] can be reduced to two-allele models if allele contribution is expressed in terms of the functions of the proteins synthesized by each allele.

Let D denote the event that an individual in the population has the disease caused by a dominant allele. Let $P(D)$ denote the probability that any individual in the population has the disease. In the literature, $P(D)$ is sometimes referred to as: (a) the *frequency* of the disease in the population; (b) the *risk* of the disease for an individual in the population; (c) the *likelihood* an individual in the population has the disease; or (d) the *prevalence* of the disease in the population [10,11].

In our two-allele model, we denote the alleles by C and c and define them as the only two options, where a C allele synthesizes a functioning protein and a c allele makes a non-functioning protein. The C allele is called a *dominant allele*, and the c allele is called a *recessive allele*. We will use the following notation for the frequency of these alleles in the population: Let $p = P(C)$ denote the frequency (probability) of the C allele in the population; let $q = P(c)$ denote the frequency (probability) of the c allele in the population. Obviously, $p + q = 1$, since C and c are the only options in our two-allele model.

2.1. Penetrance and Environmental Influence

Penetrance refers to the frequency (probability) of the disease D, given a particular genotype CC, Cc, or cc [8,12–14]. Specifically, the penetrance of a particular genotype is the corresponding conditional probability: The penetrance of CC is $P(D|CC)$; the penetrance of Cc is $P(D|Cc)$, which is the same as the penetrance of cC; the penetrance of cc is $P(D|cc)$. For example, $P(D|CC)$ is the frequency of those in the population with genotype CC who have the disease D.

In agreement with some authors [15], we say a specific genotype has *full penetrance* provided its penetrance is one; for example, $P(D|CC) = 1$ corresponds to the genotype CC having full penetrance. A specific genotype has *partial penetrance* provided its penetrance is less than one; for example, $P(D|CC) < 1$ corresponds to the genotype CC having partial penetrance.

Penetrance is often presented in an imprecise manner [8], which may lead to misunderstanding; our probability-based quantitative description is unambiguous. Indeed, because genotype penetrance indicates the *frequency* of those people with a particular genotype who have the disease, penetrance is *not* a measure of disease severity. This means genotype penetrance does not influence whether a person has a severe, moderate, or mild form of the disease. For example, $P(D|Cc) = 0.5$ means that, of those people with genotype Cc, about 50% are identified with the disease; it does *not* mean a diseased person with genotype Cc has a moderate form of the disease. Disease severity is instead related to the concepts of "complete/incomplete dominance" and "expressivity" [8].

The concept of penetrance is one way to include an environmental component in the genotype-phenotype correlation. The estimate of penetrance may include a suspected environmental effect on gene expression (e.g., eating gluten is necessary for the onset of Celiac disease [16]). Even so, it is not always possible to accurately identify a disease phenotype, though the genotype might be known. Griffiths et al. [8] describe this as an aspect of penetrance leading to the "subtlety" of the mutant phenotype; we add that incomplete diagnosis can masquerade as partial penetrance (Section 3).

In order to use genotype frequencies to accurately estimate disease prevalence, it is *essential* that penetrance be accurately estimated (Section 2.2). With that in mind, it is important to note that using clinical studies to estimate the penetrance of a particular genotype requires: (i) the use of a genetic test to identify whether a person has the genotype; (ii) the identification of the disease's phenotypes; and (iii) the use of a diagnostic test to determine whether such a person with the genotype has the disease (i.e., exhibits the disease's phenotypes). Thus, the accuracy of diagnosis plays a critical role in estimations of penetrance (Section 3).

2.2. *Prevalence of Diseases Caused by Dominant Alleles*

A person with either genotype CC or Cc might be affected with a condition sometimes called a *dominant disorder* [15]. This may occur where the genotype cc produces the wild-type phenotype, but mutation from c to C generates a new version of the c protein that may impair cellular function.

We introduce a parameter that describes the relationship between the penetrance of CC and Cc. The parameter r is the ratio of the penetrance of Cc to the penetrance of CC (Section 2.1); that is,

$$r = \frac{P(D|Cc)}{P(D|CC)}, \tag{1}$$

where $0 < r \leq 1$ because $0 < P(D|Cc) \leq P(D|CC)$. We will use the parameter r in clarifying a theoretical framework for the prevalence of diseases caused by dominant alleles.

Because the genotypes CC, Cc, cC, and cc form a partition of the population, prevalence can be written in the form

$$P(D) = p^2 P(D|CC) + 2pqP(D|Cc) + q^2 P(D|cc). \tag{2}$$

Equation (2) describes the prevalence for diseases ($P(D)$) in terms of the frequencies of the alleles (p and q) and in terms of the penetrance of the genotypes ($P(D|CC)$, $P(D|Cc)$, and $P(D|cc)$). The derivation of Equation (2) is provided in Appendix A.

For a disease caused by a dominant allele, $P(D|cc) = 0$, $P(D|CC) > 0$, and $P(D|Cc) > 0$. In this case, Equation (2) becomes

$$P(D) = p^2 P(D|CC) + 2pqP(D|Cc);$$

in other words, disease prevalence ($P(D)$) in principle equals the sum of the homozygote dominant and heterozygote genotype population frequencies (p^2 and $2pq$), where each frequency is *rescaled* according to its associated penetrance ($P(D|CC)$ and $P(D|Cc)$). This allows us to introduce a new formulation for $P(D)$. Substituting Equation (1) yields,

$$\begin{aligned} P(D) &= p^2P(D|CC) + 2pqrP(D|CC) \\ &= (p^2 + 2pqr)P(D|CC) \\ &= p(p + 2qr)P(D|CC) \\ &= p(p + 2(1 - p)r)P(D|CC) \\ &= p(p + 2r - 2pr)P(D|CC), \end{aligned}$$

which we write in the form

$$P(D) = p(2r + (1 - 2r)p)P(D|CC). \tag{3}$$

Incidentally, in the above derivation of Equation (3), we demonstrate that

$$p^2 + 2pqr = p(2r + (1 - 2r)p);$$

in other words, the expression $p(2r + (1 - 2r)p)$ is simply another way to write the sum of the homozygote dominant and (rescaled by r) heterozygote population frequencies (p^2 and $2pqr$). The advantages of using this expression will become apparent in the following discussion.

Equation (3) completely characterizes the theoretical prevalence of such a disease by describing it in terms of only three parameters: the penetrance of the genotype CC ($P(D|CC)$); the parameter r (Equation (1)); and the frequency of the C allele in the population ($p = P(C)$). It thus identifies the roles of the three important parameters in determining disease prevalence. In particular, prevalence has a different structure as a function of p in each of the three cases for r:

(i) If $1/2 < r \leq 1$, then $P(D)$ has a concave down parabolic relationship in terms of p.
(ii) If $r = 1/2$, then $P(D)$ has a linear relationship in terms of p.
(iii) If $0 < r < 1/2$, then $P(D)$ has a concave up parabolic relationship in terms of p.

Figure 1 illustrates how Equation (3) uses allele frequency and the penetrance of the genotype CC to determine disease prevalence, where graphs for the three cases of r are shown:

(i) The blue shaded region corresponds to $1/2 < r \leq 1$, where the solid blue curve is $r = 1$, and the dotted blue curve is an illustrative example ($r = 3/4$).
(ii) The black line corresponds to $r = 1/2$.
(iii) The red shaded region corresponds to $0 < r < 1/2$, where the dashed red curve is the lower limit $r = 0$, which cannot be achieved because r must be positive for diseases caused by dominant alleles. The dotted red curve is another illustrative example ($r = 1/4$).

An advantage of Equation (3) (and Figure 1) over other expressions for prevalence (e.g., Equation (2)) is that it clearly identifies the critical role r plays in determining the prevalence's different theoretical framework as a function of p in each of the three cases mentioned. Incidentally, the parameter r has an important role in our alternative new concept of disease aggregation (Section 4).

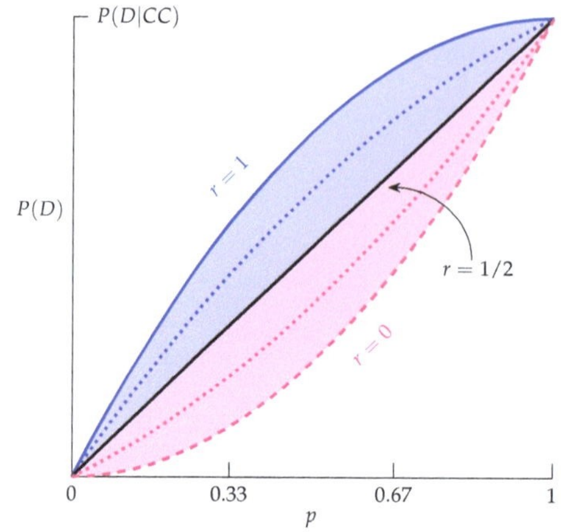

Figure 1. Graph of disease prevalence $P(D)$ versus dominant allele population frequency p for the three cases of r (Equation (3)): (i) the blue shaded region corresponds to $1/2 < r \leq 1$, where the solid blue curve is $r = 1$, and the dotted blue curve is an illustrative example ($r = 3/4$); (ii) the black line corresponds to $r = 1/2$; (iii) the red shaded region corresponds to $0 < r < 1/2$, where the dashed red curve is the lower limit $r = 0$, which cannot be achieved because $r > 0$ for dominant diseases. The dotted red curve is another illustrative example ($r = 1/4$). The theoretical prevalence of *any* disease caused by a dominant allele must be above the dashed red curve and, at most, the solid blue curve. Numerical values on the vertical axis can be assigned once a value of $P(D|CC)$ is known. Note that the largest possible value of $P(D)$ is $P(D|CC)$, which occurs at $p = 1$, where all three cases coalesce.

An important property for the prevalence of diseases caused by dominant alleles illustrated in Figure 1 is:

> The theoretical prevalence of *any* disease caused by a dominant allele must be greater than the dashed red curve ($r = 0$) and, at most, the solid blue curve ($r = 1$). That is, $P(D)$ always satisfies
>
> $$p^2 P(D|CC) < P(D) \leq p(2-p)P(D|CC).$$

Thus, if clinicians estimate a value of disease prevalence ($\widehat{P}(D)$) to be outside this interval, it should suggest to them that there likely are diagnostic errors (Section 3) with how $P(D)$ has been estimated.

Moreover, if a disease is thought to be caused by a dominant allele, then clinicians should find that prevalence estimated from diagnostic tests will be close to $P(D)$ described in Equation (3). If it is not, then that should alert clinicians that the diagnostic test is possibly not accurate (Section 3.2).

2.3. Necessary and/or Sufficient Genotypes

We develop the theoretical framework characterizing when the disease-causing genotypes are necessary and/or sufficient for the presence of the disease. Let G denote the disease-causing genotypes for a disease caused by a dominant allele; specifically, $G = \{CC\} \cup \{Cc\}$.

To define the logical concepts of "necessary" and "sufficient", we frame the discussion in terms of the events G and D representing the disease-causing genotypes and the presence of the disease, respectively. However, the concepts apply to any two events; for example, in Section 3.2, we discuss whether a positive result in a diagnostic test (denoted by T) is necessary and/or sufficient for the presence of the disease (again, denoted by D).

We say that G is *necessary* for D provided $D \Rightarrow G$. That is, the occurrence of D implies the occurrence of G. In other words, (in this context) if a person has the disease, then the person will (likely) have the disease-causing genotype.

We say that G is *sufficient* for D provided $G \Rightarrow D$. That is, the occurrence of G implies the occurrence of D. In other words, (in this context) if a person has the disease-causing genotype, then the person will (likely) have the disease.

Conditional probability formulations. We now develop equivalent conditional probability formulations for the concepts of "necessary" and "sufficient" discussed above. The formulations apply to any two events, but we will frame the discussion in terms of G and D as above (see Section 3.2 for another example). Observe that $P(G|D) = 1$ is equivalent to saying that "G is *necessary* for D". Also, observe that $P(D|G) = 1$ is equivalent to saying that "G is *sufficient* for D". The details for the equivalence of these formulations is established in Appendix B.

We now use the formulations to clearly identify when the disease-causing genotypes are necessary and/or sufficient for the presence of a disease caused by a dominant allele. In addition, we include implications for clinicians as the context.

For a disease caused by a dominant allele, $P(D|G') = 0$. Now,

$$\begin{aligned} P(D) &= P(D \cap G) + P(D \cap G') \\ &= P(D \cap G) + P(D|G')P(G') \\ &= P(D \cap G), \end{aligned}$$

which implies

$$P(G|D) = \frac{P(D \cap G)}{P(D)} = \frac{P(D)}{P(D)} = 1;$$

therefore, G is necessary for D. Moreover,

$$P(D|G) = \frac{P(D \cap G)}{P(G)} = \frac{P(D)}{P(G)};$$

hence, G is sufficient for D if and only if $P(D) = P(G)$. Recall that the frequency of the disease-causing genotypes is

$$P(G) = P(CC) + P(Cc \cup cC) = p^2 + 2pq;$$

therefore, by Equation (2) (since $0 < P(D|CC) \leq 1$ and $0 < P(D|Cc) \leq 1$), we conclude

$$P(D) = P(G) \Leftrightarrow P(D|CC) = 1 \text{ and } P(D|Cc) = 1.$$

Thus, $P(D|G) = 1$ if and only if $P(D|CC) = 1$ and $P(D|Cc) = 1$.

In summary, the disease-causing genotypes CC and Cc are *always* necessary for D; they are sufficient for D *if and only if* the disease-causing genotypes are fully penetrant ($P(D|CC) = 1$ and $P(D|Cc) = 1$).

An implication for clinicians is that if they believe the disease-causing genotypes are "necessary, but not sufficient" for the presence of the disease, then $P(D|CC) \neq 1$ and/or $P(D|Cc) \neq 1$. Two explanations are: there could be other components (e.g., environmental) affecting the presence of the disease, resulting in CC and/or Cc not being fully penetrant; or it could be that the associated diagnostic test lacks the accuracy (Section 3.2) to correctly predict that the genotypes are fully penetrant. Consequently, it is essential that clinicians not use their belief that a disease-causing genotype is partially penetrant as the justification for relying on an inaccurate diagnostic test. In all of these scenarios, it is imperative that clinicians continue their investigations, ultimately seeking a thorough understanding and explanation of the actual relationship between $P(D)$ and $P(G)$.

In Section 3, we provide a similar analysis with D and a diagnostic test's positive result, which we denote by T. Specifically, we demonstrate that accurate diagnosis is equivalent to T being necessary and sufficient for D. This allows us to develop, in Sections 2 and 3, a unified theoretical framework for identifying a genetic disease caused by a dominant allele, as summarized in Section 5.

3. The Role of Diagnostic Tests

We provide three fundamental concepts for obtaining accurate estimates of disease prevalence: (1) identifying the genetic basis for the disease (Section 3.1); (2) achieving an accurate diagnosis via appropriate tests (Section 3.2); and (3) viewing disease prevalence as a cumulative lifetime risk [11] (Section 3.3).

Before discussing the three fundamental concepts, it is important to recognize that the prevalence of genetic diseases is commonly underestimated [17–21]. This general underdiagnosis of diseases occurs because of inattention to the three fundamental concepts, and specifically because of the difficulty of identifying people with genetic diseases that are either non-lethal or that have symptoms similar to those of other diseases. Last [17] conceived of the analogy of a *disease iceberg* to describe this general disparity between the perceived and actual prevalence of a disease in the population. In his model, the entire iceberg represents the proportion of the population with the disease (actual prevalence); the "above water portion" of the iceberg corresponds to the diagnosed portion of the population with the disease (perceived prevalence); the "below water portion" of the iceberg corresponds to the portion of the population with the disease, but as yet undiagnosed (Figure 2A).

Theoretical framework. Let D denote the event that an individual from the population has the disease. Let A denote the event that an individual from the population has been diagnosed with the disease. The complement of A (denoted by A') will therefore be the event that an individual from the population has not been diagnosed with the disease for whatever reason.

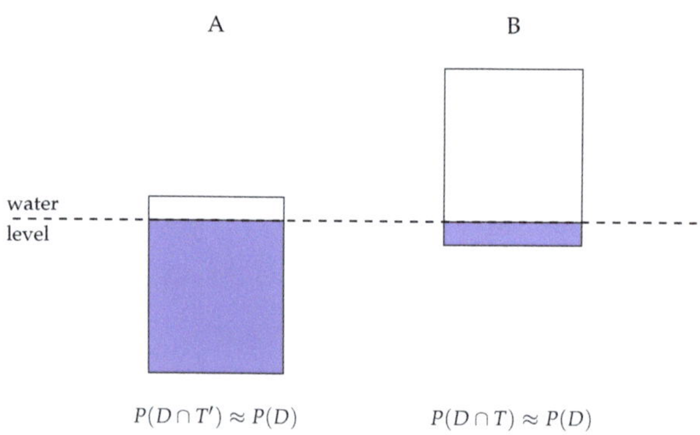

Figure 2. An extended disease iceberg analogy differentiating between various levels of identifying a disease based on a particular diagnostic test. Each rectangle (an iceberg) represents the proportion of the population with a given disease ($P(D)$) and is the same in each panel. The differences between the panels represent the various abilities that particular diagnostic tests may have in identifying the disease. The white region (above water portion) in each rectangle denotes the proportion of the population with the disease and a positive test result ($P(D \cap T)$), while the blue region (below water portion) in each rectangle denotes the proportion of the population with the disease, but unknown because they have a negative test result ($P(D \cap T')$). (**A**) A classical disease iceberg effect in which most of those with the disease are undiagnosed. (**B**) A well-identified disease in which almost all of the proportion of the population with the disease has a positive test result.

Consider a disease with a *significant iceberg effect*, that is to say, the above-water portion of the iceberg is *significantly smaller than* the below-water portion of the iceberg. For the diseases studied by Last [17], the undiagnosed cases were 2–10-times the diagnosed cases. In other words,

$$P(D \cap A) \ll P(D \cap A').$$

Now, $D = (D \cap A) \cup (D \cap A')$, and because A and A' are mutually exclusive, $P(D) = P(D \cap A) + P(D \cap A')$. Hence, for a disease experiencing a significant iceberg effect,

$$P(D \cap A) \ll P(D),$$

demonstrating that the perceived prevalence ($P(D \cap A)$) consisting of those thought to be affected by the disease will significantly underestimate the actual disease prevalence ($P(D)$).

The disease iceberg effect is common among diseases caused by dominant alleles and can be significant; indeed, disease prevalence can be underestimated by close to 90% [17,19,22]. Moreover, knowing the ratio of diagnosed-to-undiagnosed cases allows researchers and clinicians to more accurately estimate the actual disease prevalence $P(D)$ [17,19,22], which we illustrate with an example.

Consider a disease with a perceived prevalence of 3.6% ($P(D \cap A) = 0.036$). In addition, suppose it is reported that 90% of those with the disease are undiagnosed; that is, $P(D \cap A') = 0.9P(D)$. Using this information, researchers and clinicians can give a more accurate estimate of the actual disease prevalence $P(D)$. Indeed, one can show that $P(D) = 0.36$; thus, the actual disease prevalence is more accurately estimated as 36%, which is 10-times the perceived prevalence.

In Section 3.1, we extend the iceberg analogy and explain that the disease iceberg effect can be reduced by better: (i) disease identification; (ii) knowledge of disease-causing genotypes; and (iii) diagnosis (Section 3.2).

3.1. Identifying a Genetic Disease

Identifying a genetic disease requires two key approaches: (i) the assignment of a disease to a particular genotype; and (ii) the performance of accurate diagnostic tests.

The assignment of a disease to a particular genotype. Each person with the disease caused by a dominant allele has a particular genotype (CC or Cc). This genotype can be inferred from a family pedigree, and it can be directly determined by laboratory genotype tests. The genotype can be correlated via other laboratory tests with known symptoms and signs of the disease in order to discover (structurally, immunologically, or physiologically) why the particular genotype generates the disease phenotype. A combination of genetic tests and diagnostic tests is used; these tests must each be sensitive (very high true-positive rate) and specific (very high true-negative rate) for an accurate assignment (Section 3.2). If the various tests are appropriate and accurate, they should all agree with each other within reasonable error bounds. If different tests give different results regarding disease presence, clinicians should determine why the tests differ. These tests plus careful clinical examination should lead to an accurate diagnosis that minimizes the likelihood of misidentification.

The performance of accurate diagnostic tests. Clinical studies are used to estimate disease prevalence (Section 2.2), to determine which symptoms and signs are the most relevant, and to correlate these with the genotypes of disease carriers. Medical diagnoses (e.g., physical biopsies, tests for antibodies, and observation of symptoms) are combined with genotype determination [23].

Theoretical framework. Let T denote the event that a particular diagnostic test yields a positive result for the disease, which can be used to decompose $P(D)$ as

$$P(D) = P(D \cap T) + P(D \cap T').$$

We develop an *extended disease iceberg analogy* to differentiate between various levels of identifying a disease based on a particular diagnostic test. In Figure 2, the rectangle (an iceberg) in each panel represents the proportion of the population with a given disease. In our analysis, both the disease and $P(D)$ are the same in both panels. The differences between the panels represent the various abilities that particular diagnostic tests may have in identifying the disease. The white region (above water portion) in each rectangle denotes the proportion of the population with the disease and a positive test result ($P(D \cap T)$), while the blue region (below water portion) in each rectangle denotes the proportion of the population with the disease, but who are unknown because they have a negative test result ($P(D \cap T')$).

More precisely, we have the following levels of a diagnostic test identifying a disease:

- A disease is *not a well-identified disease* (with respect to the diagnostic test) provided

$$P(D \cap T') \approx P(D),$$

which is equivalent to $P(D \cap T) \approx 0$. This implies the prevalence of the disease will be significantly underestimated by the diagnostic test and is equivalent to Last's [17] concept of the *disease iceberg effect* (Figure 2A).

- A disease is *a well-identified disease* (with respect to the diagnostic test) provided

$$P(D \cap T) \approx P(D),$$

which is equivalent to $P(D \cap T') \approx 0$. This implies the diagnostic test will yield an accurate estimator, via an unbiased clinical study based on the diagnostic test, for the prevalence of the disease (Figure 2B).

The clinical understanding of diseases has progressed over time based on improvements in the understanding of disease mechanisms and also on the development of new diagnostic tools. Thus, we suggest that the panels for the hypothetical disease in Figure 2 should illustrate the progression from "not well-identified" to "well-identified" in an actual disease as diagnostic tests improve in disease identification. In Sections 3.2 and 3.3, we develop a theoretical framework for achieving this, as well as include suggestions/implications for researchers and clinicians.

Dominant fatal diseases, such as Huntington's disease, have a clear genotype-phenotype relationship and straight-forward diagnostic approaches; they should, therefore, show minimal iceberg effects—they are "well-identified" diseases (Figure 2B). For others, such as prion diseases [13], the genotype-phenotype relation is not as well identified (Figure 2A). Prion diseases are rare disorders in which abnormally folded proteins cause neural disabilities. An example is Creutzfeldt-Jacob disease [24], in which the disease-causing protein originates from an alteration in allele sequence or is obtained from an exogenous source (e.g., the diet). Only the genetic version of the disorder is relevant here.

3.2. Accurate Diagnosis

Again, we let D be the event that an individual in the population has the disease and let T be the event that a diagnostic test yields a positive result for the disease. For example, a diagnostic test might be: (i) a biopsy; (ii) a test for blood-borne substances, such as antibodies associated with the disease; or (iii) a test based on the presence of symptoms associated with the disease [2].

Recall that D and T can be used to partition a group of individuals (e.g., the population as a whole or a clinical study corresponding to a random sample of a population under consideration) of size n as shown in Table 1, where:

$$n_{11} = \text{the number with } D \text{ and } T;$$
$$n_{12} = \text{the number with } D \text{ and } T';$$
$$n_{21} = \text{the number with } D' \text{ and } T;$$
$$n_{22} = \text{the number with } D' \text{ and } T';$$

and $n = n_{11} + n_{12} + n_{21} + n_{22}$.

Table 1. The partition of a group of individuals by D and T.

	T	T'
D	n_{11}	n_{12}
D'	n_{21}	n_{22}

In addition, recall that *the accuracy of the diagnostic test* is defined to be

$$\text{Accuracy} = \frac{n_{11} + n_{22}}{n},$$

which measures the frequency of those individuals in the clinical study that are correctly diagnosed. The closer the ratio is to one, the more accurate the diagnostic test is. Only a diagnostic test with $n_{12} \approx 0$ and $n_{21} \approx 0$ will provide an accurate diagnosis (Accuracy ≈ 1). We now discuss the properties of such a test.

3.2.1. Necessary and Sufficient Diagnostic Tests

We show that accurate diagnosis is equivalent to a positive test result being *both* necessary and sufficient for the presence of the disease. Establishing this equivalence leads to several new advances: (i) we will be able to describe the theoretical mechanism for developing an accurate diagnosis (Section 3.2.2); (ii) we will be able to develop a theoretical framework for cumulative lifetime risk and its role in accurate diagnosis (Section 3.3); (iii) together with Section 2.3, we will have a unified theoretical framework for identifying a genetic disease by understanding the relationships between D, G, and T as summarized in Section 5.

Necessary diagnostic tests. An essential property of a diagnostic test is that it be effective at detecting the disease when the test is administered to an individual having the disease. More precisely, it should be the situation that $P(T|D) \approx 1$; otherwise, this particular test should not be used as a diagnostic tool. Sometimes, $P(T|D)$ is referred to as the *true-positive rate*, as well as the *sensitivity* of the diagnostic test [25].

Recall that $P(T|D) = 1$ is equivalent to saying that T is *necessary* for D (details of the equivalency are in Section 2.3 with G replaced by T); that is, "T is necessary for D" is equivalent to the diagnostic test having high sensitivity. Similarly, one can show that $P(T|D) = 1$ is equivalent to saying that the false-negative rate is zero ($P(T'|D) = 0$). Therefore, "T is necessary for D" (i.e., the diagnostic test has high sensitivity or has a small false-negative rate) means that: if a person has the disease, then the person will almost always test positive for the disease. When T is necessary for D, the population is partitioned, as shown in Table 1 with $n_{12} \approx 0$:

Sufficient diagnostic tests. A diagnostic test becomes a useful way of identifying those with the disease if $P(D|T) \approx 1$. Sometimes, $P(D|T)$ is referred to as the *positive predictive rate* [25].

Recall that $P(D|T) = 1$ is equivalent to saying that T is *sufficient* for D (details of the equivalency are in Section 2.3 with G replaced by T); that is, "T is sufficient for D" is equivalent to the diagnostic test having a high positive predictive rate. Similarly (assuming

$P(D') \neq 0$), one can show that $P(D|T) = 1$ is equivalent to saying that: the false-positive rate is zero ($P(T|D') = 0$); as well as $P(T'|D') = 1$. Sometimes, $P(T'|D')$ is called the *true-negative rate*, as well as the *specificity* of the diagnostic test [25]. Therefore, "T is sufficient for D" (i.e., the diagnostic test has a high positive predictive rate or a small false-positive rate, or high specificity) means that: if a person receives a positive test, then the person will almost always have the disease. When T is sufficient for D, the population is partitioned, as shown in Table 1 with $n_{21} \approx 0$:

Accurate diagnosis: A necessary and sufficient diagnostic test. The goal of any diagnostic test is for a positive test result to be *both* necessary and sufficient for an individual to be identified with the disease; that is, T and D partition the population as a *diagonal partition* (Table 1 with $n_{12} \approx 0$ and $n_{21} \approx 0$), and those individuals in the population under consideration with the disease are *precisely* those individuals who receive a positive result from the diagnostic test. Only if *both* sensitivity and specificity are high in a clinical study can clinicians be confident their analyses are accurate.

In summary, the result of the foregoing is that accurate diagnosis depends on T being both necessary and sufficient for D. When this is the case, $P(T) = P(D)$. Thus, an estimator for $P(T)$ based on a clinical study should be close to an estimator for $P(D)$ described by Equation (3).

An implication for clinicians is that if they choose to use a diagnostic test with a positive test result being "not necessary" for the occurrence of the disease, then that is equivalent to them accepting a significant iceberg effect and a large underestimation of the actual prevalence of the disease. Another implication for clinicians is that if they believe a diagnostic test's positive test result is "necessary, but not sufficient" for the occurrence of the disease, then that is equivalent to them accepting that the diagnostic test does not accurately predict whether a person has the disease or not. Instead, we suggest that it is imperative that clinicians continue their investigations—ultimately seeking a diagnostic test that *does* yield $P(T) = P(D)$.

3.2.2. Estimating Prevalence via a Diagnostic Test

To actually create a diagnostic test that yields $P(T) \approx P(D)$, a clinician should begin with a diagnostic test for which T is *necessary* for D (Table 1 with $n_{12} \approx 0$). Indeed, if T is not necessary for D, then the diagnostic procedure ought to be rejected outright. When diagnostic tests are first developed, they are likely to have difficulty identifying those with the disease and those without it (Table 1 with $n_{21} \not\approx 0$ and, therefore, n_{11} is underestimated). A clinician's goal is therefore to refine the diagnostic test, while keeping in mind accepted clinical study design protocols [7], so that it also ensures T is *sufficient* for D (Table 1 with $n_{12} \approx 0$ and $n_{21} \approx 0$). When this is achieved, clinicians will have created a diagnostic test that accurately predicts disease presence (i.e., the test is ready for usage as a diagnostic tool), and $P(T)$ will be close to $P(D)$.

The preceding intuitive discussion connects our theory to a clinician's practice. To our knowledge, we are the first to rigorously characterize the discussion by developing the theoretical mechanism for *how* $P(T)$ approaches $P(D)$ as the diagnostic test is refined. We demonstrate that when T is necessary for D (Section 3.2.1), $P(T)$ can be used to provide lower and upper bounds for $P(D)$; moreover, we show that as the false-positive rate ($P(T|D')$) approaches zero, the lower and upper bounds force $P(T)$ to approach $P(D)$. Thus, T will be both necessary and sufficient for D, and consequently, $P(T) \approx P(D)$. Specifically, the theoretical mechanism is described by

$$P(T) - (1 - P(T))\frac{\alpha_0}{1 - \alpha_0} \leq P(D) \leq P(T), \tag{4}$$

where α_0 is an upper bound for $P(T|D')$; in other words, the false-positive rate is at most α_0 ($0 \leq P(T|D') \leq \alpha_0$). The derivation of Equation (4) is provided in Appendix C.

Reducing α_0 improves the diagnostic test's accuracy. Moreover, Equation (4) describes the theoretical mechanism by which $P(T)$ approaches $P(D)$ as α_0 becomes smaller (because the lower bound in Equation (4) approaches $P(T)$ as α_0 approaches zero), resulting in the partition of the population induced by T and D approaching a diagonal partition, at which point, T will be both necessary and sufficient for D. The implication is crucial:

> As the false-positive rate becomes smaller, the probability increases that a positive result in the corresponding diagnostic test will more accurately predict prevalence of the disease.

Estimation procedure. The above theoretical development suggests the following four-step procedure for clinicians wanting to use a diagnostic test to accurately estimate disease prevalence:

(i) Begin with a diagnostic test for which T is necessary for D. A corresponding clinical study should consist of data resembling Table 1 with $n_{12} \approx 0$.

(ii) Estimate $P(T)$. Use Table 1 to find

$$\widehat{P}(T) = \frac{n_{11} + n_{21}}{n}.$$

(iii) Estimate the maximum value of a false-positive rate, which is denoted by α_0. Use Table 1 to compute, for example, a 95% confidence interval [5,6] for the false-positive rate, and take α_0 to be the maximum of the interval

$$\alpha_0 = \widehat{\alpha} + 1.96\sqrt{\widehat{\alpha}(1-\widehat{\alpha})/n}, \quad \text{where} \quad \widehat{\alpha} = \widehat{P}(T|D') = \frac{n_{21}}{n_{21}+n_{22}}.$$

(iv) Substitute the estimators of $P(T)$ and α_0 into Equation (4), which yields an interval estimate for $P(D)$.

Example 1. *As context, consider a disease caused by a dominant allele with $p = 0.2$, $r = 1$ and the genotype CC fully penetrant. Then $P(D) = 0.36$ (Equation (3)). In principle, an accurate diagnostic test should yield $P(T) \approx P(D) \approx 0.36$. To achieve this, begin with a diagnostic test for which T is necessary for D (Step (i)). Using a corresponding clinical study resembling Table 1 with $n_{12} \approx 0$, obtain the estimator $\widehat{P}(T) \approx 0.36$ (Step (ii)). Figure 3 is an illustration of Equation (4), where the lower bound is the blue curve and the upper bound is the black horizontal line (at $\widehat{P}(T) \approx 0.36$). The disease prevalence $P(D)$ lies inclusively between the two bounds, and interval estimates for $P(D)$ (indicated in red) are shown for $\alpha_0 = 0.3, 0.2, 0.1,$ and 0.02. Depending on the diagnostic test and how it is interpreted, false-positive results may generate uncertainty regarding $P(D)$; for example, if the false-positive rate is as high as 0.3 (i.e., $\alpha_0 = 0.3$), then $P(D)$ is estimated as being inclusively between 0.086 and 0.36 (Steps (iii) and (iv); Figure 3). An interval estimate with such a large spread makes any $P(D)$ estimate unreliable (e.g., the interval does not support claiming $P(D) \approx 0.09$). Indeed, such uncertainty should alert clinicians that the diagnostic test is not accurate (T is necessary, but not yet sufficient for D). However, as α_0 is reduced, the test's accuracy is improved; at values $\alpha_0 \leq 0.1$, the disease prevalence will be estimated more accurately (Figure 3 with $\alpha = 0.1$ and 0.02); T will become both necessary and sufficient for D, resulting in $P(T) \approx P(D) \approx 0.36$, as desired.*

Incidentally, our development of accurate diagnosis applies to *any* disease, whether it is genetically based or not.

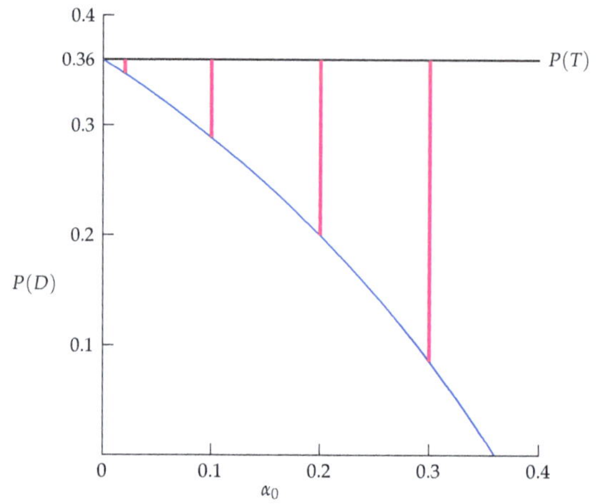

Figure 3. Illustration of Example 1, where $P(T) = 0.36$. The horizontal axis is the values for α_0, which is an upper bound for the false-positive rate; the vertical axis is the disease prevalence $P(D)$. The lower bound in Equation (4) is the blue curve, and the upper bound is the black horizontal line at $P(T) = 0.36$. $P(D)$ will lie inclusively between the two bounds. The interval estimates for $P(D)$ (indicated in red) are shown for $\alpha_0 = 0.3, 0.2, 0.1$, and 0.02. The accuracy of an interval estimate of disease prevalence increases as the false-positive rate declines; specifically, the red interval estimates become smaller as α_0 becomes smaller.

3.3. Accurate Diagnosis Requires Cumulative Lifetime Risk

For many disorders, disease prevalence is a cumulative lifetime risk; that is to say, disease prevalence is the likelihood a person from the population will be accurately diagnosed as having the disease at some point during their lifetime. For certain disorders, in particular those caused by dominant alleles, symptoms and the probability of testing positive for the disease ($P(T)$) show a peak in middle age. This leads to a steady accumulation of cases (of a particular disease) in the population [8,11,13,26,27]. Diagnostic tests for such diseases are administered to people thought to have the disease-causing genotype; these tests yield a result at a specific moment in each person's lifetime. For some disorders (e.g., Huntington's Disease (HD) [28]), the probability of a positive test result ($P(T)$) increases with age, so young people with the disease-causing genotype may not test positive for the disease. In non-fatal dominant diseases, these negative results are often misinterpreted to mean that such people will never test positive for the disease. Our analysis will make clear that this interpretation is unwarranted and is a source of underestimates of $P(D)$.

Figure 4 shows the cumulative lifetime feature of disease prevalence for people with HD. Figure 4A illustrates data for 84 people (ranging in age from 10 to over 80 years old) who at some point developed HD. The maximum proportion was diagnosed at approximately age 50, and by age 80 nearly all of those who would develop HD had been diagnosed. Figure 4B illustrates the corresponding cumulative distribution of diagnosis, indicating that it takes about 80 years for most people with the disease-causing genotype for HD to be identified. This cumulative mechanism means that a negative diagnostic test result at any age below, say 70, does not preclude either a positive diagnostic test result or actual disease itself at a later time. Therefore, HD prevalence cannot be accurately estimated by studying only those younger than age 70. This cumulative pattern of diagnosis applies to prion diseases [13] and amyotrophic lateral sclerosis [29], and in general has implications for the estimation of the prevalence of diseases that are detected only later in life.

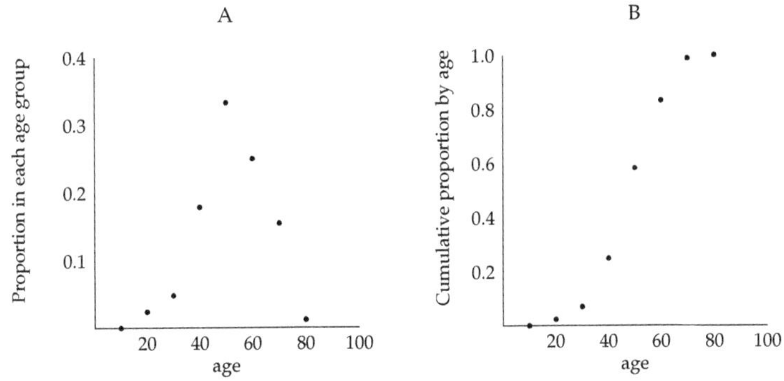

Figure 4. The cumulative lifetime feature of disease prevalence for people with Huntington's Disease (HD). (**A**) Proportion of 84 people (ranging in age from 10 to 80) with HD who are diagnosed at each of the eight age decades. The maximum proportion occurs at approximately age 50, and the distribution is bell-shaped, but not symmetric. (**B**) The cumulative proportion of the people shown in (**A**) with HD who are diagnosed at each of the eight decades. Constructed from data in [28].

Genetic tests at any time will show the presence or absence of the disease-causing genotypes. For a disease such as HD, the *CC* genotype is unlikely to be found in living people because most individuals with the *CC* genotype die before birth. The presence of the *Cc* genotype suggests that the disease will develop in severity over the lifetime of the individual and the true prevalence $P(D)$ is not accurately estimated until all ages have been accounted for [13]. Thus, for individuals with the *Cc* genotype, the variable appearance of HD over a lifespan is not necessarily a measure of the penetrance of the disease-causing genotype *Cc*, as disease prevalence may also depend on how carefully clinicians have diagnosed the condition (i.e., how likely it is to obtain a positive diagnostic test result may depend on disease severity and the diagnostic test's ability to detect mild forms of the disease).

Cumulative lifetime risk is best understood as an investigation of the accuracy of diagnosis and the identification of all people who might have the disease. Recall that an accurate diagnosis can be framed in terms of a positive diagnostic test result being both necessary and sufficient for the presence of the disease (Section 3.2.1). The implications are crucial for understanding population disease prevalence. We will show that cumulative lifetime risk is *formally and actually* equal to population-wide disease prevalence, $P(D)$:

Theoretical framework. The following is a theoretical framework for cumulative lifetime risk analysis. It describes the accuracy of a diagnosis as a function of subject age in terms of two measures of cumulative diagnosis, which we call the *cumulative age-true positive rate* and the *cumulative age-positive predictive rate*. The former is an index of the diagnostic test's true-positive rate, and thus of the degree to which the diagnostic test is *necessary* for demonstrating the disease; the latter is an index of the diagnostic test's positive predictive rate, and thus of the degree to which the diagnostic test is *sufficient* for demonstrating the disease. For simplicity, we assume that the maximum lifetime of individuals in the population is 100 years.

We define the *age-true positive rate*, denoted by $f_{tpr}(i)$, to be the conditional probability a person receives a positive test result at age i years old ($i = 1, 2, \ldots, 100$), given the person has the disease; that is to say,

$$f_{tpr}(i) = P((T \cap \{\text{age } i \text{ years old}\})|D) \quad (i = 1, 2, \ldots, 100).$$

Thus, the true-positive rate is the accumulation of all age-true positive rates,

$$P(T|D) = \sum_{i=1}^{100} f_{tpr}(i).$$

We define the *age-positive predictive rate*, denoted by $f_{ppr}(i)$, to be the conditional probability a person has the disease at age i years old, given the person receives a positive test result ($i = 1, 2, \ldots, 100$); that is to say,

$$f_{ppr}(i) = P((D \cap \{\text{age } i \text{ years old}\})|T) \quad (i = 1, 2, \ldots, 100).$$

Thus, the positive predictive rate is the accumulation of all age-positive predictive rates,

$$P(D|T) = \sum_{i=1}^{100} f_{ppr}(i).$$

Here are the properties that both the age-true positive rate and the age-positive predictive rate satisfy (to simplify the notation, the function $f(i)$ stands for both $f_{tpr}(i)$ and $f_{ppr}(i)$):

(i) The function $f(i)$ has values $0 \leq f(i) \leq 1$ for all $i = 1, 2, \ldots, 100$.

(ii) The sum of all the values of $f(i)$ must equal one, $\sum_{i=1}^{100} f(i) = 1$, which is a consequence of the diagnostic test satisfying $P(T|D) = 1$ (T is necessary for D) and $P(D|T) = 1$ (T is sufficient for D).

(iii) The function $f(i)$ is bell-shaped, but is not necessarily symmetric. That is, $f(i)$ obtains its maximum at some age denoted by m; $f(i)$ will be an increasing function for $i < m$ and a decreasing function for $i > m$. For diseases with later-in-life detection (e.g., many diseases caused by dominant alleles), m typically occurs during middle-age.

Figure 5A provides a graph of a typical f (which stands for both f_{tpr} and f_{ppr}) for diseases with later-in-life detection. For convenience, the function f has been extended to a continuous function defined for all times $0 \leq t \leq 100$. Indeed, the function $f(t)$ can be thought of as a "best fit curve" using the values $f(i)$ for $i = 1, 2 \ldots, 100$, and $f(0) = 0$.

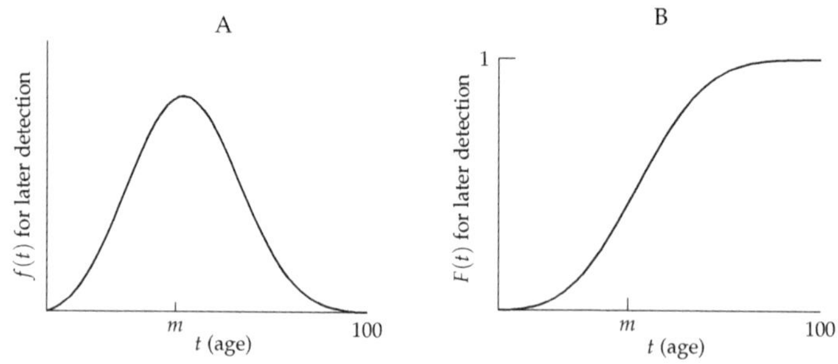

Figure 5. (**A**) Graph of a typical f, which stands for both the age-true positive rate (f_{tpr}) and the age-positive predictive rate (f_{ppr}). See the text for their descriptions. The function $f(t)$ is bell-shaped, but is not necessarily symmetric, and obtains its maximum at some age denoted by m. For a disease with later-in-life detection, m typically occurs during middle-age. (**B**) Graph of a typical F, which stands for both the cumulative age-true positive rate (F_{tpr}) and the cumulative age-positive predictive rate (F_{ppr}). See the text for their descriptions. For a disease with later-in-life detection, F is close to one only after middle age.

We define the *cumulative age-true positive rate* of the disease at age i, denoted by $F_{tpr}(i)$, to be the sum of the age-true positive rates for ages at most i; that is to say,

$$F_{tpr}(i) = \sum_{k=1}^{i} f_{tpr}(k) \quad (i = 1, 2, \ldots, 100).$$

We define the *cumulative age-positive predictive rate* of the disease at age i, denoted by $F_{ppr}(i)$, to be the sum of the age-positive predictive rate for ages at most i; that is to say,

$$F_{ppr}(i) = \sum_{k=1}^{i} f_{ppr}(k) \quad (i = 1, 2, \ldots, 100).$$

Here are properties that both the cumulative age-true positive rate and the cumulative age-positive predictive rate satisfy (to simplify the notation, the function $F(i)$ stands for both $F_{tpr}(i)$ and $F_{ppr}(i)$):

(i) The function F has values $0 \leq F(i) \leq 1$ for the ages $i = 1, 2, \ldots, 100$.
(ii) $F(i)$ is an increasing function, where $F(100) = 1$ because

$$F_{tpr}(100) = P(T|D) = 1 \quad \text{and} \quad F_{ppr}(100) = P(D|T) = 1.$$

(iii) $F(i)$ will be concave up (increasing at an increasing rate) for $1 \leq i < m$; and will be concave down (increasing at a decreasing rate) for $m < i \leq 100$.

Figure 5B provides a graph of a typical F (which stands for both F_{tpr} and F_{ppr}) for diseases with later-in-life detection. For convenience, the function F has been extended to a continuous function defined for all times $0 \leq t \leq 100$. Indeed, the function $F(t)$ can be thought of as a "best fit curve" using the values $F(i)$ for $i = 1, 2, \ldots, 100$, and $F(0) = 0$.

In summary, accurate diagnosis (Section 3.2) in the context of a cumulative lifetime risk corresponds to

$$F_{tpr}(100) = 1 \quad \text{and} \quad F_{ppr}(100) = 1.$$

Framing accurate diagnosis as a cumulative lifetime risk has implications for clinicians regarding a diagnostic test's result. For diseases with later-in-life detection (e.g., many diseases caused by dominant alleles), clinicians should be aware of three important and related concepts:

(i) A negative diagnostic test result up to middle age does not indicate that the person will never be accurately diagnosed with the disease during their lifetime. For example, a person may actually have an early form of the disease that is not detected by the diagnostic test; consequently, inadequate testing may prevent treatment for the person during their lifetime. Indeed, because $F_{tpr}(t) \approx 1$ and $F_{ppr}(t) \approx 1$ only later in life, it is essential to continue testing a person with the disease-causing genotype who receives a negative diagnostic test result well beyond middle age (Figure 5).
(ii) Clinical studies exclusively using people from a specific age group (e.g., only those from 20–30 years old) will suffer from ascertainment bias; hence, such studies will *not* produce meaningful inferences regarding population disease prevalence (Figure 5). Moreover, clinical studies consisting of people only up to middle age will suffer from ascertainment bias and result in an underestimation of the prevalence of diseases with later-in-life detection. For example, HD prevalence would be underestimated by about 30% if only people up to age 55 were included in the data in [28] (Figure 4B).
(iii) A positive diagnostic test result at any age (in a person with the disease-causing genotype) may also be a false-positive and may suggest treatments that will not be necessary. The chances of false positives should thus be minimized at all ages (Figure 5).

Cumulative lifetime risk equals disease prevalence. We now show that cumulative lifetime risk in principle equals the prevalence of the disease, $P(D)$ (Section 2). For a diagnostic test in which a positive test result is both necessary and sufficient for the presence of the disease,

$$\text{Cumulative lifetime risk} = P(T),$$

as well as

$$P(T|D) = F_{tpr}(100) = 1 \quad \text{and} \quad P(D|T) = F_{ppr}(100) = 1.$$

Now,

$$\begin{aligned} P(D) &= P(D \cap T) + P(D \cap T') \\ P(D) &= P(T|D)P(D) + P(T'|D)P(D) \\ 1 &= P(T|D) + P(T'|D), \end{aligned}$$

which implies $P(T'|D) = 0$ because $P(T|D) = 1$. Thus,

$$\begin{aligned} P(D) &= P(D \cap T) + P(D \cap T') \\ P(D) &= P(D|T)P(T) + P(T'|D)P(D), \end{aligned}$$

which implies $P(D) = P(T)$ because $P(D|T) = 1$ and $P(T'|D) = 0$. Therefore,

$$\text{Cumulative lifetime risk} = P(T) = P(D),$$

where $P(D)$ is given by Equation (3).

In summary, it is important to view the accuracy of diagnosis as a function of subject age in order to ensure that a positive diagnostic test result precisely identifies those individuals who have the disease. That is, the goal of any diagnostic test should be for $P(T)$ to accurately estimate $P(D)$.

4. Familial and Offspring-Group Aggregation

The current approach to investigating the prevalence of genetic diseases in various families relies on the concept of *familial aggregation*, in which the frequency of a disease may be higher in particular family groupings than in the general population. An initial grouping was the *hereditary family*, consisting of genetic relatives from the same family tree: grandparents, parents, siblings, cousins, etc. [8,11]. A more precise grouping is *first-degree relatives* (parents, offspring, and siblings [30]), which form a subset of the hereditary family. However, a person's genetic disease risk is not directly influenced by a non-parent in a hereditary family. Because current approaches assess a person's genetic disease risk via imprecise measures of familial aggregation, we propose they be replaced by a measure determined solely by parental genotypes; thus, we introduce a *new* approach that we call *offspring-group aggregation*. The advantages of this approach will become apparent below.

Throughout, we use standard human pedigree analysis terminology; for example, "parents" refers to genetic parents, and "siblings" refers to offspring with the same genetic parents [8].

Offspring-groups. Consider a two-allele model for a genetic disease. Table 2 illustrates all possible parental genotypes and their offspring. The entries in the individual cells are the frequencies of the corresponding offspring.

Table 2. All possible parental genotypes and frequencies of their offspring.

	CC	*Cc*	*cC*	*cc*
CC	$p^2 \times p^2$	$p^2 \times pq$	$p^2 \times qp$	$p^2 \times q^2$
Cc	$pq \times p^2$	$pq \times pq$	$pq \times qp$	$pq \times q^2$
cC	$qp \times p^2$	$qp \times pq$	$qp \times qp$	$qp \times q^2$
cc	$q^2 \times p^2$	$q^2 \times pq$	$q^2 \times qp$	$q^2 \times q^2$

Constructing all the possible matings using the parents in Table 2, we observe that there are precisely six partition subsets of the general population, which we denote by F_i (for $i = 1, 2, \ldots, 6$), and have the following probabilities:

$$\begin{aligned} &F_1: CC \times CC; && P(F_1) = p^2 \times p^2; \\ &F_2: CC \times Cc; && P(F_2) = 4(p^2 \times pq); \\ &F_3: CC \times cc; && P(F_3) = 2(p^2 \times q^2); \\ &F_4: Cc \times Cc; && P(F_4) = 4(pq \times pq); \\ &F_5: Cc \times cc; && P(F_5) = 4(pq \times q^2); \\ &F_6: cc \times cc; && P(F_6) = q^2 \times q^2. \end{aligned} \tag{5}$$

In Figure 6, we illustrate the possible offspring genotypes within each subset F_i (for $i = 1, 2, \ldots, 6$). We refer to F_i as an *offspring-group*, which consists of all people (offspring) whose parents have the genotypes that determine the partition F_i. For example, F_2 consists of all people (offspring) in the general population whose parents have genotypes $CC \times Cc$.

	C	C
C	CC	CC
C	CC	CC

F_1

	C	C
C	CC	CC
c	Cc	Cc

F_2

	C	C
c	Cc	Cc
c	Cc	Cc

F_3

	C	c
C	CC	Cc
c	Cc	cc

F_4

	C	c
c	Cc	cc
c	Cc	cc

F_5

	c	c
c	cc	cc
c	cc	cc

F_6

Figure 6. Illustration of the possible offspring genotypes within each of the six offspring-groups F_i (for $i = 1, 2, \ldots, 6$). Because offspring genotype frequencies differ among the offspring-groups, some office-spring groups may have high disease prevalence while others may have low or zero disease prevalence.

Consequently, because a person's genotype is dependent on their parents, siblings belong to the same offspring-group. Moreover, an offspring-group will include people who are not necessarily siblings; indeed, two people who are not siblings could each have parents with the same genotypes and thus be members of the same offspring-group.

Incidentally, which offspring-group a parent belongs to is determined by the genotypes of *their* parents; a parent might not belong to the same offspring-group as their children. For example, suppose you and your mate have genotypes $CC \times Cc$, then your offspring belong to F_2; in addition, suppose your parents have genotypes $Cc \times Cc$, then you belong to F_4.

At any given time, there are always exactly six offspring-groups in the general population (Figure 6), while there are a large number of hereditary families with various compositions. Most importantly, Figure 6 shows that some offspring-groups may have high $P(D)$, while others may have low or zero $P(D)$.

Clinical studies involving pairs of siblings report the likelihood that a sibling has the disease, given the other sibling has the disease. This statistic, called sibling risk, is presented as if it were a clinical characteristic of the disease. Disease risk is instead determined by the structures of the offspring-groups (Figure 6), the penetrance of disease-causing genotypes, and the frequency of the disease-causing genotypes. We will address this idea in Section 4.2. Familial aggregation is currently measured with the sibling recurrence-risk ratio, denoted by λ_s, which refers to the ratio of sibling risk to the population-wide disease prevalence (Section 4.1). An estimated high value $\widehat{\lambda}_s \gg 1$ (e.g., occasionally obtained from clinical studies) is used often as an indication that a particular disorder has familial aggregation [10,11,31]. However, as we will show, the current measure of familial aggregation is biased because it ignores a large part of the population and because it is affected by (often mistaken) estimates of population disease prevalence. Indeed, we provide several arguments that, in principle, the theoretical sibling recurrence-risk ratio is always equal to one ($\lambda_s = 1$); this gives the surprising result that any estimator $\widehat{\lambda}_s \not\approx 1$ be viewed with suspicion. Therefore, we propose that λ_s is in need of replacement.

Our new concept focuses on the six offspring-groups (Figure 6) instead of hereditary families. Because each offspring-group has its own disease risk, "familial risk" should not be represented by a population parameter with a single value such as λ_s. After demonstrating the unsuitability of λ_s, we propose an alternative that depends on the allele frequency and penetrance of disease-causing genotypes; thus, our measure differs among the possible six offspring-groups of the general population (Equation (9)). We also discuss why our new measure is likely to yield an unbiased estimator based on clinical studies—unlike estimators for the sibling recurrence-risk ratio (Section 4.2).

4.1. Sibling Recurrence-Risk Ratio

Sibling risk is defined as the probability that an individual has a disease, given that a sibling has the same disease [11,32,33]. More precisely, let S_1 and S_2 denote two (non-identical) siblings with the same parents, let D_1 denote the event that S_1 has the disease, and let D_2 denote the event that S_2 has the same disease. In the literature [10,11,33], sibling risk is often denoted by K_s; thus,

$$K_s = \text{Sibling risk} = P(D_2|D_1).$$

In addition, the population risk (frequency, prevalence, probability) of the disease in the population is often denoted by K. In particular, $P(D_1) = K$ and $P(D_2) = K$. The literature in this field [10,11] defines the *sibling recurrence-risk ratio*

$$\lambda_s = \frac{K_s}{K}$$

for use in the explanation of familial aggregation, as well as for hypothesizing a need for additional genes to describe the dependence of disease prevalence on genotype. Misunderstanding and different interpretations of the definition of K_s have led to various approaches for (inaccurately) estimating λ_s, making valid inferences and hypotheses problematic [32].

Our approach to this issue is based on the alleles of offspring being dependent on their parents, as well as on the small number of possible offspring-group types in a population and the membership of two siblings in the same offspring-group. Observe that while the siblings S_1 and S_2 are from the same offspring-group, the definition of K_s as currently used does not specify to *which* of the six offspring-groups the siblings belong (Figure 6). Thus, K_s is not defined as a conditional probability with respect to an offspring-group, forcing the general population to become the focus for determining K_s. Therefore, the heterogeneity of offspring-groups means λ_s is not an enlightening measure of familial aggregation.

Our analysis develops several biologically based probabilistic arguments leading to the demonstration that $K_s = K$ for a genetic disease; that is, $\lambda_s = 1$ (Sections 4.1.1 and 4.1.2).

Following this demonstration, we will explore its implications for the calculations of estimators for K_s and K. We also discuss why the estimator $\widehat{\lambda}_s$ experiences computational deficiencies—incorrectly predicting $\lambda_s > 1$. In addition, we discuss the implications of $K_s = K$ and the misuse of λ_s as the justification for additional gene hypotheses (Section 4.1.3).

4.1.1. Offspring Allele Independence: $\lambda_s = 1$

The genotypes of offspring are dependent on the parents, not on the siblings; consequently, whether S_1 has a particular allele is *not* affected by whether S_2 has the allele and genetic events regarding S_1 and S_2 will be independent of each other. In particular, with respect to genetic diseases, D_1 and D_2 are independent events. Therefore, $P(D_1 \cap D_2) = P(D_1)P(D_2)$, which implies

$$K_s = P(D_2|D_1) = \frac{P(D_1 \cap D_2)}{P(D_1)} = \frac{P(D_1)P(D_2)}{P(D_1)} = P(D_2) = K;$$

hence, we conclude that $\lambda_s = 1$. This means that $\lambda_s = 1$ for *any* disease in which disease status is independent in each sibling. Incidentally, the independence of D_1 and D_2 may not be the case for certain types of disorders; for example, two siblings living in the same household will likely not be independent of each other with respect to non-genetic contagious disease status [32].

As another approach showing $\lambda_s = 1$, we note that Risch [33] writes λ_s in terms of the covariance between siblings

$$\lambda_s = 1 + \frac{1}{K^2}\mathrm{Cov}(D_1, D_2).$$

Because D_1 and D_2 are independent events, $\mathrm{Cov}(D_1, D_2) = 0$ [5,6] and we again conclude that $\lambda_s = 1$.

As a third approach showing $\lambda_s = 1$, we note Risch [11] defines ϕ_s as the probability that two siblings share zero marker alleles and states that $\phi_s = 1/4$. Let $Z = \{S_1 \text{ and } S_2 \text{ share zero alleles}\}$, and observe that

$$P(Z) = \phi_s = 1/4.$$

Recall $\{S_1 \text{ and } S_2 \text{ have the disease}\} = D_1 \cap D_2$. As indicated in [11],

$$P((D_1 \cap D_2)|Z) = P(D_1)P(D_2) = K^2,$$

which implies

$$P((D_1 \cap D_2) \cap Z) = P((D_1 \cap D_2)|Z)P(Z) = K^2\phi_s;$$

moreover, $P(D_1 \cap D_2) = P(D_2|D_1)P(D_1) = K_sK$. Therefore,

$$P(Z|(D_1 \cap D_2)) = \frac{P((D_1 \cap D_2) \cap Z)}{P(D_1 \cap D_2)} = \frac{K^2\phi_s}{K_sK} = \frac{\phi_s}{K_s/K} = \frac{\phi_s}{\lambda_s}.$$

As described in [10], the expected proportion of affected sibling pairs sharing zero alleles is 0.25; that is, $P(Z|(D_1 \cap D_2)) = 0.25 = \phi_s$. Hence, $\phi_s = \phi_s/\lambda_s$, and we again conclude that $\lambda_s = 1$.

4.1.2. Siblings Are from the Same Offspring-Group: $\lambda_s = 1$

We define the *offspring-group risk* for a specific offspring-group F_i to be the probability of an individual having the disease, given that the individual is an offspring in F_i. That is, offspring-group risk is $P(D|F_i)$ (for $i = 1, 2, \ldots, 6$).

From Figure 6, using $P(D|cc) = 0$ for a disease D caused by a dominant allele (Section 2.2), we compute the offspring-group risk for each of the six offspring-groups:

$$\begin{aligned}
&P(D|F_1) = P(D|CC); \quad P(D|F_2) = \frac{1}{2}(P(D|CC) + P(D|Cc)) \\
&P(D|F_3) = P(D|Cc); \quad P(D|F_4) = \frac{1}{4}(P(D|CC) + 2P(D|Cc)) \\
&P(D|F_5) = \frac{1}{2}P(D|Cc); \quad P(D|F_6) = 0.
\end{aligned} \tag{6}$$

We are now ready to compute sibling risk using the offspring-group risks. Because the six offspring-groups form a partition of the population and because siblings are from the same offspring-group, we can write

$$\begin{aligned}
K_s = P(D_2|D_1) &= \frac{P(D_2 \cap D_1)}{P(D_1)} \\
&= \frac{1}{P(D_1)} \sum_{i=1}^{6} P(D_2 \cap D_1 \cap F_i) \\
&= \frac{1}{P(D_1)} \sum_{i=1}^{6} P(D_2 \cap F_i)P(D_1) \\
&= \sum_{i=1}^{5} P(D_2|F_i)P(F_i) \quad \text{(because } P(D_2|F_6) = 0\text{).}
\end{aligned}$$

Using the offspring-group frequencies (Equation (5)), we have that

$$\begin{aligned}
K_s = P(D_2|F_1)p^4 + P(D_2|F_2)4p^3q + P(D_2|F_3)2p^2q^2 \\
+ P(D_2|F_4)4p^2q^2 + P(D_2|F_5)4pq^3.
\end{aligned} \tag{7}$$

Substituting the offspring-group risks (Equation (6)) into Equation (7) gives the following representation

$$\begin{aligned}
K_s = P(D_2|CC)p^4 + 2[P(D_2|CC) + P(D_2|Cc)]p^3q + 2P(D_2|Cc)p^2q^2 \\
+ [P(D_2|CC) + 2P(D_2|Cc)]p^2q^2 + 2P(D_2|Cc)pq^3.
\end{aligned}$$

Finally, combining similar terms (and noting that $p + q = 1$), using Equation (1) and Section 2.2, and using Equation (3) yields

$$\begin{aligned}
K_s &= [p^4 + 2p^3q + p^2q^2]P(D_2|CC) + [2p^3q + 4p^2q^2 + 2pq^3]P(D_2|Cc) \\
&= p^2[p^2 + 2pq + q^2]P(D_2|CC) + 2pq[p^2 + 2pq + q^2]P(D_2|Cc) \\
&= p^2(p+q)^2P(D_2|CC) + 2pq(p+q)^2P(D_2|Cc) \\
&= p^2P(D_2|CC) + 2pqP(D_2|Cc) \\
&= p(2r + (1-2r)p)P(D_2|CC) \\
&= K.
\end{aligned}$$

Thus, we again conclude that $K_s = K$. This last argument has the additional utility that it provides the underlying structure for developing a new measure of aggregation (based on offspring-groups instead of hereditary families), which we discuss in Section 4.2.

Even though the values of K_s and K are identical, certain offspring-groups (and hereditary families) may have more members with a disease than other groups and may also have a higher or lower $P(D)$ than the population as a whole. The equality of K_s and K simply means that the sibling recurrence-risk ratio is not an appropriate measure of aggregation among offspring-groups or hereditary families. Before we propose an alternative measure that avoids the challenges associated with λ_s, we discuss why estimators ($\widehat{\lambda}_s$) of λ_s appear to be greater than one.

4.1.3. Estimating the Sibling Recurrence-Risk Ratio

There are two main reasons for errors in the traditional statistical construction of the estimator $\widehat{\lambda}_s$: (i) the prevalence of the disease, K, is almost always underestimated; (ii) sibling risk, K_s, is almost always overestimated.

Having already discussed the underestimation of K (Section 3), we now discuss the overestimation of K_s. Recall that

$$K_s = P(D_2|D_1) = \frac{P(D_2 \cap D_1)}{P(D_1)}.$$

Using data from a clinical study consisting of pairs of siblings, an estimator $\widehat{P}(D_2 \cap D_1)$ will likely yield an overestimation of $P(D_2 \cap D_1)$ because the clinical study will almost always not include siblings from offspring-group F_6 for which $P(D|F_6) = 0$ (Equation (6)). Hence, ascertainment bias will cause

$$\widehat{K}_s = \frac{\widehat{P}(D_2 \cap D_1)}{\widehat{P}(D_1)}$$

to be overestimated. Incidentally, the contribution of offspring-group F_6 can be significant. For example, when $p \leq 0.2$, more than 40% of all population members are in this offspring-group; thus, the same proportion (more than 40%) of the population is likely not included in computing an estimator for K_s (though F_6 is likely to be included in computing an estimator for K).

In addition, we point out that the sibling recurrence-risk ratio is particularly sensitive to underestimates of K. Indeed, observe that

$$\lambda_s = \frac{K_s}{K} = \frac{P(D_2|D_1)}{K} = \frac{P(D_1 \cap D_2)}{P(D_1)K} = \frac{P(D_1 \cap D_2)}{K^2}.$$

Because the exponent for K is two, while $P(D_1 \cap D_2)$ has exponent one, λ_s will be more sensitive to underestimates of K than to overestimates of $P(D_2 \cap D_1)$.

Similarly, an estimator for K_s based on a conditional probability approach is also almost always overestimated. Consider a clinical study consisting of pairs of siblings with one of the siblings known to have the disease. An estimator of K_s will be $\widehat{K}_s = \widehat{P}(D_2|D_1)$. In this case, the clinical study will likely consist mostly of individuals participating from offspring-groups with high offspring-group risks (Equation (6)) [32]; that is, the clinical study will suffer from ascertainment bias. Hence, the calculated value of $\widehat{K}_s$ will likely yield an overestimation of K_s.

Despite the reality that in principle $K_s = K$, several studies [10,11,31,34] have used estimators of K_s and K derived from clinical studies to suggest $\lambda_s > 1$ and propose that a more complicated genetic model is required to explain the causes of certain genetic disorders. However, as we have shown that $\lambda_s = 1$, it appears that equations using λ_s with a value other than 1 should not be used to propose alternative genetic hypotheses.

As an illustration, we now discuss an example where using λ_s is problematic. The contribution of the Human Leukocyte Antigen (HLA) region (denoted by λ_{sHLA}) to the sibling recurrence-risk ratio is the "expected proportion of affected sibling pairs sharing zero haplotypes identical-by-decent (IBD) (0.25) divided by the observed proportion [of affected sibling pairs sharing zero haplotypes IBD]" [10]; that is,

$$\lambda_{sHLA} = \frac{P(Z|(D_1 \cap D_2))}{\widehat{P}(Z|(D_1 \cap D_2))} = \frac{0.25}{\widehat{P}(Z|(D_1 \cap D_2))},$$

where $Z = \{S_1 \text{ and } S_2 \text{ share zero haplotypes}\}$.

Assuming a multiplicative model [11], the percentage of the HLA's contribution to the sibling recurrence-risk ratio (denoted by $\% \lambda_{sHLA}$) is calculated [10] using the equation

$$\% \lambda_{sHLA} = 100 \frac{\log(\lambda_{sHLA})}{\log(\lambda_s)},$$

which obviously requires $\lambda_s \neq 1$ (otherwise, the denominator is zero). However, because of our earlier discussion that $\lambda_s = 1$ (Sections 4.1.1 and 4.1.2), we conclude that this equation experiences a theoretical deficiency by always producing an undefined result—assuming the true value of λ_s is used.

In addition to the already-discussed issues with the estimator $\widehat{\lambda}_s$, it appears that estimating λ_{sHLA} also is problematic; indeed, the above equation for $\% \lambda_{sHLA}$ often is used with an estimated value of λ_s satisfying $\widehat{\lambda}_s > 1$ and an estimated value of λ_{sHLA} also satisfying $\widehat{\lambda}_{sHLA} > 1$ [10,11,31,34]. For example, Table 3 in [10] includes several clinical studies that can be used to construct $\widehat{\lambda}_{sHLA}$, where the individual studies produce values of $\widehat{P}(Z|(D_1 \cap D_2))$ ranging from a low of 0 (also the median and mode) to a high of 0.50. These values correspond to $\widehat{\lambda}_{sHLA}$ ranging from undefined (infinite) to 0.50. Combining all of the data in the clinical studies produces $\widehat{P}(Z|(D_1 \cap D_2)) = 0.07$, but due to the large spread of the data, it is not likely that this single value is meaningful (as was pointed out by the authors of the study) [10]. In any event, even if researchers wrongly use $\widehat{\lambda}_s > 1$ and $\widehat{\lambda}_{sHLA} > 1$, they will still be able to compute the quantity

$$\% \widehat{\lambda}_{sHLA} = 100 \frac{\log(\widehat{\lambda}_{sHLA})}{\log(\widehat{\lambda}_s)}.$$

However, inferences and hypotheses should not be based on such a calculated value of $\% \widehat{\lambda}_{sHLA}$ because of the previously discussed issues with the estimator $\widehat{\lambda}_s$ and because of difficulties associated with the estimator $\widehat{\lambda}_{sHLA}$. We do not dispute that, in principle, there may exist a percentage of HLA's contribution to disease risk; we are simply proposing that using $\% \widehat{\lambda}_{sHLA}$ as an indicator is suspect.

In summary, our analysis shows that λ_s experiences theoretical and computational deficiencies; in addition, its definition often is misunderstood and subject to misinterpretations [32]. These attributes lead to estimators of λ_s being greatly inflated ($\widehat{\lambda}_s \gg 1$); thus, drawing conclusions based on $\widehat{\lambda}_s$ is suspect. In particular, we propose that λ_s does not accurately indicate familial aggregation nor provide insight for the general genotype–disease relationship.

4.2. *Offspring-Group Aggregation and Its Measure*

To better account for the fact that each offspring-group has its own disease risk, we propose replacing the concept of familial aggregation with what we call *offspring-group aggregation*, which describes the aggregation of genetic diseases among the six offspring-groups (instead of among hereditary families). In addition, we propose a new measure that precisely describes the frequency distribution of genetic diseases among the six offspring-groups and yields estimators of the offspring-group aggregation of genetic diseases.

To do this, we define the *offspring-group recurrence-risk ratio* as the ratio of the offspring-group risk to the disease prevalence; specifically,

$$\mu_i = \frac{P(D|F_i)}{P(D)} \quad (\text{for } i = 1, 2, 3, 4, 5, 6).$$

It measures the likelihood that a person from offspring-group F_i has the disease, relative to a person from the general population. For example, $\mu_i = 2.5$ means that a person from F_i is about 2.5 times more likely to have the disease as a person from the general population.

Using Equations (1) and (6), we obtain the following representations of offspring-group risk (Section 4.1.2) in terms of r and $P(D|CC)$:

$$P(D|F_1) = P(D|CC), \qquad P(D|F_2) = \frac{1}{2}(1+r)P(D|CC)$$
$$P(D|F_3) = rP(D|CC), \qquad P(D|F_4) = \frac{1}{4}(1+2r)P(D|CC)$$
$$P(D|F_5) = \frac{1}{2}rP(D|CC), \qquad P(D|F_6) = 0,$$

which we collectively write in the form

$$P(D|F_i) = \beta_i(r)P(D|CC) \quad (\text{for } i = 1,2,3,4,5,6) \tag{8}$$

where the functions $\beta_i(r)$ are:

$$\beta_1(r) = 1, \qquad \beta_2(r) = \frac{1}{2}(1+r), \qquad \beta_3(r) = r,$$
$$\beta_4(r) = \frac{1}{4}(1+2r), \qquad \beta_5(r) = \frac{1}{2}r, \qquad \beta_6(r) = 0.$$

Using Equations (3) and (8), we obtain

$$\mu_i = \frac{\beta_i(r)}{p(2r+(1-2r)p)} \quad (\text{for } i = 1,2,3,4,5,6). \tag{9}$$

We propose that the values of μ_i are an appropriate way to measure the degree of offspring-group aggregation across all offspring-groups in the general population.

In Table 3, we provide illustrative examples of the offspring-group recurrence-risk ratio (Equation (9)): (i) a C allele with $p = 0.2$ and $r = 1$; (ii) a C allele with $p = 0.2$ and $r = 0.5$; (iii) a C allele with $p = 0.02$ and $r = 1$.

Table 3. Illustrative examples of the offspring-group recurrence-risk ratio.

	$p = 0.2, r = 1$	$p = 0.2, r = 0.5$	$p = 0.02, r = 1$
μ_1	2.78	5.00	25.25
μ_2	2.78	3.75	25.25
μ_3	2.78	2.50	25.25
μ_4	2.08	2.50	18.94
μ_5	1.39	1.25	12.63
μ_6	0	0	0

Table 3 illustrates several key features regarding the ability of μ_i to measure offspring-group aggregation:

(i) The disparate values of μ_i show that each offspring-group has its own contribution to offspring-group aggregation. For example, when $p = 0.2$ and $r = 1$, members of offspring-groups F_1, F_2, and F_3 are approximately three-times as likely to have the disease as members of the general population, while family F_6 will have no members with the disease.

(ii) The distribution of offspring-group aggregation is influenced by the frequency of the dominant allele C. For example, when $r = 1$, the positive values of μ_i increase markedly as p changes from $p = 0.2$ to $p = 0.02$.

(iii) The distribution of offspring-group aggregation is influenced by the parameter r. For example, when $p = 0.2$, the offspring-group aggregation is more concentrated among families F_1 and F_2 for $r = 0.5$ than for $r = 1$.

An important property of the values of the offspring-group recurrence-risk ratio μ_i is that their weighted sum is equal to 1, where the individual weights are the frequencies of the corresponding offspring-groups. Indeed, writing Equation (7) in terms of the offspring-group recurrence-risk ratios yields

$$K_s = P(D_2)\left[\,p^4\mu_1 + 4p^3q\mu_2 + 2p^2q^2\mu_3 + 4p^2q^2\mu_4 + 4pq^3\mu_5\right].$$

Recalling that $K = P(D_2)$, we obtain the following decomposition of the sibling recurrence-risk ratio λ_s in terms of the offspring-group recurrence-risk ratios μ_i

$$\lambda_s = \frac{K_s}{K} = p^4\mu_1 + 4p^3q\mu_2 + 2p^2q^2\mu_3 + 4p^2q^2\mu_4 + 4pq^3\mu_5\,.$$

Because $\lambda_s = 1$ (Sections 4.1.1 and 4.1.2), it follows that

$$p^4\mu_1 + 4p^3q\mu_2 + 2p^2q^2\mu_3 + 4p^2q^2\mu_4 + 4pq^3\mu_5 = 1\,, \tag{10}$$

where the coefficients of μ_i are the corresponding frequencies of offspring-group F_i given by Equation (5).

In addition, another key feature of the offspring-group recurrence-risk ratio is that, unlike λ_s, Equation (10) precisely describes the frequency distribution of offspring-group aggregation of the disease among the six offspring-groups (recall for family F_6 that $\mu_6 = 0$). Writing Equation (10) in the form

$$\sum_{i=1}^{6} P(F_i)\mu_i = 1$$

emphasizes that each term in the sum, $P(F_i)\mu_i$, is the offspring-group proportion of those with the disease who are in offspring-group F_i, where $P(F_i)$ is given by Equation (5).

Table 4 illustrates the offspring-group proportions when $p = 0.2$ and $r = 1$. The implication of the values is straightforward; for example, of those people with the disease, approximately 57% are from offspring-group F_5. Moreover, notice that the sum of the values equals 1, as required by Equation (10).

Table 4. Offspring-group proportions when $p = 0.2$ and $r = 1$.

$P(F_1)\mu_1$	0.004
$P(F_2)\mu_2$	0.071
$P(F_3)\mu_3$	0.142
$P(F_4)\mu_4$	0.213
$P(F_5)\mu_5$	0.569
$P(F_6)\mu_6$	0

We point out that, for diseases in which the genotype CC is lethal prior to birth or shortly thereafter (e.g., Huntington's disease and Marfan syndrome [35,36]), offspring-groups F_1, F_2, and F_3 will not appear in the (living) population. In this case, the offspring-group risk ratios μ_4 and μ_5 and the offspring-group proportions $P(F_4)\mu_4$ and $P(F_5)\mu_5$ are the most relevant.

In summary, our theoretical framework proposes replacing familial aggregation with offspring-group aggregation and replacing λ_s with the offspring-group recurrence-risk ratio μ_i, which has these advantageous properties: (i) it quantifies the clustering of the genetic disease within different offspring-groups and thus does not assume a single value of aggregation that applies across the general population; (ii) it depends on the parameters p and r, which can be estimated using unbiased clinical studies (Section 2); (iii) unlike λ_s, it does not explicitly depend on K, which is often underestimated (Section 3); (iv) it can be used to precisely describe the frequency distribution of offspring-group aggregation (Equation (10)), which cannot be done with λ_s. This emphasizes the importance for parental-sibling clinical studies of determining from which of the six offspring-groups each subject comes.

In Section 5.3, we provide a scenario illustrating how a clinician may use the theoretical framework for offspring-group aggregation as a clinical tool.

5. Discussion: Integration of Results

Researchers and clinicians who want to identify a genetic disease, including its genotype-phenotype relationship, benefit from being attentive to the three topics we have developed: (1) the relationship between the disease-causing genotypes and the presence of the associated disease (Section 2); (2) the role of diagnostic tests and their ability to identify the disease (Section 3); and (3) the frequency distribution of offspring-group aggregation among the six offspring-groups (Section 4).

Figure 7 provides an organizational diagram of our unified theoretical framework of these three topics. Recall that G, D, and T denote the events that an individual from the general population has the disease-causing genotypes, has the disease, and receives a positive test result from a diagnostic test, respectively. Their possible relationships (logical implications) are illustrated by the blue and red arrows: Section 2 discusses when G is necessary and/or sufficient for D (i.e., when the disease-causing genotypes identify the disease); Section 3 discusses when T is necessary and/or sufficient for D (i.e., when a diagnostic test identifies the disease). Section 4 investigates the frequency distribution of offspring-group aggregation among the six offspring-groups (summarized by $\sum_{i=1}^{6} P(F_i)\mu_i = 1$), which is affected by G, D, and T, as indicated by the green arrows.

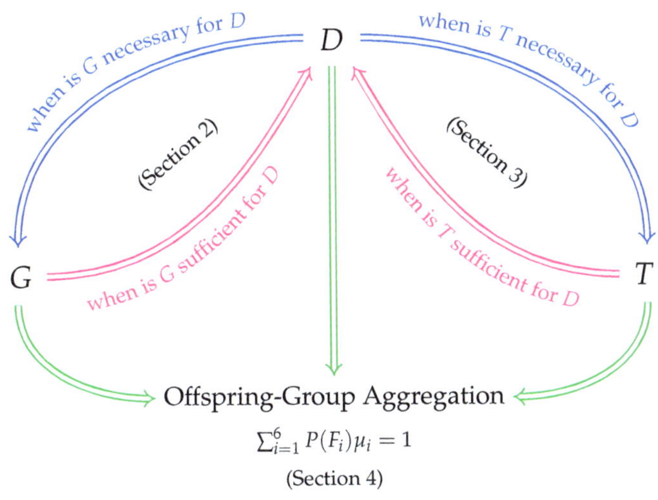

Figure 7. Organizational diagram of our unified theoretical framework of the three main topics for identifying a genetic disease. Recall that G, D, and T each denote the events that an individual from the general population has the disease-causing genotypes, has the disease, and receives a positive test result from a diagnostic test, respectively. The possible relationships between G, D, and T are illustrated by the blue and red arrows (the arrows are the notation for the logical concept "implies"). The frequency distribution of offspring-group aggregation among the six offspring-groups is summarized by the equation, which is affected by G, D, and T, as illustrated by the green arrows.

5.1. Relationship between G and D (Section 2)

Fundamental to identifying a genetic disease is determining the relationship between the disease-causing genotypes and the presence of the associated disease. For a disease caused by a dominant allele: G is *always* necessary for D; G is sufficient for D *if and only if* the disease-causing genotypes are fully penetrant. This is illustrated in Figure 7: $D \Rightarrow G$ and the corresponding blue arrow *always* occurs; $G \Rightarrow D$ and the corresponding red arrow occurs *if and only if* $P(D|CC) = 1$ and $P(D|Cc) = 1$.

In other words, the relationship between disease prevalence and the frequencies of the disease-causing genotypes is always

$$P(D) \leq P(G),$$

and

$$P(D) = P(G) \text{ only when } P(D|CC) = 1 \text{ and } P(D|Cc) = 1.$$

The theoretical framework presented in Section 2 provides guidance to researchers and clinicians with regard to determining the relationship between the disease-causing genotypes and the presence of the associated disease. In particular, if they believe "G is necessary, but not sufficient for D", then we propose that researchers and clinicians continue their investigations, being aware of the associated consequences and responsibilities (Section 2.3), with the goal of characterizing the relationship between G and D. Even so, it is essential that clinicians not use their belief that a disease-causing genotype is partially penetrant as justification for using an inaccurate diagnostic test; that is, for using a diagnostic test with low sensitivity and/or low specificity (Section 5.2).

5.2. Relationship between T and D (Section 3)

The theoretical framework presented in Section 3 provides guidance to researchers and clinicians with regard to understanding the relationship between a positive diagnostic test result and the presence of the associated disease. In summary, we recommend that researchers and clinicians:

(i) Ensure diagnostic tests have T that is both necessary and sufficient for D. Figure 7 illustrates the desired relationship: $T \Leftrightarrow D$ and the corresponding blue and red arrows both occur. When this is the case, $P(T) = P(D)$, where $P(D)$ is described in Section 2. If clinicians think that a diagnostic test's positive result is "necessary, but not sufficient" to confirm the presence of the disease, then that is equivalent to them accepting a diagnostic test that is actually inadequate at identifying the disease. The test either should be refined or replaced. We suggest it is imperative that clinicians continue their investigations—ultimately seeking a diagnostic test that consistently *does* identify the disease (Section 3.2).

(ii) Treat $P(T)$ as a cumulative lifetime risk. Framing accurate diagnosis as a cumulative lifetime risk has implications for clinicians considering the usefulness of a diagnostic test result, as well as for developing long-term clinical studies (Section 3.3).

These two essential features make it more likely that unbiased clinical studies produce an estimator $\widehat{P}(T)$ that is close to the estimator $\widehat{P}(D)$ described in Section 2.2.

In order to be useful in diagnosis, all diagnostic tests must, within reasonable error bounds, give the same diagnostic information. At present, antibody tests, pregnancy tests, and blood tests for particular substances are examples of diagnostic tests for which high sensitivity and specificity determinations are standard. This standard should be applied to all tests (e.g., tissue biopsies) that are part of the diagnostic system. Even so, for some genetic diseases, not all subjects with the disease-causing genotype will appear to have the disease. This may be because of partial penetrance, but it should also be considered that incomplete diagnosis may be at fault or that people may tend to ignore their symptoms or ascribe them to other causes. Those persons should be more carefully followed up with additional investigations and perhaps different types of diagnostic tests.

Finally, we mention that when G and T are both necessary and sufficient for D (all blue and red arrows in Figure 7 occur), then

$$P(G) = P(D) = P(T),$$

and clinical studies should produce estimators for $P(G)$ and $P(T)$ that are close; that is, $\widehat{P}(G) \approx \widehat{P}(T)$. Because genetic tests are less likely to have errors than are diagnostic tests, a discrepancy between the estimators more than likely suggests that $\widehat{P}(T)$ is not accurate, indicating that further investigation is warranted, rather than concluding simply that G is not sufficient.

5.3. *Offspring-Group Aggregation (Section 4)*

The general population can be partitioned into six offspring-groups denoted by F_i (for $i = 1, 2, \ldots, 6$), and a specific offspring-group F_i is determined by parental genotypes (Figure 6). We provide a theoretical framework for describing a genetic disease's *offspring-group aggregation* (i.e., disease aggregation among the six offspring-groups).

We discuss the theoretical and computational deficiencies of the sibling recurrence-risk ratio, whose definition often is misunderstood and subject to differing and inconsistent interpretations. This ratio typically is used as an indicator of familial aggregation even though it ignores the six offspring-groups (Section 4.1).

We propose replacing familial aggregation with offspring-group aggregation, as well as an alternative measure that does not experience the deficiencies and precisely describes the frequency distribution of offspring-group aggregation among the six offspring-groups (Section 4.2). In summary, our proposed measure is the *offspring-group recurrence-risk ratio* (denoted by μ_i), which is defined in Equation (9). It measures the likelihood a person from offspring-group F_i has the disease, relative to a person from the general population. The frequency distribution of offspring-group aggregation is described by the equation

$$\sum_{i=1}^{6} P(F_i)\mu_i = 1,$$

where $P(F_i)\mu_i$ is the offspring-group proportion of those with the disease who are in offspring-group F_i.

Finally, we note that μ_i and $P(F_i)$ depend on understanding the disease-causing genotypes and the presence of the disease (Section 2), as well as accurate diagnosis of the disease (Section 3). Thus, our theoretical framework for offspring-group aggregation fundamentally relies on an understanding of the relationships between G, D, and T, as communicated by the green arrows in Figure 7.

Offspring-group aggregation as a clinical tool. We conclude with a scenario illustrating how a clinician may use the theoretical framework for offspring-group aggregation as a clinical tool. Consider a disease caused by a dominant allele with $p = 0.2$, $r = 1$, and $P(D|CC) = 1$. Then, $P(D) = 0.36$ (Equation (3)). Suppose a person visits a clinician wanting to know the likelihood they have the disease, given the person has a sibling known to have the disease. While the clinician may not know to which offspring-group the siblings belong, it is known they are not in offspring-group F_6. As illustrated in Table 3, the clinician predicts the person is either 1.39, 2.08, or 2.78 times as likely to have the disease, compared to members of the general population, which is 0.36. Using this information, the clinician predicts the likelihood that the person has the disease is approximately either 0.50, 0.75, or 1.00, respectively, and the person's offspring-group determines which of the three values it is. However, even if the clinician does not know the person's offspring-group, it is still possible to estimate the likelihood the person has the disease. Indeed, based on Table 4, the clinician notices that, of those people with the disease, F_5 has the highest percentage (in fact, higher than the sum of all other offspring-groups); thus, the clinician may choose to only use the F_5 information and predict that the likelihood the person has the disease is about $(1.39) \times (0.36) = 0.50$. Alternatively, the clinician may choose to use a weighted average, incorporating all the information in Tables 3 and 4,

$$0.57(0.50) + 0.21(0.75) + 0.22(1.00) = 0.66$$

as a prediction of the likelihood the person has the disease. Whichever value the clinician chooses (0.50 or 0.66), the clinician concludes the person is at a higher risk than a member of the general population (0.36). This information can be used to frame a discussion between the clinician and the patient regarding the next steps to pursue (e.g., whether to test the person for the disease-causing genotypes or administer accurate diagnostic tests).

We recommend that researchers and clinicians consider using the theoretical framework for offspring-group aggregation discussed in Section 4 and summarized in Section 5.3.

To place our analysis in the context of the current state of research, it is still epidemiologically valid to say that if one person in a hereditary family has a genetic disease, other family members are at risk, should be carefully evaluated, and appropriate precautions should be taken. Though other hereditary family members often are at higher risk than are members of the population as a whole, this does not mean $K_s > K$ in the general population. We suggest this mistaken idea be replaced by an approach that carefully uses diagnostic tools to accurately evaluate K, as well as describe genetic disease aggregation in terms of the offspring-groups F_i and the offspring-group recurrence-risk ratio μ_i.

Author Contributions: The authors contributed equally to all phases of this work. All authors have read and agreed to the published version of the manuscript.

Funding: This research received no external funding.

Institutional Review Board Statement: Not applicable.

Informed Consent Statement: Not applicable.

Data Availability Statement: Not applicable.

Acknowledgments: The authors thank J. Christopher Gaiser, Linfield University Department of Biology, for the helpful advice and discussion regarding population genetics; and Nadine Grzeskowiak, Celiac Nurse Consulting, Salem, Oregon, for insightful discussions regarding clinical applications of gene-disease relationships. The authors also thank the Editor for the valuable assistance, as well as the Reviewers for their helpful comments/feedback, which improved the exposition.

Conflicts of Interest: The authors declare no conflict of interest.

Appendix A. Derivation of Equation (2)

Consider the partition of the population in terms of the genotypes CC, Cc, cC, and cc. Now,

$$D = (D \cap CC) \cup (D \cap Cc) \cup (D \cap cC) \cup (D \cap cc),$$

and because the genotypes are mutually exclusive (the intersection of any two genotypes is the empty set $\emptyset$),

$$P(D) = P(D \cap CC) + P(D \cap Cc) + P(D \cap cC) + P(D \cap cc).$$

Because $P(D \cap Cc) = P(D \cap cC)$, we obtain

$$P(D) = P(D \cap CC) + 2P(D \cap Cc) + P(D \cap cc).$$

By the definition of the probability of an intersection,

$$P(D) = P(D|CC)P(CC) + 2P(D|Cc)P(Cc) + P(D|cc)P(cc),$$

which can be written in the form shown in Equation (2).

Appendix B. Necessary and Sufficient as Conditional Probabilities

We now develop equivalent conditional probability formulations for the concepts of "necessary" and "sufficient". The formulations apply to any two events, but we will frame the discussion in terms of G and D (Section 2.3).

Observe that $P(G|D) = 1$ is equivalent to saying that "G is *necessary* for D". Indeed:

$$\begin{aligned} P(G|D) = 1 &\Leftrightarrow P(D \cap G) = P(D) \\ &\Leftrightarrow P(D \cap G') = 0 \quad (\text{because } P(D) = P(D \cap G) + P(D \cap G')) \\ &\Leftrightarrow D \cap G' = \emptyset \quad (\emptyset \text{ denotes the empty set}) \\ &\Leftrightarrow D = D \cap G \quad (\text{because } D = (D \cap G) \cup (D \cap G')) \\ &\Leftrightarrow \text{the occurrence of } D \text{ implies the occurrence of } G \\ &\Leftrightarrow G \text{ is necessary for } D. \end{aligned}$$

Furthermore, observe that $P(D|G) = 1$ is equivalent to saying that "G is *sufficient* for D." Indeed:

$$\begin{aligned} P(D|G) = 1 &\Leftrightarrow P(G \cap D) = P(G) \\ &\Leftrightarrow P(G \cap D') = 0 \quad (\text{because } P(G) = P(G \cap D) + P(G \cap D')) \\ &\Leftrightarrow G \cap D' = \emptyset; \\ &\Leftrightarrow G = G \cap D \quad (\text{because } G = (G \cap D) \cup (G \cap D')) \\ &\Leftrightarrow \text{the occurrence of } G \text{ implies the occurrence of } D \\ &\Leftrightarrow G \text{ is sufficient for } D. \end{aligned}$$

Appendix C. Derivation of Equation (4)

Because $T = (T \cap D) \cup (T \cap D')$ and because D and D' are mutually exclusive,

$$\begin{aligned} P(T) &= P(T \cap D) + P(T \cap D') \\ &= P(T|D)P(D) + P(T|D')P(D') \\ &= P(D) + P(T|D')(1 - P(D)) \quad (\text{because } P(T|D) = 1) \end{aligned}$$

which implies,

$$P(T) = (1 - P(T|D'))P(D) + P(T|D').$$

Solving for $P(D)$ yields

$$P(D) = \frac{P(T) - P(T|D')}{1 - P(T|D')}.$$

To simplify the notation in the following derivation, we let $\omega = P(T)$ and $\alpha = P(T|D')$. Then, we can write

$$\begin{aligned} P(D) &= \frac{\omega - \alpha}{1 - \alpha} \\ &= \frac{\omega(1 - \alpha) - \alpha(1 - \omega)}{1 - \alpha}, \end{aligned}$$

which implies that

$$P(D) = \omega - (1 - \omega)\frac{\alpha}{1 - \alpha}. \tag{A1}$$

Let $f(\alpha) = \alpha/(1 - \alpha)$ for $0 \leq \alpha < 1$. The derivative of f is

$$f'(\alpha) = (1 - \alpha)^{-2} > 0,$$

which implies that $f(\alpha)$ is an increasing function on the interval $0 \le \alpha < 1$. Thus, for α_0 with $0 < \alpha_0 < 1$,

$$0 \le \alpha \le \alpha_0 \Rightarrow f(0) \le f(\alpha) \le f(\alpha_0)$$
$$\Rightarrow 0 \le \frac{\alpha}{1-\alpha} \le \frac{\alpha_0}{1-\alpha_0}.$$

Therefore, using Equation (A1), we obtain the following lower and upper bounds for $P(D)$:

$$\omega - (1-\omega)\frac{\alpha_0}{1-\alpha_0} \le P(D) \le \omega .$$

Substituting $\omega = P(T)$ yields Equation (4).

References

1. Jackson, M.; Marks, L.; May, G.; Wilson, J. The genetic basis of disease. *Essays Biochem.* **2018**, *62*, 643–723. [CrossRef]
2. King, R.; Roaer, J.; Motulsky, A. (Eds.) *The Genetic Basis of Common Diseases*, 2nd ed.; Oxford University Press: Oxford, UK, 2002.
3. Garrod, A.E. The incidence of Alkaptonuria: A study in chemical individuality. *Lancet* **1902**, *160*, 1616–1620. [CrossRef]
4. Coban-Akdemir, Z.; White, J.; Song, X.; Jhangiani, S.; Fatih, J.; Gambin, T.; Bayram, Y.; Chinn, I.; Karaca, E.; Punetha, J.; et al. Identifying Genes Whose Mutant Transcripts Cause Dominant Disease Traits by Potential Gain-of-Function Alleles. *Am. J. Hum. Genet.* **2018**, *103*, 171–187. [CrossRef] [PubMed]
5. Ross, S.M. *Introduction to Probability and Statistics for Engineers and Scientists*, 5th ed.; Academic Press: San Diego, CA, USA, 2014.
6. Wackerly, D.; Mendenhall, W.; Scheaffer, R. *Mathematical Statistics with Applications*, 7th ed.; Brooks/Cole: Belmont, CA, USA, 2008.
7. Piantadosi, S. *Clinical Trials: A Methodologic Perspective*, 3rd ed.; John Wiley & Sons, Inc.: Hoboken, NJ, USA, 2017.
8. Griffiths, A.; Wessler, S.; Lewontin, R.; Carroll, S. *Introduction to Genetic Analysis*, 11th ed.; W.H. Freeman: New York, NY, USA, 2015.
9. Relethford, J.H. *Human Population Genetics*; John Wiley & Sons, Inc.: Hoboken, NJ, USA, 2012.
10. Petronzelli, F.; Bonamico, M.; Ferrante, P.; Grillo, R.; Mora, B.; Mariani, P.; Gemme, G.; Mazzilli, M. Genetic contribution of the HLA region to the familial clustering of coeliac disease. *Ann. Hum. Genet.* **1997**, *61*, 307–317. [CrossRef] [PubMed]
11. Risch, N. Assessing the role of HLA-linked and unlinked determinants of disease. *Am. J. Hum. Genet.* **1987**, *40*, 1–14.
12. Lewis, C.; Whitwell, S.; Forbes, A.; Sanderson, J.; Mathew, C.; Marteau, T. Estimating risks of common complex diseases across genetic and environmental factors: The example of Crohn disease. *J. Med. Genet.* **2007**, *44*, 689–694. [CrossRef]
13. Minikel, E. Estimation of Penetrance Using Population Allele Frequency. Available online: https://www.cureffi.org (accessed on 7 October 2018).
14. Zlotogora, J. Penetrance and expressivity in the molecular age. *Genet. Med.* **2003**, *5*, 347–352. [CrossRef]
15. Whiffin, N.; Minikel, E.; Walsh, R.; O'Donnell-Luria, A.; Karczewski, K.; Ing, A.; Barton, P.; Funke, B.; Cook, S.; MacArthur, D.; et al. Using high-resolution variant frequencies to empower clinical genome interpretation. *Genet. Med.* **2017**, *19*, 1151–1158. [CrossRef]
16. Kang, J.; Kang, A.; Green, A.; Gwee, K.; Ho, K. Systematic review: Worldwide variation in the frequency of coeliac disease and changes over time. *Aliment. Pharmacol. Ther.* **2013**, *38*, 226–245. [CrossRef]
17. Last, J.M. The iceberg: 'Completing the clinical picture' in general practice. *Lancet* **1963**, *2*, 28–31. [CrossRef]
18. Last, J.M. Commentary: The iceberg revisited. *Int. J. Epidemiol.* **2013**, *42*, 1615–1617. [CrossRef] [PubMed]
19. Rubio-Tapia, A.; Ludvigsson, J.; Brantner, T.; Murray, J.; Everhart, J. The prevalence of celiac disease in the United States. *Am. J. Gastroenterol.* **2012**, *107*, 1538–1544. [CrossRef] [PubMed]
20. Sapone, A.; Lammers, K.; Mazzarella, G.; Mikhailenko, I.; Carteni, M.; Casolaro, V.; Fasano, A. Differential mucosal IL-17 expression in two gliadin-induced disorders: Gluten sensitivity and the autoimmune enteropathy celiac disease. *Int. Arch. Allergy Immunol.* **2010**, *152*, 75–80. [CrossRef] [PubMed]
21. Spinney, L. Uncovering the true prevalence of Huntington's disease. *Lancet* **2010**, *9*, 760–761. [CrossRef] [PubMed]
22. Csizmadia, C.; Mearin, M.; von Blomberg, B.; Brand, R.; Verloove-Vanhorick, S. An iceberg of childhood coeliac disease in the Netherlands. *Lancet* **1999**, *353*, 813–814. [CrossRef] [PubMed]
23. Lerner, A.; Jeremias, P.; Matthias, T. Outside of normal limits: False positive/negative anti TG2 autoantibodies. *Int. J. Celiac Dis.* **2015**, *3*, 87–90. [CrossRef]
24. Minikel, E.; Zerr, I.; Collins, S.; Ponto, C.; Boyd, A.; Klug, G.; Karch, A.; Kenny, J.; Collinge, J.; Takada, L.; et al. Ascertainment bias causes false signal of anticipation in genetic prion disease. *Am. J. Hum. Genet.* **2014**, *95*, 371–382. [CrossRef]
25. Fawcett, T. An introduction to ROC analysis. *Pattern Recognit. Lett.* **2006**, *27*, 861–874. [CrossRef]
26. Ebers, G.; Sadovnick, A.; Risch, N.; the Canadian Collaborative Study Group. A genetic basis for familial aggregation in multiple sclerosis. *Nature* **1995**, *377*, 150–151. [CrossRef]
27. Myers, R.H. Huntington's Disease genetics. *Neurotherapeutics* **2004**, *1*, 255–262. [CrossRef]

28. Reed, T.E.; Chandler, J.H. Huntington's Chorea in Michigan. I. Demography and genetics. *Am. J. Hum. Genet.* **1958**, *10*, 201–225. [PubMed]
29. Mehta, P.; Antao, V.; Kaye, W.; Sanchez, M.; Williamson, D.; Bryan, L.; Muravov, O.; Horton, K. Prevalence of Amyotrophic Lateral Sclerosis—United States, 2010–2011. *MMWR Suppl.* **2014**, *63*, 1–14. [PubMed]
30. Talley, N.; Segal, I.; Weltman, M. *Gastroenterology and Hepatology: A Clinical Handbook*; Elsevier Publ. Co.: Amsterdam, The Netherlands, 2008.
31. Bevan, S.; Popat, S.; Braegger, C.; Busch, A.; O'Donoghue, D.; Falth-Magnusson, K.; Ferguson, A.; Godkin, A.; Hogberg, L.; Holmes, G.; et al. Contribution of the MHC region to the familial risk of coeliac disease. *J. Med. Genet.* **1999**, *36*, 687–690. [PubMed]
32. Guo, S.-W. Inflation of sibling recurrence-risk ratio, due to ascertainment bias and/or over reporting. *Am. J. Hum. Genet.* **1998**, *63*, 252–258. [CrossRef] [PubMed]
33. Risch, N. Linkage strategies for genetically complex Traits. I. Multilocus models. *Am. J. Hum. Genet.* **1990**, *46*, 222–228. [PubMed]
34. Louka, A.; Sollid, L. HLA in coeliac disease: Unravelling the complex genetics of a complex disorder. *Tissue Antigens* **2003**, *61*, 105–117. [CrossRef] [PubMed]
35. Arnaud, P.; Hanna, N.; Aubart, M.; Leheup, B.; Dupuis-Girod, S.; Naudion, S.; Lacombe, D.; Milleron, O.; Odent, S.; Faivre, L.; et al. Homozygous and compound heterozygous mutations in the FBN1 gene: Unexpected findings in molecular diagnosis of Marfan Syndrome. *J. Med. Genet.* **2017**, *54*, 125–133. [CrossRef]
36. U.S.-Venezuela Collaborative Research Project; Wexler, N. Venezuelan kindreds reveal that genetic and environmental factors modulate Huntington's disease age of onset. *Proc. Nat. Acad. Sci. USA* **2004**, *101*, 3498–3503.

life

MDPI

Article

Identifying Neutrophil Extracellular Traps (NETs) in Blood Samples Using Peripheral Smear Autoanalyzers

Kateryna Fedorov [1,2,*], Mohammad Barouqa [3], David Yin [4], Margarita Kushnir [1], Henny H. Billett [1] and Morayma Reyes Gil [3,5,*]

1 Division of Hematology, Albert Einstein College of Medicine, Bronx, NY 10467, USA
2 Division of Hematology, Department of Oncology, Montefiore Medical Center, Albert Einstein School of Medicine, 3411 Wayne Ave, Ground Floor, Bronx, NY 10467, USA
3 Department of Pathology, Albert Einstein College of Medicine, Bronx, NY 10467, USA
4 Department of Internal Medicine, Montefiore Medical Center, Albert Einstein College of Medicine, Bronx, NY 10467, USA
5 Medical Director Hemostasis and Thrombosis Laboratories Cleveland Clinic, Cleveland, OH 44195, USA
* Correspondence: kfedorov@montefiore.org (K.F.); reyesgm@ccf.org (M.R.G.); Tel.: +718-920-4137 (K.F.); +216-444-2407 (M.R.G.); Fax: +718-882-8698 (K.F.)

Abstract: Neutrophil Extracellular Traps (NETs) are large neutrophil-derived structures composed of decondensed chromatin, cytosolic, and granule proteins. NETs play an important role in fighting infection, inflammation, thrombosis, and tumor progression processes, yet their fast and reliable identification has been challenging. Smudge cells (SCs) are a subcategory of white cells identified by CellaVision®, a hematology autoanalyzer routinely used in clinical practice that uses digital imaging to generate "manual" differentials of peripheral blood smears. We hypothesize that a proportion of cells identified in the SC category by CellaVision® Hematology Autoanalyzers are actually NETs. We demonstrate that NET-like SCs are not present in normal blood samples, nor are they an artifact of smear preparation. NET-like SCs stain positive for neutrophil markers such as myeloperoxidase, leukocyte alkaline phosphatase, and neutrophil elastase. On flow cytometry, cells from samples with high percent NET-like SCs that are positive for surface DNA are also positive for CD45, myeloperoxidase and markers of neutrophil activation and CD66b. Samples with NET-like SCs have a strong side fluorescent (SFL) signal on the white count and nucleated red cells (WNR) scattergram, representing cells with high nucleic acid content. When compared to patients with low percent SCs, those with a high percentage of SCs have a significantly higher incidence of documented bacterial and viral infections. The current methodology of NET identification is time-consuming, complicated, and cumbersome. In this study, we present data supporting identification of NETs by CellaVision®, allowing for easy, fast, cost-effective, and high throughput identification of NETs that is available in real time and may serve as a positive marker for a bacterial or viral infections.

Keywords: neutrophil extracellular traps; peripheral blood; sepsis; infection; digital white blood cell differential

Citation: Fedorov, K.; Barouqa, M.; Yin, D.; Kushnir, M.; Billett, H.H.; Reyes Gil, M. Identifying Neutrophil Extracellular Traps (NETs) in Blood Samples Using Peripheral Smear Autoanalyzers. *Life* **2023**, *13*, 623. https://doi.org/10.3390/life13030623

Academic Editors: Stefanos Roumeliotis and Giuseppe Minervini

Received: 8 February 2023
Revised: 17 February 2023
Accepted: 21 February 2023
Published: 23 February 2023

1. Introduction

Neutrophils are an integral part of the immune system's first line of defense against foreign organisms. Neutrophils' antimicrobial properties encompass three processes: phagocytosis, degranulation, and release of neutrophil extracellular traps (NETs) [1–3]. NETs are large cell-derived structures composed of decondensed chromatin, cytosolic and granule proteins. They function by trapping, neutralizing, killing, and preventing dissemination of infectious pathogens such as bacteria, viruses, fungi, and parasites [4–7]. Sterile inflammatory processes have also been associated with increased NET production in which case they have been implicated in pathologic amplification of inflammation, cytokine release, and tissue damage. In addition to their antimicrobial functions, NETs are thought to play an important role in pathogenesis of autoimmunity, vaso-occlusion, thrombosis, tumor capture, and spread [2,8–10].

Since their initial discovery in 2004, the scientific community has been working on finding reliable in-vivo NET identification methods [5]. Currently, visual identification of NETs relies on the visualization of DNA, histones, myeloperoxidase, and neutrophil elastase, using advanced immunohistochemical staining and microscopic techniques [5,9,11,12]. Alternatively, cell-free DNA, MPO-DNA complexes, citrullinated histones C3, neutrophil elastase, and cathelicidin antimicrobial peptides are used as surrogate markers for NETosis [13–18]. Neutrophil activation marker CD66b has been described as positively correlating with side-fluorescent scatter (SFL) generated by the Sysmex system [18,19], with several reports suggesting that NETs are identified with Sysmex' SFL scatters [18,20]. Such techniques are time-consuming, complicated, and cumbersome, hindering expansion into clinical practice. Currently, there are no readily available tools for the rapid clinical identification of NETs in patients.

Sysmex is an automated Hematology System routinely used in clinical laboratories for quantification of cells within peripheral blood and body fluid samples. Sysmex's White Count and Nucleated Red Cell channel (WNR) uses fluorescent flow cytometry employing polymethine dye for nucleic acids and a cell-specific lyse to capture side fluorescence (SFL) measuring cell's nucleic acid content and complexity and forward scatter (FSC) assessing cell size [21]. Automated image analyzers such as the CellaVision® Hematology Autoanalyzer are frequently used together with Sysmex. Blood samples flagged by Sysmex as abnormal are routed for peripheral blood smear generation and further analysis by CellaVision®. CellaVision® takes images of the cells on the slide and categorizes them based on morphology, generating a "manual" differential. Digital images of white blood cells (WBC) on the blood smear can subsequently be accessed and reviewed by clinical personnel. One of CellaVision®'s WBC categories is termed smudge cells (SC). It contains cellular entities that have lost their structural integrity and cannot be morphologically classified any further. Classically, on the peripheral blood smear, the smudge cells have been thought to represent degenerated lymphocytes (DL), which are abundant in blood smears of patients with chronic lymphocytic leukemia (CLL) [22]. Such smudge cells are a result of breakdown of fragile leukemic lymphocytes and, therefore, represent an artifact of smear preparation [22]. We observed that a proportion of cell derived entities categorized as smudge cells by CellaVision® morphologically resembled NETs. Sysmex WNR scattergrams that corresponded to blood samples with abundant SC have an increased population of unique, cellular entities that are comparable to WBC in size (FSC), but have high nucleic acid content (SFL).

We hypothesize that, in addition to the classic degenerated lymphocytes, a proportion of SC, as identified by the CellaVision® Hematology Autoanalyzer, are actually NETs. Here, we present supporting albeit preliminary data showing that NET-like SC are not present in normal blood samples and are not specimen handling artifacts, display neutrophil and NET specific markers on immunohistochemistry and flow cytometry, and generate unique patterns on Sysmex WNR scattergrams comparable to those seen in scattergrams of samples induced with NET trigger reagents. Additionally, we show that increased percent SC in the samples of hospitalized patients correlates positively with infection rates.

2. Materials and Methods

CellaVision® peripheral smear images and Sysmex WNR scattergram analysis. Clinical laboratories at Montefiore Medical Center use Sysmex CBC analyzers (XN 9000) and CellaVision® (v6.0.3) for routine analysis of EDTA-whole blood for CBC, peripheral blood smear generation using Wright Giemsa stain, and acquisition of digital images of these smears to classify white blood cells and generate a manual differential count. The smudge cell category reported by CellaVision® includes the classic degenerated lymphocytes, but also cellular entities that resemble NETs. We initially identified NET-like SC using a set of morphologic characteristics: lack of discernible plasma membrane, no intact cytoplasm, dispersed granules, decondensed and congested nuclei, and polarized chromatin projections. To investigate whether such NET-like SC are detectable by Sysmex's WNR (White Count and Nucleated Red Blood Cells) scattergrams corresponding to samples, we assessed the area of moderate FSC and high SFL, as it is known that NETs are similar in size to WBC but have a higher nucleic acid and granulation. To quantify the fluorescence signal in the WBC and NET area of WNR scattergram we used ImageJ® software (v1.53a).

Flow cytometry characterization of NETs. To further characterize NET-like SC as of neutrophil origin, we selected samples with ≤5% SC, ≥20% with majority SC morphologically characterized as NETs, and ≥20% with majority degenerated lymphocytes. To maintain cell integrity, centrifugation and cell permeabilization was avoided. Antibodies to SYTOX green, CD45, MPO, Neutrophil Elastase (NE), and CD66b were added to the buffy coats of gravity-separated EDTA whole blood samples. All antibodies were purchased from Invitrogen, Waltham MA and were used according to manufacturer recommendations. Gating was done using the Sytox positive cell gate, since only the SC should have surface DNA and be in this category, followed by gates for CD45, MPO and CD66b.

Effects of specimen handling and slide preparation (Incubation time, smearing angle, and pressure). To determine whether NET-like SC were a product of sample handling and slide preparation, samples with no detectable morphological "NETs" or smudge cells as analyzed by the CellaVision® underwent different slide preparation techniques. Five samples were incubated for 2, 6, 8, 10 and 24 h at 37 °C. Peripheral blood smears of these samples were processed through the CellaVision® for analysis. Different angles (60°, 30°, 15°, 0°, and standard 45°) and different pressures (as hard as possible without breaking the slide and soft capillary pressure) were used in the preparation of manual slides. Smearing was performed using both push and pull techniques. As analysis of manually prepared slides by CellaVision® is not possible, morphological NET counts were performed by microscopic examination of the slides by two different, blinded pathologists.

In vitro NET formation. EDTA whole blood specimens without SC reported on CellaVision® were then incubated with 100 nM phorbol 12-myristate 13-acetate (PMA), 100 μg/mL lipopolysaccharide (LPS), and 5 μM Ionomycin at 37 °C for 2, 6, 8, 10, and 24 h before re-processing through CellaVision®. All reagents were purchased from Sigma-Aldrich, St Louis, MO, USA.

Immunofluorescent staining for NET markers. To ensure viable cell counts, 50 uL of Sytox green (Invitrogen, Waltham, MA, USA) was added directly to the EDTA whole blood tube prior to smear processing. For all other stains, blood smears were dried and permeabilized with 4% paraformaldehyde (PFA) in phosphate buffered saline (PBS) for 10 min and washed with PBS (both reagents purchased from Sigma-Aldrich, St. Louis, MO, USA). Smears were then incubated with anti-histone H3 (citrulline R2 + R8 + R17; Ab5103, from Abcam, Cambridge, UK) at 1:100 (in PBS + 1% bis(trimethylsilyl)acetamide (BSA)) followed by Alexa Fluoro 488 goat anti-rabbit IgG (purchased from Abcam, Cambridge, UK) at a 1:1000 dilution for 1 h. Immunohistochemistry staining for leukocyte alkaline phosphatase (LAP) activity and LAP scoring was performed as per manufacturer recommendations (Sigma-Aldrich, St. Louis, MO, USA). For myeloperoxidase (MPO) and neutrophil elastase staining, smears were stained with directly conjugated Alexa-Flouro488 MPO (Abcam, Cambridge, UK) at 1:1000 dilution for 1 h.

Correlating %SC in EDTA whole blood with presence of infections. The CellaVision® database was reviewed to randomly identify specimens with ≤5% and ≥20% SC between March 2018 to February 2020. After IRB approval, the corresponding electronic medical records were reviewed to collect data on demographics, %SC, WBC count, and presence of infections within 10 days of specimen collection (either confirmed by microbiology or documented as such by medical provider). Fluorescence signal of suspected NET area on Sysmex WNR scattergrams was quantified using ImageJ software (v1.53a).

Statistical Analysis. Statistical analyses of averages were performed using means and standard deviations or IQR for normal and non-normal distribution of data respectively. p values were calculated with Kruskal–Wallis test for continuous variable and Chi-Squared (or Fisher's as needed) test for categorical variables using the R Studio® software (v1.4.1717). Significance was denoted by a two tailed $\alpha = 0.05$.

3. Results

3.1. Smudge Cells Are Not Increased in Normal Samples

To establish SC reference range for normal samples, 46 consecutive CBC specimens that were not flagged by Sysmex as abnormal were identified and manually routed to CellaVision® for analysis. The median %SC on these normal samples was 4.3 [2.6; 4.3].

3.2. The CellaVision® SC Category Contains Two Distinct Entities: Degenerated Lymphocytes and NET-like SC

A proportion of cells in the SC category resembled classic degenerated lymphocytes (DL)—cellular remnants that did not retain any structural components, while other cells morphologically resembled NETs. On CellaVision® NET-like SC appear as cell remnants with no discernible plasma membrane, no intact cytoplasm, dispersed granules, decondensed and congested nuclei, and polarized chromatin projections that resemble spider nets (Figure 1).

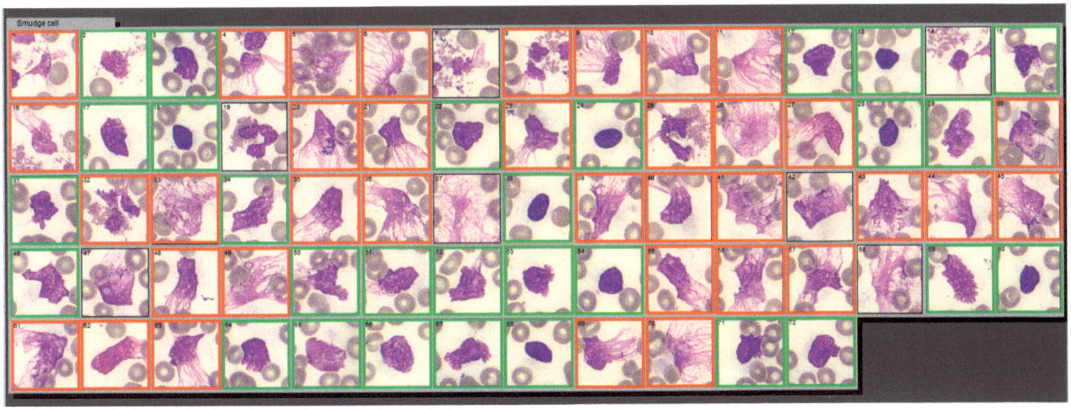

Figure 1. Example of Smudge Cell category in CellaVision® containing two distinct populations of cell derived entities: NET-like and DL-like smudge cells. This is a screenshot of Smudge Cell category from Cellavision® illustrating examples morphological differences between degenerating lymphocytes (green square) and NET-like smudge cells (red square). NET-like smudge cells are characterized by lack of discernible plasma membrane, no intact cytoplasm, dispersed granules, and polarized chromatin projections that resemble spider webs. Cellular entities that we were not able to classify as DL or NET-like were left without outline. Images are captured with a 100× magnification lens.

3.3. Sysmex WNR Scattergram Can Detect Differences in Nucleic Acid Content within WBC

To further differentiate between DL-like and NET-like SC we evaluated samples with ≤5% SC, ≥20% SC with majority morphologic NET-like SC, and ≥20% SC majority with majority morphologic DL. WNR scattergram of samples with ≤5% SC had low-to-no signal at medium FSC (size) and high SFL (nucleic acid) areas (Figure 2, panel A). Samples with ≥20% DL-like SC had a distinct pattern with a strong and broad signal at higher-than-expected FSC, yet a low-to-intermediate signal in the high SFL region (compared to the samples with ≥20% NET-like SC) (Figure 2, panel B). This pattern was characteristic to samples of patients with lymphocytosis, mainly secondary to CLL. This pattern has been described by others as prolymphocytic cell clusters that form an "inverted comma" with high FSC in the WNR scattergram in chronic lymphoproliferative disorders [23]. Scattergrams of samples with ≥20% majority NET-like SC had visibly higher SFL signals within the expected FSC range for WBC (Figure 2, panel C). This further confirms that the SC category does contain two separate populations of cells: one with cells with increased nucleic acid contents and sizes comparable to WBC—likely representing NETs—and the second with cells without increased nucleic acid contents but with likely increased clumping that is represented by a large size range—likely representing increased numbers of fragile lymphocytes turning into smudge cells during smearing (hence ≥20% SC) but staying intact during flow cytometry.

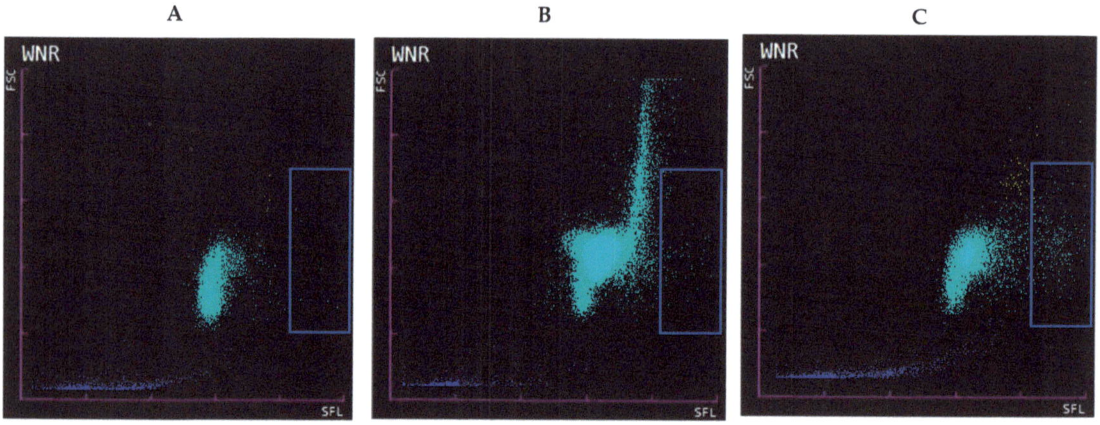

Figure 2. Sysmex WNR scattergram. WNR scattergram of EDTA-whole blood samples of hospitalized patients (**A**). Sample with ≤5% SC showing low signal in the high SFL area (blue box representing suspected NET area). (**B**). Sample with ≥20% majority DL-like SC with wide range of FSC and low-to-intermediate signal in the suspected NET area/high SFL. Such pattern is seen in samples with marked lymphocytosis secondary to CLL, high SFL signal is absent as fragile lymphocytes turn into smudge cells during smearing but stay intact during flow cytometry (**C**). Sample with ≥20% SC containing majority NET-like SC with FSC (size) within expected range for WBC but high SFL (nucleic acid content).

3.4. Identification by Immunohistochemistry: Samples with Majority NETs-like SC Stain Positively with for LAP, MPO, and NE

To further confirm our ability to identify NETs within the SC category, we assessed the cell of origin for NET-like and DL-like SC in samples with >20% SC. Twenty EDTA whole blood samples with >20% SC identified on CellaVision®, 10 with mostly NET-like SC and 10 with mostly DL-like SC, were selected for staining with LAP and blinded scoring. The samples with majority NET-like SC had LAP score of 172.1 and those with DL-like SC had a score of 103.3, $p < 0.00087$. Slides from patients with documented SC LAP scores were stained for MPO and NE; the NET-like SC cases stained strongly for MPO and NE (Figure 3).

3.5. Identification by Flow Cytometry: Samples with Majority NET-like SC Contain Surface MPO and CD66b

To confirm the two groups within SC category that we identified using routinely available WNR scattergram and morphologic identification, we used flow cytometry to further characterize our populations. We used surface DNA (Sytox), CD45, MPO, and CD66b staining to identify SC and SC subtypes. Samples with ≤5% SC by CellaVision® were usually negative by Sytox green while samples with ≥20% SC were positive. Sytox green positive cells were also positive for CD45, affirming that SC are of WBC origin. Surface MPO and CD66b within this Sytox+, CD45+ population was positive only in those samples with high NET-like SC but not in samples with high DL-like SC. This again affirms that the SC category contains both cells of neutrophil (Sytox green+/CD45+/MPO+/CD66b+) and lymphocyte origin (Sytox green+/CD45+/MPO-/CD66b−). This is demonstrated in Figure 4.

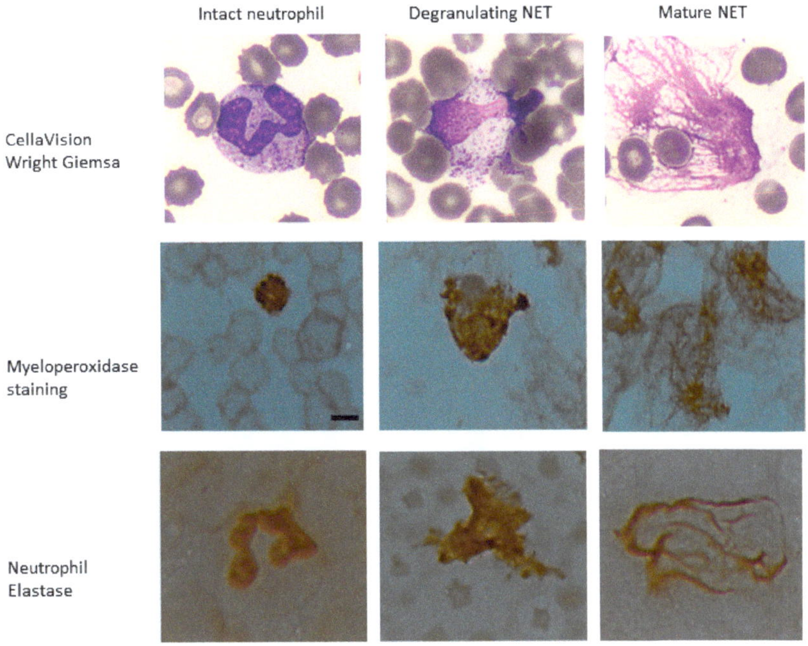

Figure 3. Myeloperoxidase and neutrophil elastase staining of samples with high LAP score. Peripheral blood samples with ≥20% NET-like smudge cells were stained and scored for leukocyte alkaline phosphatase (LAP). These samples also stained positive for neutrophil specific markers myeloperoxidase (MPO) and neutrophil elastase (NE) in intact neutrophils as well as degranulating neutrophils with features of nuclear decondensation and NET-like cells with web-like projections expressing myeloperoxidase and neutrophil elastase. Scale bar = 10 μm.

3.6. NET-like SC Are Not an Artifact of Specimen Handing

Compared to the standard smear preparation technique, neither larger or smaller angles nor increased smearing pressure resulted in greater numbers of NET-like SC ($p = 0.14$ for angle and $p = 0.07$ for pressure). When subjected to prolonged incubation times, EDTA-whole blood specimens did not develop increased number of NET-like SC ($p = 0.09$), although some vacuolation and expansion of WBC cytoplasm was observed (Figure 5, top row).

3.7. Induced NETs Have the Same Appearance as NET-like SC on CellaVision® and Produce the Same Signal on WNR Scattergram

PMA, LPS, and Ionomycin were used to determine whether NETs could be induced in routinely collected EDTA-whole blood specimens (Figure 5). In samples incubated with PMA, LPS, and Ionomycin up to 24 h, we observed vacuolation within the leukocyte cytoplasm, followed by congestion and decondensation of the nuclei. Neutrophil degranulation and ejection of chromatin and nuclear material was observed as early as 30 min and continued for up to 8 h. After 6 h of incubation, most neutrophils converted into SC, morphologically resembling NETs. Further expansion of the extracellular nuclear material and chromatin was observed up to 24 h. After 24 h, many of the neutrophil remnants disappeared. Following the stimulation of whole blood with PMA, morphologically identified induced NETs stained strongly with Sytox green, MPO, and citrullinated histone H3 (Figures 6–8).

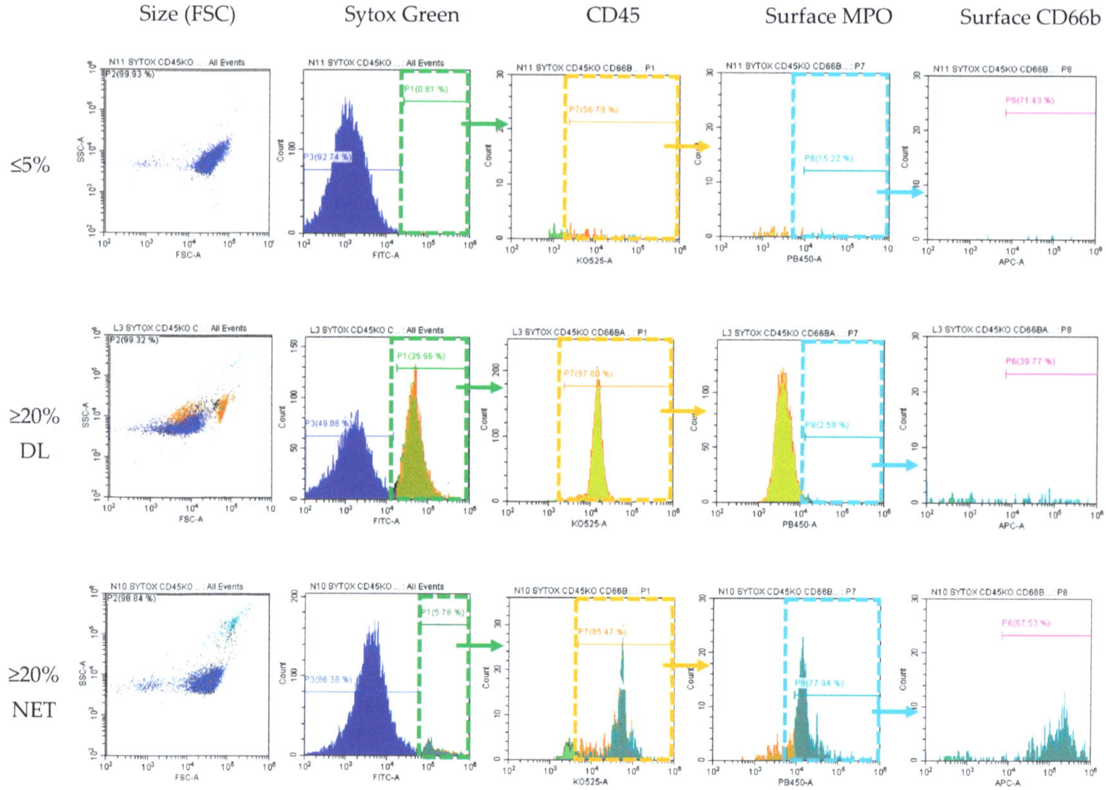

Figure 4. Flow cytometry to differentiate NETs vs. Degenerated Lymphocytes. Soft spin buffy coat samples were incubated unpermeabilized with antibodies for Sytox (surface DNA dye), CD45 (WBC marker K0525), surface MPO (PB450), surface CD66b (APC, marker for activated neutrophils). Sytox green positive cells were serially gated for CD45, then MPO, and then CD66b. Cells from sample with ≤5% SC did not express surface DNA and thus were negative for all subsequent gating. Cells from samples ≥20%SC with morphologically identified majority degenerated lymphocytes stain positive for Sytox+ and CD45+ but negative for MPO- and CD66b- (this population was back-gated and highlighted as orange in the SSC vs. FSC dot plot). Cells from samples ≥20%SC morphologically identified as majority NETs stain positive for all surface markers: Sytox+/CD45+/MPO+/CD66b+ (this population was back-gated and highlighted as cyan in the SSC vs. FSC dot plot). Note the difference in size and granulation between DL and NET-like SC.

WNR scattergrams of PMA stimulated EDTA-whole blood samples (definitively containing NETs) demonstrated signal in the same area of WNR scattergram as seen in samples with ≥20% NET-like SC. These changes in the scattergram were observed as early as 30 min, and events in the large SFL area continuously increased up to two hours (Figure 9). This further affirms the identification of a NETs area in high SFL but moderate FSC on the WNR scattergram (Figure 9, blue rectangle).

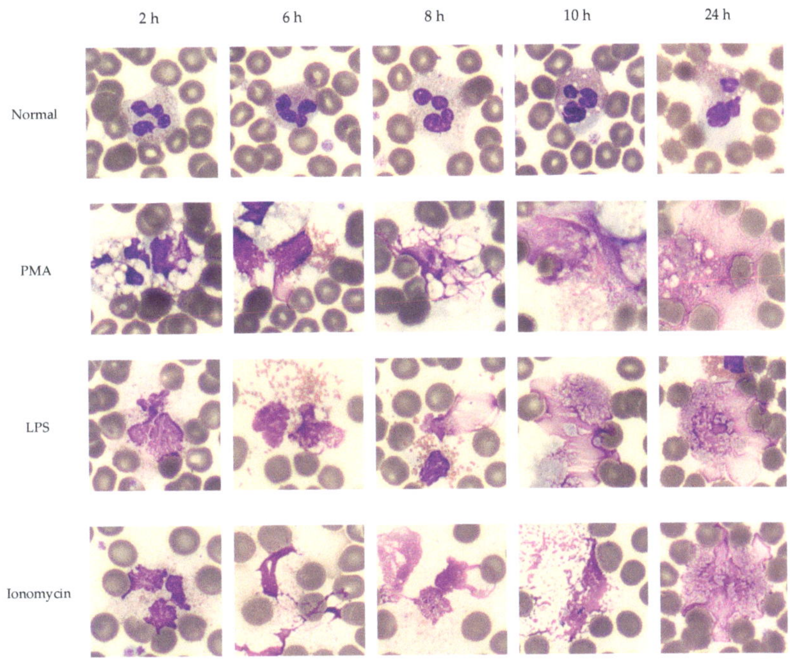

Figure 5. Effect of time on NET formation in EDTA-whole blood samples. NET formation was induced with classic triggers (PMA, LPS, Ionomycin) in EDTA whole blood from normal donors. Smears were prepared at 2, 6, 8, 10 and 24 h. WBC manual differential was performed by CellaVision® to capture NETs at different stages within the smudge cell population. NET formation followed a canonical order of morphological changes: vacuolation, nuclear decondensation, degranulation, chromatin ejection and protrusions. Images are captured with a 100× magnification lens.

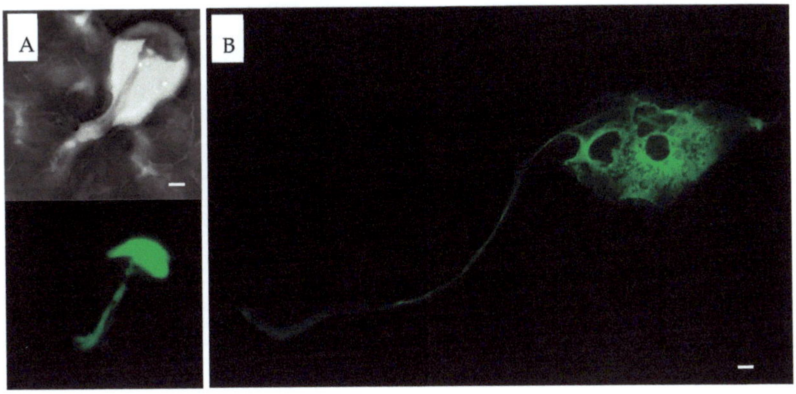

Figure 6. Sytox green staining of PMA induced NETs. EDTA-whole blood samples stimulated with PMA stained with Sytox green dye. (**A**). At 2 h, NET formation extracellular projection is seen on the hematoxylin stain (top, brightfield, grayscale). Sytox green highlights DNA projection from the center of the NET (bottom). (**B**). At 3 h, thin DNA projection as well as center of the NET are visualized with Sytox green stain. Scale bar = 10 μm.

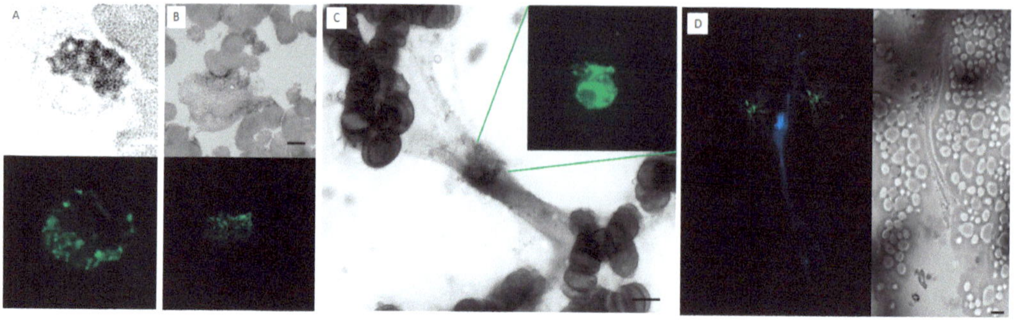

Figure 7. MPO staining of PMA induced NETs. EDTA-whole blood samples stimulated with PMA to induce NETs were stained with hematoxylin dye (brightfield, grayscale images) and MPO (fluorescent green images) at 45 min, 2 h, and 3.5 h. (**A**) At 45 min, MPO is confined within the neutrophil. (**B**) At 2 h NET formation is visible under hematoxylin stain and MPO is seen outside of cellular bounds. (**C**) At 3.5 h, on hematoxylin stain, mature NET is visualized with DNA projections extending from the center which stains strongly for MPO. (**D**) At 3.5 h MPO (fluorescent green) is seen located centrally and extending peripherally within the NET DNA projections positive for DAPI stain (fluorescent blue). Discoid, round cells in the periphery and near the scale bars are red blood cells, some forming rouleaux due to the fixation and smearing. Scale bar = 10 μm.

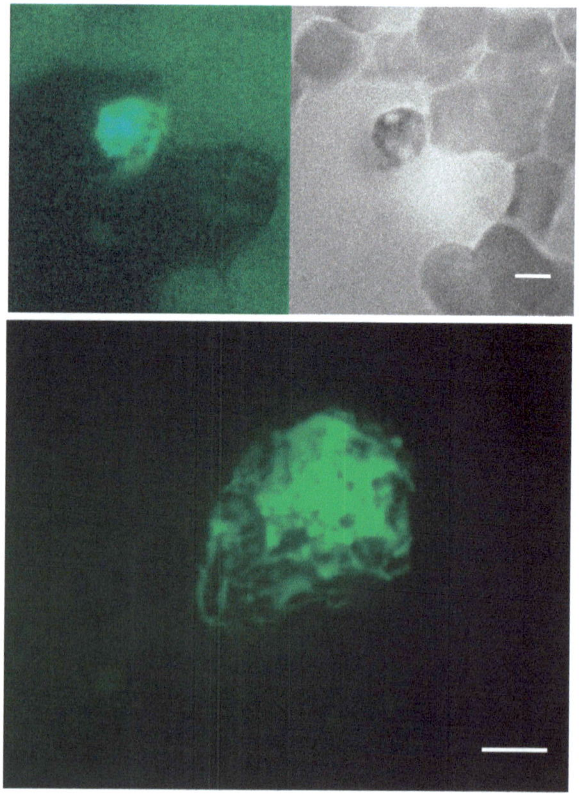

Figure 8. Citrullinated Histone3 staining of PMA induced NETs. EDTA-whole blood stimulated with PMA stained for citrullinated histone. Scale bar = 10 μm.

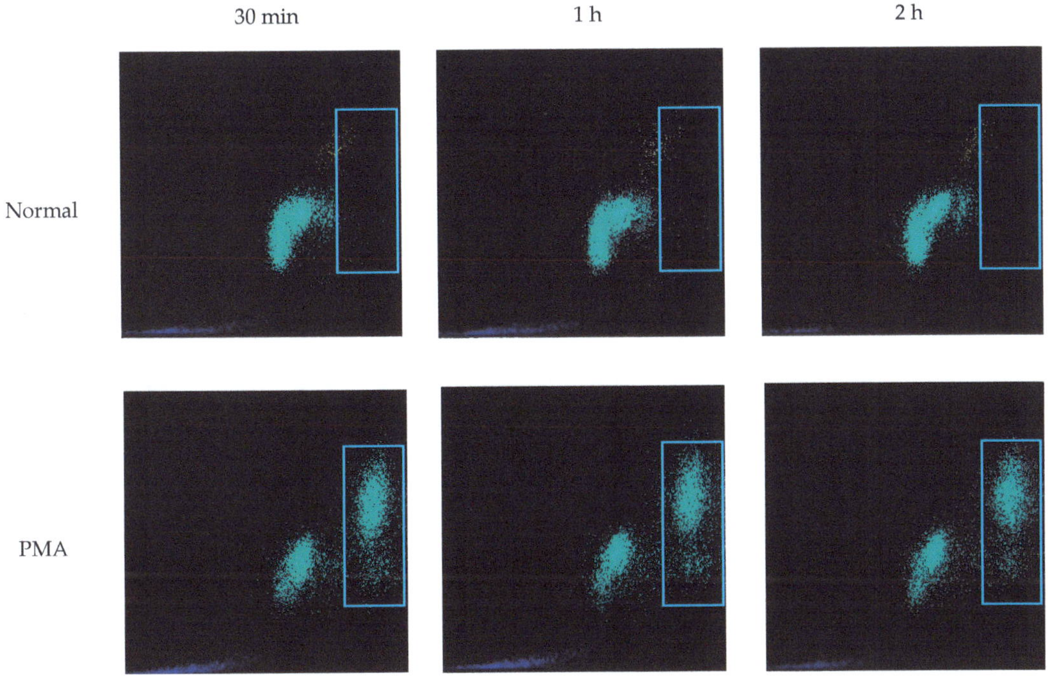

Figure 9. WNR scattergrams of PMA stimulated EDTA-whole blood samples. EDTA-whole blood samples from healthy donors were incubated with PMA to induce NETs. After 2 **h** of incubation the normal sample (no PMA added) did not have increased signal in the region of high nucleic acid content (SFL, blue rectangle). Blood samples stimulated with PMA developed progressively increasing signal at the region of high SFL. In the PMA-induced sample, as the intensity of signal in the high SFL region increased the signal for WBC cells decreased suggesting that a proportion of WBCs evolved into NETs and were now detected in high SFL region.

3.8. % SC in EDTA Whole Blood Correlates with Presence of Infections

We reviewed the electronic medical records of 200 patients with $\leq$5% and 194 patients with $\geq$20% SC on CellaVision®. As shown in Table 1, 50.5% patients with $\geq$20% SC had infections, as compared to 31.5% patients with $\leq$5% SC, $p < 0.001$. This increase was true for both bacterial ($p = 0.034$) and viral infections ($p < 0.001$). The XN scattergrams of samples with $\geq$20% SC had a significantly higher signal in the area representing high nucleic acid content than scattergrams of samples with $\leq$5% SC, 1.6 [0.67, 3.3]) vs. 0.69 [0.29, 1.7], respectively ($p < 0.001$), suggesting the presence of NETs.

Table 1. Infection rates in samples with <5% SC and >20% SC.

	Control ($\leq$5% SC) (n = 200)	**High SC ($\geq$20% SC) (n = 194)**	p
Female, n (%)	108 (54.0)	103 (53.1)	0.94
Age, median [IQR]	59.9 [46.1, 69.7]	59.3 [41.1, 70.7]	0.64
% Smudge Cells (SC), median [IQR]	2.6 [1.7, 3.5]	33.0 [24.5, 45.7]	
WBC $\times$ 10^9/L, median [IQR]	8.7 [4.60, 14.7]	7.3 [3.7, 14.3]	0.14
XN Scattergram NETs area, median [IQR]	0.69 [0.29, 1.7]	1.6 [0.67, 3.3]	<0.001

Table 1. *Cont.*

	Control (≤5% SC) (n = 200)	High SC (≥20% SC) (n = 194)	*p*
Patients with infections *, n (%)	63 (31.5)	98 (50.5)	<0.001
Bacterial infections, n (%)	44 (22.0)	62 (32.0)	0.034
Viral infections, excluding HIV, n (%)	20 (10.0)	51 (26.3)	<0.001
Acute viral infection **, n (%)	15 (7.5)	29 (14.9)	0.029
Chronic viral infection ***, n (%)	7 (3.5)	22 (11.3)	0.005
HIV ****, n (%)	10 (5.0)	14 (7.2)	0.48

* Each patient could have more than one infection, ** excluding HIV, EBV, CMV, HCV, HBV, *** CMV, EBV, HCV, HBV, **** HIV not included in total number of infections.

4. Discussion

NETs represent one of neutrophil's defense mechanisms against septic and sterile inflammatory states [1–3,8,10]. They migrate to infected or inflamed tissues and have been identified within parenchyma of the affected organs [24]. Nevertheless, a quick, reliable, and clinically meaningful identification method for circulating NETs has not been developed. In addition to the use of immunohistochemistry for the direct visualization of NETs, studies also report using surrogate markers such as cell-free DNA, MPO-DNA complexes, citrullinated histones C3, neutrophil elastase, and cathelicidin antimicrobial peptides [13–16]. Additionally, the presence of serologic NET markers has been correlated to increased SFL signals on Sysmex WDF scattergrams in patients with both acute and chronic inflammatory states [18,20].

A possible explanation for the lack of reliable visualization techniques of circulating NETs is that they are difficult to identify without using NET specific stains and markers, which have not been integrated into clinical practices and are not readily available in strictly clinical settings. On digital images of peripheral smears generated by CellaVision®, at first glance, NETs resemble the classic smudged lymphocytes seen in peripheral smears of patients with CLL. Upon closer inspection, they differ from these lymphocytes in size and by their intricate network of fine extracellular projections. With the advent of digital imaging systems for morphological WBC differential and quantification, such as the CellaVision®, we observed that the SC category contains two distinct entities: degenerated lymphocytes and cell remnants resembling NETs. Such an observation opens up a new quick, easy, and readily available avenue for NET identification. To investigate this further, we developed a set of experiments to characterize these NET-like smudge cells.

Samples classified as normal by Sysmex had on average 4.3% SC. Typical lymphocyte smudge cells, as seen in patients with CLL, are a product of smear preparation, nevertheless we did not see a significant increase in NET-like SC when we altered specimen storage conditions and slide preparation technique. As described in prior studies, nucleic acid content of WBC represented by side scatter on WDF Sysmex scattergrams correlates with NET markers [18,20]. In our study, we used the WNR scattergram to show that samples with high contents of NET-like SC also had a unique signal that localized to the high SFL and moderate FSC area. Samples of patients with CLL, expected to have smudge cells, did not have this distinct pattern on the WNR scattergram. To further confirm our ability to differentiate between NETs and DL within the SC category we used LAP staining and flow cytometry. Both techniques confirmed that NET-like SC are of neutrophil origin. Samples with ≥20% NET-like SC stained strongly for LAP, MPO, and NE by immunohistochemistry and on flow cytometry were positive for surface DNA, CD45, MPO, and CD66b which is a marker of neutrophil activation that is upregulated during NETosis [24].

Identification of NETs is further complicated by their dynamic morphology. On digital peripheral smears of CellaVision® we observed many morphologically distinct forms of NET-like SC. We hypothesize that these might represent different stages of NET formation and maturation. To test this, we developed an in-vitro model to study the morphological changes of neutrophils during NET formation using PMA, LPS, and Ionomycin. Using these triggers, we observed changes in neutrophils including vacuolation, nuclear decompensation and development of spider-web like projections in as early as 30 min. These changes were captured by the CellaVision® and appeared similar to some of the NET-like SC seen in unmanipulated EDTA whole blood samples. NETs induced in peripheral blood samples with PMA, LPS, and Ionomycin resulted in a signal similar on the WNR scattergram to that produced by samples with $\geq$20% NET-like SC.

To apply our findings clinically, we correlated % SC with the presence of documented bacterial and viral infections in hospitalized patients. When compared to patients with $\leq$5% SC, those with $\geq$20% SC have a significantly higher incidence of infections within 10 days of specimen collection. WNR scattergrams of samples with $\geq$20% SC display a strong signal in the high SFL area of the WNR scattergram—a pattern unique to samples induced with NET triggers. This suggests that patients with high %SC identified by CellaVision® may have an underlying inflammatory process driving NETosis. This study was limited to studying the correlation between % NET-like SC and infections and the sample size was not sufficiently powered to study the association of NET-like SC in other non-infectious diseases and conditions. Nonetheless, NETosis has been associated with many non-infectious conditions including cancer, thrombosis, autoimmune disorders, and chronic metabolic disorders [8,25–29]. Future studies are needed to establish the association of NET-like SC with these conditions. With the availability of automated and digitized blood cell differential count becoming routine not only in hospitals but also in community-based clinics, a pragmatic, fast, and cost-effective screen tool such as the one described herein has potential for wide applications and the early detection of NETosis in multiple diseases and disorders.

5. Conclusions

In this article, we propose that the smudge cell category of CellaVision® likely contains two distinct populations of leukocytes: degenerated lymphocytes and NETs. NET-like smudge cells are not an artifact of smear preparation, are identified in the high SFL area of the WNR scattergram, and express neutrophil markers identifiable on immunohistochemistry and flow cytometry. In hospitalized patients, the percentage of smudge cells correlated with infections. The identification of NETs on digital images of peripheral blood smears generated by routinely used automated hematology systems such as CellaVision® offers an easy, fast, cost-effective approach with a variety of possible clinical applications and potentially an early marker for infections.

6. Patents

Identifying neutrophil extracellular traps in biological samples: US20220254015A1, Publication Date: 11 August 2022.

Author Contributions: Conceptualization, K.F., D.Y., M.K., H.H.B. and M.R.G.; methodology, K.F., D.Y., M.K., H.H.B., M.B. and M.R.G.; software, M.B., D.Y., K.F., M.B., H.H.B., M.R.G.; validation, K.F., D.Y., M.K., M.B. and M.R.G.; formal analysis, K.F., D.Y., H.H.B., M.B. and M.R.G.; investigation, K.F., D.Y., H.H.B., M.B. and M.R.G.; resources, H.H.B., M.B. and M.R.G.; data curation, K.F., D.Y., H.H.B., M.B. and M.R.G.; writing—original draft preparation, K.F., H.H.B., M.B. and M.R.G.; writing—review and editing, K.F., M.K., H.H.B., M.B. and M.R.G.; visualization, K.F., M.K., H.H.B., M.B. and M.R.G.; supervision, H.H.B. and M.R.G.; project administration, H.H.B. and M.R.G.; funding acquisition, H.H.B. and M.R.G. All authors have read and agreed to the published version of the manuscript.

Funding: This research received no external funding.

Institutional Review Board Statement: The study was conducted according to the guidelines of the Declaration of Helsinki and approved by the Institutional Review Board of Albert Einstein College of Medicine (protocol 2020-11393; date of approval 18 May 2018).

Informed Consent Statement: Patient consent was waived given the nature of the retrospective design, the specimens were anonymized, and the study was deemed as minimal risk since all identifiers were removed.

Data Availability Statement: The data presented in this study are available on request from the corresponding author.

Conflicts of Interest: The authors declare no conflict of interest.

References

1. Manda, A.; Pruchniak, M.P.; Arazna, M.; Demkow, U.A. Neutrophil extracellular traps in physiology and pathology. *Cent. Eur. J. Immunol.* **2014**, *39*, 116–121. [CrossRef] [PubMed]
2. Papayannopoulos, V. Neutrophil extracellular traps in immunity and disease. *Nat. Rev. Immunol.* **2018**, *18*, 134–147. [CrossRef]
3. McDonald, B.; Urrutia, R.; Yipp, B.G.; Jenne, C.N.; Kubes, P. Intravascular neutrophil extracellular traps capture bacteria from the bloodstream during sepsis. *Cell Host Microbe* **2012**, *12*, 324–333. [CrossRef]
4. Camicia, G.; Pozner, R.; de Larranaga, G. Neutrophil extracellular traps in sepsis. *Shock* **2014**, *42*, 286–294. [CrossRef]
5. Brinkmann, V.; Reichard, U.; Goosmann, C.; Fauler, B.; Uhlemann, Y.; Weiss, D.S.; Weinrauch, Y.; Zychlinsky, A. Neutrophil extracellular traps kill bacteria. *Science* **2004**, *303*, 1532–1535. [CrossRef] [PubMed]
6. Jorgensen, I.; Rayamajhi, M.; Miao, E.A. Programmed cell death as a defence against infection. *Nat. Rev. Immunol.* **2017**, *17*, 151–164. [CrossRef] [PubMed]
7. de Oliveira, S.; Rosowski, E.E.; Huttenlocher, A. Neutrophil migration in infection and wound repair: Going forward in reverse. *Nat. Rev. Immunol.* **2016**, *16*, 378–391. [CrossRef]
8. Demers, M.; Wagner, D.D. NETosis: A new factor in tumor progression and cancer-associated thrombosis. *Semin. Thromb. Hemost.* **2014**, *40*, 277–283. [CrossRef] [PubMed]
9. Alasmari, S.Z. In Vivo Imaging of Neutrophil Extracellular Traps (NETs): Visualization Methods and Outcomes. *Biomed. Res. Int.* **2020**, *2020*, 4192745. [CrossRef]
10. Brill, A.; Fuchs, T.A.; Savchenko, A.S.; Thomas, G.M.; Martinod, K.; De Meyer, S.F.; Bhandari, A.A.; Wagner, D.D. Neutrophil extracellular traps promote deep vein thrombosis in mice. *J. Thromb. Haemost.* **2012**, *10*, 136–144. [CrossRef]
11. Gavillet, M.; Martinod, K.; Renella, R.; Harris, C.; Shapiro, N.I.; Wagner, D.D.; Williams, D.A. Flow cytometric assay for direct quantification of neutrophil extracellular traps in blood samples. *Am. J. Hematol.* **2015**, *90*, 1155–1158. [CrossRef]
12. Kolaczkowska, E.; Jenne, C.N.; Surewaard, B.G.; Thanabalasuriar, A.; Lee, W.Y.; Sanz, M.J.; Mowen, K.; Opdenakker, G.; Kubes, P. Molecular mechanisms of NET formation and degradation revealed by intravital imaging in the liver vasculature. *Nat. Commun.* **2015**, *6*, 6673. [CrossRef]
13. Margraf, S.; Logters, T.; Reipen, J.; Altrichter, J.; Scholz, M.; Windolf, J. Neutrophil-derived circulating free DNA (cf-DNA/NETs): A potential prognostic marker for posttraumatic development of inflammatory second hit and sepsis. *Shock* **2008**, *30*, 352–358. [CrossRef]
14. Donkel, S.J.; Wolters, F.J.; Ikram, M.A.; de Maat, M.P.M. Circulating Myeloperoxidase (MPO)-DNA complexes as marker for Neutrophil Extracellular Traps (NETs) levels and the association with cardiovascular risk factors in the general population. *PLoS ONE* **2021**, *16*, e0253698. [CrossRef]
15. Smith, P.; Rosell, A.; Farm, M.; Bruzelius, M.; Aguilera Gatica, K.; Mackman, N.; Odeberg, J.; Thalin, C. Markers of neutrophil activation and neutrophil extracellular traps in diagnosing patients with acute venous thromboembolism: A feasibility study based on two VTE cohorts. *PLoS ONE* **2022**, *17*, e0270865. [CrossRef]
16. Chen, X.Q.; Tu, L.; Tang, Q.; Huang, L.; Qin, Y.H. An Emerging Role for Neutrophil Extracellular Traps in IgA Vasculitis: A Mini-Review. *Front. Immunol.* **2022**, *13*, 912929. [CrossRef]
17. Middleton, E.A.; He, X.Y.; Denorme, F.; Campbell, R.A.; Ng, D.; Salvatore, S.P.; Mostyka, M.; Baxter-Stoltzfus, A.; Borczuk, A.C.; Loda, M.; et al. Neutrophil extracellular traps contribute to immunothrombosis in COVID-19 acute respiratory distress syndrome. *Blood* **2020**, *136*, 1169–1179. [CrossRef]
18. Stiel, L.; Mayeur-Rousse, C.; Helms, J.; Meziani, F.; Mauvieux, L. First visualization of circulating neutrophil extracellular traps using cell fluorescence during human septic shock-induced disseminated intravascular coagulation. *Thromb. Res.* **2019**, *183*, 153–158. [CrossRef]
19. Domer, D.; Walther, T.; Moller, S.; Behnen, M.; Laskay, T. Neutrophil Extracellular Traps Activate Proinflammatory Functions of Human Neutrophils. *Front. Immunol.* **2021**, *12*, 636954. [CrossRef]
20. Stiel, L.; Delabranche, X.; Galoisy, A.C.; Severac, F.; Toti, F.; Mauvieux, L.; Meziani, F.; Boisrame-Helms, J. Neutrophil Fluorescence: A New Indicator of Cell Activation During Septic Shock-Induced Disseminated Intravascular Coagulation. *Crit. Care Med.* **2016**, *44*, e1132–e1136. [CrossRef]
21. Sysmex America, Inc. *Multispecies Hematology Analyzers XN-V SERIES TM*; Sysmex America, Inc.: Kobe, Japan, 2019.

22. Marionneaux, S.M.; Keohane, E.M.; Lamanna, N.; King, T.C.; Mehta, S.R. Smudge Cells in Chronic Lymphocytic Leukemia: Pathophysiology, Laboratory Considerations, and Clinical Significance. *Lab. Med.* **2021**, *52*, 426–438. [CrossRef] [PubMed]
23. Ningombam, A.; Abhirup, S.; Kumar, K.; Chopra, A. Scattergram patterns of hematological malignancies on sysmex XN-series analyzer. *J. Appl. Hematol.* **2021**, *12*, 83–89.
24. Kinnare, N.; Hook, J.S.; Patel, P.A.; Monson, N.L.; Moreland, J.G. Neutrophil Extracellular Trap Formation Potential Correlates with Lung Disease Severity in COVID-19 Patients. *Inflammation* **2022**, *45*, 800–811. [CrossRef] [PubMed]
25. Chen, K.; Shao, L.H.; Wang, F.; Shen, X.F.; Xia, X.F.; Kang, X.; Song, P.; Wang, M.; Lu, X.F.; Wang, C.; et al. Netting Gut Disease: Neutrophil Extracellular Trap in Intestinal Pathology. *Oxid. Med. Cell Longev.* **2021**, *2021*, 5541222. [CrossRef] [PubMed]
26. Chen, C.; Huang, T.; Zhai, X.; Ma, Y.; Xie, L.; Lu, B.; Zhang, Y.; Li, Y.; Chen, Z.; Yin, J.; et al. Targeting neutrophils as a novel therapeutic strategy after stroke. *J. Cereb. Blood Flow Metab.* **2021**, *41*, 2150–2161. [CrossRef]
27. Fuchs, T.A.; Brill, A.; Wagner, D.D. Neutrophil extracellular trap (NET) impact on deep vein thrombosis. *Arter. Thromb. Vasc. Biol.* **2012**, *32*, 1777–1783. [CrossRef]
28. Herre, M.; Cedervall, J.; Mackman, N.; Olsson, A.K. Neutrophil extracellular traps in the pathology of cancer and other inflammatory diseases. *Physiol. Rev.* **2023**, *103*, 277–312. [CrossRef]
29. Shao, B.Z.; Yao, Y.; Li, J.P.; Chai, N.L.; Linghu, E.Q. The Role of Neutrophil Extracellular Traps in Cancer. *Front. Oncol.* **2021**, *11*, 714357. [CrossRef]

life

MDPI

Article

Modelling of Tissue Invasion in Epithelial Monolayers

Faris Saad Alsubaie [1], Hamid Khataee [1,2] and Zoltan Neufeld [1,*]

[1] School of Mathematics and Physics, The University of Queensland, Brisbane, QLD 4072, Australia
[2] Australian Bureau of Statistics, Brisbane, QLD 4000, Australia
* Correspondence: z.neufeld@uq.edu.au

Abstract: Mathematical and computational models are used to describe biomechanical processes in multicellular systems. Here, we develop a model to analyse how two types of epithelial cell layers interact during tissue invasion depending on their cellular properties, i.e., simulating cancer cells expanding into a region of normal cells. We model the tissue invasion process using the cellular Potts model and implement our two-dimensional computational simulations in the software package CompuCell3D. The model predicts that differences in mechanical properties of cells can lead to tissue invasion, even if the division rates and death rates of the two cell types are the same. We also show how the invasion speed varies depending on the cell division and death rates and the mechanical properties of the cells.

Keywords: cell competition; cellular Potts model; invasion; travelling wave

check for updates

Citation: Alsubaie, F.S.; Khataee, H.; Neufeld, Z. Modelling of Tissue Invasion in Epithelial Monolayers. *Life* **2023**, *13*, 427. https://doi.org/10.3390/life13020427

Academic Editor: Gerhard A. Holzapfel

Received: 24 November 2022
Revised: 20 January 2023
Accepted: 31 January 2023
Published: 2 February 2023

1. Introduction

A challenging question in developmental biology and cancer research is how cellular properties influence cell competition in epithelial tissues, which is crucial in normal tissue development and elimination of transformed precancerous cells [1–4]. Epithelial cell layers line organs throughout the body [5] and play important roles in tissue and organ development, yet account for about 90% of all cancers [6]. In cell competition, normal and mutant cell populations with different properties compete with each other at their interface for survival, where the winner cells invade and occupy the space held by the loser cells, which are eventually eliminated [1–3,7]. A key question is how this competition process is influenced by the cellular interactions and properties. Answers to this question can provide new information in the development of cancer treatments and regenerative medicine [2].

Theoretical models are ideal tools to assess the main mechanisms of the competitive cell invasion phenomenon [8]. Various models have been developed to study the cell competition process, including differential equations of predator–prey interactions [7,9], continuous mechanical models of cell proliferation and death [4,10], the vertex model of the evolution of cell turnover and local topology dynamics [11], and the cellular Potts model (CPM) of regulation of mechanical contact-dependent competition [12]. However, it remains elusive how cellular properties affect the speed of cell competition in which winner cells occupy the space following loser cells' apoptosis.

To fill this gap, we propose a computational model to analyse how different properties of epithelial cells determine the speed of competitive invasion. The model represents the generation and progress of the cell invasion process in a generic epithelial layer due to various differences in the cell parameters. In principle, such differences may arise due to mutations characteristic of cancer cells within the resident population that may lead to invasion of resident cells by the modified cell type. The proposed model is based on the CPM [13], a computational modelling framework that enables the simulation of epithelial cell dynamics (e.g., cell shape and cell–cell interactions), while being computationally and conceptually simpler than most off-lattice models (e.g., vertex model) [14–17]. The model simulates the competition between two cell populations with different properties. Cell shapes and interactions evolve according to the Potts energy model. Cell proliferation and death events are associated with mechanical properties of cells and modelled as stochastic events. The modelling results are discussed in the context of experiments and other theoretical studies.

This paper is organised as follows. Section 2 presents the development of the model. This section first presents how the dynamics of cellular shapes and interactions between cells are modelled. It also describes modelling cell proliferation and death processes. In Section 3, the computational results are presented and discussed. First we investigate the equilibrium state of a single cell type as a function of the parameters, then we analyse competition between cell types that differ either in their turnover rates or bio-mechanical properties. Finally, results are discussed in context with earlier findings, followed by potential future research directions.

2. Model Description

To model the effect of cellular properties on epithelial cell invasion, we propose a two-dimensional computational model that represents the competition of two cell types within an epithelial monolayer. The model is based on the CPM such that cells are represented on a lattice, where each cell covers a set of connected lattice sites (or pixels) and each pixel can only be occupied by one cell at a time.

The expansion and retraction of the cell contours is determined by stochastic minimisation of a phenomenological energy function [15,16,18–21]:

$$E = \lambda_{\text{area}} \sum_{\alpha=1}^{N} (A_\alpha - A_0)^2 + \lambda_{\text{cont}} \sum_{\alpha=1}^{N} L_\alpha^2 + \sum_{\vec{i},\vec{j}} \phi\left(\alpha_{\vec{i}}, \alpha_{\vec{j}}\right)\left(1 - \delta(\alpha_{\vec{i}}, \alpha_{\vec{j}})\right) \tag{1}$$

where A_α and L_α are the area and perimeter of each cell α, respectively, of N cells with indices $\alpha = 1, \ldots, \text{N}$. The first term represents preference of the cells to maintain a preferred area A_0, and λ_{area} is an area compressibility coefficient, which determines how easily cells can deviate from the preferred area. The second term describes the contractility of the cell perimeter, where the penalty parameter λ_{cont} represents cortical actomyosin contractility around the lateral cell membrane [22]. The last term represents cell–cell adhesion, mediated by adhesion molecules such as E-cadherin [23]. The parameters λ_{area}, λ_{cont}, and ϕ determine the relative contribution of mechanical properties of the cells to the energy function E, and thus to the configuration of cells in the monolayer. $\phi(\alpha_{\vec{i}}, \alpha_{\vec{j}})$ is the boundary energy cost at neighbouring lattice sites $\vec{i}$ and $\vec{j}$. The Kronecker δ function prevents counting pixels that belong to the same cell. When both lattice sites $\vec{i}$ and $\vec{j}$ correspond to cells, $\phi(\alpha_{\vec{i}}, \alpha_{\vec{j}}) = \lambda_{\text{adh}}$; otherwise when one or both lattice sites represent boundary walls surrounding the monolayer, the boundary energy cost ϕ is set to zero. Note that $\lambda_{\text{adh}} < 0$ to represent that cells preferentially expand their boundaries shared with neighbouring cells. This is, however, balanced by the contractility of the cell perimeter. In this paper, we use Equation (1) to model the effect of mechanical properties of cells on epithelial cell invasion in a two-dimensional space. This model considers a minimal set of parameters efficient for model analysis along with the cell proliferation and death rate parameters. The model can be extended to three-dimensional space for considering further properties, such as extracellular components [24].

A cell expands or shrinks following a stochastic series of elementary steps. The algorithm selects two adjacent lattice sites $\vec{i}$ and $\vec{j}$ that belong to different cells $\alpha_{\vec{i}} \neq \alpha_{\vec{j}}$. Then, it attempts to copy the cell index $\alpha_{\vec{i}}$ into the adjacent lattice site $\vec{j}$, which takes place with probability [25,26]:

$$P\left(\alpha_{\vec{i}} \longrightarrow \alpha_{\vec{j}}\right) = \begin{cases} 1 & \Delta E \leq 0 \\ e^{-\Delta E/T} & \Delta E > 0 \end{cases} \tag{2}$$

where ΔE is the change of energy in functional (1) due to this elementary step, and the temperature-like parameter T is a scaling factor that represents the magnitude of stochastic fluctuations in the model. Following our earlier works [15,16], we set $T = 50$ since it provides cell shapes in both the soft and hard regimes for various combinations of parameters in Equation (1). The time unit of the model is given by a Monte Carlo step (MCS) that corresponds to selecting every pixel site in the lattice once for a copy attempt described above [25]. Taken together, Equations (1) and (2) imply that cell configurations that increase the penalties in functional (1) are less likely to occur. Thus, the population of cells evolves through stochastic rearrangements in accordance with the biological factors incorporated into the effective energy function E.

To model the competition for space between two cell populations, it is also necessary to include a turnover of cells through stochastic cell birth and death events [9,12]. A crucial factor that regulates cell proliferation is cell growth factor [27,28], so that the probability of cell proliferation for individual cells increases with the cell area [29]. We therefore define cell proliferation as a stochastic event: at every MCS, a set of uniformly distributed random numbers in [0,1] are generated for each cell that reaches the target area (i.e., $A_\alpha \geq A_0$). If the random number is smaller than the cell division parameter B, the corresponding cell is divided into two cells each with area $\approx A_0/2$. Then, according to Equations (1) and (2), these two daughter cells grow and approach the target area A_0.

We model the cell death process using characteristics identified experimentally. Experiments have shown that during the death process of a cell, the cell cortical actin network, together with microtubule and intermediate filaments, become depolymerised [30,31], and the interactions of the cell with its neighbouring cells become disorganized [32], leading to the degradation of cellular components and the loss of cell volume (i.e., cell shrinkage) [32,33]. Accordingly, in our model, within every MCS, each cell can die with a probability M. The parameters of the dead cells are modified by setting the contractility and adhesion parameters to zero (i.e., $\lambda_{\text{cont}} = 0$ and $\lambda_{\text{adh}} = 0$). Also, the target area of the dead cell is set to zero ($A_0 = 0$), and the area compressibility is increased to $\lambda_{\text{area}} = 200$ so that the dead cell gradually shrinks and then disappears from the layer. Using computer simulations, we found that $\lambda_{\text{area}} = 200$ was sufficient to avoid the accumulation of a large number of partially compressed dead cells in the system over time.

We note that in a real tissue, cell division and death may be influenced by multiple factors, including signals from surrounding cells and interactions with the extracellular matrix. For simplicity, in this model we do not consider these factors, in order to focus on the main mechanisms determined by the competition for space of two cell types with different properties.

We implement computational simulations of the cell invasion model using the open-source software package CompuCell3D (CC3D) [25]. Each simulation starts with two cell types (each with 225 cells or 900 cells and different set of parameters) placed on a rectangular domain and separated by a barrier. In the initial condition, the area of each cell was set to the target area A_0, i.e., each cell occupies a square shaped area of 10×10 pixels. The simulation domain is surrounded by wall cells that prevent the cells from sticking to the lattice boundaries. The wall cells are excluded from participating in the pixel copies of the Potts model [34].

We run each simulation in three stages. First, cell death and division events are switched off, and the two cell types are separated by a barrier. In this stage, both cell types reach their equilibrium shapes according to their mechanical parameters in the energy function E. As was shown earlier, when the contractility λ_{cont} is high (or the cell–cell adhesion coefficient is low) the cells form quasi-polygonal approximately hexagonal shapes (hard regime) [18,19]. In the opposite case of low contractility, the cell shapes are more irregular, with strongly fluctuating dynamical boundaries (soft regime). This implies that the model takes into account both the shape and size of the cells in representing the invasion process. In the second stage of the cell invasion simulation, both cell death and division are allowed (according to the stochastic rules described above), while the two cell types remain separated by the barrier. During this stage, each cell type reaches their equilibrium density and the corresponding average cell size. The competition between the two cell types takes place in the third stage when the separating barrier is removed. The simulation of this stage is usually continued until one of the cell types disappears from the domain.

3. Results and Discussion

In order to calibrate the model parameters to represent a realistic epithelium, first we investigate the equilibrium state of a homogeneous monolayer composed of a single cell type. We analyse how the equilibrium cell density changes with the model parameters, such as the cell division and death probabilities and the mechanical parameters of the CPM energy function.

We then model cell competition with two different spatially separated cell types and examine how one cell type invades the region occupied by the other, depending on the model parameters. First, we will focus on competition between cells that have the same mechanical parameters but different biological properties, represented by the probabilities of cell division and death. Then we consider the case where competing cell types have the same cell turnover parameters but differ in their mechanical properties characterised by parameters in the energy function, such as cortex contractility, area compressibility, and cell–cell adhesion. Then, we will also model the cell competition of two cell types in case they have different biological and mechanical properties at the same time.

3.1. Homeostatic Equilibrium in a Homogeneous Cell Layer

To investigate how the model parameters affect the equilibrium cell density, we analyse the behaviour of a cell layer with a single cell type occupying the entire simulation domain. In the initial condition, the area of each cell was set to the target cell area $A_0 = 100$, and the domain size is 200×200 lattice sites, which is initially fully occupied by $N_0 = 400$ cells. The simulation parameters are listed in Table 1. Then, the CPM simulation is run until the total number of cells reaches a stationary state in which there is a dynamical equilibrium between the stochastic cell division and cell death processes. We checked that the domain size and cell numbers are sufficiently large so that the results of the simulations are robust and not affected by random fluctuations of individual cells.

We found that for all parameter values considered, the total number of cells at equilibrium is higher then the initial cell number N_0, corresponding to cells occupying the target area A_0. This means that the cells are slightly compressed at equilibrium, i.e., $\langle A_\sigma \rangle < A_0$, and therefore cell division is suppressed by crowding. However, random cell death events result in apoptotic shrinking cells extruded from the layer. This creates space for the neighbouring cells to grow and reach the target area, so that a cell division can take place in one of the neighbours of the dead cell.

We studied the parameter dependence of the equilibrium cell density. The numerical results show that the total number of cells at equilibrium increases with the cell mortality rate M; see Figure 1a. However, this is caused by the increasing number of dead cells within the layer that shrink over time and disappear, while the number of live cells decreases slightly with the death rate. The overall number of both live and dead cells is higher when the cell perimeter is more contractile (i.e., $\lambda_{\text{cont}} = 7$); see Figure 1a–c. Increasing cortex contractility, λ_{cont}, reduces stochastic fluctuations at the cell boundaries [15]. Therefore, in the neighbourhood of dead cells, the process of elimination of the dying cell becomes slower. In contrast, when live cells have softer boundaries (i.e., $\lambda_{\text{cont}} = 0.5$), they are more likely to change their shape and advance into the region occupied by a shrinking dead cell. This effect is more clear at lower area strain λ_{area}, where the cells area A_α can deviate more from the target cell area A_0. According to Equations (1) and (2), with strengthening λ_{area}, the cell area approaches A_0 more closely, slowing down the shrinkage of the dead cells; compare Figure 1a,c,e with Figure 1b,d,f.

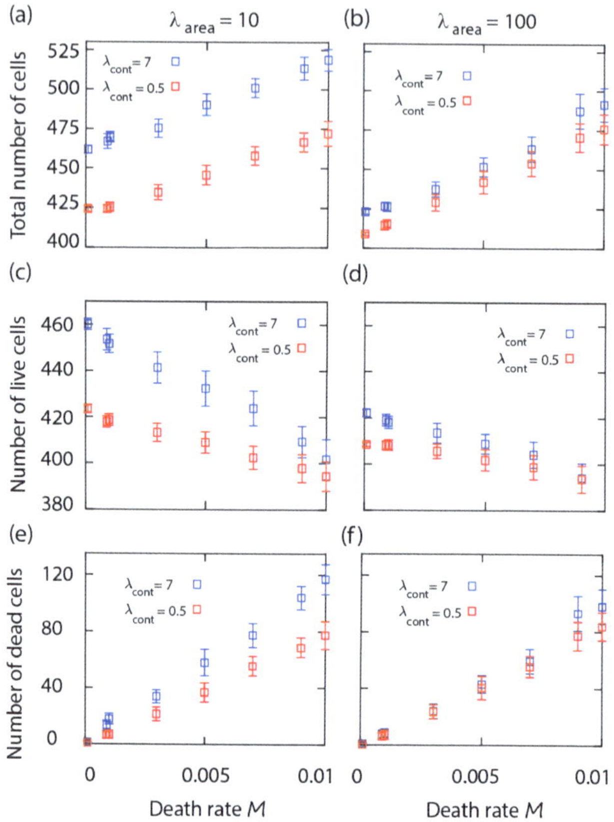

Figure 1. Number of cells at equilibrium in a cell sheet with single cell type versus cell mortality rate M. Total number of cells (top row), number of live cells (middle row), and number of dead cells (bottom row) versus M at cell area compressibility $\lambda_{area} = 10$ (**a**,**c**,**e**), 100 (**b**,**d**,**f**), and various cell perimeter contractility λ_{cont} (inset). Other simulation parameters: Birth rate $B = 0.03$ and $\lambda_{adh} = -10$ (see Movies S1–S4). Each symbol is derived from an individual simulation run and corresponds to mean ± SD calculated over time in the stationary state.

Table 1. Figure 1 parameters.

Parameter	Value
Domain size	200 × 200 pixels
Initial cells size	100 pixels
λ_{area}	100, 10
λ_{cont}	7, 0.5
λ_{adh}	−10
A_0	100 pixels
Number of cells	400
T	50
B	0.03
M	Variable

We also examined the variation of equilibrium cell density by altering the cell proliferation probability B. At small values of B, the equilibrium number of cells increases sharply and then saturates from around $B \approx 0.1$; see Figure 2a,c,d. Thus, the density is mostly unaffected by the cell division probability except when B is small. Note that in the $B \to 0$ limit, there is no well-defined equilibrium between the birth and death processes so the change around a small B may be due to very long transients. Similarly to the results in Figure 1, the cell density increases with the cell perimeter contractility; see Figure 2a–c. This is explained by the slower shrinkage of the dead cells surrounded by live cells with hard boundaries. Results in Figure 2d–f show that the cell density decreases slightly with the area compressibility λ_{area}.

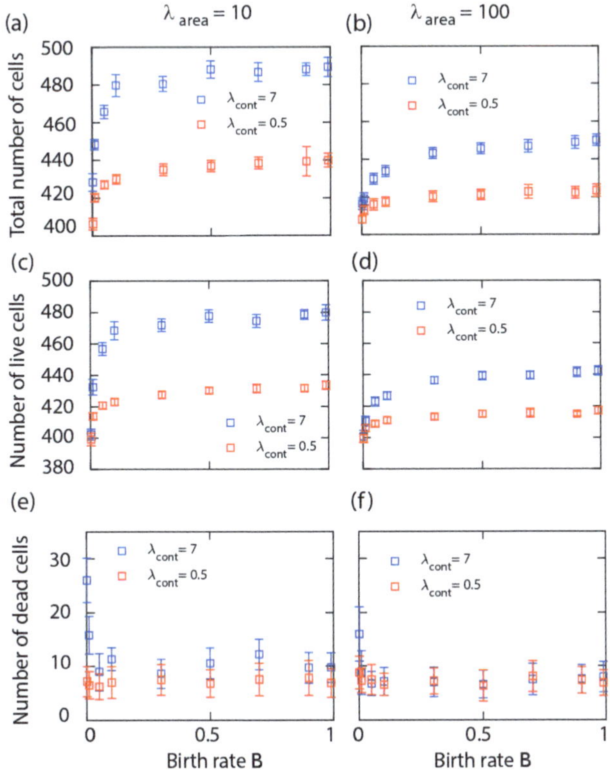

Figure 2. Number of cells at equilibrium in a cell sheet with single cell type versus cell birth rate B. Total number of cells (top row), number of live cells (middle row), and number of dead cells (bottom row) versus B at cell area compressibility $\lambda_{\text{area}} = 10$ (**a**,**c**,**e**), 100 (**b**,**d**,**f**), and various cell perimeter contractility λ_{cont} (inset). Other simulation parameters: Death rate $M = 0.001$ and $\lambda_{\text{adh}} = -10$. Each symbol is derived from an individual simulation run and corresponds to mean ± SD.

From these simulation results, we see that the proportion of the dead cells within the cell layer increases with the death rate parameter M, is relatively insensitive to the birth rate, and changes slightly with the mechanical parameters. In order to limit the proportion of dead cells within a realistic range for a biologically functional epithelial cell layer (e.g., well below 10%), in the following cell competition simulations, we will restrict the range of the death rate parameter to $0 < M \leq 0.003$; see Figure 1e,f.

3.2. Competitive Invasion due to Different Division and Death Rates

Next, we model competitive cell invasion with two cell types that initially occupy the left and right halves of the domain. This follows the three simulation stages outlined in Section 2; see Figure 3. Briefly, first, a simulation is run to reach equilibrium of cell shapes within the two sub-domains separated by a barrier. Then, cell proliferation and death are enabled to reach equilibrium cell density and size for each cell type separately. Finally, the barrier is removed, and the two cell types compete for space.

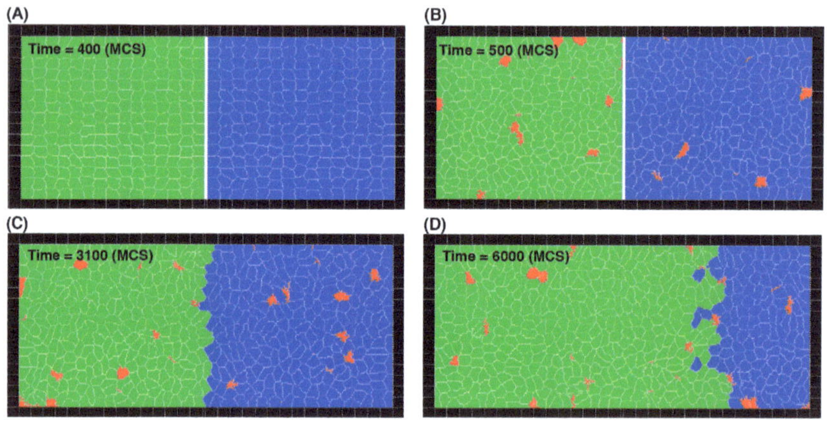

Figure 3. Three stages of the simulations of the cell invasion process. (**A**) Stage 1: cell division and death are switched off for both cell types (green and blue) to allow cells to reach their shape at mechanical equilibrium. Cell types are separated by a barrier (white). (**B**) Stage 2: cell division and death are switched on to allow cells to reach their steady density and size for both types, while separated by the barrier. Red cells indicate dead cells, which gradually shrink and disappear. (**C**,**D**) Stage 3: the separating barrier is removed, and the green cell type invades the region of the blue cell type, because in the case shown, the green cells have a greater division probability ($B = 0.9$) than the blue cells ($B = 0.1$), while the death rates are the same ($M_1 = M_2 = 0.003$). The invasion is shown at two different time points (**C**,**D**). For simulation movies, see Movies S6–S8.

To analyse the dynamics of the simulated competitive cell invasion, we first examine the effects of cell division and death rates. We consider cell types that have the same mechanical parameters, but they are different in either the cell division or death probabilities. A series of snapshots of typical cell distributions is shown in Figure 3 where green and blue represent different cell types (in this example green cells have higher division probability) and red represents dead cells.

The changes in the cell numbers over time for each type are shown in Figure 4A,B. After the barrier removal, the number of dominant cells increases approximately linearly, while at the same time the number of the other cell type decreases and eventually reaches zero. At that stage, the whole domain is fully occupied by the dominant cell type only. We find a similar change in the number of cells when the cells have different death rates; see Figure 4C,D. The simulation shows a well-defined linear regime in the numbers of each cell type during the invasion process, indicating that the front separating the invading and invaded cells progresses with an approximately constant speed.

We analysed the dependence of the invasion speed on the division and death rate parameters. The simulation parameters are shown in Table 2. First the slope of the linear growth of the total number of invading cells over time was determined, then the invasion speed was calculated as the average rate of change of the number of invading cells divided by the equilibrium density ρ corresponding to the parameters of the invading cells, which was estimated earlier from the simulations with a single cell type:

$$v = \frac{\Delta N}{\Delta t} \frac{L}{\rho} \quad (3)$$

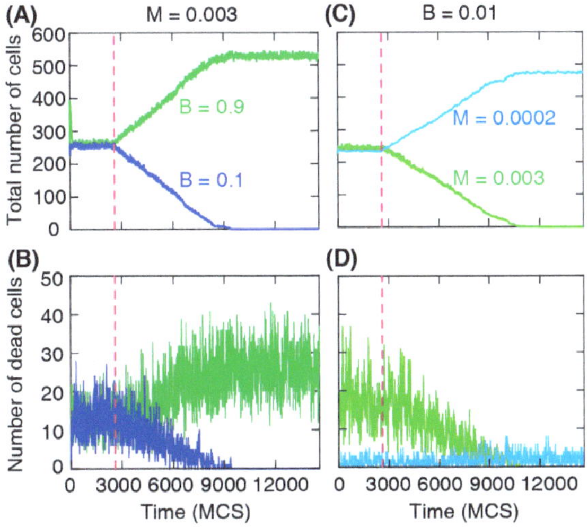

Figure 4. Total number of cells and number of dead cells for each cell type over time during the invasion. The mechanical properties are the same for both types: $\lambda_{\text{area}} = 70$, $\lambda_{\text{cont}} = 7$, and $\lambda_{\text{adh}} = -10$. (**A**,**B**) The death probability $M = 0.003$ is the same for all cells. Cells with greater division probability ($B = 0.9$) invade the region occupied by cells with lower division probability ($B = 0.1$). (**C**,**D**) When cell division probabilities are the same ($B = 0.001$), the cells with a lower death rate ($M = 0.0002$) invade the region occupied by cells with a greater death rate ($M = 0.003$). The invasion is demonstrated by the approximately linear increase of the number of invading cells (**A**,**C**). Dashed line: time of wall removal.

Table 2. Figure 5 parameters.

Parameter	Value
Domain size	600 × 300 pixels
Initial cells size	100 pixels
λ_{area}	70
λ_{cont}	7
λ_{adh}	−10
A_0	100 pixels
Number of cells	1800
T	50
B	Variable
M	Variable

We chose the width of the domain perpendicular to the direction of invasion as the length unit, $L = 1$. When one of the rates is the same for both cell types, we find that the invasion speed increases with the difference between either the cell division or death rates;

see Figure 5A–D. As expected, results in Figure 5 show that the invading cell type is the one with the higher division rate or the lower death rate.

To interpret the numerical results obtained for the invasion velocity shown in Figure 5, we compare the behavior of the CPM model to an analogous reaction–diffusion model with two competing species described by the following system of partial differential equations [35]:

$$\frac{\partial \rho_1}{\partial t} = b_1\rho_1(1-\rho_1-\rho_2) - m_1\rho_1 + D\nabla^2\rho_1$$
$$\frac{\partial \rho_2}{\partial t} = b_2\rho_2(1-\rho_1-\rho_2) - m_2\rho_2 + D\nabla^2\rho_2 \quad (4)$$

where $\rho_1(\mathbf{r},t)$ and $\rho_2(\mathbf{r},t)$ are the densities of the competing species, b_1 and b_2 are the reproduction rate constants, m_1 and m_2 are the mortality parameters, and D is the diffusion coefficient. The spatially uniform system has three steady states: $(0,0)$, $(0,1-m_2/b_2)$, and $(1-m_1/b_1,0)$. Note that in general, there is no co-existence of the two species in the uniform system (except in the special case when $b_1/m_1 = b_2/m_2$). Linear stability analysis of the uniform steady states shows that $(0,0)$ is unstable and, of the remaining two states, one is stable and the other is unstable. For the case when $b_1/m_1 > b_2/m_2$, the first species is dominant and the stable steady state is $(1-m_1/b_1,0)$, while the other steady state is unstable. In the opposite case, the second species dominates, and the only stable uniform steady state is $(0,1-m_2/b_2)$.

When the initial condition of the reaction–diffusion model is such that the two species are spatially separated, a Fisher–Kolmogorov type travelling wave solution develops, where the stable state corresponding to the dominant species propagates into the space occupied by the other species: $\rho_{1,2}(\mathbf{r},t) = f_{1,2}(x-vt)$, where v is the front velocity moving with constant speed along the x axis. For this type of so-called "pulled" front, where the stable phase is pulled into the unstable phase by the instability at the leading edge, the front velocity is determined by the linear instability near the unstable state [35–37]. For concreteness, let us assume that the first species dominates, i.e., $b_1/m_1 > b_2/m_2$. Thus, in the neighbourhood of the leading edge, the density of the invading species is small, while the second species is close to the unstable equilibrium: $\rho_1 \ll 1, \rho_2 \approx 1 - m_2/b_2$. Therefore, the reaction–diffusion equation can be linearised as:

$$\frac{\partial \rho_1}{\partial t} = \rho_1\left(m_2\frac{b_1}{b_2} - m_1\right) + D\nabla^2\rho_1. \quad (5)$$

Note that this equation is equivalent to the analogous linear approximation of the standard Fisher–Kolmogorov travelling wave problem [38], and the corresponding asymptotic wave velocity (for sufficiently sharp initial conditions, i.e., spatially separated cell types) is:

$$v = 2\sqrt{D\frac{b_1m_2 - b_2m_1}{b_2}}. \quad (6)$$

In the special case, when $m_1 = m_2 = m$, the formula simplifies to:

$$v = \sqrt{D\frac{m(b_1-b_2)}{b_1}} \quad (7)$$

or in the other case, with equal division rates $b_1 = b_2 = b$, we have

$$v = \sqrt{D(m_2-m_1)}. \quad (8)$$

Although the continuous reaction–diffusion model and the CPM represent quite different modelling approaches, the results for the invasion front speed v in Equations (6)–(8) are qualitatively consistent with our numerical results obtained from the CPM simulations.

First, in the case of equal death rates $M_1 = M_2$, we find that the invasion front speed increases with the difference between the cell division rates and also increases with the common death rate; see Figure 5A. The rescaled data in Figure 5B show that the invasion speed is an increasing function of $M(1 - B_2/B1)$ as in Equation (7). Then, in the case of equal cell division rates $B_1 = B_2$, we find that the invasion front velocity increases with the difference in the death rates and is not affected much by the common cell division rate; see Figure 5C,D. The functional form appears to be consistent with $v \sim \sqrt{M_1 - M_2}$.

We note that the CPM model does not have a simple parameter for cell motility that can be linked to the diffusion coefficient of the PDE model. This may account for the limitations of the similarity between the theoretical prediction based on the reaction–diffusion model and the simulations, since random cell motility in the CPM may depend on multiple parameters. We also note that the inherent fluctuations in the stochastic CPM model seem to play a role in the somewhat irregular variability of the front velocity shown in Figure 5. Of course, it might be possible to reduce the fluctuations by using a larger domain size with more cells; however, this leads to a much higher computational cost of the simulation.

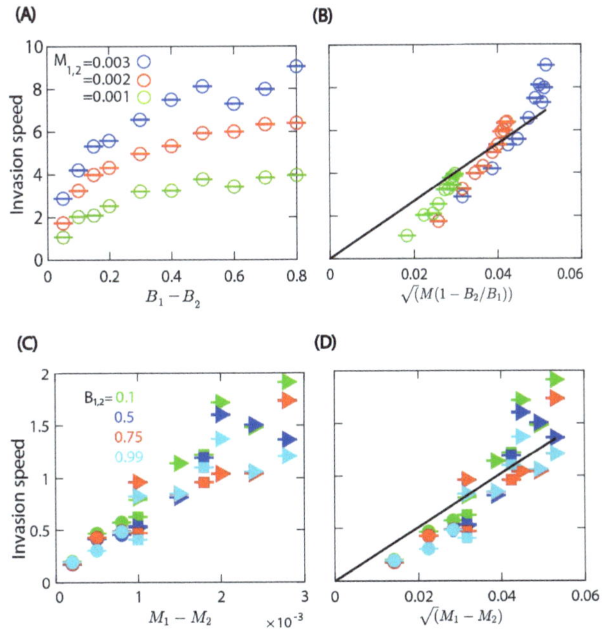

Figure 5. Cell invasion speed changes with differences in the cell division and death probabilities, when the mechanical properties are the same for both cell types: $\lambda_{area} = 70$, $\lambda_{cont} = 7$, and $\lambda_{adh} = -10$. (**A**) The invasion speed increases with the difference in cell division probabilities. The division rate parameter of cell type 2 is set to $B_2 = 0.1$. Both cell types have equal death probabilities (see color legend). (**B**) Comparison of the invasion speed with the functional form predicted by the reaction–diffusion model when the cell death probabilities M are the same; see Equation (7). Black line: linear fit $y(x) = 134.37x$. (**C**) The invasion speed increases with the difference in death probabilities when both types have equal proliferation probability $B_1 = B_2 = 0.1$. (**D**) Invasion speed versus the square root of the difference of death probabilities; see Equation (8). Black line: linear fit $y(x) = 25.55x$. Colors represent different birth rates (see color legend), and the symbols indicate the death rate of the first cell type, i.e., $M_1 = 0.001$ (circle), $M_1 = 0.002$ (square), and $M_1 = 0.003$ (triangle). In (**A**–**D**), open symbols: cell type 1 invades the area occupied by cell type 2; closed symbols: cell type 2 invades the area occupied by cell type 1. Each symbol is derived from an individual simulation run and corresponds to mean ± SD.

3.3. Invasion Due to Different Mechanical Properties

To test whether differences in mechanical properties of the cells alone can also generate invasion waves, we run simulations with cell types that have the same biological parameters (i.e., equal death and division rates) but different values for the mechanical parameters in the energy function of the CPM in Equation (1).

Through tracking the number of cells over time, results show that cells with higher perimeter contractility λ_{cont} invade softer cells with lower contractility; see Figure 6A,B. Similarly, higher area compressibility parameter λ_{area} of cells leads to invasion when all other parameters are the same for both cell types; see Figure 6C,D. In the case of cell–cell adhesion strength, we found that cells with a weaker cell–cell adhesion invade more adhesive cells; see Figure 6E,F. However, in this case, the invasion speed is much lower compared to the previous cases, indicating a weaker competitive advantage of cells with modified cell–cell adhesion.

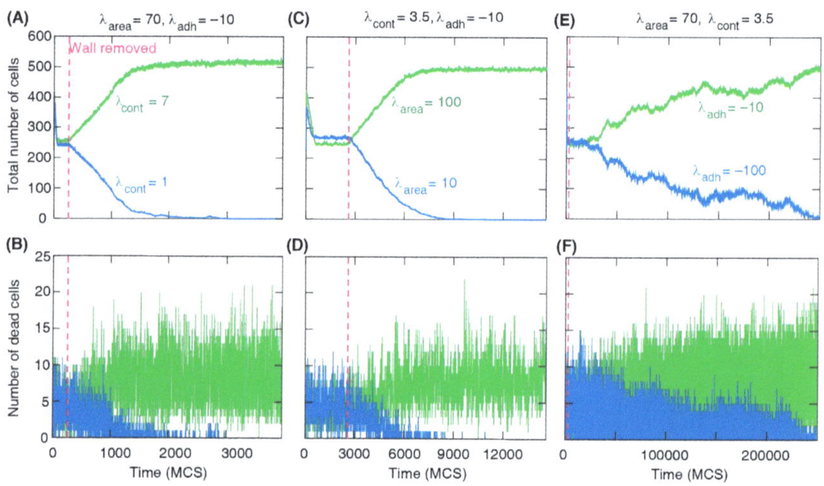

Figure 6. Total number of cells and number of dead cells vs time for competing cell types with different mechanical properties, where division and death probabilities are the same for all cells, $B = 0.99$ and $M = 0.001$. (**A**,**B**) Cells with stronger perimeter contractility ($\lambda_{\text{cont}} = 7$) invade the region occupied by cells with softer shapes ($\lambda_{\text{cont}} = 1$). The area elasticity $\lambda_{\text{area}} = 70$ and cell-cell adhesion $\lambda_{\text{adh}} = -10$ are the same for all cells. (**C**,**D**) With fixed $\lambda_{\text{cont}} = 1$ and $\lambda_{\text{adh}} = -10$, cells with greater area elasticity ($\lambda_{\text{area}} = 100$) invade the region occupied by cells with lower area elasticity ($\lambda_{\text{area}} = 10$). (**E**,**F**) With fixed $\lambda_{\text{area}} = 70$ and $\lambda_{\text{cont}} = 3.5$, cells with weaker adhesion ($\lambda_{\text{adh}} = -10$) invade the region occupied by more adhesive cells ($\lambda_{\text{adh}} = -100$). (**A**,**C**,**E**) The invasion is demonstrated by the linear increase in the total number of invading cells. (**A**–**F**) Dashed line: time of wall removal.

We then studied how the invasion speed changes with the mechanical properties of competing cell types. The invasion speed is calculated as the slope of the linear increase of the total number of invading cells divided by the equilibrium density. When the invasion is due to different area compressibility, the invasion speed increases monotonically with the difference in the area compressibility. The numerical results also show that the invasion is faster when both cell types are softer, i.e., having a weak cortex contractility; see Figure 7A. When the contractility of the cells are different, the invasion speed increases with the difference in the contractility parameters; however, it appears to be unaffected by changing the common area compressibility; see Figure 7B. In this case, we also found that the invasion speed increases with the cell death probability. This is consistent with the role of cell turnover in the cell invasion process. Even when the cell invasion is due to different mechanical properties, the turnover of cells by death and division is necessary for competitive cell invasion. Increasing the cell death probability speeds up the turnover of both types of cells, which then contributes to faster invasion. In the case with different cell–cell adhesion parameters, we see that the invasion speed is much smaller than in the previous cases and is only slightly affected by cell contractility; see Figure 7C. The numerical results in Figure 7C also show that contractility may influence the direction of the invasion. In the case of hard cells with high contractility such as $\lambda_{\text{cont}_{1,2}} = 7$, cell type 2, i.e., the more adhesive cell type, invades cell type 1, while the invasion direction changes to the opposite when both cell types are less contractile soft cells with $\lambda_{\text{cont}_{1,2}} = 0.7$.

Finally, we also studied the competitive cell invasion in the case when there are differences in both biological and biomechanical parameters at the same time. Figure 7D shows how these combined differences can enhance the invasion speed when the cell type with a higher compressibility parameter also has a higher division rate. In the opposite case, when the division rate of the cell type with a higher compressibility parameter is reduced, the invasion becomes much slower or the direction of invasion may change. Thus, biomechanical differences can compensate for the higher division rate of a competing cell type and could be used to control invading cells.

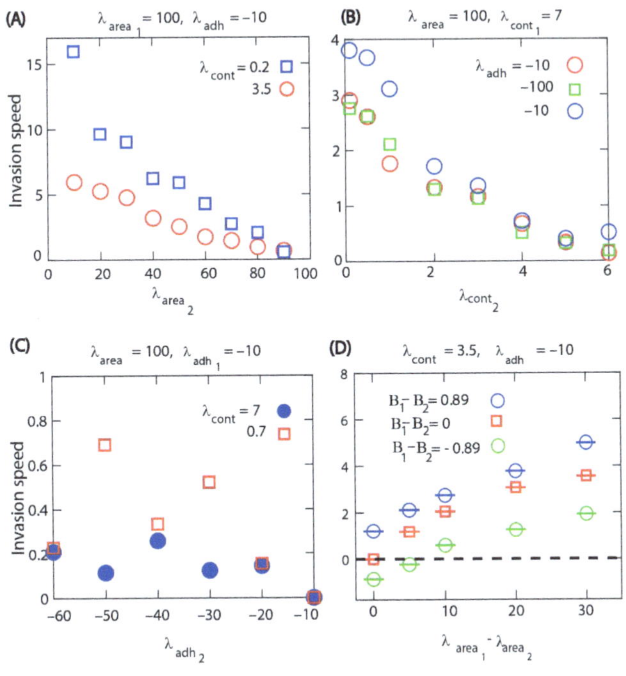

Figure 7. Cell invasion speed changes with variations in the mechanical properties and the biological properties of cells, where the cell division and death probabilities are the same for both cell types at $B = 0.99$ and $M = 0.001$ in (**A–C**). (**A**) Invasion speed versus cell area elasticity λ_{area} at different cell contractilities λ_{cont}. (**B**) Invasion speed versus λ_{cont} at different cell–cell adhesions λ_{adh}. In (**B**), we also tested the invasion velocity when we have higher death rates for both cell types such as $M_1 = M_2 = 0.003$ (blue circle). (**C**) Invasion speed versus λ_{adh} at different λ_{cont}. (**D**) Invasion speed versus the differences of cell area elasticities of the two cell types at different division rates of the cells. In (**A–C**), open symbols: cell type 1 invades the area occupied by cell type 2. Closed symbols: cell type 2 invades the area occupied by cell type 1.

4. Discussion

In the simulations presented here, we gained some insights into how cellular properties may influence the cell competition process. Our modelling results predict that differences in cell properties can generate invasion waves at the interface of two types of cells. The invasion front moves with a constant speed, and the invasion is generally faster when the differences between the parameters of the two cell types are larger.

In the case of a cell layer with a single cell type, when there is a dynamic equilibrium between cell division and cell death events, we found that the cell density is always higher than the neutral density corresponding to cells with target area A_0. Therefore, the cell division is suppressed almost everywhere except in the neighbourhood of cell death events where live cells can expand, reach the cell division threshold, and then replace the lost cell.

We can obtain a lower bound for the average equilibrium cell size, or upper bound for cell density. For the live neighbouring cells to be able to reach the threshold A_0 requires that $A_\alpha + A_\alpha/N_c \geq A_0$, where N_c is the average cell coordination number, i.e., the number of live cells surrounding a dead cell. In the hard cell boundary regime (i.e., with a large contractility parameter), the cell layer forms a hexagonal honeycomb type structure with $N_c = 6$ [19]. For lower contractility, the shape of the cells will change; however, the average number of neighbouring cells can be expected to remain similar. Thus we obtain a lower bound for the average cell size in equilibrium as $A_\alpha = A_0 N_c/(1 + N_c) \approx 5A_0/6$. This approximation is in agreement with the numerical results in Figures 1 and 2, showing that when starting the simulations with 400 cells with their area equal to A_0, at equilibrium the total number of live cells is bounded from above by $N \approx 400 \times 6/5 = 480$.

In the cell competition process at the interface between two cell types, the different cell properties result in a biased competition for replacing the missing cell after cell death. For example, when there is a difference in cell death rates, one cell type is more likely to generate some extra space at the boundary, but the neighbouring cells have an equal chance of replacing the missing cell. When the cell death rates are the same but cell division probabilities are different, the probability of replacing the dead cell is biased towards the cells with a higher division rate. This is essentially the same mechanism that leads to the invasion waves in simple lattice models (e.g., [39]) where each competitor is represented by a single lattice site. This mechanism, however, cannot explain the invasion wave induced by mechanical differences in the two cell types, and such differences cannot be represented in simple stochastic lattice models of competing populations [35,39].

The computational study presented here provides experimentally testable predictions for the process of competitive cell invasion. Although some of the model parameters are not easily accessible and modifiable in experiments, the regulation of cell cortex contractility by multiple signaling pathways may provide an option for investigating competitive cell invasion and comparing it with the predictions of our model. For our simulations, we used the computational modelling framework of the CPM. It would be interesting to test whether the same behaviour can be observed with alternative multicellular modelling approaches, e.g., the vertex model. Mechanical cell competition was also studied in simplified one-dimensional elastic spring models [10]. This type of reduced model may allow for developing analytical approaches to gain better insights into the mechanisms that determine the characteristics of cell invasion.

Here we focused on the average rate of invasion in cell competition. However, fluctuations and variability along the front interface can also be important in some biological or medical applications. Such fluctuations were studied using simple lattice models [35,39] and could be extended further multicellular models.

Supplementary Materials: The following supporting information can be downloaded at: www.mdpi.com/xxx/s1, Movie captions, Movie S1: A simulation of a monolayer with a single cell type (green). Simulation parameters are: $B = 0.03$, $M = 0.003$, $\lambda_{area} = 10$, $\lambda_{adh} = -10$, and low contractility $\lambda_{cont} = 0.5$ corresponding to "soft" cells. Red cells: dead cells that gradually shrink and disappear, Movie S2: Monolayer with a single cell type (green) in the "hard" regime. Simulation parameters are: $B = 0.03$, $M = 0.003$, $\lambda_{area} = 10$, $\lambda_{adh} = -10$, and high contractility corresponding to hard cells $\lambda_{cont} = 7$, Movie S3: A simulation of a monolayer with a single cell type (green) with high area strain and low contractility. Simulation parameters are: $B = 0.03$, $M = 0.003$, $\lambda_{area} = 100$, $\lambda_{cont} = 0.5$, and $\lambda_{adh} = -10$, Movie S4: A simulation of a monolayer with a single cell type (green) with high area strain parameter and high contractility. Simulation parameters are: $B = 0.03$, $M = 0.003$, $\lambda_{area} = 100$, $\lambda_{cont} = 7$, and $\lambda_{adh} = -10$, Movie S5: A simulation of a monolayer with two cell types. Simulation parameters are: $B = 0.9$, $M = 0.001$, $\lambda_{area} = 70$, $\lambda_{cont} = 7$, and $\lambda_{adh} = -10$ (green); $B = 0.1$, $M = 0.001$, $\lambda_{area} = 70$, $\lambda_{cont} = 7$, and $\lambda_{adh} = -10$ (blue), Movie S6: A simulation of a monolayer with two cell types. Simulation parameters are: $B = 0.99$, $M = 0.007$, $\lambda_{area} = 100$, $\lambda_{cont} = 0.2$, and $\lambda_{adh} = -10$ (green); $B = 0.99$, $M = 0.001$, $\lambda_{area} = 10$, $\lambda_{cont} = 0.2$, and $\lambda_{adh} = -10$ (blue), Movie S7: A simulation of a monolayer with two cell types. Simulation parameters are: $B = 0.99$, $M = 0.002$, $\lambda_{area} = 100$, $\lambda_{cont} = 7$, and $\lambda_{adh} = -10$ (green); $B = 0.99$, $M = 0.002$, $\lambda_{area} = 100$, $\lambda_{cont} = 1$, and $\lambda_{adh} = -10$ (blue), Movie S8: A simulation of a monolayer with two cell types. Simulation parameters are: $B = 0.99$, $M = 0.001$, $\lambda_{area} = 70$, $\lambda_{cont} = 0.7$, and $\lambda_{adh} = -10$ (green); $B = 0.99$, $M = 0.001$, $\lambda_{area} = 70$, $\lambda_{cont} = 0.7$, and $\lambda_{adh} = -60$ (blue).

Author Contributions: Conceptualization, F.S.A., H.K. and Z.N.; Methodology, F.S.A., H.K. and Z.N.; Software, F.S.A., H.K. and Z.N.; Validation, F.S.A.; Formal analysis, F.S.A., H.K. and Z.N.; Investigation, F.S.A., H.K. and Z.N.; Writing—original draft, F.S.A., H.K. and Z.N.; Writing—review & editing, F.S.A., H.K. and Z.N.; Supervision, Z.N. and H.K.; Project administration, Z.N. All authors have read and agreed to the published version of the manuscript.

Funding: This research was funded by the Australian Research Council Discovery Project No. DP160104342. F.S.A. was funded by a scholarship from Taif University (TU) and the Saudi Arabian Cultural Mission.

Data Availability Statement: The model codes used in the numerical simulations are available on request from the corresponding author.

Conflicts of Interest: The authors declare no conflict of interest.

References

1. Lima, A.; Rodriguez, T.A. MHC-I presents: Tumor surveillance in the epithelia by cell competition. *Nat. Immunol.* **2021**, *22*, 1358–1360. [CrossRef] [PubMed]
2. Ayukawa, S.; Kamoshita, N.; Nakayama, J.; Teramoto, R.; Pishesha, N.; Ohba, K.; Sato, N.; Kozawa, K.; Abe, H.; Semba, K.; et al. Epithelial cells remove precancerous cells by cell competition via MHC class I–LILRB3 interaction. *Nat. Immunol.* **2021**, *22*, 1391–1402. [CrossRef] [PubMed]
3. Kon, S.; Ishibashi, K.; Katoh, H.; Kitamoto, S.; Shirai, T.; Tanaka, S.; Kajita, M.; Ishikawa, S.; Yamauchi, H.; Yako, Y.; et al. Cell competition with normal epithelial cells promotes apical extrusion of transformed cells through metabolic changes. *Nat. Cell Biol.* **2017**, *19*, 530–541. [CrossRef] [PubMed]
4. Shraiman, B.I. Mechanical feedback as a possible regulator of tissue growth. *Proc. Natl. Acad. Sci. USA* **2005**, *102*, 3318–3323. [CrossRef]
5. Vincent, R.; Bazellières, E.; Pérez-González, C.; Uroz, M.; Serra-Picamal, X.; Trepat, X. Active Tensile Modulus of an Epithelial Monolayer. *Phys. Rev. Lett.* **2015**, *115*, 248103. [CrossRef]
6. Pedersen, S.F.; Hoffmann, E.K.; Novak, I. Cell volume regulation in epithelial physiology and cancer. *Front. Physiol.* **2013**, *4*, 1–12. [CrossRef] [PubMed]
7. Nishikawa, S.; Takamatsu, A.; Ohsawa, S.; Igaki, T. Mathematical model for cell competition: Predator–prey interactions at the interface between two groups of cells in monolayer tissue. *J. Theor. Biol.* **2016**, *404*, 40–50. [CrossRef]
8. Levayer, R. Cell competition: Bridging the scales through cell-based modeling. *Curr. Biol.* **2021**, *31*, R856–R858. [CrossRef] [PubMed]
9. Nishikawa, S.; Takamatsu, A. Effects of cell death-induced proliferation on a cell competition system. *Math. Biosci.* **2019**, *316*, 108241. [CrossRef]
10. Murphy, R.J.; Buenzli, P.R.; Baker, R.E.; Simpson, M.J. Mechanical Cell Competition in Heterogeneous Epithelial Tissues. *Bull. Math. Biol.* **2020**, *82*, 130. [CrossRef]
11. Tsuboi, A.; Ohsawa, S.; Umetsu, D.; Sando, Y.; Kuranaga, E.; Igaki, T.; Fujimoto, K. Competition for Space Is Controlled by Apoptosis-Induced Change of Local Epithelial Topology. *Curr. Biol.* **2018**, *28*, 2115–2128.e5. [CrossRef] [PubMed]

12. Gradeci, D.; Bove, A.; Vallardi, G.; Lowe, A.R.; Banerjee, S.; Charras, G. Cell-scale biophysical determinants of cell competition in epithelia. *eLife* **2021**, *10*, e61011. [CrossRef] [PubMed]
13. Graner, F.; Glazier, J.A. Simulation of biological cell sorting using a two-dimensional extended Potts model. *Phys. Rev. Lett.* **1992**, *69*, 2013–2016. [CrossRef] [PubMed]
14. Kempf, F.; Goychuk, A.; Frey, E. Tissue flow through pores: A computational study. *bioRxiv* **2021**. [CrossRef]
15. Khataee, H.; Czirok, A.; Neufeld, Z. Multiscale modelling of motility wave propagation in cell migration. *Sci. Rep.* **2020**, *10*, 8128. [CrossRef]
16. Khataee, H.; Fraser, M.; Neufeld, Z. Modelling the Collective Mechanical Regulation of the Structure and Morphology of Epithelial Cell Layers. *Front. Cell Dev. Biol.* **2022**, *10*, 767688. [CrossRef]
17. Osborne, J.M.; Fletcher, A.G.; Pitt-Francis, J.M.; Maini, P.K.; Gavaghan, D.J. Comparing individual-based approaches to modelling the self-organization of multicellular tissues. *PLoS Comput. Biol.* **2017**, *13*, e1005387. [CrossRef]
18. Farhadifar, R.; Röper, J.C.; Aigouy, B.; Eaton, S.; Jülicher, F. The influence of cell mechanics, cell-cell interactions, and proliferation on epithelial packing. *Curr. Biol.* **2007**, *17*, 2095–2104. [CrossRef]
19. Noppe, A.R.; Roberts, A.P.; Yap, A.S.; Gomez, G.A.; Neufeld, Z. Modelling wound closure in an epithelial cell sheet using the cellular Potts model. *Integr. Biol.* **2015**, *7*, 1253–1264. [CrossRef]
20. Albert, P.J.; Schwarz, U.S. Dynamics of Cell Ensembles on Adhesive Micropatterns: Bridging the Gap between Single Cell Spreading and Collective Cell Migration. *PLoS Comput. Biol.* **2016**, *12*, e1004863. [CrossRef]
21. Thüroff, F.; Goychuk, A.; Reiter, M.; Frey, E. Bridging the gap between single-cell migration and collective dynamics. *eLife* **2019**, *8*, e46842. [CrossRef]
22. Reffay, M.; Parrini, M.C.; Cochet-Escartin, O.; Ladoux, B.; Buguin, A.; Coscoy, S.; Amblard, F.; Camonis, J.; Silberzan, P. Interplay of RhoA and mechanical forces in collective cell migration driven by leader cells. *Nat. Cell Biol.* **2014**, *16*, 217–223. [CrossRef] [PubMed]
23. Charras, G.; Yap, A.S. Tensile Forces and Mechanotransduction at Cell–Cell Junctions. *Curr. Biol.* **2018**, *28*, R445–R457. [CrossRef] [PubMed]
24. Okuda, S.; Inoue, Y.; Adachi, T. Three-dimensional vertex model for simulating multicellular morphogenesis. *Biophys. Physicobiol.* **2015**, *12*, 13–20. [CrossRef]
25. Swat, M.H.; Thomas, G.L.; Belmonte, J.M.; Shirinifard, A.; Hmeljak, D.; Glazier, J.A. Multi-Scale Modeling of Tissues Using CompuCell3D. *Methods Cell Biol.* **2012**, *110*, 325–366. [CrossRef]
26. Glazier, J.A.; Graner, F. Simulation of the differential adhesion driven rearrangement of biological cells. *Phys. Rev. E* **1993**, *47*, 2128–2154. [CrossRef]
27. Schwartz, M.A.; Assoian, R.K. Integrins and cell proliferation: Regulation of cyclindependent kinases via cytoplasmic signaling pathways. *J. Cell Sci.* **2001**, *114*, 2553–2560. [CrossRef] [PubMed]
28. Brakebusch, C.; Bouvard, D.; Stanchi, F.; Sakai, T.; Fässler, R. Integrins in invasive growth. *J. Clin. Investig.* **2002**, *109*, 999–1006. [CrossRef]
29. Streichan, S.J.; Hoerner, C.R.; Schneidt, T.; Holzer, D.; Hufnagel, L. Spatial constraints control cell proliferation in tissues. *Proc. Natl. Acad. Sci. USA* **2014**, *111*, 5586–5591. [CrossRef]
30. Doncel, J.P.; de la Cruz Ojeda, P.; Oropesa-Avila, M.; Paz, M.V.; De Lavera, I.; De La Mata, M.; Cordoba, M.A.; Hidalgo, R.L.; Rivero, J.M.; Cotan, D.; et al. *Cytoskeleton Rearrangements during the Execution Phase of Apoptosis*; IntechOpen: London, UK, 2017; Chapter 8.
31. Ren, W.; Zhao, W.; Cao, L.; Huang, J. Involvement of the Actin Machinery in Programmed Cell Death. *Front. Cell Dev. Biol.* **2021**, *8*, 634849. [CrossRef]
32. Ramachandran, A.; Madesh, M.; Balasubramanian, K.A. Apoptosis in the intestinal epithelium: Its relevance in normal and pathophysiological conditions. *J. Gastroenterol. Hepatol.* **2000**, *15*, 109–120. [CrossRef] [PubMed]
33. Bortner, C.D.; Cidlowski, J.A. Apoptotic volume decrease and the incredible shrinking cell. *Cell Death Differ.* **2002**, *9*, 1307–1310. [CrossRef] [PubMed]
34. Swat, M.H.; Hester, S.D.; Balter, A.I.; Heiland, R.W.; Zaitlen, B.L.; Glazier, J.A. Multi-cell simulations of development and disease using the CompuCell3D simulation environment. *Methods Mol. Biol.* **2009**, *500*, 361–428. [CrossRef] [PubMed]
35. O'Malley, L.; Kozma, B.; Korniss, G.; Racz, Z.; Caraco, T. Fisher waves and front roughening in a two-species invasion model with preemptive competition. *Phys. Rev. E* **2006**, *74*, 041116. [CrossRef] [PubMed]
36. Ebert, U.; van Saarlos, W. Front propagation into unstable states: Universal algebraic convergence towards uniformly translating pulled fronts. *Physica D* **2000**, *146*, 1–99. [CrossRef]
37. Van Saarloos, W. Front propagation into unstable states. *Phys. Rep.* **2003**, *386*, 29–222. [CrossRef]
38. Murray, J.D. *Mathematical Biology II: Spatial Models and Biomedical Applications*; Springer: New York, NY, USA, 2001; Volume 3.
39. O'Malley, L.; Korniss, G.; Caraco, T. Ecological invasion, roughened fronts, and a competitor's extreme advance: Integrating stochastic spatial-growth models. *Bull. Math. Biol.* **2009**, *71*, 1160–1188.

life

MDPI

Review

Sepsis-Induced Coagulopathy: An Update on Pathophysiology, Biomarkers, and Current Guidelines

Andreas G. Tsantes [1,2,*,†], Stavroula Parastatidou [3,†], Emmanuel A. Tsantes [1], Elli Bonova [4], Konstantina A. Tsante [1], Petros G. Mantzios [1], Aristeidis G. Vaiopoulos [1], Stavros Tsalas [1], Aikaterini Konstantinidi [5], Dimitra Houhoula [1], Nicoletta Iacovidou [6], Daniele Piovani [4,7], Georgios K. Nikolopoulos [8] and Rozeta Sokou [5,6]

1 Laboratory of Haematology and Blood Bank Unit, "Attiko" Hospital, School of Medicine, National and Kapodistrian University of Athens, 12462 Athens, Greece
2 Microbiology Department, "Saint Savvas" Oncology Hospital, 11522 Athens, Greece
3 Neonatal Intensive Care Unit, 3rd Department of Paediatrics, "Attiko" Hospital, 12462 Athens, Greece
4 Department of Biomedical Sciences, Humanitas University, Pieve Emanuele, 20090 Milan, Italy
5 Neonatal Intensive Care Unit, "Agios Panteleimon" General Hospital of Nikea, 18454 Piraeus, Greece
6 Neonatal Department, National and Kapodistrian University of Athens, Aretaeio Hospital, 11528 Athens, Greece
7 IRCCS Humanitas Research Hospital, 20089 Rozzano, Italy
8 Medical School, University of Cyprus, Nicosia 2029, Cyprus
* Correspondence: andreas.tsantes@yahoo.com
† These authors contributed equally to this work.

Abstract: Significant cross talk occurs between inflammation and coagulation. Thus, coagulopathy is common in sepsis, potentially aggravating the prognosis. Initially, septic patients tend to exhibit a prothrombotic state through extrinsic pathway activation, cytokine-induced coagulation amplification, anticoagulant pathways suppression, and fibrinolysis impairment. In late sepsis stages, with the establishment of disseminated intravascular coagulation (DIC), hypocoagulability ensues. Traditional laboratory findings of sepsis, including thrombocytopenia, increased prothrombin time (PT) and fibrin degradation products (FDPs), and decreased fibrinogen, only present late in the course of sepsis. A recently introduced definition of sepsis-induced coagulopathy (SIC) aims to identify patients at an earlier stage when changes to coagulation status are still reversible. Nonconventional assays, such as the measurement of anticoagulant proteins and nuclear material levels, and viscoelastic studies, have shown promising sensitivity and specificity in detecting patients at risk for DIC, allowing for timely therapeutic interventions. This review outlines current insights into the pathophysiological mechanisms and diagnostic options of SIC.

Keywords: sepsis; coagulation; disseminated intravascular coagulation; sepsis-induced coagulopathy; laboratory evaluation; guidelines

check for updates

Citation: Tsantes, A.G.; Parastatidou, S.; Tsantes, E.A.; Bonova, E.; Tsante, K.A.; Mantzios, P.G.; Vaiopoulos, A.G.; Tsalas, S.; Konstantinidi, A.; Houhoula, D.; et al. Sepsis-Induced Coagulopathy: An Update on Pathophysiology, Biomarkers, and Current Guidelines. *Life* **2023**, *13*, 350. https://doi.org/10.3390/life13020350

Academic Editors: Stefanos Roumeliotis and Giuseppe Minervini

Received: 14 December 2022
Revised: 16 January 2023
Accepted: 20 January 2023
Published: 28 January 2023

1. Introduction

The traditional definition of sepsis is a systemic inflammatory response syndrome induced by infection. In 2016, this definition was updated by the Third International Consensus Definitions for Sepsis and Septic Shock to *"a life-threatening organ dysfunction caused by a host's dysfunctional response to infection"* [1]. The current concept highlights the risk of severe morbidity and mortality due to the dysregulated host response rather than the infection itself. Organ dysfunction is defined as an increase in the sequential organ failure assessment (SOFA) score by at least 2 points. Our understanding of sepsis mechanisms and pathophysiology has greatly improved over the last few years, while contemporary and more efficient diagnostic tools are currently being developed (Figure 1). However, the pathobiology of sepsis has not been fully elucidated, and there is no gold standard diagnostic test. Sepsis is a complex clinical syndrome with a prevalence of approximately

2.5 per 1000 individuals in the Western world, and an annual increase of 8.7% over the last 20 years, partly due to the aging of the population [2]. Nineteen million cases of sepsis are diagnosed annually, with almost 5 million deaths, rendering it a leading cause of mortality globally [3].

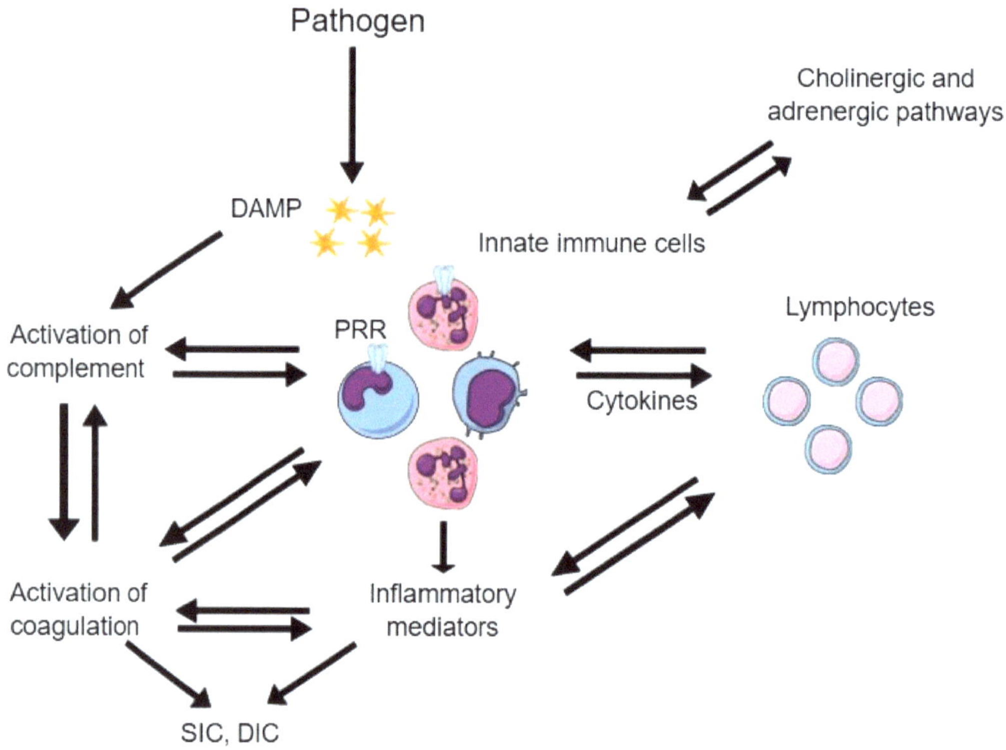

Figure 1. The main pathogenetic mechanisms involved in sepsis. Following pathogen invasion, innate immune cells recognize antigens through pattern-recognition receptors (PRRs). Activated innate immune cells release cytokines and inflammatory mediators to activate lymphocytes and the coagulation cascade, resulting in sepsis-induced coagulopathy and disseminated intravascular coagulopathy. Moreover, damage-associated molecular patterns (DAMPs) activate complement, which also results in activation of the coagulation cascade.

Infection, and sepsis, in particular, induce multiple and complex derangements in many systems, including the coagulation cascade. The vast majority of septic patients present with hemostatic abnormalities, ranging from subclinical coagulopathy to fulminant disseminated intravascular coagulation (DIC) [4]. During the initial stages of infection, coagulation operates as a natural defense mechanism, attempting to confine the responsible pathogen and prevent its spread into systematic circulation. However, in advanced and severe infections, as in sepsis, mass inflammatory cytokine production and release into the circulation lead to excessive activation of the coagulation process, fibrinolysis impairment, and suppression of anticoagulant mechanisms [5]. The hemostatic balance is significantly deranged in sepsis. The coagulation process is activated, while anticoagulant mechanisms, including fibrinolysis and anticoagulant factors, are suppressed (Figure 2). Consequently, septic patients are prone to a prothrombotic state through 4 main mechanisms: extrinsic pathway activation, cytokine-induced coagulation amplification, anticoagulant pathways suppression, and fibrinolysis impairment [6]. Laboratory assessment of hemostatic disorders in sepsis is based on conventional tests, including absolute platelet count, prothrombin time (PT), international normalized ratio (INR), fibrin degradation products (FDPs), such as d-dimers and fibrinogen levels, and nonconventional assays, including the measurement of anticoagulant proteins and nuclear material levels, and viscoelastic studies [2].

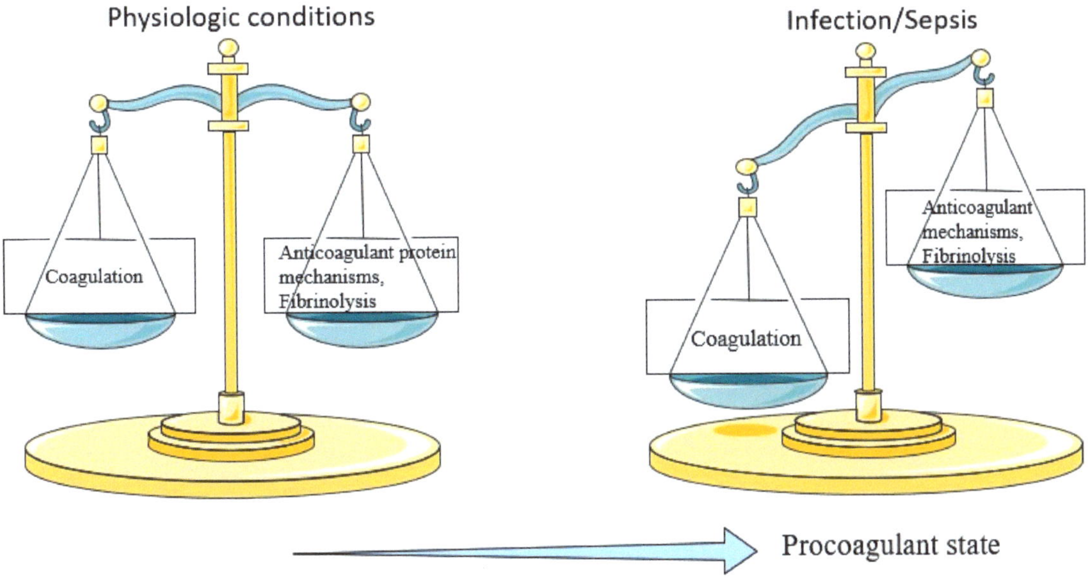

Figure 2. Derangement of the hemostatic balance in sepsis includes hyperactivation of the coagulation process and suppression of the anticoagulant mechanisms such as fibrinolysis and release of anticoagulant factors.

This review outlines current insights into the pathophysiological mechanisms and diagnostic options of sepsis-induced coagulopathy, focusing on potential biomarkers of interest and relevant existing guidelines. This study aims to review the current literature regarding the following key questions: (1) What are the main pathogenetic mechanisms involved in sepsis-induced coagulopathy? (2) What are the diagnostic criteria for sepsis-induced coagulopathy? (3) Are there any recent advances in the laboratory evaluation and treatment of sepsis-induced coagulopathy?

2. Hemostatic Abnormalities in Sepsis

The tissue factor pathway is the initial and main trigger for coagulation activation in sepsis. The tissue factor is located in the vascular endothelium, and its exposure to circulation in case of endothelial damage leads to activation of the extrinsic coagulation pathway [5]. However, this is not the primary activating mechanism in sepsis. Tissue factor is also present in inflammatory cells, mainly the monocytes and other circulating macrophages. In case of infection, these cells are activated through pattern-recognition receptors (PRRs) by pathogen-associated molecular patterns (PAMPs) and damage-associated molecular patterns (DAMPs) [7]. PAMPs are molecules that circulate following the destruction of pathogens or can be released by live pathogens, while DAMPs are host cellular components released when cells are lysed. PAMPs and DAMPs are recognized and bound to specific surface PRRs in monocytes and macrophages. Following PAMPs/DAMPs recognition by the PRRs on the surface of monocytes and macrophages, these cells are activated and release cytokines and chemokines, which subsequently activate neutrophils, platelets, and endothelial cells. Moreover, activated monocytes release extracellular vesicles that express procoagulant tissue factor and phosphatidylserine on their surfaces. Therefore, tissue factor is released into the circulation, and the extrinsic coagulation pathway is activated. Neutrophils also play a significant role in the activation of the coagulation cascade through the expression of the tissue factor and the release of chemical mediators and proteins. Another important mechanism through which neutrophils activate the coagulation cascade is the release of neutrophil extracellular traps (NETs). NETs are particles consisting of histones, procoagulant DNA, and other DAMP, released following the pathogen's invasion to limit the infection. However, these NETs are highly prothrombotic, contributing to the procoagulant state of infection.

The activation of coagulation is further enhanced via the release of inflammatory cytokines and antigenic products [2]. Bacterial endotoxins, which are circulating bacterial cell wall fragments, are strong stimuli for the activation of coagulation cascade and DIC syndrome, particularly in Gram-negative infections. Endotoxins bind to monocyte and endothelial cells, leading to the release of coagulation-inducing cytokines and triggering tissue factor pathways [8]. Endotoxins, in this case, either bind to membrane-associated PRR or Toll-like receptors of these cells, or if they are present in cytosol, bind to and are detected by Caspase 11.

In the early stages of sepsis, coagulation activation is counteracted by three anticoagulant pathways: antithrombin, protein C, and tissue factor pathway inhibitor [2]. As sepsis progresses, these three mechanisms are deranged, resulting in a hypercoagulable state. Specifically, antithrombin, an important anticoagulant mechanism that inhibits thrombin and factor Xa, is decreased in sepsis because of reduced synthesis and increased degradation through proteases and neutrophil elastases [6]. Normal activation of protein C is mediated through the thrombin–thrombomodulin complex on endothelial cells leading to inhibition of factors Va and VIIIa. Additionally, the endothelial protein C receptor (EPCR) is expressed on the surface of endothelial cells and further enhances protein C activation [9]. However, protein C levels are suppressed in sepsis. Finally, the tissue factor pathway inhibitor (TFPI) inactivates the tissue factor–factor VIIa complex and is produced by several cells, including endothelial cells, but its levels are decreased in sepsis resulting in dysregulated inactivation of the tissue factor–factor VIIa complex.

In sepsis, fibrinolytic activity depends on the balance between the tissue plasminogen activator (t-PA) and tissue plasminogen activator inhibitor PAI-1 [10]. T-PA facilitates fibrinolysis through fibrin degradation by plasmin, while PAI-1 inhibits fibrinolysis. At the early transient phase of sepsis, fibrinolysis is increased because of the conversion of plasminogen to plasmin by the enhanced effect of t-PA. Subsequently, impairment of fibrinolysis ensues as PAI-1 is increased, thrombin-activatable fibrinolysis inhibitor (TAFI) levels are elevated, and so are plasma levels of nuclear products. Impairment of fibrinolysis contributes to the hypercoagulable state observed in sepsis [11]. Since coagulation serves as a defense mechanism, bacterial pathogens are confined in a fibrin network at the infection site, limiting the spread to adjacent tissues and systemic circulation. In this context, impairment of fibrinolysis is useful to some extent, but at the same time, it bears negative consequences [12]. Pathogens are prevented from disseminating to other tissues at the expense of unburdened oxygen flow to these tissues, which leads to hypoxia.

3. Inflammation–Hemostasis Cross Talk

In sepsis, a bi-directional interplay between inflammation and coagulation is developed, resulting in a self-sustaining cycle (Figure 3) [2]. High levels of pro-inflammatory mediators are present, most of which, including tumor necrosis factor-a (TNF-a) and interleukin-6 (IL-6), induce the coagulation cascade. At the same time, various hemostatic factors further sustain and augment the inflammatory process. Coagulation proteins interact with cell receptors, resulting in the modification of inflammatory pathways [5]. This regulatory action is largely mediated by protease-activated receptors (PARs) [13]. PARs are transmembrane receptors mainly activated by thrombin and other coagulation factors to trigger the release of pro-inflammatory cytokines [14]. Additionally, interactions occur between hemostasis and the complement, which plays an important role in DIC [15].

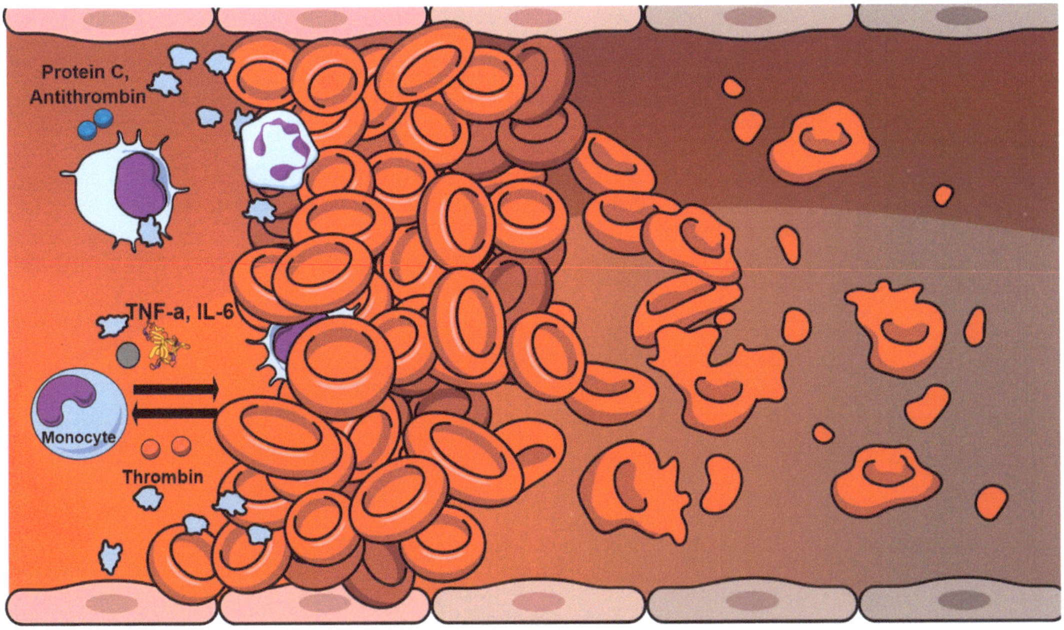

Figure 3. Main mechanisms involved in hemostasis–inflammation cross talk. Pro-inflammatory mediators such as tumor necrosis factor-a (TNF-a) and interleukin-6 (IL-6) are released by monocytes and macrophages to induce the coagulation cascade, while transmembrane receptors on monocytes can be activated by thrombin and other coagulation factors to trigger the release of pro-inflammatory cytokines. Moreover, antithrombin can directly bind to inflammatory cells and suppresses the expression of cytokine receptors, while also activated protein C downregulates endotoxin-induced production of cytokines by monocytes and macrophages.

The significant cross talk also exists between anticoagulant factors and inflammatory mediators [5]. Antithrombin directly binds to inflammatory cells and suppresses the expression of cytokine receptors. Additionally, activated protein C has been shown to downregulate endotoxin-induced production of TNF-α, IL-1β, IL-6, and IL-8 by monocytes and macrophages. Inhibition of leukocyte activation may be another role of activated protein C [16].

4. Sepsis-Induced Coagulopathy and Disseminated Intravascular Coagulation

DIC is characterized by a dysfunctional systemic activation of the coagulation cascade leading to excess thrombotic and hemorrhagic complications resulting from intravascular fibrin formation, microangiopathic thrombosis, and subsequent depletion of coagulation factors and platelets [5]. Clinically evident hemostatic disorders occur in approximately 50% to 70% of septic patients, while 35% of these patients develop DIC [17]. Over three decades ago, the Scientific Subcommittee (SSC) of the International Society on Thrombosis and Haemostasis (ISTH) on DIC defined the condition as *"an acquired syndrome characterized by the intravascular activation of coagulation with loss of localization arising from different causes"* [18]. Although triggered by different underlying disorders, including sepsis and noninfectious causes such as trauma and malignancies, the common feature of DIC is the systemic activation of coagulation. This activation is induced by endothelial damage and may culminate in tissue vascular hypoperfusion and subsequent multiple organ failure [19]. Coagulopathy in septic patients progresses from an initially compensated derangement of the hemostatic system, termed non-overt DIC, to overt DIC, a totally decompensated coagulation state [20].

The first diagnostic criteria for DIC were introduced in 1983 by the Japanese Ministry of Health and Welfare. They included both clinical characteristics and laboratory variables such as platelet count, PT, FDPs, and fibrinogen [21]. Later, the ISTH DIC SSC recommended criteria for the diagnosis of overt DIC, focusing on laboratory parameters [18]. D-dimers were included in the criteria for the first time, while the significance of platelet count was reduced, and the importance of fibrin-related markers was increased. According to the ISTH DIC SSC criteria, elevated levels of FDPs or d-dimers, decreased platelet count, prolonged PT, and decreased fibrinogen levels are consistent with overt DIC (Table 1). Other DIC scoring systems have also been employed, including the Japanese Association for Acute Medicine (JAAM) DIC diagnostic criteria [22]. Platelet count, FDP concentration, PT, and systemic inflammatory response are among the JAAM DIC criteria.

Table 1. International Society on Thrombosis and Haemostasis criteria for DIC and SIC diagnosis.

Item	Score	Overt DIC	SIC
		Range	Range
Platelet count ($\times 10^9$/L)	2 1	<50 ≥50, <100	<100 ≥100, <150
FDP/D-dimers	3 2	Strong increase Moderate increase	- -
Prothrombin time (PT ratio)	2 1	≥6 s ≥3 s, <6 s	(>1.4) (>1.2, ≤1.4)
Fibrinogen (g/mL)	1	<100	-
SOFA score	2 1	- -	≥2 1
Total score for DIC or SIC		≥5	≥4

Abbreviations: DIC—disseminated intravascular coagulation; SIC—sepsis-induced coagulopathy; FDP—fibrin degradation products; SOFA—Sequential Organ Failure Assessment.

Sepsis represents a condition where prompt diagnosis and initiation of treatment are of the utmost importance. The DIC score has shown a good predictive value for mortality; however, by the time of detection, patients are already at an advanced and irreversible stage of coagulopathy, beyond the optimal timeframe for therapeutic intervention [23]. Early identification of patients with sepsis-associated coagulopathy prior to progressing to this phase of hemostatic derangement would be ideal for the initiation of anticoagulant treatment [24]. Thus, the ISTH DIC subcommittee suggested simple diagnostic criteria for sepsis-induced coagulopathy (SIC) composed of only three parameters: platelet count, PT or INR, and SOFA score [25]. The presence of sepsis is confirmed by the inclusion of the SOFA score, reflecting the updated sepsis definition. DIC associated with sepsis is characterized by impairment of fibrinolysis, resulting from excessive production of PAI-1 [26,27]. This potentially leads to a prothrombotic state and organ dysfunction due to tissue hypoperfusion [28,29]. In contrast, in non-sepsis DIC, suppression of fibrinolysis is rare and systemic bleeding often occurs [30]. Therefore, reduced fibrinogen levels are not a common or specific finding in sepsis, in contrast to thrombocytopenia and PT prolongation. Finally, FDPs and d-dimers were not included in the SIC score as they lacked correlation with the severity of sepsis [31].

Comparing the ISTH overt DIC and SIC scoring systems, it became evident that the SIC score was twice as sensitive as the overt DIC score and that SIC always preceded overt DIC [32]. The SIC score was also validated against the JAAM DIC criteria and demonstrated similar prognostic value [33].

Diagnosis of either SIC or overt DIC may be useful in identifying patients who would benefit from therapeutic anticoagulant intervention [34]. A "two-step" sequential scoring system was developed by the ISTH for the identification of patients with sepsis-associated coagulopathy (Table 1). Patients are initially screened with the SIC score, and if the criteria for SIC are met, the overt DIC score is then calculated. This approach could increase the possibility of timely identification of suitable candidates for anticoagulant treatment [21].

5. Conventional Hemostatic Tests and Markers in Sepsis

In case of sepsis, well-established findings emerge on conventional coagulation assays. These findings include thrombocytopenia, prolongation of PT, increased levels of FDPs, and reduced fibrinogen levels. Such abnormalities often present in the setting of DIC and are not usually observed before its development, during the initial stages of sepsis.

5.1. Thrombocytopenia

Sepsis is typically associated with thrombocytopenia, despite the release of pro-inflammatory mediators and thrombopoietin, both of which induce platelet production [35,36]. The vast majority of sepsis patients develop thrombocytopenia, an established independent predictor of poor outcomes in sepsis [37,38]. In the early phase of sepsis, platelets, following their activation, aggregate with leucocytes to form platelet–leucocyte aggregates, leading to increased sequestration in the spleen [39]. Moreover, infections can stimulate platelet activation and aggregation and cause thrombocytopenia, either directly or through cell destruction, inflammation, and clot formation [40]. The phagocytosis of thrombocyte progenitors by monocytes due to macrophage colony-stimulating factor (M-CSF) further contributes to the low platelet count. In addition, altered production of platelets is observed in sepsis with a significant release of precursor cells, and the immature platelet fraction (IPF) correlates well with sepsis severity scores [41].

5.2. Fibrin Degradation Products

Assessment of fibrin-related biomarkers includes tests detecting FDPs, such as d-dimers, and assays detecting precursor fibrin formation products at an intermediate stage between fibrinogen and final stable fibrin, such as soluble fibrin monomers.

FDPs, such as protein fragments X, Y, and D, mainly result from the degradation of three components in the fibrinogen–fibrin cycle: the initial fibrinogen, the soluble precursor fibrin, and the cross-linked fibrin—the final stable form of fibrin. FDPs have been found in up to 99% of sepsis patients. However, these tests lack specificity, as they cannot discriminate degradation products deriving from final cross-linked fibrin, intermediate soluble fibrin, or initial fibrinogen [42]. FDP levels are measured by immunoenzyme assay ELISA or latex agglutination methods, allowing for point of care evaluation.

D-dimers are also FDPs, but they only result from proteolysis of the final cross-linked fibrin, and their levels are not affected by fibrinogen degradation products [5]. Consequently, d-dimers are the most specific marker among FDPs for assessing DIC. Detection of d-dimers indicates that thrombin induces the conversion of fibrinogen to fibrin monomer and that fibrin is cross-linked by activated factor XIII and subsequently degraded by plasmin [43]. Although d-dimers are FDPs and are associated with fibrinolysis, high levels reflect concomitant activation of coagulation [44]. Therefore, d-dimers may indicate increased formation rather than degradation of fibrin. In fact, increased d-dimers levels are observed in thromboses and are also included in DIC scores where severe sepsis is correlated with hypofibrinolysis. Thus, in sepsis, d-dimers are elevated because of both the activation of the coagulation cascade and the hyperfibrinolysis observed in the early phase of infection. However, in advanced sepsis, d-dimers may be normal. This is attributed to a significant inhibition of fibrinolysis, which prevents the formation of d-dimers despite increased fibrin formation. There is evidence that the use of d-dimers for the diagnosis of DIC and risk stratification in severe sepsis may be misleading, as normal levels of d-dimers were associated with higher mortality rates [43,44].

On the other hand, soluble fibrin monomers could be effective markers of intravascular fibrin formation in DIC [45]. Plasma levels of soluble fibrin monomers reflect intravascular fibrin formation and are not affected by extravascular fibrin formation that may accompany local inflammation or trauma. Available clinical trials demonstrate that soluble fibrin monomers exceeding a threshold level allow for DIC accurate diagnosis. To date, no reliable test is available for the quantification of soluble fibrin levels.

5.3. Fibrinogen

In general, low serum fibrinogen levels are considered a primary index of coagulation disorders in sepsis [46]. However, fibrinogen is an acute-phase reactant, and its levels are increased because of inflammation. As a result, fibrinogen levels may remain within the normal reference range for a long period of time after its continuing consumption. Sequential fibrinogen measurements might be more helpful, with higher diagnostic accuracy [47].

5.4. Standard Coagulation Tests

Standard coagulation tests, including PT and activated partial thromboplastin time (aPTT), have traditionally been used to assess the hemostatic system [48]. Nevertheless, they fail to fully reflect the hemostatic derangement incited by sepsis [49]. Abnormal values of standard coagulation tests are only observed late in the course of sepsis when the hypocoagulable hemostatic status emerges and is detected by these tests. Additionally, they assess part of the hemostatic mechanism, as they are based on plasmatic components of the coagulation system, while the crucial contribution of cellular components is not evaluated. Standard coagulation tests primarily assess the activity of procoagulant factors without taking into account the simultaneous activation of the anticoagulant mechanism.

6. Nonconventional Hemostatic Tests and Markers in Sepsis

Nonconventional tests have been applied in the diagnosis of coagulation derangement associated with sepsis.

6.1. Viscoelastic Tests

Thromboelastography (TEG) and rotational thromboelastometry (ROTEM) are viscoelastic, whole-blood, point of care tests that provide a comprehensive evaluation of the hemostatic process from coagulation initiation and clot formation to clot dissolution and fibrinolysis [50,51]. The contribution of both plasmatic and cellular components of coagulation are assessed through these methods. Viscoelastic tests may be useful for completing the gaps of the standard coagulation tests in evaluating the hemostatic status of septic patients [49]. Thus, numerous studies have focused on the use of viscoelastic tests for the detection of the hemostatic changes accompanying sepsis. Studies in subpopulations, including pediatric and neonatal septic patients, have also been conducted [52–54]. The prevalence of septic patients with hemostatic disorders detected by TEG/ ROTEM ranged between 43% and 100% [55]. There is heterogeneity in the design, conduction, and results of the studies [56,57]. Both hypocoagulability and hypercoagulability were reported, reflecting the pathophysiology of coagulopathy in sepsis and DIC. As a dynamic process, coagulopathy associated with sepsis evolves rapidly, and the timing of the testing greatly affects TEG/ ROTEM results. Sequential measurements may more accurately depict the progress of SIC, from hypercoagulability in the early stages to subsequent development of DIC and hypocoagulability. Viscoelastic tests can also detect impairment in fibrinolysis, as reported in several studies in sepsis patients [55,58].

Viscoelastic assays can detect the early activation of coagulation that leads to hypercoagulability when standard coagulation test results are still within normal limits [55]. ROTEM has been used to distinguish between septic patients with normal coagulability, hypercoagulability, and hypocoagulability. Both hypocoagulable and hypercoagulable hemostatic profile in ROTEM was correlated with significantly higher mortality risk [59]. In another study, patients with overt DIC presented a hypocoagulable profile in ROTEM, while septic patients without overt DIC tended to demonstrate hypercoagulability [60]. All of these patients had abnormal conventional coagulation tests, and the use of ROTEM could help prevent procoagulant interventions in patients with a hypercoagulable status not detected by standard coagulation assays. One hundred patients with sepsis, severe sepsis, or septic shock were assessed by ROTEM assay [61]. Maximum clot firmness (MCF) was higher in the sepsis and severe sepsis groups compared with the healthy control group. Normal MCF and prolonged clot development were observed in case of septic shock. These results indicate hypercoagulability in patients with sepsis or severe sepsis and hypocoagulability in the more advanced phase of septic shock. Interestingly, fibrinolytic activity was positively correlated with 28-day mortality. TEG parameters have been used for the development of a score to predict DIC [62]. Furthermore, ROTEM clotting time (CT) variable correlated strongly with the JAAM DIC score and performed well in predicting DIC [63].

A recent meta-analysis concluded that viscoelastic assays are reliable and useful for predicting DIC associated with sepsis and assessing mortality risk in severe sepsis [56]. It seems that both the hypocoagulable profile and transition towards hypocoagulability could identify patients at risk for developing DIC. Serial and combined viscoelastic and conventional coagulation testing could optimize DIC detection and management and improve survival and outcome.

6.2. Measurement of Nuclear Materials

Sepsis causes cellular activation and damage and the subsequent release of nuclear materials into circulation [15]. Nuclear materials include high mobility group box protein-1 (HMGB1), nucleosomes, histones, cell-free DNA, and neutrophil extracellular traps (NETs). Nuclear materials can directly trigger the expression of tissue factor in macrophages and endothelial cells. Tissue factor expression and subsequent activation of the extrinsic coagulation cataract is mediated by the activation of TLR2/4 receptors and the nuclear factor-kappa B (NF-κB) and activator protein 1 (AP-1) pathways [64].

HMGB1 serves as a marker of cell damage, inflammation, and thrombosis [65]. Acting on surrounding cells through receptors, it mediates the migration of leucocytes and the production of pro-inflammatory cytokines [66]. HMGB1 also promotes tissue factor expression on the surface of monocytes and reduces the anticoagulant activity of thrombomodulin, facilitating microvascular thrombosis through these pathways. High HMGB1 levels have been observed in patients with sepsis and DIC and are associated with poor prognosis and increased mortality [67].

Nucleosomes are complexes formed of 147 base pairs of DNA wrapped around a protein core of histones [68]. Nucleosomes are released into circulation with apoptotic cell death [69]. Elevated nucleosome levels were reported in various conditions, including malignancies, cerebral stroke, sepsis, and septic shock [70]. Increased plasma histone levels are observed in patients with sepsis and DIC and correlate positively with mortality [71]. In a preclinical model, extracellular histones triggered platelet aggregation, leading to consumptive coagulopathy, thrombosis, and bleeding. The prothrombotic action of histones is inhibited by recombinant thrombomodulin, which has been used therapeutically in DIC. Apart from being a biomarker of endothelial damage and activation of hemostasis, histone levels are associated with SOFA scores [72].

Plasma cell-free DNA demonstrated high prognostic value in patients with severe sepsis, superior to the multiple organ dysfunction (MODS) and the acute physiology and chronic health evaluation (APACHE) II score [73].

NETs are extracellular components of neutrophils, formed by DNA, histones, and granule proteins, and exhibit significant prothrombotic and pro-inflammatory properties [74].

6.3. Measurement of Anticoagulant Proteins

Antithrombin is one of the most important physiological anticoagulants and inhibits the intrinsic (factor XIa), extrinsic (factor VIIa), and common coagulation pathways (factor Xa, thrombin). In sepsis and DIC, antithrombin levels are decreased because of reduced synthesis, increased degradation by neutrophil elastase, and excess consumption resulting from the overproduction of thrombin [75]. Reduction in antithrombin levels is associated with disease severity in sepsis-induced DIC [76]. A decrease in antithrombin activity below

80% was reported in septic patients without multiple organ dysfunction [77]. This level reaches 60% in patients with multiple organ dysfunction, while progress to DIC further reduces antithrombin activity to approximately 40%. Increased mortality was demonstrated with low antithrombin levels in adult and pediatric septic patients [78,79].

Another anticoagulant protein, protein C, is naturally activated to inhibit thrombin formation through both extrinsic and intrinsic pathways [6]. Sepsis is characterized by the depletion of protein C and impaired production of activated protein C, rendering their levels potential prognostic biomarkers in this setting [80]. Activated protein C binds to its endothelial receptor (EPCR), which is released into the circulation following cell damage. This soluble EPCR was also studied as an index of disease progression and outcome in septic patients [81].

Thrombomodulin is an anticoagulant protein produced by endothelial cells and binds to thrombin, converting protein C into its activated form [82]. Thrombomodulin has a key anti-inflammatory, anticoagulant, and antifibrinolytic role. It inhibits leucocyte adhesion to endothelial cells, prevents complement activation, modifies cytokine generation, and degrades HMGB1 [83]. Thrombomodulin is cleaved by neutrophil elastase and circulates in its soluble form [84]. High plasma thrombomodulin levels are correlated with increased mortality in patients with sepsis and DIC [85]. Elevation of soluble plasma thrombomodulin with a concomitant decrease in endothelial surface thrombomodulin is observed in sepsis-induced DIC [86].

The natural anticoagulant TFPI inhibits the activation of tissue factor and the extrinsic coagulation pathway. Depletion of TFPI is associated with increased susceptibility to the development of DIC [6]. TFPI binds to endothelial heparin-like molecules, and its circulating levels are lower compared with antithrombin and activated protein C. Moreover, a significant part of TFPI is inactivated by binding to the lipoprotein. Consequently, TFPI has not emerged as a sensitive marker of DIC.

6.4. Other Markers of Interest

The thrombin–antithrombin (TAT) complex is a marker of thrombin generation, which could be used to identify patients with DIC, as excess thrombin formation is a key feature of this condition [46]. Higher TAT levels were reported in patients with DIC on admission or in those who developed DIC compared with patients without DIC [87]. Raised TAT levels were correlated with increased mortality in sepsis patients [26]. A combination of TAT with other markers has a higher prognostic value than each molecule alone.

Although fibrinolysis is impaired in sepsis-induced DIC, this is not detected by current coagulation parameters. The antifibrinolytic protein PAI-1 has been extensively investigated as a potential marker of hypofibrinolysis in septic patients with DIC [46]. PAH-1 levels can identify patients with DIC and predict DIC development [88,89]. Similar to TAT, combining PAI-1 with other biomarkers increased the performance ability of PAI-1 [26]. High PAI-1 was associated with increased mortality risk [90].

Endogenous thrombin potential—an assay indicative of thrombin generation—was evaluated in sepsis. Results were conflicting, and further research is warranted. However, recent evidence suggested a correlation between increased infection severity and decreased ability of thrombin generation [91]. This biomarker could possibly serve in the prediction of multiorgan dysfunction development and poor outcome in septic patients [92].

Prothrombin fragment 1.2 (F1.2) is an activation peptide generated when prothrombin is converted to thrombin [93]. Its use as a marker of thrombin generation was published and included in the DIC criteria of the Japanese Society on Thrombosis and Hemostasis (JSTH) [94].

ADAMTS-13 is a von Willebrand factor-cleaving protease regulating the size of von Willebrand factor multimers [95]. Cleaving von Willebrand multimers decrease their pro-thrombotic properties, as larger molecules have enhanced hemostatic competency [96]. ADAMTS-13 deficiency, leading to ultra large von Willebrand factor multimers and thrombotic microangiopathy in sepsis, was associated with sepsis severity and poor prognosis.

Fourteen conventional and nonconventional biomarkers, including platelet count, PT, aPTT, fibrinogen, FDPs, TAT, protein C, plasminogen, and PAI-1, were evaluated for early diagnosis of DIC in a study by Koyama et al. [26]. TAT, PAI-1, and protein C on admission discriminated well between patients with and without overt DIC, while TAT and PAI-1 were also significant predictors of 28-day mortality. Apart from predicting prognosis, certain markers can additionally be used to monitor treatment in patients with DIC [15]. Furthermore, some of them, including antithrombin and recombinant soluble thrombomodulin, were also studied and used for the treatment of DIC.

7. From Guidelines to Clinical Practice

Currently, there is no established therapy for sepsis-induced coagulopathy. International Surviving Sepsis Campaign guidelines on the management of sepsis and septic shock have recently been published [97]. On the basis of these guidelines, pharmacologic thromboprophylaxis with low molecular weight heparin is strongly recommended for patients with sepsis or septic shock. Moreover, in the latest Japanese Surviving Sepsis Campaign guidelines of 2020, the early detection of DIC is encouraged, and the use of anticoagulants for sepsis-associated DIC is weakly recommended [98].

Several treatment strategies for SIC have been evaluated, mainly directed at suppressing the prothrombotic effects, such as the administration of heparin/heparinoids or anticoagulant proteins (Table 2) [99,100]. The value of recombinant thrombomodulin in sepsis-induced coagulopathy was recently evaluated in a multinational, randomized controlled phase III trial (including patients with a platelet count $< 50 \times 10^9$/L and a prothrombin time ratio > 1.4). The authors of this study reported that the 28-day mortality improved by 2.6% in 800 septic patients, although this difference in the mortality rate was not statistically significant. [101]. During the last few years, several anticoagulant agents, including antithrombin, have been tested in an attempt to reduce mortality in patients with sepsis; however, they have largely failed to prove effective [101]. It should be noted, though, that all these trials targeted septic patients and not patients with SIC. Antithrombin is not recommended by the international sepsis guidelines. In contrast, post hoc analysis of databases has indicated the beneficial effects of anticoagulants in certain subgroups of septic patients with DIC [102]. A possible explanation for this discrepancy lies in the heterogeneity of patients and the timing of anticoagulant treatment in large-scale trials. Precision medicine principles should be applied to select suitable candidates for anticoagulation intervention among sepsis patients with SIC.

Table 2. Treatment options for sepsis-induced coagulopathy.

Treatment Options	Comments	References
Heparin and heparinoids	Their effectiveness in sepsis-induced coagulopathy is debatable and limited to preventing deep vein thrombosis.	Iba et al. [99]
Antithrombin, activated protein C, and tissue factor pathway inhibitors	Potential survival benefit with antithrombin administration.	Kienast et al. [100]
Fresh frozen plasma	No evidence supporting its use unless there are specific indications for bleeding or factor depletion beyond antithrombin	Iba et al. [99]
Recombinant thrombomodulin	It may improve overall mortality in patients with SIC	Vincent et al. [101]

8. Conclusions

This updated review consolidates all the current knowledge regarding the pathogenesis of SIC while it includes all the recent updates regarding the diagnostic criteria for SIC based on international scientific societies. Moreover, this comprehensive review includes an extensive discussion of all conventional and nonconventional biomarkers for SIC. Sepsis-induced coagulopathy often complicates the course of patients, with potentially adverse outcomes and increased mortality. Hypercoagulability is a well-established pathophysiological feature of sepsis-induced coagulopathy, with a shift towards hypocoagulability only in the late sepsis stages, after the development of DIC. Traditional coagulation tests can detect late-stage hypocoagulability but are not sensitive to identify early-phase hypocoagulability. A gap exists in the diagnosis of hemostatic derangement in sepsis. The definition of SIC was introduced to help identify septic patients before the establishment of DIC, during the early stages, which could be reversed with therapeutic interventions. In this context, investigating novel, specialized assays, such as thromboelastometry, is essential for patients with severe sepsis, as it may allow for early intervention during the hypercoagulability phase. Further research for diagnostic biomarkers and potential combinations to increase diagnostic accuracy is warranted.

Author Contributions: Conceptualization, A.G.T., S.P. and R.S.; methodology, P.G.M., S.P., A.G.T., E.B., E.A.T. and K.A.T.; validation, A.G.V., S.T. and A.K.; formal analysis, D.H.; investigation, D.P., G.K.N., N.I. and R.S.; data curation, P.G.M., A.G.T., S.P., E.B., E.A.T. and K.A.T.; writing—original draft preparation, S.P. and A.G.T.; writing—review and editing, A.G.T., S.P., E.A.T., E.B., K.A.T., A.G.V., S.T., A.K., D.H., D.P., G.K.N., N.I. and R.S.; supervision, R.S., A.G.T. and S.P. All authors have read and agreed to the published version of the manuscript.

Funding: This research received no external funding.

Data Availability Statement: Not applicable.

Conflicts of Interest: The authors declare no conflict of interest.

References

1. Singer, M.; Deutschman, C.S.; Seymour, C.W.; Shankar-Hari, M.; Annane, D.; Bauer, M.; Bellomo, R.; Bernard, G.R.; Chiche, J.-D.; Coopersmith, C.M.; et al. The Third International Consensus Definitions for Sepsis and Septic Shock (Sepsis-3). *JAMA* **2016**, *315*, 801–810. [CrossRef]
2. Giustozzi, M.; Ehrlinder, H.; Bongiovanni, D.; Borovac, J.A.; Guerreiro, R.A.; Gąsecka, A.; Papakonstantinou, P.E.; Parker, W.A. Coagulopathy and sepsis: Pathophysiology, clinical manifestations and treatment. *Blood Rev.* **2021**, *50*, 100864. [CrossRef] [PubMed]
3. Martin, G.S.; Mannino, D.M.; Eaton, S.; Moss, M. The Epidemiology of Sepsis in the United States from 1979 through 2000. *N. Engl. J. Med.* **2003**, *348*, 1546–1554. [CrossRef] [PubMed]
4. Cecconi, M.; Evans, L.; Levy, M.; Rhodes, A. Sepsis and septic shock. *Lancet* **2018**, *392*, 75–87. [CrossRef]
5. Levi, M.; van der Poll, T. Coagulation and sepsis. *Thromb. Res.* **2017**, *149*, 38–44. [CrossRef] [PubMed]
6. Sungurlu, S.; Kuppy, J.; Balk, R.A. Role of Antithrombin III and Tissue Factor Pathway in the Pathogenesis of Sepsis. *Crit. Care Clin.* **2020**, *36*, 255–265. [CrossRef] [PubMed]
7. Denning, N.-L.; Aziz, M.; Gurien, S.D.; Wang, P. DAMPs and NETs in Sepsis. *Front. Immunol.* **2019**, *10*, 2536. [CrossRef] [PubMed]
8. Levi, M.; van der Poll, T. Inflammation and coagulation. *Crit. Care Med.* **2010**, *38*, S26–S34. [CrossRef]
9. Levi, M.; Poll, T. Coagulation in patients with severe sepsis. *Semin. Thromb. Hemost.* **2015**, *41*, 9–15. [CrossRef]
10. Gando, S. Role of Fibrinolysis in Sepsis. *Semin. Thromb. Hemost.* **2013**, *39*, 392–399. [CrossRef]
11. Degen, J.L.; Bugge, T.H.; Goguen, J.D. Fibrin and fibrinolysis in infection and host defense. *J. Thromb. Haemost.* **2007**, *5*, 24–31. [CrossRef] [PubMed]
12. Bergmann, S.; Hammerschmidt, S. Fibrinolysis and host response in bacterial infections. *Thromb. Haemost.* **2007**, *98*, 512–520. [CrossRef]
13. Petros, S.; Kliem, P.; Siegemund, T. Thrombin generation in severe sepsis. *Thromb. Res.* **2012**, *129*, 797–800. [CrossRef]
14. Coughlin, S.R. Thrombin signalling and protease-activated receptors. *Nature* **2000**, *407*, 258–264. [CrossRef] [PubMed]
15. Iba, T.; Ito, T.; Maruyama, I.; Jilma, B.; Brenner, T.; Müller, M.C.; Juffermans, N.P.; Thachil, J. Potential diagnostic markers for disseminated intravascular coagulation of sepsis. *Blood Rev.* **2016**, *30*, 149–155. [CrossRef]
16. Yuksel, M.; Okajima, K.; Uchiba, M.; Horiuchi, S.; Okabe, H. Activated protein C inhibits lipopolysaccharide-induced tumor necrosis factor-alpha production by inhibiting activation of both nuclear factor-kappa B and activator protein-1 in human monocytes. *Thromb. Haemost.* **2002**, *88*, 267–273. [CrossRef] [PubMed]
17. Wheeler, A.P.; Bernard, G.R. Treating Patients with Severe Sepsis. *N. Engl. J. Med.* **1999**, *340*, 207–214. [CrossRef] [PubMed]
18. Taylor, F.B.; Toh, C.H.; Hoots, W.K.; Wada, H.; Levi, M. Towards definition, clinical and laboratory criteria, and a scoring system for disseminated intravascular coagulation. *Thromb. Haemost.* **2001**, *86*, 1327–1330. [CrossRef]
19. Gando, S.; Levi, M.; Toh, C.H. Disseminated intravascular coagulation. *Nat. Rev. Dis. Primers* **2016**, *2*, 16037. [CrossRef]
20. Iba, T.; Levy, J.H. Sepsis-induced Coagulopathy and Disseminated Intravascular Coagulation. *Anesthesiology* **2020**, *132*, 1238–1245. [CrossRef]

21. Iba, T.; Levy, J.H.; Warkentin, T.E.; Thachil, J.; van der Poll, T.; Levi, M. Diagnosis and management of sepsis-induced coagulopathy and disseminated intravascular coagulation. *J. Thromb. Haemost.* **2019**, *17*, 1989–1994. [CrossRef] [PubMed]
22. Gando, S.; Iba, T.; Eguchi, Y.; Ohtomo, Y.; Okamoto, K.; Koseki, K.; Mayumi, T.; Murata, A.; Ikeda, T.; Ishikura, H.; et al. A multicenter, prospective validation of disseminated intravascular coagulation diagnostic criteria for critically ill patients: Comparing current criteria. *Crit. Care Med.* **2006**, *34*, 625–631. [CrossRef] [PubMed]
23. Levi, M.; Sivapalaratnam, S. Disseminated intravascular coagulation: An update on pathogenesis and diagnosis. *Expert Rev. Hematol.* **2018**, *11*, 663–672. [CrossRef] [PubMed]
24. Iba, T.; Levi, M.; Levy, J.H. Sepsis-Induced Coagulopathy and Disseminated Intravascular Coagulation. *Semin. Thromb. Hemost.* **2020**, *46*, 089–095. [CrossRef]
25. Iba, T.; Di Nisio, M.; Levy, J.H.; Kitamura, N.; Thachil, J. New criteria for sepsis-induced coagulopathy (SIC) following the revised sepsis definition: A retrospective analysis of a nationwide survey. *BMJ Open* **2017**, *7*, e017046. [CrossRef]
26. Koyama, K.; Madoiwa, S.; Nunomiya, S.; Koinuma, T.; Wada, M.; Sakata, A.; Ohmori, T.; Mimuro, J.; Sakata, Y. Combination of thrombin-antithrombin complex, plasminogen activator inhibitor-1, and protein C activity for early identification of severe coagulopathy in initial phase of sepsis: A prospective observational study. *Crit. Care* **2014**, *18*, R13. [CrossRef] [PubMed]
27. Hack, C.E. Fibrinolysis in Disseminated Intravascular Coagulation. *Semin. Thromb. Hemost.* **2001**, *27*, 633–638. [CrossRef]
28. Engelmann, B.; Massberg, S. Thrombosis as an intravascular effector of innate immunity. *Nat. Rev. Immunol.* **2013**, *13*, 34–45. [CrossRef]
29. Schmitt, F.C.F.; Manolov, V.; Morgenstern, J.; Fleming, T.; Heitmeier, S.; Uhle, F.; Al-Saeedi, M.; Hackert, T.; Bruckner, T.; Schöchl, H.; et al. Acute fibrinolysis shutdown occurs early in septic shock and is associated with increased morbidity and mortality: Results of an observational pilot study. *Ann. Intensive Care* **2019**, *9*, 19. [CrossRef]
30. Asakura, H. Classifying types of disseminated intravascular coagulation: Clinical and animal models. *J. Intensive Care* **2014**, *2*, 20. [CrossRef]
31. Iba, T.; Di Nisio, M.; Thachil, J.; Wada, H.; Asakura, H.; Sato, K.; Saitoh, D. A Proposal of the Modification of Japanese Society on Thrombosis and Hemostasis (JSTH) Disseminated Intravascular Coagulation (DIC) Diagnostic Criteria for Sepsis-Associated DIC. *Clin. Appl. Thromb.* **2018**, *24*, 439–445. [CrossRef]
32. Iba, T.; Arakawa, M.; Di Nisio, M.; Gando, S.; Anan, H.; Sato, K.; Ueki, Y.; Levy, J.H.; Thachil, J. Newly Proposed Sepsis-Induced Coagulopathy Precedes International Society on Thrombosis and Haemostasis Overt-Disseminated Intravascular Coagulation and Predicts High Mortality. *J. Intensive Care Med.* **2020**, *35*, 643–649. [CrossRef] [PubMed]
33. Iba, T.; Arakawa, M.; Levy, J.H.; Yamakawa, K.; Koami, H.; Hifumi, T.; Sato, K. Sepsis-Induced Coagulopathy and Japanese Association for Acute Medicine DIC in Coagulopathic Patients with Decreased Antithrombin and Treated by Antithrombin. *Clin. Appl. Thromb.* **2018**, *24*, 1020–1026. [CrossRef] [PubMed]
34. Yamakawa, K.; Yoshimura, J.; Ito, T.; Hayakawa, M.; Hamasaki, T.; Fujimi, S. External Validation of the Two Newly Proposed Criteria for Assessing Coagulopathy in Sepsis. *Thromb. Haemost.* **2019**, *119*, 203–212. [CrossRef] [PubMed]
35. Folman, C.C.; Linthorst, G.E.; van Mourik, J.; van Willigen, G.; de Jonge, E.; Levi, M.; von dem Borne, A.E. Platelets release thrombopoietin (Tpo) upon activation: Another regulatory loop in thrombocytopoiesis? *Thromb. Haemost.* **2000**, *83*, 923–930. [CrossRef]
36. Shannon, O. The role of platelets in sepsis. *Res. Pract. Thromb. Haemost.* **2020**, *5*, 27–37. [CrossRef]
37. Venkata, C.; Kashyap, R.; Farmer, J.C.; Afessa, B. Thrombocytopenia in adult patients with sepsis: Incidence, risk factors, and its association with clinical outcome. *J. Intensive Care* **2013**, *1*, 9. [CrossRef] [PubMed]
38. Vanderschueren, S.; De Weerdt, A.; Malbrain, M.; Vankersschaever, D.; Frans, E.; Wilmer, A.; Bobbaers, H. Thrombocytopenia and prognosis in intensive care. *Crit. Care Med.* **2000**, *28*, 1871–1876. [CrossRef]
39. Gawaz, M.; Fateh-Moghadam, S.; Pilz, G.; Gurland, H.-J.; Werdan, K. Platelet activation and interaction with leucocytes in patients with sepsis or multiple organ failure. *Eur. J. Clin. Investig.* **1995**, *25*, 843–851. [CrossRef]
40. Hamzeh-Cognasse, H.; Damien, P.; Chabert, A.; Pozzetto, B.; Cognasse, F.; Garraud, O. Platelets and Infections—Complex Interactions with Bacteria. *Front. Immunol.* **2015**, *6*, 82. [CrossRef]
41. Hubert, R.M.E.; Rodrigues, M.V.; Andreguetto, B.D.; Santos, T.M.; Gilberti, M.D.F.P.; de Castro, V.; Annichino-Bizzacchi, J.M.; Dragosavac, D.; Carvalho-Filho, M.A.; De Paula, E.V. Association of the immature platelet fraction with sepsis diagnosis and severity. *Sci. Rep.* **2015**, *5*, srep08019. [CrossRef] [PubMed]
42. Horan, J.T.; Francis, C.W. Fibrin Degradation Products, Fibrin Monomer and Soluble Fibrin in Disseminated Intravascular Coagulation. *Semin. Thromb. Hemost.* **2001**, *27*, 657–666. [CrossRef] [PubMed]
43. Semeraro, F.; Ammollo, C.T.; Caironi, P.; Masson, S.; Latini, R.; Panigada, M.; Colucci, M. Low D-dimer levels in sepsis: Good or bad? *Thromb. Res.* **2019**, *174*, 13–15. [CrossRef]
44. Favresse, J.; Lippi, G.; Roy, P.M.; Chatelain, B.; Jacqmin, H.; Ten Cate, H.; Mullier, F. D-dimer: Preanalytical, analytical, postanalytical variables, and clinical applications. *Crit. Rev. Clin. Lab. Sci.* **2018**, *55*, 548–577. [CrossRef]
45. Toh, J.M.; Ken-Dror, G.; Downey, C.; Abrams, S.T. The clinical utility of fibrin-related biomarkers in sepsis. *Blood Coagul. Fibrinolysis* **2013**, *24*, 839–843. [CrossRef]
46. Adelborg, K.; Larsen, J.B.; Hvas, A. Disseminated intravascular coagulation: Epidemiology, biomarkers, and management. *Br. J. Haematol.* **2021**, *192*, 803–818. [CrossRef] [PubMed]
47. Levi, M.; Meijers, J.C. DIC: Which laboratory tests are most useful. *Blood Rev.* **2011**, *25*, 33–37. [CrossRef]

48. Kamal, A.H.; Tefferi, A.; Pruthi, R.K. How to Interpret and Pursue an Abnormal Prothrombin Time, Activated Partial Thromboplastin Time, and Bleeding Time in Adults. *Mayo Clin. Proc.* **2007**, *82*, 864–873. [CrossRef]
49. Scarlatescu, E.; Juffermans, N.P.; Thachil, J. The current status of viscoelastic testing in septic coagulopathy. *Thromb. Res.* **2019**, *183*, 146–152. [CrossRef]
50. Görlinger, K.; Pérez-Ferrer, A.; Dirkmann, D.; Saner, F.; Maegele, M.; Calatayud, Á.A.P.; Kim, T.-Y. The role of evidence-based algorithms for rotational thromboelastometry-guided bleeding management. *Korean J. Anesthesiol.* **2019**, *72*, 297–322. [CrossRef]
51. Georgiadou, P.; Sokou, R.; Tsantes, A.G.; Parastatidou, S.; Konstantinidi, A.; Houhoula, D.; Kokoris, S.; Iacovidou, N.; Tsantes, A.E. The Non-Activated Thromboelastometry (NATEM) Assay's Application among Adults and Neonatal/Pediatric Population: A Systematic Review. *Diagnostics* **2022**, *12*, 658. [CrossRef] [PubMed]
52. Sokou, R.; Ioakeimidis, G.; Piovani, D.; Parastatidou, S.; Konstantinidi, A.; Tsantes, A.G.; Lampridou, M.; Houhoula, D.; Iacovidou, N.; Kokoris, S.; et al. Development and validation of a sepsis diagnostic scoring model for neonates with suspected sepsis. *Front. Pediatr.* **2022**, *10*, 1004727. [CrossRef] [PubMed]
53. Sokou, R.; Tritzali, M.; Piovani, D.; Konstantinidi, A.; Tsantes, A.G.; Ioakeimidis, G.; Lampridou, M.; Parastatidou, S.; Iacovidou, N.; Kokoris, S.; et al. Comparative Performance of Four Established Neonatal Disease Scoring Systems in Predicting In-Hospital Mortality and the Potential Role of Thromboelastometry. *Diagnostics* **2021**, *11*, 1955. [CrossRef] [PubMed]
54. Tsantes, A.G.; Sokou, R.; Konstantinidi, A.; Ioakeimidis, G.; Lampridou, M.; Parastatidou, S.; Theodoraki, M.; Piovani, D.; Iliodromiti, Z.; Boutsikou, T.; et al. Rotational Thromboelastometry in Neonates Admitted to a Neonatal Intensive Care Unit: A Large Cross-sectional Study. *Semin. Thromb. Hemost.* **2021**, *47*, 875–884. [CrossRef] [PubMed]
55. Müller, M.C.; Meijers, J.C.; Vroom, M.B.; Juffermans, N.P. Utility of thromboelastography and/or thromboelastometry in adults with sepsis: A systematic review. *Crit. Care* **2014**, *18*, R30. [CrossRef] [PubMed]
56. Hu, Y.L.; McRae, H.L.; Refaai, M.A. Efficacy of viscoelastic hemostatic assay testing in patients with sepsis-induced disseminated intravascular coagulation. *Eur. J. Haematol.* **2021**, *106*, 873–875. [CrossRef]
57. Katsaras, G.; Sokou, R.; Tsantes, A.G.; Piovani, D.; Bonovas, S.; Konstantinidi, A.; Ioakeimidis, G.; Parastatidou, S.; Gialamprinou, D.; Makrogianni, A.; et al. The use of thromboelastography (TEG) and rotational thromboelastometry (ROTEM) in neonates: A systematic review. *Eur. J. Pediatr.* **2021**, *180*, 3455–3470. [CrossRef]
58. Lampridou, M.; Sokou, R.; Tsantes, A.G.; Theodoraki, M.; Konstantinidi, A.; Ioakeimidis, G.; Bonovas, S.; Politou, M.; Valsami, S.; Iliodromiti, Z.; et al. ROTEM diagnostic capacity for measuring fibrinolysis in neonatal sepsis. *Thromb. Res.* **2020**, *192*, 103–108. [CrossRef]
59. Adamik, B.; Gozdzik, W.; Jakubczyk, D.; Welna, M.; Kübler, A. Coagulation abnormalities identified by thromboelastometry in patients with severe sepsis: The relationship to endotoxemia and mortality. *Blood Coagul. Fibrinolysis* **2017**, *28*, 163–170. [CrossRef]
60. Sivula, M.; Pettilä, V.; Niemi, T.T.; Varpula, M.; Kuitunen, A.H. Thromboelastometry in patients with severe sepsis and disseminated intravascular coagulation. *Blood Coagul. Fibrinolysis* **2009**, *20*, 419–426. [CrossRef]
61. Davies, G.R.; Lawrence, M.; Pillai, S.; Mills, G.M.; Aubrey, R.; Thomas, D.; Williams, R.; Morris, K.; Evans, P.A. The effect of sepsis and septic shock on the viscoelastic properties of clot quality and mass using rotational thromboelastometry: A prospective observational study. *J. Crit. Care* **2018**, *44*, 7–11. [CrossRef] [PubMed]
62. Sharma, P.; Saxena, R. A Novel Thromboelastographic Score to Identify Overt Disseminated Intravascular Coagulation Resulting in a Hypocoagulable State. *Am. J. Clin. Pathol.* **2010**, *134*, 97–102. [CrossRef] [PubMed]
63. Koami, H.; Sakamoto, Y.; Ohta, M.; Goto, A.; Narumi, S.; Imahase, H.; Inoue, S. Can rotational thromboelastometry predict septic disseminated intravascular coagulation? *Blood Coagul. Fibrinolysis* **2015**, *26*, 778–783. [CrossRef]
64. Li, Y.; Wan, D.; Luo, X.; Song, T.; Wang, Y.; Yu, Q.; Jiang, L.; Liao, R.; Zhao, W.; Su, B. Circulating Histones in Sepsis: Potential Outcome Predictors and Therapeutic Targets. *Front. Immunol.* **2021**, *12*, 650184. [CrossRef] [PubMed]
65. Andersson, U.; Tracey, K.J. HMGB1 Is a Therapeutic Target for Sterile Inflammation and Infection. *Annu. Rev. Immunol.* **2011**, *29*, 139–162. [CrossRef]
66. Ito, T.; Kawahara, K.; Nakamura, T.; Yamada, S.; Nakamura, T.; Abeyama, K.; Hashiguchi, T.; Maruyama, I. High-mobility group box 1 protein promotes development of microvascular thrombosis in rats. *J. Thromb. Haemost.* **2007**, *5*, 109–116. [CrossRef]
67. Hatada, T.; Nobori, T.; Okabayashi, K.; Maruyama, K.; Abe, Y.; Uemoto, S.; Yamada, S.; Maruyama, I.; Wada, H. Plasma concentrations and importance of high mobility group box protein in the prognosis of organ failure in patients with disseminated intravascular coagulation. *Thromb. Haemost.* **2005**, *94*, 975–979. [CrossRef] [PubMed]
68. Morimont, L.; Dechamps, M.; David, C.; Bouvy, C.; Gillot, C.; Haguet, H.; Favresse, J.; Ronvaux, L.; Candiracci, J.; Herzog, M.; et al. NETosis and Nucleosome Biomarkers in Septic Shock and Critical COVID-19 Patients: An Observational Study. *Biomolecules* **2022**, *12*, 1038. [CrossRef]
69. Chen, Q.; Ye, L.; Jin, Y.; Zhang, N.; Lou, T.; Qiu, Z.; Jin, Y.; Cheng, B.; Fang, X. Circulating nucleosomes as a predictor of sepsis and organ dysfunction in critically ill patients. *Int. J. Infect. Dis.* **2012**, *16*, e558–e564. [CrossRef]
70. Xu, J.; Zhang, X.; Pelayo, R.; Monestier, M.; Ammollo, C.T.; Semeraro, F.; Taylor, F.B.; Esmon, N.L.; Lupu, F.; Esmon, C.T. Extracellular histones are major mediators of death in sepsis. *Nat. Med.* **2009**, *15*, 1318–1321. [CrossRef]
71. Nakahara, M.; Ito, T.; Kawahara, K.-I.; Yamamoto, M.; Nagasato, T.; Shrestha, B.; Yamada, S.; Miyauchi, T.; Higuchi, K.; Takenaka, T.; et al. Recombinant Thrombomodulin Protects Mice against Histone-Induced Lethal Thromboembolism. *PLoS ONE* **2013**, *8*, e75961. [CrossRef] [PubMed]

72. Abrams, S.T.; Zhang, N.; Manson, J.; Liu, T.; Dart, C.; Baluwa, F.; Toh, C.H. Circulating histones are mediators of trauma-associated lung injury. *Am. J. Respir. Crit. Care Med.* **2013**, *187*, 160–169. [CrossRef] [PubMed]
73. Dwivedi, D.J.; Toltl, L.J.; Swystun, L.L.; Pogue, J.; Liaw, K.-L.; Weitz, J.I.; Cook, D.J.; Fox-Robichaud, A.E.; Liaw, P.C.; Canadian Critical Care Translational Biology Group. Prognostic utility and characterization of cell-free DNA in patients with severe sepsis. *Crit. Care* **2012**, *16*, R151. [CrossRef] [PubMed]
74. Iba, T.; Levy, J.H. Inflammation and thrombosis: Roles of neutrophils, platelets and endothelial cells and their interactions in thrombus formation during sepsis. *J. Thromb. Haemost.* **2018**, *16*, 231–241. [CrossRef]
75. Levi, M.; de Jonge, E.; van der Poll, T. Rationale for restoration of physiological anticoagulant pathways in patients with sepsis and disseminated intravascular coagulation. *Crit. Care Med.* **2001**, *29*, S90–S94. [CrossRef]
76. Levi, M.M.; Toh, C.H.; Thachil, J.; Watson, H.G. Guidelines for the diagnosis and management of disseminated intravascular coagulation. British Committee for Standards in Haematology. *Br. J. Haematol.* **2009**, *145*, 24–33. [CrossRef]
77. Iba, T.; Kidokoro, A.; Yagi, Y. The Role of the Endothelium in Changes in Procoagulant Activity in Sepsis. *J. Am. Coll. Surg.* **1998**, *187*, 321–329. [CrossRef]
78. Warren, B.L.; Eid, A.; Singer, P.; Pillay, S.S.; Carl, P.; Novak, I.; Chalupa, P.; Atherstone, A.; Pénzes, I.; Kübler, A.; et al. High-dose antithrombin III in severe sepsis: A randomized controlled trial. *JAMA* **2001**, *286*, 1869–1878. [CrossRef]
79. Niederwanger, C.; Hell, T.; Hofer, S.; Salvador, C.; Michel, M.; Schenk, B.; Treml, B.; Bachler, M. Antithrombin deficiency is associated with mortality and impaired organ function in septic pediatric patients: A retrospective study. *PeerJ* **2018**, *6*, e5538. [CrossRef]
80. Martí-Carvajal, A.J.; Solà, I.; Gluud, C.; Lathyris, D.; Anand, V. Human recombinant protein C for severe sepsis and septic shock in adult and paediatric patients. *Cochrane Database Syst. Rev.* **2012**, *12*, CD004388. [CrossRef]
81. Guitton, C.; Gérard, N.; Sébille, V.; Bretonnière, C.; Zambon, O.; Villers, D.; Charreau, B. Early rise in circulating endothelial protein C receptor correlates with poor outcome in severe sepsis. *Intensive Care Med.* **2011**, *37*, 950–956. [CrossRef]
82. Huang, M.; Cai, S.; Su, J. The Pathogenesis of Sepsis and Potential Therapeutic Targets. *Int. J. Mol. Sci.* **2019**, *20*, 5376. [CrossRef] [PubMed]
83. Conway, E.M. Thrombomodulin and its role in inflammation. *Semin. Immunopathol.* **2011**, *34*, 107–125. [CrossRef] [PubMed]
84. Furuno, T.; Mitsuyama, T.; Hidaka, K.; Tanaka, T.; Hara, N. The Role of Neutrophil Elastase in Human Pulmonary Artery Endothelial Cell Injury. *Int. Arch. Allergy Immunol.* **1997**, *112*, 262–269. [CrossRef] [PubMed]
85. Kinasewitz, G.T.; Yan, S.B.; Basson, B.; Comp, P.; Russell, J.A.; Cariou, A.; Um, S.L.; Utterback, B.; Laterre, P.-F.; Dhainaut, J.-F. Universal changes in biomarkers of coagulation and inflammation occur in patients with severe sepsis, regardless of causative micro-organism [ISRCTN74215569]. *Crit. Care* **2004**, *8*, R82–R90. [CrossRef]
86. Boehme, M.W.; Deng, Y.; Raeth, U.; Bierhaus, A.; Ziegler, R.; Stremmel, W.; Nawroth, P.P. Release of thrombomodulin from endothelial cells by concerted action of TNF-alpha and neutrophils: In vivo and in vitro studies. *Immunology* **1996**, *87*, 134–140.
87. Kushimoto, S.; Wada, H.; Kawasugi, K.; Okamoto, K.; Uchiyama, T.; Seki, Y.; Hatada, T.; Imai, H.; Nobori, T.; Subcommittee, J.S.O.T.H. Increased Ratio of Soluble Fibrin Formation/Thrombin Generation in Patients With DIC. *Clin. Appl. Thromb.* **2012**, *18*, 628–632. [CrossRef]
88. Mei, H.; Jiang, Y.; Luo, L.; Huang, R.; Su, L.; Hou, M.; Wang, X.; Deng, J.; Hu, Y. Evaluation the combined diagnostic value of TAT, PIC, tPAIC, and sTM in disseminated intravascular coagulation: A multi-center prospective observational study. *Thromb. Res.* **2018**, *173*, 20–26. [CrossRef]
89. Hoshino, K.; Kitamura, T.; Nakamura, Y.; Irie, Y.; Matsumoto, N.; Kawano, Y.; Ishikura, H. Usefulness of plasminogen activator inhibitor-1 as a predictive marker of mortality in sepsis. *J. Intensive Care* **2017**, *5*, 67. [CrossRef]
90. Tipoe, T.L.; Wu, W.K.K.; Chung, L.; Gong, M.; Dong, M.; Liu, T.; Roever, L.; Ho, J.; Wong, M.C.S.; Chan, M.T.V.; et al. Plasminogen Activator Inhibitor 1 for Predicting Sepsis Severity and Mortality Outcomes: A Systematic Review and Meta-Analysis. *Front. Immunol.* **2018**, *9*, 1218. [CrossRef]
91. Elad, B.; Avraham, G.; Schwartz, N.; Elias, A.; Elias, M. Role of a thrombin generation assay in the prediction of infection severity. *Sci. Rep.* **2021**, *11*, 7814. [CrossRef]
92. Mihajlovic, D.; Brkic, S.; Lendak, D.; Mikic, A.N.; Draskovic, B.; Mitic, G. Endogenous thrombin potential as marker of procoagulant response that can be useful in early stage of sepsis. *Blood Coagul. Fibrinolysis* **2017**, *28*, 460–467. [CrossRef] [PubMed]
93. Levi, M.; Vincent, J.-L.; Tanaka, K.; Radford, A.H.; Kayanoki, T.; Fineberg, D.A.; Hoppensteadt, D.; Fareed, J. Effect of a Recombinant Human Soluble Thrombomodulin on Baseline Coagulation Biomarker Levels and Mortality Outcome in Patients with Sepsis-Associated Coagulopathy. *Crit. Care Med.* **2020**, *48*, 1140–1147. [CrossRef] [PubMed]
94. Asakura, H.; Takahashi, H.; Uchiyama, T.; Eguchi, Y.; Okamoto, K.; Kawasugi, K.; Madoiwa, S.; Wada, H.; DIC Subcommittee of the Japanese Society on Thrombosis and Hemostasis. Proposal for new diagnostic criteria for DIC from the Japanese Society on Thrombosis and Hemostasis. *Thromb. J.* **2016**, *14*, 42. [CrossRef] [PubMed]
95. Zheng, X.; Chung, D.; Takayama, T.K.; Majerus, E.M.; Sadler, J.E.; Fujikawa, K. Structure of von Willebrand Factor-cleaving Protease (ADAMTS13), a Metalloprotease Involved in Thrombotic Thrombocytopenic Purpura. *J. Biol. Chem.* **2001**, *276*, 41059–41063. [CrossRef]
96. Levi, M.; Scully, M.; Singer, M. The role of ADAMTS -13 in the coagulopathy of sepsis. *J. Thromb. Haemost.* **2018**, *16*, 646–651. [CrossRef]

97. Evans, L.; Rhodes, A.; Alhazzani, W.; Antonelli, M.; Coopersmith, C.M.; French, C.; Machado, F.R.; Mcintyre, L.; Ostermann, M.; Prescott, H.C.; et al. Surviving sepsis campaign: International guidelines for management of sepsis and septic shock 2021. *Intensive Care Med.* **2021**, *47*, 1181–1247. [CrossRef]
98. Egi, M.; Ogura, H.; Yatabe, T.; Atagi, K.; Inoue, S.; Iba, T.; Kakihana, Y.; Kawasaki, T.; Kushimoto, S.; Kuroda, Y.; et al. The Japanese Clinical Practice Guidelines for Management of Sepsis and Septic Shock 2020 (J-SSCG 2020). *Acute Med. Surg.* **2021**, *8*, 53. [CrossRef]
99. Inata, Y. Should we treat sepsis-induced DIC with anticoagulants? *J. Intensive Care* **2020**, *8*, 18. [CrossRef]
100. Kienast, J.; Juers, M.; Wiedermann, C.J.; Hoffmann, J.N.; Ostermann, H.; Strauss, R.; Keinecke, H.-O.; Warren, B.L.; Opal, S.M.; The KyberSept Investigators. Treatment effects of high-dose antithrombin without concomitant heparin in patients with severe sepsis with or without disseminated intravascular coagulation. *J. Thromb. Haemost.* **2006**, *4*, 90–97. [CrossRef]
101. Vincent, J.L.; Francois, B.; Zabolotskikh, I.; Daga, M.K.; Lascarrou, J.B.; Kirov, M.Y.; SCARLET Trial Group. Effect of a recombinant human soluble thrombomodulin on mortality in patients with sepsis-associated coagulopathy: The SCARLET randomized clinical trial. *JAMA* **2019**, *321*, 1993–2002. [CrossRef] [PubMed]
102. Scarlatescu, E.; Tomescu, D.; Arama, S.S. Review. Anticoagulant Therapy in Sepsis. The Importance of Timing. *J. Crit. Care Med.* **2017**, *3*, 63–69. [CrossRef] [PubMed]

life

MDPI

Review

Soluble and EV-Associated Diagnostic and Prognostic Biomarkers in Knee Osteoarthritis Pathology and Detection

Marko Moravek, Jana Matejova and Timea Spakova *

Associated Tissue Bank, Faculty of Medicine, Pavol Jozef Safarik University and Louis Pasteur University Hospital, Tr. SNP 1, 040 11 Kosice, Slovakia
* Correspondence: timea.spakova@upjs.sk; Tel.: +421-55-234-3241

Abstract: Osteoarthritis (OA) is the most common degenerative disease of the connective tissue of the human musculoskeletal system. Despite its widespread prevalence, there are many limitations in its diagnosis and treatment. OA diagnosis currently relies on the presence of clinical symptoms, sometimes accompanied by changes in joint X-rays or MRIs. Biomarkers help not only to diagnose early disease progression but also to understand the process of OA in many ways. In this article, we briefly summarize information on articular joints and joint tissues, the pathogenesis of OA and review the literature about biomarkers in the field of OA, specifically inflammatory cytokines/chemokines, proteins, miRNA, and metabolic biomarkers found in the blood, synovial fluid and in extracellular vesicles.

Keywords: osteoarthritis; knee joint; biomarkers; extracellular vesicles

check for updates

Citation: Moravek, M.; Matejova, J.; Spakova, T. Soluble and EV-Associated Diagnostic and Prognostic Biomarkers in Knee Osteoarthritis Pathology and Detection. *Life* **2023**, *13*, 342. https://doi.org/10.3390/life13020342

Academic Editors: Stefanos Roumeliotis and Giuseppe Minervini

Received: 15 December 2022
Revised: 13 January 2023
Accepted: 25 January 2023
Published: 27 January 2023

1. Introduction

Osteoarthritis (OA) of the knee joint is one of the most widespread musculoskeletal system diseases. OA is accompanied by number of symptoms, such as strong knee joint pain, articular cartilage degradation, synovial membrane inflammation and pathological enlargement of the subchondral bone [1]. OA was considered as an excessive wear and tear disease for a long time. This theory was supported by the fact that cartilage contains only one type of cell (chondrocytes), which does not have a high regenerative capacity. The regenerative process is demanding due to the fact that cartilage is not physiologically innervated or vascularized. Subsequently, the wear and tear theory was substituted by the inflammatory environment theory. The theory is based on the action of molecules such as cytokines, chemokines and prostaglandins. These inflammatory mediators significantly influence the production of matrix metalloproteinases (MMPs) and thereby contribute to the gradual degradation of joint cartilage [2].

Cytokines are secreted by chondrocytes, synovial fibroblasts and various other cell types present in the injured knee joint. Chemokines and other protein and non-protein inflammatory mediators are potential molecular biomarkers of OA. They are detectable in the blood, urine and synovial fluid (SF) of OA patients. It would be possible to predict the early stages of OA by identifying a single biomarker or group of biomarkers, which would lead to the early detection of OA and eventually reverse the disease progression.

These potential biomarkers of early-stage OA are not only detectable in soluble form in bodily fluids, but also in extracellular vesicles (EVs) produced by different cells. EVs are naturally occurring cell-derived particles that are surrounded by a lipid bilayer, are incapable of replicating, and lack a functioning nucleus. They are synthesized by several cell types and are present in various bodily fluids (serum, urine, cerebrospinal fluid and SF). EVs were formerly thought to be byproducts of cell metabolism. Nowadays, studies revealed that they perform a variety of crucial functions. Biologically active molecules found in EVs include proteins, messenger RNA (mRNA), microRNA (miRNA) and long non-coding

RNA (lncRNA). EVs are considered to be able to influence the microenvironment and offer intercellular communication because of their unique "cargo".

In this review, we intend to provide an updated overview of the OA pathogenesis, by emphasizing the currently available data and future perspectives of relevant biomarkers, which might augment the diagnosis, monitoring and prediction of this disease.

2. Osteoarthritis—Overall

The high prevalence of OA is the main cause of musculoskeletal system disabilities around the world. The disease affects weight-bearing joints, especially hip and knee joints [3]. It is the most frequent type of joint disease limiting the movement of people. Therefore, OA is associated with high health-care costs [4]. The disease is characterized by degradation of articular cartilage, osteophytes' formation, subchondral bone sclerosis and synovitis present in the injured joint. These degenerative processes cause the common clinical manifestations of OA as chronic pain, stiffness, joint instability, joint space narrowing and other various deformities regularly detected by X-ray [5]. Diagnosis of OA is possible based on typical symptoms of the disease or radiologically using X-ray, MRI or USG. Pathogenesis of OA includes focal progressive degradation of the hyaline cartilage and structural changes to the subchondral bone followed by osteophyte formation [6]. The synovial membrane is a soft tissue protecting joint capsule and is also significantly affected during the development of OA. Throughout the disease progression, immune cells are transferred from the vascular compartment into the synovium [7].

Many MRI-diagnosed osteoarthritic patients are totally asymptomatic [8]. Typical symptoms of OA combined with the occurrence of pathological processes are the most suitable method to diagnose OA [9].

In the past, OA was associated only with articular cartilage destruction caused by systematic overloading. Nowadays, it is known that synovitis as well as inflammatory mediators are crucial elements in OA pathology. Accordingly, the therapy along with the diagnosis of OA is focused on this molecular level [10].

Two types of OA are known, primary and secondary. Primary OA is a hereditary, or age-related disease. It affects predominantly the distal interphalangeal joints of hands, hips and knees. Secondary OA is characterized as a result of an injury associated with trauma, excessive overloading, or metabolic syndrome [11,12]. Injury, such as knee bending and repetitive stress on a joint, can damage a joint and increase the risk of OA in the joint. It is a complex disease as a result of the combination of systematic and biomechanical factors [13]. Although the incidence of OA increases with age it is not an indispensable effect of ageing. Age is always the strongest factor affecting the pathology of OA. Other factors include sex, biological race, bone density, estrogen level (decreasing significantly in women after menopause), nutrition and heredity. Biomechanical factors include increasingly widespread obesity, muscle weakness, various types of joint injuries and malformations [14]. Hereditary manifestation of the development of the disease does not mean the disease will develop into a pathological condition in the future [15]. Occurrences of hypertension, hypercholesterolemia and increased level of glucose in serum are usually coincidences associated with unilateral and bilateral knee OA. These facts suggest that OA is composed of systemic as well as metabolic factors [16].

2.1. Pathophysiology of Osteoarthritis

OA is a complex disease and its pathogenesis is composed of biomechanical as well as metabolic factors. Over time, these factors significantly affect the tissues present in the joint. It is well-known that genetic susceptibility is one of those factors and has an immense impact on the origin and progression of OA [17]. In the healthy synovial joint, the subchondral bone is protected by articular cartilage. Articular cartilage is composed of a dense extracellular matrix (ECM) with a rare distribution of highly specialized cells called chondrocytes. The main functions of that strong connective tissue are to spread the weight of the body and decrease the friction of contact areas during the joint motion.

Mechanical damage of articular cartilage causes rapid loss of these functions. Previously mentioned irreversible changes of the cartilage structure cause a joint space narrowing and during end-stage OA, contact of opposite bones is observed. This terminal stage of OA is accompanied by osteophytes' formation and chronic inflammation in the affected joint. During the inflammation in the joint capsule, a huge number of various cytokines and metalloproteinases are produced into the microenvironment (Figure 1) [14]. These inflammatory-associated molecules support other degradation processes in the affected joint. Studies confirmed that this molecular mechanism is the main cause of the progression of OA [17].

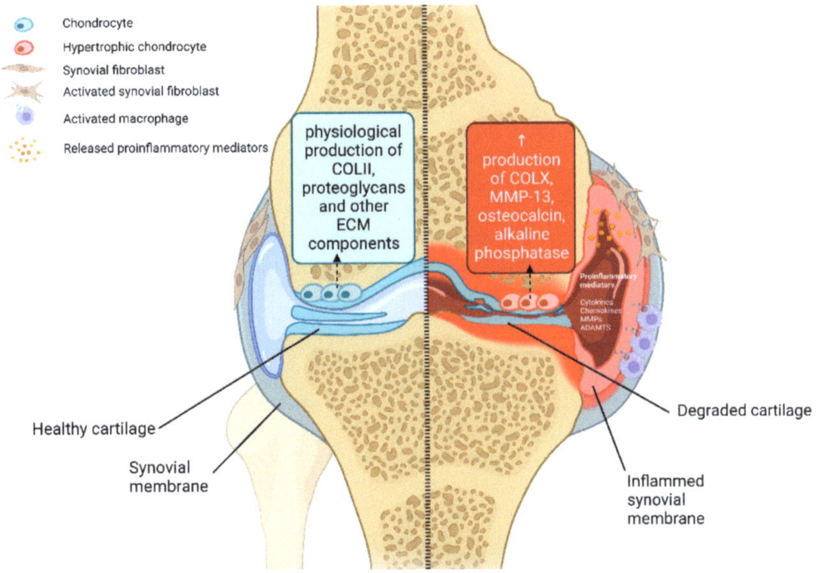

Figure 1. Structural and molecular changes during OA process. Chondrocytes present in healthy articular cartilage (**left**) produce ECM components under physiological conditions. Hypertrophic chondrocytes present in the affected OA joint (**right**) produce degradative enzymes such as MMP13 and the typical hypertrophic chondrocyte marker COLX. Created with BioRender.com.

2.2. *Structural Composition of Articular Cartilage*

The components of the ECM of mature articular cartilage are produced by specific cells—chondrocytes [18]. The ECM mainly consists of a dense grouping of collagen fibers (mainly type II, but also IX, XI, etc.), which are stored in a jelly-like environment of proteoglycans [19]. The structural composition of the matrix ensures the strength and elasticity of the cartilage and helping to maintain the correct biomechanical function of the joint [20]. Chondrocytes are the special cells present in cartilage. Their role is to ensure the synthesis of ECM components (collagens, proteoglycans) as well as the synthesis of degradative enzymes (MMPs) during the maturation of articular cartilage [17]. There is a balance between these processes under physiological conditions. In the process of the development of OA, this balance is significantly shifted to the side of degradation processes [21]. Significant structural changes occur in the subchondral bone as part of the body's reaction to inflammation. These changes are associated with the appearance of sclerosis and the formation of osteophytes, which can be detected by radiographic examination [10]. Changes in the structure of articular cartilage during the process of OA are also associated with phenotypic changes of the chondrocytes themselves [22]. In the initial phase of OA, chondrocyte hyperplasia and subsequent formation of clusters of these specific chondral cells occurs. Superficial chondrocytes synthesize molecules that are released under physiological conditions by hypertrophic chondrocytes located in the lower layer of hyaline cartilage [23]. Hypertrophic (terminally differentiated) chondrocytes are responsible for endochondral ossification, during which bone formation occurs from the original cartilage tissue. Signaling molecules produced by osteoarthritic chondrocytes (pathological state) include osteocalcin, transcription factors c-Maf and Runx2 and the specific marker of hypertrophic chondrocytes collagen type X (Figure 1) [22,24]. Furthermore, the enzyme MMP-13 is produced. This enzyme can efficiently cleave collagen type II and thereby contributes to the destruction of the cartilaginous ECM [22].

2.3. Synovial Fluid

SF is a suitable source of information for monitoring the development of the pathogenesis of OA. This type of bodily fluid directly connects and ensures communication between tissues in the joint capsule, such as the synovial membrane, cartilage, infrapatellar fat pad (IFP), etc. Pathological changes in the SF composition are detectable earlier compared to other bodily fluids (e.g., plasma) [25]. Cartilage and SF in healthy joints cooperate with each other to reduce the friction present in the joint during movement. SF provides mechanical shock absorption, lubrication and nutrition of the cartilage. It is produced by the inner membrane of the joint (synovial membrane) and mainly contains serum albumin, hyaluronan, lubricin and γ-globulins. The friction that occurs in the joint during physiological movement changes the composition of the SF. A naturally thin layer of homogeneous fluid is transformed into a thicker, heterogeneous mixture of dense fluid and precipitates due to frictional forces [26]. SF is therefore a typical example of a non-Newtonian fluid.

2.4. Synovial Membrane

The synovial membrane is a specialized connective tissue that lines the diarthrodial joints and is responsible for maintaining the volume and composition of the SF. The SF components are mainly produced by cells present in the synovial membrane [7]. These components contribute to the unique functional properties of joint surfaces and modulate the activity of chondrocytes. Lubricin and hyaluronic acid are two main molecules produced by synovial membrane cells. These molecules protect and maintain the integrity of the articular cartilage surfaces in diarthrodial joints. The synovial membrane consists of two layers. The outer layer (subintima) is up to 5 mm thick and consists of several types of connective tissues. This layer contains predominantly type I collagen and is vascularized and predominantly acellular. The inner layer (intima) is in direct contact with the joint cavity and consists of a layer of cells with a thickness of 20–40 μm. These synovial cells called synoviocytes consist mainly of fibroblasts and macrophages. Fibroblasts are the dominant cell population in the healthy synovial membrane [27]. During disease progression, the synovial membrane is a source of proinflammatory and catabolic mediators (MMPs, aggrecan, etc.) [28]. The articular cartilage is not independently vascularized. It is dependent on the neighboring tissues (synovial membrane, subchondral bone) which provide it with the nutrients necessary to maintain vitality [29]. The synovial membrane is semipermeable, i.e., it is responsible for the transfer of nutrients and waste products within the joint space. The synovial membrane is also a rich source of multipotent mesenchymal stem cells (MSCs). These cells are capable of differentiating into multiple tissue-specific lineages including cartilage, bone, muscle and adipose tissue [30]. Therefore, the synovial membrane is a suitable candidate as a source of cells and their products, which can participate in the regeneration of affected components of joint connective tissue [31].

2.5. Synovial Inflammation

The role of inflammation in the process of OA was unclear and often debated for a long time [32]. OA was not officially classified as an inflammatory disease based on the number of leukocytes present in the SF. Only articular cartilage degradation and pathological bone growth were considered as features of OA [33]. Furthermore, much higher levels of pro-inflammatory serum biomarkers and more pronounced synovial inflammation (synovitis) were found in inflammatory joint diseases such as rheumatoid arthritis (RA) compared to OA [34]. This finding contributed to the use of alternative names for the disease, such as osteoarthrosis or degenerative joint disease [35]. Increasingly, OA was associated only with mechanical damage to joint components without the direct influence of chronic inflammation [36]. Studies testing anti-inflammatory therapies that failed to modify the progression of OA confirmed that OA belongs to the group of non-inflammatory diseases [37]. However, modern laboratory techniques allowing extensive analyzes of cellular, molecular and genetic factors associated with OA showed that OA is also associated with inflammatory processes. Studies established constant low-grade inflammation and activation of innate inflammatory pathways as mediators of OA pathogenesis [2]. Synovial inflammation is a major factor associated with the risk of cartilage degradation and disease symptoms, including joint pain, swelling and stiffness. Synovitis is commonly present in OA joints. The synovitis in OA is macrophage-predominant, whereas RA synovitis is T-cell-predominant. This reflects the activation of the innate immune response in OA joints, possibly caused by damage to joint tissues that have resulted from a chronic wound in the environment. OA synovitis is more focal than in RA; in the knee, it is commonly located in the suprapatellar pouch. Synovitis plays a significant role in joint destruction in RA, while its role in OA progression may be limited to a subset of individuals. Synovitis involving infiltration of mononuclear cells into the synovial membrane and production of pro-inflammatory mediators is common in all stages of the disease [38]. Histologically, the synovial membrane of patients with OA is characterized by hyperplasia, fibrosis and increased vascularization [39]. Infiltration of leukocytes from the vascular compartment occurs in response to cytokines and cell adhesion molecules [29]. Studies confirmed that macrophages and T-lymphocytes are the most abundant immune cells in the affected synovium. Mast cells, B cells and plasma cells are present in the synovial membrane to a significantly lesser extent [40].

3. Potential Soluble Biomarkers of Osteoarthritis

Currently, the evaluation of OA is still based on radiological examinations and subjective pain assessment. Therefore, there is an effort to discover a molecular biomarker of early-stage OA. A biomarker is a characteristic that is objectively measured and evaluated as an indicator of normal biological process, pathogenic processes or pharmacological responses to a therapeutic intervention [41]. To identify early-stage OA predictors, biochemical indicators are now being investigated as the most promising disease markers [42].

Molecular biomarkers are typically measured in bodily fluids such as serum, plasma, urine or SF. Since OA develops inside the knee joint, SF is likely to be the most suitable source of information to detect early-stage OA. Engaging in the effort to detect the early-stage OA provides an opportunity to initiate appropriate therapy. The most plausible options for OA biomarkers are structural molecules or fragments associated to cartilage, bone or synovium. They may be unique to a particular kind of joint tissue or present in all joints [43]. The potential candidates for OA biomarkers discussed in this review are shown in Table 1.

Table 1. Potential OA biomarkers.

Type	Category	Molecule	Bodily Fluid/ MSCs Type	Ref.
Soluble	Inflammatory	IL-1β	plasma, SF	[44,45]
		TNFα	N/A	[46]
		IL-6	SF, serum	[47]
		CCL2	SF	[48]
		CCL3	serum	[49]

Table 1. *Cont.*

Type	Category	Molecule	Bodily Fluid/ MSCs Type	Ref.
		CCL5	SF	[50]
		CCL13	SF, serum	[51]
		CXCL12	SF	[52]
	Collagenous	CTX-II	urine	[53–55]
		Coll 2-1	urine	[56]
		C2C	urine	[57]
	Non-collagenous	COMP	SF, serum	[58,59]
		S100	serum	[60]
EV-associated	Protein	IL-1β	SF	[61]
		IL-17	SF	[61]
		IL-10	SF	[61]
		INFγ	SF	[61]
		TNFα	plasma	[62]
		haptoglobin (female)	SF	[63]
		orosomucoid (female)	SF	[63]
		ceruloplasmin (female)	SF	[63]
		β-2-glycoprotein (male)	SF	[63]
		complement component 5 (male)	SF	[63]
	Lipid	phospholipid	SF	[64]
	miRNA	miR-95-5p	MSCs-EVs	[65]
		miR-193b-3p	plasma-EVs	[66]
		miR-92a-3p	MSCs-EVs	[67]
		miR-140-5p	MSCs-EVs	[68]
		miR-26a-5p	BMSCs-EVs	[69]
		miR-100-5p	IFP-MSCs-EVs	[70]
	lncRNA	PCGEM1	SF-EVs	[71]
		KLF3 AS1	MSCs-EVs	[72]
		PVT1	serum-EVs	[73]
		LYRM4-AS1	BMSCs-EVs	[74]

IL-1β: interleukin-1 beta; TNFα: tumor necrosis factor alpha; IL-6: interleukin 6; CCL2: monocyte chemoattractant protein-1; CCL3: macrophage inflammatory protein-1 alpha; CCL5: regulated upon activation, normal T cell expressed and secreted; CCL13: CC motif chemokine ligand 13; CXCL12: CXC motif chemokine ligand 12; CTX-II: C-terminal telopeptide of collagen type II; Coll 2-1: type II collagen-specific biomarker; C2C: type II collagen cleavage product; COMP: cartilage oligomeric matrix protein; S100: proteins of S100 family; IL-17: interleukin 17; IL-10: interleukin 10; INFγ: interferon gamma; PCGEM1: prostate-specific transcript 1; KLF3 AS1: KLF3 antisense RNA 1; PVT1: Pvt1 oncogene; LYRM4-AS1: LYRM4 antisense RNA 1; SF: synovial fluid; MSCs-EVs: mesenchymal stem cell-derived extracellular vesicles; BMSCs-EVs: bone marrow mesenchymal stem cell-derived extracellular vesicles; IFP-MSCs-EVs: extracellular vesicles from infrapatellar fat pad-derived mesenchymal stem cells; SF-EVs: synovial fluid-derived extracellular vesicles; serum-EVs: serum-derived extracellular vesicles; N/A: not available.

3.1. Inflammatory Biomarkers

3.1.1. Cytokines and Chemokines

Previous studies confirmed the positive relation between the progressive degradation of articular cartilage and the presence of synovial inflammation [75–77]. Therefore, the production of pro-inflammatory cytokines/chemokines in the process of OA significantly contributes to the catabolic processes occurring in the joint capsule.

The main pro-inflammatory cytokines in the pathogenesis of OA are interleukin-1β (IL-1β)—associated with cartilage degradation, tumor necrosis factor α (TNFα)—controlling the cascade of inflammatory processes and IL-6—one of the main regulatory cytokines in inflammatory reactions in the body. IL-1β and TNFα are produced by chondrocytes, osteoblasts, synovial fibroblasts and mononuclear cells (lymphocytes, monocytes) [78]. These cytokines regulate the production of other pro-inflammatory and catabolic factors. Elevated levels of IL-1β and TNFα were confirmed in SF, synovial membrane, subchondral bone and also in cartilage in patients with OA [79].

Cytokine IL-1β can activate cells through a specific IL-1RI receptor (CD121a) located on the cell surface. Molnar et al. confirmed that expression of the IL-1RI receptor on the surface of OA chondrocytes and synovial fibroblasts was increased in vitro [80]. The binding of IL-1β to the receptor IL-1RI from the Toll-like receptor (TLR) family causes a multistep activation of transcription factors. It leads to increased gene expression and results in the production of other cytokines, chemokines, adhesion molecules and various degradation enzymes [81]. IL-1β significantly contributes to the composition of the ECM by influencing cell metabolism. It reduces the production of the two main ECM components (collagen type II and aggrecan) directly in the chondrocytes in vitro [82]. IL-1β also affects the synthesis of MMPs (MMP-1, interstitial collagenase; MMP-2, gelatinase A; MMP-3, stromelysin-1; MMP-8, neutrophil collagenase; MMP-9, gelatinase B; MMP -13, collagenase 3; MMP-14 or MMP-16) capable of degrading the cartilage ECM [83].

Together with IL-1β, TNFα is considered the main pro-inflammatory cytokine influencing the pathogenesis of OA. TNFα is one of the 19 ligands of the tumor necrosis factor superfamily and binds to two specific receptors (TNFRI and TNFRII) located on the cell membrane [84]. In the same way as IL-1β receptors, TNFα receptors are overexpressed on the surface of chondrocytes and synovial fibroblasts in OA [79]. TNFα also negatively affects the production of proteoglycan components and collagen type II by the chondrocytes [85]. TNFα-activated chondrocytes produce MMP-1, MMP-3, MMP-13 and disintegrin and metalloproteases with thrombospondin motifs (ADAMTSs) responsible for the breakdown of aggrecan [86]. TNFα activity usually corresponds with IL-1β action, and there is a notable synergism between the two cytokines in the case of many phenomena that occur throughout OA. Furthermore, IL-1β and TNFα stimulate the production of inducible nitric oxide synthase (iNOS), cyclooxygenase-2 (COX-2) and prostaglandin E2 (PGE2) synthase, increasing the quantities of their products [87]. Therefore, one of the potential therapies for OA is focused on reducing the negative effect of IL-1β and TNFα [79]. Faster senescence and more frequent apoptotic processes are shown by chondrocytes that are affected by IL-1β and TNFα [88–90].

Another main regulatory cytokine in inflammatory reactions in the body is IL-6 that can activate the immune system and strengthen the body's immune response in a wide range of inflammatory conditions. The production of IL-6 in affected tissues is the result of the action of IL-1β and TNFα. IL-6 is produced in the injured joint by chondrocytes, osteoblasts, synovial fibroblasts, macrophages and adipocytes [91]. Increased levels of IL-6 were observed in the SF and the serum of OA patients. These levels correlate with the radiographically confirmed severity of OA [47]. IL-6 regulates changes in the subchondral bone and supports the formation of osteoclasts and thus the resorption of bone tissue [92]. IL-6 in cooperation with IL-1β and TNFα reduce collagen-type II production and contributes to the overproduction of MMPs [93].

These cytokines are activators of a large number of signaling pathways that activate the production of other inflammatory mediators. This cascade also includes chemokines that can attract inflammatory cells to the affected microenvironment and thereby support the secretion of other inflammatory factors and the progression of the disease [80]. The proliferation, differentiation and activation of cellular responses are all impacted by their diverse range of activity [94]. In OA, chemokines act as mediators of dysregulated joint-tissue metabolism. Based on the position of the N-terminal cysteine residues, these small (8–12 kDa) protein ligands are grouped into four families: C, CC, CXC and CX3C. The great majority of chemokines are members of the CC and CXC families [80].

The most significant CC family chemokines that are associated with OA are CCL2 (monocyte chemoattractant protein-1, MCP-1), CCL3 (macrophage inflammatory protein-1 alpha, MIP-1α), CCL4 (macrophage inflammatory protein-1 beta, MIP-1β) and CCL5 (Regulated upon Activation, Normal T cell Expressed and Secreted (RANTES)) [94]. CC chemokines have a key role in macrophage recruitment and are increased following joint damage in OA.

CCL2 is a ligand of C-C-chemokines-receptor-2 (CCR2) that is expressed in chondrocytes, osteoblasts and synovial cells and has a function in bone metabolism and OA [78]. CCL2 functions by aggregating monocytes in the host defense and macrophages at the site of inflammation. CCL2 expression was elevated in individuals with a variety of inflammatory diseases, including OA. CCL3//MIP-1 α is a chemotactic chemokine released by macrophages. It carries out a number of biological processes, including the recruitment of inflammatory cells, wound healing, the suppression of stem cells and the maintenance of effector immune responses. Furthermore, CCL3 stimulates osteoclastogenesis, which is important in the bone remodeling process and CCL3-expressing cells are typically found in sites of inflammation and bone resorption [95]. CCL4 is a small cytokine of the CC chemokine family. CCL4 is released in response to mitogenic signals and antigens, acting as a chemoattractant for natural killer cells, monocytes and other immune cells at the site of inflamed or injured tissue [96]. CCL4 is regulated by the NF-KB signaling pathway. Due to its stimulation of OA chondrocyte apoptosis, studies have shown that the NF-KB signaling pathway is strongly associated with OA. The NF-KB signaling pathway's inactivation has been shown to be a helpful factor in the OA process of cartilage breakdown [97]. CCL5 was discovered to be a product of activated T cells and plays an important function in the inflammatory response. CCL5 has been previously linked to chronic inflammatory disorders such as RA, inflammatory bowel disease and cancer. It attracts monocytes, eosinophils and T lymphocytes while also activating eosinophils and basophils to release granule content. It has been shown that chondrocytes expressed CCL5 together with other various chemokines during OA pathological processes [98]. CXCL12 is a CXC family chemokine that is also important in the pathophysiology of OA. By interacting with a single receptor, CXCR4, CXCL12 mobilizes MSCs to sites of injury and therefore could be a potential diagnostic as well as therapeutical tool associated with OA [99].

Potential Cytokine/Chemokine Biomarkers in Synovial Fluid

OA is an expensive and debilitating disease that is frequently not detected early enough to stop its progressing. The study of SF biomarkers can advance understanding in the field of knee OA diagnosis and therapy [100]. SF is a suitable source of potential biomarkers because it is in direct contact with the cartilage and synovial layer of the injured joint. OA causes a malfunction in the crucial ECM alterations' process, which results in a significant loss of cartilage [101]. As a result of aberrant matrix turnover and altered SF composition in an OA-affected joint, numerous molecules and fragments of matrix components from tissues such as articular cartilage, bone and synovium are released into the SF. Some of these fragments can be measured in SF even before they can be found in other samples such as serum and urine [102]. Therefore, SF can more accurately represent the changes caused by OA in a specific joint. Since a pro-inflammatory environment can negatively impact the health of chondrocytes and the maintenance of a healthy ECM, local inflammatory cytokines such as IL-1β, TNF-α and IL-6 are crucial in the process of OA formation and development [103]. Additionally, there is rising evidence that the pathophysiology of OA is influenced by the local production of pro-inflammatory cytokines and chemokines [87]. Chondrocytes, osteoblasts, synovial cells and mononuclear cells present in the microenvironment of the affected joint are able to produce a large number of these inflammatory mediators. Therefore, SF is a strong candidate for discovering important OA biomarkers.

Monibi et al. used a multiplex test to examine SF samples from 18 individuals. When compared to healthy individuals, MMP-1, IL-6, IL-8 and CCL5 were all significantly higher in the SF of OA patients. They also confirmed that CCL2 was strongly linked with IL-6, IL-8 and the radiographic OA severity ratings further support the idea that it is a useful biomarker for clinical diagnosis [48]. Li et al. confirmed a positive correlation between CCL2 concentrations in SF and the Western Ontario and McMaster Universities index (WOMAC) pain, function, and overall scores [104]. CCL2 and CCL5 can stimulate MMP-3 expression in vitro, which causes proteoglycan loss and cartilage degradation in the OA inflammatory microenvironment [105]. Chemokine expression in SF, synovium and cartilage was examined in patients with and without knee OA [106]. In comparison to controls, the SF of knee OA patients had higher levels of CCL2, CCL3 and CCL4. Inflammatory mediators in the SF that are connected to nociceptive and neuropathic pain in knee OA were analyzed by Li et al. [107]. They found that expression of IL-1β and IL-6 was increased in the early-stage OA group compared with the late-stage OA group. The WOMAC pain score has no correlation with any of the inflammatory mediators analyzed. Beekhuizen et al. analyzed the levels of 47 mediators in the SF of control donors and OA patients [50]. The majority of the mediators were found in both the control and OA SF samples. Some of them, such as IL-6 and CCL5, were shown to be significantly higher in OA compared to controls. CCR2 ligands (CCL2, CCL7, CCL8) were found to be increased in SF from human OA and post-traumatic knees [108]. CCR2-expressing cells were found in higher numbers in OA synovium, and CCR2-expressing macrophages were detected by immunofluorescence at areas of damage, suggesting that this pathway is also involved.

There is evidence that articular chondrocytes express CXCR4, and CXCL12 also stimulates MMP-13 and several other catabolic mediators in addition to its effect on MSCs. The role of CXCL12/CXCR4 signaling in fracture healing and bone remodeling has been established [109]. CXCL12 levels in SF were shown to be strongly correlated with the radiographic severity of knee OA in a study that included 252 patients with the condition and 144 healthy controls [52]. The Kellgren–Lawrence (K-L) grading method was used for the radiological grading of OA in the knee. CXCL12 levels in the SF of knee OA patients with K-L grade 4 were considerably higher than those with K-L grades 2 and 3. Furthermore, individuals with knee OA with K-L grade 3 showed substantially greater SF levels of CXCL12 than those with K-L grade 2.

In-depth research in this field has been limited since many patients with degenerative OA have small volumes of SF in the intra-articular space [78]. Although SF only reaches small volumes, it is nevertheless highly likely to be the best source of OA biomarkers.

Potential Cytokine/Chemokine Biomarkers in Blood

Since peripheral blood contains tens of thousands of different proteins and many of them are produced by numerous extra-articular sites, measuring specific cytokine, chemokine or MMP levels in the peripheral blood may not accurately reflect levels in the synovial space. Blood is considered a less specific source of information when searching for a suitable OA biomarker compared to SF. Research also focuses on the study of blood because it is a much easier source to obtain from the patient. Many studies are therefore focused on the research of such biomarkers that could reveal the progression of OA in the blood.

Independent of other risk variables, the severity and development of symptomatic knee OA were marginally and causally correlated with plasma levels of IL-1 receptor antagonist (IL-1Ra) [110]. These findings are encouraging for the identification of predictive biomarkers involved in IL-1 signaling as well as the development of innovative drugs for the treatment of OA. According to Runhaar et al., variations in serum levels of IL-6, TNF-α, IL-1R and CRP throughout the intervention period explained 15% of the change in WOMAC pain ratings and 29% of the change in WOMAC function scores [111]. These findings emphasize the importance of changes in systemic inflammation as drivers of clinically significant effects following diet and exercise in overweight and obese people with knee OA. Nordahl et al. confirmed that the presence of IL-1β in plasma and SF is associated with temporomandibular joint (TMJ) radiographic alterations. The extent of erosion and the severity of radiographic alterations to the TMJ were both larger in individuals with detectable IL-1β levels in their plasma than in those without [44]. Panina et al. revealed that early post-traumatic OA was associated with the circulating level of IL-1β in serum and SF [45]. Before routine radiography, combined serum IL-6, TNF-α, and leptin levels can be used as biomarkers to differentiate between post-traumatic OA patients and healthy controls [112]. Combined levels of these three potential biomarkers positively correlated with the K-L score of post-traumatic OA patients. The peripheral blood of OA patients has higher levels of CCL2 and CCL3, which have great predictive value for the incidence, effectiveness and prognosis of recurrence of OA, suggesting their potential roles as excellent markers for OA diagnosis and therapy in the future [113]. According to the study by Zhao et al., CCL3 may be a serum biomarker for knee OA with the ability to identify alterations that are not yet visible on X-rays and classify the severity of knee injury [49]. A total of 181 subjects were included and subdivided into three subgroups (control subjects, pre-X-ray-defined knee degeneration patients and X-ray-confirmed knee OA patients). In the pre-X-ray-defined knee degeneration patients, articular cartilage loss was measured during arthroscopy using the International Cartilage Repair Society (ICRS) classification or recorded on MRI with chondral whole-organ magnetic resonance imaging score (WORMS). The radiographic severity of OA was significantly correlated with CCL13 levels in serum and SF in another study [51]. When compared to knee OA patients with K-L grades 2 and 3, those with K-L grade 4 had substantially higher serum and SF levels of CCL13.

However, many more studies comparing the level of potential cytokine/chemokine biomarkers in SF and blood will have to be carried out to create a standardized protocol for evaluating the appropriate OA biomarker.

3.2. *Collagenous Biomarkers*

3.2.1. C-Terminal Telopeptide of Collagen Type II

Type II collagen is the major component of the articular cartilage matrix [114]. Fragments of C-terminal telopeptide are released following the degradation of type II collagen. At the most common sites of radiographic OA, levels of urinary C-terminal telopeptide of collagen type II (uCTX-II) were shown to be correlated with the overall radiographic score as determined by the K-L method. It was also shown that scores at the knee, hip, facet and hand joints independently contributed to this association [53]. A significant reduction in hand pain and function in individuals with symptomatic hand OA throughout a six-month clinical study with chondroitin sulfate was not connected to a change in uCTX-II levels [115]. uCTX-II correlates strongly with early indicators of inflammatory arthritis, such as bone-mineral density loss and power Doppler ultrasonography synovitis [116]. Following six and twelve months of therapy with glucosamine and chondroitin sulfate or glucosamine, chondroitin sulfate and collagen type II, Scarpellini et al. discovered considerably reduced levels of uCTX-II [117]. Visual analogue scale (VAS) and uCTX-II mean values were considerably lower than the baseline after 6 months and 1 year of treatment. The study consisted of 129 participants (78 in the OA group and 51 in the control group) showed significantly higher levels of uCTX-II in the OA group compared to the control group [54]. Furthermore, uCTX-II levels were independently correlated with the radiographic severity of OA of the knee. The uCTX-II levels and the WOMAC index showed a positive correlation. A comparative study of uCTX-II for knee OA patients and healthy individuals revealed that late-stage OA is associated with higher levels of uCTX-II [118]. Eighty-two patients with knee OA and 20 healthy volunteers were enrolled in this study. Anteroposterior and lateral position X-rays of knee joints were collected. The images were classified using the K-L radiographic grading criteria. The molecular biomarkers CTX-II and IL-1β, which were both considerably elevated throughout the development of knee OA, can be utilized to help with early diagnosis and knee OA therapy [119]. Valdes et al. confirmed in their large-scale meta-analysis the importance of uCTX-II as a degradation product that correlates with a wide range of OA features, including hip, knee and hand OA as well as knee OA progression and radiographic severity of knee OA [55]. In several OA animal models, uCTX-II and serum CTX-II both showed promise for diagnostic and staging purposes. Significant differences in the serum CTX-II levels in rabbits were observed between the adult OA (OA induced by anterior cruciate ligament transection) and the control (unoperated) groups [120]. Csifó et al. studied the effect of meloxicam on knee cartilage degradation in an iodoacetate-induced rat OA model. Within four weeks of therapy, the high-dose group of meloxicam treatment resulted in a remarkable decrease in CTX-II compared to the low-dose and placebo groups [121]. These results suggest an interest in serum CTX-II monitoring for OA progression. Innovative techniques also propose detecting CTX-II in serum and urine simultaneously using a fluoro-microbeads guiding chip [122]. Patients with primary OA had greater concentrations of CTX-II in SF than in the reference group. The mean levels of CTX-II in SF increased above reference values following joint damage at all time points, with the greatest levels occurring shortly after the trauma [123]. Sofat et al. conducted a cross-sectional study on patients with knee OA and healthy controls. A total of 130 patients were evaluated, including 78 with advanced OA who required total knee replacement (TKR), 42 with moderate OA who received conventional therapy and 6 non-OA controls, with four drop-outs. They discovered that increased MRI-detected joint damage was related to higher levels of CTX-II, indicating that MRI and CTX-II biomarkers can be used to monitor OA disease development.

3.2.2. Type II Collagen-Specific Biomarker

Type II collagen-specific biomarker (Coll 2-1) may be described as a biomarker useful for examining the burden of disease, the prognosis and diagnosis based on the Burden of Disease, Investigative, Prognostic, Efficacy of Intervention and Diagnostic (BIPED) categorization system for OA biomarkers published by Bauer et al. [124]. According to research by Henrotin et al., a rise in urine levels of Coll 2-1 or its nitrated form (Coll 2-1NO_2) over a year was a reliable indicator of the course of joint space narrowing in OA patients [56]. The blood levels of Coll 2-1, a biomarker particular to type II collagen breakdown, can be decreased in knee OA patients by intra-articular injection of reticulated hyaluronic acid with mannitol, according to a randomized double-blind placebo controlled trial. Eligible participants were men and women between the ages of 45 and 80 who had unilateral symptomatic femoro-tibial knee OA that fulfilled clinical and radiologic American College of Rheumatology (ACR) criteria. OA must have been present for more than 6 months, with a mean global knee pain measured on a VAS over the past 24 h above 40 mm (without any analgesics for at least 48 h) [125]. One-year follow-up of Coll 2-1 serum levels in OA patients after hip or knee replacement indicates that Coll 2-1 is a disease-specific marker that is sensitive to the structural changes occurring in a single joint. Additionally, the immunohistochemical results support the idea that injured articular cartilage is the primary source of serum Coll 2-1 [126].

3.2.3. Type II Collagen Cleavage Product

One of the potential biomarkers of early-stage OA is type II collagen cleavage product (C2C). Poole et al. attempted to assess the relationship between early and late knee cartilage pathology and the evolution of cartilage damage using the C2C human urine sandwich assay (IB-C2C-HUSA), a test for cartilage collagenase-mediated degradation. In a population-based cohort of early pre-radiographic disease and radiographic OA, they showed substantial relationships between the novel urine IB-C2C-HUSA immunoassay with cartilage damage cross-sectionally and with cartilage loss longitudinally [57]. To investigate if SF biomarker concentrations corresponded with the severity of radiographic OA and were higher in joints with radiographic OA compared to controls, Coppelman et al. examined SF biomarker concentrations from distal intertarsal and tarsometatarsal joints in adult horses. They confirmed that overall radiographic scores have a positive correlation with the C2C value concentration in equine SF [127]. In addition to the correlations identified with several other injury-related biomarkers, the higher levels of C2C in SF following injury show that an acute knee injury is linked to the rapid and long-lasting local breakdown of type II collagen [128]. These results suggest that C2C could be a suitable OA biomarker.

3.3. Non-Collagenous Biomarkers

3.3.1. Cartilage Oligomeric Matrix Protein

A non-collagenous ECM glycoprotein called cartilage oligomeric matrix protein (COMP) is structurally linked to thrombospondins. Initially, COMP was believed to be the unique protein of cartilage, but further research showed that it may also be found in tendons, ligaments and menisci [129]. The cartilage breakdown in OA is measured using the biomarkers COMP and uCTX-II. Increased concentrations of these biomarkers can reveal OA's severity and prognosis [43]. It was hypothesized that a decrease in both biomarker levels reflects a cartilage recovery. According to a thorough review of OA biomarkers, the most accurate indicators of OA nowadays are COMP, osteocalcin and CTX-II [130]. COMP fragments are released into the SF during the breakdown of articular cartilage. They were discovered in elevated levels immediately following the injury and in the early stages of OA. Plsikova et al. studied SF samples aspirated from the knees of 65 OA patients (46 patients with early-stage OA and 19 patients with end-stage OA according to the K-L grading scale). When compared to the group of patients with end-stage OA, the concentration of COMP in SF was significantly lower in the early OA group of patients. Additionally, the age of the patients and the levels of COMP in the SF were shown to be significantly correlated [58]. Only the baseline level of COMP of the investigated biomarkers was able to predict later MRI-determined cartilage loss in the OA knees [131]. In this study, the WORMS semiquantitative grading method was used to assess baseline and follow-up knee MRI images for cartilage loss. According to the study of Verma et al., early on in the development of knee OA, COMP concentrations in primary OA serum samples were shown to be higher than healthy donors' values [132]. On a sample of 60 male Sprague-Dawley rats, a study was conducted to evaluate the diagnostic capability of the biomarkers COMP and chondroitin sulfate epitope 846 (CS846). Serum levels of COMP (sCOMP) and CS846 in the model group were considerably greater than those in the control group 10 weeks following surgery [133]. In patients with unilateral hip OA, a group led by Endres attempted to investigate the impact of total hip replacement on sCOMP and its relationship to joint stress during gait [134]. Unexpectedly, the excision of an OA joint had no long-term impact on sCOMP's level. Independently of age and BMI, high sCOMP levels were linked to an increased risk of incident knee OA, while synovitis was demonstrated to have the biggest impact on COMP levels in established knee OA [59].

3.3.2. S100 Proteins

S100A9 belongs to the alarmin family. It is a crucial protein in the breakdown of cartilage and synovial inflammation in OA. S100A9 expression in cartilage is only seen in hypertrophic chondrocytes and is crucial for the matrix mineralization [135]. The Cohort Hip and Cohort Knee study's analysis of arthroscopic synovial biopsy samples from patients with early symptoms of OA also uncovered elevated levels of S100A9, which significantly correlated with synovial lining thickness, cellularity in the subintima and joint degeneration [136]. Serum levels of S100A8 or S100A9 were shown to be linked with overall WOMAC scores, weight-bearing pain and physical disability in a study of 141 individuals with clinical knee OA [60].

3.3.3. C-Terminal End-Product of Vitronectin and C3f Peptide

As a ligand for the αVβ3 integrin receptor, vitronectin is degraded by a number of metalloproteinases, including MMP-1,-2,-3,-7 and -9. Vitronectin is a cell adhesion and spreading factor that is highly expressed by bone-resorbing osteoclasts. The C3f peptide is highly expressed, especially in severe forms (K-L 3 and 4). It is also seen in SF, and has a strong correlation with the C-terminal end-product of vitronectin (V65) [137]. De Seny et al. examined 284 serum samples from patients with knee OA from the Bristol OA 500 cohort and the Bristol Validation Study, together with healthy controls and individuals with RA [138]. They discovered four new biomarkers in the serum of OA patients using the SELDI-TOF MS proteomics approach: V65, C3f peptide, the 3762 protein and CTAPIII (Connective tissue-activating peptide III). When compared to controls or those with RA, V65 showed higher amounts in MS spectra in all K-L grades. These findings emphasize its specificity for OA. The C3f peptide is abundantly expressed, particularly in severe instances (K-L 3 and 4), is also seen in SF and has a strong correlation with V65 [137]. Two immunoassays have been created by Ourradi et al. to measure the biomarkers C3f and V65 peptides that were found by their prior proteomic study [139]. These assays were able to identify endogenous peptides in patient and control blood samples, but they lacked the sensitivity necessary to assess peptide levels accurately in patients.

4. Potential EV-Associated Biomarkers of Osteoarthritis

Potential biomarkers are not only found in bodily fluids as freely detectable molecules but are also widely present in EVs (EV-associated) [61]. EVs are membrane vesicles with diameters ranging from 30–5000 nm that are released by distinct cells and communicate with one another via paracrine signaling. Exosomes, microvesicles and apoptotic bodies are subtypes of EVs, and research on these EVs has grown dramatically in recent years. Apoptotic bodies are the largest EVs, with sizes ranging from 1000 to 5000 nm. The size of microvesicles ranges from 100 to 1000 nm and exosomes are vesicles typically defined by diameters of 30–150 nm [140]. According to Minimal information for studies of extracellular vesicles (MISEV), EVs should be named either in accordance with size (small EVs <200 nm, large EVs >200 nm), density (low, medium, high), biochemical composition (expression of surface markers) or the origin of the cells from which they originate (e.g., mesenchymal stem cell-derived EVs) [141]. EVs contain and protect useful biological information, including proteins, lipids, lncRNA, mRNAs, and regulatory miRNA [140]. Janockova et al. demonstrated that small EVs and their content can be taken-up by different types of cells isolated from tissues associated with OA (SF, osteoblasts and periosteum-derived MSCs) suggesting their prospective role in the treatment of OA [142]. It is thought that EVs have the ability to act as paracrine effectors and mediators of cell-to-cell communication [62]. Through their functions in intercellular transport, EVs are considered to support a variety of crucial physiological processes including immunological responses, tissue healing and neural communication [143]. EVs show therefore a promising role in tissue regeneration, especially MSCs- and platelet-derived EVs as listed in recently published articles [144,145]. It is difficult to distinguish between early and advanced OA, therefore it is important to investigate and identify sensitive and objective molecular markers of early disease.

4.1. *EV-Associated Protein/Lipid Biomarkers*

The amounts of EV-associated cytokines IL-1β, IL-17, IL-10 and INF-γ found in the SF of patients with late-stage OA were significantly higher than those found in patients with early-stage OA [61]. Zhang et al. identified plasma EVs in OA that carry the major pro-inflammatory cytokines, TNFα, IL-1β and IL-6, demonstrating their pro-inflammatory phenotype [62]. They found that the concentration of TNFα within EVs and the integrated mean fluorescence intensity of TNFα in EVs in OA plasma were associated with and strong predictors of radiographic knee OA progression, while plasma TNFα outside EVs was neither associated with nor predictive of radiographic knee OA progression. Chondrocytes may form exosome-like vesicles (ELV) that are released from cartilage during the matrix loss and cartilage degradation. These ELV may be substantially concentrated in synovial tissue and could have the ability to enter macrophages. The ELV could transfer miR-449a-5p into macrophages and reduce ATG4B expression in lipopolysaccharide-primed macrophages, resulting in autophagy inhibition. Reduced autophagy encourages the production of mitochondrial reactive oxygen species, which increases inflammasome activation and mature IL-1β production. Finally, an increase in IL-1β aggravates synovial inflammation and accelerates the progression of OA [146]. SF is a suitable source of information in monitoring the pathogenesis of OA, because it directly connects the tissues present in the joint capsule, such as the synovial membrane, cartilage or IFP [7]. Based on mass spectrometry protein profiling, Kolhe et al. identified multiple gender (male and female)-specific differential proteins in OA and non-OA EVs. They found that haptoglobin, orosomucoid, and ceruloplasmin were significantly upregulated, whereas apolipoprotein was downregulated in female OA EVs. In males, they discovered β-2-glycoprotein and complement component 5 significantly upregulated and SAGA-associated factor 29 downregulated in male OA EVs [63].

EV-associated lipids could also be a potential biomarker of OA. In the most recent study of Ben-Trad et al. an important finding was reported [64]. They compared healthy and OA samples and showed that the phospholipid (PL) amount increased in pathological samples. However, the PL/neutral lipid ratio decreased, suggesting destabilization of bilayer structures.

4.2. EV-Associated miRNA Biomarkers

The 18–25 nucleotide RNA molecules known as miRNAs can control protein translation by complementarily binding to mRNA transcripts [147]. EV-associated miRNA-92a is also involved in mitigating the negative effects of OA by increasing chondrocyte proliferation and ECM synthesis through the PI3K/AKT/mTOR pathway. EV-associated miR-95-5p was shown to enhance chondrogenesis and prevent the development of OA by directly targeting histone deacetylase (HDAC)-2/8. MiR-95-5p suppressed the expression of HDAC2/8 and promoted the formation of cartilage ECM. Therefore, EV-associated miR-95-5p may act as an inhibitor of HDAC2/8, making it a potential diagnostic biomarker of OA [65]. MiR-193b-3p affects histone deacetylase 3 (HDAC3), which in turn affects chondrogenesis and chondrocyte metabolism. Overexpression of this miRNA has been shown to significantly increase cartilage tissue formation in vivo. EV-associated miR-193b-3p plasma levels in patients with OA were shown to be lower than in control samples, thus supporting the positive effect [66].

The WNT5A protein plays a key role in the destruction and degradation of cartilage in the pathogenesis of OA. Huang et al. confirmed that WNT5A can promote chondrocyte catabolic activity through a non-canonical Wnt signaling cascade in OA cartilage [148]. EV-associated miR-92a-3p can suppress the production of WNT5A, which is largely involved in the pathogenesis of OA. Increased expression levels of miR-92a-3p in EVs from MSCs and significantly decreased levels in EVs from OA chondrocytes were confirmed. Treatment with EVs containing miR-92a-3p increased chondrocyte proliferation by suppressing WNT5A protein production [67].

Similarly, miR-140-5p found in EVs from synovial MSCs has shown promising effects. The regulation of the Wnt signaling cascade by miR-140-5p in a rat model has been demonstrated to support cartilage tissue regeneration and protect against knee OA [68]. EVs from MSCs significantly reduced the expression levels of catabolic genes in IL-1β activated human chondrocytes. Analysis of miRNA content in these EVs revealed that these particles contain chondroprotective miR-140 and miR-451 [149]. It was confirmed that miR-26a-5p specifically binds to *PTGS2* (gene encoding prostaglandin-endoperoxide synthase 2). Overexpression of miR-26a-5p in EVs from bone marrow stem cells (BMSCs) has a regenerative effect on damaged synovial fibroblasts through suppression of *PTGS2* expression [69]. Wu et al. reported in their study that miR-100-5p in EVs isolated from IFP-MSCs protects articular cartilage from damage and regulates its homeostasis through inhibition of the mTOR-autophagy pathway [70]. In the future, isolated EVs from IFP might be used as potential biomarkers of OA. Another study confirmed that EVs can promote the proliferation of chondrocytes through miR-302c and inhibit the production of MMP-13, as the main degradative enzyme of cartilage ECM [150].

4.3. EV-Associated lncRNA Biomarkers

In addition to EV-associated miRNAs, lncRNAs have been reported to be involved in promoting proliferation and inhibiting apoptosis of chondrocytes during OA. The heterogeneity of lncRNAs is due to their size, which ranges from several hundred to several thousand nucleotides. They have an important regulatory role in the processes of development, differentiation, proliferation, apoptosis and cell metabolism. However, it seems that it is not their size, but the secondary and tertiary structures that are essential in the correct performance of the functions of these molecules [151].

Three groups of participants (the control group, the early OA group, and the late OA group) were used in a research by Zhao and Xu [71]. All individuals provided blood samples from the elbow vein and knee joint SF samples. EVs were isolated using ultracentrifugation, and RT-PCR was used to assess the expression of a number of EV-associated lncRNAs. EV-associated lncRNA PCGEM1 expression progressively rises as OA progresses. This demonstrated that EV-associated lncRNA could be a novel molecular biomarker for the precise and efficient monitoring of OA development. Kohle et al. found that the miRNA content of the EVs from SF differ between OA and non-OA groups. In males, 69 miRNAs were significantly downregulated and 45 miRNAs were upregulated. In females, 91 miRNAs were downregulated and 53 miRNAs were upregulated. The data showed gender-specific differences in miRNA content in OA EVs [152]. EV-associated lncRNA KLF3 AS1 from MSCs affects chondrocyte proliferation and inhibition of chondrocyte apoptosis through the miR-206/GIT1 pathway [72]. EV-associated lncRNA PVT1 regulated OA progression by modulating HMGB1/TLR4/NF-κB pathway through miR-93-5p [73]. The experimental results confirmed that the EV-associated lncRNA LYRM4-AS1 regulated the growth of activated chondrocytes through the GRPR/miR-6515-5p pathway and alleviated the inflammation present in OA [74]. Reviewing the roles of EVs containing miRNAs and lncRNAs and the research progress of these molecules can help to better understand the pathogenesis and to discover new molecular biomarkers of OA.

5. Conclusions

Refined diagnostic approaches need to be developed that identify OA subtypes and indicators of its progression, at earlier stages of the disease. This approach may enable personalized interventions that offer patients a better chance of preserving joint function and reducing pain. Success in this field has the potential to improve the lives of the many millions of OA sufferers worldwide. The ideal biomarker could be collected non-invasively, be predictive of the outcome of the disease and also provide potential therapeutic targets. The current markers all have advantages and disadvantages. Bodily fluids such as blood or urine are easily accessible, but it is known that changes in the synovial fluid can be detected earlier suggesting that markers may have a higher sensitivity and specificity in synovial fluid. MiRNA-based diagnosis nowadays represents the most dynamic area in OA biomarker research. Several studies have identified OA-specific miRNAs but there is a need to validate these results with a large-scale sample size in preclinical and clinical studies. For early and accurate diagnosis of OA, mainly knee OA, there is a need to identify complex panels of soluble biomarkers in various biofluids (serum, urine and synovial fluid) as well as in EVs to predict early-stage OA in a more precise manner. There are several options for measuring OA biomarkers, ranging from simple and relatively inexpensive methods to complex and demanding laboratory techniques. The development of tests should prioritize multiplex marker miniaturization and chip-based measurement in order to increase the cost-effectiveness of OA diagnostics and monitoring.

Author Contributions: Conceptualization, M.M.; writing—original draft preparation, J.M.; writing—review and editing, T.S. All authors have read and agreed to the published version of the manuscript.

Funding: This study was supported by the Internal Scientific Grant System VUaVP35 UPJS No. vvgs-2022-2186 and by the Slovak Research and Development Agency under Contract No. APVV-17-0118. This publication is the result of the project implementation: "Open scientific community for modern interdisciplinary research in medicine (OPENMED)", ITMS2014+: 313011V455 supported by the Operational Programme Integrated Infrastructure, funded by the ERDF.

Institutional Review Board Statement: Not applicable.

Informed Consent Statement: Not applicable.

Data Availability Statement: Not applicable.

Conflicts of Interest: The authors declare no conflict of interest.

References

1. Malemud, C.J. Biologic basis of osteoarthritis: State of the evidence. *Curr. Opin. Rheumatol.* **2015**, *27*, 289–294. [CrossRef]
2. Berenbaum, F. Osteoarthritis as an inflammatory disease (osteoarthritis is not osteoarthrosis!). *Osteoarthr. Cartil.* **2013**, *21*, 16–21. [CrossRef] [PubMed]
3. Vina, E.R.; Kwoh, C. Epidemiology of osteoarthritis: Literature update. *Curr. Opin. Rheumatol.* **2018**, *30*, 160–167. [CrossRef] [PubMed]
4. Cross, M.; Smith, E.; Hoy, D.; Nolte, S.; Ackerman, I.; Fransen, M.; Bridgett, L.; Williams, S.; Guillemin, F.; Hill, C.; et al. The global burden of hip and knee osteoarthritis: Estimates from the Global Burden of Disease 2010 study. *Ann. Rheum. Dis.* **2014**, *73*, 1323. [CrossRef] [PubMed]
5. Abramoff, B.; Caldera, F. Osteoarthritis: Pathology, Diagnosis, and Treatment Options. *Med. Clin. North Am.* **2020**, *104*, 293–311. [CrossRef]
6. Grunz, J.P.; Gietzen, C. Osteoarthritis of the Wrist: Pathology, Radiology, and Treatment. *Semin. Musculoskelet. Radiol.* **2021**, *25*, 294–303. [CrossRef]
7. Mathiessen, A.; Conaghan, P. Synovitis in osteoarthritis: Current understanding with therapeutic implications. *Arthritis Res. Ther.* **2017**, *19*, 18. [CrossRef] [PubMed]
8. Culvenor, A.G.; Øiestad, B.; Hart, H.; Stefanik, J.J.; Guermazi, A.; Crossley, K.M. Prevalence of knee osteoarthritis featuRes. on magnetic resonance imaging in asymptomatic uninjured adults: A systematic review and meta-analysis. *Br. J. Sport. Med.* **2019**, *53*, 1268–1278. [CrossRef] [PubMed]
9. Runhaar, J.; Kloppenburg, M.; Boers, M.; Bijlsma JW, J.; Bierma-Zeinstra SM, A.; CREDO Expert Group. Towards developing diagnostic criteria for early knee osteoarthritis: Data from the CHECK study. *Rheumatology* **2021**, *60*, 2448–2455. [CrossRef]
10. Bijlsma, J.W.J.; Berenbaum, F.; Lafeber, F. Osteoarthritis: An update with relevance for clinical practice. *Lancet* **2011**, *377*, 2115–2126. [CrossRef] [PubMed]
11. Benis, S.; Vanhove, W.; Van Tongel, A.; Hollevoet, N. Non-traumatic primary and secondary osteoarthritis of the distal radioulnar joint. *J. Hand Surg. Eur. Vol.* **2019**, *44*, 951–956. [CrossRef] [PubMed]
12. Taruc-Uy, R.L.; Lynch, S. Diagnosis and treatment of osteoarthritis. *Prim Care* **2013**, *40*, 821–836. [CrossRef] [PubMed]
13. Berenbaum, F.; Griffin, T.; Liu-Bryan, R. Review: Metabolic Regulation of Inflammation in Osteoarthritis. *Arthritis Rheumatol.* **2017**, *69*, 9–21. [CrossRef] [PubMed]
14. Ashford, S.; Williard, J. Osteoarthritis: A review. *Nurse Pract.* **2014**, *39*, 1–8. [CrossRef]
15. Felson, D.T.; Lawrence, R.; Dieppe, P.; Hirsch, R.; Helmick, C.; Jordan, J.; Kington, R.; Lane, N.; Nevitt, M.; Zhang, Y.; et al. Osteoarthritis: New Insights. Part 1: The Disease and Its Risk Factors. *Ann. Intern. Med.* **2000**, *133*, 635–646. [CrossRef]
16. Berenbaum, F.; Wallace, I.; Lieberman, D.; Felson, D. Modern-day environmental factors in the pathogenesis of osteoarthritis. *Nat. Rev. Rheumatol.* **2018**, *14*, 674–681. [CrossRef]
17. Xia, B.; Di, C.; Zhang, J.; Hu, S.; Jin, H.; Tong, P. Osteoarthritis pathogenesis: A review of molecular mechanisms. *Calcif. Tissue Int.* **2014**, *95*, 495–505. [CrossRef]
18. Carballo, C.B.; Nakagawa, Y.; Sekiya, I.; Rodeo, S. Basic Science of Articular Cartilage. *Clin. Sport. Med.* **2017**, *36*, 413–425. [CrossRef]
19. Brody, L.T. Knee osteoarthritis: Clinical connections to articular cartilage structure and function. *Phys. Ther. Sport* **2015**, *16*, 301–316. [CrossRef]
20. Guilak, F.; Nims, R.; Dicks, A.; Wu, C.-L.; Meulenbelt, I. Osteoarthritis as a disease of the cartilage pericellular matrix. *Matrix Biol. J. Int. Soc. Matrix Biol.* **2018**, *71–72*, 40–50. [CrossRef]
21. Bolduc, J.A.; Collins, J.; Loeser, R. Reactive oxygen species, aging and articular cartilage homeostasis. *Free Radic. Biol. Med.* **2019**, *132*, 73–82. [CrossRef]
22. van der Kraan, P.M.; Davidson, E.B.; van den Berg, W. A role for age-related changes in TGFbeta signaling in aberrant chondrocyte differentiation and osteoarthritis. *Arthritis Res.* **2010**, *12*, 201. [CrossRef]

23. Charlier, E.; Deroyer, C.; Ciregia, F.; Malaise, O.; Neuville, S.; Plener, Z.; Malaise, M.; de Seny, D. Chondrocyte dedifferentiation and osteoarthritis (OA). *Biochem. Pharm.* **2019**, *165*, 49–65. [CrossRef]
24. He, Y.; Manon-Jensen, T.; Arendt-Nielsen, L.; Petersen, K.; Christiansen, T.; Samuels, J.; Abramson, S.; Karsdal, M.; Attur, M.; Bay-Jensen, A. Potential diagnostic value of a type X collagen neo-epitope biomarker for knee osteoarthritis. *Osteoarthr. Cartil.* **2019**, *27*, 611–620. [CrossRef]
25. Munjal, A.; Bapat, S.; Hubbard, D.; Hunter, M.; Kolhe, R.; Fulzele, S. Advances in Molecular biomarker for early diagnosis of Osteoarthritis. *Biomol. Concepts* **2019**, *10*, 111–119. [CrossRef]
26. Bonnevie, E.D.; Galesso, D.; Secchieri, C.; Cohen, I.; Bonassar, L. Elastoviscous Transitions of Articular Cartilage Reveal a Mechanism of Synergy between Lubricin and Hyaluronic Acid. *PLoS ONE* **2015**, *10*, e0143415. [CrossRef]
27. Li, N.; Gao, J.; Mi, L.; Zhang, G.; Zhang, L.; Zhang, N.; Huo, R.; Hu, J.; Xu, K. Synovial membrane mesenchymal stem cells: Past life, current situation, and application in bone and joInt. diseases. *Stem Cell Res.* **2020**, *11*, 381. [CrossRef]
28. Eymard, F.; Pigenet, A.; Citadelle, D.; Flouzat-Lachaniette, C.; Poignard, A.; Benelli, C.; Berenbaum, F.; Chevalier, X.; Houard, X. Induction of an inflammatory and prodegradative phenotype in autologous fibroblast-like synoviocytes by the infrapatellar fat pad from patients with knee osteoarthritis. *Arthritis Rheumatol.* **2014**, *66*, 2165–2174. [CrossRef]
29. Scanzello, C.R.; Goldring, S. The role of synovitis in osteoarthritis pathogenesis. *Bone* **2012**, *51*, 249–257. [CrossRef]
30. Harvanová, D.; Tóthová, T.; Sarišský, M.; Amrichová, J.; Rosocha, J. Isolation and characterization of synovial mesenchymal stem cells. *Folia Biol.* **2011**, *57*, 119–124.
31. Fox, D.B.; Warnock, J. Cell-based meniscal tissue engineering: A case for synoviocytes. *Clin. Orthop. Relat. Res.* **2011**, *469*, 2806–2816. [CrossRef] [PubMed]
32. Haubruck, P.; Pinto, M.; Moradi, B.; Little, C.; Gentek, R. Monocytes, Macrophages, and Their Potential Niches in Synovial Joints—Therapeutic Targets in Post-Traumatic Osteoarthritis? *Front. Immunol.* **2021**, *12*, 763702. [CrossRef] [PubMed]
33. Farinelli, L.; Aquili, A.; Mattioli-Belmonte, M.; Manzotti, S.; D'Angelo, F.; Ciccullo, C.; Gigante, A. Synovial mast cells from knee and hip osteoarthritis: Histological study and clinical correlations. *J. Exp. Orthop.* **2022**, *9*, 13. [CrossRef] [PubMed]
34. Altobelli, E.; Angeletti, P.; Piccolo, D.; De Angelis, R. Synovial Fluid and Serum Concentrations of Inflammatory Markers in Rheumatoid Arthritis, Psoriatic Arthritis and Osteoarthitis: A Systematic Review. *Curr. Rheumatol. Rev.* **2017**, *13*, 170–179. [CrossRef] [PubMed]
35. Dequeker, J.; Luyten, F. The history of osteoarthritis-osteoarthrosis. *Ann. Rheum. Dis.* **2008**, *67*, 5–10. [CrossRef] [PubMed]
36. Felson, D.T. Osteoarthritis as a disease of mechanics. *Osteoarthr. Cartil.* **2013**, *21*, 10–15. [CrossRef]
37. Verbruggen, G.; Wittoek, R.; Cruyssen, B.V.; Elewaut, D. Tumour necrosis factor blockade for the treatment of erosive osteoarthritis of the interphalangeal finger joints: A double blind, randomised trial on structure modification. *Ann. Rheum. Dis.* **2012**, *71*, 891–898. [CrossRef] [PubMed]
38. Sellam, J.; Berenbaum, F. The role of synovitis in pathophysiology and clinical symptoms of osteoarthritis. *Nat. Rev. Rheumatol.* **2010**, *6*, 625–635. [CrossRef] [PubMed]
39. Prieto-Potin, I.; Largo, R.; Roman-Blas, J.; Herrero-Beaumont, G.; Walsh, D. Characterization of multinucleated giant cells in synovium and subchondral bone in knee osteoarthritis and rheumatoid arthritis. *BMC Musculoskelet. Disord.* **2015**, *16*, 226. [CrossRef]
40. Klein-Wieringa, I.R.; de Lange-Brokaar, B.; Yusuf, E.; Andersen, S.; Kwekkeboom, J.; Kroon, H.; van Osch, G.; Zuurmond, A.; Stojanovic-Susulic, V.; Nelissen, R.; et al. Inflammatory Cells in Patients with Endstage Knee Osteoarthritis: A Comparison between the Synovium and the Infrapatellar Fat Pad. *J. Rheumatol.* **2016**, *43*, 771–778. [CrossRef]
41. Glyn-Jones, S.; Palmer, A.; Agricola, R.; Price, A.; Vincent, T.; Weinans, H.; Car, A.J. Osteoarthritis. *Lancet* **2015**, *386*, 376–387. [CrossRef]
42. Madry, H.; Kon, E.; Condello, V.; Peretti, G.; Steinwachs, M.; Seil, R.; Berruto, M.; Engebretsen, L.; Filardo, G.; Angele, P. Early osteoarthritis of the knee. *Knee Surg. Sport. Traumatol. Arthrosc.* **2016**, *24*, 1753–1762. [CrossRef]
43. Lotz, M.; Martel-Pelletier, J.; Christiansen, C.; Brandi, M.; Bruyère, O.; Chapurlat, R.; Collette, J.; Cooper, C.; Giacovelli, G.; Kanis, J.; et al. Republished: Value of biomarkers in osteoarthritis: Current status and perspectives. *Postgrad Med. J.* **2014**, *90*, 171–178. [CrossRef]
44. Nordahl, S.; Alstergren, P.; Eliasson, S.; Kopp, S. Interleukin-1beta in plasma and synovial fluid in relation to radiographic changes in arthritic temporomandibular joints. *Eur. J. Oral Sci.* **1998**, *106*, 559–563. [CrossRef]
45. Panina, S.B.; Krolevets, I.; Milyutina, N.; Sagakyants, A.; Kornienko, I.; Ananyan, A.; Zabrodin, M.; Plotnikov, A.; Vnukov, V. Circulating levels of proinflammatory mediators as potential biomarkers of post-traumatic knee osteoarthritis development. *J. Orthop. Traumatol.* **2017**, *18*, 349–357. [CrossRef] [PubMed]
46. Konopka, J.; Richbourgh, B.; Liu, C. The role of PGRN in musculoskeletal development and disease. *Front. Biosci. Landmark Ed.* **2014**, *19*, 662–671. [CrossRef]
47. Stannus, O.; Jones, G.; Cicuttini, F.; Parameswaran, V.; Quinn, S.; Burgess, J.; Ding, C. Circulating levels of IL-6 and TNF-α are associated with knee radiographic osteoarthritis and knee cartilage loss in older adults. *Osteoarthr. Cartil.* **2010**, *18*, 1441–1447. [CrossRef] [PubMed]
48. Monibi, F.; Roller, B.; Stoker, A.; Garner, B.; Bal, S.; Cook, J. Identification of Synovial Fluid Biomarkers for Knee Osteoarthritis and Correlation with Radiographic Assessment. *J. Knee Surg.* **2016**, *29*, 242–247. [CrossRef]

49. Zhao, X.Y.; Yang, Z.; Zhang, Z.; Zhang, Z.; Kang, Y.; Huang, G.; Wang, S.; Huang, H.; Liao, W. CCL3 serves as a potential plasma biomarker in knee degeneration (osteoarthritis). *Osteoarthr. Cartil.* **2015**, *23*, 1405–1411. [CrossRef]
50. Beekhuizen, M.; Gierman, L.; van Spil, W.; Van Osch, G.; Huizinga, T.; Saris, D.; Creemers, L.; Zuurmond, A. An explorative study comparing levels of soluble mediators in control and osteoarthritic synovial fluid. *Osteoarthr. Cartil.* **2013**, *21*, 918–922. [CrossRef]
51. Gao, F.; Tian, J.; Pan, H.; Gao, J.; Yao, M. Association of CCL13 levels in serum and synovial fluid with the radiographic severity of knee osteoarthritis. *J. Investig. Med.* **2015**, *63*, 545–547. [CrossRef]
52. Xu, Q.; Sun, X.; Shang, X.; Jiang, H. Association of CXCL12 levels in synovial fluid with the radiographic severity of knee osteoarthritis. *J. Investig. Med.* **2012**, *60*, 898–901. [CrossRef]
53. Meulenbelt, I.; Kloppenburg, M.; Kroon, H.; Houwing-Duistermaat, J.; Garnero, P.; Le Graverand, M.H.; DeGroot, J.; Slagboom, P. Urinary CTX-II levels are associated with radiographic subtypes of osteoarthritis in hip, knee, hand, and facet joints in subject with familial osteoarthritis at multiple sites: The GARP study. *Ann. Rheum. Dis.* **2006**, *65*, 360. [CrossRef] [PubMed]
54. Arunrukthavon, P.; Heebthamai, D.; Benchasiriluck, P.; Chaluay, S.; Chotanaphuti, T.; Khuangsirikul, S. Can urinary CTX-II be a biomarker for knee osteoarthritis? *Arthroplasty* **2020**, *2*, 6. [CrossRef]
55. Valdes, A.M.; Meulenbelt, I.; Chassaing, E.; Arden, N.; Bierma-Zeinstra, S.; Hart, D.; Hofman, A.; Karsdal, M.; Kloppenburg, M.; Kroon, H.; et al. Large scale meta-analysis of urinary C-terminal telopeptide, serum cartilage oligomeric protein and matrix metalloprotease degraded type II collagen and their role in prevalence, incidence and progression of osteoarthritis. *Osteoarthr. Cartil.* **2014**, *22*, 683–689. [CrossRef]
56. Henrotin, Y.; Deberg, M.; Dubuc, J.; Quettier, E.; Christgau, S.; Reginster, J. Type II collagen peptides for measuring cartilage degradation. *Biorheology* **2004**, *41*, 543–547.
57. Poole, A.R.; Ha, N.; Bourdon, S.; Sayre, E.; Guermazi, A.; Cibere, J. Ability of a Urine Assay of Type II Collagen Cleavage by Collagenases to Detect Early Onset and Progression of Articular Cartilage Degeneration: Results from a Population-based Cohort Study. *J. Rheumatol.* **2016**, *43*, 1864–1870. [CrossRef]
58. Plsikova Matejova, J.; Spakova, T. A Preliminary Study of Combined Detection of COMP, TIMP-1, and MMP-3 in Synovial Fluid: Potential Indicators of Osteoarthritis Progression. *Cartilage* **2021**, *13* (Suppl. S2), 1421s–1430s. [CrossRef]
59. Kluzek, S.; Bay-Jensen, A.; Judge, A.; Karsdal, M.; Shorthose, M.; Spector, T.; Hart, D.; Newton, J.; Arden, N. Serum cartilage oligomeric matrix protein and development of radiographic and painful knee osteoarthritis. A community-based cohort of middle-aged women. *Biomarkers* **2015**, *20*, 557–564. [CrossRef]
60. Ruan, G.; Xu, J.; Wang, K.; Zheng, S.; Wu, J.; Ren, J.; Bian, F.; Chang, B.; Zhu, Z.; Han, W.; et al. Associations between serum S100A8/S100A9 and knee symptoms, joInt. structuRes. and cartilage enzymes in patients with knee osteoarthritis. *Osteoarthr. Cartil.* **2019**, *27*, 99–105. [CrossRef]
61. Gao, K.; Zhu, W.; Li, H.; Ma, D.; Liu, W.; Yu, W.; Wang, L.; Cao, Y. Association between cytokines and exosomes in synovial fluid of individuals with knee osteoarthritis. *Mod. Rheumatol.* **2020**, *30*, 758–764. [CrossRef]
62. Zhang, X.; Hsueh, M.; Huebner, J.; Kraus, V. TNF-α Carried by Plasma Extracellular Vesicles Predicts Knee Osteoarthritis Progression. *Front. Immunol* **2021**, *12*, 758386. [CrossRef] [PubMed]
63. Kolhe, R.; Owens, V.; Sharma, A. Sex-Specific Differences in Extracellular Vesicle Protein Cargo in Synovial Fluid of Patients with Osteoarthritis. *Life* **2020**, *10*, 337. [CrossRef]
64. Ben-Trad, L.; Matei, C.; Sava, M.; Filali, S.; Duclos, M.; Berthier, Y.; Guichardant, M.; Bernoud-Hubac, N. Synovial Extracellular Vesicles: Structure and Role in Synovial Fluid Tribological Performances. *Int. J. Mol. Sci.* **2022**, *23*, 11998. [CrossRef]
65. Mao, G.; Hu, S.; Zhang, Z.; Wu, P.; Zhao, X.; Lin, R.; Liao, W.; Kang, Y. Exosomal miR-95-5p regulates chondrogenesis and cartilage degradation via histone deacetylase 2/8. *J. Cell. Mol. Med.* **2018**, *22*, 5354–5366. [CrossRef] [PubMed]
66. Meng, F.; Li, Z.; Zhang, Z.; Yang, Z.; Kang, Y.; Zhao, X.; Long, D.; Hu, S.; Gu, M.; He, S.; et al. MicroRNA-193b-3p regulates chondrogenesis and chondrocyte metabolism by targeting HDAC3. *Theranostics* **2018**, *8*, 2862–2883. [CrossRef]
67. Mao, G.; Zhang, Z.; Hu, S.; Zhang, Z.; Chang, Z.; Huang, Z.; Liao, W.; Kang, Y. Exosomes derived from miR-92a-3p-overexpressing human mesenchymal stem cells enhance chondrogenesis and suppress cartilage degradation via targeting WNT5A. *Stem Cell Res. Ther.* **2018**, *9*, 247. [CrossRef] [PubMed]
68. Tao, S.C.; Yuan, T.; Zhang, Y.; Yin, W.; Guo, S.; Zhang, C. Exosomes derived from miR-140-5p-overexpressing human synovial mesenchymal stem cells enhance cartilage tissue regeneration and prevent osteoarthritis of the knee in a rat model. *Theranostics* **2017**, *7*, 180–195. [CrossRef]
69. Jin, Z.; Ren, J.; Qi, S. Human bone mesenchymal stem cells-derived exosomes overexpressing microRNA-26a-5p alleviate osteoarthritis via down-regulation of PTGS2. *Int. Immunopharmacol.* **2020**, *78*, 105946. [CrossRef]
70. Wu, J.; Kuang, L.; Chen, C.; Yang, J.; Zeng, W.; Li, T.; Chen, H.; Huang, S.; Fu, Z.; Li, J.; et al. miR-100-5p-abundant exosomes derived from infrapatellar fat pad MSCs protect articular cartilage and ameliorate gait abnormalities via inhibition of mTOR in osteoarthritis. *Biomaterials* **2019**, *206*, 87–100. [CrossRef]
71. Zhao, Y.; Xu, J. Synovial fluid-derived exosomal lncRNA PCGEM1 as biomarker for the different stages of osteoarthritis. *Int. Orthop.* **2018**, *42*, 2865–2872. [CrossRef] [PubMed]
72. Liu, Y.; Lin, L.; Zou, R.; Wen, C.; Wang, Z.; Lin, F. MSC-derived exosomes promote proliferation and inhibit apoptosis of chondrocytes via lncRNA-KLF3-AS1/miR-206/GIT1 axis in osteoarthritis. *Cell Cycle* **2018**, *17*, 2411–2422. [CrossRef] [PubMed]

73. Meng, Y.; Qiu, S.; Sun, L.; Zuo, J. Knockdown of exosome-mediated lnc-PVT1 alleviates lipopolysaccharide-induced osteoarthritis progression by mediating the HMGB1/TLR4/NF-κB pathway via miR-93-5p. *Mol. Med. Rep.* **2020**, *22*, 5313–5325. [CrossRef] [PubMed]
74. Wang, X.; Li, Z.; Cui, Y.; Cui, X.; Chen, C.; Wang, Z. Exosomes Isolated From Bone Marrow Mesenchymal Stem Cells Exert a Protective Effect on Osteoarthritis via lncRNA LYRM4-AS1-GRPR-miR-6515-5p. *Front. Cell Dev. Biol.* **2021**, *9*, 644380. [CrossRef] [PubMed]
75. Ene, R.; Sinescu, R.; Ene, P.; Cîrstoiu, M.; Cîrstoiu, F. Synovial inflammation in patients with different stages of knee osteoarthritis. *Rom. J. Morphol. Embryol.* **2015**, *56*, 169–173.
76. Krasnokutsky, S.; Belitskaya-Lévy, I.; Bencardino, J.; Samuels, J.; Attur, M.; Regatte, R.; Rosenthal, P.; Greenberg, J.; Schweitzer, M.; Abramson, S.; et al. Quantitative magnetic resonance imaging evidence of synovial proliferation is associated with radiographic severity of knee osteoarthritis. *Arthritis Rheum.* **2011**, *63*, 2983–2991. [CrossRef]
77. Guermazi, A.; Hayashi, D.; Roemer, F.; Zhu, Y.; Niu, J.; Crema, M.; Javaid, M.; Marra, M.; Lynch, J.; El-Khoury, G.; et al. Synovitis in knee osteoarthritis assessed by contrast-enhanced magnetic resonance imaging (MRI) is associated with radiographic tibiofemoral osteoarthritis and MRI-detected widespread cartilage damage: The MOST study. *J. Rheumatol.* **2014**, *41*, 501–508. [CrossRef]
78. Meehan, R.T.; Regan, E.; Hoffman, E.; Wolf, M.; Gill, M.; Crooks, J. Synovial Fluid Cytokines, Chemokines and MMP Levels in Osteoarthritis Patients with Knee Pain Display a Profile Similar to Many Rheumatoid Arthritis Patients. *J. Clin. Med.* **2021**, *10*, 5027. [CrossRef]
79. Kapoor, M.; Martel-Pelletier, J.; Lajeunesse, D.; Pelletier, J.-P.; Fahmi, H. Role of proinflammatory cytokines in the pathophysiology of osteoarthritis. *Nat. Rev. Rheumatol.* **2011**, *7*, 33–42. [CrossRef]
80. Molnar, V.; Matišić, V. Cytokines and Chemokines Involved in Osteoarthritis Pathogenesis. *Int. J. Mol. Sci.* **2021**, *22*, 9208. [CrossRef]
81. Johnson, A.; Huang, Y.-C.; Mao, C.-F.; Chen, C.-K.; Thomas, S.; Kuo, H.-P.; Miao, S.; Kong, Z.-L. Protective effect of ethanolic extract of Echinacea purpurea contained nanoparticles on meniscal/ligamentous injury induced osteoarthritis in obese male rats. *Sci. Rep.* **2022**, *12*, 5354. [CrossRef] [PubMed]
82. Liu, Y.; Shah, K.; Luo, J. Strategies for Articular Cartilage Repair and Regeneration. *Front. Bioeng. Biotechnol.* **2021**, *9*, 770655. [CrossRef] [PubMed]
83. Slovacek, H.; Khanna, R.; Poredos, P.; Jezovnik, M.; Hoppensteadt, D.; Fareed, J.; Hopkinson, W. Interrelationship of Osteopontin, MMP-9 and ADAMTS4 in Patients With Osteoarthritis Undergoing Total JoInt. Arthroplasty. *Clin. Appl. Thromb. /Hemost. Off. J. Int. Acad. Clin. Appl. Thromb. /Hemost.* **2020**, *26*, 1076029620964864. [CrossRef] [PubMed]
84. Croft, M.; Siegel, R. Beyond TNF: TNF superfamily cytokines as targets for the treatment of rheumatic diseases. *Nat. Rev. Rheumatol.* **2017**, *13*, 217–233. [CrossRef] [PubMed]
85. Meng, X.; Grad, S.; Wen, C.; Lai, Y.; Alini, M.; Qin, L.; Wang, X. An impaired healing model of osteochondral defect in papain-induced arthritis. *J. Orthop. Transl.* **2020**, *26*, 101–110. [CrossRef] [PubMed]
86. Verma, P.; Dalal, K. ADAMTS-4 and ADAMTS-5: Key enzymes in osteoarthritis. *J. Cell Biochem.* **2011**, *112*, 3507–3514. [CrossRef]
87. Wojdasiewicz, P.; Poniatowski, L.; Szukiewicz, D. The Role of Inflammatory and Anti-Inflammatory Cytokines in the Pathogenesis of Osteoarthritis. *Mediat. Inflamm.* **2014**, *2014*, 561459. [CrossRef]
88. Huang, X.; You, Y.; Xi, Y.; Ni, B.; Chu, X.; Zhang, R.; You, H. p-Coumaric Acid Attenuates IL-1β-Induced Inflammatory Responses and Cellular Senescence in Rat Chondrocytes. *Inflammation* **2020**, *43*, 619–628. [CrossRef]
89. Chai, B.; Zheng, Z.; Liao, X.; Li, K.; Liang, J.; Huang, Y.; Tong, C.; Ou, D.; Lu, J. The protective role of omentin-1 in IL-1β-induced chondrocyte senescence. *Artif. Cells Nanomed. Biotechnol.* **2020**, *48*, 8–14. [CrossRef]
90. Wang, Q.; Chen, Q.; Sui, J. Celecoxib prevents tumor necrosis factor-α (TNF-α)-induced cellular senescence in human chondrocytes. *Bioengineered* **2021**, *12*, 12812–12820. [CrossRef]
91. Distel, E.; Cadoudal, T.; Durant, S.; Poignard, A.; Chevalier, X.; Benelli, C. The infrapatellar fat pad in knee osteoarthritis: An important source of interleukin-6 and its soluble receptor. *Arthritis Rheum.* **2009**, *60*, 3374–3377. [CrossRef] [PubMed]
92. Kwan Tat, S.; Padrines, M.; Théoleyre, S.; HeymAnn, D.; Fortun, Y. IL-6, RANKL, TNF-alpha/IL-1: Interrelations in bone resorption pathophysiology. *Cytokine Growth Factor Rev.* **2004**, *15*, 49–60. [CrossRef]
93. Porée, B.; Kypriotou, M.; Chadjichristos, C.; Beauchef, G.; Renard, E.; Legendre, F.; Melin, M.; Gueret, S.; Hartmann, D.; Malléin-Gerin, F.; et al. Interleukin-6 (IL-6) and/or soluble IL-6 receptor down-regulation of human type II collagen gene expression in articular chondrocytes requiRes. a decrease of Sp1.Sp3 ratio and of the binding activity of both factors to the COL2A1 promoter. *J. Biol. Chem.* **2008**, *283*, 4850–4865. [CrossRef] [PubMed]
94. Scanzello, C.R. Chemokines and inflammation in osteoarthritis: Insights from patients and animal models. *J. Orthop. Res.* **2017**, *35*, 735–739. [CrossRef] [PubMed]
95. Bhavsar, I.; Miller, C.; Al-Sabbagh, M. Macrophage Inflammatory Protein-1 Alpha (MIP-1 alpha)/CCL3: As a Biomarker. *Gen. Methods Biomark. Res. Appl.* **2015**, 223–249. [CrossRef]
96. Menten, P.; Wuyts, A.; Van Damme, J. Macrophage inflammatory protein-1. *Cytokine & Growth Factor Reviews* **2002**, *13*, 455–481. [CrossRef]
97. Yang, D.-W.; Qian, G.-B.; Jiang, M.-J.; Wang, P.; Wang, K.-Z. Inhibition of microRNA-495 suppresses chondrocyte apoptosis through activation of the NF-κB signaling pathway by regulating CCL4 in osteoarthritis. *Gene Ther.* **2019**, *26*, 217–229. [CrossRef]

98. Pierzchala, A.W.; Kusz, D.; Hajduk, G. CXCL8 and CCL5 Expression in Synovial Fluid and Blood Serum in Patients with Osteoarthritis of the Knee. *Arch. Immunol. Ther. Exp.* **2011**, *59*, 151–155. [CrossRef] [PubMed]
99. Marquez-Curtis, L.A.; Janowska-Wieczorek, A. Enhancing the migration ability of mesenchymal stromal cells by targeting the SDF-1/CXCR4 axis. *BioMed. Res. Int.* **2013**, *2013*, 561098. [CrossRef]
100. Boffa, A.; Merli, G.; Andriolo, L.; Lattermann, C.; SalzmAnn, G.; Filardo, G. Synovial Fluid Biomarkers in Knee Osteoarthritis: A Systematic Review and Quantitative Evaluation Using BIPEDs Criteria. *Cartilage* **2021**, *13* (Suppl. S1), 82S–103S. [CrossRef]
101. Katz, J.N.; Arant, K.; Loeser, R. Diagnosis and Treatment of Hip and Knee Osteoarthritis: A Review. *JAMA* **2021**, *325*, 568–578. [CrossRef] [PubMed]
102. Blanco, F.J. Osteoarthritis year in review 2014: We need more biochemical biomarkers in qualification phase. *Osteoarthr. Cartil.* **2014**, *22*, 2025–2032. [CrossRef] [PubMed]
103. Goldring, M.B.; Otero, M.; Plumb, D.; Dragomir, C.; Favero, M.; El Hachem, K.; Hashimoto, K.; Roach, H.; Olivotto, E.; Borzì, R.; et al. Roles of inflammatory and anabolic cytokines in cartilage metabolism: Signals and multiple effectors converge upon MMP-13 regulation in osteoarthritis. *Eur. Cell Mater.* **2011**, *21*, 202–220. [CrossRef]
104. Li, L.; Jiang, B. Serum and synovial fluid chemokine ligand 2/monocyte chemoattractant protein 1 concentrations correlates with symptomatic severity in patients with knee osteoarthritis. *Ann. Clin. Biochem.* **2015**, *52 Pt 2*, 276–282. [CrossRef]
105. Borzì, R.M.; Mazzetti, I.; Cattini, L.; Uguccioni, M.; Baggiolini, M.; Facchini, A. Human chondrocytes express functional chemokine receptors and release matrix-degrading enzymes in response to C-X-C and C-C chemokines. *Arthritis Rheum.* **2000**, *43*, 1734–1741. [CrossRef]
106. Zhao, X.; Gu, M.; Xu, X.; Wen, X.; Yang, G.; Li, L.; Sheng, P.; Meng, F. CCL3/CCR1 mediates CD14(+)CD16(-) circulating monocyte recruitment in knee osteoarthritis progression. *Osteoarthr. Cartil.* **2020**, *28*, 613–625. [CrossRef]
107. Li, L.; Li, Z.; Li, Y.; Hu, X.; Zhang, Y.; Fan, P. Profiling of inflammatory mediators in the synovial fluid related to pain in knee osteoarthritis. *BMC Musculoskelet. Disord.* **2020**, *21*, 99. [CrossRef]
108. Raghu, H.; Lepus, C.; Wang, Q.; Wong, H.; Lingampalli, N.; Oliviero, F.; Punzi, L.; Giori, N.; Goodman, S.; Chu, C.; et al. CCL2/CCR2, but not CCL5/CCR5, mediates monocyte recruitment, inflammation and cartilage destruction in osteoarthritis. *Ann. Rheum. Dis.* **2017**, *76*, 914–922. [CrossRef] [PubMed]
109. Kitaori, T.; Ito, H.; Schwarz, E.; Tsutsumi, R.; Yoshitomi, H.; Oishi, S.; Nakano, M.; Fujii, N.; Nagasawa, T.; Nakamura, T. Stromal cell-derived factor 1/CXCR4 signaling is critical for the recruitment of mesenchymal stem cells to the fracture site during skeletal repair in a mouse model. *Arthritis Rheum.* **2009**, *60*, 813–823. [CrossRef]
110. Attur, M.; Statnikov, A.; Samuels, J.; Li, Z.; Alekseyenko, A.; Greenberg, J.; Krasnokutsky, S.; Rybak, L.; Lu, Q.; Todd, J.; et al. Plasma levels of interleukin-1 receptor antagonist (IL1Ra) predict radiographic progression of symptomatic knee osteoarthritis. *Osteoarthr. Cartil.* **2015**, *23*, 1915–1924. [CrossRef]
111. Runhaar, J.; Beavers, D.; Miller, G.; Nicklas, B.; Loeser, R.; Bierma-Zeinstra, S.; Messier, S. Inflammatory cytokines mediate the effects of diet and exercise on pain and function in knee osteoarthritis independent of BMI. *Osteoarthr. Cartil.* **2019**, *27*, 1118–1123. [CrossRef]
112. Wang, P. Diagnostic Value of Combined Serum IL-6, TNF-α, and Leptin Levels in Patients with Post-Traumatic Osteoarthritis. *Clin. Lab.* **2020**, *66*. [CrossRef] [PubMed]
113. Guo, Q.; Liu, Z.; Wang, M.; Guo, S.; Cong, H.; Liu, L. Analysis on the expression and value of CCL2 and CCL3 in patients with osteoarthritis. *Exp. Mol. Pathol.* **2021**, *118*, 104576. [CrossRef]
114. Lennerová, T.; Pavelka, K.; Šenolt, L. Biomarkers of hand osteoarthritis. *Rheumatol. Int.* **2018**, *38*, 725–735. [CrossRef]
115. Gabay, C.; Medinger-Sadowski, C.; Gascon, D.; Kolo, F.; Finckh, A. Symptomatic effects of chondroitin 4 and chondroitin 6 sulfate on hand osteoarthritis: A randomized, double-blind, placebo-controlled clinical trial at a single center. *Arthritis Rheum.* **2011**, *63*, 3383–3391. [CrossRef] [PubMed]
116. Freeston, J.E.; Garnero, P.; Wakefield, R.; Hensor, E.; Conaghan, P.; Emery, P. Urinary type II collagen C-terminal peptide is associated with synovitis and predicts structural bone loss in very early inflammatory arthritis. *Ann. Rheum. Dis.* **2011**, *70*, 331–333. [CrossRef] [PubMed]
117. Scarpellini, M.; Lurati, A.; Vignati, G.; Marrazza, M.; Telese, F.; Re, K.; Bellistri, A. Biomarkers, type II collagen, glucosamine and chondroitin sulfate in osteoarthritis follow-up: The "Magenta osteoarthritis study". *J. Orthop. Traumatol.* **2008**, *9*, 81–87. [CrossRef]
118. Xin, L.; Wu, Z.; Qu, Q.; Wang, R.; Tang, J.; Chen, L. Comparative study of CTX-II, Zn2+, and Ca2+ from the urine for knee osteoarthritis patients and healthy individuals. *Medicine* **2017**, *96*, e7593. [CrossRef]
119. Liu, C.X.; Gao, G.; Qin, X.; Deng, C.; Shen, X. Correlation Analysis of C-terminal telopeptide of collagen type II and Interleukin-1β for Early Diagnosis of Knee Osteoarthritis. *Orthop. Surg.* **2020**, *12*, 286–294. [CrossRef]
120. Duclos, M.E.; Roualdes, O.; Cararo, R.; Rousseau, J.; Roger, T.; Hartmann, D. Significance of the serum CTX-II level in an osteoarthritis animal model: A 5-month longitudinal study. *Osteoarthr. Cartil.* **2010**, *18*, 1467–1476. [CrossRef] [PubMed]
121. Csifó, E.; Nagy, E.; Horváth, E.; Farr, A.; Muntean, D. Mid-term effects of meloxicam on collagen type II degradation in a rat osteoarthritis model induced by iodoacetate. *Farmacia* **2015**, *63*, 556–560.
122. Park, Y.M.; Kim, S.; Lee, K.; Yang, S.; Min, B.-H.; Yoon, H. Detection of CTX-II in serum and urine to diagnose osteoarthritis by using a fluoro-microbeads guiding chip. *Biosens. Bioelectron.* **2015**, *67*, 192–199. [CrossRef] [PubMed]

123. Lohmander, L.S.; Atley, L.; Pietka, T.; Eyre, D. The release of crosslinked peptides from type II collagen into human synovial fluid is increased soon after joInt. injury and in osteoarthritis. *Arthritis Rheum.* **2003**, *48*, 3130–3139. [CrossRef]
124. Bauer, D.C.; Hunter, D.; Abramson, S.; Attur, M.; Corr, M.; Felson, D.; Heinegård, D.; Jordan, J.; Kepler, T.; Lane, N.; et al. Classification of osteoarthritis biomarkers: A proposed approach. *Osteoarthr. Cartil.* **2006**, *14*, 723–727. [CrossRef] [PubMed]
125. Henrotin, Y.; Berenbaum, F.; Chevalier, X.; Marty, M.; Richette, P.; Rannou, F. Reduction of the Serum Levels of a Specific Biomarker of Cartilage Degradation (Coll 2-1) by Hyaluronic Acid (KARTILAGE®CROSS) Compared to Placebo in Painful Knee Osteoarthritis Patients: The EPIKART Study, a Pilot Prospective Comparative Randomized Double Blind Trial. *BMC Musculoskelet. Disord.* **2017**, *18*, 222. [CrossRef]
126. Deberg, M.; Dubuc, J.; Labasse, A.; Sanchez, C.; Quettier, E.; Bosseloir, A.; Crielaard, J.; Henrotin, Y. One-year follow-up of Coll 2-1, Coll 2-1NO2 and myeloperoxydase serum levels in osteoarthritis patients after hip or knee replacement. *Ann. Rheum. Dis.* **2008**, *67*, 168–174. [CrossRef] [PubMed]
127. Coppelman, E.B.; David, F.; Tóth, F.; Ernst, N.; Trumble, T. The association between collagen and bone biomarkers and radiographic osteoarthritis in the distal tarsal joints of horses. *Equine Vet. J.* **2020**, *52*, 391–398. [CrossRef]
128. Kumahashi, N.; Swärd, P.; Larsson, S.; Lohmander, L.; Frobell, R.; Struglics, A. Type II collagen C2C epitope in human synovial fluid and serum after knee injury–associations with molecular and structural markers of injury. *Osteoarthr. Cartil.* **2015**, *23*, 1506–1512. [CrossRef]
129. Posey, K.L.; Coustry, F.; Hecht, J. Cartilage oligomeric matrix protein: COMPopathies and beyond. *Matrix Biol.* **2018**, *71–72*, 161–173. [CrossRef]
130. Bay-Jensen, A.C.; Reker, D.; Kjelgaard-Petersen, C.; Mobasheri, A.; Karsdal, M.; Ladel, C.; Henrotin, Y.; Thudium, C. Osteoarthritis year in review 2015: Soluble biomarkers and the BIPED criteria. *Osteoarthr. Cartil.* **2016**, *24*, 9–20. [CrossRef] [PubMed]
131. Hunter, D.J.; Li, J.; LaValley, M.; Bauer, D.; Nevitt, M.; DeGroot, J.; Poole, R.; Eyre, D.; Guermazi, A.; Gale, D.; et al. Cartilage markers and their association with cartilage loss on magnetic resonance imaging in knee osteoarthritis: The Boston Osteoarthritis Knee Study. *Arthritis Res.* **2007**, *9*, R108. [CrossRef] [PubMed]
132. Verma, P.; Dalal, K. Serum cartilage oligomeric matrix protein (COMP) in knee osteoarthritis: A novel diagnostic and prognostic biomarker. *J. Orthop. Res.* **2013**, *31*, 999–1006. [CrossRef] [PubMed]
133. Ma, T.; Zhang, Z.; Song, X.; Bai, H.; Li, Y.; Li, X.; Zhao, J.; Ma, Y.; Gao, L. Combined detection of COMP and CS846 biomarkers in experimental rat osteoarthritis: A potential approach for assessment and diagnosis of osteoarthritis. *J. Orthop. Surg. Res.* **2018**, *13*, 230. [CrossRef] [PubMed]
134. Endres, E.; van Drongelen, S.; Meurer, A.; Zaucke, F.; Stief, F. Effect of total joInt. replacement in hip osteoarthritis on serum COMP and its correlation with mechanical-functional parameters of gait analysis. *Osteoarthr. Cart. Open* **2020**, *2*, 100034. [CrossRef] [PubMed]
135. Lambert, C.; Dubuc, J.; Montell, E.; Vergés, J.; Munaut, C.; Noël, A.; Henrotin, Y. Gene expression pattern of cells from inflaMed. and normal areas of osteoarthritis synovial membrane. *Arthritis Rheumatol.* **2014**, *66*, 960–968. [CrossRef] [PubMed]
136. Van Lent, P.L.; Blom, A.; Schelbergen, R.; Slöetjes, A.; Lafeber, F.; Lems, W.; Cats, H.; Vogl, T.; Roth, J.; van den Berg, W. Active involvement of alarmins S100A8 and S100A9 in the regulation of synovial activation and joInt. destruction during mouse and human osteoarthritis. *Arthritis Rheum.* **2012**, *64*, 1466–1476. [CrossRef] [PubMed]
137. Nagy, E.E.; Nagy-Finna, C.; Popoviciu, H. Soluble Biomarkers of Osteoporosis and Osteoarthritis, from Pathway Mapping to Clinical Trials: An Update. *Clin. Interv. Aging* **2020**, *15*, 501–518. [CrossRef]
138. De Seny, D.; Sharif, M.; Fillet, M.; Cobraiville, G.; Meuwis, M.; Marée, R.; Hauzeur, J.; Wehenkel, L.; Louis, E.; Merville, M.; et al. Discovery and biochemical characterisation of four novel biomarkers for osteoarthritis. *Ann. Rheum. Dis.* **2011**, *70*, 1144–1152. [CrossRef]
139. Ourradi, K.; Xu, Y.; de Seny, D.; Kirwan, J.; Blom, A.; Sharif, M. Development and validation of novel biomarker assays for osteoarthritis. *PloS ONE* **2017**, *12*, e0181334. [CrossRef]
140. Yin, B.; Ni, J.; Witherel, C.; Yang, M.; Burdick, J.; Wen, C.; Wong, S. Harnessing Tissue-derived Extracellular Vesicles for Osteoarthritis Theranostics. *Theranostics* **2022**, *12*, 207–231. [CrossRef] [PubMed]
141. Théry, C.; Witwer, K. Minimal information for studies of extracellular vesicles 2018 (MISEV2018): A position statement of the International Society for Extracellular Vesicles and update of the MISEV2014 guidelines. *J. Extracell. Vesicles* **2018**, *7*, 1535750. [CrossRef] [PubMed]
142. Janockova, J.; Matejova, J.; Moravek, M.; Homolova, L.; Slovinska, L.; Nagyova, A.; Rak, D.; Sedlak, M.; Harvanova, D.; Spakova, T.; et al. Small Extracellular Vesicles Derived from Human Chorionic MSCs as Modern Perspective towards Cell-Free Therapy. *Int. J. Mol. Sci.* **2021**, *22*, 13581. [CrossRef] [PubMed]
143. Murphy, C.; Withrow, J.; Hunter, M.; Liu, Y.; Tang, Y.; Fulzele, S.; Hamrick, M. Emerging role of extracellular vesicles in musculoskeletal diseases. *Mol. Asp. Med.* **2018**, *60*, 123–128. [CrossRef] [PubMed]
144. Janockova, J.; Slovinska, L.; Harvanova, D.; Spakova, T.; Rosocha, J. New therapeutic approaches of mesenchymal stem cells-derived exosomes. *J. Biomed. Sci.* **2021**, *28*, 39. [CrossRef] [PubMed]
145. Spakova, T.; Janockova, J. Characterization and Therapeutic Use of Extracellular Vesicles Derived from Platelets. *Int. J. Mol. Sci.* **2021**, *22*, 9701. [CrossRef]

146. Ni, Z.; Kuang, L.; Chen, H.; Xie, Y.; Zhang, B.; Ouyang, J.; Wu, J.; Zhou, S.; Chen, L.; Su, N.; et al. The exosome-like vesicles from osteoarthritic chondrocyte enhanced mature IL-1β production of macrophages and aggravated synovitis in osteoarthritis. *Cell Death Dis.* **2019**, *10*, 522. [CrossRef] [PubMed]
147. Foers, A.D.; Garnham, A.; Chatfield, S.; Smyth, G. Extracellular Vesicles in Synovial Fluid from Rheumatoid Arthritis Patients Contain miRNAs with Capacity to Modulate Inflammation. *Int. J. Mol. Sci.* **2021**, *22*, 4910. [CrossRef] [PubMed]
148. Huang, G.; Chubinskaya, S.; Liao, W.; Loeser, R. Wnt5a induces catabolic signaling and matrix metalloproteinase production in human articular chondrocytes. *Osteoarthr. Cartil.* **2017**, *25*, 1505–1515. [CrossRef]
149. Mihanfar, A.; Shakouri, S.; Khadem-Ansari, M.; Fattahi, A.; Latifi, Z.; Nejabati, H.; Nouri, M. Exosomal miRNAs in osteoarthritis. *Mol. Biol. Rep.* **2020**, *47*, 4737–4748. [CrossRef] [PubMed]
150. Sun, H.; Hu, S.; Zhang, Z.; Lun, J.; Liao, W.; Zhang, Z. Expression of exosomal microRNAs during chondrogenic differentiation of human bone mesenchymal stem cells. *J. Cell Biochem.* **2019**, *120*, 171–181. [CrossRef]
151. Kazimierczyk, M.; Kasprowicz, M.; Kasprzyk, M.; Wrzesinski, J. Human Long Noncoding RNA Interactome: Detection, Characterization and Function. *Int. J. Mol. Sci.* **2020**, *21*, 1027. [CrossRef] [PubMed]
152. Kolhe, R.; Hunter, M.; Liu, S.; Jadeja, R. Gender-specific differential expression of exosomal miRNA in synovial fluid of patients with osteoarthritis. *Sci. Rep.* **2017**, *7*, 2029. [CrossRef] [PubMed]

life

MDPI

Article

Nematode-Induced Growth Factors Related to Angiogenesis in Autoimmune Disease Attenuation

Marta Maruszewska-Cheruiyot [1], Katarzyna Krawczak-Wójcik [1], Martyna Michniowska [2], Michael James Stear [3], Maja Machcińska [4], Maria Doligalska [2] and Katarzyna Donskow-Łysoniewska [1,*]

1 Laboratory of Parasitology, General Karol Kaczkowski Military Institute of Hygiene and Epidemiology, 01-163 Warsaw, Poland
2 Department of Parasitology, Institute of Functional Biology and Ecology, Faculty of Biology, University of Warsaw, 02-096 Warsaw, Poland
3 Department of Animal, Plant and Soil Science, Agribio, La Trobe University, Bundoora 3086, Australia
4 Department of Experimental Immunotherapy, Faculty of Medicine, Lazarski University, 02-662 Warsaw, Poland
* Correspondence: k.donskow-lysoniewska@lazarski.edu.pl

Simple Summary: Helminths are parasitic worms that influence their host in a variety of ways, including the production of growth factors and the creation of blood vessels (angiogenesis). Parasites are used to control autoimmune diseases and parasite-derived molecules are widely studied for their therapeutic potential. Accordingly, the objective of this study was to evaluate the influence of parasitic nematode infection on growth factors related to angiogenesis in murine colitis and multiple sclerosis. We observed significant changes in both models of autoimmune disorders. In addition, parasitic infection remodeled the creation of vessels in the brains of mice with multiple sclerosis. Nematode-derived factors are promising tools to fight autoimmune diseases and to study angiogenesis.

check for updates

Citation: Maruszewska-Cheruiyot, M.; Krawczak-Wójcik, K.; Michniowska, M.; Stear, M.J.; Machcińska, M.; Doligalska, M.; Donskow-Łysoniewska, K. Nematode-Induced Growth Factors Related to Angiogenesis in Autoimmune Disease Attenuation. *Life* **2023**, *13*, 321. https://doi.org/10.3390/life13020321

Academic Editors: Marcel Ramirez, Stefanos Roumeliotis and Giuseppe Minervini

Received: 29 November 2022
Revised: 29 December 2022
Accepted: 18 January 2023
Published: 23 January 2023

Abstract: Accumulating data suggest an important role of growth factors in autoimmune diseases and parasitic nematode infections. Nematodes are used in clinical studies of autoimmune diseases and parasite-derived molecules are widely studied for their therapeutic potential in various types of disorders. However, the effect of nematode infection on growth factors in autoimmune disorders has not been studied. The objective of this study was to evaluate the influence of infection with the intestinal nematode *Heligmosomoides polygyrus* in murine autoimmune models on the production of growth factors. Here, the level of a variety of growth factors related mainly to angiogenesis was evaluated by protein array in the intestinal mucosa of C57BL/6 dextran sodium sulfate-induced colitic mice and in cerebral spinal fluid of experimental autoimmune encephalomyelitis (EAE) mice infected with nematodes. In addition, vessel formation was evaluated in the brains of EAE mice infected with *H. polygyrus*. A significant influence of nematode infection on the level of angiogenic factors was observed. Parasitic infection of colitic mice resulted in upregulation of mucosal AREG, EGF, FGF-2, and IGFBP-3 in the intestine of the host and better adaptation (infectivity). In EAE mice, infection increased the level of FGF-2 and FGF-7 in CSF. In addition, remodeling of brain vessels was observed, with a higher density of long vessels. Nematode-derived factors are promising tools to fight autoimmune diseases and to study angiogenesis.

Keywords: experimental autoimmune encephalomyelitis; colitis; growth factors; nematode adaptation; angiogenesis

1. Introduction

Autoimmune diseases (ADs) are characterized by immune-mediated damage. Growth factors related to angiogenesis can contribute to pathogenesis [1]. Angiogenesis is an important process in the body in normal development and during repair processes, as well as in disease [2]. Angiogenesis is a complex, multistep process including cell proliferation, differentiation, migration and cell–cell interactions, and requires appropriate regulation [3]. Angiogenic processes create new vessels from already functioning ones. Various growth factors are involved in angiogenesis, including vascular endothelial growth factors (VEGF), fibroblast growth factors (FGF), epidermal growth factors (EGF), hepatocyte growth factor (HGF), insulin-like growth factors (IGF), and platelet-derived growth factors (PDGF) [4].

Multicellular parasites, including nematodes, have developed multiple immunoregulatory molecules. Consequently, parasites and their products are being tested as treatments for autoimmune diseases [5]. Clinical studies on patients with inflammatory bowel diseases such as ulcerative colitis and Crohn's disease have shown that nematode infection can reduce inflammation of the intestine and colon [6,7]. Similarly, in patients suffering from multiple sclerosis, a positive outcome of helminth therapy has been observed [8]. The therapeutic effect is mainly correlated with inhibition of the proinflammatory response associated with Th1 and Th17 T cells and induction of regulatory activity of Treg cells [9]. However, the host–parasite relationship is extremely complex, and processes that take place in the host during infection are not well explored. Nematodes need nutrition and to eliminate waste products. The formation of a network of blood vessels by parasites during infection is one of their adaptation strategies [10]. Nematodes can influence angiogenesis by modulating the production of angiogenic factors or by producing molecules that mimic host molecules or homologues of proteins with roles in angiogenesis.

The aim of this study was to evaluate the influence of infection with the intestinal nematode *Heligmosomoides polygyrus* during autoimmune diseases on growth factors related to angiogenesis. Infection with *H. polygyrus* is a model for human infection with *Necator americanus*. This hookworm is a significant cause of disease and is used as a treatment for autoimmune disorders (helminth therapy) in clinical studies [11]. Amphiregulin (AREG), epidermal growth factor (EGF), fibroblast growth factor 2 (FGF-2), FGF-7, granulocyte-macrophage colony-stimulating factor (GM-CSF), hepatocyte growth factor (HGF), insulin-like growth factor binding protein-3 (IGFBP-3), platelet-derived growth factor-AA (PDGF-AA), PDGF-BB, and vascular endothelial growth factor (VEGF) were evaluated in the intestinal mucosa of C57BL/6 colitic mice and in the cerebral spinal fluid (CSF) of EAE mice with *H. polygyrus* infection. In addition, the creation of new vessels in the brains of mice with EAE was evaluated by expression of CD31. Here, we examine angiogenesis in a model with both inflammatory and parasitic disease; a state corresponding to human helminth therapy.

2. Materials and Methods

2.1. Colitis Model

Eight-week-old pathogen-free C57BL/6 males were allowed to adapt to laboratory environment one week before the experiment began (n = 48). Severe colitis was provoked by the administration of 3% dextran sulphate sodium (DSS) (TdB Consultancy AB, Uppsala, Sweden), a 35–50 kDa sulphated polymer, in drinking water; it was administered two days before oral infection with 300 L3 of *H. polygyrus*, and administration of DSS was continued until the end of the experiment. The following clinical symptoms confirmed the successful induction of colitis: reduced body weight, soft stools, fecal bleeding, and diarrhea. The disease activity index (DAI) was calculated as the sum of weight loss compared to baseline weight, stool consistency, and bleeding [12]. The same researcher assessed all indications of colitis, including changes in body weight, stool consistency, and the presence of occult blood in the stools using a paper test (HemoActive, Diagnosis, Białystok, Poland). Mice were divided into four experimental groups. One of the groups received DSS (COL), the second group of mice was infected with *H. polygyrus* (HP), and the third group received both DSS and *H. polygyrus* (HP COL). Uninfected, untreated mice constituted the control group (CTR). The mice were euthanized and samples were obtained six days after infection, when the parasite was in its fourth larval stage.

2.2. Burden of Parasitic Infection

The small intestines of colitic mice were removed, ligated at both ends with cotton twine to prevent digested matter from contaminating the medium, and incubated for two hours at 37 °C in Petri dishes containing RPMI-1640 Medium with L-glutamine (2 mM), penicillin (100 U/mL) and streptomycin (100 µg/mL) (Biowest, Lakewood Ranch, FL, USA). The existence of the bursa at the caudal end of pre-male larvae was used to determine the sex of the L4 stage. The larvae were counted separately in each mouse.

2.3. Preparation of Blood, Small Intestine and Colon Mucosa Samples

Blood samples taken after heart puncture from animals with colitis were used to make serum. The small intestine and colon were removed, opened longitudinally, and washed in cold PBS, pH 7.4. Mucosa samples were prepared by scraping the inner layer of the small intestine and colon with a microscope slide. The samples were diluted in 2 mL of cold PBS, pH 7.4, including protease inhibitor cocktail tablets (Roche Applied Science, Indianapolis, IN, USA), mixed with disposable needles of decreasing diameter, then centrifuged at 4000× *g* at 4 °C for 45 min. Prior to cytokine and growth factor analysis, the supernatant was kept at −80 °C.

2.4. ELISA

ELISA was used to determinate the levels of IL-1β, IL-6, TNF-α, IL-10, and TGF-β in the serum, small intestine, and colonic mucosa of mice with induced colitis according to the manufacturer's guidelines (eBiosciences, Thermo Fisher, Waltham, MA, USA). The colorimetric reaction was defined at 450 nm with a Synergy™ H1 Microplate Reader (BioTek, Winooski, VT, USA). The mean optical densities (OD) of triplicate cultures were compared to recombinant cytokine-prepared standard curves.

2.5. EAE Model

Eight-week-old pathogen-free C57BL/6 males were allowed to adapt to laboratory environment week before the experiment began (n = 48). Experimental autoimmune encephalomyelitis (EAE) was induced by subcutaneous injection in the rear flanks with 200 µg of myelin oligodendrocyte glycoprotein $MOG_{35–55}$ (purity > 95%) per mouse emulsified in complete Freund's adjuvant (CFA) containing 300 µg of *Mycobacterium tuberculosis* H37RA strain. Immediately afterwards and again 2 days later, the animals received an intraperitoneal injection of 400 ng of *Bordetella pertussis* toxin (PTX; Sigma, St. Louis, MO, USA) in 100 µL of PBS, pH 7.2. Mice were orally infected with 300 L3 of *H. polygyrus* 21 days postimmunization. Clinical signs and ascending paralysis in EAE were assessed as described before [13]. Four experimental groups of mice were formed. The first group was immunized with EAE (EAE), the second group of mice was infected with *H. polygyrus* (HP), and the third group was immunized with EAE and infected with *H. polygyrus* (HP EAE). The control group consisted of uninfected, untreated mice (CTR). The mice were euthanized and samples were obtained six days after infection, when the parasite was in its fourth larval stage.

2.6. Cerebral Spinal Fluid (CSF)

Cerebrospinal fluid (CSF) from EAE mice was collected as described before [13]. Briefly, a syringe was gently introduced into the atlanto-occipital membrane between the occipital protuberance and the spine of the atlas. Slow aspiration of CSF produced roughly 20 µL of clear liquid with no blood contamination. The samples were centrifuged at 2000× *g* for 15 min at 4 °C.

2.7. Visualization of the Vascular Endothelium

For histological evaluation, the brains of EAE mice were removed and placed in 10% sucrose solution for 24 h. The specimens were subsequently immersed in sucrose solution (Sigma, St. Louis, MO, USA) at escalating concentrations for three days to prepare the tissue for cryosectioning. Sections eight micrometers thick were incubated with primary rat anti-CD31 monoclonal antibody [ER-MP12] (Invitrogen, Thermo Scientific, Waltham, MA, USA) and secondary rabbit anti-rat IgG (Alexa Fluor 594) (Invitrogen, Thermo Scientific). The CD31 protein is a well-characterized marker of angiogenesis. Nikon Eclipse Ti-S microscope images were captured and analyzed with NIS Elements F2.30 software (Nikon, Tokyo, Japan).

2.8. Antibody Arrays

Proteins associated with angiogenesis in CSF isolated from mice with induced EAE or in the mucosa of the small intestine isolated from mice with induced colitis were analyzed with the Angiogenesis Array (Proteome Profiler Mouse Angiogenesis Array Kit; R&D Systems, Minneapolis, MN, USA) and Mouse Growth Factor Array (Ray Biotech, Peachtree Corners, GA, USA), respectively, according to the manufacturer's instructions. The exposure time was 5 min, and the examination took 20 min since chemiluminescence signals degrade over time. The Syngene G-Box was used to scan the membranes, and the signal values were evaluated using Image J software. The array's internal positive and negative controls were used to normalize the signals.

2.9. Statistical Analysis

All experiments and tests were performed in triplicate to ensure reliable results. The significance of differences was defined with Student's t test (two-tailed unpaired) or the Mann–Whitney test. When more than two groups were analyzed, analysis of variance was caried out (one- or two-way ANOVA; GraphPad Software Inc., La Jolla, CA, USA). When the p-value was less than 0.05, the ANOVA was followed by post hoc analysis using Tukey's multiple comparisons method. The data were presented as mean $\pm$ SEM or mean $\pm$ SD. A p value of <0.05 was considered to be statistically significant.

3. Results

3.1. Symptoms of Colitis

C57BL/6 mice that received DSS and were infected with *H. polygyrus* developed colitis. Weight was significantly lower from day 7 of the experiment, four days after infection with nematodes. DAI based on weight change, diarrhea, and fecal blood was significantly higher from day 3 of the experiment (1 day before infection with *H. polygyrus*) in comparison with control mice infected with nematodes but without colitis. At the end of the experiment, mice treated with DSS and infected with nematodes had DAI around 8 compared to 0 for the control group (Figure 1A). The weight decreased to around 80% of the starting value, when the control group was around 100% of the original weight (Figure 1B).

3.2. Nematodes Adapt to Colitis in C57BL/6 Mice

H. polygyrus adapts to the colitis milieu in BALB/c mice strain [13]. To evaluate if colitis promoted adaptation of *H. polygyrus* in C57BL/6 mice, parasites were counted and the sex of the L4 stage was determined for each mouse. The number of L4 stage *H. polygyrus* present in submucosal tissue was significantly enhanced in mice with colitis compared to untreated mice (Figure 1C). The number of pre-male and pre-female parasites was also counted. Similarly, the ratio of male to female was significantly higher in mice with colitis in comparison with control animals (Figure 1D).

3.3. Nematode Adaptation to Colitis Correlate with Changes in Immune Response

To evaluate how the immune response correlates with adaptation of nematodes to the inflammatory conditions, the level of proinflammatory cytokines (IL-1β, IL-6, TNF-α) and regulatory (TGF-β, IL-10) was evaluated. Treatment of mice with DSS and infection with parasites resulted in increased levels of IL-6, TNF-α, and IL-10 in serum; IL-1β and IL-6 in the colon; and IL-6 in the small intestine. Differences of IL-1β and TGF-β in serum; TNF-α,

IL-10, and TGF-β in the colon; and IL-1β, TNF-α, IL-10, and TGF-β in the small intestine were not statistically significant (Table 1).

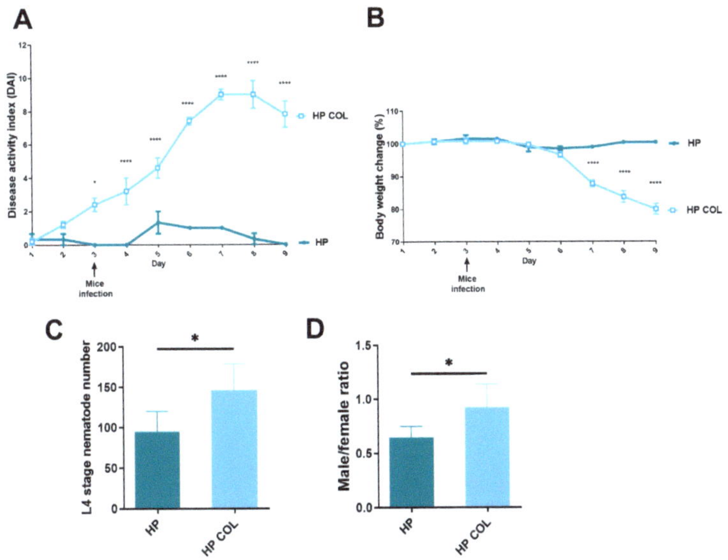

Figure 1. Symptoms of colitis after infection with *H. polygyrus*. C57BL/6 male mice were given 3% dextran sulphate sodium (DSS) in drinking water for two days before being infected orally with 300 L3 *H. polygyrus*. Disease activity index (**A**) was determined using weight change, stool consistency, and blood content. The mice were weighed every day for 9 days until the end of the experiment. Weight change (**B**) is expressed as a percentage of the initial weight. The number of L4 stage nematodes (**C**) was counted for each mouse. Ratio (**D**) was counted as the number of male nematodes divided by the number of female nematodes in each mouse. HP—mice infected with *H. polygyrus*; HP COL—mice with colitis infected with *H. polygyrus*. Data are expressed as mean values ± SEM or SD from one representative of three independent experiments (n = 5 mice/group). * $p < 0.05$ and **** $p < 0.0001$.

Table 1. Level of cytokines in serum, colon, and small intestine of C57BL/6 mice with induced colitis and parasitic infection. C57BL/6 male mice were given 3% dextran sulphate sodium (DSS) in drinking water for two days before being infected orally with 300 L3 *H. polygyrus*. Levels of IL-1β, IL-6, TNF-α, IL-10, and TGF-β were measured by ELISA. HP—mice infected with *H. polygyrus*; HP COL—colitis mice infected with *H. polygyrus*. Data are shown as means ± SD from one of three independent experiments (n = 3–5 mice/group).

Cytokine		Serum	Colon	Small Intestine
IL-1β	HP	2.9 ± 1.1	154.5 ± 54	113.5 ± 64
	HP COL	7.5 ± 7.5	2518 ± 638 *	144.3 ± 38.4
IL-6	HP	1.2 ± 2.8	206.9 ± 66.2	not detected
	HP COL	241 ± 363.1 *	360.3 ± 89.7 *	150 ± 120.1 *
TNF-α	HP	28.8 ± 4.5	148.5 ± 40.2	222.6 ± 144.8
	HP COL	73.4 ± 22.2 *	130.7 ± 32	921 ± 608.3
IL-10	HP	3685.1 ± 1829.8	8973.6 ± 3336.7	4854.2 ± 1362
	HP COL	6735.6 ± 2101.2 *	9833.1 ± 3740.8	5471.3 ± 2256.6
TGF-β	HP	977.7 ± 418.4	19.7 ± 18.5	4655 ± 1267.7
	HP COL	479.7 ± 167	38 ± 22.7	5099.9 ± 4049.9

* $p < 0.05$ compared to HP; pg/mL; Mean ± SD; Student's t-test or Mann–Whitney test.

3.4. Colitis Induction and Parasitic Infection Influence Level of Angiogenic Factors in the Intestine

To evaluate how nematode infection during colitis influenced the production of angiogenic factors in the intestine, we examined in the intestinal mucosa of mice molecules related to angiogenesis: Amphiregulin (AREG), EGF, FGF-2, FGF-7, GM-CSF, HGF, IGFBP-3, PDGF-AA, PDGF-BB, and VEGF. Colitis induction resulted in a significant reduction in GM-CSF, IGFBP-3, and both PDGF molecules compared to control mice. *H. polygyrus* infection alone resulted in an increased level of EGF, FGF-7, VEGF-A, and decreased IGFBP-3, PDGF-AA, and PDGF-BB in the intestine of mice compared to control animals. Parasitic infection during colitis was associated with elevated levels of AREG, EGF, IGFBP-3, and reduced levels of both PDGF-AA and -BB. Production of AREG, EGF, FGF-2, and IGFBP-3 was significantly higher in the intestinal mucosa of colitic mice with parasitic infection than in the intestine of mice without induced disease but infected with *H. polygyrus*. On the other hand, the levels of VEGF-A and FGF-7 were decreased in this group of mice (Figure 2).

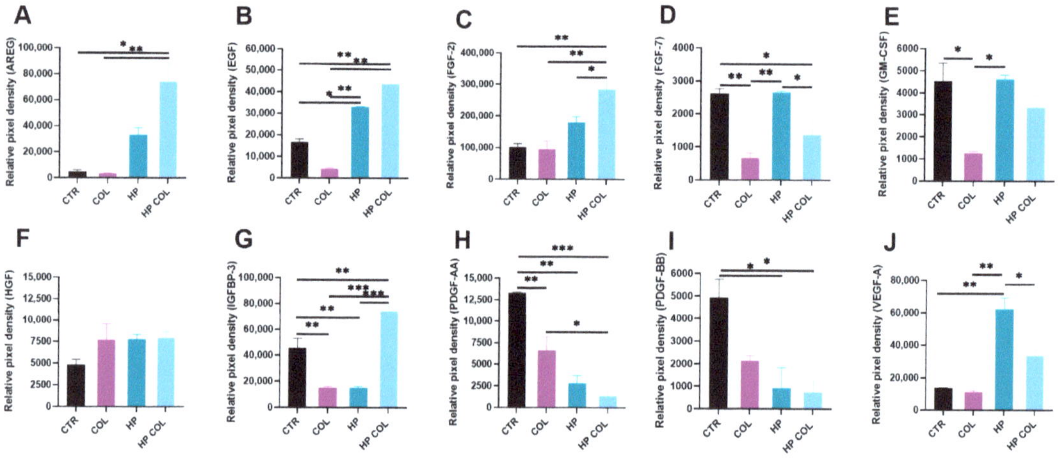

Figure 2. Level of angiogenic factors in the small intestine of C57BL/6 mice with induced colitis and parasitic infection. C57BL/6 male mice were given 3% dextran sulphate sodium (DSS) in drinking water for two days before being infected orally with 300 L3 *H. polygyrus*. Mean relative pixel density of AREG (**A**), EGF (**B**), FGF-2 (**C**), FGF-7 (**D**), GM-CSF (**E**), HGF (**F**), IGFBP-3 (**G**), PDGF-AA (**H**), PDGF-BB (**I**), VEGF-A (**J**). Data are presented as mean pixel density ± SD of two technical replicates. Data are representative of three independent experiments (n = 3). * $p < 0.05$, ** $p < 0.01$ and *** $p < 0.001$.

3.5. Nematode Infection Influences Angiogenesis in the Brain

To assess the effect of parasite infestation on the formation and growth of blood vessels in the brains of EAE mice, sections of the brain tissue were stained with the CD31 antibody. There were visible differences between groups in the number and density of vessels in brain tissue (Figure 3A). Mean vessel length was significantly decreased in brain tissue of EAE mice, mice infected with *H. polygyrus*, as well as EAE mice with parasitic infection in comparison to controls. In addition, vessels in EAE mice infected with *H. polygyrus* were significantly shorter than vessels in EAE mice without parasitic infection (Figure 3B). Induction of EAE in mice resulted in an increased density of short vessels. Mice infected with *H. polygyrus* had a higher density when only short vessels were analyzed as well as when the density of all vessels was taken into account. In addition, the density of long vessels in brain tissue was significantly higher in mice infected with parasites in comparison to EAE mice. Total and short vessel density in the brains of EAE mice infected with *H. polygyrus* was significantly lower than in mice infected with parasites, but without disease. In contrast, infection of EAE mice resulted in significantly higher density of long vessels compared to uninfected EAE (Figure 3C–E).

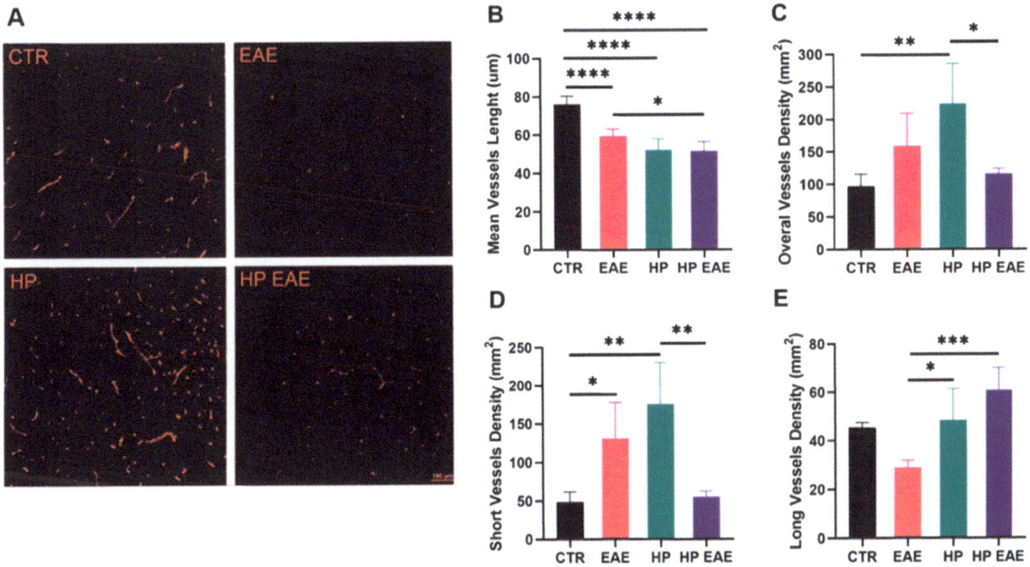

Figure 3. Vessels in the brains of EAE mice infected with *H. polygyrus*. C57BL/6 female mice were immunized with myelin oligodendrocyte glycoprotein (MOG35–55) 21 days before oral infection with 300 L3 *H. polygyrus*. Brain slices were stained with anti-CD31 (**A**); Mean vessel length is expressed in µm (**B**); total (**C**); short (**D**); and long (**E**) vessel densities were counted in 1 mm^2 based on CD31 staining. Data are expressed as mean values ± SD from one representative of three independent experiments ($n = 5$ mice/group). * $p < 0.05$, ** $p < 0.01$, *** $p < 0.001$ and **** $p < 0.0001$.

3.6. EAE Induction and Parasitic Infection Influence Level of Angiogenic Factors in the Brain

The levels of the same angiogenic factors as in the intestinal mucosa of colitic mice infected with nematode parasites were evaluated in the CSF of EAE mice with *H. polygyrus* infection. EAE development resulted in a slightly decreased level of most factors similar to colitis. However, most differences were not significant, but the level of IGFBP-3 was significantly higher in the CSF of EAE mice than of control mice (Figure 4G). *H. polygyrus* infection resulted in a significantly increased level of all evaluated growth factors: AREG, EGF, FGF-2, FGF-7, GM-CSF, HGF, IGFBP-3, PDGF-AA, PDGF-BB, and VEGF-A. Production of all molecules except FGF-2 and FGF-7 was significantly reduced in the CSF of EAE mice with parasitic infection. Levels of FGF-2 and FGF-7 were also significantly higher than in uninfected EAE mice (Figure 4C,D).

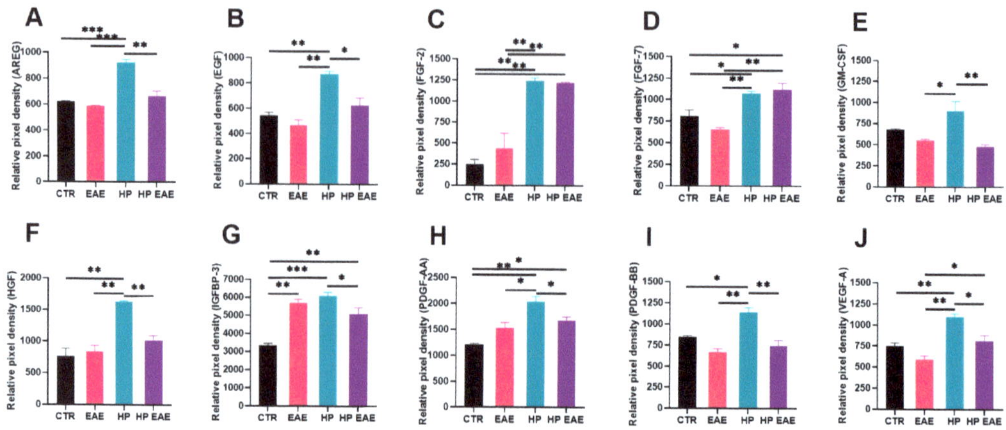

Figure 4. Level of angiogenic factors in cerebral spinal fluid (CSF) of C57BL/6 EAE mice infected with *H. polygyrus*. C57BL/6 female mice were immunized with myelin oligodendrocyte glycoprotein (MOG35–55) 21 days before oral infection with 300 L3 *H. polygyrus*. Mean relative pixel density of AREG (**A**), EGF (**B**), FGF-2 (**C**), FGF-7 (**D**), GM-CSF (**E**), HGF (**F**), IGFBP-3 (**G**), PDGF-AA (**H**), PDGF-BB (**I**) and VEGF-A (**J**). Data are presented as mean pixel density ± SD of two technical replicates. Data are representative for three independent experiments (n = 3). * $p < 0.05$, ** $p < 0.01$ and *** $p < 0.001$.

4. Discussion

This study has shown a significant influence of *H. polygyrus* infection on a variety of growth factors related mainly to angiogenesis in the intestinal mucosa of C57BL/6 colitic mice and in the cerebral spinal fluid of C57BL/6 mice with experimental autoimmune encephalomyelitis:VEGF, EGF, amphiregulin (AREG), FGF-2, FGF-7, GM-CSF, HGF, IGFBP-3, PDGF-AA, PDGF-BB.

The course of EAE in mice infected with parasites and animals without infection was analogous to that observed in our previous experiments [13]. Symptoms of colitis induced with DSS in C57BL/6 mice are similar to that observed in the BALB/c strain: both strains of animals had diarrhea, considerable weight loss, and rectal bleeding [14]. However, in the C57BL/6 mice, we observed more severe symptoms of colitis compared to the BALB/c strain [14]. This is consistent with observations reported in the literature [15].

The effectiveness of the immune response to *H. polygyrus* differs among strains of mice. We used the C57BL/6 mouse strain, which is often used, especially in experiments on the parasite–host relationship and immunity against nematode infection. During our previous studies, we observed parasite adaptation to the inflammatory milieu in BALB/c strain mice with colitis induced by DSS. Adaptation was expressed by increased growth, survival, and reproduction, as well as a significantly higher male-to-female ratio [16]. The adaptation of *H. polygyrus* in C57BL/6 mice was reflected in the increased number of L4 as well as in the higher male-to-female ratio. The results are in line with previous observations made for BALB/c mouse strain [16]. BALB/c and C57BL/6 strains differ genetically. Those differences are reflected in various immune responses, including protection against multicellular parasites. In BALB/c there is a Th2 type immune response, but in C57BL/6 a stronger Th1 immune response is observed. In addition, BALB/c produces a stronger humoral response than C57BL/6. In our study adaption of *H. polygyrus* to the colitic microenvironment in C57BL/6 mice resulted in significant changes in cytokine levels. Localization of nematodes was similar to that observed in BALB/c mice. Larvae in control mice clustered in the duodenum, whereas larvae in mice with colitis invaded more distal regions of the small intestine (data not shown) [16]. Conversely to colitis, inflammation in the central nervous system under EAE induction in the same strain of C57BL/6 mice reduced the number of parasites compared with control infection [13]. Nematode adaptation and growth are connected with nutrition and the elimination of waste products. The formation of a network of blood vessels is an adaptation strategy [10].

Growth factors play a significant role in development of both vertebrate and invertebrate animals. Basically, they influence cell division or differentiation [17]. Growth signaling can be transmitted by various pathways and affects various biological processes. In the host, growth factors influence regeneration and wound healing [18]. Repair of the tissues frequently accompanies inflammatory and autoimmune pathology as well as multicellular parasitic infection [19]. Hence, helminths are regularly exposed to host growth factors and they have evolved appropriate responses. Helminths are strong modulators of the host milieu. Studies on the transforming growth factor beta (TGF-β) confirmed that immune response to helminths is strongly dependent on both host and parasite factors [20]. Neutralization of TGF-β affected the concentration of cytokines and their pattern of production and resulted in a reduction in worm numbers and fecal egg counts [21]. Further, nematodes produce ligands for host growth factors such as TGF-β mimics [22]. Molecular interactions between mammals and helminths are the result of the host response to the parasite, as well as parasitic activity to increase their viability and reproduction success [23]. Understanding the host–parasite relationship is important in many aspects from looking for new drugs against helminthic infection to designing new therapies based on parasite-derived products.

Angiogenesis is one of the processes involved in the pathogenesis of autoimmune diseases [24]. Capillary formation is observed in the course of multiple sclerosis. This is correlated with the release of angiogenic factors. In addition, angiogenesis has been demonstrated in EAE, an experimental model of multiple sclerosis [25]. Angiogenetic processes are important in the pathogenesis and course of inflammatory bowel diseases, with promising potential as therapeutic targets [26,27]. On the other hand, parasite infection is also associated with the influence on angiogenic processes in the host's organism [10]. This study demonstrates the significant impact of intestinal nematode infection on growth factors related to angiogenesis in autoimmune disease attenuation.

Vascular endothelial growth factor, VEGF-A, is considered the most important regulator of angiogenesis. In our study, EAE induction resulted in increased level of VEGF-A in CSF; this is in line with previous observations in mice and multiple sclerosis patients [28]. The release of vascular permeability factor (VPF)/vascular endothelial growth factor (VEGF) is the main, although not the only, cause of the enhanced BBB permeability [29]. In EAE, astrocytes, monocytes, and activated Th1 lymphocytes all express VEGF, which leads to the disruption of the BBB [30,31]. Here, we observed the highest level of VEGF-A in the CSF during *H. polygyrus* infection, but interestingly, this level was lower when EAE mice were infected with nematodes. A similar effect of nematodes was observed in the intestinal mucosa of mice with DSS-induced colitis. Indeed, enhanced level of VEGF-A in IBD patients is associated with a worse course of the disease [32]. Helminths modulate the level of VEGF family factors. These results are in line with others. The soluble egg antigen of the liver fluke, *Schistosoma mansoni,* promotes angiogenesis by enhancing VEGF-A production by human endothelial cells [33]. The nematode *Trichinella spiralis* induces production of VEGF-A in nurse cells [34]. The free-living soil nematode *Caenorhabditis elegans* produces a PDGF/VEGF-like ligand, also called PVF1, which binds to mammalian VEGF receptors and induces angiogenesis [35].

The epidermal growth factor (EGF) family is also called epithelial cell-derived factors. EGF signaling is involved in angiogenesis both directly and indirectly [36]. In our study, we observed a very strong induction of EGF-pathway components during nematode infection, with even higher expressions of AREG and EGF, ligands for EGFR in mice infected with parasites and with induced colitis. Amphiregulin (AREG) is produced by many immune cells such mast cells, basophils, eosinophils, neutrophils, dendritic cells, group 2 innate lymphoid cells, and T cells. The primary role of AREG is to direct the repair damage caused by inflammation [37]. Lack of AREG in mice infected with *Trichuris muris* decreased the ability of the host to expel parasites. Lowered proliferation of colonic epithelial cells indicated a crucial role of AREG in tissue protection [38]. Our results are in line with results of Minutti [39], where infection of mice with *H. polygyrus* resulted in an increased number of $CD4^+$ T cells with EGFR expression in duodenum, MLN, and spleen. EGF-pathway is important in Treg activity [40]. As a method to modulate the immune response higher levels of EGF-signaling proteins could be responsible for increased numbers of adapted nematodes. Moreover, the protozoan *Toxoplasma gondii* induces EGFR autophosphorylation to avoid the destructive autophagic process [41].

Fibroblast growth factors (FGFs) are a group of molecules involved in various developmental and metabolic processes [42]. FGF-2, also called basic FGF, is a potent mitogen and chemotactic factor for fibroblasts and endothelial cells. FGF-2 is also an angiogenic factor involved in tissue repair and wound healing [43]. FGF-2 has a protective effect on the nervous tissue [44]. We observed a significantly increased level of FGF-2 in the CSF of EAE mice infected with *H. polygyrus*. In addition, the level of FGF-2 was elevated in the intestines of colitic mice infected with the parasite, while the FGF-7 level was highest in the intestines of infected mice without induced disease. During colitis, FGF-2 signaling is essential for maintaining gut homeostasis [45]. FGF-7 ameliorates DSS colitis in mice [46]. Knowledge of the role of FGF molecules in the parasite–host relationship is very limited. Host FGF signaling influences development of the larval stage of the tapeworm *Echinococcus multilocularis* [47].

Granulocyte-macrophage colony-stimulating factor, GM-CSF, is a multifunctional factor produced by various cells, involved in immunity. GM-CSF can also influence wound healing as an angiogenesis promotor [48]. The effect of GM-CSF on autoimmunity depends on the disease entity [49]. We observed significantly increased levels of GM-CSF during nematode infection, with lower levels during inflammation. As GM-CSF seems not to be involved in the immune response against nematodes [50], participation in tissue remodeling and VEGF signaling modification may promote parasitic invasion.

Hepatocyte growth factor (HGF) shows pleiotropic activity, including angiogenesis, by stimulating VEGF activity [51]. In our study, we observed elevated levels of HGF in the CSF of *H. polygyrus*-infected mice. So far, no studies on the involvement of HGF in the helminth–host relationship have been published.

The Insulin-like growth factor (IGF) pathway's major protein is IGF-binding protein 3 (IGFBP-3). IGFBP-3 is a growth factor downregulating angiogenesis [52]. In addition, upregulation of IGFBP-3 is correlated with the improvement of colitic mice, and IGFBP-3 knockout animals are resistant to DSS-induced inflammation of the colon [53,54]. Interestingly, the level of IGFBP-3 in the intestine did not change under the influence of *H. polygyrus* in healthy mice. However, IGFBP-3 was significantly increased when the parasite developed in mice with colitis. This may indicate a crucial contribution of IGFBP-3 to helminth therapy. IGFBP-3 in CSF is highest in mice infected with *H. polygyrus*.

The PDGF growth factor family controls proliferation, differentiation, chemotaxis, and angiogenesis and is involved in wound healing. A low level of PDGF-AA and -BB was observed in the intestines of mice infected with *H. polygyrus*, with an even lower level in colitis mice with parasitic infection. Elevated levels of PDGFs are associated with a worse course of inflammatory bowel diseases [55]. On the other hand, the highest level of PDGF factors in CSF was observed in mice infected with nematodes. This is in line with observations that higher production of PDGF molecules in human CSF correlates with anti-inflammatory microenvironment during multiple sclerosis [56].

In our study, we also observed significant differences in vessels in EAE mice brains. The shortest vessels were observed in EAE mice infected with parasites. In contrast, in this group of mice, the density of long vessels was the highest. This observation suggests that angiogenesis in helminth therapy proceeds in a different way. Although this hypothesis needs to be confirmed, future therapeutic efforts against MS should perhaps focus more on developing new vasculature with functional integration and less on total angiogenesis blockade [25].

5. Conclusions

Intestinal nematode infection altered the angiogenic growth factor response. There was an increase in VEGF, EGF, amphiregulin (AREG), FGF-2, FGF-7, GM-CSF, HGF, IGFBP-3, PDGF-AA, and PDGF-BB. The parasite's promotion of growth factors related to angiogenesis increases vascular permeability and could inhibit the host's immunological response and assist helminth survival. Parasitic nematodes are very well adapted, hence their influence on growth factors is not surprising. Interestingly, nematode infection altered the growth factor response in inflammatory conditions, such as in murine colitis and multiple sclerosis. Although more research is needed, nematode-derived growth factors appear to be promising tools to control autoimmune diseases.

Author Contributions: Conceptualization, K.D.-Ł. and M.M.-C.; investigation, M.M.-C., K.K.-W., M.M. (Martyna Michniowska), and M.D.; writing—original draft preparation, M.M.-C; K.D.-Ł.; writing—review and editing, K.D.-Ł., M.J.S., K.K.-W., and M.M. (Maja Machcińska); visualization, M.M.-C. and K.K.-W. All authors have read and agreed to the published version of the manuscript.

Funding: This research was funded by the Ministry of Science and Higher Education through the Military Institute of Hygiene and Epidemiology, Young Scientist Grant, Information No. 4562/E-290/M/2018 and supported by TEAM TECH/2017-4/22 project carried out within the TEAM TECH programme of the Foundation for Polish Science, co-financed by the European Union under the European Regional Development Fund.

Institutional Review Board Statement: All experimental procedures were performed in accordance with the Polish Law on Animal Experimentation and Directive 2010/63/UE. The study was approved by the Warsaw Local Ethics Committee for Animal Experimentation, with ID numbers WAW1/536/2014 and WAW2/186/2018.

Informed Consent Statement: Not applicable.

Data Availability Statement: Not applicable.

Conflicts of Interest: The authors declare no conflict of interest. The funders had no role in the design of the study; in the collection, analyses, or interpretation of data; in the writing of the manuscript; or in the decision to publish the results.

References

1. Zhan, H.; Li, H.; Liu, C.; Cheng, L.; Yan, S.; Li, Y. Association of circulating vascular endothelial growth factor levels with Autoimmune diseases: A systematic review and meta-analysis. *Front. Immunol.* **2021**, *27*, 674343. [CrossRef] [PubMed]
2. Carmeliet, P.; Jain, R.K. Molecular mechanisms and clinical applications of angiogenesis. *Nature* **2011**, *473*, 298–307. [CrossRef] [PubMed]
3. Adams, R.; Alitalo, K. Molecular regulation of angiogenesis and lymphangiogenesis. *Nat. Rev. Mol. Cell Biol.* **2007**, *8*, 464–478. [CrossRef]
4. Ucuzian, A.A.; Gassman, A.A.; East, A.T.; Greisler, H.P. Molecular mediators of angiogenesis. *J. Burn. Care Res.* **2010**, *31*, 158–175. [CrossRef]
5. Sobotková, K.; Parker, W.; Levá, J.; Růžková, J.; Lukeš, J.; Jirků Pomajbíková, K. Helminth Therapy—From the Parasite Perspective. *Trends Parasitol.* **2019**, *35*, 501–515. [CrossRef]
6. Maruszewska-Cheruiyot, M.; Donskow-Łysoniewska, K.; Doligalska, M. Helminth Therapy: Advances in the use of Parasitic Worms Against Inflammatory Bowel Diseases and its Challenges. *Helminthologia* **2018**, *27*, 1–11. [CrossRef]
7. Shields, V.; Cooper, J. Use of helminth therapy for management of ulcerative colitis and Crohn's disease: A systematic review. *Parasitology* **2022**, *149*, 145–154. [CrossRef] [PubMed]
8. Fleming, J.O. Helminth therapy and multiple sclerosis. *Int. J. Parasitol.* **2013**, *43*, 259–274. [CrossRef]
9. Gazzinelli-Guimaraes, P.H.; Nutman, T.B. Helminth parasites and immune regulation. *F1000Research* **2018**, *7*, 1685. [CrossRef]
10. Dennis, R.D.; Schubert, U.; Bauer, C. Angiogenesis and parasitic helminth-associated neovascularization. *Parasitology* **2011**, *138*, 426–439. [CrossRef]
11. Wammes, L.J.; Mpairwe, H.; Elliott, A.M.; Yazdanbakhsh, M. Helminth therapy or elimination: Epidemiological, immunological, and clinical considerations. *Lancet Infect. Dis.* **2014**, *14*, 1150–1162. [CrossRef]
12. Maruszewska-Cheruiyot, M.; Donskow-Łysoniewska, K.; Krawczak, K.; Machcińska, M.; Doligalska, M. Immunomodulatory potential of nematodes against dendritic cells is dependent on intestinal inflammation. *Dev. Comp. Immunol.* **2021**, *115*, 103879. [CrossRef]

13. Donskow-Łysoniewska, K.; Krawczak, K.; Doligalska, M. *Heligmosomoides polygyrus*: EAE remission is correlated with different systemic cytokine profiles provoked by L4 and adult nematodes. *Exp. Parasitol.* **2012**, *132*, 243–248. [CrossRef]
14. Donskow-Łysoniewska, K.; Majewski, P.; Brodaczewska, K.; Jóźwicka, K.; Doligalska, M. *Heligmosmoides polygyrus* fourth stages induce protection against DSS-induced colitis and change opioid expression in the intestine. *Parasite Immunol.* **2012**, *34*, 536–546. [CrossRef] [PubMed]
15. Melgar, S.; Karlsson, A.; Michaëlsson, E. Acute colitis induced by dextran sulfate sodium progresses to chronicity in C57BL/6 but not in BALB/c mice: Correlation between symptoms and inflammation. *Am. J. Physiol. Gastrointest. Liver Physiol.* **2005**, *288*, G1328–G1338. [CrossRef] [PubMed]
16. Donskow-Łysoniewska, K.; Bien, J.; Brodaczewska, K.; Krawczak, K.; Doligalska, M. Colitis promotes adaptation of an intestinal nematode: A *Heligmosomoides polygyrus* mouse model system. *PLoS ONE* **2013**, *22*, e78034. [CrossRef] [PubMed]
17. Cross, M.; Dexter, T.M. Growth factors in development, transformation, and tumorigenesis. *Cell* **1991**, *25*, 271–280. [CrossRef]
18. Werner, S.; Grose, R. Regulation of wound healing by growth factors and cytokines. *Physiol. Rev.* **2003**, *83*, 835–870. [CrossRef]
19. Allen, J.E.; Sutherland, T.E. Host protective roles of type 2 immunity: Parasite killing and tissue repair, flip sides of the same coin. *Semin. Immunol.* **2014**, *26*, 329–340. [CrossRef]
20. Maruszewska-Cheruiyot, M.; Stear, M.J.; Machcińska, M.; Donskow-Łysoniewska, K. Importance of TGFβ in Cancer and Nematode Infection and Their Interaction-Opinion. *Biomolecules* **2022**, *26*, 1572. [CrossRef]
21. Doligalska, M.; Rzepecka, J.; Drela, N.; Donskow, K.; Gerwel-Wronka, M. The role of TGF-beta in mice infected with *Heligmosomoides polygyrus. Parasite Immunol.* **2006**, *28*, 387–395. [CrossRef] [PubMed]
22. Coakley, G.; Buck, A.H.; Maizels, R.M. Host parasite communications—Messages from helminths for the immune system: Parasite communication and cell-cell interactions. *Mol. Biochem. Parasitol.* **2016**, *208*, 33–40. [CrossRef]
23. King, I.L.; Li, Y. Host-parasite interactions promote disease tolerance to intestinal helminth infection. *Front. Immunol.* **2018**, *9*, 2128. [CrossRef]
24. Szekanecz, Z.; Koch, A.E. Mechanisms of Disease: Angiogenesis in inflammatory diseases. *Nat. Clin. Pract. Rheumatol.* **2007**, *3*, 635–643. [CrossRef] [PubMed]
25. Girolamo, F.; Coppola, C.; Ribatti, D.; Trojano, M. Angiogenesis in multiple sclerosis and experimental autoimmune encephalomyelitis. *Acta Neuropathol. Commun.* **2014**, *2*, 84. [CrossRef] [PubMed]
26. Alkim, C.; Alkim, H.; Koksal, A.R.; Boga, S.; Sen, I. Angiogenesis in Inflammatory Bowel Disease. *Int. J. Inflam.* **2015**, *2015*, 970890. [CrossRef]
27. Tas, S.W.; Maracle, C.X.; Balogh, E.; Szekanecz, Z. Targeting of proangiogenic signalling pathways in chronic inflammation. *Nat. Rev. Rheumatol.* **2016**, *12*, 111–122. [CrossRef]
28. Tham, E.; Gielen, A.W.; Khademi, M.; Martin, C.; Piehl, F. Decreased expression of VEGF-A in rat experimental autoimmune encephalomyelitis and in cerebrospinal fluid mononuclear cells from patients with multiple sclerosis. *Scand. J. Immunol.* **2006**, *64*, 609–622. [CrossRef]
29. Mayhan, W.G. VEGF increases permeability of the blood-brain barrier via a nitric oxide synthase/cGMP-dependent pathway. *Am. J. Physiol.* **1999**, *276*, C1148–C1153. [CrossRef]
30. Argaw, A.T.; Asp, L.; Zhang, J.; Navrazhina, K.; Pham, T.; Mariani, J.N.; Mahase, S.; Dutta, D.J.; Seto, J.; Kramer, E.G.; et al. Astrocyte-derived VEGF-A drives blood–brain barrier disruption in CNS inflammatory disease. *J. Clin. Investig.* **2012**, *122*, 2454–2468. [CrossRef]
31. Quintana, F.J.; Cohen, I.R. Angiogenesis-inflammation cross-talk: Vascular endothelial growth factor is secreted by activated T cells and induces Th1 polarization. *J. Immunol.* **2004**, *172*, 4618–4623. [CrossRef]
32. Scaldaferri, F.; Vetrano, S.; Sans, M.; Arena, V.; Straface, G.; Stigliano, E.; Repici, A.; Sturm, A.; Malesci, A.; Panes, J. VEGF-A links angiogenesis and inflammation in inflammatory bowel disease pathogenesis. *Gastroenterology* **2009**, *136*, 585–595.e5. [CrossRef] [PubMed]
33. Loeffler, D.A.; Lundy, S.K.; Singh, K.P.; Gerard, H.C.; Hudson, A.P.; Boros, D.L. Soluble egg antigens from *Schistosoma mansoni* induce angiogenesis-related processes by up-regulating vascular endothelial growth factor in human endothelial cells. *J. Infect. Dis.* **2002**, *185*, 1650–1656. [CrossRef]
34. Capó, V.A.; Despommier, D.D.; Polvere, R.I. *Trichinella spiralis*: Vascular endothelial growth factor is up-regulated within the nurse cell during the early phase of its formation. *J. Parasitol.* **1998**, *84*, 209–214. [CrossRef] [PubMed]
35. Tarsitano, M.; De Falco, S.; Colonna, V.; McGhee, J.D.; Persico, M.G. The *C. elegans* pvf-1 gene encodes a PDGF/VEGF-like factor able to bind mammalian VEGF receptors and to induce angiogenesis. *FASEB J.* **2006**, *20*, 227–233. [CrossRef]
36. Hirata, A.; Ogawa, S.; Kometani, T.; Kuwano, T.; Naito, S.; Kuwano, M.; Ono, M. ZD1839 (Iressa) induces antiangiogenic effects through inhibition of epidermal growth factor receptor tyrosine kinase. *Cancer Res.* **2002**, *62*, 2554–2560.
37. Zaiss, D.M.W.; Gause, W.C.; Osborne, L.C.; Artis, D. Emerging functions of amphiregulin in orchestrating immunity, inflammation, and tissue repair. *Immunity* **2015**, *42*, 216–226. [CrossRef] [PubMed]
38. Zaiss, D.M.; Yang, L.; Shah, P.R.; Kobie, J.J.; Urban, J.F.; Mosmann, T.R. Amphiregulin, a TH2 cytokine enhancing resistance to nematodes. *Science* **2006**, *15*, 1746. [CrossRef]
39. Minutti, C.M.; Drube, S.; Blair, N.; Schwartz, C.; McCrae, J.C.; McKenzie, A.N.; Kamradt, T.; Mokry, M.; Coffer, P.J.; Sibilia, M.; et al. Epidermal Growth Factor Receptor Expression Licenses Type-2 Helper T Cells to Function in a T Cell Receptor-Independent Fashion. *Immunity* **2017**, *17*, 710–722.e6. [CrossRef]

40. Zaiss, D.M.; van Loosdregt, J.; Gorlani, A.; Bekker, C.P.; Gröne, A.; Sibilia, M.; van Bergen en Henegouwen, P.M.; Roovers, R.C.; Coffer, P.J.; Sijts, A.J. Amphiregulin Enhances Regulatory T Cell-Suppressive Function via the Epidermal Growth Factor Receptor. *Immunity* **2013**, *38*, 275–284. [CrossRef]
41. Lopez Corcino, Y.; Gonzalez Ferrer, S.; Mantilla, L.E.; Trikeriotis, S.; Yu, J.S.; Kim, S.; Hansen, S.; Portillo, J.C.; Subauste, C.S. *Toxoplasma gondii* induces prolonged host epidermal growth factor receptor signalling to prevent parasite elimination by autophagy: Perspectives for in vivo control of the parasite. *Cell. Microbiol.* **2019**, *21*, e13084. [CrossRef] [PubMed]
42. Itoh, N.; Ornitz, D.M. Functional evolutionary history of the mouse Fgf gene family. *Dev. Dyn.* **2008**, *237*, 18–27. [CrossRef] [PubMed]
43. Okada-Ban, M.; Thiery, J.P.; Jouanneau, J. Fibroblast growth factor-2. *Int. J. Biochem. Cell Biol.* **2000**, *32*, 263–267. [CrossRef]
44. Klimaschewski, L.; Claus, P. Fibroblast Growth Factor Signalling in the Diseased Nervous System. *Mol. Neurobiol.* **2021**, *58*, 3884–3902. [CrossRef] [PubMed]
45. Song, X.; Dai, D.; He, X.; Zhu, S.; Yao, Y.; Gao, H.; Wang, J.; Qu, F.; Qiu, J.; Wang, H.; et al. Growth Factor FGF2 Cooperates with Interleukin-17 to Repair Intestinal Epithelial Damage. *Immunity* **2015**, *15*, 488–501. [CrossRef]
46. Egger, B.; Procaccino, F.; Sarosi, I.; Tolmos, J.; Büchler, M.W.; Eysselein, V.E. Keratinocyte growth factor ameliorates dextran sodium sulfate colitis in mice. *Dig. Dis. Sci.* **1999**, *44*, 836–844. [CrossRef] [PubMed]
47. Förster, S.; Koziol, U.; Schäfer, T.; Duvoisin, R.; Cailliau, K.; Vanderstraete, M.; Dissous, C.; Brehm, K. The role of fibroblast growth factor signalling in *Echinococcus multilocularis* development and host-parasite interaction. *PLoS Negl. Trop. Dis.* **2019**, *8*, e0006959. [CrossRef] [PubMed]
48. Eubank, T.D.; Roberts, R.; Galloway, M.; Wang, Y.; Cohn, D.E.; Marsh, C.B. GM-CSF induces expression of soluble VEGF receptor-1 from human monocytes and inhibits angiogenesis in mice. *Immunity* **2004**, *21*, 831–842. [CrossRef]
49. Lotfi, N.; Thome, R.; Rezaei, N.; Zhang, G.X.; Rezaei, A.; Rostami, A.; Esmaeil, N. Roles of GM-CSF in the Pathogenesis of Autoimmune Diseases: An Update. *Front. Immunol.* **2019**, *4*, 1265. [CrossRef]
50. Shim, D.S.; Schilter, H.C.; Knott, M.L.; Almeida, R.A.; Short, R.P.; Mackay, C.R.; Dent, L.A.; Sewell, W.A. Protection against *Nippostrongylus brasiliensis* infection in mice is independent of GM-CSF. *Immunol. Cell Biol.* **2012**, *90*, 553–558. [CrossRef]
51. Xin, X.; Yang, S.; Ingle, G.; Zlot, C.; Rangell, L.; Kowalski, J.; Schwall, R.; Ferrara, N.; Gerritsen, M.E. Hepatocyte growth factor enhances vascular endothelial growth factor-induced angiogenesis in vitro and in vivo. *Am. J. Pathol.* **2001**, *158*, 1111–1120. [CrossRef] [PubMed]
52. Varma Shrivastav, S.; Bhardwaj, A.; Pathak, K.A.; Shrivastav, A. Insulin-Like Growth Factor Binding Protein-3 (IGFBP-3): Unraveling the Role in Mediating IGF-Independent Effects Within the Cell. *Front. Cell Dev. Biol.* **2020**, *5*, 286. [CrossRef]
53. Kim, S.C.; Hwang, P.H. Up-regulation of IGF Binding Protein-3 Inhibits Colonic Inflammatory Response. *J. Korean Med. Sci.* **2018**, *26*, e110. [CrossRef] [PubMed]
54. Yancu, D.; Blouin, M.J.; Birman, E.; Florianova, L.; Aleynikova, O.; Zakikhani, M.; VanderMeulen, H.; Seidman, E.; Pollak, M. A phenotype of IGFBP-3 knockout mice revealed by dextran sulfate-induced colitis. *J. Gastroenterol. Hepatol.* **2017**, *32*, 146–153. [CrossRef] [PubMed]
55. Kumagai, S.; Ohtani, H.; Nagai, T.; Funa, K.; Hiwatashi, N.O.; Shimosegawa, T.; Nagura, H. Platelet-derived growth factor and its receptors are expressed in areas of both active inflammation and active fibrosis in inflammatory bowel disease. *Tohoku J. Exp. Med.* **2001**, *195*, 21–33. [CrossRef]
56. Stampanoni Bassi, M.; Iezzi, E.; Marfia, G.A.; Simonelli, I.; Musella, A.; Mandolesi, G.; Fresegna, D.; Pasqualetti, P.; Furlan, R.; Finardi, A.; et al. Platelet-derived growth factor predicts prolonged relapse-free period in multiple sclerosis. *J. Neuroinflam.* **2018**, *15*, 108. [CrossRef]

life

MDPI

Review

Effectiveness of a Therapeutic Exercise Program to Improve the Symptoms of Peripheral Neuropathy during Chemotherapy: Systematic Review of Randomized Clinical Trials

Snehil Dixit [1], Valentina Tapia [2], Carolina Sepúlveda [2], Daniela Olate [2], Lily Berríos-Contreras [2], Luz Alejandra Lorca [3], Abdulfattah S. Alqahtani [4] and Ivana Leão Ribeiro [2,*]

1 Department of Medical Rehabilitation Sciences, College of Applied Medical Sciences, King Khalid University, Abha 61471, Saudi Arabia
2 Department of Kinesiology, Faculty of Healthy Sciences, Universidad Católica del Maule, Talca 3460000, Chile
3 Hospital del Salvador, Servicio de Salud Metropolitano Oriente, Santiago de Chile 13123, Chile
4 Department of Rehabilitation Sciences, College of Applied Medical Sciences, King Saud University, Riyadh 11433, Saudi Arabia
* Correspondence: ileao@ucm.cl; Tel.: +56-712413622

Abstract: Background: Therapeutic exercise has an important role to manage chemotherapy-induced peripheral neuropathy symptoms. However, there is little evidence of its effectiveness. Objective: To synthesize the evidence regarding therapeutic exercise during chemotherapy to improve peripheral neuropathy symptoms. Databases: PubMed, CINAHL, Cochrane Library, PEDro, ScienceDirect, Scopus, Web of Science and BIREME. Methodology: Randomized clinical trials were included. GRADE was used to synthesize evidence and an inverse variance model for meta-analysis. Results: Up to May 2022, 2172 references were analyzed and 14 studies that evaluated 1094 participants were included. The exercises were highly effective in improving pain threshold and moderately effective in improving peripheral neuropathy symptoms at the 8-week follow-up and the 4–24 weeks. Furthermore, the evidence was low in improving thermal threshold, tactile and vibratory sensitivity. Conclusion: Therapeutic exercise generates a significant reduction in peripheral neuropathy symptoms in patients in short- and long-term follow-up with a moderate level of evidence quality.

Keywords: Neoplasia; exercise; sensitivity; chemotherapy; measurement of results reported by the patient

Citation: Dixit, S.; Tapia, V.; Sepúlveda, C.; Olate, D.; Berríos-Contreras, L.; Lorca, L.A.; Alqahtani, A.S.; Ribeiro, I.L. Effectiveness of a Therapeutic Exercise Program to Improve the Symptoms of Peripheral Neuropathy during Chemotherapy: Systematic Review of Randomized Clinical Trials. *Life* **2023**, *13*, 262. https://doi.org/10.3390/life13020262

Academic Editors: Stefanos Roumeliotis and Giuseppe Minervini

Received: 20 December 2022
Revised: 6 January 2023
Accepted: 14 January 2023
Published: 18 January 2023

1. Introduction

Cancer is a global health issue with an increasing incidence and mortality. It is estimated that there will be 18.1 million new cases worldwide and 9.6 million deaths due to this disease [1].

Cancer therapy involves various treatments, such as surgery, chemotherapy, radiation therapy, immunotherapy and hormone therapy [2]. Chemotherapy, being one of the most widely used therapies, uses cytotoxic drugs with the aim of damaging the genetic material of neoplastic cells and preventing their replication [3]. This therapy is not selective; therefore, it damages both tumor cells and healthy cells. As a result of the damage, many side effects are manifested either in the short term such as nausea, neuropathy and fatigue, or in the long term such as premature menopause and cardiac and cognitive dysfunction [4].

Chemotherapy-induced peripheral neuropathy is one of the most debilitating side effects of chemotherapy, since the manifestation of symptoms is linked to the delivered dose of the different chemotherapeutic agents such as platinum compounds, taxanes vinca alkaloids, proteasome inhibitors and epothilones, among others [5].

The prevalence of developing peripheral neuropathy one month after completing chemotherapy is around 68%. The symptoms develop mainly in the hands and feet, with sensory alterations associated with numbness and paresis, motor generating balance and balance problems and autonomous problems with orthostatic hypotension.

Peripheral neuropathy can be evaluated objectively using quantitative sensory tests by performing clinical examinations, as well as subjective measurements such as questionnaires, scales and evaluations of nerve function [6,7]. However, there is no evaluation guideline that is used as a "gold standard", which generates a great limitation for proper clinical applicability for these patients [5].

Conservative management of chemotherapy-induced peripheral neuropathy involves physical exercise with different types of training, whether aerobic, endurance, motor sensory or balance. Only one systematic review was found, in which it evidenced that a training plan combined with resistance, strength and motor sensory exercises, which should last 36 weeks, at moderate intensities, with a frequency of 2 to 5 days a week and a duration 60 min has been effective in reducing symptoms of chemotherapy-induced peripheral neuropathy [8].

However, studies are lacking that address specific exercise programs for this particular condition [9] and that their results provide clinical applicability. While many studies were found specifying different types of training and subjective measurements of symptoms caused by chemotherapy-induced peripheral neuropathy, many did not identify specific objective and subjective measurements such as the perception of peripheral neuropathy, pressure pain threshold and thermal, tactile and vibration sensitivity.

Considering the above, this systematic review aims to synthesize the evidence regarding interventions with therapeutic exercises during chemotherapy to improve the symptoms produced by peripheral neuropathy with respect to the variables described above.

2. Materials and Methods

2.1. Study Designation

This systematic review was written according to the preferred reporting model for these study types and meta-analysis (PRISMA) and the recommendations of the Cochrane Collaborations for systematic reviews [10]. The review was registered in PROSPERO with the following number: CRD42020188275. On 9 April 2020, the search began in different databases, regarding various components of the research question considering population, intervention, comparison and results, to identify the knowledge gap; the search was performed until May 2022.

2.2. Literature Search

An electronic search of various articles indexed in the following databases was performed: PubMed, CINAHL Plus, Cochrane Central Register of Controlled Trials, Physiotherapy Evidence Database, Science Direct, Scopus and Web of Science y BIREME. The search strategy was adapted for each database. In PubMed, a combination of words was used: ("Neoplasms" [Mesh]) OR cancer AND (exercise) OR "Resistance Training" [Mesh] AND chemotherapy AND ("Peripheral Nervous System Diseases" [Mesh] OR peripheral neuropathy OR pressure pain threshold OR thermal sensitivity OR tactile sensitivity OR vibration sensitivity).

The Start program (version 3.4 BETA, sourced by the Research Laboratory in Software Engineering (LaPES) of the Federal University of São Carlos, Brazil) was used, which was held in the selection of titles, abstracts and full text, considering the analysis between evaluators and consensus criteria. Two independent reviewers (V.T. and D.O.) performed the selection process and two (C.S. and I.L.) participated in the consensus.

2.3. Inclusion Criteria

This systematic review included only randomized clinical trials that included therapeutic exercise with a variable related to symptoms of peripheral neuropathy in patients who underwent chemotherapy. The language of the publications was unlimited and should contain a pre-post comparison exercise and that the beginning of the training program was during chemotherapy.

2.4. Evaluation of Methodological Quality of the Studies

To Physiotherapy Evidence Database, a PEDro (www.pedro.org.au, accessed on 1 May 2022) scale was used to assess the methodological quality of the studies based on the Delphi list [11]. The studies that were included in this database were previously qualified; if there were no studies, they were manually evaluated by two examiners with a possible consensus by two evaluators. Clinical trials with scores greater than or equal to 6 were considered high methodological, 4 to 5 were rated as moderate quality and lastly, less than or equal to 3 were classified as low methodological quality [12,13].

Data of participants and methodology of the studies were extracted using a standardized form adapted from the Cochrane Collaboration model [10]. Moreover, effect size (ES) with a 95% confidence interval (CI) for continuous outcomes in each comparison group was calculated and the values before and after the intervention were considered. The treatment was classified as small (<0.3), moderate (between 0.4 and 0.7) and large (>0.8) according to Cohen's index interpretation [14].

The results of the primary studies were interpreted according to the effectiveness of the training programs to improve the symptoms of perception of peripheral neuropathy and increase the pain threshold to pressure, thermal, tactile and vibratory sensitivity. They were considered positive when comparing the intervention and the control groups presented a statistically significant improvement in the primary outcomes.

The preventive effects of therapeutic exercise were rated with an equal sign when there was no difference between the pre and post intervention. Finally, studies that presented a significant reduction in the variables of interest of the intervention were classified as having no effect. The effect size was calculated for studies that presented descriptive ideas, represented by means and standard deviation for the main variables such as pressure, thermal, tactile and vibratory pain threshold.

The synthesis of evidence for each intervention was calculated with the Grading of Recommendations Assessment, Development and Evaluation (GRADE) that considers high, moderate, low or very low evidence level based on the following factors: limitations, indirectness, inconsistency, imprecision and lastly bias risk. In this review, the GRADEpro software (https://gradepro.org, accessed on 1 May 2022) [15] was used to create tables with the synthesis of evidence.

2.5. Statistical Analysis

A meta-analysis was performed using means and standard deviations from each selected clinical trial. The difference of standardized means and the 95% confidence interval were calculated using an inverse variance model of random effects for the meta-analysis, considering the data after the intervention. Data heterogeneity between studies were assessed using the I statisitic^2. The p values were calculated and statistical significance was set at <0.05. Statistical analysis was performed using the RevMan five-revision management software (version 5.3, 11-13 Cavendish Square, London, UK).

3. Results

The studies obtained based on the search with the keywords totaled 2.172 articles, which were examined by title and abstracts; after reading the full text of 42 studies, 14 articles were selected that met the inclusion criteria. The flow diagram used is presented in Figure 1.

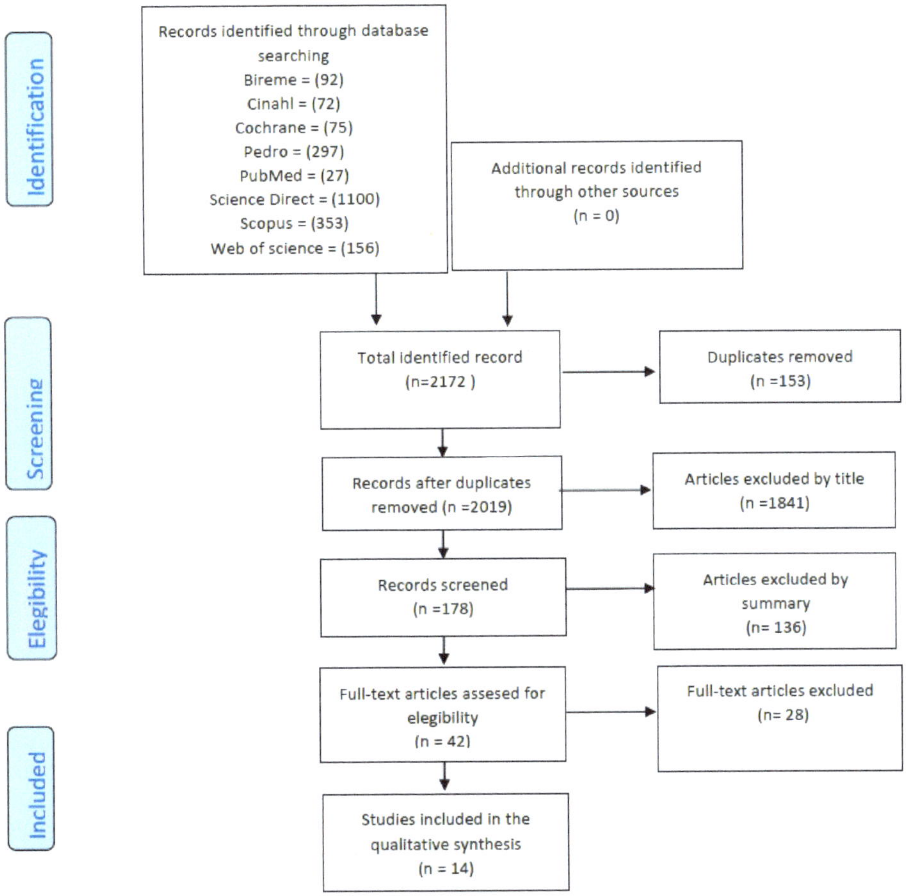

Figure 1. PRISMA flow diagram for the systematic review.

3.1. Evaluation of the Methodological Quality of the Studies

Of the 14 studies collected, 13 were indexed in the PEDro scale [7,16–26]. One [27] was performed manually using the same scale between two evaluators (V.T. and C.S.) in consensus with a third party (D.O.) in case of disagreement. Table 1 shows PEDro scale scores from studies.

Eight of the studies obtained a score equal to or greater than six; therefore, they were classified as having high methodological quality [8,17,18,22,23,26–28]. On the other hand, three studies [7,19,20] reached a score between four and five and were categorized as moderate quality. Finally, three studies [16,21,24] obtained a score of three and were therefore cataloged as having low methodological quality. None of the studies scored on the blind allocation criteria for both participants and therapists. In addition, only five studies [17,20,25,27,28] reported that the evaluators who measured at least one key result were blinded. Only six studies [7,19,23,25,26,28] presented results for all subjects who received treatment or were assigned to the control group, or when this could not be, data for at least one key outcome were analyzed by intention to treat (Table 1).

Table 1. Identification of the 14 studies included in the review classified according to the PEDro scale.

Author	1	2	3	4	5	6	7	8	9	10	11	Total
Henke, et al., 2014 [16]	1	1	-	-	-	-	-	-	-	1	1	3
Bahar-Ozdemir Y et al., 2020 [27]	1	-	1	1	-	-	1	1	-	1	1	6
Hammond E et al., 2020 [17]	1	1	1	1	-	-	1	-	-	1	1	6
Bland, K. A et al., 2019 [18]	1	1	1	1	-	-	-	1	-	1	1	6
Mijwel et al., 2018 [19]	-	1	-	1	-	-	-	-	1	1	1	4
Schönsteiner et al., 2017 [20]	-	1	-	1	-	-	1	1	-	1	1	5
Kleckner IR et al., 2017 [7]	-	1	1	1	-	-	-	-	1	1	1	5
Vollmers, P et al., 2018 [21]	1	1	-	-	-	-	-	-	-	1	1	3
Schwenk et al., 2016 [22]	1	1	1	1	-	-	-	1	-	1	1	6
Visovsky et al., 2014 [23]	1	1	1	1	-	-	-	-	1	1	1	6
Stuecher, K. et al., 2018 [24]	1	1	-	-	-	-	-	-	-	1	1	3
Streckmann F et al., 2014 [25]	-	1	-	1	-	-	1	1	1	1	1	6
Dhawan S et al., 2020 [26]	1	1	1	1	-	-	-	1	1	1	1	7
Saraboon, C et al., 2021 [28]	1	1	1	1	-	-	1	1	1	1	1	8
	10/14	13/14	8/14	11/14	0/14	0/14	5/14	7/14	6/14	14/14		

1. Were the eligibility criteria specified? 2. Were the participants randomly allocated between the groups? 3. Was the allocation blinded? 4. Were the groups similar at the baseline for the most important prognostic indicators? 5. Were the participants blinded? 6. Were the therapists who performed the intervention blinded? 7. Were the evaluators who measured at least one measure of response blinded? 8. Did the measures of at least one outcome affect >85% of the participants initially allocated to the groups? 9. Did all the participants receive the treatment or a control condition; if not, were the data analyzed with intention-to-treat analysis? 10. Did the statistical comparison results between groups report at least one key response variable? 11. Did the study present reliability measures for at least one variable response?

3.2. Characteristics of Included Studies

Table 2 describes the main characteristics of the 14 included studies, of which 1094 people participated, having an average age range of 19 to 79 years old, with solid and hematological cancer diagnoses. The comparison was made between a control group, which was based on standard care mainly focused on evaluations and education to patients, and an intervention group, where the main type of exercises that were performed were aerobic training, strengthening of both lower and upper limbs and balance exercises, that began from the first day of chemotherapy treatment or weeks after it. Among the most used equipment in these were the elastic bands, treadmill and pedometer. From 14 studies, five mentioned that intervention was supervised by a physiotherapist [16,17,27,28], one by a nurse [23], one by a sport scientist [21], one by a certified investigator by the ACSM [7], one by an exercise physiologist or oncology nurse [19] and one by a specialist in prescribing exercises for cancer patients [18]. Four studies did not mention the profession of the trainer [20,22,24,26].

The training frequency ranged from 2 to 7 days a week with a duration of 5 to 60 min depending on the exercise performed, a moderate intensity depending on the chemotherapy cycle in which the patients were, and the duration of the protocol varied between 4 and 56 weeks. A physiotherapist supervised 23% of the programs, while the others were supervised by a professional trained to carry out this work. The main variables analyzed were peripheral neuropathy perception, pressure pain threshold and thermal, tactile and vibratory sensitivity. The follow-up was carried out in a period where the minimum range was 4 weeks and the maximum was approximately 36 weeks. The effect size range varied from 0.05 to 0.93 for peripheral neuropathy perception; as for pressure pain threshold, it ranged from 0.44 to 0.57, thermal threshold was 0.06 to 0.28, tactile sensitivity presented a value of 0.01 and vibratory sensitivity presented a value of 0.15.

Table 2. Characteristics of the studies included in the review.

Study	Participants, Mean ± DE of Age	Start of Intervention	Comparison Groups and Training Type	Frequency and Duration of Training/Protocol	Outcomes	Follow-Up	Main Results/Magnitude of Effect
Henke, et al., 2014 [16]	29 Participants IG: 18 CG: 11 IG: NI CG: NI	First day of Che	IG: Aerobic and whole body strength training CG: Conventional physical therapy (breathing techniques and manual therapy)	Aerobic: 6 min a day/5 times per week Strengthening: 2 times per week, 10 repetitions per exercise at their maximum capacity/NF	Quality of life (Peripheral neuropathy) Questionnaire	NF	Peripheral neuropathy (+)/ES PI = −0.81 (−1.52; 0.02); ES IG = −0.64 (−1.25; 0.08); ES CG = −0.41 (−1.22; 0.46)
Bahar-Ozdemir et al., 2020 [27]	60 Participants IG: 24 CG: 36 IG: 52 ± 9.99 years CG: 53.58 ± 11.92 years	Started together with Che	IG: Strengthening with LL resistance exercises and equilibrium/ balance exercises. CG: Guidance regarding PA	Strengthening: 2 sets/10 rep. 5 times per week Equilibrium: 10 min of exercise/5 days a week/10 weeks	Neuropathic pain Questionnaire	Post. Third round of Che	Neuropathic pain (+), IG: 26.3%, CG: 47.2% Pain (=)/ES PI = 0.47 (−0.09; 0.95)
Hammond E et al., 2020 [17]	48 Participants IG1: 22 CG: 26 IG2: 56.3 ± 9.9 years CG: 53.0 ± 10.3 years	Started together with Che	IG: Nerve gliding exercises, stretching, ROM. and education CG: Standard care and nerve reevaluations	5 to 10 min./3 times a day/24 weeks	Pain report, neuropathic pain, vibratory threshold, pressure pain threshold. Numerical scale, survey, The TSAII Vibration Sensory Analyzer, algomeESr	Baseline, PChe, 12 weeks and 24 weeks	Pain (+), no pain report, IG: 70.1%; CG: 51% Neuropathic pain (=)/ES = NI Vibratory threshold (=)/ES = NI Pain pressure threshold (+)/ES PI = 0.54 (−0.08; 1.07) ES PI 3 months = 0.65 (0.01; 1.18); ES PI 6 months = 0.23 (−0.37; 0.79)
Bland, K. A et al., 2019 [18]	27 Participants IG1: 12, CG: 15 IG2: 51.0 ± 8.1 CG: 49.5 ± 11	IG: 1 week before Che. CG: 2 to 3 weeks post Che	Aerobic and LL strengthening exercises in both groups	Aerobic: 5 days/week, 50% to 75% HRR and Borg of 12 to 14 in a classification of 6 to 20, 15 to 30 min, progressive. Strengthening: 1 to 2 sets of 10 rep. at 50% to 65% 1RM, progressive/10 weeks	CIPN, Vibratory threshold, Tactile threshold. Questionnaire, Diapason, Esthesiometer	10 to 15 weeks	CIPN, sensory symptoms PI (=)/ES = −0.11 (−0.86; 0.66); (=) follow-up, ES = 0.34 (−0.45; 1.07)/CIPN, motor symptoms PI (=)/ES = 0.14 (−0.63; 0.89); (=) follow-up, ES < 0.01 (−0.76; 0.76)/CIPN, autonomic symptoms PI (=)/ES = 0.30 (−0.48; 1.04); (=) follow-up, ES = 0.54 (−0.27; 1.27)/ Vibratory threshold PI (=)/IG, 59% with vibratory symptoms; CG, 68% with vibratory symptoms/Tactile sensitivity (=)/NI

Table 2. *Cont.*

Study	Participants, Mean ± DE of Age	Start of Intervention	Comparison Groups and Training Type	Frequency and Duration of Training/Protocol	Outcomes	Follow-Up	Main Results/Magnitude of Effect
Mijwel et al., 2018 [19]	206 Participants IG1: 74 IG2: 72 CG:60 IG1: 52.7 ± 10.3 years IG2: 54.4 ± 10.3 years CG: 52.6 ± 10.2 years	3 days after second Che Session	IG1: conventional resistance exercises with high intensity intervals IG2: Continuous aerobic exercises of moderate intensity CG: Standard care	IG1: 2 days per week, 2 or 3 sets of 8 to 12 rep. at an intensity of 80% of 1RM. IG2: 20 min of continuous aerobic exercise, 2 days per week IG1 y IG2: 3 × 3 min HIIT with an of RPE 16–18 interspersed with 1 min recovery/16 weeks	Pain pressure threshold. Algometer	Baseline and 16 weeks	Trapezium PPT, taxanes (=)/ES IG1xCG = 0.27 (−0.20; 0.71); ES IG2xCG = −0.16 (−0.59; 0.29) Gluteal PPT, taxanes (=)/ES IG1xCG = 0.14 (−0.32; 0.58); ES IG2xCG = −0.12 (−0.56; 0.34) Trapezium PPT, without taxanes (+)/ES IG1xCG = 1.30 (0.61; 1.79)/ES IG2xCG = 0.66 (0.04; 1.19) Gluteal PPT, without taxanes (+)/ES IG1xCG = 1.03 (0.38; 1.52)/ES IG2xCG = 0.82 (0.18; 1.34)
Schönsteiner et al., 2017 [20]	131 Participants IG: 66 CG: 65 IG: 59 (range: 28–70) years CG: 62 (range: 24–71) years	NI	IG: Training with whole body vibration platform. CG: Posture and transport movements training. IG + CG: Massages and passive mobilization	15 sessions, 2 times/week, with warm-up of 3 min per session, 9–23 Hz with progressive increments of 12 min with progression of 9–13 Hz during 9 min. Massage and passive mobilization for 30 min./15 weeks	Peripheral neuropathy, Quantitative evaluation of paresthesia, Thermal and Tactile threshold. Questionnaire Diapason. Quantitative sensory tests	Baseline, 4 weeks, 8 weeks post last intervention	Peripheral neuropathy symptoms in LL PI (+)/reduction of numbness from 97 to 81% and discomfort from 98 to 71%; Thermal threshold to hot PI (=)/ES = −0.15 (−0.56; 0.28); Heat pain threshold PI (=)/ES = −0.01 (−0.43; 0.41); Thermal threshold to cold PI (=)/ES = 0.02 (−0.40; 0.44); Tactile sensitivity (=)/ES = 0.01 (−0.41; 0.43)
Kleckner IR et al., 2017 [7]	355 Participants IG: 170 CG: 185 IG: 55.6 ± 11.8 years CG: 55.9 ± 9.7 years	First day of Che	IG: Standard care and exercise (aerobic and strengthening of UL and LL) CG: Standard care (completed all assessments and intervention at the end of the study)	60 min/week Aerobic: 60–85% HRR, progressing 5–20% each week. Strengthening: Low to moderate intensity, dependent on elastic bands, RPE valued at 3 to 5./6 weeks	Peripheral neuropathy, numbness and tingling, hot/cold. Scales	Baseline and post 6 weeks	Peripheral neuropathy, numbness and tingling (+)/ ES PI = −0.29 (−0.47; −0.06); hot and cold in extremities (+)/ES PI = −0.28 (−0.47; −0.05)
Vollmers P et al., 2018 [21]	36 participants IG: 17 CG: 19 IG:48.56 ± 11.94 years CG: 52.39 ± 10.14 years	At the start of Che	IG: Regular physical training and motor sensitive exercises. CG: Brochure with information and suggestion of PA	Intensity depends on the physical state of the participant/56 weeks	Neuropathic symptoms. Questionnaire	Baseline and PAter 6 weeks post Che	Neuropathic symptoms. (=)/NI

Table 2. *Cont.*

Study	Participants, Mean ± DE of Age	Start of Intervention	Comparison Groups and Training Type	Frequency and Duration of Training/Protocol	Outcomes	Follow-Up	Main Results/Magnitude of Effect
Schwenk et al., 2016 [22]	19 Participants IG: 9 CG: 10 IG: 68.73 ± 8.72 years CG: 71.82 ± 8.85 years	NF	IG: Equilibrium and balance exercises CG: Encouraged to remain active	2 45 min. sessions/week for 4 weeks./4 weeks	Pain, Vibratory threshold: Numbness in feet. Scales	Ev. Baseline and after 4 weeks	Pain (=)/ES PI = 0.31 (−0.55; 1.13); Vibratory threshold (=)/ES PI = −0.15 (−0.98; 0.69); Numbness in feet (=)/ES PI = 0.31 (−0.55; 1.13)
Visovsky et al., 2014 [23]	19 Participants IG: NE CG: NE 48.8 (range 24–65) years	Before starting Che	IG: Aerobic and resistance exercises for LL and UL. CG: ACS standardized brochures	5–7 days for 20 min in intervals with a light to moderate intensity Strengthening: 3 times per week, 1–3 sets of 8–12 progressive strength exercises./12 weeks	Peripheral neuropathy. Questionnaire	Baseline, 4, 8, 12 and 24 weeks	Peripheral neuropathy (=)/ES PI 4 weeks = 0.96 (−0.06; 1.83); ES PI 8 weeks = 0.14 (−0.77; 1.03); ES PI 12 weeks = 0.34 (−0.60; 1.22); ES PI 24 weeks = 0.73 (−0.25; 1.60)
Stuecher, K. et al., 2018 [24]	28 Participants IG: 13 CG: 15 IG: 66.8 ± 7.8 years CG: 65.9 ± 7.9 years	During Che	IG: Aerobic training. CG: Standard care based on hospital oncologist guidelines	IG: moderate intensity, RPE + Borg, classification of 11–13 on the 6–20 scale, progressive until reaching 150 min per week./12 weeks	Vibratory threshold. Diapason	From 4 to 6 weeks and after week 12	Peripheral neuropathy (=)/NI
Streckmann F et al., 2014 [25]	61 Participants IG: 30 CG: 31 IG: 44 (range: 20–67) years CG: 48 (range: 19–73) years	In the first round of chemotherapy	IG: Standard care and training (aerobic, motor sensory and strengthening) CG: Standard routine care	Frequency: 2 times per week Aerobic: Start: (60%−70% of HRM) Final: 10 to 30 min. (70%–80% of HRM) Motor sensory: postural stabilization, progressive, in 3 sets/20 s. between each set and 1 min between exercise. Strengthening: 4 exercises during 1 min with maximum force./36 weeks	Vibratory threshold. Diapason	Baseline, 12, 24 and 36 week follow-ups	Vibratory threshold PI 36 weeks (+)/IG reduced 87.5% of the symptoms compared to CG (0%)
Dhawan S et al., 2020 [26]	45 participants GE: 19 CG: 22 GE: 50.5 ± 7.9 years CG: 52.5 ± 6.6 years	NF	GE: Muscle strengthening and balance exercises. CG: Standard routine care	30 min. a day/convenience./ 10 weeks	Neuropathic pain. Peripheral neuropathy symptoms experience. Questionnaire	Baseline, 10 week follow-up	Neuropathic pain (+)/ES PI = −0.28 (−0.85; 0.33); Peripheral neuropathy symptoms experience (+)/ES PI = −0.37 (−0.93; 0.25)

Table 2. *Cont.*

Study	Participants, Mean ± DE of Age	Start of Intervention	Comparison Groups and Training Type	Frequency and Duration of Training/Protocol	Outcomes	Follow-Up	Main Results/Magnitude of Effect
Saraboon C et al., 2021 [28]	30 participants GE: 45.07 ± 3.88 years GC: 45.53 ± 4.64 years	Before starting Che	GE: Balance, aerobic and stretching exercises, plus 10 min rest between each exercise. GC: conventional therapy plus balance exercise program if desired	Frequency: 2 times per week for 6 weeks balance 10 rep at 40 min, aerobic 5 min of cycling, 5 min of stretching once a day./6 weeks	Symptoms of peripheral neuropathy (Michigan Diabetic Neuropathy Score: MDNS) Quality of life (FACT scale -Taxane)	Baseline, 4 and 6 week follow-up	Symptoms of peripheral neuropathy (+)/0.30 (−0.44; 0.99) Quality of life (=)/0.19 (−0.54; 0.89)

±: Standard deviation; PI: Post intervention; Che: Chemotherapy; CIPN: Chemotherapy-induced peripheral neuropathy; IG: Intervention group; CG: Control group; NF: Not found; Post.: Posterior; HRM: Maximum heart rate; min: Minutes; s: Seconds; rep.: Repetitions; ROM: Range of motion; LL: Lower limbs; UL: Upper limbs; RM: Maximum repetition; RPE: Scale of perceived exertion; ACS: American cancer society; Ev.: Evaluation; PPT: Pressure pain threshold; HIIT: *High Intensity Interval Training*; PA: Physical activity; (+): Positive effect of the treatment; (=): Treatment with no effect; ES: Effect size.

3.3. Synthesis of Evidence

The evidence regarding therapeutic exercises to improve symptoms of peripheral neuropathy, pressure pain threshold, thermal threshold, and tactile and vibratory sensitivity was synthesized according to GRADE with follow-up times of 8 weeks (Table 3) and between 4 weeks and 24 weeks (Table 4). For the synthesis of evidence, two studies were excluded [16,23] because they did not present the necessary data to form part of this analysis, such as control group, intervention, follow-up and the duration of the protocol.

3.4. Peripheral Neuropathy Perception

3.4.1. Follow-Up 4 to 24 Weeks

Eight studies [7,17,18,20–22,26–28] evaluated the peripheral neuropathy perception using questionnaires and scales; with a total of 747 participants in these trials, 52.7% were part of the control group, while 47.2% belonged to the exercise group. According to the factors that can lower the level of quality of the evidence, a score of not serious was presented for risk bias, indirect evidence, imprecision and publication bias, while the inconsistency was categorized as serious since four of the studies were classified as serious and one as very serious, while three of them were not serious. Finally, the therapeutic exercises of strengthening, aerobics, equilibrium and balance presented moderate evidence to improve the symptoms of peripheral neuropathy during chemotherapy for cancer treatment.

3.4.2. Follow-Up at 8 Weeks

Seven studies [7,18,21,22,26,27] evaluated the peripheral neuropathy perception through scales and questionnaires, which included a total of 538 participants of which 53.3% were from the control group and 46.6% from the exercise group. According to factors that may lower the level of quality of the evidence, risk of bias, imprecision and publication bias were categorized as non-serious.

The inconsistency was serious since three studies were classified as serious, one study was classified as very serious and two studies as not serious. Eight weeks of therapeutic exercises to strengthen the upper and lower limbs, equilibrium, aerobics and balance, presented moderate evidence to improve the symptoms of peripheral neuropathy during chemotherapy for cancer treatment.

3.5. Pressure Pain Threshold

Two studies [17,19] with a follow-up range of 16 to 18 weeks in which pressure pain threshold was evaluated with an algometer had a total of 254 participants, where 33.8% belonged to the control group and 66.1% to the group with exercises. None of the factors that may lower the level of quality of the evidence were considered serious or very serious. A 16–18-week follow-up with therapeutic nerve gliding, stretching, aerobic and interval resistance exercises presented high evidence for increasing the pressure pain threshold in the trapezium, quadriceps and gluteal areas.

3.6. Thermal Threshold

Two studies [7,20] with a follow-up that ranged from 6 to 19 weeks and where thermal threshold was evaluated through questionnaires and scales included 486 participants, of which 51.4% were from the control group and 48.5% from the exercise groups. According to the factors that can lower the level of quality of the evidence, the risk of bias, imprecision, inconsistency and publication bias were categorized as non-serious; however, the indirect evidence was stated as very serious, since both included studies using tools that are not objective for measurement, such as quantitative sensory testing and a numerical scale of 0 to 10.

Along with the above, a follow-up of 6–19 weeks with therapeutic exercises on a vibration platform for the whole body, aerobics and strengthening exercises in the upper and lower limbs presented low evidence to improve the thermal threshold in the lower limb area.

Table 3. Summary of the evidence for the perception of peripheral neuropathy with an 8-week follow-up according to GRADE.

Certainty Assessment							Summary of the Results			
							Study Event Rates (%)		Anticipated Absolute Effects	
Participants (Studies) Follow-Up	Risk of Bias	Inconsistency	Indirect Evidence	Imprecision	Risk of Publication	Overall Certainty of Evidence	Control Group	Exercise Group	Control Group Risk	The Risk Difference with Exercises
Peripheral Neuropathy Symptoms (Evaluated with: Questionnaire and Scale)										
538 (6 Random trials)	Not serious	Serious [a]	Not serious	Not serious	Neither	⊕⊕⊕○ **MODERATE**	287/538 (53.34%)	251/538 (46.65%)	The mean symptoms of peripheral neuropathy Follow-up 2 months was 0	Mean 0.33 (Range: 0.7 to 0.7)

GRADE: Grading of Recommendations Assessment, Development and Evaluation. Event rates: number of patients in the intervention or comparison group/total study participants (% of patients in each intervention or comparison group used according to the GRADE recommendation). The term in bold refers to the level of evidence according to GRADE. [a]: <75% of the studies report that the intervention presented positive or negative results.

Table 4. Summary of the evidence for the variables of perception of peripheral neuropathy, pressure pain threshold, vibratory pain, tactile and thermal sensitivity in a follow-up of 4 to 24 weeks according to GRADE.

Certainty Assessment							Summary of the Results			
							Study Event Rates (%)		Anticipated Absolute Effects	
Participants (Studies) Follow-Up	Risk of Bias	Inconsistency	Indirect Evidence	Imprecision	Risk of Publication	Overall Certainty of Evidence	Control Group	Exercise Group	Control Group Risk	The Risk Difference with Exercises
Peripheral Neuropathy Symptoms (Assessed with: Questionnaires and Scales)										
747 (9 Random trials)	Not serious	Serious [a]	Not serious	Not serious	Neither	⊕⊕⊕○ **MODERATE**	393/747 (52.71%)	354/747 (47.28%)	The mean peripheral neuropathy symptoms was **0**	Mean 0.33 (Range: 0.93 to 1.13)
Pressure Pain Threshold (Evaluated with: Algometer)										
254 (2 Random trials)	Not serious	Not serious	Not serious	Not serious	Neither	⊕⊕⊕⊕ **HIGH**	86/254 (33.85%)	168/254 (66.14%)	The mean pressure pain threshold was **0**	Mean 0.37 (Range: 0.59 to 1.34)

Table 4. *Cont.*

Certainty Assessment							Summary of the Results			
							Study Event Rates (%)		Anticipated Absolute Effects	
Participants (Studies) Follow-Up	**Risk of Bias**	**Inconsistency**	**Indirect Evidence**	**Imprecision**	**Risk of Publication**	**Overall Certainty of Evidence**	**Control Group**	**Exercise Group**	**Control Group Risk**	**The Risk Difference with Exercises**
Vibratory Threshold (Evaluated with: Sensitive Quantitative Test and Tuning Fork)										
183 (5 Random trials)	Not serious	Serious [b]	Not serious	Serious [c]	Neither	⊕⊕○○ **LOW**	97/183 (53%)	86/183 (46.99%)	The mean vibratory threshold was **0**	Mean 0.15 (0.98 to 0.69)
Tactile Sensitivity (Evaluated with: Questionnaire and Esthesiometer)										
158 (2 Random trials)	Not serious	Serious [d]	Not serious	Serious [e]	Neither	⊕⊕○○ **LOW**	80/158 (50.63%)	78/158 (49.36%)	The mean tactile sensitivity was **0**	Mean 0.01 (Range: 0.41 to 0.43)
Thermal Sensitivity (Evaluated with: Questionnaire and Scale)										
486 (2 Random trials)	Not serious	Not serious	Very serious [f]	Not serious	Neither	⊕⊕○○ **LOW**	250/486 (51.44%)	236/486 (48.55%)	The mean thermal threshold was **0**	Mean 0.17 (Range: 0.56 to 0.44)

GRADE: *Grading of Recommendations Assessment, Development and Evaluation*. Event rates: number of patients in the intervention or comparison group/total study participants (% of patients in each intervention or comparison group used according to the GRADE recommendation). The term in bold refers to the level of evidence according to GRADE. [a,b,d]: <75% of the studies report that the intervention presented positive or negative results. [f]: Heterogeneity in relation to the intervention protocols used. [c,e]: Results based on a total sample of <200 participants.

3.7. Tactile Sensitivity

Two studies [18,20] with a follow-up range of 12 to 19 weeks evaluated the effects of the therapeutic exercises on tactile sensitivity with questionnaires and Esthesiometer; a total of 158 participants were included, of which 50.6% were from the control and 49.3% were from the exercise group. Regarding the factors that can reduce the level of quality of the evidence, the risk of bias, indirect evidence and publication bias were not serious, while the inconsistency was categorized as serious because two studies were categorized as serious, as well as imprecise because the included studies considered less than 200 participants. Thus, a 12–19-week follow-up with therapeutic exercises to strengthen the lower limbs, aerobics and with a whole-body vibration platform presented low evidence to improve tactile sensitivity in the lower limb area.

3.8. Vibratory Sensitivity

Five studies [17,18,22,24,25] with a follow-up range of 4 to 36 weeks evaluated the effectiveness of therapeutic exercises on the vibratory threshold using a quantitative sensitive test and diapason; a total of 183 participants were included, of which 53% were from the control group and 46.9% from the exercise group. According to the factors that can lower the level of quality of the evidence, the risk of bias, indirect evidence and publication bias were not serious, while inconsistency was classified as serious. Only one was not serious, as well as imprecise because the included studies considered less than 200 participants. A follow-up of 4–36 weeks of therapeutic exercises to strengthen the lower limbs, aerobics, balance and motor sensory showed low evidence to increase the vibratory threshold in the lower limb area, such as phalangeal metatarsus, medial malleolus and phalanges, as well as upper limbs such as hands and wrists.

3.9. Meta-Analysis

Ten of the fourteen selected studies presented the mean and standard deviation to calculate the effect size (TE) of the intervention [7,16–19,22,23,26–28]. Estimates of the grouped standardized mean difference (DME) showed significant reduction in the symptoms of peripheral neuropathy after a therapeutic exercise program in people with cancer compared to the control group (DME = −0.31; IC 95% = −0.61 to −0.02; $p = 0.04$) (Figure 2), with significant heterogeneity ($I^2 = 86\%$; $p \leq 0.00001$).

Study or Subgroup	Therapeutic Exercise Mean	SD	Total	Non-intervention Mean	SD	Total	Weight	Mean Difference IV, Fixed, 95% CI
Bahar-ozdemir et al., 2020	34.3	36.1	24	18.8	28.4	36	0.0%	15.50 [-1.67, 32.67]
Bland et al., 2019	20.9	5	15	11.5	5.6	16	0.6%	9.40 [5.67, 13.13]
Dhawan et al., 2020	10.7	16.7	22	15.8	20	23	0.1%	-5.10 [-15.85, 5.65]
Hammond et al., 2020	906	437	22	818	343	26	0.0%	88.00 [-137.23, 313.23]
Henkeet al., 2013	20.8	26.8	18	46.2	37.4	11	0.0%	-25.40 [-50.73, -0.07]
Kleckner et al., 2017	1.1	1.4	170	1.63	2	185	69.9%	-0.53 [-0.89, -0.17]
Mijwel et al., 2018	457.9	115.6	29	314.8	102.7	24	0.0%	143.10 [84.29, 201.91]
Saraboon and Siriphorn, 2021	155.2	7.39	15	148.8	8.98	15	0.3%	6.40 [0.51, 12.29]
Schwenk et al., 2015	5.9	3.25	11	4.91	3.08	11	1.3%	0.99 [-1.66, 3.64]
Visovsky et al., 2014	0.65	0.32	10	0.77	0.81	9	27.9%	-0.12 [-0.69, 0.45]
Total (95% CI)			**336**			**356**	**100.0%**	**-0.31 [-0.61, -0.02]**

Heterogeneity: $Chi^2 = 65.04$, df = 9 ($P < 0.00001$); $I^2 = 86\%$
Test for overall effect: Z = 2.06 (P = 0.04)

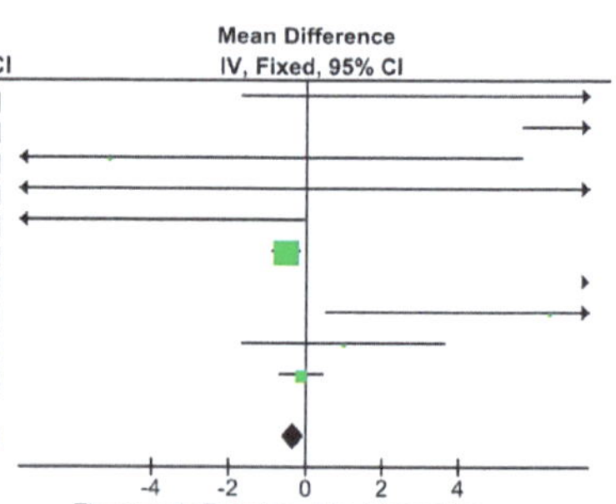

Figure 2. Forest plot of therapeutic exercise program versus control for peripheral neuropathy symptoms [7,16–19,22,23,26–28].

The sensitivity analysis revealed that heterogeneity was influenced by the studies by Bland et al. 2019 [18] and Mijwel et al. 2019 [19]. There were no changes in the results in favor of therapeutic exercise compared to the control groups and the DME was reduced to −0.40 with changes in heterogeneity from moderate to significant ($I^2 = 45\%$; $p = 0.09$).

4. Discussion

With respect to the quantitative analysis of this systematic review, the findings of the meta-analysis show that a therapeutic exercise program of 4 to 56 weeks generates significant changes, reducing the symptoms of peripheral neuropathy in subjects with cancer compared to the control group with short-term and long-term follow-up. However, given the significant heterogeneity presented, these results should be viewed with caution.

Of the main studies selected, two of them reported improvement of pressure pain threshold after a therapeutic exercise program [17,19]. The study by Mijwel et al., 2018 [13] reported that resistance exercise associated with HIIT significantly improves muscle strength and reduces pain sensitivity; these studies had a moderate effect size with a range of 0.44 to 0.57 and with a high level of evidence.

Regarding the evaluation of neuropathy symptoms through questionnaires, six studies [7,18,21,22,26–28] presented moderate evidence with an effect size of 0.27 to 0.47, categorizing them as small to moderate. Three of these studies [7,26,28] reported improvement of peripheral neuropathy symptoms, while two other studies [21,22] kept their symptoms. There was one study [27] that reported an improvement in neuropathic pain symptoms while maintaining generalized pain symptoms after a therapeutic exercise program. The studies that evaluated neuropathic symptoms through thermal threshold [7,20], tactile sensitivity [18,20] and vibratory sensitivity [17,18,22,24,25] presented a low level of evidence.

In regard to the studies that evaluated tactile sensitivity [18,20] and thermal threshold [7,20], no significant differences were obtained. The effect size of the studies [7,20] that evaluated thermal was 0.28 and 0.06, considered small. Likewise, the study [20] that evaluated tactile sensitivity had a small effect size of 0.01. The study that evaluated the vibratory threshold [22] presented a small effect size with a value of 0.15. Those results could be explained by the fact that symptoms of peripheral neuropathy induced by chemotherapy should be assessed by both objective methods and from a patient perspective [29]. Moreover, the heterogeneity of evaluation tools used in those studies negatively impacts these results.

The findings reported in this review are similar to the study by Dobson et al., 2014 [30] that evaluated the effects of balance and aerobic exercise training on neuropathy symptoms, sensory dysfunctions and increased peripheral nerve conduction velocity. However, the review by Dobson et al., 2014 [30] did not determine the quality of evidence and included studies that focus on diabetic neuropathy and its neuro-inflammatory etiology and did not incorporate studies where the neuropathy is the result of exposure to chemotherapy.

The present systematic review determines that strengthening, aerobic and motor sensory exercises for a total average time of 14 weeks (considering a standard deviation of 9 weeks) 2 to 5 days per week and with low to moderate intensities present a moderate level of evidence for the improvement of neuropathy symptoms. These facts coincide with the results of the study by Kneis et al., 2019 [31] that reported that resistance and equilibrium exercises reduced sensitivity symptoms, with an improvement in the physical function of the cancer survivors.

According to the above and considering that there is still controversy regarding the effectiveness of drugs in the management of peripheral neuropathy [32], multimodal exercise emerges as an effective and safe therapeutic tool to reduce peripheral symptoms induced by chemotherapy.

Some limitations of the present study should be considered: (1) three studies showed poor methodological quality [10,15,18]; (2) different therapeutic exercise protocols were used; (3) significant heterogeneity (I^2 = 86%) which is due to the different types of exercises between studies and different evaluation tools used, providing variability; (4) the selected studies used distant tools to evaluate peripheral neuropathy; (5) two studies [7,20] used methods to evaluate the peripheral neuropathy that were inadequate, since they lacked reliability and objectivity; (6) non-specificity of therapeutic exercise in terms of its dosage; (7) the beginning of the therapeutic exercise program was nonspecific since some studies began together with the chemotherapy [17,27], on the first day of chemotherapy [7,16], before starting it [18,23], during this therapy [24,25] or on subsequent days to the start of chemotherapy [18,19]. In addition, three studies [20,22,26] did not specify the beginning of the intervention protocol; (8) Three studies [20,22,24] did not identify any supervisor, which may limit the correct execution of the exercises; (9) different follow-up times between studies can generate a bias in the results.

5. Conclusions

In general, this systematic review and meta-analysis suggest that therapeutic exercise generates a significant reduction in peripheral neuropathy symptoms in patients in short and long-term follow-up with a moderate level of evidence quality. However, these results must be viewed with caution due to the significant heterogeneity of the studies analyzed. The available studies are diverse in terms of methodology, exercise dosage, and tools to assess peripheral neuropathy; therefore, further research is warranted. Future clinical trials must present adequate methodological quality and use valid and reliable evaluation methods.

Author Contributions: S.D.: Formal analysis; validation; visualization; roles/writing—original draft; writing—review and editing. V.T.: Formal analysis; methodology; data curation; validation; visualization; roles/writing—original draft. C.S.: Formal analysis; methodology; data curation; validation; visualization; roles/writing—original draft. D.O.: Formal analysis; methodology; data curation; validation; visualization; roles/writing—original draft. I.L.R.: Conceptualization; formal analysis; methodology; project administration; resources; supervision; validation; visualization; roles/writing—original draft; writing—review and editing. L.B.-C.: Data curation; formal analysis; methodology; resources; roles/writing—original draft. L.A.L.: Formal analysis; validation; visualization; roles/writing—original draft; writing—review and editing. A.S.A.: Visualization; roles/writing—original draft; writing—review and editing. All authors have read and agreed to the published version of the manuscript.

Funding: King Khalid University; Project number: RGP 2/134/43.

Informed Consent Statement: Not applicable.

Data Availability Statement: All data are from the primary included studies in this systematic review and are referenced in the article.

Conflicts of Interest: The authors declare no conflict of interest.

References

1. Bray, F.; Ferlay, J.; Soerjomataram, I.; Siegel, R.L.; Torre, L.A.; Jemal, A. Global cancer statistics 2018: GLOBOCAN estimates of incidence and mortality worldwide for 36 cancers in 185 countries. *CA A Cancer J. Clin.* **2018**, *68*, 394–424. [CrossRef]
2. Cáncer SACE. *Biopsia Del Seno*; American Cancer Society: Atlanta, GA, USA, 2019.
3. Ramírez, K.; Acevedo, F.; Herrera, M.E.; Ibáñez, C.; Sánchez, C. Actividad física y cáncer de mama: Un tratamiento dirigido. *Rev. Médica Chile* **2017**, *145*, 75–84. [CrossRef] [PubMed]
4. Furmaniak, A.C.; Menig, M.; Markes, M.H. Exercise for women receiving adjuvant therapy for breast cancer. *Cochrane Database Syst. Rev.* **2016**, *9*, CD005001. [CrossRef] [PubMed]
5. Colvin, L.A. Chemotherapy-induced peripheral neuropathy: Where are we now? *Pain* **2019**, *160* (Suppl. S1), S1–S10. [CrossRef] [PubMed]
6. McCrary, J.M.; Goldstein, D.; Boyle, F.; Cox, K.; Grimison, P.; Kiernan, M.C.; Krishnan, A.V.; Lewis, C.R.; Webber, K.; Baron-Hay, S.; et al. Optimal clinical assessment strategies for chemotherapy-induced peripheral neuropathy (CIPN): A systematic review and Delphi survey. *Support. Care Cancer* **2017**, *25*, 3485–3493. [CrossRef] [PubMed]
7. Kleckner, I.R.; Kamen, C.; Gewandter, J.S.; Mohile, N.A.; Heckler, C.E.; Culakova, E.; Fung, C.; Janelsins, M.C.; Asare, M.; Lin, P.-J.; et al. Effects of exercise during chemotherapy on chemotherapy-induced peripheral neuropathy: A multicenter, randomized controlled trial. *Support Care Cancer* **2018**, *26*, 1019–1028. [CrossRef]
8. Streckmann, F.; Zopf, E.M.; Lehmann, H.C.; May, K.; Rizza, J.; Zimmer, P.; Gollhofer, A.; Bloch, W.; Baumann, F.T. Exercise Intervention Studies in Patients with Peripheral Neuropathy: A Systematic Review. *Sport. Med.* **2014**, *44*, 1289–1304. [CrossRef]
9. Knoerl, R.; Gilchrist, L.; Kanzawa-Lee, G.A.; Donohoe, C.; Bridges, C.; Lavoie Smith, E.M. Proactive Rehabilitation for Chemotherapy-Induced Peripheral Neuropathy. *Semin. Oncol. Nurs.* **2020**, *36*, 150983. [CrossRef]
10. Higgins, J.P.T.T.J.; Chandler, J.; Cumpston, M.; Li, T.; Page, M.J.; Welch, V.A. *Cochrane Handbook for Systematic Reviews of Interventions*, 2nd ed.; Cochrane: London, UK, 2019.
11. Verhagen, A.; De Vet, H.; Bie, R.; Kessels, A.G.; Boers, M.; Bouter, L.; Knipschild, P. The Delphi List: A Criteria List for Quality Assessment of Randomized Clinical Trials for Conducting Systematic Reviews Developed by Delphi Consensus. *J. Clin. Epidemiol.* **1999**, *51*, 1235–1241. [CrossRef]

12. Maher, C.G.; Sherrington, C.; Herbert, R.D.; Moseley, A.M.; Elkins, M. Reliability of the PEDro scale for rating quality of randomized controlled trials. *Phys. Ther.* **2003**, *83*, 713–721. [CrossRef] [PubMed]
13. Ribeiro, I.L.; Carreira, F.M.; Ferrari, A.V.; Alburquerque-Sendín, F.; Camargo, P.R.; Salvini, F.T. Effectiveness of early rehabilitation on range of motion, muscle strength and arm function after breast cancer surgery: A systematic review of randomized controlled trials. *Clin. Rehabil.* **2019**, *33*, 1876–1886. [CrossRef] [PubMed]
14. Cohen, J. *The concepts of power analysis. In Statistical Power Analysis for the Behavioral Sciences*; Lawrence Erlbaum Associates: New Brunswick, NJ, Canada, 1988.
15. Guyatt, G.; Oxman, A.D.; Akl, E.A.; Kunz, R.; Vist, G.; Brozek, J.; Norris, S.; Falck-Ytter, Y.; Glasziou, P.; DeBeer, H.; et al. GRADE guidelines: 1. Introduction-GRADE evidence profiles and summary of findings tables. *J. Clin. Epidemiol.* **2011**, *64*, 383–394. [CrossRef]
16. Henke, C.C.; Cabri, J.; Fricke, L.; Pankow, W.; Kandilakis, G.; Feyer, P.C.; de Wit, M. Strength and endurance training in the treatment of lung cancer patients in stages IIIA/IIIB/IV. *Support. Care Cancer* **2014**, *22*, 95–101. [CrossRef] [PubMed]
17. Andersen Hammond, E.; Pitz, M.; Steinfeld, K.; Lambert, P.; Shay, B. An Exploratory Randomized Trial of Physical Therapy for the Treatment of Chemotherapy-Induced Peripheral Neuropathy. *Neurorehabilit. Neural Repair* **2020**, *34*, 235–246. [CrossRef] [PubMed]
18. Bland, K.A.; Kirkham, A.A.; Bovard, J.; Shenkier, T.; Zucker, D.; McKenzie, D.C.; Davis, M.K.; Gelmon, K.A.; Campbell, K.L. Effect of Exercise on Taxane Chemotherapy-Induced Peripheral Neuropathy in Women With Breast Cancer: A Randomized Controlled Trial. *Clin. Breast Cancer* **2019**, *19*, 411–422. [CrossRef]
19. Mijwel, S.; Backman, M.; Bolam, K.A.; Olofsson, E.; Norrbom, J.; Bergh, J.; Sundberg, C.J.; Wengström, Y.; Rundqvist, H. Highly favorable physiological responses to concurrent resistance and high-intensity interval training during chemotherapy: The OptiTrain breast cancer trial. *Breast Cancer Res. Treat.* **2018**, *169*, 93–103. [CrossRef]
20. Schönsteiner, S.S.; Bauder Mißbach, H.; Benner, A.; Mack, S.; Hamel, T.; Orth, M.; Landwehrmeyer, B.; Süßmuth, S.D.; Geitner, C.; Mayer-Steinacker, R.; et al. A randomized exploratory phase 2 study in patients with chemotherapy-related peripheral neuropathy evaluating whole-body vibration training as adjunct to an integrated program including massage, passive mobilization and physical exercises. *Exp. Hematol. Oncol.* **2017**, *6*, 5. [CrossRef]
21. Vollmers, P.L.; Mundhenke, C.; Maass, N.; Bauerschlag, D.; Kratzenstein, S.; Röcken, C.; Schmidt, T. Evaluation of the effects of sensorimotor exercise on physical and psychological parameters in breast cancer patients undergoing neurotoxic chemotherapy. *J. Cancer Res. Clin. Oncol.* **2018**, *144*, 1785–1792. [CrossRef]
22. Schwenk, M.; Grewal, G.S.; Holloway, D.; Muchna, A.; Garland, L.; Najafi, B. Interactive Sensor-Based Balance Training in Older Cancer Patients with Chemotherapy-Induced Peripheral Neuropathy: A Randomized Controlled Trial. *Gerontology* **2016**, *62*, 553–563. [CrossRef]
23. Visovsky, C.; Bovaird, J.A.; Tofthagen, C.; Rice, J. Heading off Peripheral Neuropathy with Exercise: The Hope Study. *Nurs. Health* **2014**, *2*, 115–121. [CrossRef]
24. Stuecher, K.; Bolling, C.; Vogt, L.; Niederer, D.; Schmidt, K.; Dignaß, A.; Banzer, W. Exercise improves functional capacity and lean body mass in patients with gastrointestinal cancer during chemotherapy: A single-blind RCT. *Support. Care Cancer* **2019**, *27*, 2159–2169. [CrossRef]
25. Streckmann, F.; Kneis, S.; Leifert, J.A.; Baumann, F.T.; Kleber, M.; Ihorst, G.; Herich, L.; Grüssinger, V.; Gollhofer, A.; Bertz, H. Exercise program improves therapy-related side-effects and quality of life in lymphoma patients undergoing therapy. *Ann. Oncol.* **2014**, *25*, 493–499. [CrossRef] [PubMed]
26. Dhawan, S.; Andrews, R.; Kumar, L.; Wadhwa, S.; Shukla, G. A Randomized Controlled Trial to Assess the Effectiveness of Muscle Strengthening and Balancing Exercises on Chemotherapy-Induced Peripheral Neuropathic Pain and Quality of Life Among Cancer Patients. *Cancer Nurs.* **2020**, *43*, 269–280. [CrossRef] [PubMed]
27. Bahar-Ozdemir, Y.; Akyuz, G.; Kalkandelen, M.; Yumuk, P.F. The Effect of Therapeutic Exercises on Balance, Quality of Life, and Pain in Patients Who Were Receiving Neurotoxic Chemotherapy. *Am. J. Phys. Med. Rehabil.* **2020**, *99*, 291–299. [CrossRef]
28. Saraboon, C.; Siriphorn, A. Effects of foam pad balance exercises on cancer patients undergoing chemotherapy: A randomized control trial. *J. Bodyw. Mov. Ther.* **2021**, *28*, 164–171. [CrossRef]
29. Park, S.B.; Goldstein, D.; Krishnan, A.V.; Lin, C.S.; Friedlander, M.L.; Cassidy, J.; Koltzenburg, M.; Kiernan, M.C. Chemotherapy-induced peripheral neurotoxicity: A critical analysis. *CA Cancer J. Clin.* **2013**, *63*, 419–437. [CrossRef] [PubMed]
30. Dobson, J.L.; McMillan, J.; Li, L. Benefits of exercise intervention in reducing neuropathic pain. *Front. Cell Neurosci.* **2014**, *8*, 102. [CrossRef]
31. Kneis, S.; Wehrle, A.; Müller, J.; Maurer, C.; Ihorst, G.; Gollhofer, A.; Bertz, H. It's never too late-balance and endurance training improves functional performance, quality of life, and alleviates neuropathic symptoms in cancer survivors suffering from chemotherapy-induced peripheral neuropathy: Results of a randomized controlled trial. *BMC Cancer* **2019**, *19*, 414. [CrossRef]
32. Hu, L.-Y.; Mi, W.-L.; Wu, G.-C.; Wang, Y.-Q.; Mao-Ying, Q.-L. Prevention and Treatment for Chemotherapy-Induced Peripheral Neuropathy: Therapies Based on CIPN Mechanisms. *Curr. Neuropharmacol.* **2019**, *17*, 184–196. [CrossRef]

life

MDPI

Article

Effects of Obesity on Medial Tibiofemoral Cartilage Mechanics in Females—An Exploration Using Musculoskeletal Simulation and Probabilistic Cartilage Failure Modelling

Jonathan Sinclair [1,*], Holly Lynch [1], Nachiappan Chockalingam [2] and Paul John Taylor [3]

[1] School of Sport & Health Sciences, Faculty of Allied Health & Wellbeing, University of Central Lancashire, Preston PR1 2HE, UK
[2] School of Life Sciences and Education, Staffordshire University, Stoke on Trent ST4 2DE, UK
[3] School of Psychology & Computer Sciences, Faculty of Science & Technology, University of Central Lancashire, Preston PR1 2HE, UK
* Correspondence: jksinclair@uclan.ac.uk

Abstract: This study examined the effects of obesity on cartilage mechanics and longitudinal failure probability at the medial tibiofemoral compartment, using combined musculoskeletal simulation and probabilistic failure modelling approaches. The current investigation examined twenty obese females (BMI > 30.0 kg/m^2) and 20 healthy weight (BMI < 25.0 kg/m^2) females. Walking kinematics were obtained via an 8-camera optoelectric system, and a force plate was used to collect ground reaction forces. Musculoskeletal simulation and probabilistic failure modelling were utilized to explore medial tibiofemoral forces and cartilage probability. Comparisons between groups were undertaken using linear mixed-effects models. Net peak cartilage forces, stress and strain were significantly larger in the obese group (force = 2013.92 N, stress = 3.03 MPa & strain = 0.25), compared to health weight (force = 1493.21 N, stress 2.26 MPa & strain = 0.19). In addition, medial tibiofemoral cartilage failure probability was also significantly larger in the obese group (42.98%) compared to healthy weight (11.63%). The findings from the current investigation show that obesity has a profoundly negative influence on longitudinal medial knee cartilage health and strongly advocates for the implementation of effective weight management programs into long-term musculoskeletal management strategies.

Keywords: biomechanics; obesity; osteoarthritis; cartilage; musculoskeletal simulation; probabilistic modelling

Citation: Sinclair, J.; Lynch, H.; Chockalingam, N.; Taylor, P.J. Effects of Obesity on Medial Tibiofemoral Cartilage Mechanics in Females—An Exploration Using Musculoskeletal Simulation and Probabilistic Cartilage Failure Modelling. *Life* **2023**, *13*, 270. https://doi.org/10.3390/life13020270

Academic Editor: Christine Chappard

Received: 8 November 2022
Revised: 1 December 2022
Accepted: 27 December 2022
Published: 18 January 2023

1. Introduction

Obesity is present in over a third of the adult population in the United States [1] and continues to escalate at an alarming rate [2]. Increased adiposity is linked to the aetiology of heart disease, diabetes, stroke and many forms of cancer [3] and also regarded as the fifth leading risk factor for mortality, causing over 2.8 million deaths annually [4]. In addition, obesity also increases the risk for comorbidities, including chronic musculoskeletal pathologies [5]. Therefore, the rapidly accelerating rates of global obesity raise concerns regarding associated increases in the prevalence of musculoskeletal disorders.

Osteoarthritis (OA) is the most frequently experienced chronic musculoskeletal pathology and represents the foremost cause of enduring disability among older adults [6]. Tibiofemoral OA the most frequently experienced form of OA, is the principal cause of international musculoskeletal disability [7] and has a negative fiscal influence on global healthcare systems [8]. Knee OA is representative of a degenerative articular cartilage disease, illustrated by deterioration of the cartilage itself within the knee joint [9]. Affected individuals importantly experience enduring pain and dysfunction [10], and knee joint OA has been shown have an incidence rate of almost 10% in individuals aged 60 and above [11]. Knee OA cases are most frequent in females and predominantly detected at the medial compartment of the tibiofemoral joint, as loads borne by this joint predominantly pass through the medial aspect of the knee [12].

Longitudinal analyses have shown that obesity may be a significant risk factor for the instigation and advancement of symptomatic and radiographic tibiofemoral OA, but have not conclusively exposed the mechanisms responsible for this link [13]. Multiple hypotheses have been advocated that expound the association between obesity and chronic musculoskeletal disorders [14]. Mechanically it is advocated that excessive axial loading mediated through increased body mass in obese individuals, promotes degeneration of lower extremity joint structures [15]. However, whilst mechanical inferences predominate, metabolic factors associated with obesity including hormonal and biochemical alterations have also been proposed as being responsible for the incidence of musculoskeletal disorders in obese individuals [16]. Furthermore, accumulating evidence also shows that obesity mediates systemic low-grade inflammation, that contributes to metabolic dysfunction [17]. Adipose tissue itself is functional as an active endocrine organ by releasing bioactive substances known adipokines, which are able to mediate either pro or anti-inflammatory activities [18]. There has been considerable research interest concerning the potential role of adipokines in the pathogenesis of OA [19]. Previous analyses have confirmed that levels of leptin and resistin were greater in obese individuals with knee OA in relation to healthy controls and that levels of these adipokines were also associated with radiographic OA stage [20], indicating that they may play a significant role in the multifactorial nature of knee OA pathophysiology [21].

Currently, the implications of obesity during everyday tasks such as walking, remain poorly understood. Obese individuals exhibit a reduced self-selected walking velocity [22,23]; alongside shorter absolute stride and step lengths [22,24]. Kinematically, obese individuals have been shown to adopt a significantly increased hip adduction angle [24], hip extension angle [25] and peak hip extension moment [26]. At the knee joint, obese individuals exhibit reduced knee flexion at initial contact [26], peak flexion [25], and an enhanced knee extension moment [26,27]. In the coronal plane, obese individuals are associated with a greater knee adduction moment (KAM) during weight acceptance [28], peak KAM [26] and KAM impulse [27]. At the ankle joint, obese individuals are associated with increased dorsiflexion throughout the stance phase [24], greater inversion at footstrike [29], an increased peak eversion angle [23] and increased toe-out throughout the stance phase [22,29,30]. In addition, obese individuals also exhibited a statistically greater ankle plantarflexion moment [25,26].

However, joint moments are not characteristic of localized joint loading [31], and it is the tibiofemoral joint contact forces that are linked to the initiation and progression of cartilage breakdown. Considerable advances in musculoskeletal simulation modelling have been made [32], allowing skeletal muscle driven indices of lower extremity joint reaction forces to be calculated [12]. Lerner et al. [33] examined the effects of paediatric obesity on tibiofemoral joint compressive loading and showed that obese children had significantly greater compressive forces and that body mass index (BMI) predicted the percentage of total tibiofemoral load borne by the medial compartment. Harding et al. [34] examined the effects of overweight (BMI > 25.0) and obese (BMI > 30.0) individuals on muscle and medial tibiofemoral compartment forces compared to healthy weight (BMI < 25.0) participants. Their findings showed that in relation to healthy weight participants, obese individuals exhibited greater quadriceps and medial tibiofemoral compartment forces.

However, although quantification of tibiofemoral joint kinetics is now feasible, there remain difficulties in exploring the influence of distinct mechanical and physiological conditions on the instigation, progression and temporal profile of knee OA. Therefore, probabilistic modelling of cartilage of stress and strain induced accumulative damage may be valuable for determining the effects of obesity on probability of osteoarthritic degeneration over a lifetime of cyclic loading [35]. However, probabilistic cartilage modelling has not been adopted to explore differences in medial tibiofemoral cartilage failure probability between obese and healthy weight individuals.

The aim of the current investigation was to explore the effects of obesity on medial tibiofemoral cartilage mechanics and lifetime failure probability in relation to healthy weight individuals using a combined musculoskeletal simulation and computational modelling approach. The findings from this investigation will yield new information firstly on the effects of obesity on medial tibiofemoral cartilage mechanics during walking, but also on lifetime failure probability in relation to healthy individuals. This study tests the hypothesis that medial-tibiofemoral cartilage loading mechanics and lifetime failure probability will be significantly greater in the obese group compared to healthy individuals.

2. Materials and Methods

2.1. Participants

Twenty healthy weight and twenty obese female participants volunteered to take part in this study. Participants not eligible for this study if they had a current lower extremity pathology or had previously undergone lower extremity surgery. Body mass index (BMI) was utilized to define obesity (BMI > 30.00 kg/m^2) and healthy weight groups (BMI < 25.00 kg/m^2) due to its adoption in clinical practice, as well as its correlation with more accurate measures of adiposity [36]. Using data from previous work in obese and healthy weight adults [34] and mean $\pm$ SD values for the peak net medial tibiofemoral force of 1227.30 $\pm$ 521.30 N in healthy weight and 1812.90 $\pm$ 703.80 N in obese individuals, it was determined using GPower software (GPower 3.1) that for between group comparisons, to achieve α = 5% and β = 80%, that 40 total participants would be required. All participants provided consent in written form in accordance with the ideologies outlined in the Declaration of Helsinki. The methodological approach adopted in the current study was approved by an institutional ethics panel (STEMH 1013).

Body segments were modelled in 6 degrees of freedom using the calibrated anatomical system technique [37], using a marker/ model configuration utilized previously to quantify the biomechanics of walking [12]. (Figure 1). Intra rater reliability for the individual responsible for positioning of the anatomical markers has been shown to be high (ICC $\geq$ 0.931) [38]. The centres of the ankle and knee joints were the midpoints between the malleoli and the femoral epicondyle markers [39,40] and the hip joint centre was established via a regression approach using the locations of the anterior superior iliac spine markers [41].

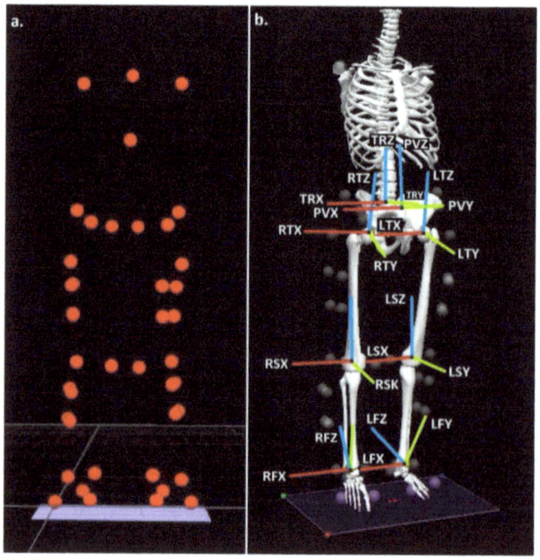

Figure 1. (**a**) Anatomical landmark locations and (**b**) modelled segments, with segment co-ordinate axes (R = right & L = left), (TR = trunk, P = pelvis, T = thigh, S = shank & F = foot), (X = sagittal, Y = coronal & Z = transverse planes).

2.2. Procedure

Retroreflective marker data were obtained using an 8-camera optoelectric motion capture system (Qualisys Medical, Gothenburg, Sweden) operating at 250 Hz. Dynamic calibration of the camera system was undertaken prior to each testing session. A piezoelectric force plate (Kistler Instruments, Winterthur, Switzerland) operating at 1000 Hz was utilized to capture ground reaction forces (GRF). Kinematic and GRF data were collected in a synchronous manner.

The calibrated anatomical system technique (CAST) [37], was adopted to reconstruct body segments in 6 degrees of freedom. A marker/ modelling configuration that has been previously utilized to quantify walking biomechanics was adopted [12] (Figure 1). Intra rater reliability for the individual in control of placing the anatomical markers has been shown through previous publication to be very high (ICC $\geq$ 0.931) [38]. The ankle and knee joint centres were located at the centre point of the malleoli and the femoral epicondyle markers [39,40] and centre of the hip joint was ascertained using the locations of the anterior superior iliac spine markers via a regression based approach [41].

2.3. Processing

Digitization of the dynamic walking trials was undertaken using Qualisys Track Manager (QTM) (Qualisys Medical AB, Gothenburg, Sweden) software. Digitized QTM files were then exported in.C3D file format into Visual 3D (C-Motion, Germantown, MD, USA). Data were time normalized within Visual 3D to identify the stance phase, which was defined as the period over which the force plate measured > 20 N of vertical GRF [42]. Three-dimensional marker trajectories and GRF's were smoothed with cut-off frequencies of 6 and 50 Hz, respectively, via a 4th-order low-pass zero-lag Butterworth filter. Cut-off frequencies were optimized using residual analysis for both kinetic and kinematics data [43]. The velocity of walking (m/s) was calculated as mean linear velocity of the model centre of mass in the anterior direction during the stance phase using Visual 3D [44]. Stride length (m) was determined as the linear anterior distance in the foot centre of mass location at footstrike between initial and subsequent ipsilateral footfalls [45].

2.3.1. Medial Tibiofemoral Forces

Walking data during the stance phase were exported into bespoke musculoskeletal simulation software (OpenSim v3.3, Simtk.org). A validated musculoskeletal model [46] was firstly scaled to account for the anthropometrics of each participant. Dynamic inconsistency was solved using a residual reduction algorithm function within OpenSim [32]. Muscle kinetics were then quantified using a weighted static optimization process [47]. A joint reaction analysis process within OpenSim was then utilized, using muscle force data generated via static optimization [32]. The peak net (N) and normalized medial tibiofemoral forces (BW) were calculated using data derived from the joint reaction analysis. The cumulative medial tibiofemoral load was computed as the quotient of the mean stance phase medial tibiofemoral force and the stride length [35]. Pilot walking data shows a minimal detectable difference (MDC) of 0.27 BW and a high level of reliability (ICC = 0.951) for the peak medial tibiofemoral force (Table S1). Sinclair et al. [45] also importantly showed that vastus intermedius, vastus lateralis and vastus medialis muscle forces at the instance of peak joint force, were the strongest predictors of peak medial tibiofemoral joint loading during walking. Therefore, to determine the mechanisms responsible for any alterations in peak medial tibiofemoral kinetics between footwear conditions, the peak net (N) and normalized forces (BW) quantified during static optimization for the aforementioned muscles were quantified at the instance of peak joint force and extracted for statistical analysis.

2.3.2. Medial Tibiofemoral Contact Mechanics

The medial tibiofemoral contact forces obtained from OpenSim were input into a model of medial knee contact mechanics which was utilized to calculate tibiofemoral cartilage stress and strain via adapted MATLAB source code [35]. Pilot walking data shown MDCs of 0.01 and 0.16 MPa and high reliability (ICC $\geq$ 0.945) for indices of medial tibiofemoral stress and strain (Table S1). The tibiofemoral contact model is based on that outlined by Nuño and Ahmed [48]. Medial tibiofemoral stresses (σ) and strains (ε) were quantified using the formulae outlined in Equations (1) and (2).

$$\text{EQ1: } \sigma = -\text{ Mean tibiofemoral cartilage modulus} * (\text{Log}\ (1 - \varepsilon)) \quad (1)$$

$$\text{EQ2: } \varepsilon = \text{Cartilage element compression} - \text{modelled cartilage height} \quad (2)$$

The medial femoral condyle was modelled from a sagittal viewpoint as two convex curves denoting its anterior and posterior components, and from a coronal posterior perspective as a single arc. Conversely, the tibial plateau was denoted as a concave arc. The radii of the anterior and posterior components of the femoral arc in the sagittal plane were 35.0 mm and 18.9 mm, whereas that of the tibial arc in the frontal plane was modelled as 21 mm. In accordance with the Nuno & Ahmed [48] model, the tibia was considered to-be held in a fixed position-in space and the femur featured two modifiable components: the-axial height of the knee flexion axis relative to the tibia and the knee flexion angle itself. The tibiofemoral joint cartilage itself was modelled as a series of elements on the tibial plateau, with an unloaded height of 5.0 mm [49]. The cartilage elements were assumed to display a nonlinear elastic stress-strain relationship [50].

Contact stress (MPa) and strain at the medial tibiofemoral compartment were obtained using modelled indices for cartilage moduli, compression magnitude of the modelled cartilage contact elements as well as the quantity of contact elements. The modelled contact elements were 7326, which reflected a distance of 0.5 mm between elements, and the aforementioned tibiofemoral radii. The moduli of the cartilage included in the model were distinct for the different locations as some were covered by the medial meniscus. The femoral cartilage, unconcealed tibial cartilage and concealed tibial cartilage, were considered to have moduli values of 8.6, 4.0 and 10.1 MPa [51]. The medial meniscus modulus was included into the model as 1.3 MPa, and the meniscus itself considered to obscure 46 % of the tibial plateau [52,53]. The cartilage and menisci elements were described with a modelled Poisson's ratio of 0.45 [54].

The angle of knee flexion was included into the contact model as that at which the peak medial tibiofemoral contact force (obtained using musculoskeletal simulation) occurred. The axial elevation of the knee flexion axis was incrementally decreased until the modelled peak medial tibiofemoral contact force matched that provided from musculoskeletal simulation. As the modelled tibiofemoral radii are distinct, the location of the loaded articular cartilage also differed alongside changes in the angle of knee flexion [55]. As the medial femoral condyle has been shown to remain close to the centre of the tibial plateau with alterations in the angle of knee flexion, it was determined that inclusion of translational knee joint mechanics were not necessary for this model [56].

2.3.3. Medial Tibiofemoral Cartilage Failure Probabilistic Modelling

Medial tibiofemoral cartilage failure was defined as macroscopical plastic deformation typically observed in early-stage OA cartilage deterioration [57]. As 55 years has been demonstrated as the median age for knee OA diagnosis, and 9.29% of the US population is diagnosed with symptomatic knee OA by age 60 [11]; probability of cartilage failure was quantified across a duration of 42 years, from anatomical musculoskeletal maturity aged 18 until 60 years of age [58]. Probability of cartilage failure was quantified using probabilistic modelling; incorporating indices of both damage and repair [59–61], with cartilage strain the primary input parameter for damage. Sensitivity analyses were undertaken to determine the sensitivity of the key cartilage failure determinant, i.e., peak tibiofemoral strain to alterations (within feasible biological/anthropometric ranges) of each modelled parameter separately whilst maintaining the others at their modelled values (Tables S2 and S3 and Figures S1–S8).

Cartilage failure probability across the quantified duration, was obtained as a collective function of the aforementioned articular cartilage properties experiencing loading cycles over the daily modelled distance, using the stride length from the initial processing section to determine the daily number of loading cycles using Equation (3).

EQ3: Probability of cartilage failure = 1 − Exp − [(Volume of stressed cartilage / Reference stressed cartilage volume)(time − time until failure)Weibull exponent /Power law exponent] (3)

In Equation (3), constants in the probabilistic cartilage failure model were the reference cartilage volume (78.5 mm^3), Weibull exponent (14.3) and power law exponent (12.9). Time until failure of the articular cartilage was quantified using Equation (4).

EQ4: Time to failure = (Power law coefficient ∗ Stride length / Distance-per day) (Weibull coefficient ∗ ε) − Power law exponent (4)

In Equation (4), the time until failure is representative of the duration at which 63.2% of cases would experience failure after undergoing the magnitude and volume of cartilage strains. Daily distance travelled was included in the model as 6.0 km, which represents the approximate distance covered, had 7000 steps (the number now considered optimal for health and wellbeing [62] been completed per day, taking into account the stride lengths obtained from the current investigation. The power law coefficient (1.0), Weibull coefficient (1.03) and power law exponent (12.9) were incorporated as constants in the quantification of time until failure. These parameters were extracted from Miller & Krupenevich, [35], who fit a power law function to the loading cycles to failure data of Riemenschneider et al. [63].

Equation (3) shows in vitro failure probability. As living cartilage does possess limited innate ability to recover from strain-induced damage over time [64], the probability of medial tibiofemoral cartilage repair included into the failure model using Equation (5).

EQ5: Probability of repair = 1 − Exp − [− (time / time until repair) Cartilage repair exponent] (5)

In Equation (5), the cartilage repair exponent (5.2) and time until repair (5.0 years) were modelled as constants [35], and the repair duration was correspondingly included as the time after which repair would be anticipated in 63.2% of cases of damage.

A probability density function determining the instantaneous probability of failure at a given time, was utilized to encompass repair into Equation 3 [35]. This is delineated in Equation (6).

EQ6: Probability density function = (Volume of stressed cartilage ∗ Weibull exponent / Power law-exponent ∗ Reference stressed cartilage volume ∗ time until failure) (time / time until failure) Weibull exponent / Power law exponent − 1 Exp [− (Volume of stressed cartilage / Reference stressed cartilage volume) (time / time until failure) Weibull exponent / Power law exponent] (6)

The product of the probability density function and the communal probability that repair had not yet occurred, was integrated as a function of time in order to ascertain failure probability with repair. This procedure is described in Equation 7.

EQ7: Probability of failure with repair = ∫ (time 0) [Probability density function ∗ (1 − Probability of repair)] Modelled distance between contact elements ∗ time (7)

2.4. Statistical Analyses

For each biomechanical and cartilage failure outcome variable; means, standard deviations (SD) and 95% confidence intervals (95% CI) around the mean were calculated. To compare participant characteristics, biomechanical and cartilage failure outcomes between healthy weight and obese groups, between groups linear mixed effects models were adopted using the restricted maximum-likelihood method, with group (i.e., obese/healthy weight) included as a fixed factor and random intercepts modelled by participants [44]. Linear regression analysis was also adopted in both groups to determine the relationship between BMI and peak force, peak stress and peak strain. All statistical analyses were conducted using SPSS v27 (IBM, SPSS). For linear mixed models, the mean difference (b), t-value, and 95% CI of the difference are presented. Statistical significance for all analyses was accepted at the $p < 0.05$ level.

3. Results

3.1. Participant Characteristics

There were no differences in between groups for age (b = 1.32 $_{(95\%\ CI = -1.07–3.70)}$, t = 1.12, p = 0.27) and stature (b = 0.00 $_{(95\%\ CI = -0.03–0.03)}$, t = 0.03, p = 0.98) between groups. However, both body mass (b = 29.64 $_{(95\%\ CI = 26.78–32.49)}$, t = 20.97, p < 0.001) and BMI (b = 11.16 $_{(95\%\ CI = 10.01–12.31)}$, t = 19.54, p < 0.001) were significantly greater in the obese group (Table 1).

Table 1. Participant characteristic values for the obese and healthy weight groups.

	Healthy Weight				Obese				
	Mean	SD	95% CI Lower	95% CI Upper	Mean	SD	95% CI Lower	95% CI Upper	
Age (years)	25.50	4.53	23.49	27.51	24.18	3.19	22.77	25.59	
Mass (kg)	63.18	3.55	61.61	64.76	92.82	5.59	90.34	95.30	*
Stature (m)	1.63	0.05	1.61	1.66	1.63	0.05	1.61	1.66	
BMI (kg/m^2)	23.71	1.27	23.14	24.27	34.87	2.36	33.82	35.91	*

Notes: * = significant difference between healthy-weight and obese groups.

3.2. Initial Kinematic Processing

No significant differences in walking velocity were found between the two groups (b = 0.07 $_{(95\%\ CI = -0.07–0.21)}$, t = 0.98, p = 0.33). In addition, there were no significant differences between groups for stride length was (b = 0.06 $_{(95\%\ CI = -0.06–0.19)}$, t = 0.99, p = 0.31) (Table 2).

Table 2. Kinematic temporal parameters from normal weight and obese groups.

	Healthy Weight				Obese			
	Mean	SD	95% CI Lower	95% CI Upper	Mean	SD	95% CI Lower	95% CI Upper
Walking velocity (m/s)	1.45	0.24	1.34	1.56	1.38	0.21	1.28	1.48
Stride length (m)	1.61	0.21	1.51	1.70	1.55	0.18	1.46	1.63

3.3. Medial Tibiofemoral Forces and Muscle Forces

There were no differences in peak normalized medial tibiofemoral force (b = 0.00 $_{(95\%\ CI = -0.31–0.32)}$, t = 0.02, p = 0.98) or normalized cumulative load (b = 0.14 $_{(95\%\ CI = -0.07–0.34)}$, t = 1.32, p = 0.19) between groups. However, peak net medial tibiofemoral force (b = 520.71 $_{(95\%\ CI = 212.70–828.72)}$, t = 3.42, p < 0.001) and net medial tibiofemoral cumulative load were shown to be significantly greater in the obese group (b = 452.19 $_{(95\%\ CI = 270.36–634.02)}$, t = 5.03, p < 0.001) (Table 3).

Table 3. Medial tibiofemoral and muscle forces from normal weight and obese groups.

	Healthy Weight				Obese				
	Mean	SD	95% CI Lower	95% CI Upper	Mean	SD	95% CI Lower	95% CI Upper	
Peak medial tibiofemoral force (BW)	2.22	0.52	1.98	2.46	2.22	0.46	2.01	2.44	
Medial tibiofemoral cumulative load (BW/m)	1.43	0.33	1.28	1.58	1.56	0.32	1.41	1.71	
Net peak medial tibiofemoral force (N)	1493.21	370.19	1319.96	1666.47	2013.92	570.91	1746.72	2281.12	*
Net medial tibiofemoral cumulative load (N/m)	956.11	194.39	865.13	1047.09	1408.30	351.50	1243.79	1572.81	*
Vastus intermedius force (BW)	0.56	0.25	0.44	0.68	0.57	0.19	0.47	0.66	
Vastus lateralis force (BW)	0.49	0.22	0.39	0.60	0.50	0.17	0.42	0.58	
Vastus medialis force (BW)	0.42	0.19	0.33	0.51	0.42	0.15	0.35	0.49	
Net vastus intermedius force (N)	375.85	172.24	295.24	456.47	529.08	272.59	401.50	656.66	*
Net vastus lateralis force (N)	330.71	151.40	259.85	401.56	465.39	239.61	353.25	577.53	*
Net vastus medialis force (N)	280.17	128.23	220.16	340.18	394.00	203.59	298.71	489.28	*

Notes: * = significant difference between healthy-weight and obese groups.

There were no differences in normalized vastus intermedius (b = 0.00 $_{(95\%\ CI\ =\ -0.31–0.32)}$, t = 0.02, p = 0.98), vastus lateralis (b = 0.00 $_{(95\%\ CI\ =\ -0.31–0.32)}$, t = 0.02, p = 0.98) or vastus medialis (b = 0.00 $_{(95\%\ CI\ =\ -0.31–0.32)}$, t = 0.02, p = 0.98) forces. However, net vastus intermedius (b = 153.23 $_{(95\%\ CI\ =\ 7.26–299.19)}$, t = 2.17, p = 0.04), vastus lateralis (b = 134.69 $_{(95\%\ CI\ =\ 6.39–262.99)}$, t = 2.13, p = 0.04) and vastus medialis (b = 113.82 $_{(95\%\ CI\ =\ 4.91–222.74)}$, t = 2.12, p = 0.04) forces were significantly greater in the obese group (Table 3).

3.4. Medial Tibiofemoral Contact Mechanics

Peak medial tibiofemoral stress was significantly greater in the obese group (b = 0.77 $_{(95\%\ CI\ =\ 0.23–1.31)}$, t = 2.90, p = 0.01), Furthermore, peak tibiofemoral strain was also found to be significantly greater in the obese group (b = 0.06 $_{(95\%\ CI\ =\ 0.02–0.09)}$, t = 2.97, p = 0.01) (Table 4).

Table 4. Medial tibiofemoral contact mechanics from normal weight and obese groups.

	Healthy Weight				Obese				
	Mean	SD	95% CI Lower	95% CI Upper	Mean	SD	95% CI Lower	95% CI Upper	
Peak medial tibiofemoral stress (MPa)	2.26	0.61	1.98	2.55	3.03	1.02	2.56	3.51	*
Peak medial tibiofemoral strain	0.19	0.05	0.17	0.22	0.25	0.07	0.22	0.28	*

Notes: * = significant difference between healthy-weight and obese groups.

3.5. Medial Tibiofemoral Cartilage Failure Probabilistic Modelling

Probability of failure was significantly greater in the obese group (b = 31.35 $_{(95\%\ CI\ =\ 5.81–56.90)}$, t = 2.48, p = 0.02). Furthermore, Probability of failure with repair was also found to be significantly greater in the obese group (b = 22.66 $_{(95\%\ CI\ =\ 1.26–44.05)}$, t = 2.14, p = 0.04) (Table 5; Figure 2).

Table 5. Medial tibiofemoral cartilage failure probabilistic parameters from normal weight and obese groups.

	Healthy Weight				Obese				
	Mean	SD	95% CI Lower	95% CI Upper	Mean	SD	95% CI Lower	95% CI Upper	
Probability of failure (%)	11.63	30.32	3.11	25.82	42.98	47.61	20.70	65.26	*
Probability of failure with repair (%)	7.58	22.84	2.56	18.26	30.23	41.38	10.87	49.60	*

Notes: * = significant difference between healthy-weight and obese groups.

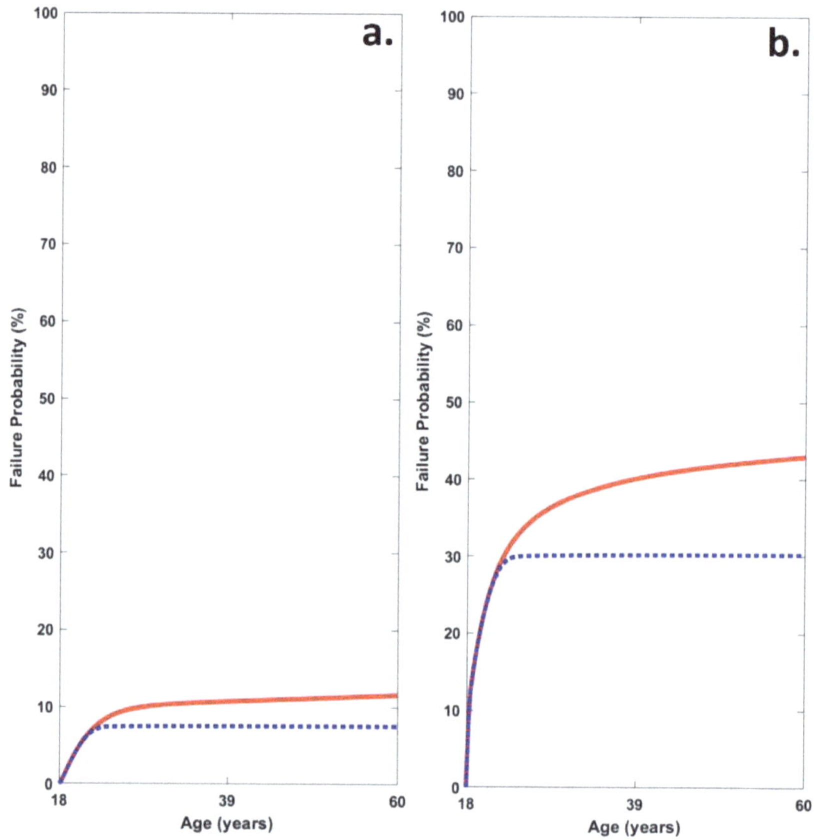

Figure 2. Average medial tibiofemoral cartilage failure time series probabilities in (**a**) healthy weight and (**b**) obese groups (red line = failure probability without adaptation and blue line = failure probability with adaptation).

3.6. Regression Analyses

In obese individuals BMI significantly predicted peak net medial tibiofemoral joint force, peak stress and peak strain. The regression models showed that peak forces, stress and strains at the medial tibiofemoral compartment were augmented by 47.73 N, 0.005 and 0.07 MPa, respectively, for every 1 unit increase in BMI (Figure 3).

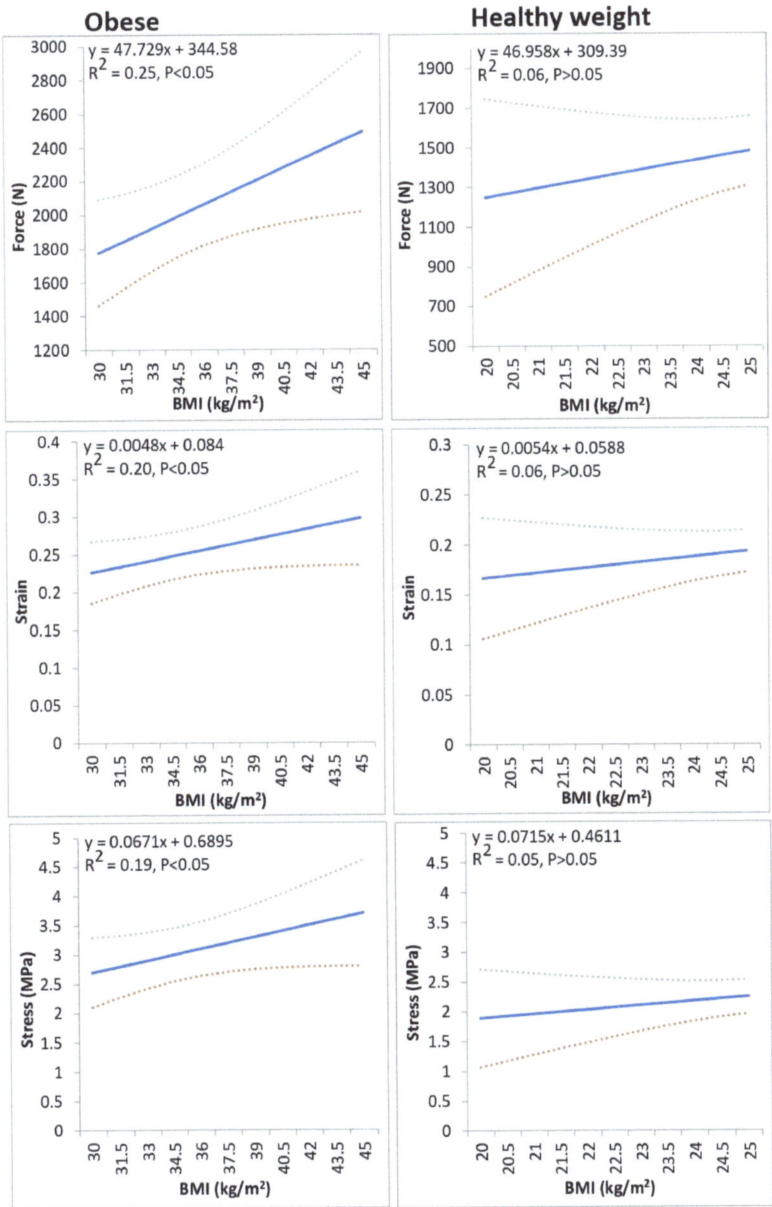

Figure 3. The relationship between BMI and indices of medial tibiofemoral loading. The solid line denotes the linear regression, and the dashed lines characterize its 95% confidence intervals.

4. Discussion

The current study aimed to explore the effects of obesity on medial tibiofemoral cartilage mechanics and longitudinal failure probability, in comparison to healthy individuals using both musculoskeletal simulation and computational modelling approaches. This represents the first investigation to examine the influence of obesity using the aforementioned approaches and may thus yield more comprehensive evidence concerning the influence of obesity on medial knee OA risk.

The plausibility of the medial tibiofemoral mechanical outcomes was inspected through comparisons against previously presented in vivo and other biomechanical modelling information. Taking into account the experimental walking velocities, the peak normalized medial tibiofemoral forces in the healthy weight group were analogous to those using both musculoskeletal modelling (2.90 BW, 1.52 m/s [35]) and simulation techniques (2.73 BW, 1.50 m/s [12]) and also to participant K8L (2.59 BW, 1.39 m/s) from in vivo data [65]. Furthermore, values in obese individuals were also similar to the normalized values obtained from musculoskeletal simulation in asymptomatic obese individuals (2.00 BW, 1.35 m/s [34]). Similarly, the strains experienced by the medial tibiofemoral cartilage were similar to those of Miller & Krupenevich, [35] (0.23) at 1.52 m/s. In comparison to the longitudinal medial tibiofemoral cartilage failure indices, the values in the healthy group are similar to those of Miller & Krupenevich, [35] (13.4%), and in line with the epidemiological literature in the general public for medial tibiofemoral OA aged 60 [11]. Furthermore, the cartilage failure probability values in the obese group are in line with incidence rates presented within the literature [13], and the increased risk for medial knee OA in this group compared to the healthy weight are in agreement with published relative risk indices of 3.78 [66].

In agreement with our hypotheses, the observations from this study importantly revealed that peak net medial tibiofemoral joint forces, stresses and strains were significantly greater in obese individuals in comparison to healthy weight participants. As previous analyses [45] have shown the vastus intermedius, vastus lateralis and vastus medialis muscle forces to be the strongest predictors of medial tibiofemoral joint compartment loading during walking, it is probable that the findings in relation to medial tibiofemoral joint mechanics, were arbitrated as a result of the corresponding increases in vasti muscle kinetics. Our observations support those of Harding et al. [34] who showed that medial tibiofemoral forces were greater in obese individuals. Notably our regression models also showed that in obese individuals BMI significantly predicted indices of medial tibiofemoral joint loading. It is interesting to note that BMI was significantly associated with medial tibiofemoral loading only in obese individuals and not in those who are a healthy weight. Previous analyses have shown significant associations between BMI and medial tibiofemoral strains [67], but this investigation is the first to undertake separate regression models in both obese and healthy weight groups. Therefore, this indicates that there appears to be a threshold above which, BMI appears to have a more pronounced influence on medial tibiofemoral loading indices. Nonetheless, this study does confirm that obesity appears to augment the risk of from the mechanical indices connected to the aetiology of medial knee OA [68].

Notably, in addition to the aforementioned observations concerning medial tibiofemoral loading indices experienced as a function of each footfall, the findings from the current investigation also showed that net medial tibiofemoral cumulative load was also significantly augmented in obese individuals. This observation also supports our hypothesis and allied to the enhanced indices of medial knee joint loading per footfall in the obese group, it would appear that the cumulative joint loads were further exacerbated by the reduced (although not significantly) stride lengths that were found. This importantly meant that a larger number of footfalls with increased medial tibiofemoral loads were required to complete the same modelled distance, which had unequivocal implications for lifetime cartilage failure probability.

Once again in line with our hypotheses, this investigation most importantly revealed, that failure probability was statistically greater in the obese group in comparison to healthy-weight individuals. It is noteworthy that the average failure probability indices of the obese group were 3.99 times greater than in the healthy weight participant group. Taking into account the parameters included in the probabilistic failure model [35], such increases were mediated as a combined function of the significantly greater cartilage strains allied with the increased number of steps required to complete the required daily distance in the obese group. This investigation therefore strongly supports the long-held notion regarding the negative effects of obesity on tibiofemoral cartilage health. This investigation showed BMI to be a significant predictor of cartilage loading indices in obese individuals and previous analyses importantly having revealed that weight loss is able to mediate significant reductions in medial tibiofemoral loading [69,70]. Taking into account the debilitating and painful presentation of knee OA [7] as well as its fiscal healthcare implications [10], the findings from this study therefore strongly advocate for the implementation of effective weight management programs into long-term musculoskeletal management strategies.

Taking into account the modelled walking volume and measured velocity, the current investigation produced similar axial joint forces and cartilage strains to previous musculoskeletal modelling, simulation and in vivo analyses [12,34,35] as well as medial tibiofemoral failure probabilities to epidemiological incidence rates in both healthy weight and obese groups [11,13,35,66]. However, OA is recognized as a multifactorial joint disease [14] in which chronic low-grade inflammation plays an important role [17,18,20,21], therefore as the computational model of medial tibiofemoral cartilage failure probability adopted in the current investigation did not account for adipokine levels, may serve as a limitation to this investigation. Future developmental analyses are necessary to develop a more complex and computationally heavy probabilistic model, capable of quantifying the interaction between mechanical and biochemical mechanisms of medial tibiofemoral OA. A more robust and pathophysiologically relevant probabilistic model of knee OA may allow future disease-modifying therapeutic interventions to be examined more readily. Taking into the debilitating nature of knee OA [10] in addition to its fiscal implications [8], this is an avenue of significant interest for future computational modelling research.

5. Conclusions

In conclusion, though walking biomechanics in obese individuals has received considerable research attention, there has not yet been an exploration of the longitudinal effects of obesity using a cumulative musculoskeletal simulation and probabilistic modelling approach. The present study, therefore, enhances current clinical knowledge, by examining the effects of obesity on medial tibiofemoral cartilage failure probability. Importantly, medial tibiofemoral cartilage force, stress and strain were statistically greater in obese individuals in comparison to those of healthy weight. The findings from the current investigation also importantly showed that obesity has a profoundly negative influence on longitudinal knee cartilage health and strongly advocate for the implementation of effective weight management programs into long-term musculoskeletal management strategies.

Supplementary Materials: The following supporting information can be downloaded at: https://www.mdpi.com/article/10.3390/life13020270/s1, Figure S1: Anterior femoral arc in sagittal plane; Figure S2: Femoral cartilage modulus; Figure S3: Covered tibial cartilage modulus; Figure S4: Uncovered tibial cartilage modulus; Figure S5: Meniscus modulus; Figure S6: Unloaded cartilage height; Figure S7: Frontal tibial arc; Figure S8: Poisson's ratio; Table S1: Reliability and MDC values; Table S2: Walking velocity; Table S3: Input peak medial tibiofemoral forces.

Author Contributions: Conceptualization, J.S. and H.L.; methodology, J.S. and H.L.; formal analysis, J.S., P.J.T. and N.C.; data curation, H.L.; writing—original draft preparation, J.S., P.J.T. and N.C.: writing—review and editing, J.S., H.L., P.J.T. and N.C. All authors have read and agreed to the published version of the manuscript.

Funding: This investigation received no external funding.

Institutional Review Board Statement: The procedure utilized for this investigation was approved by a university ethical committee (STEMH 1013).

Informed Consent Statement: Participants provided informed consent in written form.

Data Availability Statement: Not applicable.

Acknowledgments: We thank Gareth Shadwell for his technical support.

Conflicts of Interest: The authors declare no conflict of interest.

References

1. Imes, C.C.; Burke, L.E. The obesity epidemic: The USA as a cautionary tale for the rest of the world. *Curr. Epidemiol. Rep.* **2014**, *1*, 82–88. [CrossRef] [PubMed]
2. Flegal, K.M.; Carroll, M.D.; Kit, B.K.; Ogden, C.L. Prevalence of obesity and trends in the distribution of body mass index among US adults, 1999–2010. *JAMA* **2012**, *307*, 491–497. [CrossRef] [PubMed]
3. Formica, V.; Morelli, C.; Riondino, S.; Renzi, N.; Nitti, D.; Di Daniele, N.; Tesauro, M. Obesity and common pathways of cancer and cardiovascular disease. *Endocr. Metab. Sci.* **2020**, *1*, 100065. [CrossRef]
4. Frühbeck, G.; Toplak, H.; Woodward, E.; Yumuk, V.; Maislos, M.; Oppert, J.M. Obesity: The gateway to ill health-an EASO position statement on a rising public health, clinical and scientific challenge in Europe. *Obes. Facts* **2013**, *6*, 117–120. [CrossRef] [PubMed]
5. Anandacoomarasamy, A.; Caterson, I.; Sambrook, P.; Fransen, M.; March, L. The impact of obesity on the musculoskeletal system. *Int. J. Obes.* **2008**, *32*, 211–222. [CrossRef] [PubMed]
6. Zhang, Y.; Jordan, J.M. Epidemiology of osteoarthritis. *Clin. Geriatr. Med.* **2010**, *26*, 355–369. [CrossRef]
7. Heidari, B. Knee osteoarthritis prevalence, risk factors, pathogenesis and features: Part I. *Casp. J. Intern. Med.* **2011**, *2*, 205–212.
8. Martins, R.; Kotsopoulos, N.; Kließ, M.K.; Beck, C.; Abraham, L.; Large, S.; Connolly, M.P. Comparing the fiscal consequences of controlled and uncontrolled osteoarthritis pain applying a UK public economic perspective. *J. Health Econ. Outcomes Res.* **2021**, *8*, 127–136. [CrossRef]
9. Chen, D.I.; Shen, J.; Zhao, W.; Wang, T.; Han, L.; Hamilton, J.L.; Im, H.J. Osteoarthritis: Toward a comprehensive understanding of pathological mechanism. *Bone Res.* **2017**, *5*, 16044. [CrossRef]
10. Alshami, A.M. Knee osteoarthritis related pain: A narrative review of diagnosis and treatment. *Int. J. Health Sci.* **2014**, *8*, 85–104. [CrossRef]
11. Losina, E.; Weinstein, A.M.; Reichmann, W.M.; Burbine, S.A.; Solomon, D.H.; Daigle, M.E.; Katz, J.N. Lifetime risk and age at diagnosis of symptomatic knee osteoarthritis in the US. *Arthritis Care Res.* **2013**, *65*, 703–711. [CrossRef] [PubMed]
12. Sinclair, J.; Brooks, D.; Butters, B. Effects of different heel heights on lower extremity joint loading in experienced and in-experienced users: A musculoskeletal simulation analysis. *Sport Sci. Health* **2019**, *15*, 237–248. [CrossRef]
13. Felson, D.T.; Anderson, J.J.; Naimark, A.; Walker, A.M.; Meenan, R.F. Obesity and knee osteoarthritis: The Framingham Study. *Ann. Intern. Med.* **1988**, *109*, 18–24. [CrossRef]
14. Coaccioli, S.; Sarzi-Puttini, P.; Zis, P.; Rinonapoli, G.; Varrassi, G. Osteoarthritis: New insight on its pathophysiology. *J. Clin. Med.* **2022**, *11*, 6013. [CrossRef]
15. Andriacchi, T.P.; Mündermann, A.; Smith, R.L.; Alexander, E.J.; Dyrby, C.O.; Koo, S. A framework for the in vivo pathomechanics of osteoarthritis at the knee. *Ann. Biomed. Eng.* **2004**, *32*, 447–457. [CrossRef] [PubMed]
16. Sharma, L.; Lou, C.; Cahue, S.; Dunlop, D.D. The mechanism of the effect of obesity in knee osteoarthritis: The mediating role of malalignment. *Arthritis Rheum. Off. J. Am. Coll. Rheumatol.* **2000**, *43*, 568–575. [CrossRef]
17. Dell'Isola, A.; Allan, R.; Smith, S.L.; Marreiros, S.S.P.; Steultjens, M. Identification of clinical phenotypes in knee osteoarthritis: A systematic review of the literature. *BMC Musculoskelet. Disord.* **2016**, *17*, 425. [CrossRef] [PubMed]
18. Ouchi, N.; Parker, J.L.; Lugus, J.J.; Walsh, K. Adipokines in inflammation and metabolic disease. *Nat. Rev. Immunol.* **2011**, *11*, 85–97. [CrossRef] [PubMed]
19. Azamar-Llamas, D.; Hernandez-Molina, G.; Ramos-Avalos, B.; Furuzawa-Carballeda, J. Adipokine contribution to the pathogenesis of osteoarthritis. *Mediat. Inflamm.* **2017**, *2017*, 5468023. [CrossRef]
20. Lambova, S.N.; Batsalova, T.; Moten, D.; Stoyanova, S.; Georgieva, E.; Belenska-Todorova, L.; Kolchakova, D.; Dzhambazov, B. Serum Leptin and Resistin Levels in Knee Osteoarthritis—Clinical and Radiologic Links: Towards Precise Definition of Metabolic Type Knee Osteoarthritis. *Biomedicines* **2021**, *9*, 1019. [CrossRef]
21. Ilia, I.; Nitusca, D.; Marian, C. Adiponectin in Osteoarthritis: Pathophysiology, Relationship with Obesity and Presumptive Diagnostic Biomarker Potential. *Diagnostics* **2022**, *12*, 455. [CrossRef] [PubMed]
22. De Souza, S.A.F.; Faintuch, J.; Valezi, A.C.; Sant'Anna, A.F.; Gama-Rodrigues, J.J.; de Batista Fonseca, I.C.; Senhorini, R.C. Gait cinematic analysis in morbidly obese patients. *Obes. Surg.* **2005**, *15*, 1238–1242. [CrossRef] [PubMed]
23. Lai, P.P.; Leung, A.K.; Li, A.N.; Zhang, M. Three-dimensional gait analysis of obese adults. *Clin. Biomech.* **2008**, *23*, 2–6. [CrossRef] [PubMed]
24. Spyropoulos, P.; Pisciotta, J.C.; Pavlou, K.N.; Cairns, M.A.; Simon, S.R. Biomechanical gait analysis in obese men. *Arch. Phys. Med. Rehabil.* **1991**, *72*, 1065–1070. [PubMed]
25. DeVita, P.; Hortobágyi, T. Obesity is not associated with increased knee joint torque and power during level walking. *J. Biomech.* **2003**, *36*, 1355–1362. [CrossRef]
26. Browning, R.C.; Kram, R. Effects of obesity on the biomechanics of walking at different speeds. *Med. Sci. Sport. Exerc.* **2007**, *39*, 1632. [CrossRef]
27. MacLean, K.F.; Callaghan, J.P.; Maly, M.R. Effect of obesity on knee joint biomechanics during gait in young adults. *Cogent Med.* **2016**, *3*, 1173778. [CrossRef]
28. Segal, N.A.; Yack, H.J.; Khole, P. Weight, rather than obesity distribution, explains peak external knee adduction moment during level gait. *Am. J. Phys. Med. Rehabil./Assoc. Acad. Physiatr.* **2009**, *88*, 180–188. [CrossRef]

29. Messier, S.P.; Davies, A.B.; Moore, D.T.; Davis, S.E.; Pack, R.J.; Kazmar, S.C. Severe obesity: Effects on foot mechanics during walking. *Foot Ankle Int.* **1994**, *15*, 29–34. [CrossRef]
30. Vismara, L.; Romei, M.; Galli, M.; Montesano, A.; Baccalaro, G.; Crivellini, M.; Grugni, G. Clinical implications of gait analysis in the rehabilitation of adult patients with" Prader-Willi" Syndrome: A cross-sectional comparative study ("Prader-Willi" Syndrome vs. matched obese patients and healthy subjects). *J. Neuroeng. Rehabil.* **2007**, *4*, 17734317. [CrossRef]
31. Herzog, W.; Clark, A.; Wu, J. Resultant and local loading in models of joint disease. *Arthritis Care Res. Off. J. Am. Coll. Rheumatol.* **2003**, *49*, 239–247. [CrossRef] [PubMed]
32. Delp, S.L.; Anderson, F.C.; Arnold, A.S.; Loan, P.; Habib, A.; John, C.T.; Thelen, D.G. OpenSim: Open-Source software to create and analyze dynamic simulations of movement. *IEEE Trans. Biomed. Eng.* **2007**, *54*, 1940–1950. [CrossRef] [PubMed]
33. Lerner, Z.F.; Board, W.J.; Browning, R.C. Pediatric obesity and walking duration increase medial tibiofemoral compartment contact forces. *J. Orthop. Res.* **2016**, *34*, 97–105. [CrossRef] [PubMed]
34. Harding, G.T.; Dunbar, M.J.; Hubley-Kozey, C.L.; Stanish, W.D.; Wilson, J.L.A. Obesity is associated with higher absolute tibiofemoral contact and muscle forces during gait with and without knee osteoarthritis. *Clin. Biomech.* **2016**, *31*, 79–86. [CrossRef]
35. Miller, R.H.; Krupenevich, R.L. Medial knee cartilage is unlikely to withstand a lifetime of running without positive adaptation: A theoretical biomechanical model of failure phenomena. *PeerJ* **2020**, *8*, e9676. [CrossRef]
36. Gutin, I. In BMI we trust: Reframing the body mass index as a measure of health. *Soc. Theory Health* **2018**, *16*, 256–271. [CrossRef]
37. Cappozzo, A.; Catani, F.; Della Croce, U.; Leardini, A. Position and orientation in space of bones during movement: Anatomical frame definition and determination. *Clin. Biomech.* **1995**, *10*, 171–178. [CrossRef]
38. Sinclair, J.; Hebron, J.; Taylor, P.J. The influence of tester experience on the reliability of 3D kinematic information during running. *Gait Posture* **2014**, *40*, 707–711. [CrossRef]
39. Graydon, R.W.; Fewtrell, D.J.; Atkins, S.; Sinclair, J.K. The test-retest reliability of different ankle joint center location techniques. *Foot Ankle Online J.* **2015**, *1*, 26–31.
40. Sinclair, J.; Hebron, J.; Taylor, P.J. The test-retest reliability of knee joint center location techniques. *J. Appl. Biomech.* **2015**, *31*, 117–121. [CrossRef]
41. Sinclair, J.; Taylor, P.J.; Currigan, G.; Hobbs, S.J. The test-retest reliability of three different hip joint centre location techniques. *Mov. Sport Sci.-Sci. Mot.* **2014**, *83*, 31–39. [CrossRef]
42. Sinclair, J.K.; Edmundson, C.J.; Brooks, D.; Hobbs, S.J. Evaluation of kinematic methods of identifying gait Events during running. *Int. J. Sport. Sci. Eng.* **2011**, *5*, 188–192.
43. Sinclair, J.; Taylor, P.J.; Hobbs, S.J. Digital filtering of three-dimensional lower extremity kinematics: An assessment. *J. Hum. Kinet.* **2013**, *39*, 25–36. [CrossRef]
44. Sinclair, J.; Chockalingam, N.; Taylor, P.J. Lower Extremity Kinetics and Kinematics in Runners with Patellofemoral Pain: A Retrospective Case–Control Study Using Musculoskeletal Simulation. *Appl. Sci.* **2022**, *12*, 585. [CrossRef]
45. Sinclair, J.; Brooks, D.; Taylor, P.J.; Liles, N. Effects of toe-in/out toe-in gait and lateral wedge orthoses on lower extremity joint kinetics; an exploration using musculoskeletal simulation and Bayesian contrasts. *Sport Sci. Health* **2021**, *17*, 781–795. [CrossRef]
46. Lerner, Z.F.; DeMers, M.S.; Delp, S.L.; Browning, R.C. How tibiofemoral alignment and contact locations affect predictions of medial and lateral tibiofemoral contact forces. *J. Biomech.* **2015**, *48*, 644–650. [CrossRef] [PubMed]
47. Steele, K.M.; DeMers, M.S.; Schwartz, M.H.; Delp, S.L. Compressive tibiofemoral force during crouch gait. *Gait Posture* **2012**, *35*, 556–560. [CrossRef]
48. Nuno, N.; Ahmed, A.M. Sagittal profile of the femoral condyles and its application to femorotibial contact analysis. *J. Biomech. Eng.* **2001**, *123*, 18–26. [CrossRef]
49. Liu, F.; Kozanek, M.; Hosseini, A.; Van de Velde, S.K.; Gill, T.J.; Rubash, H.E.; Li, G. In Vivo tibiofemoral cartilage deformation during the stance phase of gait. *J. Biomech.* **2010**, *43*, 658–665. [CrossRef]
50. Blankevoort, L.; Kuiper, J.H.; Huiskes, R.; Grootenboer, H.J. Articular contact in a three-dimensional model of the knee. *J. Biomech.* **1991**, *24*, 1019–1031. [CrossRef]
51. Shepherd, D.E.; Seedhom, B.B. The'instantaneous' compressive modulus of human articular cartilage in joints of the lower limb. *Rheumatology* **1999**, *38*, 124–132. [CrossRef] [PubMed]
52. Danso, E.K.; Mäkelä, J.T.A.; Tanska, P.; Mononen, M.E.; Honkanen, J.T.J.; Jurvelin, J.S.; Korhonen, R.K. Characterization of site-specific biomechanical properties of human meniscus—Importance of collagen and fluid on me-chanical nonlinearities. *J. Biomech.* **2015**, *48*, 1499–1507. [CrossRef] [PubMed]
53. Blöcker, K.; Guermazi, A.; Wirth, W.; Benichou, O.; Kwoh, C.K.; Hunter, D.J.; Englund, M.; Resch, H.; Eckstein, F.; OAI investigators. Tibial coverage, meniscus position, size and damage in knees discordant for joint space narrowing–data from the Osteoarthritis Initiative. *Osteoarthr. Cartil.* **2013**, *21*, 419–427. [CrossRef] [PubMed]
54. Thambyah, A.; Nather, A.; Goh, J. Mechanical properties of articular cartilage covered by the meniscus. *Osteoarthr. Cartil.* **2006**, *14*, 580–588. [CrossRef] [PubMed]
55. Henderson, C.E.; Higginson, J.S.; Barrance, P.J. Comparison of MRI-based estimates of articular cartilage contact area in the tibiofemoral joint. *J. Biomech. Eng.* **2011**, *133*, 014502. [CrossRef]
56. DeFrate, L.E.; Sun, H.; Gill, T.J.; Rubash, H.E.; Li, G. In Vivo tibiofemoral contact analysis using 3D MRI-based knee models. *J. Biomech.* **2004**, *37*, 1499–1504. [CrossRef]
57. Weightman, B.O.; Freeman, M.A.R.; Swanson, S.A.V. Fatigue of articular cartilage. *Nature* **1973**, *244*, 303–304. [CrossRef]

58. Johnson, W.; Stovitz, S.D.; Choh, A.C.; Czerwinski, S.A.; Towne, B.; Demerath, E.W. Patterns of linear growth and skeletal maturation from birth to 18 years of age in overweight young adults. *Int. J. Obes.* **2012**, *36*, 535–541. [CrossRef]
59. Taylor, D. Fatigue of bone and bones: An analysis based on stressed volume. *J. Orthop. Res.* **1998**, *16*, 163–169. [CrossRef]
60. Taylor, D.; Kuiper, J.H. The prediction of stress fractures using a 'stressed volume'concept. *J. Orthop. Res.* **2001**, *19*, 919–926. [CrossRef]
61. Taylor, D.; Casolari, E.; Bignardi, C. Predicting stress fractures using a probabilistic model of damage, repair and adaptation. *J. Orthop. Res.* **2004**, *22*, 487–494. [CrossRef] [PubMed]
62. Paluch, A.E.; Gabriel, K.P.; Fulton, J.E.; Lewis, C.E.; Schreiner, P.J.; Sternfeld, B.; Carnethon, M.R. Steps per day and all-cause mortality in middle-aged adults in the Coronary Artery Risk Development in Young Adults study. *JAMA Netw. Open* **2021**, *4*, e2124516. [CrossRef] [PubMed]
63. Riemenschneider, P.E.; Rose, M.D.; Giordani, M.; McNary, S.M. Compressive fatigue and endurance of juvenile bovine articular cartilage explants. *J. Biomech.* **2019**, *95*, 109304. [CrossRef]
64. Nakamura, N.; Horibe, S.; Toritsuka, Y.; Mitsuoka, T.; Natsuume, T.; Yoneda, K.; Shino, K. The location-specific healing response of damaged articular cartilage after ACL reconstruction: Short-term follow-up. *Knee Surg. Sport. Traumatol. Arthrosc.* **2008**, *16*, 843–848. [CrossRef]
65. Bergmann, G.; Bender, A.; Graichen, F.; Dymke, J.; Rohlmann, A.; Trepczynski, A.; Kutzner, I. Standardized loads acting in knee implants. *PLoS ONE* **2014**, *9*, e86035. [CrossRef] [PubMed]
66. Anderson, J.J.; Felson, D.T. Factors associated with osteoarthritis of the knee in the first national Health and Nutrition Examination Survey (HANES I) evidence for an association with overweight, race, and physical demands of work. *Am. J. Epidemiol.* **1988**, *128*, 179–189. [CrossRef]
67. Collins, A.T.; Kulvaranon, M.L.; Cutcliffe, H.C.; Utturkar, G.M.; Smith, W.A.; Spritzer, C.E.; DeFrate, L.E. Obesity alters the in vivo mechanical response and biochemical properties of cartilage as measured by MRI. *Arthritis Res. Ther.* **2018**, *20*, 232. [CrossRef] [PubMed]
68. Simonsen, E.B.; Svendsen, M.B.; Nørreslet, A.; Baldvinsson, H.K.; Heilskov-Hansen, T.; Larsen, P.K.; Henriksen, M. Walking on high heels changes muscle activity and the dynamics of human walking significantly. *J. Appl. Biomech.* **2012**, *28*, 20–28. [CrossRef]
69. Messier, S.P.; Gutekunst, D.J.; Davis, C.; DeVita, P. Weight loss reduces knee-joint loads in overweight and obese older adults with knee osteoarthritis. *Arthritis Rheum.* **2005**, *52*, 2026–2032. [CrossRef]
70. DeVita, P.; Rider, P.; Hortobágyi, T. Reductions in knee joint forces with weight loss are attenuated by gait adaptations in class III obesity. *Gait Posture* **2016**, *45*, 25–30. [CrossRef]

life

Article

Rice Intake Is Associated with Longer Reaction Time and Interacts with Blood Lipids and Hypertension among Qatari Adults

Arwa Elrahmani, Farah Youssef, Haidi Elsayed, Nada Mohamed, Tahra El-Obeid and Zumin Shi *

Human Nutrition Department, College of Health Sciences, QU Health, Qatar University, Doha 2713, Qatar
* Correspondence: zumin@qu.edu.qa; Tel.: +974-4403-6037

Abstract: We aimed to assess the association between rice intake and cognitive function among Qatari adults and test the interactions with health conditions. Data from 1000 adults aged ≥18 years old who attended the Qatar Biobank (QBB) study were used. Rice dietary intake was measured by a food frequency questionnaire (FFQ), and mean reaction time (MRT) was used as an indicator of cognitive function. Linear regression and structure equation models were used. The mean rice consumption was 7.6 times/week (SD 2.0). The sample had a mean MRT of 717 milliseconds (SD 205). Rice consumption was positively associated with MRT. Across the quartiles of rice intake, the regression coefficients (95% CI) for MRT were 0.0 (reference), 22.4 (−7.8, 52.6), 36.3 (5.1, 67.5), and 34.5 (2.6, 66.4). There was a significant interaction between rice intake and hypertension, BMI, and blood lipids in relation to MRT. The association between rice intake and MRT was only observed among those with hypertension, overweight/obesity, low LDL, and low total cholesterol levels. Serum magnesium did not mediate the association. High rice consumption was associated with a higher MRT, especially among those with hypertension, overweight/obesity, low LDL, and or low total cholesterol levels. Further longitudinal studies are needed to confirm the findings.

Keywords: cognition; rice intake; adults; Qatar Biobank study

Citation: Elrahmani, A.; Youssef, F.; Elsayed, H.; Mohamed, N.; El-Obeid, T.; Shi, Z. Rice Intake Is Associated with Longer Reaction Time and Interacts with Blood Lipids and Hypertension among Qatari Adults. *Life* **2023**, *13*, 251. https://doi.org/10.3390/life13010251

Academic Editor: Jonathan Foster

Received: 21 December 2022
Revised: 4 January 2023
Accepted: 9 January 2023
Published: 16 January 2023

1. Introduction

Reaction time (RT) is a measure of processing speed or efficiency in the central nervous system [1]. It is a major determinant of higher cognitive function [2]. In addition to older age, men, lower education, and smoking are also associated with RT in some population studies [3]. Population studies suggest that diet is one of the important determinants for cognition function [4–6].

Rice is the main staple food for almost two billion people (~50%) in Asia [7,8]. The association between rice consumption and health outcomes has been examined in a limited number of studies with inconsistent findings [9–12]. In Asian populations specifically, two meta-analyses found that higher rice consumption is associated with an increased risk of type 2 diabetes [9,10]. While rice consumption increases the risk of diabetes and abnormal blood lipids in some populations, rice consumption has been shown to be inversely associated with obesity, hypertension, and cardiovascular diseases in other studies [11,12]. Chronic diseases such as diabetes and hypertension are associated with a higher risk of mild cognitive impairment (MCI) [13]. Only two population studies have examined the association between rice intake and cognition [14,15]. Studies in China found that higher rice intake was associated with a higher likelihood of functional impairment, difficulties in decision making, and a decline in cognitive function [14,15]. In the Shanghai Women's Health Study and the Shanghai Men's Health Study, those with high rice intake were over 20% more likely to have memory problems [14]. A 2-year cohort study conducted in the Chinese population concluded that weekly higher white rice intake was directly associated with an increased risk of incident mild cognitive impairment (MCI) [15]. In the study, a total of 471 participants without cognitive impairment at baseline developed incident MCI during the two-year follow up. High white rice consumption was associated with an increased risk of MCI (HR = 1.051, 95% CI: 1.008~1.096) and was independent of education, age, and drinking [15]. A randomized clinical trial that recruited 52 Japanese elderly participants aged 65 and above (25 men and 27 women) showed that the group that consumed white rice required more time to answer questions in the computerized cognitive function test compared with the brown rice group. Furthermore, the mean change in the total time required to answer all questions of the test was shorter in the brown rice group than in the white rice group [16]. However, the association between rice consumption and cognition has not been studied in countries with different food cultures. The mechanisms linking rice intake and cognition have not been tested. Furthermore, there is a lack of studies on the interaction between rice intake and chronic diseases. Blood lipids are associated with cognitive function. While higher total cholesterol and low-density lipoprotein cholesterol (LDL-C) are related to a higher risk of Alzheimer's disease in the 3C study [17], high-density lipoprotein cholesterol (HDL-C) and triglycerides were positively associated with cognitive function in overweight and obese individuals in China [18].

In Qatar, rice is the staple food [19]. Data from the Qatari Planning and Statistics Authority showed that the mean household purchase of rice was 56 kg/month [20], which is comparable to the consumption level in China [12]. The high consumption of rice among the Qatari population is partly because it is part of the subsidized monthly food rations, which also include oils, condensed milk, and sugar. Expenditure on rice was 49% of the cereals category in the food basket composition of Qatari households [19].

Refined grain (such as rice) consumption has been shown to contribute to a low magnesium consumption [21]. In many countries, magnesium consumption decreased over the past decades due to the low consumption of whole grains and fresh fruits and vegetables. Low serum magnesium is related to a poor cognitive function in Qatari adults [22]. It is unknown whether low serum magnesium mediates the association between rice intake and cognitive function.

To address the above knowledge gap, the aims of the study were to (1) assess the association between rice consumption and cognitive function among Qatari adults; (2) test the interaction between rice intake and hypertension, BMI, diabetes, and blood lipids; and (3) test whether serum magnesium mediates the association between rice intake and cognition. We have three hypotheses: (1) rice intake was positively associated with reaction time; (2) there was an interaction between rice intake and chronic diseases; and (3) magnesium mediated the association between rice intake and reaction time.

2. Materials and Methods

2.1. Study Design and Study Sample

Data from 1000 (500 men and 500 women) randomly selected Qatari adults aged 18 years old and above who attended the Qatar Biobank study (QBB) were analyzed. The details of the QBB study have been published elsewhere [23]. In short, Qatari adults or long-term residents (aged $\geq$18 years) were invited to participate in the study with a goal to include 60,000 participants, with follow ups planned for every 5 years. To be eligible for the analysis, participants were required to have data on food intake and attend the cognition test. By using a self-administered questionnaire, the sociodemographic data, dietary habits, and lifestyle factors were obtained. The biomarkers in the QBB cohort consisted of 66 clinical biomarkers which were routinely measured on the participants' blood samples [24]. The sample size in the current analysis was determined by the fact that QBB provides 1000 samples to research projects conducted at Qatar University for free. This study was conducted according to the guidelines in the Declaration of Helsinki and all procedures involving human subjects/patients were approved by the Hamad Medical Corporation Ethics Committee in 2011 and continued with the QBB Institutional Review Board from 2017 onward. Written informed consent was obtained from all subjects/patients.

For the current study, the ethical approval was obtained from QBB (Ex-2021-QF-QBB-RES-ACC-00035-0164).

2.2. Outcome Variable: Cognitive Function (Mean Reaction Time)

Mean reaction time (MRT) was used as an indicator for cognitive function. The MRT test is a computer-based, self-administered touch screen test and consists of 60 tasks using a visual stimulus [24,25]. It was designed by the Cambridge Neuropsychological Test Automated Battery (CANTAB) (https://www.cambridgecognition.com/cantab, accessed on 27 December 2022). The task generates 60 presentations of one of two targets. The target is presented as a small white box within one of two larger black boxes. The location of the target within the black box varies. During each trial, the participant has to select the box where the target appears as quickly as possible. The reaction time each individual took to complete each of the 60 tasks was measured. The mean value of the reaction time of the 60 tasks was calculated and used in the current study. A higher MRT represents a worse cognitive function. MRT was used to measure cognitive function in population studies [25,26].

2.3. Exposure Variable: Rice Intake

Rice dietary intake was assessed by a food frequency questionnaire (FFQ) that was self-administered and computerized. The participants were asked about their intake frequency as well as their dietary habits [23]. The FFQ contained 102 food items and was adapted from the European Perspective Investigation into the Cancer and Nutrition (EPIC) study; however, it has not been validated in Qatar. However, the food items included in the FFQ were similar to a recent validated FFQ in Qatar [27].

2.4. Covariates

The following covariates were used in the study: gender, age, BMI (categorical, overweight 25.0–29.9 kg/m^2 and obesity $\geq$30 kg/m^2), level of education (below or above university education), medication use, smoking (non-smokers, ex-smokers, and current smokers), intake of fruit and vegetable, total leisure time physical activity level (MET hours/week) [28], and self-reported chronic conditions. Fruit and vegetable intake (times/week) were self-reported. The criteria for diagnosing diabetes were: HbA1c $\geq$ 6.5%, random blood glucose (RBG) of $\geq$11.1 mmol/L, fasting blood glucose (FBG) of $\geq$7 mmol/L, or self-reported diabetes [29]. Hypertension was defined as systolic blood pressure $\geq$140 mmHg or diastolic is $\geq$90 mmHg or previous doctor diagnosis. Total cholesterol, HDL-C, and triglyceride levels were measured using standard laboratory enzymatic methods. LDL-C was calculated using the Friedewald formula [30]. Serum magnesium was measured by an automated colorimetric method (Magnesium Gen. 2 from Roche Diagnostics, Indianapolis, IN, USA) [22].

2.5. Statistical Analysis

Rice intake was categorized into quartiles. Sample characteristics were presented as percentage or mean (SD). Chi-squared test and ANOVA were used to test the differences in continuous variables and categorical variables by quartiles of rice intake. For our research aim 1, three multiple linear regression models were used to examine the association between rice intake and MRT. Model 1 was adjusted for gender and age. Model 2 was further adjusted for smoking, education, fruit and vegetable intake, and physical activity. Model 3 was further adjusted for BMI (continuous), hypertension, diabetes, and medication use. The variables adjusted were either sociodemographic factors or known risk factors for cognitive impairment. For our research aim 2, by adding the product terms of the two variables in the linear regression model, the interactions between rice intake, chronic diseases (diabetes and hypertension), BMI, and blood lipids were tested in the corresponding multivariable model. The interaction was visualized using the marginsplot command. For our research aim 3, the structural equation model was used to test the direct and indirect effect (via serum magnesium) of rice on cognitive function. STATA (Version 17, Stata Corporation,

College Station, TX, USA) was used for all the analysis. *p*-values < 0.05 (2-tailed) were considered significant.

3. Results

3.1. Sample Characteristics

The mean age of the sample taken was 35.8 (SD 10.4) years (Table 1). More than half of the participants had a high educational level (65.9%). Most of the participants were non-smokers (67.1%), while smokers made up 18.8% of the sample, and 14.1% were former smokers. The mean BMI was 28.2 (SD 5.7) kg/m^2. The majority of the participants were either overweight or obese, making up almost 70.5% of the sample. The sample had a mean MRT of 717 (SD 205) milliseconds. The mean serum magnesium was 0.84 (SD 0.06) mmol/L.

Table 1. Sample characteristics by quartiles of rice consumption among participants attending the Qatar Biobank study (N = 1000).

	Q1 (n = 306)	Q2 (n = 244)	Q3 (n = 219)	Q4 (n = 231)	*p*-Value *
Rice intake (times/week)	1.8 (1.0)	5.2 (0.8)	8.1 (0.9)	15.1 (5.4)	<0.001
Age (years)	36.1 (9.6)	35.4 (11.0)	36.9 (10.8)	34.8 (10.0)	0.167
Gender					0.581
Male	147 (48.0%)	117 (48.0%)	115 (52.5%)	121 (52.4%)	
Female	159 (52.0%)	127 (52.0%)	104 (47.5%)	110 (47.6%)	
Education					0.001
Low (below university)	94 (30.7%)	73 (30.0%)	68 (31.1%)	103 (44.8%)	
High (university or above)	212 (69.3%)	170 (70.0%)	151 (68.9%)	127 (55.2%)	
Smoking					0.785
Non	213 (69.6%)	162 (66.4%)	145 (66.2%)	153 (66.2%)	
Smoker	52 (17.0%)	45 (18.4%)	40 (18.3%)	50 (21.6%)	
Ex-smoker	41 (13.4%)	37 (15.2%)	34 (15.5%)	28 (12.1%)	
Leisure time physical activity (MET hours/week)	5.8 (17.9)	5.2 (15.0)	6.3 (17.0)	7.9 (35.5)	0.598
BMI (kg/m^2)	28.8 (5.6)	27.8 (5.5)	28.0 (6.0)	28.1 (5.8)	0.212
BMI categories					0.784
Normal	79 (25.8%)	76 (31.1%)	67 (30.6%)	71 (30.7%)	
Overweight	118 (38.6%)	93 (38.1%)	83 (37.9%)	88 (38.1%)	
Obese	109 (35.6%)	75 (30.7%)	69 (31.5%)	72 (31.2%)	
Supplement use	189 (61.8%)	158 (64.8%)	141 (64.4%)	126 (54.5%)	0.087
Vitamin D and calcium use	119 (38.9%)	105 (43.0%)	85 (38.8%)	74 (32.0%)	0.101
Vegetable intake (times/week)	14.2 (12.0)	15.3 (11.5)	17.5 (11.8)	23.1 (18.1)	<0.001
Fruit intake (times/week)	5.7 (5.5)	6.9 (6.4)	7.1 (6.0)	7.9 (6.8)	<0.001
Magnesium (mmol/L)	0.84 (0.05)	0.84 (0.06)	0.83 (0.06)	0.83 (0.06)	0.046
LDL (mmol/L)	3.0 (0.8)	3.0 (0.8)	2.9 (0.8)	2.9 (0.9)	0.461
HDL (mmol/L)	1.4 (0.4)	1.4 (0.4)	1.3 (0.4)	1.3 (0.4)	0.322
Total cholesterol (mmol/L)	5.0 (0.9)	4.9 (0.9)	4.9 (0.9)	4.9 (0.9)	0.697
HbA1C (%)	5.5 (0.9)	5.5 (0.8)	5.5 (0.8)	5.7 (1.1)	0.137
Hypertension	30 (9.8%)	20 (8.2%)	29 (13.2%)	17 (7.4%)	0.154
Diabetes	31 (10.5%)	25 (10.5%)	24 (11.3%)	36 (16.5%)	0.149
Insulin use	4 (1.3%)	3 (1.2%)	4 (1.8%)	8 (3.5%)	0.241
Diabetes medication other than insulin	8 (2.6%)	14 (5.7%)	17 (7.8%)	16 (6.9%)	0.046
Hypertension medication use	12 (3.9%)	11 (4.5%)	18 (8.2%)	14 (6.1%)	0.159
Mean reaction time (millisecond)	693.72 (175.83)	711.85 (194.49)	734.41 (250.92)	729.35 (197.96)	0.089

* One-way ANOVA was used for continuous variables; Chi-square test was used for other categorical variables listed in the table.

The mean rice consumption was 7.6 times/week, ranging from 1.8 times/week in quartile 1 (Q1) to 15.1 times/week in quartile 4 (Q4). Across the quartiles of rice intake, the intake of fruits and vegetables increased but the education level decreased. The prevalence of diabetes was higher in the high rice consumption group compared with low intake

(16.5% vs. 10.5%). There was no difference in age, smoking, physical activity, BMI, and hypertension across the quartiles of rice intake.

3.2. Association between Rice Consumption and MRT

Rice consumption was directly associated with a higher MRT (Table 2). After adjusting for age, gender, and lifestyle factors, the regression coefficients for MRT were 0.0 (reference), 22.4 (−7.8, 52.6), 36.3 (5.1, 67.5), and 34.5 (2.6, 66.4) across the quartiles of rice consumption. After further adjusting for BMI, diabetes, and hypertension, the above association was attenuated and became borderline significant. The association was independent of serum magnesium level (model 4). In the structure equation model, there was no mediating effect by serum magnesium (Table 3). Excluding participants with extreme values of MRT (i.e., <1st or >99th), the above findings remained.

Table 2. Association between quartiles of rice intake and cognitive function as measured by mean reaction time.

	Q1 (n = 306)	Q2 (n = 244)	Q3 (n = 219)	Q4 (n = 231)	*p* for Trend
Model 1	Ref	23.6 (−7.0, 54.1)	38.6 (7.2, 70.1)	50.1 (19.0, 81.1)	0.001
Model 2	Ref	22.4 (−7.8, 52.6)	36.3 (5.1, 67.5)	34.5 (2.6, 66.4)	0.017
Model 3	Ref	17.1 (−13.5, 47.8)	26.6 (−5.3, 58.4)	26.3 (−6.5, 59.0)	0.079
Model 4	Ref	21.9 (−8.3, 52.1)	33.7 (2.4, 65.0)	33.0 (1.1, 64.9)	0.024

Values are regression coefficients (95% CI) from linear regression. Model 1 adjusted for age and gender. Model 2 further adjusted for education, smoking, physical activity, fruit, and vegetable intake. Model 3 further adjusted for BMI, hypertension, and medication use for diabetes and hypertension. Model 4 is Model 2 plus further adjustment for serum magnesium.

Table 3. Direct and indirect effect of rice intake on cognitive function measured by mean reaction time.

	β (95% CI)	*p* Value
Total effect	3.13 (1.13–5.12)	0.002
Direct effect	3.00 (1.01–5.00)	0.003
Indirect effect (via serum magnesium)	0.13 (−0.05–3.09)	0.160

Model was adjusted for age and gender. Rice intake was modeled as a continuous variable in the structure equation model analysis.

3.3. Interactions between Rice Intake and Chronic Conditions

There was a significant two-way interaction ($p = 0.032$) between hypertension and rice in relation to cognitive function. High consumption of rice was associated with higher MRT among those with hypertension (Figure 1). However, no interaction between rice consumption and diabetes was found.

A significant interaction ($p = 0.041$) was found between rice intake and BMI in relation to MRT. No association between rice intake and MRT was found among people who had a normal BMI. However, among those with overweight/obesity, higher rice intake had a higher MRT.

Values were marginal means (SD). Models were adjusted for age, gender, education, smoking, leisure time and physical activity, and intake of fruit and vegetable.

LDL cholesterol level had a significant interaction with rice intake in relation to MRT. Figure 2 shows that among people with a low LDL level, there was a positive association between rice intake and MRT. However, there was no similar association among those with a high LDL. A borderline significant ($p = 0.051$) interaction was found with total cholesterol levels. However, no such interaction was found with HDL levels.

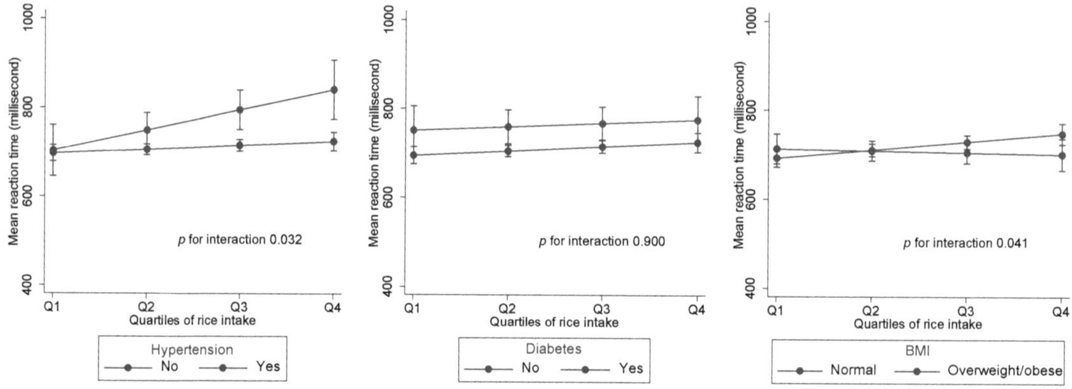

Figure 1. Interaction between rice intake and hypertension, diabetes, and BMI in relation to MRT.

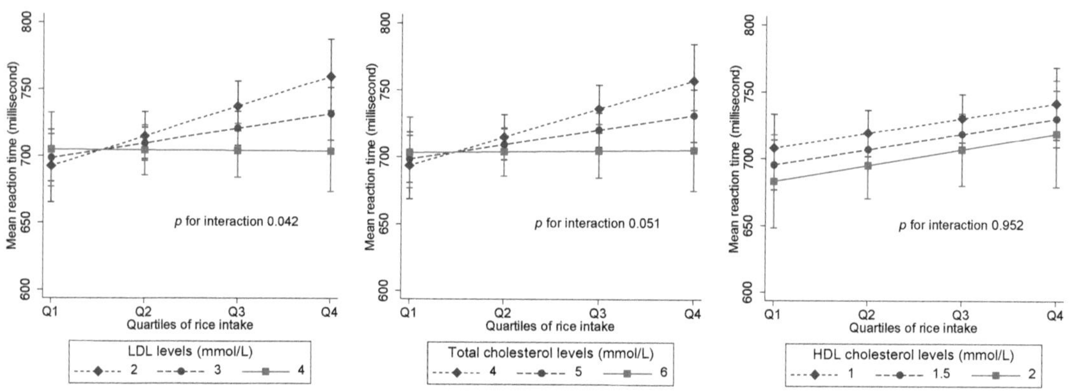

Figure 2. Interaction between rice intake and blood lipids in relation to MRT. Values were marginal means (SD). Models were adjusted for age, gender, education, smoking, leisure time and physical activity, and intake of fruit and vegetable. Values for LDL, HDL, and total cholesterol presented were around 10, 50, and 90 percentiles.

4. Discussion

In this cross-sectional study, we found that rice consumption is positively associated with MRT. There was an interaction between rice consumption and hypertension, BMI, LDL, and total cholesterol levels in relation to MRT. The positive association between rice intake and MRT was only observed among those with hypertension, high BMI, low LDL, and low total cholesterol levels.

Most of the studies on rice consumption and cognitive function were conducted in Asian populations [14–16,31]. Direct comparison between our study and other population studies is difficult due to the difference in the outcome measures. Our findings on the positive association between rice consumption and MRT are in line with other studies [14–16,31].

4.1. Potential Mechanisms

Several mechanisms may explain the link between rice intake and cognitive function impairment including low magnesium levels in refined rice, the positive association between rice and diabetes, the high glycemic index, and heavy metal contamination.

Inadequate micronutrients (e.g., magnesium) may also explain the link. Magnesium is an important nutrient that can affect cognition [24]. Magnesium is found in limited amounts in refined grains; and the Qatari dietary pattern is characterized by high consumption of refined grains such as rice and wheat [24]. A study in Qatar showed that there is an association between the concentrations of serum magnesium and cognitive function. It suggested that low serum magnesium is associated with increased MRT especially in women with diabetes and hypertension [24]. However, in our study, serum magnesium is not a mediator between rice intake and cognitive function. Further research is needed to validate the finding.

Evidence from meta-analyses suggests that high rice consumption increases the risk of diabetes in Asian populations [9,10]. It has been shown that diabetes increases the risk of cognitive function impairment [32]. Rice, especially refined white rice, has a high glycemic index. Based on a systematic review, consumption of a low glycemic index diet may favor cognitive function in adults [33]. High consumption of a high-glycemic-index rice-based diet may increase the risk of stroke in some populations [34]. It is well known that stroke increases the risk of cognitive impairment. The prevalence of post-stroke cognitive impairment is estimated to range from 20% to 80% [35].

The interaction between rice intake and hypertension may be because hypertension is a risk factor for cognitive impairment. For example, in a cross-sectional study of Chinese adults aged 60 years and above (n = 46,011), hypertension was associated with both dementia (OR 1.86 (95% CI 1.70–2.03) and mild cognitive impairment (MCI) (OR 1.62 (1.54–1.7) [36].

The interaction between blood lipids and rice intake is intriguing. The mechanisms are yet to be studied. A study involving 789 men and 1105 women from the Framingham Heart Study cohort indicated a positive direct association between total cholesterol (TC) and cognitive measures such as attention, abstract reasoning, and several cognitive domains [37]. It could be due to the need of TC for neural cells to perform normal metabolic processes [38]. Some studies suggested that high TC in older adults is associated with improved cognitive function [37,38]. It would be possible that under the condition of low cholesterol level, high rice consumption aggravates the impairment of cognitive function.

Oxidative stress (OS) is a main factor contributing to cognitive impairment as it has a role in the pathophysiology and neuronal degeneration that leads to diseases such as dementia, mild cognitive impairment (MCI), and eventually Alzheimer's disease [39]. Rice consumption may increase oxidative stress by various mechanisms including reducing liver function [40] and increasing the risk of non-communicable chronic diseases.

The bioaccumulation of arsenic in rice and the subsequent consumption by consumers can lead to adverse health effects [41]. Chronic arsenic exposure decreases serum brain-derived neurotrophic factor (sBDNF) and cognitive function in adults [42].

Finally, rice-related dietary patterns may also explain the link. Based on Qatari cuisine, foods high in saturated fat such as lamb meat are often eaten as an accompaniment to rice [19]. In Qatar, rice is also consumed as a dessert with high amounts of sugar and ghee added to it. A cross-sectional study on middle-aged adults found that intake of saturated fat was associated with an increased risk of cognitive function impairment [43].

4.2. Strengths and Limitations

This research has several strengths. Firstly, the participants were selected from Qatar's general population using data from the Qatar Biobank study. Secondly, we were able to adjust for many confounding variables. Thirdly, the large variation in rice intake in the sample allowed us to examine the association with cognitive function. However, there are several limitations. First, MRT was the only outcome measurement used to assess cognition, thus it could not represent other aspects of cognition. As QBB has started to conduct MRI brain scans, in the future we will be able to examine the relationship between rice intake and brain images. Second, we have information on the frequency of rice intake but not the absolute intake. However, the frequency of intake may reflect the eating habit.

Third, the study lacks comprehensive information on medication use. Moreover, due to its cross-sectional research methodology, the study cannot indicate a cause–effect link. In the study, a high intake of rice was associated with a low education level. Although we have adjusted for education, residual confounding is possible. Furthermore, we do not have information on heavy metal levels in the blood or urine. Future studies should measure heavy metals in blood or urine and examine whether heavy metals mediate the association between rice intake and cognitive function. Cohort studies are warranted to validate our exploratory findings.

5. Conclusions

In conclusion, rice consumption was directly associated with cognitive function as measured by the mean reaction time. High rice consumption was associated with a higher MRT among those with hypertension, overweight/obesity, low LDL, and low total cholesterol levels. Further studies are needed to validate the findings.

Author Contributions: A.E., F.Y., H.E. and N.M. contributed to the conception, analysis, and interpretation of data and drafted the manuscript. Z.S. conceived the study, analyzed the data, interpreted the results, and critically revised the manuscript. T.E.-O. critically reviewed and revised the manuscript. Z.S. was responsible for the work and supervised the study. All authors have read and agreed to the published version of the manuscript.

Funding: The study was funded by the Qatar University Student Grant (QUST-1-CHS-2022-349).

Institutional Review Board Statement: The institutional review committees of the Qatar Biobank Study approved the survey.

Informed Consent Statement: The Institutional Review Board (IRB) from the Hamad Medical Corporation Ethics Committee ethically approved the current study, and the QBB study approval is under the IRB exempted category (Ex-2021-QF-QBB-RES-ACC-00035-0164). Prior to participation, written informed consent was obtained from the participants.

Data Availability Statement: The data can be requested from the Qatar Biobank study data management team.

Acknowledgments: We would like to thank the staff and members of Qatar Biobank for providing the data for this study.

Conflicts of Interest: The authors declare no conflict of interest.

References

1. Boisgontier, M.P.; Wittenberg, G.F.; Fujiyama, H.; Levin, O.; Swinnen, S.P. Complexity of Central Processing in Simple and Choice Multilimb Reaction-Time Tasks. *PLoS ONE* **2014**, *9*, e90457. [CrossRef] [PubMed]
2. Deary, I.J.; Der, G. Reaction Time, Age, and Cognitive Ability: Longitudinal Findings from Age 16 to 63 Years in Representative Population Samples. *Aging Neuropsychol. Cogn.* **2005**, *12*, 187–215. [CrossRef]
3. Talboom, J.S.; De Both, M.D.; Naymik, M.A.; Schmidt, A.M.; Lewis, C.R.; Jepsen, W.M.; Håberg, A.K.; Rundek, T.; Levin, B.E.; Hoscheidt, S.; et al. Two separate, large cohorts reveal potential modifiers of age-associated variation in visual reaction time performance. *npj Aging Mech. Dis.* **2021**, *7*, 14. [CrossRef] [PubMed]
4. Spencer, S.J.; Korosi, A.; Layé, S.; Shukitt-Hale, B.; Barrientos, R.M. Food for thought: How nutrition impacts cognition and emotion. *npj Sci. Food* **2017**, *1*, 7. [CrossRef]
5. Shi, Z.; El-Obeid, T.; Li, M.; Xu, X.; Liu, J. Iron-related dietary pattern increases the risk of poor cognition. *Nutr. J.* **2019**, *18*, 48. [CrossRef]
6. Xu, X.; E Byles, J.; Shi, Z.; Hall, J.J. Dietary patterns, dietary lead exposure and hypertension in the older Chinese population. *Asia Pac. J. Clin. Nutr.* **2018**, *27*, 451–459.
7. Baldwin, K.; Childs, N.; Dyck, J.; Hansen, J. *Southeast Asia's Rice Surplus. Outlook No.(RCS-121-01)*; USDA ERS: Washington, DC, USA, 2012.
8. Toriyama, K. (Ed.) *Rice is Life: Scientific Perspectives for the 21st Century*; International Rice Research Institute: Los Baños, Philippines, 2005.
9. Ren, G.; Qi, J.; Zou, Y. Association between intake of white rice and incident type 2 diabetes—An updated meta-analysis. *Diabetes Res. Clin. Pract.* **2021**, *172*, 108651. [CrossRef]

10. A Hu, E.; Pan, A.; Malik, V.; Sun, Q. White rice consumption and risk of type 2 diabetes: Meta-analysis and systematic review. *BMJ* **2012**, *344*, e1454.
11. Shi, Z.; Ganji, V. Dietary patterns and cardiovascular disease risk among Chinese adults: A prospective cohort study. *Eur. J. Clin. Nutr.* **2020**, *74*, 1725–1735. [CrossRef]
12. Shi, Z.; Taylor, A.W.; Hu, G.; Gill, T.; Wittert, G.A. Rice intake, weight change and risk of the metabolic syndrome development among Chinese adults: The Jiangsu Nutrition Study (JIN). *Asia Pac. J. Clin. Nutr.* **2012**, *21*, 35–43.
13. Reitz, C.; Tang, M.-X.; Manly, J.; Mayeux, R.; Luchsinger, J. Hypertension and the Risk of Mild Cognitive Impairment. *Arch. Neurol.* **2007**, *64*, 1734–1740. [CrossRef] [PubMed]
14. Zhu, J.; Xiang, Y.-B.; Cai, H.; Li, H.; Gao, Y.-T.; Zheng, W.; Shu, X.-O. A Prospective Investigation of Dietary Intake and Functional Impairments Among the Elderly. *Am. J. Epidemiol.* **2018**, *187*, 2372–2386. [CrossRef] [PubMed]
15. Li, W.; Yue, L.; Li, G.; Xiao, S. Higher weekly white rice consumption is associated with an increased risk of incident MCI: A two-year follow-up study of elderly people in Shanghai Community. *Res. Sq.* **2021**.
16. Kuroda, Y.; Matsuzaki, K.; Wakatsuki, H.; Shido, O.; Harauma, A.; Moriguchi, T.; Sugimoto, H.; Yamaguchi, S.; Yoshino, K.; Hashimoto, M. Influence of Ultra-High Hydrostatic Pressurizing Brown Rice on Cognitive Functions and Mental Health of Elderly Japanese Individuals: A 2-Year Randomized and Controlled Trial. *J. Nutr. Sci. Vitaminol.* **2019**, *65*, S80–S87. [CrossRef]
17. Schilling, S.; Tzourio, C.; Soumaré, A.; Kaffashian, S.; Dartigues, J.-F.; Ancelin, M.-L.; Samieri, C.; Dufouil, C.; Debette, S. Differential associations of plasma lipids with incident dementia and dementia subtypes in the 3C Study: A longitudinal, population-based prospective cohort study. *PLoS Med.* **2017**, *14*, e1002265. [CrossRef]
18. Li, J.; Cao, Y.; Xiao, C. Subgroup analysis of the influence of body mass index on the association between serum lipids and cognitive function in Chinese population. *Lipids Health Dis.* **2020**, *19*, 130. [CrossRef]
19. Al-Thani, M.; Al-Thani, A.-A.; Al-Mahdi, N.; Al-Kareem, H.; Barakat, D.; Al-Chetachi, W.; Tawfik, A.; Akram, H. An Overview of Food Patterns and Diet Quality in Qatar: Findings from the National Household Income Expenditure Survey. *Cureus* **2017**, *9*, e1249. [CrossRef]
20. Planning and Statistics Authority. *Final Results of Household Expenditure and Income Survey (HEIS)*; Planning and Statistics Authority: Doha, Qatar, 2013; p. 206.
21. Costello, R.; Wallace, T.; Rosanoff, A. Magnesium. *Adv. Nutr.* **2016**, *7*, 199–201. [CrossRef]
22. Al-Ghazali, K.; Eltayeb, S.; Musleh, A.; Al-Abdi, T.; Ganji, V.; Shi, Z. Serum Magnesium and Cognitive Function Among Qatari Adults. *Front. Aging Neurosci.* **2020**, *12*, 101. [CrossRef]
23. Al Thani, A.; Fthenou, E.; Paparrodopoulos, S.; Al Marri, A.; Shi, Z.; Qafoud, F.; Afifi, N. Qatar Biobank Cohort Study: Study Design and First Results. *Am. J. Epidemiol.* **2019**, *188*, 1420–1433. [CrossRef]
24. Al Kuwari, H.; Al Thani, A.; Al Marri, A.; Al Kaabi, A.; Abderrahim, H.; Afifi, N.; Qafoud, F.; Chan, Q.; Tzoulaki, I.; Downey, P.; et al. The Qatar Biobank: Background and methods. *BMC Public Health* **2015**, *15*, 1208. [CrossRef] [PubMed]
25. Lyall, D.M.; Cullen, B.; Allerhand, M.; Smith, D.J.; Mackay, D.; Evans, J.; Anderson, J.; Fawns-Ritchie, C.; McIntosh, A.M.; Deary, I.J.; et al. Cognitive Test Scores in UK Biobank: Data Reduction in 480,416 Participants and Longitudinal Stability in 20,346 Participants. *PLoS ONE* **2016**, *11*, e0154222.
26. Jakobsen, L.H.; Sorensen, J.M.; Rask, I.K.; Jensen, B.S.; Kondrup, J. Validation of reaction time as a measure of cognitive function and quality of life in healthy subjects and patients. *Nutrition* **2011**, *27*, 561–570. [CrossRef] [PubMed]
27. Bawadi, H.; Akasheh, R.; Kerkadi, A.; Haydar, S.; Tayyem, R.; Shi, Z. Validity and Reproducibility of a Food Frequency Questionnaire to Assess Macro and Micro-Nutrient Intake among a Convenience Cohort of Healthy Adult Qataris. *Nutrients* **2021**, *13*, 2002. [CrossRef] [PubMed]
28. Ainsworth, B.E.; Haskell, W.L.; Whitt, M.C.; Irwin, M.L.; Swartz, A.M.; Strath, S.J.; O'Brien, W.L.; Bassett, D.R., Jr.; Schmitz, K.H.; Emplaincourt, P.O.; et al. Compendium of Physical Activities: An update of activity codes and MET intensities. *Med. Sci. Sport. Exerc.* **2000**, *32*, S498–S516. [CrossRef] [PubMed]
29. American Diabetes Association. Diagnosis and Classification of Diabetes Mellitus. *Diabetes Care* **2014**, *37* (Suppl. 1), S81–S90. [CrossRef]
30. Friedewald, W.T.; Levy, R.I.; Fredrickson, D.S. Estimation of the Concentration of Low-Density Lipoprotein Cholesterol in Plasma, Without Use of the Preparative Ultracentrifuge. *Clin. Chem.* **1972**, *18*, 499–502. [CrossRef]
31. Kaur, B.; Ranawana, V.; Henry, J. The Glycemic Index of Rice and Rice Products: A Review, and Table of GI Values. *Crit. Rev. Food Sci. Nutr.* **2013**, *56*, 215–236. [CrossRef]
32. Zilliox, L.A.; Chadrasekaran, K.; Kwan, J.Y.; Russell, J.W. Diabetes and Cognitive Impairment. *Curr. Diabetes Rep.* **2016**, *16*, 87. [CrossRef]
33. Philippou, E.; Constantinou, M. The Influence of Glycemic Index on Cognitive Functioning: A Systematic Review of the Evidence. *Adv. Nutr. Int. Rev. J.* **2014**, *5*, 119–130.
34. Oba, S.; Nagata, C.; Nakamura, K.; Fujii, K.; Kawachi, T.; Takatsuka, N.; Shimizu, H. Dietary glycemic index, glycemic load, and intake of carbohydrate and rice in relation to risk of mortality from stroke and its subtypes in Japanese men and women. *Metabolism* **2010**, *59*, 1574–1582. [CrossRef] [PubMed]
35. Sun, J.-H.; Tan, L.; Yu, J.-T. Post-stroke cognitive impairment: Epidemiology, mechanisms and management. *Ann. Transl. Med.* **2014**, *2*, 80. [PubMed]

36. Jia, L.; Du, Y.; Chu, L.; Zhang, Z.; Li, F.; Lyu, D.; Li, Y.; Zhu, M.; Jiao, H.; Song, Y.; et al. Prevalence, risk factors, and management of dementia and mild cognitive impairment in adults aged 60 years or older in China: A cross-sectional study. *Lancet Public Health* **2020**, *5*, e661–e671. [CrossRef]
37. Elias, P.K.; Elias, M.F.; D'Agostino, R.B.; Sullivan, L.M.; Wolf, P.A. Serum Cholesterol and Cognitive Performance in the Framingham Heart Study. *Psychosom. Med.* **2005**, *67*, 24–30. [CrossRef] [PubMed]
38. Muldoon, M.F.; Flory, J.D.; Ryan, C.M. Serum cholesterol, the brain, and cognitive functioning. In *Neuropsychology of Cardiovascular Disease*; Taylor & Francis Group: New York, NY, USA, 2001; pp. 53–76.
39. Li, J.; Wuliji, O.; Li, W.; Jiang, Z.-G.; Ghanbari, H.A. Oxidative Stress and Neurodegenerative Disorders. *Int. J. Mol. Sci.* **2013**, *14*, 24438–24475. [CrossRef] [PubMed]
40. Imam, M.U.; Musa, S.N.A.; Azmi, N.H.; Ismail, M. Effects of White Rice, Brown Rice and Germinated Brown Rice on Antioxidant Status of Type 2 Diabetic Rats. *Int. J. Mol. Sci.* **2012**, *13*, 12952–12969. [CrossRef]
41. Fakhri, Y.; Bjørklund, G.; Bandpei, A.M.; Chirumbolo, S.; Keramati, H.; Pouya, R.H.; Asadi, A.; Amanidaz, N.; Sarafraz, M.; Sheikhmohammad, A.; et al. Concentrations of arsenic and lead in rice (*Oryza sativa* L.) in Iran: A systematic review and carcinogenic risk assessment. *Food Chem. Toxicol.* **2018**, *113*, 267–277. [CrossRef]
42. Karim, Y.; Siddique, A.E.; Hossen, F.; Rahman, M.; Mondal, V.; Banna, H.U.; Hasibuzzaman, M.; Hosen, Z.; Islam, S.; Sarker, K.; et al. Dose-dependent relationships between chronic arsenic exposure and cognitive impairment and serum brain-derived neurotrophic factor. *Environ. Int.* **2019**, *131*, 105029. [CrossRef]
43. Kalmijn, S.; van Boxtel, M.P.; Ocke, M.; Verschuren, W.M.; Kromhout, D.; Launer, L.J. Dietary intake of fatty acids and fish in relation to cognitive performance at middle age. *Neurology* **2004**, *62*, 275–280. [CrossRef]

life

MDPI

Article

A Voxel-Based Morphometric Study of Gray Matter in Specific Phobia

Francisco Rivero [1,2], Rosario J. Marrero [1,3], Teresa Olivares [1], Wenceslao Peñate [1,3], Yolanda Álvarez-Pérez [4], Juan Manuel Bethencourt [1] and Ascensión Fumero [1,3,*]

1 Departamento de Psicología Clínica, Psicobiología y Metodología, Facultad de Psicología, Universidad de La Laguna, 38200 La Laguna, Tenerife, Spain
2 Departamento de Psicología, Facultad de Ciencias de la Salud, Universidad Europea de Canarias, 38300 La Orotava, Tenerife, Spain
3 Instituto Universitario de Neurociencia (IUNE), Universidad de La Laguna, 38200 La Laguna, Tenerife, Spain
4 Fundación Canaria Instituto de Investigación Sanitaria de Canarias (FIISC), 38109 El Rosario, Tenerife, Spain
* Correspondence: afumero@ull.edu.es

Abstract: The objective of this study was to analyze the neurostructural abnormalities of brain areas responsible for the acquisition and maintenance of fear in small animal phobia by comparing gray matter volume (GMV) in individuals with phobia and non-fearful controls. Structural magnetic resonance imaging was obtained from 62 adults (79% female) assigned to one of two groups: 31 were diagnosed with small animal phobia and 31 were non-fearful controls. To investigate structural alterations, a whole-brain voxel-based morphometry analysis was conducted to compare the GMV of the brain areas involved in fear between both groups. The results indicated that individuals with a small animal specific phobia showed smaller GMV in cortical regions, such as the orbitofrontal (OFC) and medial frontal cortex, and greater GMV in the putamen than non-fearful controls. These brain areas are responsible for avoidant behavior (putamen) and emotional regulation processes or inhibitory control (prefrontal cortex (PFC)), which might suggest a greater vulnerability of phobic individuals to acquiring non-adaptive conditioned responses and emotional dysregulation. The findings provide preliminary support for the involvement of structural deficits in OFC and medial frontal cortex in phobia, contributing to clarify the neurobiological substrates for phobias.

Keywords: MRI; prefrontal areas; putamen; gray matter volume; specific phobia

Citation: Rivero, F.; Marrero, R.J.; Olivares, T.; Peñate, W.; Álvarez-Pérez, Y.; Bethencourt, J.M.; Fumero, A. A Voxel-Based Morphometric Study of Gray Matter in Specific Phobia. *Life* **2023**, *13*, 119. https://doi.org/10.3390/life13010119

Academic Editor: Georg Kranz

Received: 24 November 2022
Revised: 28 December 2022
Accepted: 29 December 2022
Published: 31 December 2022

1. Introduction

Anxiety disorders (ADs) have been shown to be one of the mental disorders with the highest prevalence rate [1]. Different types of ADs include generalized anxiety disorder (GAD), panic disorder, agoraphobia, social anxiety disorder (social phobia), specific phobias (SP), obsessive-compulsive disorder (OCT), and post-traumatic stress disorder (PTSD) [2]. These disorders share characteristics of excessive, disproportionate, and persistent worries and fears that interfere with activities of daily living. Biological, psychological, or cultural approaches have proposed different models in an attempt to identify the nature and conditions in which these disorders develop [2–4]. The biological approach suggests that particular genes and deficits of some neurotransmitters, such as serotonin, could be the cause of certain emotional disorders [5,6]. Accordingly, some people show greater vulnerability to developing ADs [7]. The psychological approach emphasizes fear learning processes associated with threat detection and defensive responses [3]. In this sense, theories about Pavlovian conditioning have had the greatest explanatory power [8].

Neuroimaging techniques have made it possible to identify the neurobiological substrates underlying ADs [9]. The neural basis of fear, in particular, has been extensively studied [10,11]. Fear not only implies a defensive response to a threatening stimulus but also a subjective experience of fear [8]. Fear neural systems are associated with the functional interaction of subcortical (amygdala, thalamus, and basal ganglia) and cortical (insular cortex, anterior cingulate cortex (ACC), OFC, and PFC) regions [12]. In functional studies, the left amygdala and insula, as well as the left dorsolateral PFC, left ACC, and fusiform gyrus, have shown greater brain activity in individuals with phobia, suggesting a double processing of phobic stimuli: a rapid emotional processing pathway through the limbic areas and a slow pathway involving an interaction of the limbic (emotional) and frontal (rational) areas [11]. Hence, imbalanced limbic-prefrontal processing is associated with a failure to regulate emotions, which may, in turn, contribute to maintaining fear [13]. Studies on transcranial magnetic stimulation have shown that fear lessens when the dorsolateral PFC is stimulated [14]. The stimulation of this area seems to prevent the reconsolidation of fear memory. However, the pathophysiology of ADs remains an ongoing debate, since the processes underlying anxiety and fear-related disorders are more complex. In fact, common and specific factors have been identified with the various diagnoses related to anxiety to the extent that different features of the phobic stimulus activate different brain areas. Thus, stimuli presenting near activated areas were associated with a motor response, whereas a greater number of phobic stimuli activated sensory areas [15], suggesting a different emotion regulation strategy.

Therefore, the main focus of this study was to deepen current understanding of neuromorphometric abnormalities in participants with SP. Voxel-based morphometry (VBM) studies provide additional information to functional studies on the emergence and maintenance of ADs; in other words, identifying neuroanatomical abnormalities of brain development could explain the pathologic condition [16]. The procedure mainly applied is gray matter volume (GMV) analysis. Thus, alterations in brain structures associated with dysfunctions in the processing and regulation of emotion, as well as fear conditioning processes, can be explored. In this regard, contradictory results have been found for both larger and smaller GMV in the areas traditionally linked to ADs [17–20]. Smaller subcortical and larger cortical GMVs have been associated with social anxiety disorder (SAD) compared with healthy controls [21,22]. In particular, reductions in GMV in the right thalamus, the left parahippocampus, and the bilateral putamen were found in SAD [22,23]. A reverse pattern of larger subcortical and smaller cortical GMVs has also been reported [24]. Specifically, an increased right putamen volume, and decreased lateral/medial PFC and left insula volumes have been found in generalized anxiety disorder (GAD) compared with fear-related AD [19]. Furthermore, smaller volume and altered activity patterns of the ventromedial PFC have been observed in patients with ADs [25]. On the other hand, a different pattern was revealed of both smaller cortical, such as PFC and temporal-parietal cortices, and subcortical GMVs, such as the striatum, thalamus and brain stem, in anxiety and panic disorder versus healthy controls [20,26]. The larger volume of cortical areas has been interpreted as a result of greater efforts to regulate emotions in individuals with AD. The smaller volume of subcortical areas, however, has been related to greater sensitivity to emotional stimuli and sustained emotional dysregulation that may lead to the progressive impairment of these areas [22]. Conversely, a smaller volume of cortical areas has been interpreted as deficits in top-down control [19], and a larger GMV of subcortical areas, such as the putamen, could facilitate the saliency of stimuli and be associated with fear conditioning [27].

Despite the findings on the structural alterations underlying ADs, the data are inconclusive, and studies on SPs are scant. To our knowledge, few morphometric studies on SPs have been reported. Spider-phobic individuals show smaller left amygdala volume than healthy controls [28]. In addition, the dorsomedial and dorsolateral PFC volume of individuals with dental phobia is smaller than that of non-phobic controls [29]. However, Hilbert et al. [30] found increased GMVs in left medial OFC, right subgenual ACC, and areas in the occipital cortex and cerebellum in individuals with dental and snake phobia compared with non-phobic controls. The greatest structural differences appeared between the group with dental phobia and the control group, mainly with increased GMV in OFC, dorsomedial PFC, subgenual ACC, occipital cortex, as well as the insula. Therefore, it seems that dental phobia requires more cognitive anxiety and fear processing compared to animal phobias. By contrast, in another study no statistically significant differences in GMV were found between individuals with dental phobia and healthy controls [31].

In the light of these findings, a significant heterogeneity for the brain structures involved in several ADs has been noted across studies. Moreover, the dearth of studies in SPs and the reduced number of participants highlight the need for further exploration of the VBM of the brain areas involved in SPs. The main aim of this study was to analyze whether the GMV of brain areas responsible for the acquisition and maintenance of fear was different between individuals with an SP of small animals (cockroaches, spider, mouses, and lizards) compared with non-fearful controls. The GMV of brain areas could be a cue of greater vulnerability to anxiety and fear-related disorders.

2. Materials and Methods

2.1. Participants

Participants included in the sample were 62 adults (21% male and 79% female) resident in Tenerife (Canary Islands, Spain) who were assigned to one of two groups: 31 were diagnosed with small animal phobia (19.4% males, ranging in age from 19 to 56 years, mean age = 35.16 years, SD = 11.10) and 31 were non-fearful controls (22.6% males, ranging in age from 18 to 41 years, mean age = 22.00 years, SD = 5.09).

2.2. Instruments

The Composite International Diagnostic Interview (CIDI), Version 2.1 [32], was used to test the diagnosis of phobia, and questions were asked about an SP, agoraphobia, social phobia, and panic attacks. In addition, participants' sociodemographic features (sex and age) were assessed.

The S–R (Situation–Response) Inventory of Anxiousness [33] was administered to participants of both groups with and without phobia. This inventory was composed of 14 items with a 5-point Likert-type scale that assessed the most frequent symptoms (i.e., physiological, cognitive, and behavioral) associated with the response to an anxiogenic stimulus (i.e., cockroaches, spiders, lizards or mice). The inventory showed high internal consistency (0.95) and adequate convergent validity [34].

The Edinburgh Handedness Inventory [35] was used to determine that all participants were right-handed.

2.3. Design

A cross-sectional quasi-experimental design was carried out to assess the GMV of brain areas responsible for the acquisition and maintenance of fear in small animal phobia in individuals with phobia and non-fearful controls. A whole-brain voxel-wise analysis was performed to identify the brain regions in which there were structural differences between both groups.

All participants were right-handed, and none had any visual problems. The sample with phobia fulfills the following inclusion criteria: participants showed no impediment to undergoing a magnetic resonance imaging (MRI) session; all were adults with a diagnosis of SP, according to the scores in questionnaires on SP and anxiety and through a clinical interview, and were receiving no treatment for SP at the time of the study; the phobia had to be the primary psychological disorder that could not be explained by another health condition. The inclusion criteria for sample non-fearful controls were the same as for the phobia group, except that their score in the assessment questionnaire on SP was low.

2.4. Procedure

Participants with phobia were recruited from April to July 2018 through advertisements in the press, on websites, with flyers, and on TV. Concurrently, the control group was made up of psychology students who voluntarily participated in the research, which granted them additional credit in the subjects taught by the researchers. The procedure was explained to participants before they gave their informed consent. In morphometric experimental studies with ADs, there is some variability in terms of sample size. In a meta-analysis study in which 24 papers were identified, only four slightly exceeded 30 participants per group [24]. Particularly in the case of SPs, the sample size is usually below the 30 subjects for each experimental and control group [30,31]. In this study, the effect size was calculated through r^2 for each of the differences found between the groups to identify the power of the study. This study adhered to the ethical standards of the Declaration of Helsinki and was approved by the Ethics Committee for Research and Animal Welfare of the University of La Laguna (CEIBA2013-0086).

2.5. MRI Data Acquisition

Whole-brain structural and functional MRI images were acquired on a 3.0 T MR scanner (GE 3.0T Sigma Excite HD) with a 12-channel head coil. During the scans, the subjects were instructed to keep their eyes closed, to relax but not to sleep, and to lie as still as possible. High-resolution three-dimensional T1-weighted images were acquired: repetition time (TR)/echo time (TE) = 8852 ms/1756 ms, flip angle = 10°, 172 sagittal slices, slice thickness = 1 mm, field of view (FOV) = 256 × 256 mm^2, data matrix = 256 × 256 × 172, the voxel size was 1 × 1 × 1 mm and TI = 650 ms. Each scan was inspected by an experienced neuroradiologist to rule out visible movement artifacts and gross structural abnormalities before image processing.

2.6. MRI Processing

Processing of structural images was performed using the Computational Anatomy Toolbox for Statistical Parametric Mapping software (CAT12 for SPM12; http://www.fil.ion.ucl.ac.uk/spm/ (accessed on 1 September 2022)) [36]. First, all MRI images were manually reoriented on the anterior posterior commissure line for better registration. Second, the high-resolutionT1-weighted images were segmented into gray matter (GM), white matter and cerebral spinal fluid in CAT12. The GMV were analyzed using VBM. T2 images were obtained at the end of the protocol, in the event of a clinical finding appearing by chance. Third, registered images were transformed to the MNI space using the FORWARD strategy that allows for data to be transformed to MNI coordinates. The GM data were aligned and modulated for the preservation of GMV and smoothed with an 8 mm full width at half-maximum Gaussian kernel, using SPM12 [37]. After the normalized modulation, the resulting modulated images were preserved for the total amount of the GM signal, and the total TIV was applied as a correction measure.

2.7. Statistical Analysis

2.7.1. Demographic and Clinical Data Analyses

The differences between groups in the demographic, normalization measure, and clinical data were conducted through a chi-square test for discrete variables (i.e., sex) and two-sample t-tests for continuous variables (i.e., age, total intracranial volume, TIV, SR), using IBM SPSS Statistics 25. The TIV was calculated as the sum of GMVs, white matter, and cerebrospinal fluid.

2.7.2. VBM Analyses

The between-group differences in GMV were examined using VBM [38]. Whole-brain voxel-wise comparisons of GMV between groups were performed using two-sample t-tests to compare participants with and without phobia, using age, sex, and TIV as covariates in CAT12. The Gaussian random field theory [39,40] was performed to control for multiple comparisons with a significance threshold of a voxel-wise value of $p < 0.001$ and cluster probability of $p < 0.05$ [41]. In addition, all reported results were corrected for multiple comparisons using the false discovery rate (FDR). To assess the differences in total GMV between both groups with and without phobia, an ANOVA was used. Pearson correlation coefficients were calculated to evaluate the relationship between total GMV and SR scores.

Nevertheless, an ANCOVA was applied to contrast the GMV between both phobic and non-fearful control groups, and to control for SR scores and age.

3. Results

3.1. Demographic, Normalization, and Clinical Characteristics

Significant differences between with and without phobia groups appeared in terms of age (group with phobia: mean = 35.16, SD = 11.11; group without phobia: mean = 22, SD = 5.09, t (60) = 6, $p < 0.001$) and anxiety symptoms (group with phobia: mean = 38.65, SD = 6.94; group without phobia: mean = 4.45, SD = 0.80, t (60) = 21.63, $p < 0.001$). The participants with phobia had significantly higher scores for anxiety symptoms and were older than those without phobia. Moreover, there were no significant differences in TIV—the normalization measure—between the two groups with and without phobia (group with phobia mean = 1466.29 cm^3, SD = 26.27 cm^3; group without phobia mean = 1515.39 cm^3, SD = 154.41 cm^3; t (60) = −1.27, $p = 0.209$). However, differences were found between males and females in TIV ($F_{1,60} = 19.843$, $p < 0.001$, mean males = 1636.23 cm^3, SD = 135.789 cm^3; mean females = 1452.61 cm^3, SD = 131.195 cm^3).

3.2. Groups Differences in GMV

Significant differences between with and without phobia groups appeared in total GMV (group with phobia: mean = 673,26 cm^3, SD = 70.85 cm^3; group without phobia: mean = 718.81 cm^3, SD = 62.49 cm^3, $F_{1,60} = 7.20$, $p = 0.009$). Total GMV correlated negatively with SR scores (r = −0.384, $p = 0.002$). ANCOVA revealed no significant effects of SR or age and did not exceed the cut-off point for considering them statistically significant ($F_{1,60} = 33.56$, $p < 0.05$). The whole-brain voxel-wise analysis showed that, compared with individuals without phobia, individuals with phobia had significantly smaller GMV in the right insula (t (60) = 5.18, $p < 0.001$); a cluster of right lateral, anterior, and inferior OFC (t (60) = 4.98, $p < 0.001$); a cluster of left posterior, medial, and lateral OFC, and left insula (t (60) = 4.86, $p < 0.001$); and a cluster of left superior medial frontal, right superior frontal, and right ACC (t (60) = 4.48, $p < 0.001$) (Table 1 and Figure 1). In all contrasts, the effect size was moderate.

Table 1. GMV differences between individuals with phobia and non-fearful controls.

Brain Structures	**MNI Coordinates**			k	t	*p*	r^2
	x	y	z				
Non-fearful controls > Individuals with phobia							
R Insula	45	9	−9	961	5.18	<0.001	0.31
R Lateral OFC R Anterior OFC R Inferior OFC	24	48	−21	948	4.98	<0.001	0.29
L Posterior OFC L Middle OFC L Lateral OFC L Insula	−19	27	−13	2924	4.86	<0.001	0.28
L Superior Medial Frontal R ACC R Superior Frontal	−25	51	28	7104	4.48	<0.001	0.25
Individuals with phobia > Non-fearful controls							
L Putamen	−26	−15	15	60	3.58	<0.001	0.18

Note: L = Left, R = Right, OFC = Orbitofrontal cortex, ACC = Anterior cingulate cortex, k = Cluster size, t = Peak of t score, *p* = Probability for peak voxel (FDR corr.), r^2 = effect size.

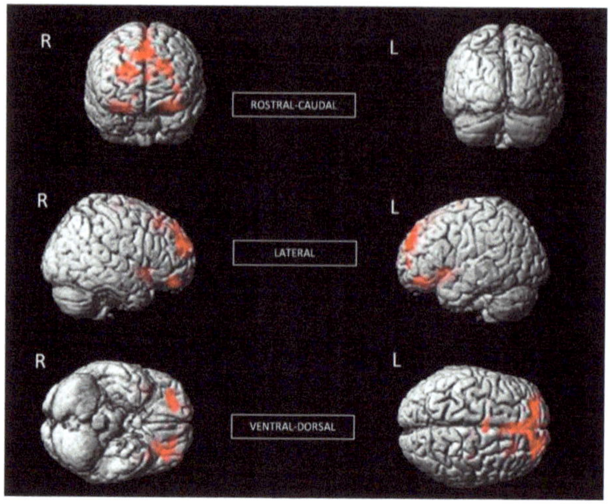

Figure 1. Significant differences in GMV of brain regions between non-fearful controls (larger) and individuals with phobia (corrected with Gaussian random field theory with a significance threshold of a voxel-wise value of $p < 0.001$ and cluster probability of $p < 0.05$).

Additionally, individuals with phobia showed a larger GMV in the left putamen than non-fearful controls (t (60) = 3.48, $p < 0.001$) (Table 1 and Figure 2), with a moderate effect size. The putamen is related to complex motor regulation and the facilitation of different types of learning.

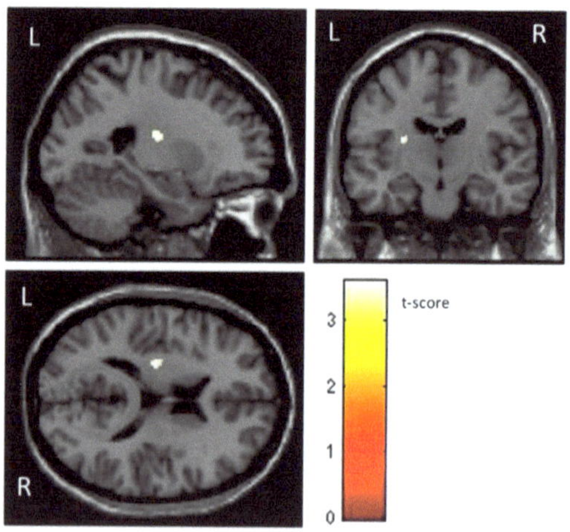

Figure 2. Significant differences in GMV of the putamen between individuals with phobia (larger) and non-fearful controls (corrected with Gaussian random field theory with a significance threshold of a voxel-wise value of $p < 0.001$ and cluster probability of $p < 0.05$). T-score is represented on a color bar.

4. Discussion

The aim of this study was to analyze whether certain areas responsible for acquiring and maintaining fear were structurally different between individuals with small animal specific phobia and non-fearful controls. The morphometric differences could suggest a greater vulnerability of phobic individuals to acquiring non-adaptive conditioned responses. Accordingly, individuals with small animal specific phobia showed smaller GMVs in cortical regions, such as the OFC and medial frontal cortex, and greater GMVs in the putamen than participants without phobia. The superior/medial frontal areas and ACC are involved in the elaboration of strategies for problem-solving and emotional regulation, while the OFC exerts cognitive control by reducing automatic responses from the amygdala, and the insula integrates interoceptive information.

Morphometric analysis revealed that a cluster of superior/medial frontal areas and ACC were diminished in phobic participants. In the same vein, decreased volumes in the lateral/medial PFC cortex have been found in GAD and panic disorder [19,26]. However, an increased volume in the left PFC, OFC, and ACC has been found when individuals with phobia were compared with non-fearful controls [30]. The superior/medial frontal areas and ACC are involved in planning and creating strategies for problem-solving and emotional regulation [42]. Therefore, decreased volume in these areas could be interpreted as an alteration to emotional regulation strategy planning to reduce fear in the face of the negative impact of phobias. These results should be interpreted with caution, because individuals with phobia could have a smaller innate GMV in these areas and therefore experience fear when confronted with a phobic stimulus (cause), or the continuous avoidance of such phobic stimuli could potentially lead to brain structure changes (consequence).

Additionally, our results showed smaller OFC and insula volumes in individuals with phobias compared with non-fearful controls, which is consistent with previous studies [19]. An increased GMV of the OFC has been associated with a high capacity for emotional self-regulation [43]. The OFC is responsible for top-down processes, exerting cognitive control by reducing automatic responses from the amygdala [44,45]. In young adults with social anxiety, an altered amygdala–orbitofrontal functional connectivity explains the effort of the PFC to control amygdala overactivity [46]. On the other hand, according to the fear network model, the insula integrates interoceptive information [47]. Taken together, the findings indicate that individuals with phobia would have difficulty integrating external information that would enhance learning new behaviors and would be carried away by the automatic triggers of emotion. Recent research suggests that the salience network and inhibitory control are altered in ADs [48]. Thus, individuals with phobia assign greater importance to the emotion generated by the feared stimulus than the regulatory mechanisms. Indeed, interventions based on exposure to the feared stimulus support the functional importance of the PFC which could suggest an attempt at emotional regulation or even the activity of other cognitive processes involved [49]. Therefore, phobias could be better explained by a model focusing on the control exerted by frontal areas as opposed to the dual model that emphasizes the effect of the deactivation of limbic areas.

However, in our study we found no significant GMV differences in amygdala. In this line, a meta-analysis reported no variations in the volume of the amygdala of individuals with SAD compared with healthy controls [22]. However, it did indicate diminished amygdala GMV in patients with spider phobia associated with higher anxiety symptom severity [28] and in GAD patients [50]. Treatment studies applying cognitive behavior therapy for SAD patients revealed a reduced GMV in amygdala and PFC, parietal–occipital regions after intervention [51]. Although functional studies found that interventions with exposure to real and virtual phobic stimuli were effective in decreasing anxiety responses and brain prefrontal activity after treatment, the amygdala remained activated [52].

Furthermore, the most striking finding of this study was a larger left putamen GMV that might be specific to phobias. This structure is related to complex motor regulation and the facilitation of different types of learning, namely, the operational learning associated with avoidance behavior [53]. Although most studies indicate a smaller putamen in ADs [20,22], a larger putamen volume has been identified in GAD [54] and SAD [27] compared with healthy controls. An increased putamen volume has also been found in individuals with anxious vulnerability [19,55]. During structural maturation in the brain, larger GMVs might reflect a lack of synaptic pruning and myelination, which could interfere with the efficiency of the corresponding psychological processes involved in this brain area [56]. Taken together, these results suggest that a pre-existing altered volume in certain brain areas could link learning impairment to anxious-fearful stimuli. Some authors suggest that atrophy in PFC areas could be a biomarker of vulnerability for the occurrence of ADs. The smaller size of these areas could interfere with emotional processing through top-down executive control mechanisms maintaining fear in the presence of the phobic stimulus [24]. Therefore, neurodevelopmental vulnerabilities would lead to the emergence of the disorder in the year prior to adolescence [7]. On the other hand, the increased putamen volume may be due to increased reactivity to threat cues or resistance to extinction. A possible explanation is that lengthy reinforcement of the behavior of escape from phobic stimulus would lead to a larger putamen volume [57]. In small animal phobia, cognitive behavioral therapy has shown efficacy in changing the emotional response, resulting in decreased severity of anxiety, as well as a reduced volume in brain areas, such as the supplementary motor area and PFC [31,52].

4.1. Limitations and Future Directions

This study has several limitations. First, the sample is small, and male individuals are underrepresented. In any case, the prevalence of phobias is more than double in females than in males [58]. Moreover, previous studies on GAD found no gender differences in GMVs [54]. Second, although both participant groups differed in age, most participants were over 20 years old. Hence brain maturity had already been reached. The GM volume increases until the age of four to six years, with development peaking at four years, whereas white matter increases until the age of 20 [59]. In the same line, Lebel et al. [60] found that deep GM structures, such as the putamen, thalamus, caudate nucleus, and globus pallidus reach maturity between 21 and 24 years. Although cortical and subcortical volume has also been found to decrease with age after the peaks [61]. However, in our study the total age span of both groups was similar so it is unlikely that a decrease in GM volume could occur due to the time course. In addition, the decrease in GMV was observed in specific areas linked to emotional regulation and appeared in the control group which was the youngest. Third, this study has not distinguished between different subtypes of animal phobias or recorded the possible comorbidity with other ADs. The results should therefore be taken with caution. Structural alterations may reflect neuroanatomical variations between different types of ADs [19]. Fourth, since the study is cross-sectional, the structural differences between individuals with phobia and non-fearful controls would be due to the pathogenesis of the disorder, a consequence of the disorder or other uncontrolled factors. Future research is needed to identify the structural changes and functional connectivity in order to establish a model that will explain both the shared elements and those specific to each type of phobia. It would be interesting to develop more precise techniques to identify structural variations in cortical and subcortical areas in fear-related disorders.

4.2. Conclusions

In sum, from our knowledge, this study is the first to examine the volumetric differences between participants with small animal phobia and non-fearful controls. The findings support the importance of the PFC regulatory role and the insula to a greater extent than limbic system deactivation. In other words, non-fearful controls showed a larger cortical GMV in areas associated with emotional regulation than individuals with phobia, although the subcortical areas linked to the limbic system showed no differences between either group (except for small differences in the putamen). Our findings have theoretical implications which contribute to a better understanding of the mechanisms underlying phobias that emphasize the predominant role of the PFC and the insula in fear regulation, both of which are diminished in individuals with phobia. On the other hand, brain areas linked to operational learning barely showed volumetric differences. These results would imply that specific phobia acquisition depends more on emotional regulatory processes than an alteration in areas associated with non-adaptive learning processes. The practical implications of these findings could be to improve the development of neuroimaging-based diagnostic markers to support clinical decisions, thereby improving diagnosis and prognosis. The prediction of an adaptive clinical response will depend on the different neural mechanisms involved in the conscious experience of fear, as well as in the defensive reaction to threat.

Supplementary Materials: The following supporting information can be downloaded at: https://drive.google.com/drive/folders/1wVOdPCafjJWesA_iqVgl84rffCCfrWad?usp=sharing (accessed on 25 July 2022).

Author Contributions: Conceptualization, methodology, formal analysis, and writing—original draft preparation: F.R., R.J.M., T.O., W.P., Y.Á.-P., J.M.B. and A.F.; project administration and funding acquisition: W.P. All authors have read and agreed to the published version of the manuscript.

Funding: This research was funded by the Ministry of Science, Innovation, and Universities of Spain, projects PSI2013-42912-R and PSI2017-83222-R, and by the European Commission, project E-MOTION 1808341802 Erasmus project.

Institutional Review Board Statement: This study was approved by the Research Ethics and Animal Welfare Committee of the University of La Laguna (Reference CEIBA2017-0245, dated 21 July 2017) and conducted according to the guidelines of the Helsinki Declaration (2008).

Informed Consent Statement: Informed consent was obtained from all subjects involved in the study.

Data Availability Statement: The data presented in this study are available in the Supplementary Materials.

Acknowledgments: The authors thank the participants, therapists, and MRI technical team (SEGAI) for their participation and involvement in this study.

Conflicts of Interest: The authors declare no conflict of interest.

References

1. Santomauro, D.F.; Herrera, A.M.M.; Shadid, J.; Zheng, P.; Ashbaugh, C.; Pigott, D.M.; Hay, S.I.; Vos, T.; Murray, C.J.L.; Whiteford, H.A.; et al. Global prevalence and burden of depressive and anxiety disorders in 204 countries and territories in 2020 due to the COVID-19 pandemic. *Lancet* **2021**, *398*, 1700–1712. [CrossRef]
2. Craske, M.G.; Rauch, S.L.; Ursano, R.; Prenoveau, J.; Pine, D.S.; Zinbarg, R.E. What is an anxiety disorder? *Focus* **2011**, *9*, 369–388. [CrossRef]
3. Olatunji, B. *The Cambridge Handbook of Anxiety and Related Disorders*; Cambridge University Press: Cambridge, UK, 2019.
4. Mah, L.; Szabuniewicz, C.; Fiocco, A.J. Can anxiety damage the brain? *Curr. Opin. Psychiatry* **2016**, *29*, 56–63. [CrossRef]
5. Mufford, M.S.; van der Meer, D.; Andreassen, O.A.; Ramesar, R.; Stein, D.J.; Dalvie, S. A review of systems biology research of anxiety disorders. *Braz. J. Psychiatry.* **2020**, *43*, 414–423. [CrossRef]
6. Tanaka, M.; Bohár, Z.; Martos, D.; Telegdy, G.; Vécsei, L. Antidepressant-like effects of kynurenic acid in a modified forced swim test. *Pharmacol. Rep.* **2020**, *72*, 449–455. [CrossRef]
7. Vargas, T.G.; Mittal, V.A. Brain morphometry points to emerging patterns of psychosis, depression, and anxiety vulnerability over a 2-year period in childhood. *Psychol. Med.* **2022**, 1–13. [CrossRef]
8. Zhou, F.; Zhao, W.; Qi, Z.; Geng, Y.; Yao, S.; Kendrick, K.M.; Wager, T.D.; Becker, B. A distributed fMRI-based signature for the subjective experience of fear. *Nat. Commun.* **2021**, *12*, 1–16. [CrossRef]
9. Holzschneider, K.; Mulert, C. Neuroimaging in anxiety disorders. *Dialogues Clin. Neurosci.* **2022**, *13*, 453–461. [CrossRef]
10. Madonna, D.; Delvecchio, G.; Soares, J.C.; Brambilla, P. Structural and functional neuroimaging studies in generalized anxiety disorder: A systematic review. *Braz. J. Psychiatry* **2019**, *41*, 336–362. [CrossRef]
11. Peñate, W.; Fumero, A.; Viña, C.; Herrero, M.; Marrero, R.J.; Rivero, F. A meta-analytic review of neuroimaging studies of specific phobia to small animals. *Eur. J. Psychiatry* **2017**, *31*, 23–36. [CrossRef]
12. Ipser, J.C.; Singh, L.; Stein, D.J. Meta-analysis of functional brain imaging in specific phobia. *Psychiatry Clin. Neurosci.* **2013**, *67*, 311–322. [CrossRef] [PubMed]
13. Wittfoth, D.; Beise, J.; Manuel, J.; Bohne, M.; Wittfoth, M. Bifocal emotion regulation through acupoint tapping in fear of flying. *Neuroimage Clin.* **2022**, *34*, 102996. [CrossRef] [PubMed]
14. Borgomaneri, S.; Battaglia, S.; Avenanti, A.; di Pellegrino, G. Don't Hurt Me No More: State-dependent Transcranial Magnetic Stimulation for the treatment of specific phobia. *J. Affect. Disord.* **2021**, *286*, 78–79. [CrossRef] [PubMed]
15. Fumero, A.; Marrero, R.J.; Rivero, F.; Alvarez-Pérez, Y.; Bethencourt, J.M.; González, M.; Peñate, W. Neuronal Correlates of Small Animal Phobia in Human Subjects through fMRI: The Role of the Number and Proximity of Stimuli. *Life* **2021**, *11*, 275. [CrossRef]
16. Ashburner, J.; Friston, K.J. Why voxel-based morphometry should be used. *Neuroimage* **2001**, *14*, 1238–1243. [CrossRef]

17. Brandl, F.; Weise, B.; Mulej Bratec, S.; Jassim, N.; Hoffmann-Ayala, D.; Bertram, T.; Ploner, M.; Sorg, C. Common and specific large-scale brain changes in major depressive disorder, anxiety disorders, and chronic pain: A transdiagnostic multimodal meta-analysis of structural and functional MRI studies. *Neuropsychopharmacology* **2022**, *47*, 1071–1080. [CrossRef]
18. Kolesar, T.A.; Bilevicius, E.; Wilson, A.D.; Kornelsen, J. Systematic review and meta-analyses of neural structural and functional differences in generalized anxiety disorder and healthy controls using magnetic resonance imaging. *Neuroimage Clin.* **2019**, *24*, 102016. [CrossRef]
19. Liu, X.; Klugah-Brown, B.; Zhang, R.; Chen, H.; Zhang, J.; Becker, B. Pathological fear, anxiety and negative affect exhibit distinct neurostructural signatures: Evidence from psychiatric neuroimaging meta-analysis. *Transl. Psychiatry* **2022**, *12*, 1–19. [CrossRef]
20. Wang, X.; Cheng, B.; Wang, S.; Lu, F.; Luo, Y.; Long, X.; Kong, D. Distinct grey matter volume alterations in adult patients with panic disorder and social anxiety disorder: A systematic review and voxel-based morphometry meta-analysis. *J. Affect. Disord.* **2021**, *281*, 805–823. [CrossRef]
21. Tükel, R.; Aydın, K.; Yüksel, Ç.; Ertekin, E.; Koyuncu, A.; Taş, C. Gray matter abnormalities in patients with social anxiety disorder: A voxel-based morphometry study. *Psychiatry Res. Neuroimaging* **2015**, *234*, 106–112. [CrossRef]
22. Wang, X.; Cheng, B.; Luo, Q.; Qiu, L.; Wang, S. Gray matter structural alterations in social anxiety disorder: A voxel-based meta-analysis. *Front. Psychiatry* **2018**, *9*, 449. [CrossRef] [PubMed]
23. Zhang, X.; Suo, X.; Yang, X.; Lai, H.; Pan, N.; He, M.; Li, Q.; Kuang, W.; Wang, S.; Gong, Q. Structural and functional deficits and couplings in the cortico-striato-thalamo-cerebellar circuitry in social anxiety disorder. *Transl. Psychiatry* **2022**, *12*, 1–11. [CrossRef]
24. Shang, J.; Fu, Y.; Ren, Z.; Zhang, T.; Du, M.; Gong, Q.; Lui, S.; Zhang, W. The common traits of the ACC and PFC in anxiety disorders in the DSM-5: Meta-analysis of voxel-based morphometry studies. *PLoS ONE* **2014**, *9*, e93432. [CrossRef]
25. Battaglia, S.; Harrison, B.J.; Fullana, M.A. Does the human ventromedial prefrontal cortex support fear learning, fear extinction or both? A commentary on subregional contributions. *Mol. Psychiatry.* **2022**, *27*, 784–786. [CrossRef] [PubMed]
26. Serra-Blasco, M.; Radua, J.; Soriano-Mas, C.; Gómez-Benlloch, A.; Porta-Casteràs, D.; Carulla-Roig, M.; Albajes-Eizagirre, A.; Arnone, D.; Klauser, P.; Canales-Rodríguez, E.J.; et al. Structural brain correlates in major depression, anxiety disorders and post-traumatic stress disorder: A voxel-based morphometry meta-analysis. *Neurosci. Biobehav. Rev.* **2021**, *129*, 269–281. [CrossRef]
27. Bas-Hoogendam, J.M.; van Steenbergen, H.; Pannekoek, J.N.; Fouche, J.P.; Lochner, C.; Hattingh, C.J.; Henk, R.; Cremers, H.R.; Furmark, T.; Månsson, K.N.T.; et al. Voxel-based morphometry multi-center mega-analysis of brain structure in social anxiety disorder. *Neuroimage Clin.* **2017**, *16*, 678–688. [CrossRef]
28. Fisler, M.S.; Federspiel, A.; Horn, H.; Dierks, T.; Schmitt, W.; Wiest, R.; Quervain, D.; Soravia, L.M. Spider phobia is associated with decreased left amygdala volume: A cross-sectional study. *BMC Psychiatry* **2013**, *13*, 1–7. [CrossRef]
29. Wabnegger, A.; Scharmüller, W.; Schienle, A. Sex-specific associations between grey matter volume and phobic symptoms in dental phobia. *Neurosci. Lett.* **2014**, *580*, 83–87. [CrossRef]
30. Hilbert, K.; Evens, R.; Maslowski, N.I.; Wittchen, H.U.; Lueken, U. Neurostructural correlates of two subtypes of specific phobia: A voxel-based morphometry study. *Psychiatry Res. Neuroimaging* **2015**, *231*, 168–175. [CrossRef]
31. Schienle, A.; Scharmüller, W.; Leutgeb, V.; Schäfer, A.; Stark, R. Sex differences in the functional and structural neuroanatomy of dental phobia. *Brain Struct. Funct.* **2013**, *218*, 779–787. [CrossRef]
32. Kessler, R.C.; Üstün, T.B. The world mental health (WMH) survey initiative version of the world health organization (WHO) composite international diagnostic interview (CIDI). *Int. J. Meth. Psych. Res.* **2004**, *13*, 93–121. [CrossRef] [PubMed]
33. Endler, N.S.; Hunt, J.M.; Rosenstein, A.J. An S-R Inventory of Anxiousness. *Psychol. Monogr.* **1962**, *76*, 143–146. [CrossRef]
34. Kameoka, V.A.; Tanaka-Matsumi, J. The appropriateness of using the S-R Inventory of Anxiousness to measure sources ofbehavioral variability. *Appl. Psych. Meas.* **1981**, *5*, 229–235. [CrossRef]
35. Oldfield, R. The assessment and analysis of handedness: The Edinburgh inventory. *Neuropsychologia* **1971**, *9*, 97–113. [CrossRef]
36. Ashburner, J.; Friston, K.J. Unified segmentation. *Neuroimage* **2005**, *26*, 839–851. [CrossRef] [PubMed]
37. Ashburner, J. A fast diffeomorphic image registration algorithm. *Neuroimage* **2007**, *38*, 95–113. [CrossRef] [PubMed]
38. Ashburner, J.; Friston, K.J. Voxel-based morphometry—The methods. *Neuroimage* **2000**, *11*, 805–821. [CrossRef]
39. Friston, K.J.; Worsley, K.J.; Frackowiak, R.S.; Mazziotta, J.C.; Evans, A.C. Assessing the significance of focal activations using their spatial extent. *Hum. Brain Mapp.* **1994**, *1*, 210–220. [CrossRef]
40. Nichols, T.; Hayasaka, S. Controlling the familywise error rate in functional neuroimaging: A comparative review. *Stat. Methods Med. Res.* **2003**, *12*, 419–446. [CrossRef]
41. Worsley, K.J.; Marrett, S.; Neelin, P.; Vandal, A.C.; Friston, K.; Evans, A.C. A unified statistical approach for determining significant signals in images of cerebral activation. *Hum. Brain Mapp.* **1996**, *4*, 58–73. [CrossRef]
42. Cohen, M.X.; Heller, A.S.; Ranganath, C. Functional connectivity with anterior cingulate and orbitofrontal cortices during decision-making. *Cog. Brain Res.* **2005**, *23*, 61–70. [CrossRef]
43. Petrovic, P.; Ekman, C.J.; Klahr, J.; Tigerström, L.; Rydén, G.; Johansson, A.G.; Sellgren, C.; Golkar, A.; Olsson, A.; Öhman, A.; et al. Significant grey matter changes in a region of the orbitofrontal cortex in healthy participants predicts emotional dysregulation. *Soc. Cogn. Affect. Neurosci.* **2016**, *11*, 1041–1049. [CrossRef] [PubMed]
44. Adhikari, A.; Lerner, T.N.; Finkelstein, J.; Pak, S.; Jennings, J.H.; Davidson, T.J.; Ferenczi, E.; Gunaydin, L.A.; Mirzabekov, J.J.; Ye, L.; et al. Basomedial amygdala mediates top-down control of anxiety and fear. *Nature* **2015**, *527*, 179–185. [CrossRef] [PubMed]

45. Blackmon, K.; Barr, W.B.; Carlson, C.; Devinsky, O.; DuBois, J.; Pogash, D.; Quinn, B.T.; Kuzniecky, R.; Halgren, E.; Thesen, T. Structural evidence for involvement of a left amygdala-orbitofrontal network in subclinical anxiety. *Psychiatry Res. Neuroimaging* **2011**, *194*, 296–303. [CrossRef] [PubMed]
46. Hasler, G.; Haynes, M.; Müller, S.T.; Tuura, R.; Ritter, C.; Buchmann, A. The association between adolescent residential mobility and adult social anxiety, BDNF and amygdala-orbitofrontal functional connectivity in young adults with higher education. *Front. Psychiatry.* **2020**, *11*, 561464. [CrossRef] [PubMed]
47. Lai, C.H. Fear network model in panic disorder: The past and the future. *Psychiatry Investig.* **2019**, *16*, 16–26. [CrossRef]
48. Xiong, H.; Guo, R.J.; Shi, H.W. Altered default mode network and salience network functional connectivity in patients with generalized anxiety disorders: An ICA-based resting-state fMRI study. *Evid. Based Complement. Altern. Med.* **2020**, *2020*, 4048916. [CrossRef] [PubMed]
49. Fumero, A.; Marrero, R.J.; Olivares, T.; Rivero, F.; Alvarez-Pérez, Y.; Pitti, C.; Peñate, W. Neuronal Activity during Exposure to Specific Phobia through fMRI: Comparing Therapeutic Components of Cognitive Behavioral Therapy. *Life* **2022**, *12*, 1132. [CrossRef]
50. Chen, Y.; Cui, Q.; Tang, Q.; Sheng, W.; Yang, Y.; Chen, H. Amygdala-Based Structural Covariance and Functional Connectivity Alterations in Patients with Generalized Anxiety Disorder. In Proceedings of the Fourth International Symposium on Image Computing and Digital Medicine, Shenyang, China, 5–7 December 2020; pp. 192–196. [CrossRef]
51. Steiger, V.R.; Brühl, A.B.; Weidt, S.; Delsignore, A.; Rufer, M.; Jäncke, L.; Herwig, U.; Hänggi, J. Pattern of structural brain changes in social anxiety disorder after cognitive behavioral group therapy: A longitudinal multimodal MRI study. *Mol. Psychiatry* **2017**, *22*, 1164–1171. [CrossRef]
52. Álvarez-Pérez, Y.; Rivero, F.; Herrero, M.; Viña, C.; Fumero, A.; Betancort, M.; Peñate, W. Changes in brain activation through cognitive-behavioral therapy with exposure to virtual reality: A neuroimaging study of specific phobia. *J. Clin. Med.* **2021**, *10*, 3505. [CrossRef]
53. Howells, F.M.; Hattingh, C.J.; Syal, S.; Breet, E.; Stein, D.J.; Lochner, C. 1H-magnetic resonance spectroscopy in social anxiety disorder. *Prog. Neuro-Psychopharmacol. Biol. Psychiatry.* **2015**, *58*, 97–104. [CrossRef] [PubMed]
54. Liao, M.; Yang, F.; Zhang, Y.; He, Z.; Su, L.; Li, L. Lack of gender effects on gray matter volumes in adolescent generalized anxiety disorder. *J. Affect. Disord.* **2014**, *155*, 278–282. [CrossRef] [PubMed]
55. Günther, V.; Ihme, K.; Kersting, A.; Hoffmann, K.T.; Lobsien, D.; Suslow, T. Volumetric associations between amygdala, nucleus accumbens, and socially anxious tendencies in healthy women. *Neuroscience* **2018**, *374*, 25–32. [CrossRef]
56. Kanai, R.; Rees, G. The structural basis of inter-individual differences in human behaviour and cognition. *Nat. Rev. Neurosci.* **2011**, *12*, 231–242. [CrossRef] [PubMed]
57. Hormigo, S.; Vega-Flores, G.; Castro-Alamancos, M.A. Basal ganglia output controls active avoidance behavior. *J. Neurosci.* **2016**, *36*, 10274–10284. [CrossRef]
58. Fredrikson, M.; Annas, P.; Fischer, H.; Wik, G. Gender and age differences in the prevalence of specific fears and phobias. *Behav. Res. Ther.* **1996**, *34*, 33–39. [CrossRef] [PubMed]
59. Pfefferbaum, A.; Mathalon, D.H.; Sullivan, E.V.; Rawles, J.M.; Zipursky, R.B.; Lim, K.O. A quantitative magnetic resonance imaging study of changes in brain morphology from infancy to late adulthood. *Arch. Neurol.* **1994**, *51*, 874–887. [CrossRef] [PubMed]
60. Lebel, C.; Walker, L.; Leemans, A.; Phillips, L.; Beaulieu, C. Microstructural maturation of the human brain from childhood to adulthood. *Neuroimage* **2008**, *40*, 1044–1055. [CrossRef]
61. Narvacan, K.; Treit, S.; Camicioli, R.; Martin, W.; Beaulieu, C. Evolution of deep gray matter volume across the human lifespan. *Hum. Brain Mapp.* **2017**, *38*, 3771–3790. [CrossRef] [PubMed]

life

Article

Lack of Skeletal Effects in Mice with Targeted Disruptionof Prolyl Hydroxylase Domain 1 (*Phd1*) Gene Expressed in Chondrocytes

Weirong Xing [1,2], Destiney Larkin [1], Sheila Pourteymoor [1], William Tambunan [1], Gustavo A. Gomez [1], Elaine K. Liu [1] and Subburaman Mohan [1,2,*]

1 Musculoskeletal Disease Center, Loma Linda VA Healthcare System, Loma Linda, CA 92357, USA
2 Department of Medicine, Loma Linda University, Loma Linda, CA 92354, USA
* Correspondence: subburaman.mohan@va.gov; Tel.: +1-909-825-7084 (ext. 6180); Fax: +1-909-796-1680

Abstract: The critical importance of hypoxia-inducible factor (HIF)s in the regulation of endochondral bone formation is now well established. HIF protein levels are closely regulated by the prolyl hydroxylase domain-containing protein (PHD) mediated ubiquitin-proteasomal degradation pathway. Of the three PHD family members expressed in bone, we previously showed that mice with conditional disruption of the *Phd2* gene in chondrocytes led to a massive increase in the trabecular bone mass of the long bones. By contrast, loss of *Phd3* expression in chondrocytes had no skeletal effects. To investigate the role of *Phd1* expressed in chondrocytes on skeletal development, we conditionally disrupted the *Phd1* gene in chondrocytes by crossing *Phd1 floxed* mice with *Collagen 2α1-Cre* mice for evaluation of a skeletal phenotype. At 12 weeks of age, neither body weight nor body length was significantly different in the Cre^{+}; $Phd1^{flox/flox}$ conditional knockout (cKO) mice compared to Cre^{-}; $Phd1^{flox/flox}$ wild-type (WT) control mice. Micro-CT measurements revealed significant gender differences in the trabecular bone volume adjusted for tissue volume at the secondary spongiosa of the femur and the tibia for both genotypes, but no genotype differences were found for any of the trabecular bone measurements of either femur or tibia. Similarly, cortical bone parameters were not affected in the *Phd1* cKO mice compared to control mice. Histomorphometric analyses revealed no significant differences in bone area, bone formation rate or mineral apposition rate in the secondary spongiosa of femurs between cKO and WT control mice. Loss of *Phd1* expression in chondrocytes did not affect the expression of markers of chondrocytes (*collage 2*, *collagen 10*) or osteoblasts (*alkaline phosphatase*, *bone sialoprotein*) in the bones of cKO mice. Based on these and our published data, we conclude that of the three PHD family members, only *Phd2* expressed in chondrocytes regulates endochondral bone formation and development of peak bone mass in mice.

Keywords: prolyl hydroxylase domain-containing protein; PHD protein; *Phd1* gene; osteoblast; chondrocyte; knockout mice; phenotype; hypoxia-inducible factor; endochondral bone formation

Citation: Xing, W.; Larkin, D.; Pourteymoor, S.; Tambunan, W.; Gomez, G.A.; Liu, E.K.; Mohan, S. Lack of Skeletal Effects in Mice with Targeted Disruptionof Prolyl Hydroxylase Domain 1 (*Phd1*) Gene Expressed in Chondrocytes. *Life* **2023**, *13*, 106. https://doi.org/10.3390/life13010106

Academic Editor: Nicola Smania

Received: 30 November 2022
Revised: 16 December 2022
Accepted: 28 December 2022
Published: 30 December 2022

1. Introduction

Previous studies have uncovered that the prolyl hydroxylase domain-containing proteins (PHDs) are negative regulators of the hypoxia-inducible transcription factor (HIF)1α [1,2]. The hydroxylation of specific proline residues (Pro-402 and Pro-564) in the C-terminal oxygen-dependent degradation domains of the HIF1α by PHDs, primarily the PHD2 isoform, leads to the targeting of HIF1α for ubiquitination through an E3 ligase complex initiated by the binding of the Von Hippel Lindau protein (pVHL) and subsequent proteasomal degradation [1,2]. When the oxygen level is low in the cells, the *Phd* gene expression is suppressed, and the HIF1α degradation is reduced and the protein is accumulated in the cytoplasm from where it traffics to nucleus and binds to HIF regulatory elements in the promoter regions of the hypoxia-responsive genes including VEGF, Runx2 and osterix to regulate the target gene expression and subsequently bone formation [3,4].

In mammals, PHD enzymes include PHD1, PHD2, and PHD3 [5]. Both PHD1 and PHD2 contain more than 400 amino acid residues while PHD3 has less than 250. All three members contain the highly conserved hydroxylase domain in the catalytic carboxy-terminal region and are expressed in bones. However, PHD1 and PHD2 preferably hydroxylate the N-terminal oxygen-dependent degradation domains (NODD) but are less active for the C-terminal oxygen-dependent degradation domains (CODD) whereas PHD3 almost exclusively hydroxylates the CODD [6,7]. Mice with deletion of *Phd1* and *Phd3* genes grow normal, but *Phd2* gene knockout (KO) in mice causes embryonic lethality because the placenta is underdeveloped [8]. The structural difference among the PHD proteins and the data from mouse genetic studies suggest they may have tissue specific functions.

We previously unveiled that PHD2 was highly expressed in bone cells and contributed to an indispensable role in regulating bone homeostasis by upregulating the transcription of genes critical for osteoblast differentiation and function [9]. Mice with targeted deletion of *Phd2* in osteoblasts were smaller and died 12 to 14 weeks after birth. Bone mineral density (BMD) in femurs and the ratio of trabecular bone volume to the tissue volume (BV/TV) in the secondary spongiosa regions of the long bones of the osteoblast-specific conditional knockout (cKO) mice were dramatically low [9]. Mice lacking PHD2 protein in chondrocytes born normally, but the growth after birth were retarded because of elevated mineralization of the cartilage matrix. The chondrocyte-specific cKO mice manifested an increased endochondral bone formation in the femur, tibia and spine, resulting from increased HIF signaling in chondrocytes [10]. While the expression level of *Phd3* in the bones in chondrocyte specific *Phd2* KO mice was dramatically elevated, loss of *Phd3* in chondrocytes did not affect endochondral bone formation and skeletal phenotypes [11]. To investigate the role of *Phd1* expressed in chondrocytes on skeletal development, we conditionally disrupted the *Phd1* gene in chondrocytes by crossing *Phd1 floxed* mice with *Col2α1-Cre* mice for evaluation of skeletal phenotypes.

2. Materials and Methods

2.1. Breeding Strategy of cKO Mice

Phd1 floxed mice were bred with mice overexpressing *Cre* under the control of the Collagen 2α1 (*Col2α1*) promoter to produce *Cre* positive, *Phd1 floxed* heterozygous mice ($Phd1^{flox/+}$; $Col2\alpha1\text{-}Cre^{+}$) according to the breeding strategy described previously [11–13]. The $Phd1^{flox/+}$; $Col2\alpha1\text{-}Cre^{+}$ mice were then backcrossed with $Phd1^{flox/flox}$ mice to generate *Cre*-positive, *loxP*-homozygous ($Phd1^{flox/flox}$; *Col2α1-Cre+*) cKO and *Cre*-negative, *Phd1 loxP*-homozygous or heterozygous ($Phd1^{flox/flox}$; $Phd1^{flox/+}$) wild-type (WT) littermates (Figure 1A). The genetic background of these mice is C57BL/6. Both sex mice were used in this study. Mice were housed at the Loma Linda VA Healthcare System (Loma Linda, CA, USA) at 22 °C and with 14 h light and 10 h dark, as well as free access to food and water. Experiments were carried out according to the protocol approved by the Institutional Animal Care and Use Committee (IACUC) of the Loma Linda VA Healthcare System (CA, USA). Mice were anesthetized using isoflurane before tail clipping. Mice were euthanized by exposing to CO_2 gas proceeded by cervical dislocation.

2.2. Evaluation of Bone Phenotypes

Areal BMD of the total body, long and lumbar bones (L4–6) of 12-week-old mice were quantified by the FAXITRON UltraFocus^{DXA} 1000 as reported [11,14,15]. Trabecular and cortical bones of the femur and the tibia were scanned and quantified by microcomputed tomography (μCT) in 12-week old mice described previously [16]. The formalin-fixed bones in PBS were scanned by μCT with 55 kVp volts and a voxel size of 10.5 μm. A 1.05 mm cortical bone in the mid-diaphysis of the femur and the tibia were analyzed for cortical bone parameters. A 2.1 mm of the secondary spongiosa of the distal femur and the proximal tibia beginning 0.3675 mm from the growth plates were assessed for TV(mm^3), BV(mm^3), and BV/TV, as described [17–19].

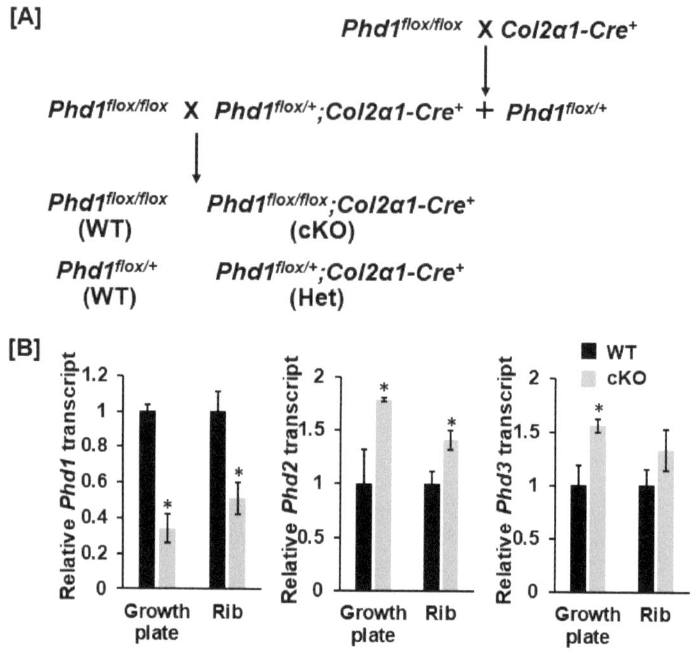

Figure 1. Breeding strategy of *Phd1* conditional knockout (cKO) mice. (**A**) A breeding strategy of *Phd1* cKO mice, heterozygous (Het) and wild-type (WT) mice. (**B**) *Phd1* expression was partially disrupted in chondrocyte cultures derived from the cKO mice. Total RNA was extracted from primary chondrocytes derived from the femur growth plates and the ribs of 10-day old mice for quantitative PCR ($n = 3$). Star (*): $p < 0.01$.

2.3. Double Labeling and Histomorphometric Analyses

Twelve-week-old mice were injected intraperitoneally with calcein (20 mg/kg) eight and two days before euthanization by CO_2 to label mineralizing bone surfaces. Mouse right femurs were fixed in 10% formalin for 3 days, washed 3 times with PBS, dehydrated, and embedded in methyl methacrylate resin for sectioning. The sampling sites and histomorphometric analyses were performed as described [19]. The first and the second calcein labeling of the trabecular bone in the secondary spongiosa region of the distal femurs were blindly quantified with OsteoMeasure V3.1.0.2 computer software (OsteoMetrics, Decatur, GA, USA) [20,21]. The mineral apposition rate (MAR) and bone formation rate/bone surface (BFR/BS) were calculated as described previously [22].

2.4. Primary Chondrocyte Culture

Primary chondrocytes isolated from the rib cartilage and the growth plates of the femurs and the tibias of 10-day old WT and cKO mice (3 female and 3 male littermate mice) were cultured as previously described [23]. Cells were grown in DMEM/F12 medium containing 10% fetal bovine serum (FBS), penicillin (100 U/mL), and streptomycin (100 μg/mL) to approximately 90% confluence before harvesting for RNA extraction.

2.5. RNA Extraction and Real-Time PCR

Total RNA was extracted from the femurs and the tibias of the WT and cKO mice or primary chondrocyte cultures derived from WT and cKO mice with the Trizol as described [24,25]. An aliquot of RNA (300 ng) was reverse-transcribed into cDNA in 20 μL volume of reaction by oligo(dT)$_{12–18}$ primer. A real-time PCR contained 0.5 μL template cDNA, 1x SYBR GREEN master mix (Qiagen), and 100 nM of specific forward and reverse primers in a 25 μL volume of reaction. Primers used for real-time PCR are listed in Table 1. Relative gene expression was calculated by using the $^{\Delta\Delta}$CT method [26].

Table 1. Primer Sequence for Real-Time PCR.

Gene	Forward Primer	Reverse Primer
Ppia	5′-CCATGGCAAATGCTGGACCA	5′-TCCTGGACCCAAAACGCTCC
Phd1	5′-GGAACCCACATGAGGTGAAG	5′-AACACCTTTCTGTCCCGATG
Phd3	5′-GGGACGCCAAGTTACACGGA	5′-GGGCTCCACGTCTGCTACAA
Phd2	5′-GAAGCTGGGCAACTACAGGA	5′-CATGTCACGCATCTTCCATC
Alp	5′-ATGGTAACGGGCCTGGCTACA	5′-AGTTCTGCTCATGGACGCCGT
Bsp	5′-AACGGGTTTCAGCAGACAACC	5′-TAAGCTCGGTAAGTGTCGCCA
Col2	5′-TGGCTTCCACTTCAGCTATG	5′-AGGTAGGCGATGCTGTTCTT
Col10	5′-ACGGCACGCCTACGATGT	5′-CCATGATTGCACTCCCTGAA

Note: *Ppia, peptidylprolyl isomerase A; Phd, prolyl hydroxylase domain-containing protein; Alp, alkaline phosphatase; Bsp, bone sialoprotein; Col2, collagen 2; Col10, collagen 10.*

2.6. Statistical Analysis

Student's *t*-test was used for data analyses. Data are Mean ± SEM (n = 6–10).

3. Results

3.1. Expression of Phd1 Was Partially Disrupted in Chondrocytes in cKO Mice

To test if loss of *Phd1* expression in chondrocytes impairs endochondral bone formation, we produced chondrocyte-specific *Phd1* cKO mice by breeding the *Phd1 floxed* mice with the *Col2α-Cre* mice, in which the Cre recombinase is overexpressed in *Col2α*-expressing chondrocytes [13,27]. After 2 generations of breeding, the *Phd1 floxed, Cre*$^{+}$ cKO mice (*Phd1*$^{flox/flox}$; *Col2α-Cre*$^{+}$) were produced and compared to *Cre* negative WT littermates (*Phd1*$^{flox/flox}$ or *Phd1*$^{lox/+}$; *Cre*$^{-}$). The cKO mice born and developed normally. To investigate if PHD1 protein exists in bone cells of cKO mice, RNA was isolated from chondrocytes derived from the growth plates of the femurs and the tibias, and the ribs of 10-day old WT and cKO mice for real-time PCR with specific primers to *Phd1, 2* and *3*. As shown in Figure 1B, the expression levels of *Phd1* transcript were reduced by 66% and 45% in the growth plate and rib chondrocytes, respectively, in the cKO mice compared to WT mice. By comparison, *Phd2* was increased in chondrocytes of both growth plates and ribs of *Phd1* cKO mice by 79% and 41%, respectively. While the expression levels of Phd3 were 56% and 33% higher, respectively, in the growth plate and rib chondrocytes of *Phd1* cKO mice, only *Phd3* expression level in growth plate chondrocytes was significantly higher compared to WT mice.

3.2. Deletion of Phd1 in Col2α-Expressing Chondrocytes Does Not Affect Skeletal Growth in Mice at 12 Weeks of Age

To analyze the bone phenotypes, we performed DXA screening and μCT scanning. At 12 weeks after birth, neither body weight nor body length was significantly different in the cKO mice compared to gender-matched control mice for either gender (Figure 2A). DXA measurements revealed no significant changes in total body, femur, tibia, and lumbar BMDs between the two genotypes for either gender (Figure 2B,C). Concurred with DXA data, μCT scanning of the femoral trabecular bone uncovered no significant changes in either BV/TV or any of the trabecular bone parameters including BMD, trabecular number (Tb. N), trabecular thickness (Tb. Th) and trabecular spacing (Tb. Sp) in *Phd1* cKO from the gender-matched WT mice for either gender (Figure 3A–C). The tibial BMD, BV/TV, Tb. N, Tb. Th, and Tb. Sp in cKO mice were also comparable to WT mice in either gender mice (Figure 4A–C). Deletion of the *Phd1* gene in chondrocytes had no impact on either cortical BV/TV ratio or BMD (Figure 5A). The deficiency of PHD1 expression had no effect on cortical BV/TV and BMD in the tibia either (Figure 5B).

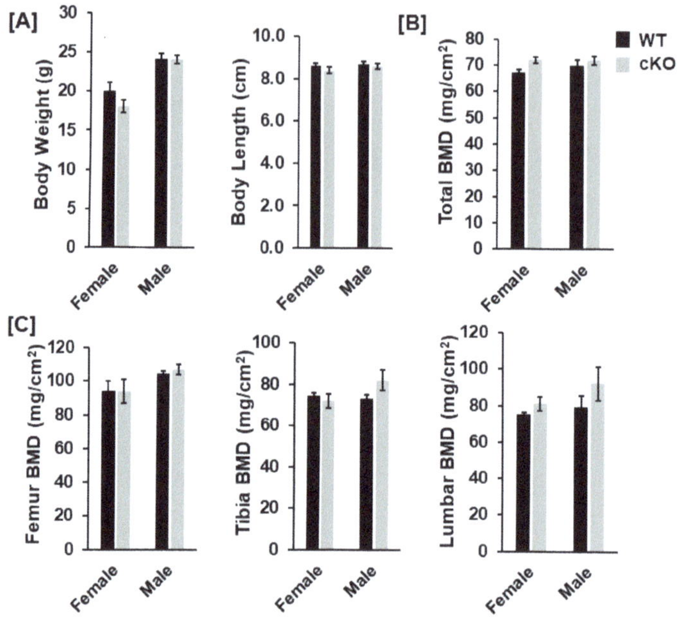

Figure 2. Bone parameters were not significantly altered in the *Phd1* cKO mice at 12 weeks after birth. (**A**) Body weight and length of the mice, as indicated in the figure. (**B**,**C**) Bone mineral density (BMD) for total body, the femur, the tibia, and the lumbar bone, respectively, quantified by DXA (n = 6–10).

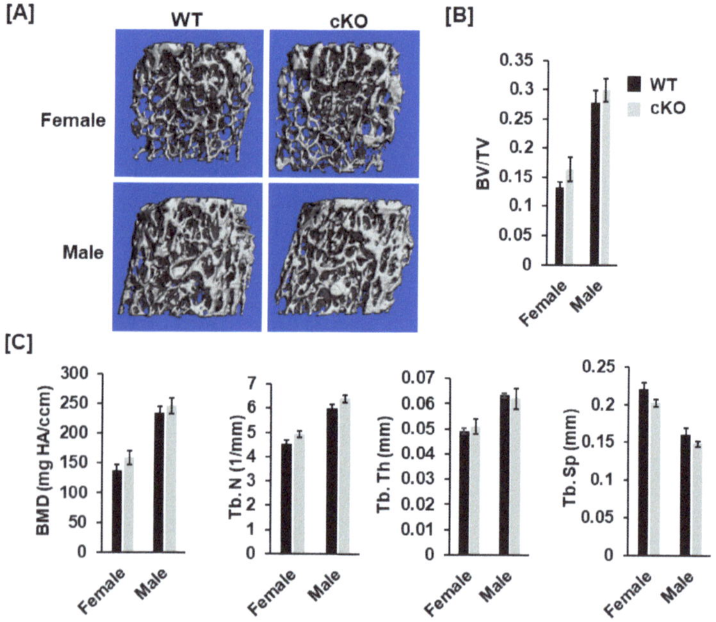

Figure 3. Trabecular parameters were not significantly altered in the femur of the *Phd1* cKO mice at 12 weeks after birth. (**A**) Representative μCT images of the distal femurs. (**B**,**C**) Trabecular bone data of the femurs (BV/TV, BMD, Tb.N, Tb. Th, and Tb. Sp) measured by μCT (n = 6–10). BV, bone volume; TV, tissue volume; Tb. N, trabecular number; Tb. Th, trabecular thickness; Th. Sp, Trabecular spacing.

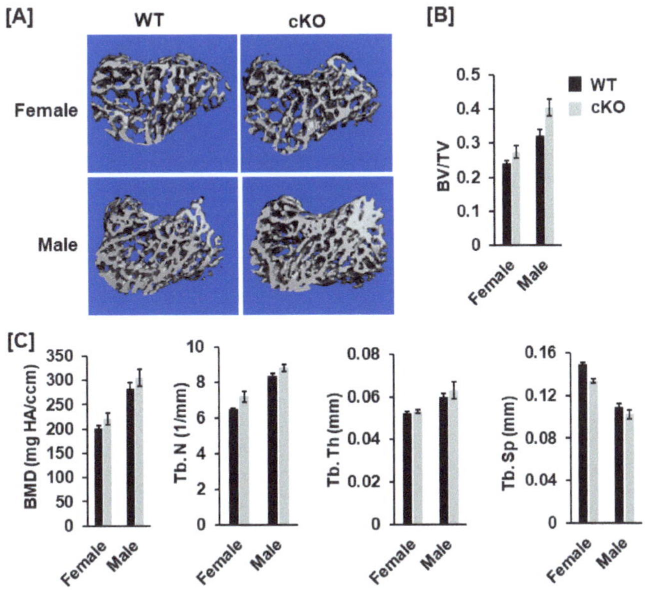

Figure 4. No changes in trabecular parameters were found in the proximal metaphysis of the tibia in the *Phd1* cKO mice at 12 weeks after birth. (**A**) Representative μCT images of the proximal tibias. (**B**,**C**) Trabecular bone data of the tibias (BV/TV, BMD, Tb.N, Tb. Th, and Tb. Sp) measured by μCT (*n* = 6–10).

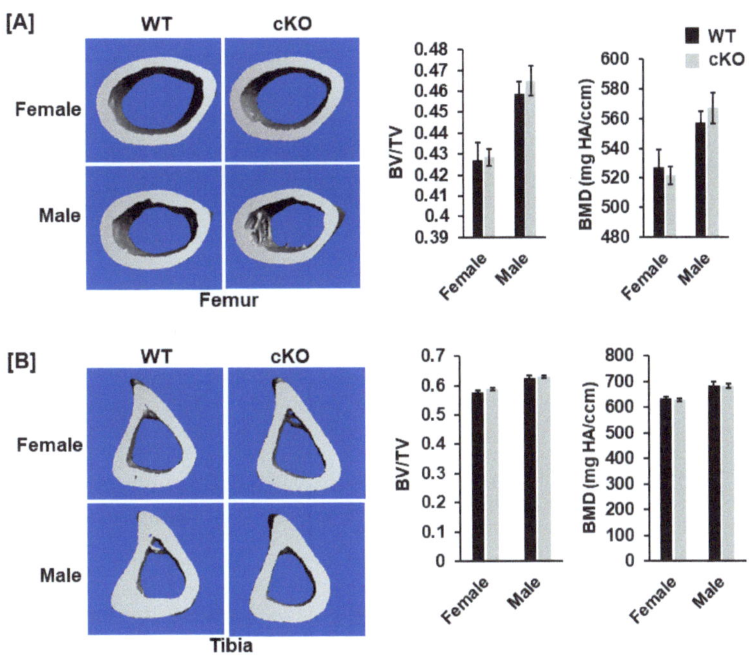

Figure 5. No changes were found in cortical bone parameters of the femur and the tibia in the *Phd1* cKO mice at 12 weeks after birth. (**A**) Representative μCT images of the cortical bone of the femurs and the quantitative data of the cortical bones of the femurs (BV/TV, BMD). (**B**) Images of the cortical bone of the tibias and the cortical bone data of the tibias (BV, BMD) (*n* = 6–10).

3.3. Knockout of *Phd1* in Chondrocytes Neither Influences Bone Formation Nor Expression of Marker Genes of Osteoblast/Chondrocyte Differentiation

To determine if the deletion of *Phd1* in *Col2α1* expressing cells impacts osteoblast formation, and trabecular bone formation in the femur, we performed histomorphometry analyses and examined the bone marker genes expression in long bones of the cKO mice. We uncovered that knockdown of *Phd1* expression in chondrocytes neither affected the MAR) nor the BFR/BS in cKO mice as compared to the WT control littermates (Figure 6A). Consistent with the histomorphometric data, lack of *Phd1* in chondrocytes had no impact on the differentiation of both osteoblasts and chondrocytes as evidenced by comparable expression levels of marker genes, *alkaline phosphatase (Alp), bone sialoprotein (Bsp), collagen 2 (Col2)*, and *collagen 10 (Col10)* in long bones in the cKO mice compared with the WT mice (Figure 6B).

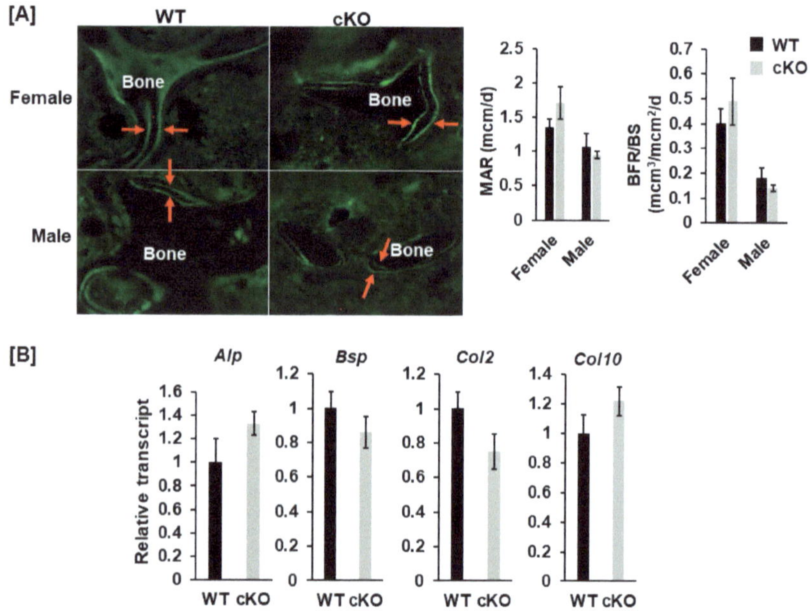

Figure 6. Knockout of *Phd1* in chondrocytes neither influences bone formation nor expression of markers of osteoblast/chondrocyte differentiation. (**A**) Representative images of the calcein-labeled trabecular bone of the distal femurs and the quantitative data of mineral apposition rate (MAR) and bone formation rate/bone surface (BFR/BS), respectively. The bone indicated by two red arrows is the double-labeled, newly formed bone ($n = 6$). (**B**) Expression levels of the marker genes of osteoblast and chondrocyte differentiation in long bones measured by RT-real-time PCR. *Alp, alkaline phosphatase; Bsp, bone sialoprotein; Col2, collagen 2; Col10: collagen 10.*

4. Discussion

Of three family members, the PHD2 protein is the most abundant in bones [28]. PHD2 is believed to be the critical oxygen sensor during hypoxia, which is emphasized by the fact that mice with global deletion of the *Phd2* gene are embryonically lethal [8]. By contrast, mice with global disruption of either the *Phd1* or *Phd3* gene develop normally. Consistent with an important role for PHD2 in bones, we and others have shown that disruption of the *Phd2* gene in osteoblasts and chondrocytes influenced bone formation and development of peak bone mass [9,27,29]. Mice with deletion of *Phd2* in osteoblasts were smaller and died twelve to fourteen weeks after birth. Femoral BMD and trabecular BV/TV of osteoblast-specific cKO mice were notably diminished. By contrast, mice lacking *Phd2* were born normally, but the development was retarded after birth resulted from abnormal mineralization of the cartilage matrix. Endochondral bone formation was enhanced in the femur, tibia, and spine of the *Phd2* chondrocyte-specific cKO mice [10]. While the expression level of *Phd3* elevated 7-fold in chondrocytes of *Phd2*-cKO mice, targeted disruption of *Phd3* gene in mice had no impact on bone cell differentiation, endochondral bone formation, and bone development [11]. Our previous studies indicate that *Phd3*, unlike *Phd2*, does not play an important role in regulating chondrocyte differentiation and bone growth.

PHD enzymes function through hydroxylation of the specific proline and asparagine residues of HIF-α and negatively regulate HIF-α protein stability [30]. Both HIF1α and HIF2α contain two prolyl hydroxylation sites in a central degradation domain of HIF1α. Hydroxylation of these sites promotes HIF1α interaction with the ubiquitin ligase for ubiquitination and subsequent degradation [5,31]. Hydroxylation of an asparagine residue in the C-terminals prevents HIFα transcription factor from cooperation with the co-activator, p300/CBP, leading to HIF1α inactivation [32]. Recent studies suggest that the PHD1/2 proteins specifically and preferentially hydroxylate their substrates. Although both PHD1 and PHD2 are active on CODD and NODD, PHD1 appears to act more effectively on substrate HIF2α, whereas PHD2 more actively hydroxylates on substrate HIF1α [7]. These studies indicate the PHD1 vs. PHD2 hydroxylate HIFα in a CODD sequence-dependent manner. Congruent with these studies, *Phd2* deletion mice had an increased level of HIF1α in the liver and the kidneys but no increase in the HIF2α protein was noted. In contrast, PHD1/3 double deficient mice had elevated level of HIF2α protein only in the liver [28,33]. On the other hand, loss of *Hif1α* in osteoblasts impaired skeletal growth [34,35]. Mice without HIF1α protein in the condensing mesenchymal stem cells had shorter bones, impaired mineralized skulls and wider sutures because of severe chondrocyte apoptosis and impaired chondrocyte proliferation in the growth plate [34]. By contrast, loss of *HIF2α* protein in mice only resulted in a modest decrease in trabecular BV [36]. However, recent mouse genetics studies demonstrated that HIF2 is a negative regulator of osteoblastogenesis and bone mass accrual by upregulating the transcription factor SOX9 to impair osteoblast differentiation [37]. Loss of HIF2 in mesenchymal progenitors increases bone mass by promoting bone formation without affecting bone resorption [37,38]. Since SOX9 is also a master transcription factor in chondrocyte differentiation, we assumed that if the PHD1/HIF/SOX9 signaling axis in chondrocytes is important in endochondral bone formation, then loss of the *Phd1* gene in chondrocytes should influence trabecular bone mass because PHD1 hydroxylates target HIF proteins and promotes ubiquitin-mediated protein degradation. To test the hypothesis, *Phd1* was deleted in chondrocytes by breeding *Phd1 floxed* mice with *Col2α1-Cre* mice, and the effects of knocking out the *Phd1* gene in chondrocytes on the development of peak bone mass was evaluated. Surprisingly, no significant changes in either body weight or body length was observed in the cKO mice compared to gender- and age-matched WT littermates. Micro-CT measurements unveiled significant gender differences in the trabecular BV/TV at the metaphysis of either the femur or the tibia of WT and cKO mice. We did not observe a genotype difference for any of the trabecular measurements of the long bones. Similarly, cortical bone parameters were not affected in the *Phd1* cKO mice compared to control mice. Histomorphometric analyses observed no significant differences in bone formation rate or mineral apposition rate in the secondary spongiosa of femurs between cKO and WT control mice. These data suggest that *Phd1* expressed in chondrocytes exert no major role in regulating the skeletal phenotype.

We found that *Phd1* expression was reduced only by 66% and 45%, respectively, in cultured growth plate and rib chondrocytes derived from the long bones of 10-day old cKO mice. The magnitude of reduction in *Phd1* expression in growth plate chondrocytes of *Phd1* cKO mice was similar to the 60% reduction in *Phd2* expression reported previously in the growth plate chondrocytes of *Phd2* cKO mice [27]. One potential explanation for the partial reduction in *Phd1* expression in the cKO mice is the possibility that the cultures used were not entirely homogeneous for chondrocytes and might contain other cell types (fibroblasts, osteoblasts) which remains to be examined. In any case, our data show that 66%-45% loss of *Phd1* transcript in the growth plate and rib chondrocytes had no impact on the transcription of chondrocyte markers, *Col2* and *Col10*, or osteoblast markers, *Alp*, *Bsp2*, in the bones of cKO mice. By contrast, we found that the expression levels of *Phd2* and *Phd3* were increased in the chondrocytes derived from *Phd1* cKO mice which could represent a compensatory response to the loss of *Phd1* expression. In previous studies, we reported that PHD2 was a negative regulator of chondrocyte differentiation since disruption of *Phd2* gene in chondrocytes, promoted chondrocyte differentiation and increased trabecular bone formation [27,39]. We, therefore, anticipated an increased *Phd2* expression to reduce chondrocyte differentiation, and trabecular bone volume in the *Phd1* cKO mice. However, that was not the case. Further studies comparing the skeletal phenotypes *Phd1*, *Phd2* and *Phd1/2 cKO* mice are needed to verify if the compensatory increase in *Phd2* expression has any role in the *Phd1* cKO mice. While expression of *Phd3* was elevated by 56% in the growth plate chondrocytes, this compensatory increase in the expression of *Phd3* is unlikely to play a significant role in regulating bone formation based on our previous findings on the lack of skeletal phenotype in chondrocyte specific *Phd3* cKO mice. Consistent with our interpretation, Wu et al. found that the trabecular bone phenotype was unaffected in mice with disruption of both *phd1* and *Phd3* genes in osterix expressing cells [40]. Our data, together with our previous reports, imply that *Phd2* transcribed in chondrocytes is a major contributor to endochondral bone formation [27]. PHD2 expressed in chondrocytes can functionally compensate for the loss of PHD1 in *Phd1* cKO mice.

5. Conclusions

Phd1 expressed in chondrocytes does not regulate endochondral bone formation. Of the *Phd1/2/3 genes*, only *Phd2* transcribed in chondrocytes contributes to the endochondral bone formation and the peak bone mass in mice.

Author Contributions: Conceptualization, S.M.; methodology, D.L., S.P., W.T. and G.A.G.; formal analysis, W.X., S.P., W.T. and E.K.L.; data curation, W.X., S.P., W.T. and E.K.L.; writing—original draft preparation, W.X.; writing—review and editing, W.X. and S.M.; supervision, S.M.; funding acquisition, S.M. All authors have read and agreed to the published version of the manuscript.

Funding: This work was supported by funding from Department of Veterans Affairs (VA) BLR&D merit review grants, 1-101-BX-001396, 1-101-BX-005263 and IK6BX005381 awarded to S.M.; S.M. is a recipient of Senior Research Career Scientist Award from the VA. All work was performed in facilities provided by the VA.

Institutional Review Board Statement: The study was conducted according to the guidelines of the National Institutes of Health (USA) and approved by the Institutional Animal Care and Use Committee of the Jerry L. Pettis Memorial Veterans Affairs Medical Center (0047/1165).

Informed Consent Statement: Not applicable.

Data Availability Statement: Raw data are available upon request.

Acknowledgments: The authors thank Donna Strong for her proofreading.

Conflicts of Interest: The authors declare no conflict of interest.

References

1. Lando, D.; Peet, D.J.; Whelan, D.A.; Gorman, J.J.; Whitelaw, M.L. Asparagine hydroxylation of the HIF transactivation domain a hypoxic switch. *Science* **2002**, *295*, 858–861. [CrossRef] [PubMed]
2. Berra, E.; Ginouves, A.; Pouyssegur, J. The hypoxia-inducible-factor hydroxylases bring fresh air into hypoxia signalling. *EMBO Rep.* **2006**, *7*, 41–45. [CrossRef] [PubMed]
3. Huang, L.E.; Bunn, H.F. Hypoxia-inducible factor and its biomedical relevance. *J. Biol. Chem.* **2003**, *278*, 19575–19578. [CrossRef] [PubMed]
4. Wan, C.; Shao, J.; Gilbert, S.R.; Riddle, R.C.; Long, F.; Johnson, R.S.; Schipani, E.; Clemens, T.L. Role of HIF-1alpha in skeletal development. *Ann. N. Y. Acad. Sci.* **2010**, *1192*, 322–326. [CrossRef]
5. Epstein, A.C.; Gleadle, J.M.; McNeill, L.A.; Hewitson, K.S.; O'Rourke, J.; Mole, D.R.; Mukherji, M.; Metzen, E.; Wilson, M.I.; Dhanda, A.; et al. *C. elegans* EGL-9 and mammalian homologs define a family of dioxygenases that regulate HIF by prolyl hydroxylation. *Cell* **2001**, *107*, 43–54. [CrossRef]

6. Villar, D.; Vara-Vega, A.; Landazuri, M.O.; Del Peso, L. Identification of a region on hypoxia-inducible-factor prolyl 4-hydroxylases that determines their specificity for the oxygen degradation domains. *Biochem. J.* **2007**, *408*, 231–240. [CrossRef] [PubMed]
7. Appelhoff, R.J.; Tian, Y.M.; Raval, R.R.; Turley, H.; Harris, A.L.; Pugh, C.W.; Ratcliffe, P.J.; Gleadle, J.M. Differential function of the prolyl hydroxylases PHD1, PHD2, and PHD3 in the regulation of hypoxia-inducible factor. *J. Biol. Chem.* **2004**, *279*, 38458–38465. [CrossRef] [PubMed]
8. Takeda, K.; Ho, V.C.; Takeda, H.; Duan, L.J.; Nagy, A.; Fong, G.H. Placental but not heart defects are associated with elevated hypoxia-inducible factor alpha levels in mice lacking prolyl hydroxylase domain protein 2. *Mol. Cell. Biol.* **2006**, *26*, 8336–8346. [CrossRef]
9. Cheng, S.; Xing, W.; Pourteymoor, S.; Mohan, S. Conditional disruption of the prolyl hydroxylase domain-containing protein 2 (Phd2) gene defines its key role in skeletal development. *J. Bone Miner. Res.* **2014**, *29*, 2276–2286. [CrossRef] [PubMed]
10. Laperre, K.F.P.; Van Looveren, R.; Bouillon, R.; Carmeliet, P.; Carmeliet, G. Deletion of the oxygen-sensor PHD2 in chondrocytes results in increased cartilage and bone mineralization. *J. Bone Miner. Res.* **2008**, *23* (Suppl. S1), S44.
11. Xing, W.; Pourteymoor, S.; Gomez, G.A.; Chen, Y.; Mohan, S. Prolyl Hydroxylase Domain-Containing Protein 3 Gene Expression in Chondrocytes Is Not Essential for Bone Development in Mice. *Cells* **2021**, *10*, 2200. [CrossRef] [PubMed]
12. Duan, L.J.; Takeda, K.; Fong, G.H. Hematological, hepatic, and retinal phenotypes in mice deficient for prolyl hydroxylase domain proteins in the liver. *Am. J. Pathol.* **2014**, *184*, 1240–1250. [CrossRef] [PubMed]
13. Ovchinnikov, D.A.; Deng, J.M.; Ogunrinu, G.; Behringer, R.R. Col2a1-directed expression of Cre recombinase in differentiating chondrocytes in transgenic mice. *Genesis* **2000**, *26*, 145–146. [CrossRef]
14. Xing, W.; Pourteymoor, S.; Chen, Y.; Mohan, S. Targeted Deletion of the Claudin12 Gene in Mice Increases Articular Cartilage and Inhibits Chondrocyte Differentiation. *Front. Endocrinol.* **2022**, *13*, 931318. [CrossRef]
15. Xing, W.; Pourteymoor, S.; Kesavan, C.; Gomez, G.A.; Mohan, S. Mice with Targeted Knockout of Tetraspanin 3 Exhibit Reduced Trabecular Bone Mass Caused by Decreased Osteoblast Functions. *Cells* **2022**, *11*, 977. [CrossRef]
16. Xing, W.; Liu, J.; Cheng, S.; Vogel, P.; Mohan, S.; Brommage, R. Targeted disruption of leucine-rich repeat kinase 1 but not leucine-rich repeat kinase 2 in mice causes severe osteopetrosis. *J. Bone Miner. Res.* **2013**, *28*, 1962–1974. [CrossRef]
17. Bouxsein, M.L.; Boyd, S.K.; Christiansen, B.A.; Guldberg, R.E.; Jepsen, K.J.; Muller, R. Guidelines for assessment of bone microstructure in rodents using micro-computed tomography. *J. Bone Miner. Res.* **2010**, *25*, 1468–1486. [CrossRef]
18. Xing, W.; Pourteymoor, S.; Mohan, S. Ascorbic acid regulates osterix expression in osteoblasts by activation of prolyl hydroxylase and ubiquitination-mediated proteosomal degradation pathway. *Physiol. Genom.* **2011**, *43*, 749–757. [CrossRef]
19. Xing, W.; Kim, J.; Wergedal, J.; Chen, S.T.; Mohan, S. Ephrin B1 regulates bone marrow stromal cell differentiation and bone formation by influencing TAZ transactivation via complex formation with NHERF1. *Mol. Cell. Biol.* **2010**, *30*, 711–721. [CrossRef]
20. Beamer, W.G.; Donahue, L.R.; Rosen, C.J.; Baylink, D.J. Genetic variability in adult bone density among inbred strains of mice. *Bone* **1996**, *18*, 397–403. [CrossRef]
21. Qin, X.; Wergedal, J.E.; Rehage, M.; Tran, K.; Newton, J.; Lam, P.; Baylink, D.J.; Mohan, S. Pregnancy-associated plasma protein-A increases osteoblast proliferation in vitro and bone formation in vivo. *Endocrinology* **2006**, *147*, 5653–5661. [CrossRef] [PubMed]
22. Parfitt, A.M.; Drezner, M.K.; Glorieux, F.H.; Kanis, J.A.; Malluche, H.; Meunier, P.J.; Ott, S.M.; Recker, R.R. Bone histomorphometry: Standardization of nomenclature, symbols, and units: Report of the ASBMR Histomorphometry Nomenclature Committee. *J. Bone Miner. Res.* **1987**, *2*, 595–610. [CrossRef] [PubMed]
23. Cheng, S.; Xing, W.; Zhou, X.; Mohan, S. Haploinsufficiency of osterix in chondrocytes impairs skeletal growth in mice. *Physiol. Genom.* **2013**, *45*, 917–923. [CrossRef] [PubMed]
24. Xing, W.; Singgih, A.; Kapoor, A.; Alarcon, C.M.; Baylink, D.J.; Mohan, S. Nuclear factor-E2-related factor-1 mediates ascorbic acid induction of osterix expression via interaction with antioxidant-responsive element in bone cells. *J. Biol. Chem.* **2007**, *282*, 22052–22061. [CrossRef] [PubMed]
25. Xing, W.; Baylink, D.; Kesavan, C.; Hu, Y.; Kapoor, S.; Chadwick, R.B.; Mohan, S. Global gene expression analysis in the bones reveals involvement of several novel genes and pathways in mediating an anabolic response of mechanical loading in mice. *J. Cell. Biochem.* **2005**, *96*, 1049–1060. [CrossRef] [PubMed]
26. Livak, K.J.; Schmittgen, T.D. Analysis of relative gene expression data using real-time quantitative PCR and the 2(-Delta Delta C(T)) Method. *Methods* **2001**, *25*, 402–408. [CrossRef] [PubMed]
27. Cheng, S.; Xing, W.; Pourteymoor, S.; Schulte, J.; Mohan, S. Conditional Deletion of Prolyl Hydroxylase Domain-containing Protein 2 (Phd2) Gene Reveals its Essential Role in Chondrocyte Function and Endochondral Bone Formation. *Endocrinology* **2015**, *157*, en20151473. [CrossRef]
28. Takeda, K.; Aguila, H.L.; Parikh, N.S.; Li, X.; Lamothe, K.; Duan, L.J.; Takeda, H.; Lee, F.S.; Fong, G.H. Regulation of adult erythropoiesis by prolyl hydroxylase domain proteins. *Blood* **2008**, *111*, 3229–3235. [CrossRef]
29. Zhu, K.; Song, P.; Lai, Y.; Liu, C.; Xiao, G. Prolyl hydroxylase domain proteins regulate bone mass through their expression in osteoblasts. *Gene* **2016**, *594*, 125–130. [CrossRef]
30. Fong, G.H.; Takeda, K. Role and regulation of prolyl hydroxylase domain proteins. *Cell Death Differ.* **2008**, *15*, 635–641. [CrossRef]
31. Bruick, R.K.; McKnight, S.L. A conserved family of prolyl-4-hydroxylases that modify HIF. *Science* **2001**, *294*, 1337–1340. [CrossRef] [PubMed]

32. Metzen, E.; Berchner-Pfannschmidt, U.; Stengel, P.; Marxsen, J.H.; Stolze, I.; Klinger, M.; Huang, W.Q.; Wotzlaw, C.; Hellwig-Burgel, T.; Jelkmann, W.; et al. Intracellular localisation of human HIF-1 alpha hydroxylases: Implications for oxygen sensing. *J. Cell Sci.* **2003**, *116 Pt 7*, 1319–1326. [CrossRef]
33. Takeda, K.; Cowan, A.; Fong, G.H. Essential role for prolyl hydroxylase domain protein 2 in oxygen homeostasis of the adult vascular system. *Circulation* **2007**, *116*, 774–781. [CrossRef]
34. Provot, S.; Zinyk, D.; Gunes, Y.; Kathri, R.; Le, Q.; Kronenberg, H.M.; Johnson, R.S.; Longaker, M.T.; Giaccia, A.J.; Schipani, E. Hif-1alpha regulates differentiation of limb bud mesenchyme and joint development. *J. Cell. Biol.* **2007**, *177*, 451–464. [CrossRef] [PubMed]
35. Wan, C.; Gilbert, S.R.; Wang, Y.; Cao, X.; Shen, X.; Ramaswamy, G.; Jacobsen, K.A.; Alaql, Z.S.; Eberhardt, A.W.; Gerstenfeld, L.C.; et al. Activation of the hypoxia-inducible factor-1alpha pathway accelerates bone regeneration. *Proc. Natl. Acad. Sci. USA* **2008**, *105*, 686–691. [CrossRef] [PubMed]
36. Shomento, S.H.; Wan, C.; Cao, X.; Faugere, M.C.; Bouxsein, M.L.; Clemens, T.L.; Riddle, R.C. Hypoxia-inducible factors 1alpha and 2alpha exert both distinct and overlapping functions in long bone development. *J. Cell. Biochem.* **2010**, *109*, 196–204. [CrossRef] [PubMed]
37. Merceron, C.; Ranganathan, K.; Wang, E.; Tata, Z.; Makkapati, S.; Khan, M.P.; Mangiavini, L.; Yao, A.Q.; Castellini, L.; Levi, B.; et al. Hypoxia-inducible factor 2alpha is a negative regulator of osteoblastogenesis and bone mass accrual. *Bone Res.* **2019**, *7*, 7. [CrossRef] [PubMed]
38. Lee, S.Y.; Park, K.H.; Yu, H.G.; Kook, E.; Song, W.H.; Lee, G.; Koh, J.T.; Shin, H.I.; Choi, J.Y.; Huh, Y.H.; et al. Controlling hypoxia-inducible factor-2alpha is critical for maintaining bone homeostasis in mice. *Bone Res.* **2019**, *7*, 14. [CrossRef]
39. Cheng, S.; Pourteymoor, S.; Alarcon, C.; Mohan, S. Conditional Deletion of the Phd2 Gene in Articular Chondrocytes Accelerates Differentiation and Reduces Articular Cartilage Thickness. *Sci. Rep.* **2017**, *7*, 45408. [CrossRef]
40. Wu, C.; Rankin, E.B.; Castellini, L.; Alcudia, J.F.; LaGory, E.L.; Andersen, R.; Rhodes, S.D.; Wilson, T.L.; Mohammad, K.S.; Castillo, A.B.; et al. Oxygen-sensing PHDs regulate bone homeostasis through the modulation of osteoprotegerin. *Genes Dev.* **2015**, *29*, 817–831. [CrossRef]

life

MDPI

Review

NF-kB in Signaling Patterns and Its Temporal Dynamics Encode/Decode Human Diseases

Sanaa Almowallad [1], Leena S. Alqahtani [2,*] and Mohammad Mobashir [3,4,5,*]

1 Department of Biochemistry, Faculty of Sciences, University of Tabuk, Tabuk 71491, Saudi Arabia
2 Department of Biochemistry, College of Science, University of Jeddah, Jeddah 23445, Saudi Arabia
3 SciLifeLab, Department of Oncology and Pathology, Karolinska Institutet, P.O. Box 1031, S-17121 Stockholm, Sweden
4 Department of Biosciences, Faculty of Natural Science, Jamia Millia Islamia, New Delhi 110025, India
5 Special Infectious Agents Unit—BSL3, King Fahd Medical Research Center, King Abdulaziz University, Jeddah 21362, Saudi Arabia
* Correspondence: lsalqahtani@uj.edu.sa (L.S.A.); m.mobashir@cdslifesciences.com (M.M.)

Abstract: Defects in signaling pathways are the root cause of many disorders. These malformations come in a wide variety of types, and their causes are also very diverse. Some of these flaws can be brought on by pathogenic organisms and viruses, many of which can obstruct signaling processes. Other illnesses are linked to malfunctions in the way that cell signaling pathways work. When thinking about how errors in signaling pathways might cause disease, the idea of signalosome remodeling is helpful. The signalosome may be conveniently divided into two types of defects: phenotypic remodeling and genotypic remodeling. The majority of significant illnesses that affect people, including high blood pressure, heart disease, diabetes, and many types of mental illness, appear to be caused by minute phenotypic changes in signaling pathways. Such phenotypic remodeling modifies cell behavior and subverts normal cellular processes, resulting in illness. There has not been much progress in creating efficient therapies since it has been challenging to definitively confirm this connection between signalosome remodeling and illness. The considerable redundancy included into cell signaling systems presents several potential for developing novel treatments for various disease conditions. One of the most important pathways, NF-κB, controls several aspects of innate and adaptive immune responses, is a key modulator of inflammatory reactions, and has been widely studied both from experimental and theoretical perspectives. NF-κB contributes to the control of inflammasomes and stimulates the expression of a number of pro-inflammatory genes, including those that produce cytokines and chemokines. Additionally, NF-κB is essential for controlling innate immune cells and inflammatory T cells' survival, activation, and differentiation. As a result, aberrant NF-κB activation plays a role in the pathogenesis of several inflammatory illnesses. The activation and function of NF-κB in relation to inflammatory illnesses was covered here, and the advancement of treatment approaches based on NF-κB inhibition will be highlighted. This review presents the temporal behavior of NF-κB and its potential relevance in different human diseases which will be helpful not only for theoretical but also for experimental perspectives.

Keywords: NF-κB signaling; signaling dynamics; cell-fate decision; encoding and decoding; cellular information; human diseases

check for updates

Citation: Almowallad, S.; Alqahtani, L.S.; Mobashir, M. NF-kB in Signaling Patterns and Its Temporal Dynamics Encode/Decode Human Diseases. *Life* **2022**, *12*, 2012. https://doi.org/10.3390/life12122012

Academic Editor: Sanda M. Cretoiu

Received: 14 November 2022
Accepted: 30 November 2022
Published: 2 December 2022

1. Introduction

The idea that structure reflects function is a recurring one in biology. The genome is arguably the most well-known example of a biological structure that foretells physiological activity. One can determine whether coding DNA encodes a protein domain, binding site, conserved motif, or hairpin structure by understanding the sequence structure of the DNA [1–5]. These illustrations show that the structural elements of a cell contain functional information that is encoded. If we could measure cellular structures in enough detail, one may claim that they contain all the necessary information. Is this the only possible method for encoding biological information or is it possible to learn about the features of biological activity that cannot be learned by studying static structures alone? Here, the main concern is about the recent development in cell biology that provides a different way for information to be sent in cells such as by the motion of signaling molecules. As per the nomenclature, dynamics refers to the form of the curve that shows how a molecule's concentration, activity, modification state, or localization alters over time (temporal dynamics) [6–10]. This kind of signaling stores data in the temporal signal's frequency, amplitude, duration, or other characteristics. As a result, it is richer and more complicated than communicating through the state of a signaling molecule instantly. We have focused on the comprehensive overview of what is known about the dynamics of many biological systems, concentrating on systems that have been well investigated and have undergone analysis using a variety of quantitative measurement and perturbation techniques. Through these illustrations, we are able to draw broad conclusions regarding the function of dynamics in biology and the potential benefits of transferring information via the dynamics of signaling molecules [11–19].

Since Sen and Baltimore's discovery of nuclear factor kappa B (NF-κB) in 1986, a great deal of work has been put forward to clarify the roles that this transcription factor plays in the body. NF-κB is a member of the Rel-homology-domain family of transcription factors. The transactivation of numerous target genes involved in immunity, inflammation, and proliferation mostly depends on its component p65/RelA. Its activity is strictly controlled by the B protein inhibitors (IBs) and the B kinase proteins (IKKs), and as a result, growth factors, cytokines, and cell proliferation are expressed. The main functions of NF-κB are to trigger immunological and inflammatory reactions as well as to control apoptosis [20–24]. Its targets include the genes that make cytokines, chemokines, and anti-apoptotic substances as well as cell adhesion molecules. By hiding its RHD, the inhibitory (inhibitor B (IB)) molecules (such as IκBα) confine NF-κB to the cytoplasm. A second complex known as IkappaB kinase (IKK) is activated when cytokines such as interleukin-1 (IL-1) or tumor necrosis factor (TNF) excite a cell [25,26].

The cytosolic IκB kinase activity was initially linked to a massive protein complex of 700–900 kDa that was capable of precisely phosphorylating IκBα on serines 32 and 36. The regulatory subunit IKKγ (NEMO) and two catalytically active kinases, IKKα and IKKβ, were found in this complex after it was purified. IKKα and IKKβ are ubiquitously expressed proteins with leucine zippers, carboxy-terminal helix–loop–helix domains, and amino-terminal kinase domains (HLH). The kinases dimerize through the leucine zipper, and mutations in this region leave the kinases inactive. In contrast, the HLH is not required for dimerization but is crucial for optimal kinase activity. The connection between the regulatory subunit IKKα and IKKβ, which is regulated by a hexapeptide sequence (LDWSWL) on IKKs known as the NEMO binding domain (NBD), depends on the carboxy-terminal parts of IKKα and IKKβ. The phosphorylation of two serines in the sequence motif SLCTS of the T-loop sections in at least one of the IκB kinases is required for the activation of the IKK complex [27].

IB is made ready for proteolysis by ubiquitin by being phosphorylated by the active IKK complex. Following this, NF-κB moves into the nucleus to start the transcription of the target genes. Due to a lack of linkages to specific human disorders, NF-κB signaling has not received much attention in the human setting despite being involved in essential cellular processes. Nevertheless, a number of publications over the last year have identified faulty NF-κB function in a number of hereditary illnesses, including ectodermal dysplasia (ED), familial expansile osteolysis (FEO), primary lymphedema (PL), and incontinentia pigmenti (IP). In this study, we have discussed the precise abnormalities in the NF-κB pathway as well as the genetic mutations that result from these four illnesses [20,28].

Since abnormalities in NF-κB function influence a variety of physiological systems and organs in mice, including the immune system, fetal liver, skin, limbs, and the osteoclast lineage, so we have discussed broad-spectrum role for it. The etiology of ED,

FEO, PL, and IP has been explained in part by our understanding of the NF-κB pathway, but the phenotypes of human diseases have also shed light on the route itself. An old protein transcription factor known as NF-κB is thought to control innate immunity. By connecting pathogenic signals and cellular danger signals, the NF-κB signaling pathway organizes cellular defenses against encroaching pathogens (Figure 1). In reality, several studies have demonstrated that NF-κB functions as a network hub for intricate biological signaling [29–31]. To this purpose, it has been proposed that NF-κB is a master regulator of metabolic cascades that have been preserved throughout evolution.

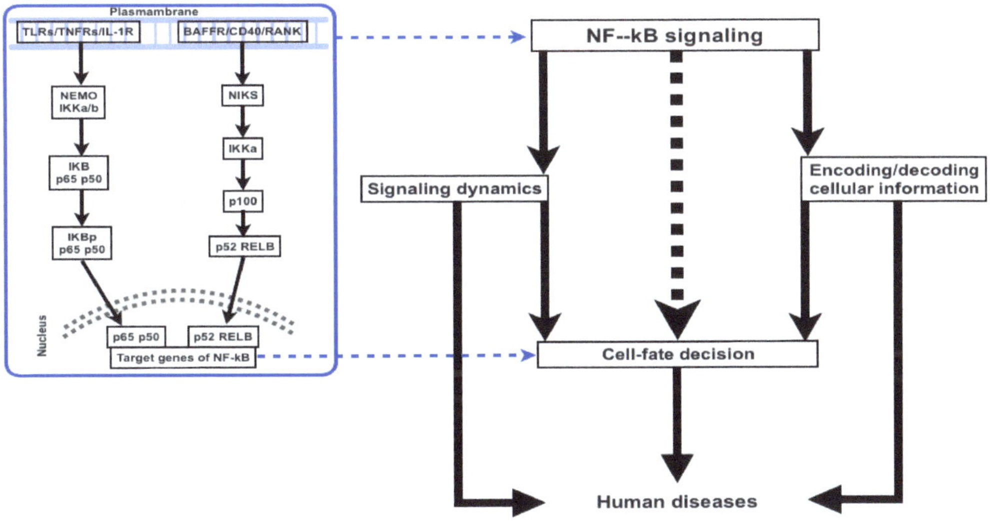

Figure 1. An overview of the work presented in this review.

Physiologist Claud Bernard proposed in 1854 that complex systems such as the human body require the ability to self-regulate their internal environment in order to live. Almost 60 years later, Walter B. Cannon used the term "homeostasis" to describe this essential characteristic of living things. Homeostasis, despite its origin, is a very dynamic process in which only a small number of internal physicochemical parameters are kept within a specific range, or are homeostatically managed. Homeostatic regulation is crucial at the system, tissue, and cellular levels in complex organisms. For instance, the blood's pH is regulated by the brain, lungs, kidneys, and red blood cells; adult stem cells renew tissues to preserve their integrity; and cells keep the baseline concentrations of Ca^{2+}, Na^{+}, and K^{+} within certain ranges [31–33]. Homeostatic regulation depends on biochemical networks known as cell signaling, which provide cells with the capacity to detect physicochemical stimuli, analyze information, and carry out the best biological reactions. Here, we focus on the new conceptual and methodological developments that are improving our knowledge of the molecular processes underlying homeostatic regulation [7,34,35].

Progenitors are the ancestors of all cells. Cellular variety and specialization can be established throughout development through the differentiation of progenitor cells. Additionally, in recent years, we know that the majority of tissues reserve undifferentiated progenitors that probably contribute to the tissue's homeostasis during the course of its lifespan. These cells' differentiation during homeostasis is probably a tightly controlled process. Progenitor growth and differentiation may become dysregulated in illness, but this is not well understood. For instance, the cancer stem cell theory contends that populations of tumor cells that resemble healthy adult stem cells biologically are the source of malignant tumors [36–38]. These might be endogenous stem cells that have developed somatic mutations over time that lead to cancer. Another illustration is fibrosis, which is characterized by an overgrowth of myofibroblasts that produce components of the extracellular matrix that render tissues non-compliant. The origins of myofibroblasts in fibrotic tissues are poorly known, but it has long been assumed that these cells come from nearby regions. Thus, cell fate decisions in development and disease could be of potential interest and this could update on the processes that regulate cell destiny differentiation, techniques for studying and quantifying cell fate differentiation, and evaluations of the current understanding of how cell fate differentiation goes haywire in illness or disease models. Cells can transmit and receive information by managing the temporal behavior (dynamics) of their signaling molecules, according to an increasing number of studies. We go through what is known about the dynamics of various signaling networks and how they affect cellular responses in this review.

We discuss the emerging general principles in the field, paying particular attention to how the type and amount of stimulus are represented in temporal patterns, how signaling dynamics affect cellular outcomes, and how particular dynamical patterns are both generated and interpreted by the organization of molecular networks. In order to conclude, we also discussed about probable functions for signaling molecules' dynamics in transferring cellular information and prospective applications for disease therapy. To achieve our goal for this review study, most relevant review and research works as well as the recent work were studied and have also cited them in the required places.

2. NF-κB Signaling

Controlling inflammation is one of the main functions of NF-κB proteins, which suggests that they focus on the body's intricate defensive systems when inflammation is present [28,39–41]. This is accomplished by controlling the expression of several crucial genes involved in the crucial process, including chemokines and pro-inflammatory cytokines, in both a positive and negative manner. IL-1, for example, and tumor necrosis factor alpha (TNF-α) are powerful inducers of NF-κB. Additionally, NF-κB aids reduce inflammation, which subsequently impairs NF-κB activity [42–44]. The anti-inflammatory, pro-autophagy, and anti-insulin resistance protein Sirtuin 1 is less abundant as people age and become obese because NF-κB is produced more frequently. By attaching to the promoter region of the microRNA miR-34a, which prevents the formation of nicotinamide adenine dinucleotides (NAD), NF-κB raises its levels in the body, causing Sirtuin 1 levels to drop. Senescence-associated secretory phenotype (SASP) factors are produced by senescent cells as a result of a positive feedback loop between NF-κB and IL-1α. NF-κB and CD38, an enzyme that breaks down nicotinamide adenine dinucleotides, also mutually induce one another [45–48].

With this review, we want to better understand how NF-κB activation affects mitochondrial function. It is expected that the reader is already familiar with the fundamentals of mitochondrial biology. RelA, RelB, c-Rel, p100, and p150 are the five different proteins that make up the NF-κB transcription factor family. For dimerization, DNA binding, and interaction with l-B inhibitors, they have RHD, which are crucial. The v-rel oncogene from the T-strain of the reticuloendotheliosis virus (REV), which produces the embryonic lymphatic tumor, is the source of the domain's name due to their same sequence. Additionally, the transcription activation domain is present in RelA, RelB, and c-Rel (transcription activation domain (TAD)) [44,49–52]. Additionally, TADs are missing from p100 and p105, which are precursor proteins for NF-kB, which, following proteolysis, creates the p50 and p52 subunits. As a result, NF-κB is a general term that can refer to a family of dimer proteins made by various substances. Additionally, they all contain the RelA, RelB, c-Rel, p50, and p52 subunits. The majority of cells express the NF-κB dimer p50/RelA, for which many research works have been performed in the past. P100 is processed to create p52 by the two serine residues (in the phosphorylation areas) and the lysine residues (in the ubiquitination region). Ankyrin (ANK) repeats: ANK IkB dysregulation has been known to include serine residues (phosphorylation sites) and lysine residues (ubiquitination sites).

The NF-κB is activated by the two signaling pathways, canonical/classical and non-canonical/alternative (Figure 1). The canonical/classical pathway is activated by extracellular stimuli such as TNF-alpha, RANK (receptor activator of nuclear factor kappa B), TCR (T-cell receptor), CD30, CD40, and LPS (bacterial lipopolysaccharides). These extracellular stimuli change the IKK trimetric complex, which is made up of two catalytic subunits of IKKα and IKKβ and a regulatory subunit of IKKγ (also known as NF-κB essential modulator or NEMO) leads to the phosphorylation of IKB inhibitor (IKB-α) at different sites (i.e., Ser 32 and Ser 36) as a result of the continued ubiquitination of IKBα [53,54]. The p50/p65-containing free NF-kB dimer is activated, translocates to the nucleus, and binds to the promoter region of responsive genes to trigger their transcription. The B-cell activator receptor (BAFF-R), lymphotoxin beta receptor (LTBR), CD40 activating NIK kinase phosphorylating the IKK complex containing IKB dimerized complex, further activating the RelB/p100 to RelB/p52, and transcription are just a few extracellular stimuli that can activate the non-canonical/alternative pathway [28,44,55].

The ability to receive and interpret information from both the intracellular and external environments, initiate and carry out biological reactions, and interact with one another is created through cell signaling. Cell signaling is ultimately in charge of preserving homeostasis at the cellular, tissue, and systemic levels. In order to understand how cells coordinate the transitions between states under developing and adult organisms in healthy and pathological settings, cell signaling is the focus of considerable study efforts. With an emphasis on how single-cell analytical tools uncover processes driving cell-to-cell variability, signaling plasticity, and collective cellular responses, we summarized current knowledge of how cell signaling functions at various spatial and temporal scales in this article [8,56–60].

Eukaryotic cells frequently employ NF-κB as a regulator of genes that govern cell survival and proliferation. As a result, NF-κB has been misregulated in a wide variety of human tumor types, making it constitutively active. Inactive NF-κB prevents the production of genes that would otherwise lead the cell to undergo apoptosis and maintain cell proliferation. Cancer is characterized by mutations or the abnormal expression of proteins that regulate NF-κB signaling, which impair the ability of the malignant cell to coordinate with the rest of the body. This is demonstrated by metastasis as well as by the immune system's ineffective removal of the tumor. When a normal cell is removed from the tissue to which it belongs or when its genome cannot function in harmony with tissue function, it might die. These events rely on the feedback control of NF-κB, which is defective in cancer. Increased apoptosis sensitivity and subsequent cell death are caused by NF-κB defects [29,61–64]. This is due to the fact that NF-κB controls genes that prevent apoptosis, particularly TRAF1 and TRAF2, and as a result, suppresses the activities of the caspase family of enzymes, which are essential to the majority of apoptotic processes. As in 41% of nasopharyngeal carcinoma, colorectal cancer, prostate cancer, and pancreatic tumors, tumor cells have increased NF-κB activity. This is caused by mutations in the genes that code for the NF-κB transcription factors or in the genes that regulate NF-κB activity (such the IB genes); in addition, certain tumor cells produce substances that activate NF-κB. By inhibiting NF-κB, tumor cells may cease growing, perish, or develop increased sensitivity to the effects of anti-tumor medications. As a result, pharmaceutical companies are actively researching NF-κB as a target for anti-cancer treatment [65–69].

The development of antitumor therapy based on the suppression of NF-κB activity is justified by convincing experimental data that identify NF-κB as a key promoter of tumorigenesis; however, care should be taken when considering anti-NF-κB activity as a general therapeutic strategy in the treatment of cancer because data also show that NF-κB activity increases tumor cell sensitivity to apoptosis and senescence. Furthermore, it has been demonstrated that the alternative NF-κB is a Fas transcription repressor and that conventional NF-κB is a Fas transcription activator. Because NF-κB encourages Fas-mediated apoptosis in cancer cells, inhibiting NF-κB may restrict Fas-mediated apoptosis and reduce the ability of host immune cells to prevent tumor growth [70–74]. Here, we have explained the role of NF-κB in different human diseases, which covers a wide range of NF-κB activation mechanisms and potentially associated SMs [1,75–77].

3. Signaling Dynamics and the Association with Signaling Parameters

Information must be transferred from a receptor to the nucleus through a process called signal transduction. This procedure is essential for regulating cellular activity and destiny. Apoptosis, proliferation, and differentiation are influenced by the dynamics of signaling activation and inhibition (Figure 2). Therefore, it is crucial to comprehend the variables that affect both transient and persistent reaction. Using a mathematical method, we investigated the variables that can change how downstream signaling molecules are activated in order to answer this issue. Loops (feedforward and feedback loops), crosstalk of signal transduction pathways, and changes in the concentration of signaling molecules are the aspects that we looked into. According to our findings, the feedback loop and cross-talks that directly block the target protein dominate in regulating the temporary cellular response [75–77]. The ability to receive and interpret information from both the intracellular and external environments, initiate and carry out biological reactions, and interact with one another is created through cell signaling. Cell signaling is ultimately in charge of preserving homeostasis at the cellular, tissue, and systemic levels. In order to understand how the cell coordinates the transitions between states under developing and adult organisms in healthy and pathological settings, cell signaling is the focus of considerable study efforts. With an emphasis on how single-cell analytical tools uncover processes driving cell-to-cell variability, signaling plasticity, and collective cellular responses, we summarize current knowledge of how cell signaling functions at various spatial and temporal scales in this article [28,78–81]. Cell signaling therefore coordinates the transition between cellular states with the molecular machinery (such as ERBB-dependent cytoskeletal rearrangements or DNA damage repair) in response to a stimulus in order to maintain cell homeostasis and function. Similar to this, signaling affects cellular choices that control the development of multicellular animals and the homeostasis of adult tissues by combining cell-autonomous and non-cell-autonomous pathways. We are able to deterministically explain each step of these mechanisms, but it is becoming more and more clear that stochastic models are better able to capture the behavior of cells within a population. For instance, stem cells that, while proliferating, demonstrate a specific likelihood to either differentiate or self-renew, maintain the homeostasis of skin and the esophageal epithelium. To ensure tissue regeneration, this likelihood is precisely calibrated. However, the disruption of cell signaling by cell-autonomous pathways or cell-to-cell communication can change this equilibrium, resulting in illnesses such as cancer [82–86].

In recent decades, phospholipid-based signal sensing has seen significant advancements. Numerous studies have shown that the homeostasis of phospholipids is maintained by an intricate and dynamic network of metabolic processes that are controlled by a number of enzymes, whose activities are extremely sensitive to external and intracellular stimuli. A sizable and structurally complex collection of signaling molecules is formed as a result of the multiplicity of phospholipid metabolic pathways. Even within a single cell, the sheer number of effectors leads to the development of a highly intricate network of signaling pathways that follow the activation of phospholipid signaling. Recent studies have uncovered crucial facets of phospholipid signaling, the relevance of their spatiotemporally diverse and dynamic molecular profile, and their multiple locations in various extracellular fluids, as well as specific membrane microdomains, distinct intramembrane pools, and various subcellular sites and compartments. Phospholipids, along with the metabolic products they produce, are essential for signaling events that are involved in a variety of biological processes, including those that control survival, growth, differentiation, shape, motility, activation, and death. Recent evidence that numerous phospholipids and their derivatives play a crucial role as transcriptional regulators of complicated nuclear signaling pathways revealed an intriguing feature of phospholipid signaling. In fact, certain phospholipid species have the ability to operate as non-membrane associated lipids to precisely bind to and functionally control the activation of particular nuclear receptors. In addition, several nuclear receptors have the ability to attach phospholipid head groups to essential phospholipid signaling enzymes, which can subsequently change the phospholipid head group with special kinetic features. Thus, phospholipid signaling is a network of metabolic pathways that is intricately regulated and crucial for the management of homeostasis, intercellular communication, and efficient cellular responses [87–90].

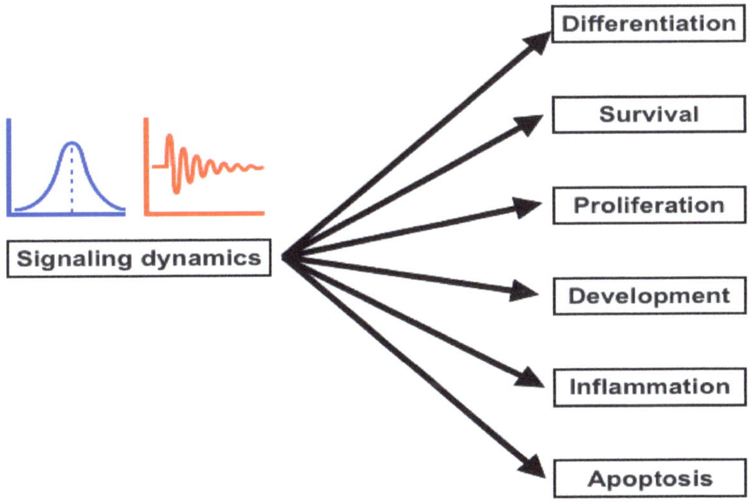

Figure 2. Signaling dynamics controlling various cellular decisions.

Recent research also demonstrated that the role of phospholipid signaling in the control of extracellular vesicles added yet another layer of intricacy to its already intricate processes. These tiny, secreted vesicular structures, which play a role in intercellular communication and the preservation of physiological homeostasis, are becoming a new frontier in signal transduction. These vesicles seem to carry particular phospholipid enzymes or signals, offering a method of efficiently transporting them across long distances to various cells without dilution or destruction. Given the importance of phospholipid signaling and the variety of cell regulatory functions it performs, it should come as no surprise that its dysregulation is the root of many diseases. The onset of a number of human diseases is driven by defects in phospholipid signaling, according to recently accumulated evidence. Numerous studies have shown that changes in phospholipid signaling can accelerate the development of a number of illnesses, including cancer, cardiovascular, and neurological problems, as well as developmental and degenerative diseases. Understanding the triggers that cause the signaling transition to a pathogenic function and developing innovative treatment techniques are two pertinent, ongoing research areas [80,91–93].

It has been demonstrated in earlier research that the temporal dynamics may be related to signaling factors such as signal molecule concentration, feedback/feedforward (positive/negative), crosstalk (positive/negative) between the pathways, and reaction rate [18,75,76,94,95]. These analyses into many parameters have been conducted for various signaling pathways, including MAPK. The strength of the receptor and input signals could perhaps have an impact on the nature of the temporal response of the downstream signaling molecules, according to the prior research. Similarly to this, while the rate of reaction (kinetic parameters) can simply increase or decrease the response strength, feedback loops and route crosstalk can entirely change the nature of the signaling response [76,77,96–102].

4. Cell-Fate Decision

Understanding the mechanisms that control cell fate decisions is a core objective of developmental and stem cell biology. The contributions of alterations in transcriptional programming, epigenetic modifications, and biochemical differentiation signals are covered in the majority of studies on the regulation of cell destiny decisions. Recent research has discovered that the regulation of cell destiny decisions is also significantly influenced by other facets of cell biology. Intracellular molecular regulatory networks and external environmental factors interact intricately to control the destiny of cells. We are able to analyze the molecular specifics of these regulatory mechanisms in ever-greater depth because of recent improvements in experimental technology. These cues serve both upstream and downstream of developmental signaling pathways and can play either a permissive or instructional role. They are a part of a wider network of signaling (Figures 1 and 2) and for detailed relevance, Figure 3 has been shown which infers the aberration to cell-fate decision. Regulation of cell destiny has a direct impact on human health and tissue homeostasis. Research on cell fate choice identifies important regulators, aids in comprehending the mechanisms, and offers fresh ideas for treating clinical disorders associated with aberrant cell development [21,22,103–109].

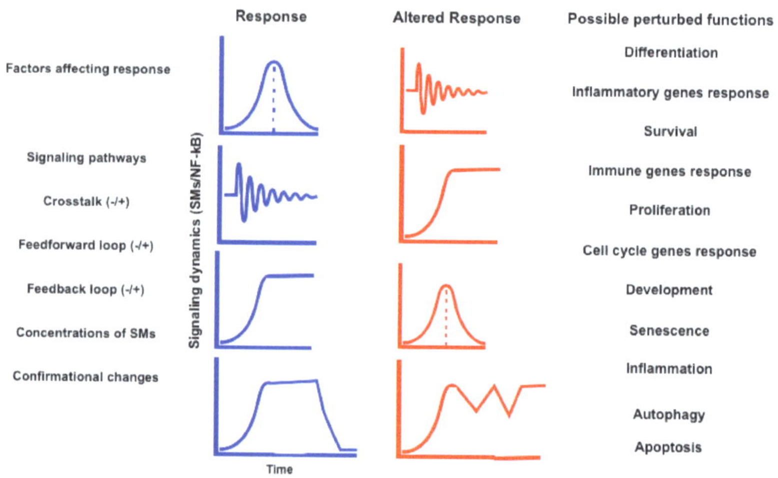

Figure 3. Signaling dynamics are known to control various cellular/cell-fate decisions. Signaling dynamics are associated with specific responses (downstream SMs). Targeted perturbations reveal the role of dynamics in cellular responses.

A specialized organelle for protein folding and trafficking, the endoplasmic reticulum (ER) is extremely sensitive to changes in intracellular homeostasis and external stimuli. Misfolded proteins build up in the ER as a result of changes in the protein-folding environment, which has a significant impact on a number of cellular signaling processes, such as energy generation, inflammation, differentiation, and death. The unfolded protein response (UPR) is a group of adaptive signaling pathways that have developed to address protein misfolding and re-establish a favorable environment for protein folding. Recent developments: The UPR and ER stress have both been connected to the production of reactive oxygen species (ROS). ROS, which can be formed in the cytosol and a number of organelles, including the ER and mitochondria, are important for many cellular activities. According to studies, ER stress, which may in turn trigger the formation of ROS in the ER and mitochondria, can be brought on by a change in the ER's redox equilibrium. Despite the fact that oxidative stress and ER stress frequently occur in pathologic situations, it is unclear whether or how these stressors interact. Additionally, it is not known how modifications to the ER's protein-folding environment result in oxidative stress. Additionally, it is uncertain how the creation of ROS and protein misfolding cause apoptosis in cells and contribute to a number of degenerative disorders. In terms of future perspectives, the discovery of innovative therapies for many human diseases will benefit from a deeper knowledge of the underlying processes that maintain the homeostasis and redox state of protein folding [16,110–113].

Through progenitor cell differentiation, cellular diversity and specialization can be established throughout development. The majority of tissues reserve undifferentiated progenitors, which are likely involved in the tissue's homeostasis during the duration of its existence, as we have also learnt in recent years. The differentiation of these cells during homeostasis is probably a carefully regulated process [114–116]. Although this is not well understood, progenitor development and differentiation may become dysregulated in disease. For instance, the cancer stem cell theory claims that the biological origin of malignant tumors is populations of tumor cells that resemble healthy adult stem cells. These could be endogenous stem cells that, over time, underwent somatic mutations that result in cancer. Another example is fibrosis, which is characterized by an overabundance of myofibroblasts that create extracellular matrix components that make tissues less flexible. Although little is known about the origins of myofibroblasts in fibrotic tissues, it has long been believed that these cells originate from the immediate area [117–121].

5. Encoding and Decoding Cellular Information

Cells modulate the dynamics of intracellular signaling molecules (SMs) to transmit and receive information through the signal transduction process. Cellular decision making critically depends on the temporal dynamics of SMs. For instance, prolonged Erk activation following NGF administration causes PC-12 cells to differentiate, whereas transient Erk activation results in proliferation. According to previously published research, a number of serious illnesses seem to be brought on by abnormalities in the signal transduction pathway. The crucial factor is the length or kind of cellular response, which appears to be directly related to the choice of the cell's fate. The cells go through apoptosis, proliferation, or differentiation depending on the kind of biological response (transient, sustained, or partly adapted) [1,16,122–126]. Understanding how the signaling pathways interact to produce a temporary or long-lasting physiological response is thus a crucial stage in the signal transduction process. A cascade of linked biochemical processes that finally control the elements in charge of cellular phenotypic activities influence the response of a cell to environmental inputs. The signaling apparatus was first envisioned as a combination of separate, linear routes. However, the present perception of the system as a complex network has supplanted the more recent elaboration of the breadth and diversity of intra-pathway crosstalk. These days, it is believed that the cell's signaling network serves as the primary functional module, which is coupled to a number of additional modules that control phenotypic function. These latter ones include those that control the cell's secretory, motile, and translational activities. A noteworthy feature of signaling is that transmission and information processing are intertwined. Through intra-cascade feedback control and cross-talk with other channels, the interactions between individual components serve as the interfaces for information computing. The context-specificity of the cellular response is a result of the signaling network's capacity to process information [85,90,127–131].

Within certain cell types, the kinetics of cell signaling and transcriptional regulatory activity vary in response to the same stimulus. There is a lot of interest in using single-cell-size data in addition to researching network connections to clarify the non-random parts of the variability involved in cellular decision making. Based on an immediate link between the molecular processes, previous studies have taken into account the information flow between the signaling and transcriptional domains. These results suggest a restricted binary on/off encoding technique that undervalues the complexity of biological information processing and, thus, the value of data at the single-cell scale. Here, instead of focusing on chemical abundances, we adopt a unique approach that reframes the information transmission problem as incorporating the dynamic aspects of signaling (Figure 3). We use a computational method to investigate whether and how the patterns of transcriptional regulatory activity might provide insight into the temporal evolution of signaling. This work also summarizes two methodological factors: (1) the dynamic characteristics of signaling that significantly change transcriptional regulatory patterns (encoding); and (2) the temporal history of signaling that can be inferred from snapshots of transcriptional activity taken at the single-cell scale (decoding). In contrast to transcription factor activity patterns, which were instructive of the activation and deactivation kinetics of signaling, immediate early gene expression patterns were indicative of signaling peak retention kinetics. Additionally, the network's information processing characteristics fluctuated, with each component encoding a particular portion of the dynamic signaling qualities. In order to understand the dynamic multiplexing of the signaling properties at each of these network components, we created unique sensitivity and information transfer maps. Two groups that corresponded with network patterns and could be separated by transcriptional feedforward vs. feedback interactions were discovered by the unsupervised clustering of the maps. By finding the downstream snapshot measurements necessary for deducing particular dynamical aspects of upstream signals important in the control of cellular responses, our novel computational technique has an influence on the single-cell size investigations [9,16,132–137].

In order to identify the functional feedback influencing the observed dynamics, it might be useful to examine the dynamics of signaling molecules in response to various stimuli. For instance, a negative feedback between ERK and Son of Sevenless (SOS) in the EGF pathway contributes to the variations in ERK dynamics in response to EGF or NGF. Additionally, NGF signaling, but not EGF signaling, persists after receptor internalization, which helps maintain ERK activation. Positive feedback on ERK activation through PKC is also supported by research. The inference is that changes in the identity and the connection of different route components are what cause the different responses to EGF and NGF, which are mediated by the dynamics of ERK [13,111,138–141].

6. NF-κB Signaling and Molecular Targets for Therapeutic Purpose of Human Diseases

Numerous factors that contribute to human diseases such as different types of cancers include NF-κB. The development of cancer is known to be linked to inflammation, which depends on the reciprocal activation of NF-κB and inflammatory cytokines. The anticancer effects of therapy are diminished by both constitutive and therapeutic-induced NF-κB activation. Understanding the functions of NF-κB in cancer aids the development of methods for cancer therapy and prevention [25,26]. A thorough analysis of NF-κB in each type of disease is essential in this regard due to the complexity of NF-κB involvement in many human diseases. To increase efficacy and lower systemic toxicity, more disease-specific NF-κB inhibiting techniques are sought. NF-κB potentially regulates the transcription process, apoptosis, and proliferation by interacting/affecting with/the critical biological pathways via their components (genes/proteins). These pathway components are targeted for therapeutic purposes. Bcl-2 family members, IAP family members, ROS, p53, MDM2, MDR1, DR5, FASL, Bax, and more are well-known targets for therapeutic purposes. Furthermore, the targeting approach may differ such as the application nanoparticles coated herbal drugs and/or pure herbal drugs [25,26,142,143].

Potential NF-κB blockers include non-steroidal anti-inflammatory drugs (NSAIDs) such as sulindac, aspirin, ibuprofen, indomethacin, and COX-2 inhibitors. These either directly suppress NF-κB at critical junctures along the NF-κB activation pathway or indirectly suppress the inflammatory cell response to do so. It has been thoroughly investigated whether combining these medications with anticancer medicines will promote chemoprevention or chemosensitization. Curcumin (diferuloylmethane), eicosapentaenoic acid (EPA), luteolin, and other naturally occurring anti-inflammatory chemicals are also able to block NF-κB, making them another class of NF-κB-blocking medications for cancer therapy and prevention. These substances obstruct NF-κB at various points along the route. Celestrol blocks NF-DNA B's binding, apigenin and anacardic acid block IKK, resveratrol blocks p65 phosphorylation, epicatechin blocks p65 translocation to the nucleus, and p65 phosphorylation, respectively. It is important to highlight that these compounds are mostly antioxidants, and their potential role in the prevention of cancer may include controlling the redox state of the cell. The modification of redox, however, might be a factor in NF-κB blocking. It is also known that luteolin inhibits TNF-α-induced NF-κB in lung cancer cells by activating superoxide. Luteolin's inhibition of NF-κB causes TNF-α-induced cancer cell survival to switch to apoptosis. Luteolin may function as a possible chemopreventive agent due to its capacity to change TNF-α from a tumor promoter to a tumor suppressor due to its ability to block NF-κB. TNF-α is engaged in inflammation-associated carcinogenesis [144–146].

7. Conclusions and Future Perspectives

When thinking about dynamics' functional role, the next question that comes to mind is how cells understand various dynamical patterns. What molecular processes, in other words, are required to recognize time-dependent patterns and convert these patterns into distinctive phenotypic responses? Identifying the mechanisms that decode dynamics continues to be one of the field's most difficult objectives despite the fact that numerous studies have identified functional roles for particular temporal behaviors, and only a small portion of these have precisely determined how different dynamical patterns are distinguished at the molecular level to cause different downstream responses. When addressing the functional relevance of dynamics, the difficult topic is how cells understand various dynamical patterns. Which molecular processes are required to recognize time-dependent patterns and convert them into different phenotypic responses? We have presented details about the NF-κB signaling roles in human diseases, details of signaling dynamics, cell-fate decision, and encoding/decoding of cellular information into final cell-fate decision. We consider it to be of potential interest which could be helpful in not only understanding and exploring the dynamics of different signaling pathway for multiple purposes, including in precise therapeutic approach for different human diseases.

Author Contributions: Conceptualization, S.A., L.S.A. and M.M.; methodology, S.A., L.S.A. and M.M.; software, S.A., L.S.A. and M.M.; validation, S.A., L.S.A. and M.M.; formal analysis, S.A., L.S.A. and M.M.; investigation, M.M.; resources, S.A., L.S.A. and M.M.; data curation, M.M.; writing—original draft preparation, S.A., L.S.A. and M.M.; writing—review and editing, S.A., L.S.A. and M.M.; visualization, S.A., L.S.A. and M.M.; supervision, M.M.; project administration, S.A., L.S.A. and M.M.; funding acquisition, S.A. and L.S.A. All authors have read and agreed to the published version of the manuscript.

Funding: This research received no external funding.

Institutional Review Board Statement: Not applicable.

Informed Consent Statement: Not applicable.

Data Availability Statement: Not applicable.

Acknowledgments: We are grateful for the facilities and support offered by the Department of Biochemistry, Faculty of Sciences, University of Tabuk, Tabuk 71491, Saudi Arabia; the Department of Biochemistry, College of Science, University of Jeddah, Jeddah 23445, Saudi Arabia; and SciLifeLab, Department of Oncology and Pathology, Karolinska Institutet, Box 1031, S-17121 Stockholm.

Conflicts of Interest: The authors declare no conflict of interest. The funders had no role in the design of the study; in the collection, analyses, or interpretation of data; in the writing of the manuscript; or in the decision to publish the results.

References

1. Purvis, J.E.; Lahav, G. Encoding and Decoding Cellular Information through Signaling Dynamics. *Cell* **2013**, *152*, 945–956. [CrossRef] [PubMed]
2. Klil-Drori, A.J.; Azoulay, L.; Pollak, M.N. Cancer, obesity, diabetes, and antidiabetic drugs: Is the fog clearing? *Nat. Rev. Clin. Oncol.* **2016**, *14*, 85–99. [CrossRef] [PubMed]

3. Davis, D.M.; Purvis, J.E. Computational analysis of signaling patterns in single cells. *Semin Cell Dev Biol.* **2015**, *37*, 35–43. [CrossRef] [PubMed]
4. Garcia-Bernardo, J.; Eppstein, M.J. Evolving modular genetic regulatory networks with a recursive, top-down approach. *Syst. Synth. Biol.* **2015**, *9*, 179–189. [CrossRef] [PubMed]
5. Batchelor, E.; Loewer, A.; Mock, C.; Lahav, G. Stimulus-dependent dynamics of p53 in single cells. *Mol. Syst. Biol.* **2011**, *7*, 488. [CrossRef] [PubMed]
6. Regev-Rudzki, N.; Wilson, D.W.; Carvalho, T.G.; Sisquella, X.; Coleman, B.M.; Rug, M.; Bursac, D.; Angrisano, F.; Gee, M.; Hill, A.F.; et al. Cell-Cell Communication between Malaria-Infected Red Blood Cells via Exosome-like Vesicles. *Cell* **2013**, *153*, 1120–1133. [CrossRef]
7. Ruch, R.J. Intercellular communication, homeostasis, and toxicology. *Toxicol. Sci.* **2002**, *68*, 265–266. [CrossRef]
8. Cotari, J.W.; Voisinne, G.; Dar, O.E.; Karabacak, V.; Altan-Bonnet, G. Cell-to-Cell Variability Analysis Dissects the Plasticity of Signaling of Common Chain Cytokines in T Cells. *Sci. Signal.* **2013**, *6*, ra17. [CrossRef]
9. Poltorak, M.; Arndt, B.; Kowtharapu, B.S.; Reddycherla, A.V.; Witte, V.; Lindquist, J.A.; Schraven, B.; Simeoni, L. TCR activation kinetics and feedback regulation in primary human T cells. *Cell Commun. Signal.* **2013**, *11*, 4. [CrossRef]
10. Lim, W.A.; Pawson, T. Phosphotyrosine Signaling: Evolving a New Cellular Communication System. *Cell* **2010**, *142*, 661–667. [CrossRef]
11. Matolcsi, M.; Giordano, N. A Novel Explanation for Observed CaMKII Dynamics in Dendritic Spines with Added EGTA or BAPTA. *Biophys. J.* **2015**, *108*, 975–985. [CrossRef] [PubMed]
12. El-Kafrawy, S.A.; El-Daly, M.M.; Bajrai, L.H.; Alandijany, T.A.; Faizo, A.A.; Mobashir, M.; Ahmed, S.S.; Ahmed, S.; Alam, S.; Jeet, R.; et al. Genomic profiling and network-level understanding uncover the potential genes and the pathways in hepatocellular carcinoma. *Front. Genet.* **2022**, *13*, 880440. [CrossRef]
13. Orton, R.J.; Sturm, O.E.; Vyshemirsky, V.; Calder, M.; Gilbert, D.R.; Kolch, W. Computational modelling of the receptor-tyrosine-kinase-activated MAPK pathway. *Biochem. J.* **2005**, *392*, 249–261. [CrossRef] [PubMed]
14. Hogenesch, J.B.; Ueda, H.R. Understanding systems-level properties: Timely stories from the study of clocks. *Nat. Rev. Genet.* **2011**, *12*, 407–416. [CrossRef]
15. Stelzl, U.; Worm, U.; Lalowski, M.; Haenig, C.; Brembeck, F.H.; Goehler, H.; Stroedicke, M.; Zenkner, M.; Schoenherr, A.; Koeppen, S.; et al. A Human Protein-Protein Interaction Network: A Resource for Annotating the Proteome. *Cell* **2005**, *122*, 957–968. [CrossRef]
16. Yao, G.; Lee, T.J.; Mori, S.; Nevins, J.R.; You, L. A bistable Rb–E2F switch underlies the restriction point. *Nat. Cell Biol.* **2008**, *10*, 476–482. [CrossRef]
17. Sobie, E.A. Bistability in Biochemical Signaling Models. *Sci. Signal.* **2011**, *4*, tr10. [CrossRef]
18. Kholodenko, B.N. Cell-signalling dynamics in time and space. *Nat. Rev. Mol. Cell Biol.* **2006**, *7*, 165–176. [CrossRef]
19. Schleich, K.; Lavrik, I.N. Mathematical modeling of apoptosis. *Cell Commun. Signal.* **2013**, *11*, 44. [CrossRef]
20. Prashar, Y.; Ritu; Gill, N.S. Emerging role of various signaling pathways in the pathogenesis and therapeutics of atherosclerosis. *Rev. Vasc. Med.* **2017**, *10*, 1–12. [CrossRef]
21. Loewer, A.; Lahav, G. Cellular Conference Call: External Feedback Affects Cell-Fate Decisions. *Cell* **2006**, *124*, 1128–1130. [CrossRef] [PubMed]
22. Niiro, H.; Clark, E.A. Decision making in the immune system: Regulation of B-cell fate by antigen-receptor signals. *Nat. Rev. Immunol.* **2002**, *2*, 945–956. [CrossRef] [PubMed]
23. White, K.L.; Rider, D.N.; Kalli, K.R.; Knutson, K.L.; Jarvik, G.P.; Goode, E.L. Genomics of the NF-κB signaling pathway: Hypothesized role in ovarian cancer. *Cancer Causes Control* **2011**, *22*, 785–801. [CrossRef] [PubMed]
24. Ricaño-Ponce, I.; Wijmenga, C. Mapping of Immune-Mediated Disease Genes. *Annu. Rev. Genom. Hum. Genet.* **2013**, *14*, 325–353. [CrossRef] [PubMed]
25. Habashy, N.H.; Kodous, A.S.; Abu-Serie, M.M. Targeting ROS/NF-κB signaling pathway by the seedless black Vitis vinifera polyphenolsin CCl. *Sci. Rep.* **2021**, *11*, 16575. [CrossRef] [PubMed]
26. Abu-Serie, M.M.; Hamouda, A.F.; Habashy, N.H. Acacia senegal gumattenuates systemic toxicityin CCl. *Sci. Rep.* **2021**, *11*, 20316. [CrossRef]
27. Oeckinghaus, A.; Ghosh, S. The NF-kappaB family of transcription factors and its regulation. *Cold Spring Harb. Perspect. Biol.* **2009**, *1*, a000034. [CrossRef]
28. Manning, B.D.; Cantley, L.C. AKT/PKB Signaling: Navigating Downstream. *Cell* **2007**, *129*, 1261–1274. [CrossRef]
29. Mostafizar, M.; Cortes-Pérez, C.; Snow, W.; Djordjevic, J.; Adlimoghaddam, A.; Albensi, B.C. Challenges with Methods for Detecting and Studying the Transcription Factor Nuclear Factor Kappa B (NF-κB) in the Central Nervous System. *Cells* **2021**, *10*, 1335. [CrossRef]
30. Yan, F.; Liu, L.; Wang, Q. Combinatorial dynamics of protein synthesis time delay and negative feedback loop in NF-κB signalling pathway. *IET Syst. Biol.* **2020**, *14*, 284–291. [CrossRef]
31. Prescott, J.A.; Mitchell, J.P.; Cook, S.J. Inhibitory feedback control of NF-κB signalling in health and disease. *Biochem. J.* **2021**, *478*, 2619–2664. [CrossRef] [PubMed]
32. ARAUJO, R.; LIOTTA, L. A control theoretic paradigm for cell signaling networks: A simple complexity for a sensitive robustness. *Curr. Opin. Chem. Biol.* **2006**, *10*, 81–87. [CrossRef]

33. Restifo, N.P.; Smyth, M.J.; Snyder, A. Acquired resistance to immunotherapy and future challenges. *Nat. Rev. Cancer* **2016**, *16*, 121–126. [CrossRef] [PubMed]
34. Inoki, K.; Kim, J.; Guan, K.-L. AMPK and mTOR in Cellular Energy Homeostasis and Drug Targets. *Annu. Rev. Pharmacol. Toxicol.* **2012**, *52*, 381–400. [CrossRef] [PubMed]
35. Buszczak, M.; Signer, R.A.J.; Morrison, S.J. Cellular Differences in Protein Synthesis Regulate Tissue Homeostasis. *Cell* **2014**, *159*, 242–251. [CrossRef]
36. Furusawa, C.; Kaneko, K. A Dynamical-Systems View of Stem Cell Biology. *Science* **2012**, *338*, 215–217. [CrossRef]
37. de Souza, N. A systems view of cellular reprogramming. *Nat. Meth.* **2014**, *11*, 987. [CrossRef]
38. Burzyn, D.; Kuswanto, W.; Kolodin, D.; Shadrach, J.L.; Cerletti, M.; Jang, Y.; Sefik, E.; Tan, T.G.; Wagers, A.J.; Benoist, C.; et al. A Special Populationof Regulatory T Cells Potentiates Muscle Repair. *Cell* **2013**, *155*, 1282–1295. [CrossRef]
39. Gutierrez-Arcelus, M.; Rich, S.S.; Raychaudhuri, S. Autoimmune diseases—Connecting risk alleles with molecular traits of the immune system. *Nat. Rev. Genet.* **2016**, *17*, 160–174. [CrossRef]
40. Kurosaki, T.; Shinohara, H.; Baba, Y. B Cell Signaling and Fate Decision. *Annu. Rev. Immunol.* **2010**, *28*, 21–55. [CrossRef]
41. Baxt, L.A.; Garza-Mayers, A.C.; Goldberg, M.B. Bacterial Subversion of Host Innate Immune Pathways. *Science* **2013**, *340*, 697–701. [CrossRef] [PubMed]
42. Shalkami, A.S.; Hassan, M.; Bakr, A.G. Anti-inflammatory, antioxidant and anti-apoptotic activity of diosmin in acetic acid-induced ulcerative colitis. *Hum. Exp. Toxicol.* **2017**, *37*, 78–86. [CrossRef] [PubMed]
43. Bouwmeester, T.; Bauch, A.; Ruffner, H.; Angrand, P.-O.; Bergamini, G.; Croughton, K.; Cruciat, C.; Eberhard, D.; Gagneur, J.; Ghidelli, S.; et al. A physical and functional map of the human TNF-α/NF-κB signal transduction pathway. *Nat. Cell Biol.* **2004**, *6*, 97–105. [CrossRef] [PubMed]
44. Helmi, N.; Alammari, D.; Mobashir, M. Role of potential COVID-19 immune system associated genes and the potential pathways linkage with type-2 diabetes. *Combinatorial Chemistry & High Throughput Screening.* **2022**, *25*, 2452–2462.
45. Zhou, T.; Hu, Z.; Yang, S.; Sun, L.; Yu, Z.; Wang, G. Review Article Role of Adaptive and Innate Immunity in Type 2 Diabetes Mellitus. *J. Diabetes Res.* **2018**, *2018*, 7457269. [CrossRef]
46. Stephenson, E.; Reynolds, G.; Botting, R.A.; Calero-Nieto, F.J.; Morgan, M.D.; Tuong, Z.K.; Bach, K.; Sungnak, W.; Worlock, K.B.; Yoshida, M.; et al. Single-cell multi-omics analysis of the immune response in COVID-19. *Nat. Med.* **2021**, *27*, 904–916. [CrossRef]
47. Chalkiadaki, A.; Guarente, L. The multifaceted functions of sirtuins in cancer. *Nat. Rev. Cancer* **2015**, *15*, 608–624. [CrossRef]
48. Machado-Oliveira, G.; Ramos, C.; Marques, A.R.A.; Vieira, O.V. Cell Senescence, Multiple Organelle Dysfunction and Atherosclerosis. *Cells* **2020**, *9*, 2146. [CrossRef]
49. Long, E.O.; Sik Kim, H.; Liu, D.; Peterson, M.E.; Rajagopalan, S. Controlling Natural Killer Cell Responses: Integration of Signals for Activation and Inhibition. *Annu. Rev. Immunol.* **2013**, *31*, 227–258. [CrossRef]
50. Kuballa, P.; Nolte, W.M.; Castoreno, A.B.; Xavier, R.J. Autophagy and the Immune System. *Annu. Rev. Immunol.* **2012**, *30*, 611–646. [CrossRef]
51. Bezbradica, J.S.; Medzhitov, R. Integration of cytokine and heterologous receptor signaling pathways. *Nat. Immunol.* **2009**, *10*, 333–339. [CrossRef] [PubMed]
52. Tigno-Aranjuez, J.T.; Bai, X.; Abbott, D.W. A Discrete Ubiquitin-Mediated Network Regulates the Strength of NOD2 Signaling. *Mol. Cell. Biol.* **2012**, *33*, 146–158. [CrossRef] [PubMed]
53. Källstig, E.; McCabe, B.D.; Schneider, B.L. The Links between ALS and NF-κB. *Int. J. Mol. Sci.* **2021**, *22*, 3875. [CrossRef] [PubMed]
54. Bagaev, A.V.; Garaeva, A.Y.; Lebedeva, E.S.; Pichugin, A.V.; Ataullakhanov, R.I.; Ataullakhanov, F.I. Elevated pre-activation basal level of nuclear NF-κB in native macrophages accelerates Lps- induced translocation of cytosolic NF-κB into the cell nucleus. *Sci. Rep.* **2019**, *9*, 4563. [CrossRef] [PubMed]
55. Hernandez, L.; Kim, M.K.; Noonan, A.M.; Sagher, E.; Kohlhammer, H.; Wright, G.; Lyle, L.T.; Steeg, P.S.; Anver, M.; Bowtell, D.D.; et al. A dual role for Caspase8 and NF. *Nat. Publ. Group* **2015**, *1*, 15053.
56. Martin, G.S. Cell signaling and cancer. *Cancer Cell* **2003**, *4*, 167–174. [CrossRef]
57. Schlessinger, J. Cell signaling by receptor tyrosine kinases. *Cell* **2000**, *103*, 211–225. [CrossRef]
58. Yang, J.-M.; Chi, W.-Y.; Liang, J.; Takayanagi, S.; Iglesias, P.A.; Huang, C.-H. Deciphering cell signaling networks with massively multiplexed biosensor barcoding. *Cell* **2021**, *184*, 6193–6206. [CrossRef]
59. Tyson, J.J.; Chen, K.C.; Novák, B. Sniffers, buzzers, toggles and blinkers: Dynamics of regulatory and signaling pathways in the cell. *Current Opinion in Cell Biology* **2003**, *15*, 221–231. [CrossRef]
60. Danko, C.G.; Hah, N.; Luo, X.; Martins, A.L.; Core, L.; Lis, J.T.; Siepel, A.; Kraus, W.L. Signaling Pathways Differentially Affect RNA Polymerase II Initiation, Pausing, and Elongation Rate in Cells. *Mol. Cell* **2013**, *50*, 212–222. [CrossRef]
61. Han, B.; Li, X.; Ai, R.-S.; Deng, S.-Y.; Ye, Z.-Q.; Deng, X.; Ma, W.; Xiao, S.; Wang, J.-Z.; Wang, L.-M.; et al. Atmospheric particulate matter aggravates cns demyelination through involvement of TLR-4/NF-kB signaling and microglial activation. *eLife* **2022**, *11*, e72247. [CrossRef] [PubMed]
62. Heltberg, M.L.; Krishna, S.; Jensen, M.H. On chaotic dynamics in transcription factors and the associated effects in differential gene regulation. *Nat. Commun.* **2018**, *10*, 71. [CrossRef] [PubMed]
63. Dorrington, M.G.; Fraser, I.D.C. NF-κB Signaling in Macrophages: Dynamics, Crosstalk, and Signal Integration. *Front. Immunol.* **2019**, *10*, 705. [CrossRef] [PubMed]

64. Kuznetsova, T.; Prange, K.H.M.; Glass, C.K.; Winther, M.P.J. Transcriptional and epigeneticregulation of macrophagesin atherosclerosis. *Nat. Rev. Cardiol.* **2019**, *17*, 216–228. [CrossRef]
65. Moore, K.E.; Carlson, S.M.; Camp, N.D.; Cheung, P.; James, R.G.; Chua, K.F.; Wolf-Yadlin, A.; Gozani, O. A General Molecular Affinity Strategy for Global Detection and Proteomic Analysis of Lysine Methylation. *Mol. Cell* **2013**, *50*, 444–456. [CrossRef] [PubMed]
66. Fabbri, G.; Rasi, S.; Rossi, D.; Trifonov, V.; Khiabanian, H.; Ma, J.; Grunn, A.; Fangazio, M.; Capello, D.; Monti, S.; et al. Analysis of the chronic lymphocytic leukemia coding genome: Role of NOTCH1mutational activation. *J. Exp. Med.* **2011**, *208*, 1389–1401. [CrossRef]
67. Ma, Y.; Galluzzi, L.; Zitvogel, L.; Kroemer, G. Autophagy and Cellular Immune Responses. *Immunity* **2013**, *39*, 211–227. [CrossRef]
68. Khan, N.; Mukhtar, H. Biochemical Pharmacology. *Biochem. Pharmacol.* **2013**, *85*, 667–672. [CrossRef]
69. Bui, J.D.; Schreiber, R.D. Cancer immunosurveillance, immunoediting and inflammation: Independent or interdependent processes? *Curr. Opin. Immunol.* **2007**, *19*, 203–208. [CrossRef]
70. Koosha, S.; Alshawsh, M.A.; Looi, C.Y.; Seyedan, A.; Mohamed, Z. An Association Map on the Effect of Flavonoids on the Signaling Pathways in Colorectal Cancer. *Int. J. Med. Sci.* **2016**, *13*, 374–385. [CrossRef]
71. Visvader, J.E. Cells of origin in cancer. *Nature* **2011**, *469*, 314–322. [CrossRef] [PubMed]
72. Gonda, T.J.; Ramsay, R.G. Directly targeting transcriptional dysregulation in cancer. *Nat. Rev. Cancer* **2015**, *15*, 686–694. [CrossRef] [PubMed]
73. da Silva, H.B.; Amaral, E.P.; Nolasco, E.L.; de Victo, N.C.; Atique, R.; Jank, C.C.; Anschau, V.; Zerbini, L.F.; Correa, R.G. Dissecting Major Signaling Pathways throughout the Development of Prostate Cancer. *Prostate Cancer* **2013**, *2013*, 920612. [CrossRef]
74. Feinberg, A.P.; Koldobskiy, M.A.; Göndör, A. Epigenetic modulators, modifiers and mediators in cancer aetiology and progression. *Nat. Rev. Genet.* **2016**, *17*, 284–299. [CrossRef] [PubMed]
75. Mobashir, M.; Madhusudhan, T.; Isermann, B.; Beyer, T.; Schraven, B. Negative Interactions and Feedback Regulations Are Required for Transient Cellular Response. *Sci. Rep.* **2014**, *4*, 3718. [CrossRef]
76. Mobashir, M.; Schraven, B.; Beyer, T. Simulated evolution of signal transduction networks. *PLoS ONE* **2012**, *7*, e50905. [CrossRef]
77. Mobashir, M. Mathematical Modeling and Evolution of Signal Transduction Pathways and Networks. Ph.D. Thesis, Otto-von-Guericke-University Magdeburg, Magdeburg, Germany, 2013.
78. Vafai, S.B.; Mootha, V.K. A Common Pathway for a Rare Disease? *Science* **2013**, *342*, 1453–1454. [CrossRef]
79. Pant, D.K.; Ghosh, A. A systems biology approach for the study of cumulative oncogenes with applications to the MAPK signal transduction pathway. *Biophys. Chem.* **2006**, *119*, 49–60. [CrossRef]
80. Rousseau, F.; Schymkowitz, J. A systems biology perspective on protein structural dynamics and signal transduction. *Curr. Opin. Struct. Biol.* **2005**, *15*, 23–30. [CrossRef]
81. Mosaddeghi, P.; Eslami, M.; Farahmandnejad, M.; Akhavein, M.; Ranjbarfarrokhi, R.; Khorraminejad-Shirazi, M.; Shahabinezhad, F.; Taghipour, M.; Dorvash, M.; Sakhteman, A.; et al. A systems pharmacology approach to identify the autophagy-inducing effects of Traditional Persian medicinal plants. *Sci. Rep.* **2020**, *11*, 336. [CrossRef]
82. Werner, H.M.J.; Mills, G.B.; Ram, P.T. Cancer Systems Biology: A peek into the future of patient care? *Nat. Rev. Clin. Oncol.* **2014**, *11*, 167–176. [CrossRef] [PubMed]
83. Wang, E.; Zou, J.; Zaman, N.; Beitel, L.K.; Trifiro, M.; Paliouras, M. Seminars in Cancer Biology. *Semin. Cancer Biol.* **2013**, *23*, 279–285. [CrossRef] [PubMed]
84. Wang, E.; Zaman, N.; Mcgee, S.; Milanese, J.-S.; Masoudi-Nejad, A.; O'Connor-McCourt, M. Seminars in Cancer Biology. *Semin. Cancer Biol.* **2015**, *30*, 4–12. [CrossRef]
85. Finley, S.D.; Chu, L.-H.; Popel, A.S. Computational systems biology approaches to anti-angiogenic cancer therapeutics. *Drug Discov. Today* **2014**, *20*, 187–197. [CrossRef]
86. Qutub, A.A. Systems approaches for synthetic biology: A pathwaytoward mammalian design. *Front. Physiol.* **2013**, *4*, 285.
87. Lin, Y.C.; Huang, D.Y.; Chu, C.L.; Lin, Y.L.; Lin, W.W. The Tyrosine Kinase Syk Differentially Regulates Toll-like Receptor Signaling Downstream of the Adaptor Molecules TRAF6 and TRAF3. *Sci. Signal.* **2013**, *6*, ra71. [CrossRef] [PubMed]
88. Lillemeier, B.F. How membrane structures control T cell signaling. 2012, 3, 291. *3*.
89. Zhang, Y.; Du, Y.; Le, W.; Wang, K.; Kieffer, N.; Zhang, J. Redox Control of the Survival of Healthy and Diseased Cells. *Antioxid. Redox Signal.* **2011**, *15*, 2867–2908. [CrossRef] [PubMed]
90. Breinig, M.; Klein, F.A.; Huber, W.; Boutros, M. A chemical-genetic interaction map of small molecules using high-throughput imaging in cancer cells. *Mol. Syst. Biol.* **2015**, *11*, 846. [CrossRef]
91. Reinartz, S.; Finkernagel, F.; Adhikary, T.; Rohnalter, V.; Schumann, T.; Schober, Y.; Nockher, W.A.; Nist, A.; Stiewe, T.; Jansen, J.M.; et al. A transcriptome-based global map of signaling pathways in the ovarian cancer microenvironment associated with clinical outcome. *Genome Biol.* **2016**, *17*, 108. [CrossRef]
92. Speer, T.; Rohrer, L.; Blyszczuk, P.; Shroff, R.; Kuschnerus, K.; Kränkel, N.; Kania, G.; Zewinger, S.; Akhmedov, A.; Shi, Y.; et al. Abnormal High-Density Lipoprotein Induces Endothelial Dysfunctionvia Activation of Toll-like Receptor-2. *Immunity* **2013**, *38*, 754–768. [CrossRef]
93. Smyth, J.T.; Hwang, S.-Y.; Tomita, T.; DeHaven, W.I.; Mercer, J.C.; Putney, J.W. Activation and regulation of store-operated calcium entry. *J. Cell. Mol. Med.* **2010**, *14*, 2337–2349. [CrossRef] [PubMed]

94. McClean, M.N.; Mody, A.; Broach, J.R.; Ramanathan, S. Cross-talk and decision making in MAP kinase pathways. *Nat. Genet.* **2007**, *39*, 409–414. [CrossRef] [PubMed]
95. Stuart, R.O.; Wachsman, W.; Berry, C.C.; Wang-Rodriguez, J.; Wasserman, L.; Klacansky, I.; Masys, D.; Arden, K.; Goodison, S.; McClelland, M.; et al. In silico dissection of cell-type-associated patterns of gene expression in prostate cancer. *Proc. Natl. Acad. Sci. USA* **2004**, *101*, 615–620. [CrossRef] [PubMed]
96. Kholodenko, B.; Yaffe, M.B.; Kolch, W. Computational Approaches for Analyzing Information Flow in Biological Networks. *Sci. Signal.* **2012**, *5*, re1. [CrossRef]
97. Kholodenko, B.N. Four-dimensional organization of protein kinase signaling cascades: The roles of diffusion, endocytosis and molecular motors. *J. Exp. Biol.* **2003**, *206*, 2073–2082. [CrossRef]
98. Kholodenko, B.N.; Demin, O.V.; Markevich, N.I.; Kiyatkin, A.; Moehren, G.; Hoek, J.B. Signal processing at the Ras circuit: What shapes Ras activation patterns? *Syst. Biol.* **2004**, *1*, 104–113.
99. Boris, N. Kholodenko Spatially distributed cell signalling. *FEBS Lett.* **2009**, *583*, 4006–4012.
100. Kholodenko, B.N.; Kiyatkin, A.; Bruggeman, F.J.; Sontag, E.; Westerhoff, H.V.; Hoek, J.B. Untangling the wires: A strategy to trace functional interactions in signaling and gene networks. *Proc. Natl. Acad. Sci. USA* **2002**, *99*, 12841–12846. [CrossRef]
101. Aksamitiene, E.; Kiyatkin, A.; Kholodenko, B.N. Cross-talk between mitogenic Ras/MAPK and survival PI3K/Akt pathways: A fine balance. *Biochm. Soc. Trans.* **2012**, *40*, 139–146. [CrossRef]
102. Bluthgen, N.; Bruggeman, F.J.; Legewie, S.; Herzel, H.; Westerhoff, H.V.; Kholodenko, B.N. Effects of sequestration on signal transduction cascades. *FEBS J.* **2006**, *273*, 895–906. [CrossRef]
103. Winstead, C.J.; Weaver, C.T. Dwelling on T Cell Fate Decisions. *Cell* **2013**, *153*, 739–741. [CrossRef] [PubMed]
104. Nguyen, L.K.; Matallanas, D.G.; Romano, D.; Kholodenko, B.N.; Kolch, W. Competing to coordinate cell fate decisions: The MST2-Raf-1 signaling device. *Cell Cycle* **2015**, *14*, 189–199. [CrossRef] [PubMed]
105. Reiterer, V.; Fey, D.; Kolch, W. Pseudophosphatase STYX modulates cell-fate decisions and cell migration by spatiotemporal regulation of ERK1/2. *Proc. Natl. Acad. Sci. USA* **2013**, *110*, E2934–E2943. [CrossRef]
106. Kumar, D.; Srikanth, R.; Ahlfors, H.; Lahesmaa, R.; Rao, K.V.S. Capturing cell-fate decisions from the molecular signatures of a receptor-dependent signaling response. *Mol. Syst. Biol.* **2007**, *3*, 150. [CrossRef] [PubMed]
107. Formosa-Jordan, P.; Ibañes, M. Competition in Notch Signaling with Cis Enriches Cell Fate Decisions. *PLoS ONE* **2014**, *9*, e95744. [CrossRef] [PubMed]
108. Li, C.; Wang, J. Quantifying Cell Fate Decisions for Differentiation and Reprogramming of a Human Stem Cell Network: Landscape and Biological Paths. *PLoS Comput. Biol.* **2013**, *9*, e1003165. [CrossRef]
109. Huang, W.; Cao, X.; Biase, F.H.; Yu, P.; Zhong, S. Time-variant clustering model for understanding cell fate decisions. *Proc. Natl. Acad. Sci. USA* **2014**, *111*, E4797–E4806. [CrossRef]
110. Wang, F.; Durfee, L.A.; Huibregtse, J.M. A Cotranslational Ubiquitination Pathway for Quality Control of Misfolded Proteins. *Mol. Cell* **2013**, *50*, 368–378. [CrossRef]
111. Cui, Q.; Ma, Y.; Jaramillo, M.; Bari, H.; Awan, A.; Yang, S.; Zhang, S.; Liu, L.; Lu, M.; O'Connor-McCourt, M.; et al. A map of human cancer signaling. *Mol. Syst. Biol.* **2007**, *3*, 152. [CrossRef]
112. Sanchez-Vega, F.; Mina, M.; Armenia, J.; Chatila, W.K.; Luna, A.; La, K.C.; Dimitriadoy, S.; Liu, D.L.; Kantheti, H.S.; Saghafinia, S.; et al. Oncogenic Signaling Pathways in The Cancer Genome Atlas. *Cell* **2018**, *173*, 321–337.e10. [CrossRef]
113. Khosravi, M.; Poursaleh, A.; Ghasempour, G.; Farhad, S.; Najafi, M. The effects of oxidative stress on the development of atherosclerosis. *Biol. Chem.* **2019**, *400*, 711–732. [CrossRef] [PubMed]
114. Tata, P.R.; Rajagopal, J. Plasticity in the lung: Making and breaking cell identity. *Development* **2017**, *144*, 755–766. [CrossRef] [PubMed]
115. Loukovaara, S.; Gucciardo, E.; Repo, P.; Lohi, J.; Salven, P.; Lehti, K. A Case of Abnormal Lymphatic-Like Differentiation and Endothelial Progenitor Cell Activation in Neovascularization Associated with Hemi-Retinal Vein Occlusion. *Case Rep. Ophthalmol.* **2015**, *6*, 228–238. [CrossRef] [PubMed]
116. Baylin, S.B.; Jones, P.A. A decade of exploring the cancer epigenome—Biological and translational implications. *Nat. Rev. Cancer* **2011**, *11*, 726–734. [CrossRef]
117. Michelini, R.H.; Doedens, A.L.; Goldrath, A.W.; Hedrick, S.M. Differentiation of CD8 memory T cells depends on Foxo1. *J. Exp. Med.* **2013**, *210*, 1189–1200. [CrossRef]
118. Chen, B.; Xue, Z.; Yang, G.; Shi, B.; Yang, B.; Yan, Y.; Wang, X.; Han, D.; Huang, Y.; Dong, W. Akt-Signal Integration Is Involved in the Differentiation of Embryonal Carcinoma Cells. *PLoS ONE* **2013**, *8*, e64877. [CrossRef]
119. Rebhahn, J.A.; Deng, N.; Sharma, G.; Livingstone, A.M.; Huang, S.; Mosmann, T.R. An animated landscape representation of CD4 +T-cell differentiation, variability, and plasticity: Insights into the behavior of populations versus cells. *Eur. J. Immunol.* **2014**, *44*, 2216–2229. [CrossRef]
120. Moustakas, A.; Pardali, K.; Gaal, A.; Heldin, C.H. Mechanisms of TGF-β signaling in regulation of cell growth and differentiation. *Immunol. Lett.* **2002**, *82*, 85–91. [CrossRef]
121. Ma, Y.; Adjemian, S.; Mattarollo, S.R.; Yamazaki, T.; Aymeric, L.; Yang, H.; Catani, J.P.P.; Hannani, D.; Duret, H.; Steegh, K.; et al. Anticancer Chemotherapy-Induced Intratumoral Recruitment and Differentiationof Antigen-Presenting Cells. *Immunity* **2013**, *38*, 729–741. [CrossRef]

122. Quann, E.J.; Liu, X.; Altan-Bonnet, G.; Huse, M. A cascade of protein kinase C isozymes promotes cytoskeletal polarization in T cells. *Nat. Publ. Group* **2011**, *12*, 647–654. [CrossRef]
123. Thomas, J.D.; Lee, T.; Suh, N.P. A function-based framework for understanding biological systems. *Annu. Rev. Biophys. Biomol. Struct.* **2004**, *33*, 75–93. [CrossRef] [PubMed]
124. Santos, S.D.M.; Verveer, P.J.; Bastiaens, P.I.H. Growth factor-induced MAPK network topology shapes Erk response determining PC-12 cell fate. *Nat. Cell Biol.* **2007**, *9*, 324–330. [CrossRef] [PubMed]
125. Orton, R.J.; Adriaens, M.E.; Gormand, A.; Sturm, O.E.; Kolch, W.; Gilbert, D.R. Computational modelling of cancerous mutations in the EGFR/ERK signalling pathway. *BMC Syst. Biol.* **2009**, *3*, 100. [CrossRef] [PubMed]
126. Krishnan, J.; Floros, I. Adaptive information processing of network modules to dynamic and spatial stimuli. *BMC Syst. Biol.* **2019**, *13*, 32. [CrossRef]
127. Zhang, R.; Lahens, N.F.; Ballance, H.I.; Hughes, M.E.; Hogenesch, J.B. A circadian gene expression atlas in mammals: Implications for biology and medicine. *Proc. Natl. Acad. Sci. USA* **2014**, *111*, 16219–16224. [CrossRef] [PubMed]
128. Cheung, K.J.; Ewald, A.J. A collective route to metastasis: Seeding by tumor cell clusters. *Science* **2016**, *352*, 167–169. [CrossRef]
129. Klein, E.A.; Cooperberg, M.R.; Magi-Galluzzi, C.; Simko, J.P.; Falzarano, S.M.; Maddala, T.; Chan, J.M.; Li, J.; Cowan, J.E.; Tsiatis, A.C.; et al. A 17-gene Assay to Predict Prostate Cancer Aggressiveness in the Context of Gleason Grade Heterogeneity, Tumor Multifocality, and Biopsy Undersampling. *Eur. Urol.* **2014**, *66*, 550–560. [CrossRef]
130. Kitano, H. Computational systems biology. *Nature* **2002**, *420*, 206–210. [CrossRef]
131. Wang, D.Y.; Cardelli, L.; Phillips, A.; Piterman, N.; Fisher, J. Computational modeling of the EGFR network elucidates control mechanisms regulating signal dynamics. *BMC Syst. Biol.* **2009**, *3*, 118. [CrossRef]
132. Klingmüller, U. Heterogeneous kinetics of AKT signaling in individual cells are accounted for by variable protein concentration. *Front. Physiol.* **2012**, *3*, 451.
133. Kozer, N.; Barua, D.; Orchard, S.; Nice, E.C.; Burgess, A.W.; Hlavacek, W.S.; Clayton, A.H.A. Exploring higher-order EGFR oligomerisation and phosphorylation–a combined experimental and theoretical approach. *Mol. BioSyst.* **2013**, *9*, 1849–1863. [CrossRef] [PubMed]
134. Di Camillo, B.; Toffolo, G.; Cobelli, C. A Gene Network Simulator to Assess Reverse Engineering Algorithms. *Ann. N. Y. Acad. Sci.* **2009**, *1158*, 125–142. [CrossRef] [PubMed]
135. Stoevesandt, O.; Kohler, K.; Wolf, S.; Andre, T.; Hummel, W.; Brock, R. A Network Analysis of Changes in Molecular Interactions in Cellular Signaling. *Mol. Cell. Proteom.* **2006**, *6*, 503–513. [CrossRef]
136. Murphy, L.O.; MacKeigan, J.P.; Blenis, J. A Network of Immediate Early Gene Products Propagates Subtle Differences in Mitogen-Activated Protein Kinase Signal Amplitude and Duration. *Mol. Cell. Biol.* **2003**, *24*, 144–153. [CrossRef]
137. Kim, S.; Elbaum, M. A Simple Kinetic Model with Explicit Predictions for Nuclear Transport. *Biophys. J.* **2013**, *105*, 565–569. [CrossRef] [PubMed]
138. Sontag, E.; Kiyatkin, A.; Kholodenko, B.N. Inferring dynamic architecture of cellular networks using time series of gene expression, protein and metabolite data. *Bioinformatics* **2004**, *20*, 1877–1886. [CrossRef] [PubMed]
139. Vera, J.; Rath, O.; Balsa-Canto, E.; Banga, J.R.; Kolch, W.; Wolkenhauer, O. Investigating dynamics of inhibitory and feedback loops in ERK signalling using power-law models. *Mol. BioSyst.* **2010**, *6*, 2174. [CrossRef] [PubMed]
140. Gonzalez, J.M.; Portillo, M.C.; Piñeiro-Vidal, M. Latitude-dependent underestimation of microbial extracellular enzyme activity in soils. *Int. J. Environ. Sci. Technol.* **2015**, *12*, 2427–2434. [CrossRef]
141. Varusai, T.M.; Kolch, W.; Kholodenko, B.N.; Nguyen, L.K. Molecular BioSystems. *Mol. BioSyst.* **2015**, *11*, 2750–2762. [CrossRef]
142. Mobasheri, A. Biosensors for the Multiplex Detection of Inflammatory Disease Biomarkers. *Biosensors* **2020**, *11*, 11. [CrossRef] [PubMed]
143. Anwer, S.T.; Mobashir, M.; Fantoukh, O.I.; Khan, B.; Imtiyaz, K.; Naqvi, I.H.; Rizvi, M.M.A. Synthesis of Silver Nano Particles Using Myricetin and the In-Vitro Assessment of Anti-Colorectal Cancer Activity: In-Silico Integration. *Int. J. Mol. Sci.* **2022**, *23*, 11024. [CrossRef]
144. Baud, V.; Karin, M. Is NF-kappaB a good target for cancer therapy? Hopes and pitfalls. *Nat. Rev. Drug Disc.* **2009**, *8*, 33–40. [CrossRef]
145. Lin, Y.; Bai, L.; Chen, W.; Xu, S. The NF-kappaB activation pathways, emerging molecular targets for cancer prevention and therapy. *Expert Opin. Ther. Targets* **2010**, *14*, 45–55. [CrossRef]
146. Mobashir, M. The Understanding of the Potential Linkage between COVID-19, Type-2 Diabetes, and Cancer (s) Could Help in Better Drug Targets and Therapeutics. *Comb. Chem. High Throughput Screen.* **2022**, *25*, 2370–2371. [CrossRef]

life

MDPI

Article

A Polymorphism in the Gene Encoding Heat Shock Factor 1 (*HSF1*) Increases the Risk of Type 2 Diabetes: A Pilot Study Supports a Role for Impaired Protein Folding in Disease Pathogenesis

Elena Klyosova [1,2,*], Iuliia Azarova [1,3] and Alexey Polonikov [2,4]

1 Laboratory of Biochemical Genetics and Metabolomics, Research Institute for Genetic and Molecular Epidemiology, Kursk State Medical University, 18 Yamskaya Street, 305041 Kursk, Russia
2 Department of Biology, Medical Genetics and Ecology, Kursk State Medical University, 3 Karl Marx Street, 305041 Kursk, Russia
3 Department of Biological Chemistry, Kursk State Medical University, 3 Karl Marx Street, 305041 Kursk, Russia
4 Laboratory of Statistical Genetics and Bioinformatics, Research Institute for Genetic and Molecular Epidemiology, Kursk State Medical University, 18 Yamskaya Street, 305041 Kursk, Russia
* Correspondence: ecless@yandex.ru

Abstract: The aim of this pilot study was to investigate whether polymorphisms in the gene encoding heat shock factor 1 (*HSF1*), a transcriptional activator of molecular chaperones, play a role in the development of type 2 diabetes (T2D). A total of 3229 unrelated individuals of Slavic origin, including 1569 T2D patients and 1660 age- and sex-matched healthy controls, were enrolled for the study. Five common single nucleotide polymorphisms (SNPs) of the *HSF1* gene were genotyped using the MassArray-4 system. SNPs rs7838717 ($p = 0.002$) and rs3757971 ($p = 0.005$) showed an association with an increased risk of T2D in females with a body mass index ≥ 25 kg/m^2. The rs7838717T-rs4279640T-rs3757971C and rs7838717T-rs4279640T-rs3757971T haplotypes were associated with increased and decreased disease risk in overweight or obese females, respectively. The associations were replicated as disease susceptibility genes in large cohorts from the UK Biobank ($p = 0.008$), DIAMANTE ($p = 2.7 \times 10^{-13}$), and DIAGRAM ($p = 0.0004$) consortiums. The functional annotation of the SNPs revealed that the rs7838717-T and rs3757971C alleles correlated with increased expression of the genes involved in unfolded protein response. The present study showed, for the first time, that genetic variation of *HSF1* is associated with the risk of type 2 diabetes, supporting a role for impaired protein folding in disease pathogenesis.

Keywords: type 2 diabetes mellitus; genetic susceptibility; molecular chaperons; heat shock factor 1 (HSF1); single nucleotide polymorphism; gene expression; protein folding; unfolded protein response; body mass index; obesity; sex dimorphism

check for updates

Citation: Klyosova, E.; Azarova, I.; Polonikov, A. A Polymorphism in the Gene Encoding Heat Shock Factor 1 (*HSF1*) Increases the Risk of Type 2 Diabetes: A Pilot Study Supports a Role for Impaired Protein Folding in Disease Pathogenesis. *Life* **2022**, *12*, 1936. https://doi.org/10.3390/life12111936

Academic Editor: Giuseppe Paolisso

Received: 27 October 2022
Accepted: 17 November 2022
Published: 20 November 2022

1. Introduction

Diabetes mellitus is one of the largest global health problems of the 21st century [1]. The International Diabetes Federation (IDF) has predicted that the prevalence of diabetes mellitus will increase from 10.5% in 2021 to 12.2% by 2045, affecting 537 million people between the ages of 20 and 79 [1]. Russia places second among all European nations in terms of the prevalence of diabetes, with 90% of patients having type 2 diabetes [1]. Type 2 diabetes (T2D) is a chronic disease characterized by hyperinsulinemia, insulin resistance, and pancreatic β-cell failure, with up to 50% cell loss at diagnosis [2]. T2D is a multifactorial disorder determined by interactions between environmental and genetic factors [3].

Preproinsulin serves as the starting point for insulin production in pancreatic β-cells, and it has been estimated that the cell is capable of producing 6000 preproinsulin molecules per second [4]. Newly synthesized proinsulin is folded by introducing the nascent polypeptide into the endoplasmic reticulum (ER), cleaving the signal peptide, and forming three proinsulin disulfide bonds that are known to be evolutionally conserved across vertebrates [5,6]. Proinsulin folding begins in the ER, where the local environment supports proinsulin folding overall and favors its disulfide bonds formation [7]. This process is tightly regulated by the ER stress-response pathways, whose effects on pancreatic β-cells could be beneficial or potentially harmful depending on the state of cellular proteostasis. These pathways represent a part of the unfolded protein response (UPR), activated as a result of an accumulation of unfolded or misfolded proteins in the endoplasmic reticulum, the mechanism by which cells control protein homeostasis [8].

Excessive biosynthesis of proinsulin in the ER and mutations in the coding sequence of the insulin gene affect the ER folding environment, leading to misfolding of the proinsulin molecule [6]. It is assumed that proinsulin misfolding represents a phenotype closely related to an insufficient insulin synthesis and associated with diabetes risk [9]. This association has been observed in rodent models having the proinsulin-misfolding mutants, in humans with Mutant INS-gene-induced Diabetes of Youth (MIDY), and with mutations in the critical ER-resident proteins [10], as well as in patients with type 2 diabetes [9].

It is well known that any protein including proinsulin must be appropriately folded into its three-dimensional structure in order to possess biological function, and protein folding happens naturally without the need for external energy sources [11]. Molecular chaperones, or heat shock proteins (HSP), are special types of proteins that represent a part of the sturdy machinery used by cells to cope with the issue of protein folding, thereby keeping proteins in their functional condition. Molecular chaperones help newly generated proteins to be folded correctly, prevent them from aggregating, and thus maintain cellular protein homeostasis [12].

Expression of chaperones is controlled by the transcription factor heat shock factor protein 1 (HSF1), which coordinates the cellular response to ER stress through the activation of the heat shock response (HSR), increasing the expression of numerous molecular chaperones [13–15]. HSF1 is also a significant transcriptional activator of co-chaperones [16] and ubiquitin [17], as well as a coordinating factor in the production of transcriptional and translational regulators, signaling molecules, and mitogens in response to stress [18,19]. Moreover, HSF1 is assumed to act as a cellular defender against protein deterioration, misfolding, and aggregation in both the cytoplasm and nucleus [20]. Despite the fact that HSF1 activates almost all chaperones and regulates UPR, the genetic variability of this chaperone has never been considered as a potential factor that may contribute to the development of type 2 diabetes. Taking into account the critical role of heat shock factor protein 1 in proteostasis, polymorphisms in the *HSF1* gene represent attractive targets for investigation of their association with the risk of T2D. Therefore, the aim of this pilot study is to investigate whether single nucleotide polymorphisms (SNP) of the *HSF1* gene are associated with the risk of type 2 diabetes.

2. Materials and Methods

2.1. Study Population

The study was conducted on an ethnically homogeneous population of Central Russia, including unrelated residents who were all of Slavic origin. The study was designed in accordance with the STREGA (STrengthening the REporting of Genetic Association Studies) guidelines. The overall sample size is 3229 individuals, of which 1569 patients with T2D (586 males and 983 females) were on treatment at the Endocrinology Division of the Kursk City Clinical Emergency Hospital from November 2016 to October 2019. T2D patients' mean age was 61.1 ± 6.9 years. The control group included 1660 healthy donors (631 males and 1029 females) recruited at the Regional Blood Transfusion Station in our previous studies [21,22] with an average age of 60.8 ± 5.7 years.

Each participant signed their informed consent prior to being included in the study. The regional ethics committee of the Kursk State Medical University approved the study protocol (protocol No. 10, dated 12 December 2016). The diagnosis of type 2 diabetes mellitus was verified by experienced endocrinologists according to the WHO guidelines [23,24].

The validated questionnaire was used to interview all participants for disease-related risk factors [25].

2.2. Genetic Analysis

Five milliliters of fasting venous blood were drawn from all study patients into Vacuette vacuum tubes containing 0.5 mM EDTA for genetic analysis. Isolation of genomic DNA was carried out by phenol-chloroform extraction and a column-based method with the QIAamp DNA blood mini kit (QIAGEN, Germany). The purity, quality, and concentration of the isolated DNA solution were assessed using a NanoDrop spectrophotometer (Thermo Fisher Scientific, Waltham, MA, USA). The SNPinfo bioinformatics tools such as GenePipe and FuncPred (https://snpinfo.niehs.nih.gov (accessed on 9 February 2022)) were used for selection of SNPs of the *HSF1* gene. SNPs were selected based on GenePipe's tool default settings (genotype data from HapMap, the CEU population, and a minor allele frequency cutoff value of 0.10), with a minimum of two SNPs ($r^2 \geq 0.8$) being tagged by each tag SNP (date of access 15 January 2022). The FuncPred tool (date of access 10 February 2022) was used for functional SNP annotation. In total, five common SNPs of the *HSF1* gene, namely rs12542298, rs7838717, rs4279640, rs3757971, and rs7827865 were selected for the genotyping. SNP rs4279640 was selected as a tagSNP. The combination of selected SNPs satisfied the conditions for their iPLEX-based co-genotyping in a single multiplex panel. Genotyping of the polymorphisms was done using the MassARRAY-4 genetic analyzer (Agena Bioscience, San Diego, CA, USA). To assure quality control, 95 randomly selected DNA samples were chosen without knowledge of the case-control status for repeat genotyping on the same platform, and the repeatability test yielded a 100% concordance rate. Since SNPs such as rs12542298 and rs7827865 yielded too low a genotyping call rate (<50%), they were excluded from the statistical analysis.

2.3. Biochemical Analysis

Six mL of fasting venous blood from 426 T2D patients and 136 healthy subjects was drawn for biochemical investigations of glutathione and reactive oxygen/nitrogen species using the Varioscan Flash microplate reader (Thermo Fisher Scientific, USA). Glutathione levels were measured using the OxiSelectTM Total Glutathione (GSSG/GSH) Assay Kit (Cell Biolabs, San Diego, CA, USA). The ROS/RNS levels were measured using the OxiSelectTM In Vitro ROS/RNS Assay Kit (Cell Biolabs, USA). The concentration of glucose, glycated hemoglobin, total cholesterol, high- and low-density lipoproteins, and triglycerides were assessed using the semi-automatic biochemical analyzer Clima MC-15 (RAL, Sevilla, Spain) and reagent kits from Diacon-DS (Moscow, Russia). The Cobas 6000 Roche Diagnostics (Basel, Switzerland) analyzer was used for measuring the plasma concentration of C-peptide by a competitive solid-phase chemiluminescent enzyme immunoassay.

2.4. Statistical Methods

The genetic association study power calculator, accessible online at http://csg.sph.umich.edu/abecasis/gaspowercalculator/ (accessed on 11 January 2022), was used to calculate the statistical power for the study. Association analysis between the *HSF1* gene polymorphisms and the risk of T2D could detect the genotype relative risk of 1.24–1.49 assuming 0.85–0.95 power and a 5% type I error ($\alpha = 0.05$) on the sample size of 1569 cases and 1660 controls. Allele and genotype frequencies in cases and controls were counted and compared by the chi-square test with the values predicted by the assumption of the Hardy–Weinberg equilibrium. Associations between SNPs and T2D risk were evaluated by multiple logistic regression analysis with adjustments for covariates such as sex, age, and body mass index (BMI) using the SNPStats statistical software (https://snpstats.net (accessed on 20 May 2022)). All sex- and BMI-stratified calculations were adjusted for age. Replication analysis of SNP–T2D associations was performed using large scale genomic data from UK Biobank (http://geneatlas.roslin.ed.ac.uk, date of access 21 September 2022) and the T2D Knowledge Portal (https://t2d.hugeamp.org, date of access 21 September

2022). Linkage disequilibrium (LD) measures such as Lewontin's D and D' were calculated with the LDpair Tool (https://ldlink.nci.nih.gov, accessed on 27 September 2022) using genotype data from the 1000 Genomes Project. The quantitative biochemical parameters were initially examined for normality by the Kolmogorov–Smirnov test using the STATISTICA software (v13.3, USA). Since the biochemical parameters showed a deviation from normal distribution, they were expressed as median (Me) and first and third quartiles [Q1; Q3]. Associations between polymorphisms of the *HSF1* gene and rank-based inversely normal transformed biochemical parameters were analyzed by linear regression analysis using software SNPStats; $p \leq 0.05$ was considered statistically significant.

2.5. Functional Annotation of SNPs

The eQTL analysis of the SNPs was performed using genome–transcriptome data from the following databases: (1) the eQTLgen consortium (https://www.eqtlgen.org, date of access 3 October 2022), which includes data from 30,847 blood samples from relatively healthy donors; and (2) the GTEx portal database (https://www.gtexportal.org, date of access 3 October 2022). Tissues of interest that were related to T2D pathogenesis, namely the pancreas, skeletal muscle, and visceral adipose tissue, were selected for the eQTL analysis. The *Enrichr* bioinformatics tools (https://maayanlab.cloud/Enrichr, date of access 12 October 2022) were used to identify biological functions of molecular chaperones of interest using Gene-Ontology-based overrepresentation analysis.

3. Results

3.1. Association of HSF1 Gene Polymorphisms with the Risk of Type 2 Diabetes

The baseline, clinical, and laboratory characteristics of the study participants are described previously [26]. Genotype frequencies for all polymorphisms were in Hardy–Weinberg equilibrium in both cases and controls. Table 1 presents the results of association analysis of alleles and genotypes of the *HSF1* gene polymorphisms with susceptibility to type 2 diabetes in both entire and sex-stratified groups. The rs3757971-C/C genotype is associated with an increased risk of T2D (OR = 1.30, 95% CI 1.03–1.64, $p = 0.026$). A sex-stratified analysis showed that a carriage of both the rs3757971-C/C genotype (OR = 1.42, 95% CI 1.04–1.95, $p = 0.027$) and the rs7838717-T/T genotype (OR = 1.53, 95% CI 1.12–2.08, $p = 0.0078$) was associated with disease risk only in females. Moreover, the rs3757971-C and rs7838717-T alleles showed significant associations with T2D susceptibility.

Table 1. Genotype and allele frequencies of the HSF1 gene in T2D patients and controls.

SNP	Genotype/ Allele	Healthy Controls n (%) [1]	Patients with T2D n (%) [1]	OR [2] (95% CI)	p-Value [3]
		Entire group			
rs7838717 C>T	C/C-C/T	1467 (88.4)	1345 (85.7)	1.00	0.05
	T/T	193 (11.6)	224 (14.3)	1.26 (1.00–1.59)	
	T	0.36	0.38	1.09 (0.98–1.20)	0.10
rs4279640 T>C	T/T-T/C	1260 (75.9)	1199 (76.4)	1.00	0.65
	C/C	400 (24.1)	370 (23.6)	1.04 (0.87–1.25)	
	C	0.49	0.48	0.97 (0.88–1.07)	0.61
rs3757971 T>C	T/T-C/T	1467 (88.5)	1337 (85.3)	1.00	**0.026**
	C/C	190 (11.5)	231 (14.7)	**1.30 (1.03–1.64)**	
	C	0.35	0.37	1.11 (1.00–1.23)	0.05

Table 1. *Cont.*

SNP	Genotype/ Allele	Healthy Controls n (%) [1]	Patients with T2D n (%) [1]	OR [2] (95% CI)	*p*-Value [3]
		Males			
rs7838717 C>T	C/C-C/T T/T	542 (87.8) 75 (12.2)	513 (87.5) 73 (12.5)	1.00 1.08 (0.75–1.56)	0.68
	T	0.38	0.36	0.94 (0.80–1.11)	0.49
rs4279640 T>C	T/T-T/C C/C	485 (78.6) 132 (21.4)	437 (74.6) 149 (25.4)	1.00 1.34 (1.00–1.78)	0.05
	C	0.47	0.50	1.11 (0.95–1.30)	0.20
rs3757971 T>C	T/T-C/T C/C	541 (87.8) 75 (12.2)	505 (86.2) 81 (13.8)	1.00 1.16 (0.81–1.67)	0.42
	C	0.37	0.36	0.97 (0.82–1.15)	0.74
		Females			
rs7838717 C>T	C/C-C/T T/T	911 (88.5) 118 (11.5)	832 (84.6) 151 (15.4)	1.00 **1.53 (1.12–2.08)**	**0.0078**
	T	0.35	0.39	**0.17 (1.03–1.33)**	**0.016**
rs4279640 T>C	T/T-T/C C/C	767 (74.5) 262 (25.5)	762 (77.5) 221 (22.5)	1.00 0.87 (0.68–1.12)	0.28
	C	0.49	0.47	0.91 (0.80–1.03)	0.13
rs3757971 T>C	T/T-C/T C/C	912 (88.8) 115 (11.2)	832 (84.7) 150 (15.3)	1.00 **1.42 (1.04–1.95)**	**0.027**
	C	0.34	0.38	**1.19 (1.05–1.36)**	**0.008**

[1] Absolute number and percentage of individuals/chromosomes with a particular genotype/allele. [2] Odds ratio with 95% confidence intervals (crude analysis) with one degree of freedom. [3] *p*-Value—significance level. Bold indicates statistically significant *p*-values.

Since obesity is a well-recognized confounding risk factor for T2D [27], it would be reasonable to analyze associations in groups stratified by body mass index. Pursuing this interest, the study patients were subdivided into the two groups. The first included subjects with BMI $\leq$ 25 kg/m^2 (i.e., normal body weight), while the second comprised subjects who were overweight or obese (i.e., BMI $\geq$ 25 kg/m^2). Following this, a BMI-stratified analysis adjusted for age (Table 2), revealed significant associations between genotypes such as rs7838717-T/T (OR = 1.62, 95% CI 1.20–2.19, p = 0.0016) and rs3757971-C/C (OR = 1.54, 95% CI 1.14–2.09, p = 0.0047) and an increased risk T2D, but only in overweight and obese females. In males, no statistically significant associations were observed. Linear regression analysis allowed associations to be revealed between polymorphisms of the *HSF1* gene and some biochemical parameters in T2D patients (Supplementary Table S1). A decrease in blood glucose after the first meal (i.e., breakfast) was associated with the rs7838717-T/T genotype (p = 0.027) in the entire group analysis.

The rs3757971-C/C genotype in females was associated with a decreased level of plasma low-density lipoproteins (p = 0.033). The rs4279640-C/C genotype was associated with decreased levels of triglycerides in females (p = 0.039). In addition, an association of genotype rs4279640-C/C with a decreased glomerular filtration rate was established in both entire (p = 0.035) and female (p = 0.021) groups. As can be seen from Supplementary Table S1, the above associations were weak in their strength. No statistically significant associations of HSF1 polymorphisms with biochemical parameters were found in males.

Table 2. Genotype and allele frequencies of the *HSF1* gene in T2D patients and controls stratified by sex and BMI.

SNP.	Genotype/ Allele	Healthy Controls n (%) [1]	Patients with T2D n (%) [1]	OR [2] (95% CI)	*p*-Value [3]	Healthy Controls n (%) [1]	Patients with T2D n (%) [1]	OR [2] (95% CI)	*p*-Value [3]
		Males				Females			
BMI ≤ 25 kg/m^2 norm									
rs7838717 C>T	C/C-C/T T/T	104 (90.4) 11 (9.6)	102 (87.2) 15 (12.8)	1 1.37 (0.60–3.12)	0.46	167 (86.1) 27 (13.9)	73 (83.9) 14 (16.1)	1 1.02 (0.48–2.14)	0.96
	T	0.35	0.34	0.99 (0.68–1.45)	0.97	0.35	0.42	1.35 (0.94–1.95)	0.10
rs4279640 T>C	T/T-T/C C/C	90 (78.3) 25 (21.7)	86 (73.5) 31 (26.5)	1 1.26 (0.69–2.31)	0.46	138 (71.1) 56 (28.9)	70 (80.5) 17 (19.5)	1 0.62 (0.33–1.17)	0.14
	C	0.49	0.47	0.95 (0.66–1.36)	0.77	0.50	0.42	0.72 (0.51–1.04)	0.08
rs3757971 T>C	T/T-C/T C/C	101 (87.8) 14 (12.2)	100 (85.5) 17 (14.5)	1 1.21 (0.57–2.59)	0.62	168 (86.6) 26 (13.4)	71 (81.6) 16 (18.4)	1 1.17 (0.57–2.42)	0.67
	C	0.38	0.33	0.82 (0.56–1.20)	0.31	0.33	0.43	1.50 (1.04–2.17)	**0.029**
BMI ≥ 25 kg/m^2 overweight and obesity									
rs7838717 C>T	C/C-C/T T/T	425 (87.3) 62 (12.7)	411 (87.6) 58 (12.4)	1 1.01 (0.69–1.49)	0.95	735 (89.2) 89 (10.8)	759 (84.7) 137 (15.3)	1 **1.62 (1.20–2.19)**	**0.0016**
	T	0.38	0.37	0.93 (0.78–1.12)	0.46	0.35	0.38	1.15 (1.00–1.32)	0.05
rs4279640 T>C	T/T-T/C C/C	386 (79.3) 101 (20.7)	351 (74.8) 118 (25.2)	1 1.29 (0.95–1.75)	0.11	621 (75.4) 203 (24.6)	692 (77.2) 204 (22.8)	1 0.90 (0.71–1.14)	0.38
	C	0.47	0.50	1.14 (0.95–1.37)	0.15	0.49	0.477	0.94 (0.82–1.08)	0.38
rs3757971 T>C	T/T-C/T C/C	426 (87.7) 60 (12.3)	405 (86.3) 64 (13.7)	1 1.13 (0.77–1.65)	0.54	734 (89.3) 88 (10.7)	761 (85) 134 (15)	1 **1.54 (1.14–2.09)**	**0.0047**
	C	0.37	0.73	1.00 (0.83–1.21)	0.97	0.34	0.37	**1.16 (1.01–1.33)**	**0.038**

[1] Absolute number and percentage of individuals/chromosomes with a particular genotype/allele. [2] Odds ratio with 95% confidence intervals (crude analysis) with one degree of freedom. [3] *p*-Value—significance level. Bold indicates statistically significant *p*-values.

3.2. *HSF1 Haplotypes and T2D Susceptibility*

The frequencies of *HSF1* haplotypes in T2D patients and healthy controls are shown in Table 3. Three common haplotypes of *HSF1* with a frequency of more than 13% were identified. As can be seen from Table 3, the rare haplotype TTT (H6) of *HSF1* was associated with decreased risk of T2D in the entire group (OR = 0.51, 95% CI 0.27–0.98, p = 0.043). Sex-stratified analysis showed that the common haplotype TTC (*H2*) was associated with increased risk of T2D in females (OR = 1.24, 95% CI 1.04–1.48, p = 0.014). A joint BMI- and sex-stratified analysis (Table 4) showed associations of *HSF1* haplotypes with T2D risk in both males and females who were overweight or obese. In particular, the *H2* haplotype was associated with increased risk of type 2 diabetes in females (OR = 1.21, 95% CI 1.02–1.43, p = 0.02). In addition, haplotype *H6* showed an association with decreased disease risk in females with BMI more than 25 kg/m^2 (OR = 0.35, 95% CI 0.15–0.83, p = 0.02). In males who were overweight or obese, the CTT haplotype (*H3*) was found to be associated with decreased risk of T2D (OR = 0.74, 95% CI 0.56–0.98, p = 0.02).

Table 3. Haplotype frequencies of the *HSF1* gene and their associations with type 2 diabetes.

N	rs7838717	rs4279640	rs3757971	Healthy Controls	Patients with T2D	OR [1] (95 CI)	*p*-Value [2]
				Entire group			
H1	C	C	T	0.4506	0.4472	1	—
H2	T	T	C	0.3065	0.339	1.07 (0.94–1.21)	0.33
H3	C	T	T	0.1571	0.1485	0.92 (0.78–1.08)	0.31
H4	C	T	C	0.0284	0.0232	0.87 (0.60–1.25)	0.44
H5	T	C	T	0.0246	0.0252	1.00 (0.67–1.49)	1
H6	T	T	T	0.0192	0.0069	**0.51 (0.27–0.98)**	**0.043**
				Global p-Value haplotype association: 0.082			
				Males			
H1	C	C	T	0.43	0.4682	1	—
H2	T	T	C	0.3279	0.3301	0.89 (0.72–1.08)	0.24
H3	C	T	T	0.1585	0.1394	0.81 (0.62–1.05)	0.11
H4	C	T	C	0.0281	0.0231	0.82 (0.46–1.44)	0.49
H5	T	C	T	0.0274	0.019	0.65 (0.34–1.25)	0.19
H6	T	T	T	0.0122	0.0083	0.84 (0.31–2.26)	0.73
				Global p-Value haplotype association: 0.44			
				Females			
H1	C	C	T	0.4607	0.4348	1	—
H2	T	T	C	0.296	0.3442	**1.24 (1.04–1.48)**	**0.014**
H3	C	T	T	0.1567	0.1539	1.00 (0.80–1.25)	0.99
H4	C	T	C	0.0279	0.0232	0.80 (0.49–1.30)	0.37
H5	T	C	T	0.0235	0.0288	1.32 (0.78–2.22)	0.3
H6	T	T	T	0.0233	0.0061	0.43 (0.18–1.05)	0.064
				Global *p*-Value haplotype association: **0.027**			

[1] Odds ratio with 95% confidence intervals (crude analysis) with one degree of freedom. [2] *p*-Value—significance level. Gray shading shows minor alleles of SNPs. Bold indicates statistically significant *p*-values.

Table 5 shows the values of linkage disequilibrium between SNPs in the *HSF1* gene. The studied SNPs were in linkage disequilibrium with each other to varying degrees, and strong differences in the LD values were observed between the Russian and European populations of the 1000 Genomes Project. The rs3757971 and rs7838717 polymorphisms are negatively linked to each other in our population, but positively linked in Europeans. A strong inter-population difference was also seen in the *D*-values between SNPs rs3757971 and rs4279640, which were in the negative linkage disequilibrium in our population and positive in the European population. Furthermore, both in our population and in Europeans from the 1000 Genomes Project, the rs7838717 polymorphism was found to be in negative linkage disequilibrium with rs4279640.

Table 4. Haplotype frequencies of the *HSF1* gene in T2D patients and controls stratified by sex and BMI.

N	rs7838717	rs4279640	rs3757971	Healthy Controls n (%) [1]	Patients with T2D n (%) [1]	OR [2] (95% CI)	*p*-Value [3]	Healthy Controls n (%) [1]	Patients with T2D n (%) [1]	OR [2] (95% CI)	*p*-Value [3]
				Males				Females			
				BMI ≤ 25 kg/m² norm							
H1	C	C	T	0.4482	0.4670	1	—	0.4726	0.4184	1	—
H2	T	T	C	0.3090	0.3068	0.96 (0.63–1.48)	0.87	0.2878	0.4017	1.42 (0.94–2.15)	0.09
H3	C	T	T	0.1456	0.1603	1.07 (0.62–1.83)	0.80	0.1414	0.1327	0.98 (0.54–1.78)	0.95
H4	C	T	C	0.0435	0.0218	0.44 (0.14–1.37)	0.16	0.0350	0.0293	0.62 (0.21–1.85)	0.39
H5	T	C	T	0.0000	0.0155	0.69 (0.17–2.75)	0.60	0.0204	0.0069	0.27 (0.03–2.26)	0.23
H6	T	T	T	0.0279	0.0239	0.95 (0.30–3.07)	0.94	0.0306	0.0110	0.32 (0.06–1.70)	0.18
			Global *p*-Value haplotype association: 0.77					Global *p*-Value haplotype association: 0.09			
				BMI ≥ 25 kg/m² overweight and obesity							
H1	C	C	T	0.4241	0.4678	1	—	0.4566	0.4363	1	—
H2	T	T	C	0.3332	0.3360	0.91 (0.74–1.12)	0.39	0.2997	0.3386	**1.21 (1.02–1.43)**	**0.02**
H3	C	T	T	0.1618	0.1349	**0.74 (0.56–0.98)**	**0.036**	0.1606	0.1561	1.02 (0.83–1.26)	0.83
H4	C	T	C	0.0255	0.0234	0.85 (0.45–1.59)	0.61	0.0258	0.0226	0.91 (0.56–1.47)	0.70
H5	T	C	T	0.0312	0.0205	0.54 (0.28–1.04)	0.06	0.0242	0.0310	1.40 (0.85–2.31)	0.18
H6	T	T	T	0.0103	0.0036	0.69 (0.33–1.44)	0.32	0.0218	0.0056	**0.35 (0.15–0.83)**	**0.02**
			Global *p*-Value haplotype association: 0.13					Global *p*-Value haplotype association: 0.03			

[1] Absolute number and percentage of individuals/chromosomes with a particular genotype/allele. [2] Odds ratio with 95% confidence intervals (crude analysis) with one degree of freedom. [3] *p*-Value—significance level. Gray shading shows minor alleles. Bold indicates statistically significant *p*-values.

Table 5. Linkage disequilibrium measures between SNPs of the *HSF1* gene in the Russian population and populations of the 1000 Genomes Project.

SNP ID	rs4279640	rs3757971
	the Russian population	
rs7838717	−0.1474 0.8253	0.1972 0.8662
rs4279640	- -	−0.1630 0.9321
	European populations of 1000 G	
rs7838717	−0.0739 0.8586	−0.0213 0.8784
rs4279640	- -	−0.1630 0.9417

Matrices show LD measures, such as a nonstandardized *D* (upper part) and a standardized *D′* (lower part). LD-values were calculated with the LDpair Tool (https://ldlink.nci.nih.gov (accessed on 27 September 2022)) using genotype data from the 1000 Genomes Project (1000 G) and GRCh37 human genome assembly. Each pair of SNPs includes two LD values calculated for the following populations: the Russian population (upper cells); the European populations of 1000 G (middle cells). All LD values $p < 0.0001$.

3.3. The Replication Analysis for SNP–T2D Associations in Independent Populations

Replication analysis of associations between the studied *HSF1* gene variants and T2D phenotypes was carried out in large populations from the T2D Knowledge portal and the UK Biobank. The results of the replication analysis are presented in Table 6. It is important to note that associations of SNPs rs3757971 and rs7838717 with T2D susceptibility, originally established in our population, were successfully replicated in independent populations. However, associations of these SNPs have not been confirmed as T2D susceptibility markers in a subpopulation of the type 2 diabetics from the UK Biobank. Moreover, the rs4279640 polymorphism showed association with a decreased risk of T2D in some of the studied cohorts, whereas we did not see such an association in our population.

Table 6. Replication for SNP associations with different T2D phenotypes in large independent cohorts.

			rs7838717 [1] C>T		rs4279640 T>C		rs3757971 T>C	
		Phenotype	*p*-Value [2]	Beta/Odds Ratio	*p*-Value	Beta/Odds Ratio	*p*-Value	Beta/Odds Ratio
UK Biobank [1]		Non-insulin dependent diabetes n (cases/controls) 19,860/432,404	**0.008**	▼ 0.973	**0.01**	▼ 0.977	**3.5×10^{-5}**	▲ 1.04
		Type 2 diabetes n (cases/controls) 2889/449,375	0.43	▼ 0.979	0.41	▼ 0.979	0.08	▲ 1.05
T2D Knowledge Portal [2]	Type 2 diabetes adj BMI	DIAMANTE (European) T2D GWAS n = 157,384	**2.70×10^{-13}**	▼ 0.944	**5.1×10^{-6}**	▼ 0.966	**8.2×10^{-16}**	▲ 1.065
		DIAGRAM 1000G GWAS n = 54,365	**0.00039**	▼ 0.941	**8.6×10^{-5}**	▼ 0.941	**1.10×10^{-6}**	▲ 1.083
	Fasting glucose adj BMI	MAGIC 2021 glycemic traits GWAS: Europeans n = 160,378	**0.00004**	▼ −0.009	**2.7×10^{-4}**	▼ −0.007	**4.9×10^{-7}**	▲ 0.011
		TOPMed fasting glucose whole genome sequence analysis n =26,807	**0.004**	▼ −0.014	0.17	▼ −0.006	**0.03**	▲ 0.009

[1] Values are for allele C rs7838717. [2] *p*-Value—significance level; values that reached the genome-wide significance level are bolded. ▲ depicts an increased value, ▼ depicts a decreased value. Genomic data obtained at the CVD Knowledge Portal (https://t2d.hugeamp.org), date of access 21 September 2022.

3.4. Functional SNP Annotation

The results of the eQTL analysis for the studied *HSF1* gene polymorphisms are shown in Table 7. SNPs rs7838717 and rs3757971 were associated with increased expression of the *VPS28* gene both in the blood (p = 1.9 × 10^{-57} and p = 1.7 × 10^{-66}, respectively) and skeletal muscles (p = 2.6 × 10^{-5} and p = 1.3 × 10^{-4}, respectively). Polymorphisms rs7838717 and rs3757971 were associated with a decrease in the *DGAT1* gene expression (p = 8.7 × 10^{-33} and p = 1.1 × 10^{-35}, respectively). SNP rs7838717 was also associated with decreased levels of the *SHARPIN* gene (p = 7.8 × 10^{-8}). Increased blood expression of the *MAF1* gene was associated with SNP rs7838717 (p = 8.8×10^{-6}). In subcutaneous adipose tissue, polymorphisms rs7838717 (p = 4.9 × 10^{-5}) and rs3757971 (p = 9.7 × 10^{-8}) were associated with increased expression of the *SCX* gene, whereas polymorphism rs4279640 (p = 3.3 × 10^{-6}) was negatively correlated with expression levels of the *SCX* gene.

The GTEx-calculator (https://gtexportal.org/home/testyourown, date of access 3 October 2022) was used to assess the effects of the T2D-asociated SNPs on the expression levels of molecular chaperones representing the Hsp70 and Hsp90 families, which are known targets of *HSF1* in T2D-related tissues such as the pancreas, skeletal muscle, and adipose tissue (Table 8). We found that a decrease in expression levels of chaperones such as *HSP90B1*, *RPS19BP1*, and *HSPA5* was associated with a carriage of the rs3757971-C and/or rs7838717-T alleles that were found to be associated with the risk of T2D in our study. Interestingly, these chaperones are directly involved in many biological processes such as ATF6-mediated UPR (GO:0036500), de novo post-translational protein folding (GO:0051084), cellular response to glucose starvation (GO:0042149), cellular response to topologically incorrect protein (GO:0035967), proteasome-mediated ubiquitin-dependent protein catabolic process (GO:0043161), negative regulation of apoptotic process (GO:0043066), post-translational protein modification (GO:0043687), and some others. The disease-associated allele rs7838717-T correlated with increased expression of the *NFE2L2* gene (transcription factor playing a key role in the response to oxidative stress by binding to antioxidant response elements in the promoters of many cytoprotective genes), which is involved in the activation of UPR and responsible for multiple biological functions, such as cytokine stimulus (GO:0071345), hydrogen peroxide (GO:0070301), oxidative stress (GO:0034599), ER-associated ubiquitin-dependent protein catabolic process (GO:0000058), positive regulation of the ERAD pathway (GO:1904294), and response to tumor necrosis factor (GO:0034612).

Table 7. Relationship between studied SNPs and expression levels of genes in T2D-related tissues.

SNP	Allele	eQTL (Blood)			GTEx-Portal								
		Gene	Z-Score	*p*-Value	Pancreas Gene	Pancreas NES	Pancreas *p*-Value	Skeletal Muscle Gene	Skeletal Muscle NES	Skeletal Muscle *p*-Value	Adipose—Subcutaneous Gene	Adipose—Subcutaneous NES	Adipose—Subcutaneous *p*-Value
rs7838717	T	*VPS28*	15.97	1.9 ×10^{-57}	*CPSF1*	0.33	10^{-6}	*CPSF1*	0.15	1.8 × 10^{-4}	*CPSF1*	0.26	2.1 × 10^{-9}
	T	*DGAT1*	−11.92	8.7 × 10^{-33}				*VPS28*	0.13	2.6 × 10^{-5}	*SCX*	0.23	4.9 × 10^{-5}
	T	*KIAA1875*	11.75	7.2 × 10^{-32}									
	T	*CPSF1*	10.29	8.1 × 10^{-25}									
	T	*TONSL*	7.56	4.1 × 10^{-14}									
	T	*EPPK1*	7.27	3.5 × 10^{-13}									
	T	*BOP1*	6.69	2.2 × 10^{-11}									
	T	*SHARPIN*	−5.37	7.8 × 10^{-8}									
	T	*MAF1*	4.44	8.8 × 10^{-6}									
rs4279640	C	*DGAT1*	0.10	2.1 × 10^{-6}	*CPSF1*	−0.32	3.5 × 10^{-6}	*CPSF1*	−0.16	1.7 × 10^{-6}	*CPSF1*	−0.22	2.1 × 10^{-5}
	C	*HSF1*	−0.06	2.7 × 10^{-6}				*SCRT1*	0.15	4.5 × 10^{-5}	*SCX*	−0.18	3.3 × 10^{-6}
	C	*CPSF1*	−0.13	3.8 × 10^{-6}									
rs3757971	C	*VPS28*	17.23	1.7 × 10^{-66}	*CPSF1*	0.39	1.4 × 10^{-7}	*CPSF1*	0.16	1.3 × 10^{-4}	*CPSF1*	0.29	2.9 × 10^{-7}
	C	*DGAT1*	−12.46	1.1 × 10^{-35}				*VPS28*	0.13	1.3 × 10^{-4}	*SCX*	0.22	9.7 × 10^{-8}
	C	*CPSF1*	11.28	1.5 × 10^{-29}									
	C	*TONSL*	8.23	1.9 × 10^{-16}									
	C	*KIAA1875*	7.09	1.3 × 10^{-12}									
	C	*EPPK1*	6.94	3.9 × 10^{-12}									
	C	*BOP1*	6.36	2.1 × 10^{-10}									
	C	*PPP1R16A*	4.90	9.6 × 10^{-7}									

Table 8. Relationship between T2D-associated SNPs and expression levels of HSF1-targeted chaperons and their biological functions.

SNP [1]	Gene [2]	*p*-Value [3]	NES [4]	Gene Ontologies [5]
rs7838717-T	*NFE2L2*	**0.020**	0.071 ▲	GO:0062197 response to chemical stress; GO:0071345 response to cytokine stimulus; GO:0070301response to hydrogen peroxide; GO:0034599 response to oxidative stress; GO:0071356 response to tumor necrosis factor; GO:0140467 integrated stress response signaling; GO:0036499 PERK-mediated UPR; GO:1903071 positive regulation of ER-associated ubiquitin-dependent protein catabolic process; GO:1904294 positive regulation of ERAD pathway; GO:0010498 proteasomal protein catabolic process; GO:0032446 protein modification by small protein conjugation; GO:1903205 regulation of hydrogen peroxide-induced cell death; GO:1902175 regulation of oxidative stress-induced intrinsic apoptotic signaling pathway; GO:0034612 response to tumor necrosis factor;
rs3757971-C		**0.018**	0.072 ▲	
rs7838717-T	*FKBP4*	**0.0098**	−0.11 ▼	GO:0031345 regulation of cell projection organization; GO:0051494 regulation of cytoskeleton organization; GO:0031111regulation of microtubule polymerization or depolymerization; GO:0018208 peptidyl-proline modification; GO:0000413 protein peptidyl-prolyl isomerization; GO:1900034 regulation of cellular response to heat GO:0080135 regulation of cellular response to stress;
rs7838717-T	*HSP90B1*	**0.0044**	−0.11 ▼	GO:0036500 ATF6-mediated UPR; GO:0044267 protein metabolic process; GO:0006464 protein modification process; GO:0071318 response to ATP; GO:0071345 response to cytokine stimulus; GO:1901701 response to oxygen-containing compound; GO:0019221 cytokine-mediated signaling pathway; GO:1903513 ER to cytosol transport; GO:0036503 ERAD pathway; GO:0043066 regulation of apoptotic process; GO:0043687 post-translational protein modification; GO:0043161 proteasome-mediated ubiquitin-dependent protein catabolic process; GO:0032527 protein exit from ER; GO:0015031 protein transport; GO:0006898 receptor-mediated endocytosis; GO:0042981 regulation of apoptotic process; GO:0010921 regulation of phosphatase activity; GO:0043666 regulation of phosphoprotein phosphatase activity; GO:0034976 response to ER stress; GO:0030970 ER to cytosol; GO:0030433 ubiquitin-dependent ERAD pathway;
rs3757971-C		**0.0012**	−0.12 ▼	

Table 8. *Cont.*

SNP [1]	Gene [2]	*p*-Value [3]	NES [4]	Gene Ontologies [5]
rs3757971-C	*HSPA5*	**0.036**	−0.073 ▼	GO:0051084 de novo post-translational protein folding; GO:0036500 ATF6-mediated unfolded protein response; GO:0042149 cellular response to glucose starvation; GO:0035967 response to topologically incorrect protein; GO:0034620 cellular response to unfolded protein; GO:0051085 chaperone-cofactor-dependent protein refolding; GO:0036503 ERAD pathway; GO:0140467 integrated stress response signaling; GO:0065002 intracellular protein transmembrane transport; GO:0036498 IRE1-mediated UPR; GO:0035437 maintenance of protein localization in ER; GO:0072595 maintenance of protein localization in organelle; GO:0043066 negative regulation of apoptotic process; GO:0051129 regulation of cellular component organization; GO:1900102 regulation of endoplasmic reticulum UPR; GO:0043069 negative regulation of programmed cell death; GO:0031333 negative regulation of protein-containing complex assembly; GO:0036499 PERK-mediated UPR; GO:0030335 positive regulation of cell migration; GO:0006620 post-translational protein targeting to endoplasmic reticulum membrane; GO:0043161 proteasome-mediated ubiquitin-dependent protein catabolic process; GO:0070972 protein localization to ER; GO:0042981 regulation of apoptotic process; GO:0043254 regulation of protein-containing complex assembly; GO:0034976 response to ER stress; GO:0006986 response to unfolded protein;

[1] SNPs associated with the risk of developing DM2 according to the results of this study; [2] Genes involved in metabolic pathways «Protein folding» and «Chaperone» according to databases Reactome (https://reactome.org (accessed on 2 June 2022)), Kegg (https://www.genome.jp/kegg (accessed on 5 June 2022)), and Wikipathways (https://www.wikipathways.org) date of access 8 June 2022; [3] *p*-Value—significance level; [4] Normalized effect size according to GTEx-calculator (https://www.gtexportal.org), date of access 3 October 2022; [5] Gene Ontologies' biological process according to Enrichr dataset (https://maayanlab.cloud/Enrichr/), date of access 12 October 2022. Bold indicates statistically significant *p*-values.

4. Discussion

The present study found, for the first time, that polymorphisms of gene encoding heat shock factor 1 are associated with an increased risk of type 2 diabetes. However, sex and body mass index were found to be confounding factors, modifying the associations between the polymorphisms and T2D risk. In particular, SNPs such as rs7838717 and rs3757971 were found to be associated with an increased risk of T2D in females with a BMI $\geq$ 25 kg/m^2. The observed associations were successfully replicated as disease-susceptibility markers in large cohorts from the UK Biobank, DIAMANTE, and DIAGRAM consortiums. In the MAGIC and TOPMed consortiums, these SNPs were also found to be associated with increased fasting blood glucose (FBG) adjusted by BMI, although we did not see an association of the SNPs with FBG in our population. Two haplotypes, such as rs7838717T-rs4279640T-rs3757971C and rs7838717T-rs4279640T-rs3757971T of *HSF1*, showed associations with increased and decreased risk of type 2 diabetes in overweight or obese females, respectively. In contrast, the rs7838717C-rs4279640T-rs3757971T haplotype was associated with decreased disease risk in males with a BMI $\geq$ 25 kg/m^2. The functional annotation of T2D-associated polymorphisms showed that the T2D-associated alleles such as rs7838717-T and rs3757971C were correlated with increased expression of the *CPSF1* gene in the pancreas, skeletal muscle, subcutaneous adipose tissue, and whole blood. In addition, these SNPs were associated with increased expression of *VPS28* in skeletal muscle and blood, as well as with expression levels of some other genes in the blood.

Many studies have shown that mutations in genes encoding chaperones and co-chaperones may cause different diseases, such as neuromuscular diseases [28], neurodegenerative disease [29], and Alzheimer's disease [30]. Studies investigating the association between *HSF1* gene polymorphisms and T2D susceptibility have not been done so far. Nonetheless, several studies have been undertaken to assess the relationship between polymorphisms of molecular chaperones and the development of type 2 diabetes. In particular, Synofzik et al. have shown that loss-of-function mutations of the *DNAJC3* (DnaJ heat shock protein family (Hsp40) member C3) gene contribute to the development of diabetes mellitus in humans [29]. In a study by Moniruzzaman M et al., it was found that the +2437T/C polymorphism (rs2227956) of *HSPA1L* is significantly associated with the incidence of type 2 diabetes in the population of Bangladesh [31]. Elshahed O.M. et al. observed significant differences in the prevalence of haplotypes such as CGGT, CCGT, AGGT, and AGAT of the *HSPA1A* gene between diabetic patients with nephropathy and healthy controls [32].

It is known that heat shock factor 1 is a transcription factor that promotes UPR and binds to heat shock elements (HSEs) in the promoter regions of HSPs, which are necessary for directing damaged and misfolded proteins toward proteasomal degradation [33]. Certain data in the literature indicate changes in the expression levels of HSF1 in type 2 diabetes mellitus. Kavanagh et al. [34] experimentally show that pancreatic cells of monkeys with T2D have increased expression of *Hsf1*. This finding was confirmed by the study of Marselli L et al. [35], who investigated the expression profile of pancreatic β-cells from 9 patients with T2D and 10 non-diabetic controls. The authors revealed that expression of *HSF1* in pancreatic β-cells was significantly increased in patients with T2D compared to controls. We hypothesize that the increased expression of the *HSF1* gene may mirror the need of the β-cells in the synthesis of more molecules of heat shock factor 1. It is known that *HSF1* is required to ensure normal protein folding through the activation of the molecular chaperone cascade, including the Hsp70 and Hsp90 families [20,36]. This assumption is in line with studies highlighting the importance of impaired protein folding for the development of type 2 diabetes [37–39]. The pancreas is an organ with increased rates of protein synthesis, and therefore higher chaperone levels are required to ensure proper folding of proteins, including proinsulin. Notably, the decreased transcriptional activity of *HSF1* was found to enhance glucolipotoxicity-induced apoptosis in both rat and human β-cells [40], suggesting a role of heat shock factor 1 in the initial mechanisms underlying type 2 diabetes mellitus.

As can be seen from Table 5, SNPs rs7838717 and rs3757971 are in positive LD with each other, whereas these SNPs are correlated negatively with rs4279640, a polymorphism which did not show association with T2D. The T2D-associated variant alleles (rs7838717-T and rs3757971-C) are correlated with the wild-type rs4279640-T allele. Apparently, the association of rs7838717 and rs3757971 with T2D risk can be explained by the relationship of these polymorphisms with the expression levels of genes such as *VPS28*, *KIAA1875*, *TONSL*, *EPPK1*, and *BOP1* (these genes were not correlated with SNP rs4279640). However, this assumption should be investigated in experimental studies.

Although the disease-associated alleles were not correlated with changes in *HSF1* gene expression, they showed correlations with the expression of genes involved in the regulation of proteostasis and unfolded protein response. In particular, it is known that *VPS28* is a component of the ubiquitin–proteasome pathway and is important for lysosomal targeting [41]. *VPS28* is also involved in protein transport into vesicles and ubiquitin-dependent catabolism through the sorting of multivesicular bodies [42]. Thus, *VPS28* eliminates dysfunctional/misfolded proteins through the ubiquitin–proteasome pathway, thereby regulating cellular proteostasis. Thus, we suggest that an increase in the expression of the *VPS28* gene in subjects with the T2D-associated alleles may demonstrate the increased activation of the ubiquitin–proteasome pathway, a part of the unfolded protein response directed at the degradation of unfolded or misfolded proteins in the ER, the conditions playing a role in the pathogenesis of type 2 diabetes [43–45].

The rs7838717-T and rs3757971-C alleles were also correlated with a decreased expression of *DGAT1*, which encodes the enzyme diacylglycerol O-acyltransferase 1, catalyzing the synthesis of triacylglycerol from diacylglycerol (DAG) and acyl-CoA as substrates [46]. Interestingly, DAG is known to be a lipid signal molecule playing a physiological role in β-cells; in particular, in the regulation of insulin secretion [47] and also participating in the induction of apoptosis [48].

The *SHARPIN* gene was also of interest, whose decreased expression was associated with the carriage of allele rs7838717-T. This gene is a component of the LUBAC complex, which conjugates linear polyubiquitin chains in a head-to-tail manner to substrates and plays a key role in NF–kappa B activation and regulation of inflammation [49–51]. The NF–kappa B (NF–κB) pathway is known to play a crucial role in the pathogenesis of T2D and its complications. This transcription factor is activated by a number of pro-inflammatory cytokines to regulate β-cell survival and death in T2D [52]. The LUBAC complex regulates canonical Wnt signaling [53], a pathway linked to insulin resistance, inflammatory response regulation, and dysfunction of pancreatic β-cells and endothelial cells [54].

The expression of the *MAF1* gene in blood was correlated with the T2D-associated alleles of *HSF1*. It is known that *MAF1* is a global repressor of RNA polymerase III transcription that regulates the expression of highly abundant noncoding RNAs in response to nutrient availability and cellular stress [55]. Bonhoure N. et al. showed that the knockout of *Maf1* in mice conferred resistance to diet-induced obesity and nonalcoholic fatty liver disease by reducing food intake and increasing metabolic inefficiency [55]. These findings suggest that the increased levels of the *MAF1* gene may be linked to the changes in lipid metabolism occurring in diabetes mellitus and obesity.

Finally, it was a very interesting finding that the rs3757971-C and rs7838717-T alleles of *HSF1* were also correlated with decreased expression of molecular chaperones such as *HSP90B1, HSPA5,* and *FKBP4*—members of the Hsp70 and Hsp90 families and the primary targets for heat shock factor 1 [56]. This finding may suggest that the carriage of T2D-associated alleles of *HSF1* may lead to the decreased expression of these chaperones responsible for efficient folding of proteins, including proinsulin in the pancreas. However, experimental studies are required to reproduce these molecular consequences of *HSF1* deficiency and to draw definitive conclusions about the causal relationship between the *HSF1* gene, molecular chaperones *HSP90B1, HSPA5,* and *FKBP4,* and impaired proinsulin folding in type 2 diabetes.

There are some limitations in the study that should be addressed. We examined a limited number of polymorphisms in the *HSF1* gene, which do not cover all functionally significant sequence variants that may influence expression or activity of this gene. Therefore, further studies with a larger number of SNPs are required to assess the comprehensive contribution of the gene to the risk of T2D. The limited number of male subjects in the sub-group analysis did not allow us to reproduce SNP–disease associations in males. Because the observed associations were relatively weak, more research is needed to assess the relationship between *HSF1* gene polymorphisms and susceptibility to type 2 diabetes in other populations around the world.

In conclusion, the present pilot study found, for the first time, that genetic variations of heat shock transcription factor 1 contribute to type 2 diabetes susceptibility in females with body mass index ≥ 25 kg/m^2. The observed associations of polymorphisms rs7838717 and rs3757971 with T2D risk have been successfully replicated in three independent European populations from the UK Biobank, DIAMANTE, and DIAGRAM consortiums. Moreover, two haplotypes such as rs7838717T-rs4279640T-rs3757971C and rs7838717T-rs4279640T-rs3757971T of *HSF1* showed significant associations with T2D risk in overweight or obese females, whereas the rs7838717C-rs4279640T-rs3757971T haplotype was associated with disease risk in males with a BMI ≥ 25 kg/m^2. A comprehensive bioinformatics analysis showed that the T2D-associated polymorphisms of the *HSF1* genes are linked with the changes in expression of genes involved in the unfolded protein response, a hallmark of the pathogenesis of type 2 diabetes mellitus. The present study provided additional evidence for the role of heat shock transcription factor 1 in the pathogenesis of type 2 diabetes mellitus, and its impact on the disease's development can be attributed to the impaired folding of proteins, including proinsulin, ultimately leading to the activation of the unfolded protein response. Our study shows that chaperone gene polymorphisms appear to contribute to the development of T2D through disturbances in protein folding and activation of the unfolded protein response, a condition responsible for β-cell loss due to apoptosis [16]. This suggests that heat shock factor 1 could be a promising target for the treatment of type 2 diabetes by improving protein folding and decreasing ER overload from unfolded and misfolded proteins. Further research is warranted to substantiate the molecular mechanisms by which *HSF1* gene polymorphisms are linked to the pathogenesis of type 2 diabetes.

Supplementary Materials: The following supporting information can be downloaded at: https://www.mdpi.com/article/10.3390/life12111936/s1, Table S1: Association of the studied polymorphic gene Variants with clinical and laboratory parameters in T2D patients.

Author Contributions: Conceptualization, A.P.; methodology, I.A., E.K. and A.P.; software, E.K., I.A. and A.P.; validation, A.P.; formal analysis, E.K. and A.P.; investigation, E.K., I.A. and A.P.; resources, E.K.; data curation, I.A., E.K. and A.P.; writing—original draft preparation, E.K. and A.P.; writing—review and editing, A.P. and E.K.; visualization, A.P. and E.K.; supervision, A.P.; project administration, A.P.; funding acquisition, E.K., I.A. and A.P. All authors have read and agreed to the published version of the manuscript.

Funding: This research was funded by Russian Science Foundation (No. 22-25-00585).

Institutional Review Board Statement: The study was conducted according to the guidelines of the Declaration of Helsinki and approved by the Ethics Committee of Kursk State Medical University (protocol 10, date of approval 12 December 2016).

Informed Consent Statement: Informed consent was obtained from all subjects involved in the study.

Data Availability Statement: Data supporting reported results are available upon request.

Acknowledgments: We are grateful to all patients with type 2 diabetes, the healthy volunteers, and the staff of the Kursk Emergency Hospital who participated in this study.

Conflicts of Interest: The authors declare no conflict of interest.

References

1. Sun, H.; Saeedi, P.; Karuranga, S.; Pinkepank, M.; Ogurtsova, K.; Duncan, B.B.; Stein, C.; Basit, A.; Chan, J.C.; Mbanya, J.C.; et al. IDF Diabetes Atlas: Global, regional and country-level diabetes prevalence estimates for 2021 and projections for 2045. *Diabetes Res. Clin. Pract.* **2022**, *183*, 109119. [CrossRef] [PubMed]
2. Holman, R.R.; Paul, S.K.; Bethel, M.A.; Matthews, D.R.; Neil, H.A. 10-year follow-up of intensive glucose control in type 2 diabetes. *N. Engl. J. Med.* **2008**, *359*, 1577–1589. [CrossRef] [PubMed]
3. Tremblay, J.; Hamet, P. Environmental and genetic contributions to diabetes. *Metabolism* **2019**, *100*, 153952. [CrossRef] [PubMed]
4. Schuit, F.C.; Kiekens, R.; Pipeleers, D.G. Measuring the balance between insulin synthesis and insulin release. *Biochem. Biophys. Res. Commun.* **1991**, *178*, 1182–1187. [CrossRef]
5. Weiss, M.A. Proinsulin and the Genetics of Diabetes Mellitus. *J. Biol. Chem.* **2009**, *284*, 19159–19163. [CrossRef]
6. Liu, M.; Wan, Z.-L.; Chu, Y.-C.; Aladdin, H.; Klaproth, B.; Choquette, M.; Hua, Q.-X.; Mackin, R.B.; Rao, J.S.; De Meyts, P.; et al. Crystal Structure of a "Nonfoldable" Insulin: Impaired folding efficiency despite native activity. *J. Biol. Chem.* **2009**, *284*, 35259–35272. [CrossRef]
7. Weiss, M.; Steiner, D.F.; Philipson, L.H. Insulin biosynthesis, secretion, structure, and structure-activity relationships. In *EndoText [Internet]*; MDText.com Inc.: South Dartmouth, MA, USA, 2015.
8. Read, A.; Schröder, M. The Unfolded Protein Response: An Overview. *Biology* **2021**, *10*, 384. [CrossRef] [PubMed]
9. Støy, J.; Steiner, D.F.; Park, S.-Y.; Ye, H.; Philipson, L.H.; Bell, G.I. Clinical and molecular genetics of neonatal diabetes due to mutations in the insulin gene. *Rev. Endocr. Metab. Disord.* **2010**, *11*, 205–215. [CrossRef]
10. Hua, Q.-X.; Liu, M.; Hu, S.-Q.; Jia, W.; Arvan, P.; Weiss, M.A. A Conserved Histidine in Insulin Is Required for the Foldability of Human Proinsulin: Structure and Function of an Alab5 Analog. *J. Biol. Chem.* **2006**, *281*, 24889–24899. [CrossRef]

11. Chaturvedi, S.; Siddiqi, M.K.; Alam, P.; Khan, R.H. Protein misfolding and aggregation: Mechanism, factors and detection. *Process Biochem.* **2010**, *51*, 1183–1192. [CrossRef]
12. Dahiya, V.; Buchner, J. Functional principles and regulation of molecular chaperones. *Adv. Protein Chem. Struct. Biol.* **2019**, *114*, 1–60. [CrossRef] [PubMed]
13. Barna, J.; Csermely, P.; Vellai, T. Roles of heat shock factor 1 beyond the heat shock response. *Cell. Mol. Life Sci.* **2018**, *75*, 2897–2916. [CrossRef] [PubMed]
14. Prince, T.L.; Lang, B.J.; Guerrero-Gimenez, M.E.; Fernandez-Muñoz, J.M.; Ackerman, A.; Calderwood, S.K. HSF1: Primary Factor in Molecular Chaperone Expression and a Major Contributor to Cancer Morbidity. *Cells* **2020**, *9*, 1046. [CrossRef] [PubMed]
15. Li, J.; Labbadia, J.; Morimoto, R.I. Rethinking HSF1 in Stress, Development, and Organismal Health. *Trends Cell Biol.* **2017**, *27*, 895–905. [CrossRef]
16. Dai, Q.; Zhang, C.; Wu, Y.; McDonough, H.; Whaley, R.A.; Godfrey, V.; Chunlian, Z.; Madamanchi, N.; Xu, W.; Neckers, L.; et al. CHIP activates HSF1 and confers protection against apoptosis and cellular stress. *EMBO J.* **2003**, *22*, 5446–5458. [CrossRef]
17. Trinklein, N.D.; Murray, J.I.; Hartman, S.J.; Botstein, D.; Myers, R.M. The Role of Heat Shock Transcription Factor 1 in the Genome-wide Regulation of the Mammalian Heat Shock Response. *Mol. Biol. Cell* **2004**, *15*, 1254–1261. [CrossRef]
18. Hahn, J.-S.; Hu, Z.; Thiele, D.J.; Iyer, V.R. Genome-Wide Analysis of the Biology of Stress Responses through Heat Shock Transcription Factor. *Mol. Cell. Biol.* **2004**, *24*, 5249–5256. [CrossRef]
19. Mendillo, M.L.; Santagata, S.; Koeva, M.; Bell, G.W.; Hu, R.; Tamimi, R.M.; Fraenkel, E.; Ince, T.A.; Whitesell, L.; Lindquist, S. HSF1 Drives a Transcriptional Program Distinct from Heat Shock to Support Highly Malignant Human Cancers. *Cell* **2012**, *150*, 549–562. [CrossRef]
20. Mahat, D.B.; Salamanca, H.H.; Duarte, F.M.; Danko, C.G.; Lis, J.T. Mammalian Heat Shock Response and Mechanisms Underlying Its Genome-wide Transcriptional Regulation. *Mol. Cell* **2016**, *62*, 63–78. [CrossRef]
21. Polonikov, A.; Bocharova, I.; Azarova, I.; Klyosova, E.; Bykanova, M.; Bushueva, O.; Polonikova, A.; Churnosov, M.; Solodilova, M. The Impact of Genetic Polymorphisms in Glutamate-Cysteine Ligase, a Key Enzyme of Glutathione Biosynthesis, on Ischemic Stroke Risk and Brain Infarct Size. *Life* **2022**, *12*, 602. [CrossRef]
22. Azarova, I.E. The relationship between polymorphism rs12449964 of the phosphatidylethanolamine- N-methyltransferase gene and hypertriglyceridemia and obesity in patients with type 2 diabetes. *Res. Results Biomed.* **2021**, *7*, 245–256. [CrossRef]
23. World Health Organization. *Definition, Diagnosis and Classification of Diabetes Mellitus and Its Complications: Report of a WHO Consultation. Part 1: Diagnosis and Classification of Diabetes Mellitus*; WHO: Geneva, Switzerland, 1999.
24. World Health Organization. *Global Report on Diabetes: Executive Summary (no. Who/nmh/nvi/16.3)*; World Health Organization: Geneva, Switzerland, 2016.
25. Klyosova, E.Y.; Azarova, I.E.; Sunyaykina, O.A.; Polonikov, A.V. Validity of a brief screener for environmental risk factors of age-related diseases using type 2 diabetes and coronary artery disease as examples. *Res. Results Biomed.* **2022**, *8*, 130–137. [CrossRef]
26. Azarova, I.; Klyosova, E.; Polonikov, A. The Link between Type 2 Diabetes Mellitus and the Polymorphisms of Glutathione-Metabolizing Genes Suggests a New Hypothesis Explaining Disease Initiation and Progression. *Life* **2021**, *11*, 886. [CrossRef] [PubMed]
27. Malone, J.I.; Hansen, B.C. Does obesity cause type 2 diabetes mellitus (T2DM)? Or is it the opposite? *Pediatr. Diabetes* **2019**, *20*, 5–9. [CrossRef] [PubMed]
28. Sarparanta, J.; Jonson, P.H.; Kawan, S.; Udd, B. Neuromuscular Diseases Due to Chaperone Mutations: A Review and Some New Results. *Int. J. Mol. Sci.* **2020**, *21*, 1409. [CrossRef] [PubMed]
29. Synofzik, M.; Haack, T.B.; Kopajtich, R.; Gorza, M.; Rapaport, D.; Greiner, M.; Schönfeld, C.; Freiberg, C.; Schorr, S.; Holl, R.W.; et al. Absence of BiP Co-chaperone DNAJC3 Causes Diabetes Mellitus and Multisystemic Neurodegeneration. *Am. J. Hum. Genet.* **2014**, *95*, 689–697. [CrossRef] [PubMed]
30. Koren, J., 3rd; Jinwal, U.K.; Lee, D.C.; Jones, J.; Shults, C.L.; Johnson, A.G.; Anderson, L.J.; Dickey, C.A. Chaperone signalling complexes in Alzheimer's disease. *J. Cell. Mol. Med.* **2009**, *13*, 619–630. [CrossRef]
31. Moniruzzaman; Ahmed, I.; Huq, S.; Mahmud, S.A.; Begum, S.; Amin, U.M.; Rahman, H.; Sarker, P.K.; Hossain, M.U.; Das, K.C.; et al. Association of polymorphism in heat shock protein 70 genes with type 2 diabetes in Bangladeshi population. *Mol. Genet. Genom. Med.* **2020**, *8*, e1073. [CrossRef]
32. Elshahed, O.M.; Shaker, O.G. Heat Shock Protein 70 Gene Polymorphism in Egyptian Patients with Type 2 Diabetes Mellitus, with and without Nephropathy. *Saudi J. Kidney Dis. Transplant.* **2020**, *31*, 787–795. [CrossRef]
33. Mathew, A.; Morimoto, R.I. Role of the Heat-Shock Response in the Life and Death of Proteins. *Ann. N. Y. Acad. Sci.* **1998**, *851*, 99–111. [CrossRef]
34. Kavanagh, K.; Zhang, L.; Wagner, J.D. Tissue-specific regulation and expression of heat shock proteins in type 2 diabetic monkeys. *Cell Stress Chaperon.* **2009**, *14*, 291–299. [CrossRef] [PubMed]
35. Marselli, L.; Thorne, J.; Dahiya, S.; Sgroi, D.C.; Sharma, A.; Bonner-Weir, S.; Marchetti, P.; Weir, G.C. Gene Expression Profiles of Beta-Cell Enriched Tissue Obtained by Laser Capture Microdissection from Subjects with Type 2 Diabetes. *PLoS ONE* **2010**, *5*, e11499. [CrossRef] [PubMed]

36. Solís, E.J.; Pandey, J.P.; Zheng, X.; Jin, D.X.; Gupta, P.B.; Airoldi, E.M.; Pincus, D.; Denic, V. Defining the Essential Function of Yeast Hsf1 Reveals a Compact Transcriptional Program for Maintaining Eukaryotic Proteostasis. *Mol. Cell* **2016**, *63*, 60–71. [CrossRef] [PubMed]
37. Hayden, M.R.; Tyagi, S.C.; Kerklo, M.M.; Nicolls, M.R. Type 2 diabetes mellitus as a conformational disease. *JOP J. Pancreas* **2005**, *6*, 287–302.
38. Mukherjee, A.; Morales-Scheihing, D.; Butler, P.C.; Soto, C. Type 2 diabetes as a protein misfolding disease. *Trends Mol. Med.* **2015**, *21*, 439–449. [CrossRef]
39. Moreno-Gonzalez, I.; Edwards, G., III; Salvadores, N.; Shahnawaz, M.; Diaz-Espinoza, R.; Soto, C. Molecular interaction between type 2 diabetes and Alzheimer's disease through cross-seeding of protein misfolding. *Mol. Psychiatry* **2017**, *22*, 1327–1334. [CrossRef]
40. Purwana, I.; Liu, J.J.; Portha, B.; Buteau, J. HSF1 acetylation decreases its transcriptional activity and enhances glucolipotoxicity-induced apoptosis in rat and human beta cells. *Diabetologia* **2017**, *60*, 1432–1441. [CrossRef]
41. Chin, G. Membrane sorting. *Cell Biol. Sci.* **2002**, *295*, 1975–1976.
42. Katzmann, D.J.; Odorizzi, G.; Emr, S.D. Receptor downregulation and multivesicular-body sorting. *Nat. Rev. Mol. Cell Biol.* **2002**, *3*, 893–905. [CrossRef]
43. Kaufman, R.J.; Back, S.H.; Song, B.; Han, J.; Hassler, J. The unfolded protein response is required to maintain the integrity of the endoplasmic reticulum, prevent oxidative stress and preserve differentiation inβ-cells. *Diabetes Obes. Metab.* **2010**, *12* (Suppl. S2), 99–107. [CrossRef]
44. Engin, F.; Nguyen, T.; Yermalovich, A.; Hotamisligil, G.S. Aberrant islet unfolded protein response in type 2 diabetes. *Sci. Rep.* **2014**, *4*, 4054. [CrossRef] [PubMed]
45. Pandey, V.K.; Mathur, A.; Kakkar, P. Emerging role of Unfolded Protein Response (UPR) mediated proteotoxic apoptosis in diabetes. *Life Sci.* **2019**, *216*, 246–258. [CrossRef] [PubMed]
46. Orland, M.D.; Anwar, K.; Cromley, D.; Chu, C.-H.; Chen, L.; Billheimer, J.T.; Hussain, M.M.; Cheng, D. Acyl coenzyme A dependent retinol esterification by acyl coenzyme A: Diacylglycerol acyltransferase 1. *Biochim. Biophys. Acta* **2005**, *1737*, 76–82. [CrossRef] [PubMed]
47. Kaneko, Y.K.; Ishikawa, T. Diacylglycerol Signaling Pathway in Pancreatic β-Cells: An Essential Role of Diacylglycerol Kinase in the Regulation of Insulin Secretion. *Biol. Pharm. Bull.* **2015**, *38*, 669–673. [CrossRef] [PubMed]
48. Yang, C.; Kazanietz, M.G. Divergence and complexities in DAG signaling: Looking beyond PKC. *Trends Pharmacol. Sci.* **2003**, *24*, 602–608. [CrossRef] [PubMed]
49. Gerlach, B.; Cordier, S.M.; Schmukle, A.C.; Emmerich, C.H.; Rieser, E.; Haas, T.L.; Webb, A.I.; Rickard, J.A.; Anderton, H.; Wong, W.W.-L.; et al. Linear ubiquitination prevents inflammation and regulates immune signalling. *Nature* **2011**, *471*, 591–596. [CrossRef]
50. Tokunaga, F.; Nakagawa, T.; Nakahara, M.; Saeki, Y.; Taniguchi, M.; Sakata, S.-I.; Tanaka, K.; Nakano, H.; Iwai, K. SHARPIN is a component of the NF-κB-activating linear ubiquitin chain assembly complex. *Nature* **2011**, *471*, 633–636. [CrossRef]
51. Ikeda, F.; Deribe, Y.L.; Skånland, S.S.; Stieglitz, B.; Grabbe, C.; Franz-Wachtel, M.; van Wijk, S.J.L.; Goswami, P.; Nagy, V.; Terzic, J.; et al. SHARPIN forms a linear ubiquitin ligase complex regulating NF-κB activity and apoptosis. *Nature* **2011**, *471*, 637–641. [CrossRef]
52. Indira, M.; Abhilash, P. Role of NF-Kappa B (NF-κB) in Diabetes. *Onco Ther.* **2013**, *4*, 111–132. [CrossRef]
53. Rivkin, E.; Almeida, S.M.; Ceccarelli, D.F.; Juang, Y.-C.; MacLean, T.A.; Srikumar, T.; Huang, H.; Dunham, W.H.; Fukumura, R.; Xie, G.; et al. The linear ubiquitin-specific deubiquitinase gumby regulates angiogenesis. *Nature* **2013**, *498*, 318–324. [CrossRef]
54. Jin, T. Current Knowledge on the Role of Wnt Signaling Pathway in Glucose Homeostasis. *Mol. Nutr. Diabetes* **2016**, 357–369. [CrossRef]
55. Bonhoure, N.; Byrnes, A.; Moir, R.D.; Hodroj, W.; Preitner, F.; Praz, V.; Marcelin, G.; Chus, S.C., Jr.; Martinez-Lopez, N.; Singh, R.; et al. Loss of the RNA polymerase III repressor MAF1 confers obesity resistance. *Genes Dev.* **2015**, *29*, 934–947. [CrossRef] [PubMed]
56. Yang, Z.; Zhuang, L.; Szatmary, P.; Wen, L.; Sun, H.; Lu, Y.; Xu, Q.; Chen, X. Upregulation of Heat Shock Proteins (HSPA12A, HSP90B1, HSPA4, HSPA5 and HSPA6) in Tumour Tissues Is Associated with Poor Outcomes from HBV-Related Early-Stage Hepatocellular Carcinoma. *Int. J. Med Sci.* **2015**, *12*, 256–263. [CrossRef] [PubMed]

life

MDPI

Article

Assessment of the Association of Vitamin D and the Risk of Tuberculosis among End-Stage Kidney Disease Population

Sithembiso Tiyandza Dlamini [1], Kyaw Moe Htet [1], Ei Chue Chue Theint [1], Wei-Ming Li [2,3,4], Hsin-Wen Chang [5,6,*,†] and Hung-Pin Tu [7,8,*,†]

1 Graduate Institute of Medicine, College of Medicine, Kaohsiung Medical University, Kaohsiung 80708, Taiwan
2 Department of Urology, Kaohsiung Medical University Hospital, Kaohsiung 80708, Taiwan
3 Department of Urology, School of Medicine, College of Medicine, Kaohsiung Medical University, Kaohsiung 80708, Taiwan
4 Department of Urology, Ministry of Health and Welfare, Pingtung Hospital, Pingtung 900, Taiwan
5 Department of Applied Psychology, Hsuan Chuang University, 48 Hsuan Chuang Rd., Hsinchu City 30092, Taiwan
6 Center for General Education, Hsuan Chuang University, Hsinchu City 30092, Taiwan
7 Department of Public Health and Environmental Medicine, School of Medicine, College of Medicine, Kaohsiung Medical University, 100 Shih-Chuan 1st Road, Kaohsiung 80708, Taiwan
8 Department of Medical Research, Kaohsiung Medical University Hospital, Kaohsiung 80708, Taiwan
* Correspondence: hsinwen@hcu.edu.tw (H.-W.C.); p915013@kmu.edu.tw (H.-P.T.); Tel.: +886-3-5302255 (ext. 5222) (H.-W.C.)
† These authors contributed equally to this work.

Abstract: We investigated the role of vitamin D in the risk of tuberculosis (TB) among patients with end-stage kidney disease (ESKD). The retrospective cohort was conducted with data of 20,985 patients with kidney disease and 20,985 controls without kidney disease (1:1 matching on age of cohort entry and sex) in the duration of 1997–2010 from the Taiwan National Health insurance database. Then, by a case–cohort study, among 20,985 kidney disease, 3194 ESKD patients were identified with matched 3194 non-ESKD patients. Multivariate analyses revealed a significant association between kidney disease and tuberculosis (adjusted incidence rate ratio (IRR) 1.57 (1.33–1.86)), and the risk increased after 3 years of follow-up the (adjusted IRR 3.79 (2.55–5.62)), but after more years of follow-up no significance was observed. We also found that ESKD increases the risk of tuberculosis (adjusted IRR 3.67 (2.27–5.93)). However, vitamin D usage was not related with the tuberculosis risk in ESKD patients ($p > 0.1783$). Our study showed increased risk of tuberculosis in kidney disease and ESKD patients, and vitamin D was not beneficial in ESKD.

Keywords: retrospective cohort study; kidney disease; end-stage kidney disease; vitamin D; tuberculosis

check for updates

Citation: Dlamini, S.T.; Htet, K.M.; Theint, E.C.C.; Li, W.-M.; Chang, H.-W.; Tu, H.-P. Assessment of the Association of Vitamin D and the Risk of Tuberculosis among End-Stage Kidney Disease Population. *Life* **2022**, *12*, 1881. https://doi.org/10.3390/life12111881

Academic Editor: Panagiotis Georgianos

Received: 24 October 2022
Accepted: 11 November 2022
Published: 14 November 2022

Publisher's Note: MDPI stays neutral with regard to jurisdictional claims in published maps and institutional affiliations.

1. Introduction

End-stage kidney disease (ESKD) inflicts significant health and economic burdens on both individuals and the public population [1]. Chronic kidney disease (CKD) is a structural and functional progressive kidney damage lasting for more than 3 months. When kidney disease reaches the end stage, that is, stage 4 and 5, high levels of fluid, electrolytes and wastes products can build up in the body; this might cause severe decline of GFR over the periods of months or years [2]. The symptoms of worsening kidney function might include leg swelling, vomiting and confusion and reduced appetite; however, this disease can complicate to hypertension, heart failure, bone disease and anemia. CKD has since been an increasing endemic, with a worldwide prevalence of 8% to 16% [3]. Taiwan has the highest prevalence of CKD, and the reported prevalence of ESKD is 6.9% in adult populations in Taiwan [4]. The major causes of CKD in Taiwan are older age, diabetes, hypertension, smoking, obesity, regular use of herbal medicine, chronic lead exposure and hepatitis C, chronic glomerulonephritis and chronic interstitial nephritis [5]. There has since been a gap on the findings about the relationship between CKD and pulmonary TB. Not many studies have reported on the high prevalence of TB among patients with CKD.

According to the World Health Organization (WHO), tuberculosis (TB) remains one of the most leading infectious diseases in the world. The World Health Organization estimates 10.4 million new TB cases worldwide and 1.3 million related deaths in 2016. The relationship between active tuberculosis (TB) and chronic kidney disease (CKD) was first reported in a 1974 case reported on a dialysis patient. According to the National Institute for Health and Care Excellence guidelines, the relative risk for developing active TB is 10% to 25% in patients with CKD at any stage [6]. This relationship has since been an emerging global syndemic. There is a hypothesis that CKD may increase the risk of developing TB and related immunosuppression, especially in kidney transplants recipients. Due to this fact, diagnosis may be challenging because of the nonspecific symptoms, which are the same as extrapulmonary TB and peritoneal disease in patients receiving renal replacement therapy. This circumstance may cause TB diagnosis in dialysis patients to be delayed because of the extrapulmonary manifestations. Initially, it was believed that hemodialysis patients have a higher incidence of latent tuberculosis than peritoneal dialysis. Studies have argued this phenomenon is caused by the fact that hemodialysis patients have more frequent hospital visits and longer hospital stays. A study in Pakistan reported that low vitamin D levels were associated with a five-fold increased risk for progression to tuberculosis [7]. Given the rising scientific evidence regarding vitamin D's multisystem role, the association between chronic kidney disease [8] with the loss of functional renal function to convert 25(OH)D to 1,25(OH)2D, calcitriol is reduced leading to a decline in plasma 1,25(OH)2D [9]. Vitamin D status in CKD patients is most commonly assessed on the basis of the plasma concentration of 25-hydroxyvitamin D or calcidiol. Vitamin D deficiency thresholds for population health are defined as 25(OH)D serum levels $<$ 25 or 30 nmol/L [10,11] The effects were shown to depend on the stage of the disease.

Observational studies in patients treated with hemodialysis showed that the use of active vitamin D sterols was associated with lower risk of all-cause mortality, regardless of parathyroid hormone levels [12]. Vitamin D supplementation in CKD is to prevent and treat the complications associated with secondary hyperparathyroidism in ESKD [13]. However, in the Japan Dialysis Active Vitamin D (J-DAVID) trial, treatment with alfacalcidol did not reduce the risk of composite cardiovascular events or the risk of all-cause mortality in hemodialysis patients without secondary hyperparathyroidism [14]. Some studies have conducted research on the effectiveness of vitamin D supplementation on plasma parathormone (PTH) concentrations, and it has been discovered to reduce the PTH concentrations. Some studies have argued that this effect depends on the patient's characteristics [15], the dose–response of vitamin D supplementation and the response in PTH. The optimal concentration ranges of PTH and 25(OH)D for the management and prevention of CKD–MBD are not well established for each stage of CKD [16]. Some studies suggest that vitamin D supplementation, especially calcidiol, is not effective in CKD patients with hyperthyroidism due to the interacting of the medication cinacalcet, which reduces the parathyroid hormone (PTH) [16,17]. Studies have shown that there was a negative correlation between 25(OH)D and PTH levels [18].

Patients with ESKD are increasing, and they need dialysis; this is a major health problem because even TB is a commonly associated infectious disease. Many studies have argued that hemodialysis patients visit the hemodialysis room frequently, so they are more likely to acquire a Mycobacterium tuberculosis infection than peritoneal dialysis patients through airborne transmission in the HD rooms [19]. It is believed that vitamin D insufficiency arises at an early stage of the disease and tends to worsen with the progressive loss of renal function [20].

In this study, the main objective is to see through this research gap by conducting a cohort study using data from the National Health Insurance database in Taiwan to assess the relationship between patients with CKD and TB and more knowledge on the outcomes in patients taking vitamin D in ESKD renal patients.

2. Materials and Methods

2.1. Source of Data and Study Population

We conducted a nationwide, population-based retrospective cohort study to clarify the role of renal disease in the risk of tuberculosis, taking advantage of a well-established and large-size data set available from the Taiwan National Health Insurance Research Database (NHIRD). The Longitudinal Health Insurance Database 2010 (LHID2010) constitutes registration and claims data collected by the NHIRD program for a nationally representative group of 1 million individuals. The NHIRD contains all claims-related data, including patient personal information (e.g., age and gender), clinical diagnoses, prescribed medicines and health-care use. Disease diagnosis is assigned according to the International Classification of Diseases, 9th Revisions, and the Clinical Modification (ICD-9-CM) diagnostic codes. To protect patient confidentiality, all their identification numbers and medical institutions were encrypted before the release of the data for research purposes. Because no patient could be identified, informed consent was waived. The study protocol was reviewed and approved by the Institutional Review Committee of Kaohsiung Medical University Hospital (KMUHIRB-EXEMPT (I)-20190011), Taiwan.

The flowchart illustrating the selection process of participants is shown in Figure 1. From 1,000,023 people (LHID 2010), we excluded 445,173 people, due to birth after 1 January 1977 (age < 20) (n = 444,812), tuberculosis diagnosed before 1 January 1997 (n = 8), kidney disease diagnosed before 1 January 1997 (n = 348) and vitamin D used before 1 January 1997 (n = 5), respectively. A total of 554,850 people are enrolled with kidney disease (n = 35,617) and the compared group (n = 519,233). From the kidney disease patients, we excluded those with prior diagnosis of tuberculosis (n = 520), kidney disease and incidence of tuberculosis with follow-up of less than 1 month (n = 33), kidney disease patients with follow-up of less than 1 month (n = 221), kidney disease patients with clinic visits < 2 (n = 13,584), tuberculosis patients with drug use less than 60 days (n = 105) and vitamin D drug use before kidney disease (n = 169), respectively. From the compared group, incidence of tuberculosis with follow-up of less than 1 month (n = 28), tuberculosis patients with drug use of less than 60 days (n = 1059) and vitamin D drug use (n = 1724) were excluded. The final kidney disease patients (n = 20,985) were matched with the compared group (matched 1:1 on age of cohort entry and sex). Presence of kidney disease and tuberculosis were defined on the basis of the fulfillment of the following criteria: tuberculosis—3 or more clinic visits. The index date was the date of the first diagnosis of kidney disease. The main study outcome was TB diagnosed. We considered incident TB from the first kidney disease diagnosis to the date of TB diagnosis or the end of the study. The follow-up period began on 1 January 1997 and ended on the date of the first TB events, the end of the study (31 December 2010) or the end of the follow-up, whichever occurred first.

2.2. Ascertainment of Kidney Diseases and Tuberculosis

In total, 20,985 patients with kidney disease and 20,985 without kidney disease (matched 1:1 on age of cohort entry and sex) were included in this study. The outcome of interest was the documentation of tuberculosis by a physician. Assessment of renal disease (by ICD-9-CM code 403.01, 403.11, 403.91, 404.02, 404.03, 404.12, 404.13, 404.92, 404.93, 582.x, 583.0–583.7, 585.x, 586.x, 588.0, V42.0, V45.1, V56.x) was carried out during an outpatient or inpatient visit. Assessment of TB was conducted with ICD-9-CM codes of TB (010-018) plus the prescription of more than two anti-tuberculosis medications (i.e., isoniazid, rifampin, pyrazinamide, ethambutol, rifater, rifinah, streptomycin, cycloserine, prothionamide, amikacin, kanamycin, ciprofloxacin, moxifloxacin and levofloxacin) for more than 60 days. Subjects with kidney disease were followed from the index date to the date of first diagnosis of kidney disease. The ESKD patients were divided into hemodialysis (HD) and peritoneal dialysis (PD) cohorts according to the dialysis modalities with different operation codes (HD, 3995; PD, 5498), and the administration code was used to define renal dialysis (D8, hemodialysis and D9, peritoneal dialysis). The primary case definition of renal transplant recipients was having a physician-recorded primary diagnosis of a kidney replaced by transplant (ICD-9-CM V420) or having complications of the transplanted kidney (996.81) at either an outpatient or inpatient visit in NHIRD data sets. The ESKD patients receiving a prescription of vitamin D included alfacalcidol and calcitriol (Anatomical Therapeutic Chemical [ATC] code A1CC03 and A11CC04).

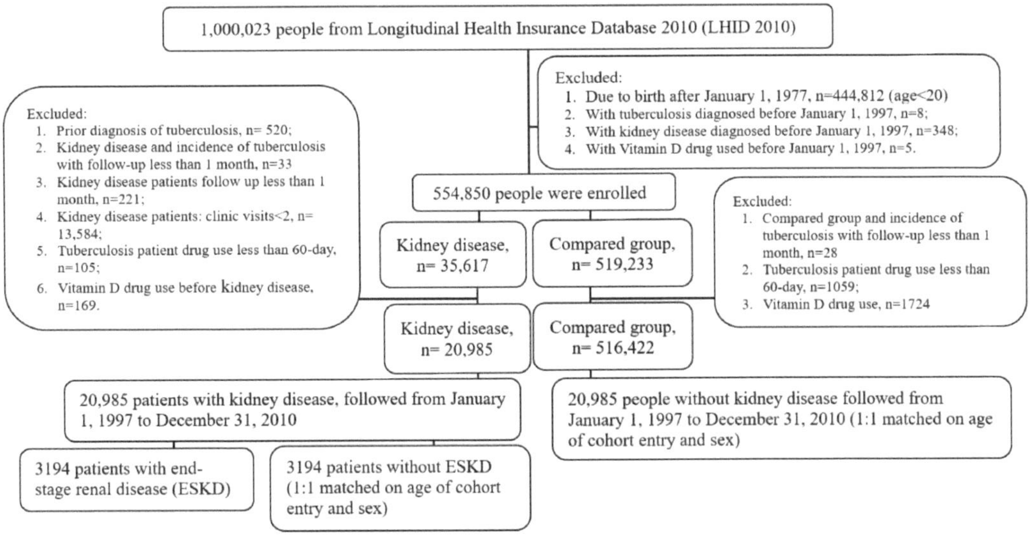

Figure 1. Flow chart for the selection of study patients.

2.3. Comorbidities

In addition to the demographic risk factors of age, sex and region, we evaluated other potentially confounding factors for alcohol abuse, lipid disorders, obesity, hypertension, myocardial infarction, congestive heart failure, peripheral vascular disease, cerebrovascular disease, chronic pulmonary disease, rheumatologic disease, liver disease, diabetes mellitus and any malignancy. These comorbidities were diagnosed according to ICD-9-CM codes [21].

2.4. Statistical Analysis

A propensity analysis was performed to obtain a match of the propensity score for each patient with the covariates, such as age of cohort entry and sex. Continuous and categorical variables were analyzed using a t-test or Wilcoxon rank sum test and a chi-squared test, respectively, and the values obtained for the renal disease group and matched non-renal disease group were compared. The Kaplan–Meier method was used to estimate the survival curves for each group and the log-rank test was used to test for homogeneity among the survival curves. The incident rate ratio (IRR) was calculated using the PROC GENMOD generalized linear model to perform Poisson regression analysis, which is a log-linear model. Potential risk factors, such as comorbidities, were incorporated into the model. Significant results were those with $p \leq 0.05$. All statistical analyses were performed using SAS statistical software (version 9.4, SAS Institute, Cary, NC, USA).

3. Results

Table 1 presents the demographic characteristics of the study population. This retrospective cohort study included 20,985 patients with chronic kidney disease and 20,985 with non-chronic kidney controls. In the 20,985 patients with renal disease, 2780 (13.2%) patients were undergoing hemodialysis only, and 291 (1.4%) were undergoing both hemodialysis and peritoneal dialysis. In patients with kidney disease, 290 developed tuberculosis (incidence rate 2.05, 95% confidence interval (CI) 2.04–2.06 per 1000-person years), and 334 of the patients without kidney disease had TB (incidence rate 1.14 95% CI 1.14–1.15 per 1000-person years). In the study, sex and age were distributed equally between the CKD and non-CKD and were matched in the participant's characteristics. Most of the participants lived in the northern region. A higher proportion of participants with CKD than without CKD were diagnosed with hypertension (72.8% vs. 47.6%). Those with lipid disorder were more prevalent in the group with CKD than in the group with non-CKD (10,780, 51.4%).

Table 1. Characteristics of patients with kidney disease and the comparison group.

	Kidney Disease	Compared Group	*p* Value
N	20,985	20,985	
Dialysis, *n* (%)			
Hemodialysis alone	2780 (13.2)	-	-
Peritoneal dialysis alone	80 (0.4)	-	-
Hemodialysis and peritoneal dialysis	291 (1.4)	-	-
Kidney transplant recipients	192 (0.9)	-	-
Tuberculosis *, *n* (%)	290 (1.4)	334 (1.6)	0.0760
Follow-up duration median (IQR), years	3.7 (1.7–6.6)	8.0 (4.9–11.2)	<0.0001
Follow-up duration groups, *n* (%)			
≤3 years	120 (41.4)	34 (10.2)	
>3 to 6 years	86 (29.7)	79 (23.7)	
>6 to 9 years	53 (18.3)	70 (21.0)	
>9 years	31 (10.7)	151 (45.2)	<0.0001
Age of cohort entry mean (SD), years	51.8 (14.2)	51.8 (14.2)	0.9501
Age group, *n* (%)			
20 to 30	1578 (7.5)	1578 (7.5)	
>30 to 40	3177 (15.1)	3177 (15.1)	
>40 to 50	4751 (22.6)	4751 (22.6)	
>50 to 60	4525 (21.6)	4525 (21.6)	
>60 to 70	4901 (23.4)	4901 (23.4)	
>70	2053 (9.8)	2053 (9.8)	1.0000
Sex, *n* (%)			
Males	11,242 (53.6)	11,242 (53.6)	
Females	9743 (46.4)	9743 (46.4)	1.0000
Residential region, *n* (%)			
Northern	9597 (45.7)	9748 (46.5)	
Central	4678 (22.3)	4899 (23.3)	
Southern	6038 (28.8)	5594 (26.7)	
Eastern and other region	672 (3.2)	744 (3.5)	<0.0001
Comorbidities, *n* (%)			
Alcohol abuse	404 (1.9)	214 (1.0)	<0.0001
Lipid disorders	10,780 (51.4)	5993 (28.6)	<0.0001
Obesity	306 (1.5)	149 (0.7)	<0.0001
Hypertension	15,274 (72.8)	9986 (47.6)	<0.0001
Myocardial infarction	380 (1.8)	176 (0.8)	<0.0001
Congestive heart failure	2709 (12.9)	1009 (4.8)	<0.0001
Peripheral vascular disease	1418 (6.8)	712 (3.4)	<0.0001
Cerebrovascular disease	3552 (16.9)	2253 (10.7)	<0.0001
Chronic pulmonary disease	5330 (25.4)	3859 (18.4)	<0.0001
Rheumatologic disease	1011 (4.8)	501 (2.4)	<0.0001
Liver disease	5083 (24.2)	2726 (13.0)	<0.0001
Diabetes mellitus	5286 (25.2)	2768 (13.2)	<0.0001
Any malignancy	1720 (8.2)	1061 (5.1)	<0.0001
Vitamin D drugs (ATC code), *n*(%)			
A11CC03 (alfacalcidol)	297 (1.4)	-	-
A11CC04 (calcitriol)	1138 (5.4)	-	-
A11CC03 or A11CC04	1306 (6.2)	-	-

IQR: interquartile range; SD: standard deviation; ATC: Anatomical Therapeutic Chemical Classification. Comorbidities were defined as more than two outpatient claims. Data of continuous and categorical variables were analyzed using the *t*-test or Wilcoxon rank sum test and chi-squared test to compare the data of kidney disease and the comparison group. * Active TB: ICD-9-CM codes of TB (010-018) plus the prescription of more than two anti-tuberculosis medications (i.e., isoniazid, rifampin, pyrazinamide, ethambutol, rifater, rifinah, streptomycin, cycloserine, protionamide, amikacin, kanamycin, ciprofloxacin, moxifloxacin and levofloxacin) for more than 60 days.

Increased risk of development of tuberculosis was observed in our study (adjusted IRR 1.57 95% CI 1.33–1.86; Table 2). After 3 years follow-up, the risk of tuberculosis in chronic kidney disease was higher (adjusted IRR 3.79 (2.55–5.62)). However, after more years of follow-up, no significance was observed (adjusted IRR 1.33 95% CI 0.96–1.84; $p = 0.0824$). The Kaplan–Meier curves for the incidence of tuberculosis in individuals with and without kidney disease differed significantly (log-rank test $p < 0.0001$) (Figure 2a).

Table 2. Association of kidney disease with the risk of incident tuberculosis.

	Tuberculosis/ Total Subjects, %	Person–Years	Events Per 1000 Person–Years (95% CI)	IRR (95% CI)	*p* Value	Adjusted IRR (95% CI)	*p* Value
Compared group	334/20,985, 1.59	291,773.08	1.14 (1.14–1.15)	1.00		1.00	
Kidney disease	290/20,985, 1.38	141,549.53	2.05 (2.04–2.06)	1.79 (1.53–2.09)	<0.0001	1.57 (1.33–1.86)	<0.0001
Follow-up duration *							
≤3 years							
Compared group	34/20,985, 0.16	62,920.18	0.54 (0.54–0.54)	1.00		1.00	
Kidney disease	120/20,985, 0.57	56,041.95	2.14 (2.12–2.16)	3.96 (2.71–5.80)	<0.0001	3.79 (2.55–5.62)	<0.0001
>3 to 6 years							
Compared group	79/20,951, 0.38	125,588.8	0.63 (0.63–0.63)	1.00		1.00	
Kidney disease	86/16,303, 0.53	91,174.27	0.94 (0.94–0.95)	1.50 (1.10–2.04)	0.0093	1.33 (0.96–1.84)	0.0824

Incidence rate ratio (IRR) was calculated by using generalized linear model (PROC GENMOD) to perform Poisson regression analysis (a log-linear model). Adjusted IRRs were calculated after adjustment for residential region and comorbidities of alcohol abuse, lipid disorders, obesity, hypertension, myocardial infarction, congestive heart failure, peripheral vascular disease, cerebrovascular disease, chronic pulmonary disease, rheumatologic disease, liver disease, diabetes mellitus and any malignancy by using a cox proportional-hazards regression model. * For follow-up period analysis, kidney disease and risk of incident tuberculosis at the more than 3 to 6 years as excluded subjects of less than 3 years were calculated.

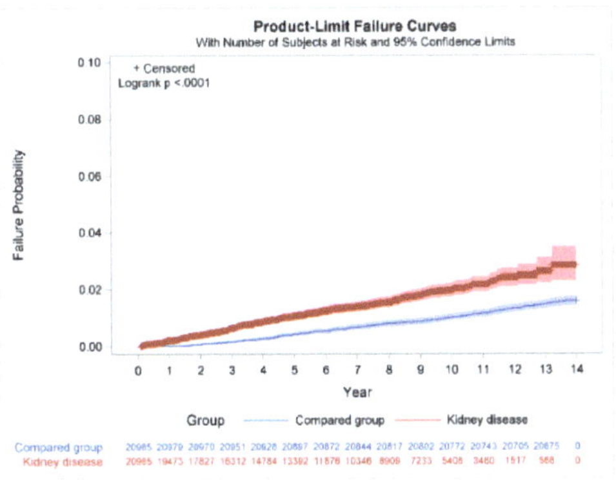

(a)

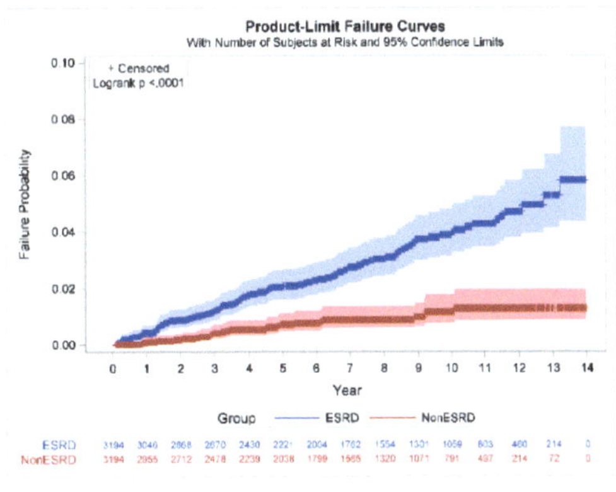

(b)

Figure 2. Cumulative incidence rates of tuberculosis: (**a**) with and without kidney disease; (**b**) with and without end-stage kidney disease (ESKD) in kidney disease patients.

Table 3 presents the demographic characteristics of the ESKD population. This retrospective cohort study included 3194 patients with ESKD and 3194 non-ESKD. In the 3194 patients with ESKD, 2657 (83.2%) patients were undergoing hemodialysis only, 74 (2.3%) peritoneal dialysis, 271 (8.5%) both hemodialysis and peritoneal dialysis as well as 192 kidney transplant recipients (6.0%), respectively. In patients with ESKD, 98 developed tuberculosis (incidence rate 4.08, 95% confidence interval (CI) 4.03–4.13 per 1000-person years) and 25 of the patients without kidney disease had TB (incidence rate 1.17, 95% CI 1.16–1.19 per 1000-person years). We also found that ESKD increases the risk of tuberculosis (adjusted IRR 3.67 95% CI 2.27–5.93). The Kaplan–Meier curves for the incidence of tuberculosis in individuals with and without ESKD differed significantly (log-rank test $p < 0.0001$; Figure 2b).

Table 3. Characteristics of end-stage kidney disease patients and kidney disease patients.

	ESKD	NonESKD	p Value
N	3194	3194	
Dialysis, n (%)			
Hemodialysis alone	2657 (83.2)	-	-
Peritoneal dialysis alone	74 (2.3)	-	-
Hemodialysis and peritoneal dialysis	271 (8.5)	-	-
Kidney transplant recipients	192 (6.0)	-	-
Tuberculosis, n (%)	98 (3.1)	25 (0.8)	<0.0001
Follow-up duration median (IQR), years	3.9 (1.7–7.4)	3.3 (2.4–5.3)	0.6085
Follow-up duration groups, n (%)			
≤3 years	36 (36.7)	11 (44.0)	
>3 to 6 years	26 (26.5)	8 (32.0)	
>6 to 9 years	24 (24.5)	3 (12.0)	
>9 years	12 (12.2)	3 (12.0)	0.5919
Age of cohort entry mean (SD), years	50.3 (13.1)	50.4 (13.3)	0.8923
Age group, n (%)			
20 to 30	199 (6.2)	199 (6.2)	
>30 to 40	519 (16.2)	519 (16.2)	
>40 to 50	908 (28.4)	908 (28.4)	
>50 to 60	726 (22.7)	726 (22.7)	
>60 to 70	629 (19.7)	629 (19.7)	
>70	213 (6.7)	213 (6.7)	1.0000
Sex, n (%)			
Males	1575 (49.3)	1575 (49.3)	
Females	1619 (50.7)	1619 (50.7)	1.0000
Residential region, n (%)			
Northern	1372 (43.0)	1476(46.2)	
Central	737 (23.1)	752(23.5)	
Southern	981 (30.7)	893(28)	
Eastern and other	104 (3.3)	73(2.3)	0.0037
Comorbidities, n (%)			
Alcohol abuse	39 (1.2)	64 (2.0)	0.0130
Lipid disorders	1648 (51.6)	1650 (51.7)	0.9601
Obesity	23 (0.7)	53 (1.7)	0.0005
Hypertension	2851 (89.3)	2172 (68.0)	<0.0001
Myocardial infarction	77 (2.4)	49 (1.5)	0.0118
Congestive heart failure	642 (20.1)	341 (10.7)	<0.0001
Peripheral vascular disease	282 (8.8)	174 (5.4)	<0.0001
Cerebrovascular disease	586 (18.3)	481 (15.1)	0.0004
Chronic pulmonary disease	683 (21.4)	751 (23.5)	0.0414
Rheumatologic disease	111 (3.5)	169 (5.3)	0.0004
Liver disease	668 (20.9)	780 (24.4)	0.0008
Diabetes mellitus	1048 (32.8)	725 (22.7)	<0.0001
Any malignancy	314 (9.8)	247 (7.7)	0.0031
Vitamin D drugs (ATC code), n(%)			
A11CC03 (alfacalcidol)	240 (7.5)	8 (0.3)	<0.0001
Patient visits median (IQR), frequency	6.5 (3.0–16.0)	4.0 (1.5–6.0)	0.0587
Total dose median (IQR)	51.9 (17.3–171.6)	29.0 (21.0–96.3)	0.3592
A11CC04 (calcitriol)	996 (31.2)	19 (0.6)	<0.0001
Patient visits median (IQR), n	9.0 (4.0–22.0)	6.0 (2.0–16.0)	0.1516
Total dose median (IQR)	54.1 (17.6–137.0)	38.5 (14.0–117.5)	0.5898
A11CC03 or A11CC04	1113 (34.8)	27 (0.8)	<0.0001
Patient visits median (IQR)	10.0 (4.0–23.0)	5.0 (2.0–11.0)	0.0061
Total dose median (IQR)	60.3 (18.8–152.1)	31.5 (14.0–117.5)	0.1975

ESKD: end-stage kidney disease; IQR: interquartile range; SD: standard deviation. Comorbidities were defined as more than three outpatient claims. Data of continuous and categorical variables were analyzed using the t-test or Wilcoxon rank sum test and chi-squared test to compare the data of ESKD and the non-ESKD patients.

However, Vitamin D uses and dosages were not related with the reduced risk of tuberculosis in ESKD patients (Table 3). Vitamin D supplementation has no significance in ESKD (adjusted IRR 0.77, 95% CI 0.49–1.19; $p = 0.2351$). Moreover, we also observed that there was no dosage effect on ESKD patients (adjusted IRR > 0.56; $p > 0.1783$). Figure 3 shows the overall cumulative incidence of TB at the end of the follow-up period in ESKD patients with and without vitamin D use. The results show no significant differences in the cumulative incidence rate of tuberculosis between vitamin D use and non-use in the ESKD group log-rank test, $p = 0.0613$.

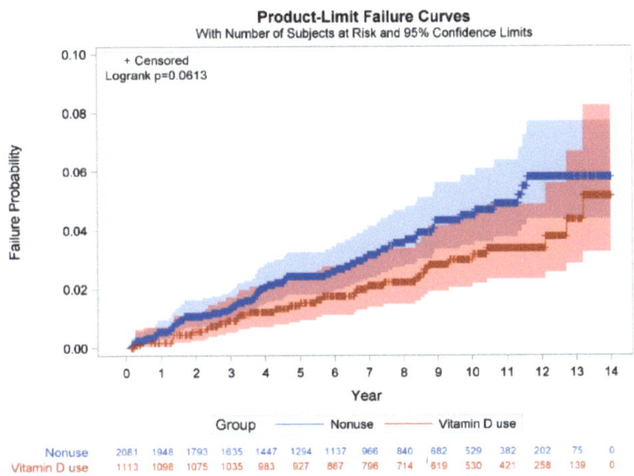

Figure 3. Cumulative incidence rates of tuberculosis in ESKD patients with and without vitamin D use. Differences in the cumulative incidence rates of tuberculosis in in ESKD patients with and without vitamin D use were compared using the log-rank test and Kaplan–Meier analysis. ESKD: end-stage kidney disease.

4. Discussion

This is a large cohort study conducted in 41,970 matched populations in Taiwan. The overall findings suggested that people with chronic kidney disease have a three-fold increased risk of developing tuberculosis compared with people without chronic kidney diseases. The important finding is that tuberculosis occurs early in chronic kidney disease patients, when at less than 3 years follow-up, the incident rate ratio of the patient with tuberculosis has already increased to (adjusted IRR 3.79 95% CI 2.55–5.62; the incident ratio of patients with tuberculosis gradually decreases in the longer follow-up year. Moreover, an increased risk of development of tuberculosis was observed in ESKD patients. Our results revealed that vitamin D uses and dosages were not related to the reduced risk of tuberculosis in ESKD patients, which is coincided withthe Lin et al. study [22]. The relationship between vitamin D level and TB seems to be controversial in ESKD at this current period, as some studies have stated that vitamin D has anti-mycobacterial activities [23]. Therefore, we need more molecular studies to evaluate the roles of vitamin D in the risk of TB.

In a study performed in Taiwan, the incidence rate of TB was similar in CKD stage 1 and stage 2 [24]. However, our findings may suggest that, indeed, the alteration in immunity during CKD may increase the risk of tuberculosis. A study also found that TB was significantly higher among those with CKD than among those without CKD [25]. This usually occurs in advance CKD patients because of the immunodeficiency status resulting from impaired T cells, B cell, neutrophils, monocytes and natural killer. The study results suggest that with the increasing severity of CKD, there is also a progressive increase in the risk of tuberculosis. There are many risk factors of tuberculosis that are also comorbidities of CKD that may also have increased TB infection in this cohort; these comorbidities may include diabetes and hypertension, which was found to be more prevalent in the CKD group than the non-CKD group. The association between diabetes mellitus and tuberculosis is mostly observed in countries where there is a high incidence of TB and the incidence of diabetes mellitus is also increasing.

However, there are still no studies to elucidate on the real mechanism of the effect of diabetes mellitus as a risk factor for TB. Some studies have suggested impaired cellular immunity, impairment of alveolar macrophages in the lungs, low levels of interferon gamma, pulmonary microangiopathy and micronutrient deficiency [26].

The number of participants on hemodialysis was high in the ESKD, which might increase the incidence of TB; previous studies have suggested that patients with chronic kidney disease and on dialysis are at risk of active tuberculosis (Table 2). A study performed in India suggested that TB in dialysis is associated with a poor prognosis and high mortality due to the delay in diagnosis and adverse effects of anti-TB drugs [27,28]. A study conducted in Northern Taiwan on patients with long-term dialysis had a hazard ratio of 2.041 [24]. Some also suggest that even after kidney transplantation, risk of tuberculosis is increased. Other cohort studies have found the IRR of TB to be 3.4 to 25.3 in dialysis patients compared to the general population. [29]. This is a very high risk on this patient, and they should be monitored closely for early diagnosis of tuberculosis. A study performed in Southern England found a higher incidence of TB in hemodialysis patients compared with patients on peritoneal dialysis. However, there were other studies that found the risk is not different from those with peritoneal dialysis [30].

This study also shows that vitamin D drug use in patients is not effective in reducing the incidence of tuberculosis in ESKD (Table 4).

Table 4. Vitamin D use did not reduce the incidence of tuberculosis risk in patients with end-stage kidney disease.

	Tuberculosis /Total Subjects, %	Person–Years	Events Per 1000 Person–Years (95% CI)	IRR (95% CI)	*p* Value	Adjusted IRR (95% CI)	*p* Value
ESKD							
None	25/3194, 0.78	21,330.40	1.17 (1.16–1.19)	1.00		1.00	
Yes	98/3194, 3.07	24,041.22	4.08 (4.03–4.13)	3.48 (2.24–5.40)	<0.0001	3.67 (2.27–5.93)	<0.0001
ESKD with vitamin D use							
Nonuse	66/2081, 3.17	14,006.34	4.71 (4.63–4.79)	1.00		1.00	
Use	32/1113, 2.88	10,034.88	3.19 (3.13–3.25)	0.68 (0.44–1.03)	0.0699	0.77 (0.49–1.19)	0.2351
Vitamin D use							
Nonuse	66/2081, 3.17	14,006.34	4.71 (4.63–4.79)	1.00			
0–6750	6/279, 2.15	2334.04	2.57 (2.47–2.68)	0.55 (0.24–1.26)	0.1553	0.56 (0.24–1.30)	0.1783
6751–21,690	8/275, 2.91	2304.91	3.47 (3.33–3.62)	0.74 (0.35–1.53)	0.4141	0.83 (0.39–1.74)	0.6183
21,691–54,810	8/281, 2.85	2663.54	3.00 (2.89–3.12)	0.64 (0.31–1.33)	0.2290	0.75 (0.36–1.58)	0.4520
>54,810	10/278, 3.60	2732.38	3.66 (3.53–3.80)	0.78 (0.40–1.51)	0.4564	0.95 (0.48–1.89)	0.8795

ESKD: end-stage kidney disease. Incidence rate ratio (IRR) was calculated by using generalized linear model (PROC GENMOD) to perform Poisson regression analysis (a log-linear model). Adjusted IRRs were calculated after adjusted covariates of residential region and comorbidities of alcohol abuse, lipid disorders, obesity, hypertension, myocardial infarction, congestive heart failure, peripheral vascular disease, cerebrovascular disease, chronic pulmonary disease, rheumatologic disease, liver disease, diabetes mellitus and any malignancy by using a generalized linear model. We classified the average vitamin D dose by using two approaches: stratifying the vitamin D exposure into yes or no and categorizing the per day milligram (mg) according to a quartile method. Daily exposure vitamin D of alfacalcidol and calcitriol dose: the accumulate vitamin D dose divided by the total follow-up days (by the first use vitamin D date until the index date of tuberculosis or to study end). The vitamin D dose–response (daily exposure dose) was analyzed after adjusted covariates using a by using generalized linear model.

Host genetic susceptibility has been suggested as one of the most important explanations for inter-individual differences in tuberculosis (TB) risk. The vitamin D receptor gene is located at chromosome 12 (12q13.11) [31]. Vitamin D can be obtained from nutrition, and it can also be synthesized by the human body during sunlight exposure. This form of vitamin D is biologically inactive, and then it is delivered into the liver, where it undergoes hydroxylation to become 25-hydroxy vitamin D. From the liver, it is taken to the kidneys, where it undergoes another hydroxylation to become 1α-25-dihydroxy vitamin D. This active form of vitamin D affects the immune function and regulates the activity of the defense immune system. During a tuberculosis infection, vitamin D binds to the vitamin D receptor gene in macrophages, and this binding activates synthesis of the antimicrobial peptide cathelicidin, which restricts M. tuberculosis intracellular growth in macrophages [32]. Vitamin D deficiency, which is commonly observed in ESKD [33], impairs monocyte function, reducing the production of cathelicidin, a peptide that is capable of destroying mycobacteria; hence, patients with CKD are given vitamin D supplementation to prevent the deficiency.. The main issue about the long-term use of vitamin D derivatives in patients with impaired renal function is the risk of inducing or accelerating the progression of renal failure [34]. Due to dietary restrictions in patients with ESKD on dialysis, and the presence of comorbidities that may result in longer hospitalization and less exposure to natural sunlight, CKD patients usually require vitamin D supplementation, especially cholecalciferol- and calcifediol-based supplements [33]. There is also a significant role in patients with lipid disorder, who seemed to also have a protective benefit from acquiring tuberculosis. The mechanism of these two is still unknown; however, some studies have suggested that host lipids act as a major source of carbon and energy for mycobacterium tuberculosis (M. tb), creating a favorable environment for it. They are important for the slow metabolizing population of the bacilli in the host [35]. Therefore, in our study, the findings suggest that the alteration in the lipids was beneficial for protection against M. TB survival in the host; however, the mechanism for this remains elusive and needs further investigations, since lipid disorders are supposed to make mycobacterium tuberculosis strive more in the host.

The strength of this study was that it was performed using data from a large population-based database in Taiwan. Therefore, the findings are likely applicable to the general population. However, electronic health databases with coding errors could be a problem of NHIRD. Health-care providers might resort to upcoding the diagnoses to more severe ones. Misclassification bias may thus become an issue if those diagnosis codes have not been properly validated. Although large data sets could potentially overcome this problem, the real impact of the incorrect coding awaits further elucidation [36].

A limitation of our study is that database-driven studies have greater potential for bias in observational studies. If we had combined multiple databases, the researcher would have been able to access more variables than those available in the NHIRD, such as physical examination results, laboratory data, stage of cancer, level of disability, quality of life, body mass index, smoking, marital status, education and household income, which were not included in our study [36]. Other important information was also unable to be obtained, such as hours of sun exposure and use of sunscreen. Analysis from NHANES III (the Third National Health and Nutrition Examination Survey) reported an inverse association between BMI and 25(OH)D levels in persons with CKD [37]. In this study, laboratory data from our participants were not retrieved from the database, which may be of importance to validate the immunological status of our study participants. This study did not include biochemical indices of bone metabolism and markers of bone and mineral disorders in patients who were given vitamin D therapeutic intervention, which can affect the PTH [38]. However, in the case of the suboptimal vitamin D levels and vitamin D deficiency in ESKD, vitamin D supplementation will be essential for those patients.

5. Conclusions

The study findings were that patients have an increased risk of early development of tuberculosis in chronic kidney diseases. Importantly, the risk was more increased in end-stage kidney diseases (ESKD), and vitamin D supplementation use might not be helpful to reduce the incidence of tuberculosis in this group. This leaves a gap in the health system in the treatment guidelines of chronic kidney disease, and these patients should be screened routinely and carefully for early detection of TB infection. This study provides the current actual knowledge and addresses the questions regarding vitamin D supplementation in ESKD, and its clinical benefit remains elusive in the scientific community.

Author Contributions: All authors were involved in drafting the article or revising it critically for important intellectual content, and all authors approved the final version to be published. H.-P.T. had full access to all the data in the study and takes responsibility for the integrity of the data and the accuracy of the data analysis. Study conception and design and final approval of the version: H.-W.C. and H.-P.T. Drafting the article: S.T.D., K.M.H., E.C.C.T., W.-M.L. and H.-P.T. Analysis and interpretation of the data: S.T.D., K.M.H., H.-W.C. and H.-P.T. All authors have read and agreed to the published version of the manuscript.

Funding: This work was supported by a grant from the Kaohsiung Medical University Research Foundation (KMU-M111007).

Institutional Review Board Statement: The study protocol was reviewed and approved by the Institutional Review Committee of Kaohsiung Medical University Hospital (KMUHIRB-EXEMPT (I)-20190011), Taiwan.

Informed Consent Statement: To protect patient confidentiality, all their identification numbers and medical institutions were encrypted before the release of the data for research purposes. Because no patient could be identified, informed consent was waived.

Data Availability Statement: Not applicable.

Acknowledgments: We thank the National Health Insurance Administration, Ministry of Health and Welfare, Taiwan, for its support. This study is based on data from the National Health Insurance Research Database (NHIRD) provided by the National Health Insurance Administration and managed by the Health and Welfare Data Science Center, Ministry of Health and Welfare (HWDC, MOHW). This manuscript was edited by Wallace Academic Editing.

Conflicts of Interest: None of the authors have any conflict of interest to declare.

References

1. Xu, L.; Wan, X.; Huang, Z.; Zeng, F.; Wei, G.; Fang, D.; Deng, W.; Li, Y. Impact of vitamin D on chronic kidney diseases in nondialysis patients: A meta-analysis of randomized controlled trials. *PLoS ONE* **2013**, *8*, e61387. [CrossRef] [PubMed]
2. Basile, D.P.; Anderson, M.D.; Sutton, T.A. Pathophysiology of acute kidney injury. *Compr. Physiol.* **2012**, *2*, 1303–1353. [CrossRef] [PubMed]
3. Pradhan, R.R.; Sigdel, M.R. Prevalence, clinical presentation, and outcome of tuberculosis in patients with chronic kidney disease at a tertiary care hospital in Nepal. *Int. J. Nephrol.* **2020**, *2020*, 7401541. [CrossRef] [PubMed]
4. Hill, N.R.; Fatoba, S.T.; Oke, J.L.; Hirst, J.A.; O'Callaghan, C.A.; Lasserson, D.S.; Hobbs, F.D. Global prevalence of chronic kidney disease—A systematic review and meta-analysis. *PLoS ONE* **2016**, *11*, 158–765. [CrossRef]
5. Yang, W.C.; Hwang, S.J.; Taiwan Society of Nephrology. Incidence, prevalence and mortality trends of dialysis end-stage renal disease in Taiwan from 1990 to 2001: The impact of national health insurance. *Nephrol. Dial. Transplant.* **2008**, *23*, 3977–3982. [CrossRef]
6. Cahuayme-Zuniga, L.J.; Brust, K.B. Mycobacterial infections in patients with chronic kidney disease and kidney transplantation. *Adv. Chronic Kidney Dis.* **2019**, *26*, 35–40. [CrossRef]
7. Talat, N.; Perry, S.; Parsonnet, J.; Dawood, G.; Hussain, R. Vitamin D deficiency and tuberculosis progression. *Emerg. Infect. Dis.* **2010**, *16*, 853–855. [CrossRef]
8. Graidis, S.; Papavramidis, T.S.; Papaioannou, M. Vitamin D and acute kidney injury: A two-way causality relation and a predictive, prognostic, and therapeutic role of vitamin D. *Front. Nutr.* **2020**, *7*, 630951. [CrossRef]
9. Christakos, S.; Ajibade, D.V.; Dhawan, P.; Fechner, A.J.; Mady, L.J. Vitamin D: Metabolism. *Endocrinol. Metab. Clin. N. Am.* **2010**, *39*, 243–253. [CrossRef]
10. Holick, M.F.; Binkley, N.C.; Bischoff-Ferrari, H.A.; Gordon, C.M.; Hanley, D.A.; Heaney, R.P.; Murad, M.H.; Weaver, C.M. Guidelines for preventing and treating vitamin D deficiency and insufficiency revisited. *J. Clin. Endocrinol. Metab.* **2012**, *97*, 1153–1158. [CrossRef]
11. Griffin, G.; Hewison, M.; Hopkin, J.; Kenny, R.A.; Quinton, R.; Rhodes, J.; Subramanian, S.; Thickett, D. Preventing vitamin D deficiency during the COVID-19 pandemic: UK definitions of vitamin D sufficiency and recommended supplement dose are set too low. *Clin. Med.* **2021**, *21*, e48–e51. [CrossRef]
12. Investigators, J.D.; Shoji, T.; Inaba, M.; Fukagawa, M.; Ando, R.; Emoto, M.; Fujii, H.; Fujimori, A.; Fukui, M.; Hase, H.; et al. Effect of oral alfacalcidol on clinical outcomes in patients without secondary hyperparathyroidism receiving maintenance hemodialysis: The J-DAVID randomized clinical trial. *JAMA* **2018**, *320*, 2325–2334. [CrossRef]
13. Hu, L.; Napoletano, A.; Provenzano, M.; Garofalo, C.; Bini, C.; Comai, G.; La Manna, G. Mineral bone disorders in kidney disease patients: The ever-current topic. *Int. J. Mol. Sci.* **2022**, *23*, 12223. [CrossRef] [PubMed]
14. Iseki, K.; Kabata, D.; Shoji, T.; Inaba, M.; Emoto, M.; Mori, K.; Morioka, T.; Nakatani, S.; Shintani, A. Dialysate calcium, alfacalcidol, and clinical outcomes: A post-hoc analysis of the J-DAVID trial. *PLoS ONE* **2022**, *17*, e0273195. [CrossRef] [PubMed]

15. Christodoulou, M.; Aspray, T.J.; Schoenmakers, I. Vitamin D supplementation for patients with chronic kidney disease: A systematic review and meta-analyses of trials investigating the response to supplementation and an overview of guidelines. *Calcif. Tissue Int.* **2021**, *109*, 157–178. [CrossRef] [PubMed]
16. Finch, J.L.; Tokumoto, M.; Nakamura, H.; Yao, W.; Shahnazari, M.; Lane, N.; Slatopolsky, E. Effect of paricalcitol and cinacalcet on serum phosphate, FGF-23, and bone in rats with chronic kidney disease. *Am. J. Physiol. Ren. Physiol.* **2010**, *298*, F1315–F1322. [CrossRef]
17. Banon, S.; Rosillo, M.; Gomez, A.; Perez-Elias, M.J.; Moreno, S.; Casado, J.L. Effect of a monthly dose of calcidiol in improving vitamin D deficiency and secondary hyperparathyroidism in HIV-infected patients. *Endocrine* **2015**, *49*, 528–537. [CrossRef]
18. Martins, J.S.; Palhares, M.O.; Teixeira, O.C.; Gontijo Ramos, M. Vitamin D status and its association with parathyroid hormone concentration in Brazilians. *J. Nutr. Metab.* **2017**, *2017*, 9056470. [CrossRef]
19. Bonkain, F.; De Clerck, D.; Dirix, V.; Singh, M.; Locht, C.; Mascart, F.; Corbiere, V. Early diagnosis of miliary tuberculosis in a hemodialysis patient by combining two interferon-gamma-release assays: A case report. *BMC Nephrol.* **2020**, *21*, 214. [CrossRef]
20. Cardoso, M.P. Native vitamin D in pre-dialysis chronic kidney disease. *Nefrología* **2019**, *39*, 18–28. [CrossRef]
21. Quan, H.; Sundararajan, V.; Halfon, P.; Fong, A.; Burnand, B.; Luthi, J.C.; Saunders, L.D.; Beck, C.A.; Feasby, T.E.; Ghali, W.A. Coding algorithms for defining comorbidities in ICD-9-CM and ICD-10 administrative data. *Med. Care* **2005**, *43*, 1130–1139. [CrossRef]
22. Lin, S.Y.; Chiu, Y.W.; Yang, H.R.; Chen, T.C.; Hsieh, M.H.; Wang, W.H.; Chen, Y.H. Association of vitamin D levels and risk of latent tuberculosis in the hemodialysis population. *J. Microbiol. Immunol. Infect.* **2021**, *54*, 680–686. [CrossRef] [PubMed]
23. Todoriko, L.D.; Toderika, Y.I.; Shevchenko, O.S.; Pidverbetska, O.V.; Pidverbetskyi, O.Y. The role of vitamin D deficiency in antituberculous protection. *Infus. Chemother.* **2021**, *4*, 38–44. [CrossRef]
24. Shu, C.C.; Wei, Y.F.; Yeh, Y.C.; Lin, H.H.; Chen, C.Y.; Wang, P.H.; Cheng, S.L.; Wang, J.Y.; Yu, C.J. The impact on incident tuberculosis by kidney function impairment status: Analysis of severity relationship. *Respir. Res.* **2020**, *21*, 51. [CrossRef] [PubMed]
25. Bardenheier, B.H.; Pavkov, M.E.; Winston, C.A.; Klosovsky, A.; Yen, C.; Benoit, S.; Gravenstein, S.; Posey, D.L.; Phares, C.R. Prevalence of Tuberculosis disease among adult US-bound refugees with chronic kidney disease. *Immigr. Minor. Health* **2019**, *21*, 1275–1281. [CrossRef]
26. Baghaei, P.; Marjani, M.; Javanmard, P.; Tabarsi, P.; Masjedi, M.R. Diabetes mellitus and tuberculosis facts and controversies. *J. Diabetes Metab. Disord.* **2013**, *12*, 58. [CrossRef]
27. Prasad, R.; Singh, A.; Balasubramanian, V.; Gupta, N. Extensively drug-resistant tuberculosis in India: Current evidence on diagnosis & management. *Indian J. Med. Res.* **2017**, *145*, 271–293. [CrossRef]
28. Segall, L.; Covic, A. Diagnosis of tuberculosis in dialysis patients: Current strategy. *Clin. J. Am. Soc. Nephrol.* **2010**, *5*, 1114–1122. [CrossRef]
29. Dobler, C.C.; McDonald, S.P.; Marks, G.B. Risk of tuberculosis in dialysis patients: A nationwide cohort study. *PLoS ONE* **2011**, *6*, e29563. [CrossRef]
30. Ostermann, M.; Palchaudhuri, P.; Riding, A.; Begum, P.; Milburn, H.J. Incidence of tuberculosis is high in chronic kidney disease patients in South East England and drug resistance common. *Ren. Fail.* **2016**, *38*, 256–261. [CrossRef]
31. Gao, L.; Tao, Y.; Zhang, L.; Jin, Q. Vitamin D receptor genetic polymorphisms and tuberculosis: Updated systematic review and meta-analysis. *Int. J. Tuberc. Lung Dis.* **2010**, *14*, 15–23. [PubMed]
32. Hu, Q.; Chen, Z.; Liang, G.; Mo, F.; Zhang, H.; Xu, S.; Wang, Y.; Kang, L.; Jin, T. Vitamin D receptor gene associations with pulmonary tuberculosis in a Tibetan Chinese population. *BMC Infect. Dis.* **2016**, *16*, 469. [CrossRef] [PubMed]
33. Zappulo, F.; Cappuccilli, M.; Cingolani, A.; Scrivo, A.; Chiocchini, A.L.C.; Nunzio, M.D.; Donadei, C.; Napoli, M.; Tondolo, F.; Cianciolo, G.; et al. Vitamin D and the Kidney: Two players, one console. *Int. J. Mol. Sci.* **2022**, *23*, 9135. [CrossRef] [PubMed]
34. Hamdy, N.A.; Kanis, J.A.; Beneton, M.N.; Brown, C.B.; Juttmann, J.R.; Jordans, J.G.; Josse, S.; Meyrier, A.; Lins, R.L.; Fairey, I.T. Effect of alfacalcidol on natural course of renal bone disease in mild to moderate renal failure. *BMJ* **1995**, *310*, 358–363. [CrossRef]
35. Chang, D.P.S.; Guan, X.L. Metabolic versatility of mycobacterium tuberculosis during infection and dormancy. *Metabolites* **2021**, *11*, 88. [CrossRef] [PubMed]
36. Hsieh, C.Y.; Su, C.C.; Shao, S.C.; Sung, S.F.; Lin, S.J.; Kao Yang, Y.H.; Lai, E.C. Taiwan's National health insurance research database: Past and future. *Clin. Epidemiol.* **2019**, *11*, 349–358. [CrossRef]
37. Navaneethan, S.D.; Schold, J.D.; Arrigain, S.; Jolly, S.E.; Jain, A.; Schreiber, M.J., Jr.; Simon, J.F.; Srinivas, T.R.; Nally, J.V., Jr. Low 25-hydroxyvitamin D levels and mortality in non-dialysis-dependent CKD. *Am. J. Kidney Dis.* **2011**, *58*, 536–543. [CrossRef] [PubMed]
38. Pagani, F.; Francucci, C.M.; Moro, L. Markers of bone turnover: Biochemical and clinical perspectives. *J. Endocrinol. Investig.* **2005**, *28*, 8–13.

life

MDPI

Article

An In-Silico Identification of Potential Flavonoids against Kidney Fibrosis Targeting TGFβR-1

MD. Hasanur Rahman [1,2,†], Partha Biswas [1,3,†], Dipta Dey [1,4], Md. Abdul Hannan [1,5], Md. Sahabuddin [2], Yusha Araf [6], Youngjoo Kwon [7], Talha Bin Emran [8,9], Md. Sarafat Ali [2,*] and Md Jamal Uddin [1,7,*]

1 ABEx Bio-Research Center, East Azampur, Dhaka 1230, Bangladesh
2 Department of Biotechnology and Genetic Engineering, Faculty of Life Sciences, Bangabandhu Sheikh Mujibur Rahman Science and Technology University, Gopalganj 8100, Bangladesh
3 Laboratory of Pharmaceutical Biotechnology and Bioinformatics, Department of Genetic Engineering and Biotechnology, Jashore University of Science and Technology, Jashore 7408, Bangladesh
4 Department of Biochemistry and Molecular Biology, Faculty of Life Sciences, Bangabandhu Sheikh Mujibur Rahman Science and Technology University, Gopalganj 8100, Bangladesh
5 Department of Biochemistry and Molecular Biology, Bangladesh Agricultural University, Mymensingh 2202, Bangladesh
6 Department of Genetic Engineering and Biotechnology, School of Life Sciences, Shahjalal University of Science and Technology, Sylhet 3114, Bangladesh
7 Graduate School of Pharmaceutical Sciences, College of Pharmacy, Ewha Womans University, Seoul 03760, Korea
8 Department of Pharmacy, BGC Trust University Bangladesh, Chittagong 4381, Bangladesh
9 Department of Pharmacy, Faculty of Allied Health Sciences, Daffodil International University, Dhaka 1207, Bangladesh
* Correspondence: sarafatbiotech@bsmrstu.edu.bd (M.S.A.); hasan800920@gmail.com (M.J.U.); Tel.: +880-1714775662 (M.S.A.); +880-1943760028 (M.J.U.)
† These authors contributed equally to the work.

Citation: Rahman, M.H.; Biswas, P.; Dey, D.; Hannan, M.A.; Sahabuddin, M.; Araf, Y.; Kwon, Y.; Emran, T.B.; Ali, M.S.; Uddin, M.J. An In-Silico Identification of Potential Flavonoids against Kidney Fibrosis Targeting TGFβR-1. *Life* **2022**, *12*, 1764. https://doi.org/10.3390/life12111764

Academic Editors: Ju-Seop Kang, Stefanos Roumeliotis and Giuseppe Minervini

Received: 8 October 2022
Accepted: 27 October 2022
Published: 2 November 2022

Abstract: Fibrosis is a hallmark of progressive kidney diseases. The overexpression of profibrotic cytokine, namely transforming growth factor β (TGF-β) due to excessive inflammation and tissue damage, induces kidney fibrosis. The inhibition of TGF-β signaling is markedly limited in experimental disease models. Targeting TGF-β signaling, therefore, offers a prospective strategy for the management of kidney fibrosis. Presently, the marketed drugs have numerous side effects, but plant-derived compounds are relatively safer and more cost-effective. In this study, TGFβR-1 was targeted to identify the lead compounds among flavonoids using various computational approaches, such as ADME/T (absorption, distribution, metabolism, and excretion/toxicity) analysis, molecular docking, and molecular dynamics simulation. ADME/T screening identified a total of 31 flavonoids with drug-like properties of 31 compounds, a total of 5 compounds showed a higher binding affinity to TGFβR-1, with Epicatechin, Fisetin, and Luteolin ranking at the top three (−13.58, −13.17, and −10.50 kcal/mol, respectively), which are comparable to the control drug linagliptin (−9.074 kcal/mol). The compounds also exhibited outstanding protein–ligand interactions. The molecular dynamic simulations revealed a stable interaction of these compounds with the binding site of TGFβR-1. These findings indicate that flavonoids, particularly Epicatechin, Fisetin, and Luteolin, may compete with the ligand-binding site of TGFβR-1, suggesting that these compounds can be further evaluated for the development of potential therapeutics against kidney fibrosis. Further, *in-vitro* and *in-vivo* studies are recommended to support the current findings.

Keywords: kidney fibrosis; chronic kidney disease; TGFβR-1; flavonoids; pharmacokinetics; molecular docking; molecular dynamics simulations

1. Introduction

Chronic kidney disease (CKD) is a worldwide public health concern, with a growing incidence and frequency of patients requiring replacement therapy [1]. Fibrosis is a major factor in the advancement of practically all types of CKD [2]. Additionally, various other factors, including diabetes, hypertension, infection, ureter obstruction, and genetic alterations, are associated with CKD [3]. In kidney fibrosis, an abnormally large amount of extracellular matrix (ECM) proteins is deposited within the kidney interstitium, glomerular capillaries, and around arterioles in association with inflammatory cell infiltration, tubular epithelial cell loss, and fibroblast accumulation, which can impair the normal physiological functions of the kidney and lead to CKD [2]. Current pharmaceutical interventions for diabetic and non-diabetic CKD patients include angiotensin-converting enzyme inhibitors and angiotensin II receptor antagonists, which offer only modest renoprotection [4]. Thus, there is an unmet need of exploring other potential pharmacological options to treat CKD patients targeting kidney fibrosis.

Transforming growth factor (TGF) is a protein that affects several biological processes, including cell proliferation, differentiation, and immune response. The TGF superfamily consists of 33 members and three TGF isoforms (TGF-1, TGF-2, and TGF-3), with the majority of members being dimeric, secreted polypeptides. TGF, among other things, plays a significant role in renal fibrosis [5,6]. TGF-1 promotes epithelial-to-mesenchymal transition (EMT), which is being more recognized as an important component of renal tissue fibrogenesis [7]. TGFR-1 is also one of the most important receptors in the serine/threonine protein kinase family [8]. TGFR-1 has been shown in studies to contribute to EMT by activating the TGFR-1/Smad signaling pathway. TGFR-1 and its downstream signaling components, such as smad2, smad3, collagen I, collagen IV, and α-SMA, are all increased during EMT [9]. TGFR-1 activation increases profibrotic genes and mediates renal fibrosis, whereas TGF-1 inhibition may minimize kidney injury and fibrosis [10]. As a result, inhibiting the TGF-1/Smad pathway is thought to be a therapeutic strategy for treating renal fibrosis [11]. Diverse therapeutic compounds have been used in kidney fibrosis, but most of the marketed drugs have different side effects; however, plant-based therapeutics, especially flavonoids, have a more reliable history of safer treatment.

From ancient times, plant-derived bioactive phytochemicals have been used as therapeutic agents to treat numerous pathological conditions, including inflammation, oxidative stress, fungal contamination, viral disease, cancer, mutagenic toxicity, neurodegenerative disorders, cardiovascular diseases, and kidney diseases [12–19]. Although alkaloids, flavonoids, terpenoids, and lignans, the major classes of bioactive phytochemicals, are one of the most promising and alternative options in new drug discovery as well as development, flavonoid-based phytochemicals have shown different biological activity towards disease conditions, including kidney disease [20–22] and liver disease [23,24]. Epigallocatechin-3-gallate is one of the major flavonoid phytochemicals that is closely associated with the improvement of kidney fibrosis [20]. Additionally, Luteolin was shown to be effective against nephropathy in streptozotocin (STZ)-induced diabetic rats [25]. Recently, resveratrol showed the most significant effects against various kidney diseases along with minimizing mortality risk [26,27]. In addition, (-)-Epicatechin possesses beneficial properties in the rat kidney [28]. Ethyl acetate extract of *Coreopsis tinctoria* Nutt has enriched potential flavonoids and possesses anti-fibrotic activity in STZ-induced diabetic rats via targeting the TGFβ-1 [29,30]. Consequently, quercetin is a major flavonoid compound, which directly suppresses the overexpression of TGFβ-1 and ameliorates the severity of diabetic nephropathy in STZ-induced diabetic rats [31]. However, the functional role of flavonoids targeting TGFβR-1 in kidney fibrosis has not yet been explored.

Considering the emerging need for a therapeutic option to treat kidney fibrosis, we performed an In-Silico identification of potential natural flavonoids targeting TGFβR-1 (Figure 1). In this present In-Silico workflow, we selected 51 natural flavonoids from the published literature, where phytochemicals have a potential role against kidney disease, and subsequently, we chose the best 31 compounds based on their pharmacokinetic properties, including ADMET (absorption, distribution, metabolism, elimination, and toxicity). Additionally, to find out the best ligands (i.e., phytochemicals), we conducted a molecular docking study against the targeted protein TGFβR-1 (PDB ID: 6B8Y) and found the best five compounds based on their docking score. The top five compounds with protein receptor interactions were also analyzed via the BIOVIA Discovery Studio Visualizer, which produced more positive results than the control. Finally, the Desmond (Schrödinger Release 2020-3) paid simulator package was applied to validate the "protein–ligand complex" files and produced more acceptable results.

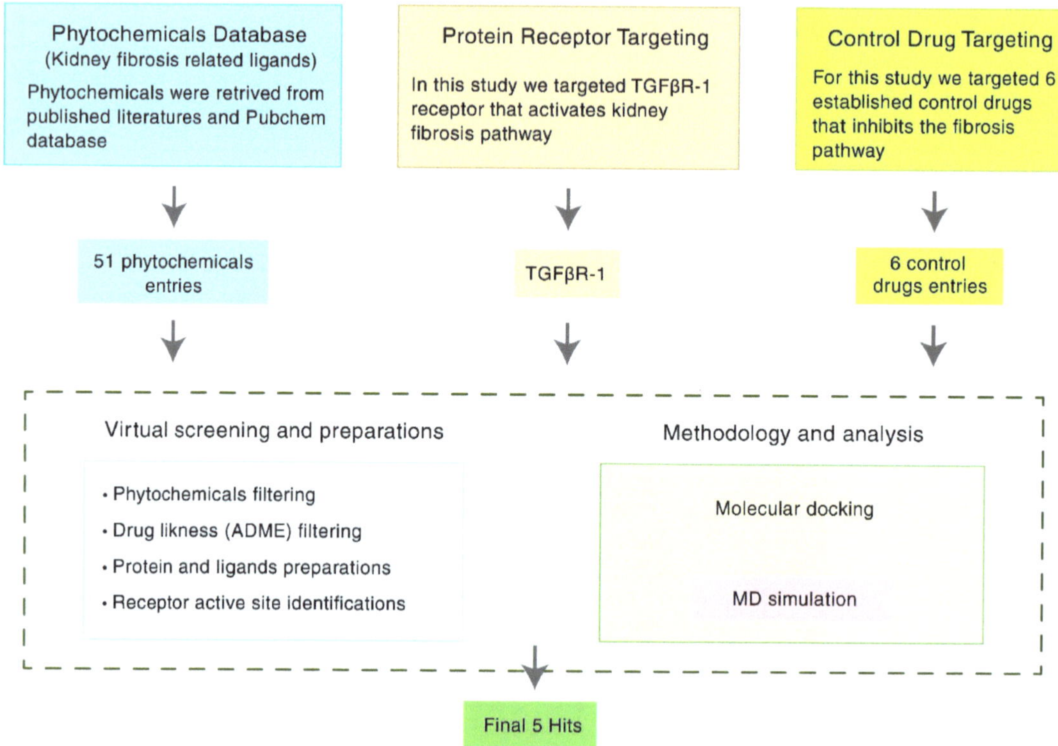

Figure 1. Schematic overview of the strategies targeting TGFβR-1 (PDB ID: 6B8Y) signaling. TGFβR-1 = Transforming growth factor beta receptor 1; MD simulation = Molecular dynamics simulation; ADME = Absorption, distribution, metabolism, and excretion.

2. Materials and Methods

2.1. Receptor and Ligand Selection

For the docking study, phytochemicals with potential anti-kidney fibrosis effects were considered. Heterobicyclic inhibitors of TGFβR-1 [32] and drugs, such as Losartan, Sitagliptin, Vildagliptin, Saxagliptin, Linagliptin, and Alogliptin, were considered as the standard references for the study.

2.2. Compound Screening and ADMET Prediction

In clinical trials, QikProp (Schrödinger Release 2020-3, Schrödinger, LLC, New York, NY, USA, 2020) finds lead compounds that perform better in terms of ADMET. QikProp is a powerful ADMET prediction tool for pharmaceutical companies. The number of attributes that extend outside the 95 percent range of similar values for recognized medications is indicated by the #stars (Supplementary Table S1). The researchers looked at 51 bioactive ligand molecules linked to kidney fibrosis. The chemicals were all derived from a variety of published sources.

2.3. Protein Preparation

According to the RCSB Protein Data Bank (PDB) (https://www.rcsb.org/, accessed on 24 July 2021) database information, TGFβR-1 has five existing inhibitors and the PDB ID 6B8Y shows the highest resolution and highest reliability [33]. The crystal structure of 6B8Y was downloaded using the RCSB PDB and preprocessed using Protein Preparation Wizard (Maestro Desmond version 12.5). The default parameters of assigned bond orders, CCD database, addition of hydrogens, creation of zero-order bonds to metals, creation of disulfide bonds, and filled missing side chains and loops were used by Prime (Maestro Desmond version 12.5). Additionally, the missing cap termini was fixed, and waters beyond 5 was deleted, as well as generating heat states of pH 7.0 +/− 2.0 were used by Epik (Maestro Desmond version 12.5). The H-bond was assigned in PROPKA with pH level 7.0 and the degradation was limited with the coverage heavy atom to RMSD 0.30 Å by using the refine tab with force field of OPLS3e.

2.4. Ligand Preparation

The three-dimensional structure SDF file format of the phytochemicals and the standard drugs were downloaded from the open-source PubChem database (https://pubchem.ncbi.nlm.nih.gov/, accessed on 24 July 2021). LigPrep (Schrödinger Release ver. 2020-3) was used to prepare the ligand structures for this study. At the time of preparing the ligands, the default ligprep parameters were used with a standard pH of 7.0 to (+/−) 2.0, a maximum number of conformers per structure was 32, and RMSD value was 1.0 Å. Additionally, a minimization was performed using the OPLS3e force field and the Epik ionizer.

2.5. Active Site (ASs) Identification and Receptor Grid Generation

After the protein preparation of 6B8Y was performed, the possible binding site of the TGFβR-1 domain was developed using the Schrödinger Sitemap (Maestro version 12.5). The SiteMap in Maestro is a method for locating putative binding sites on a protein for small-molecule ligands. It plots and scores regions on the protein surface that are likely to contain a ligand. The new SiteMap is a development of Maestro's initial SiteMap facility (formerly known as hppmap) [34,35]. Site mapping works similarly to Goodford's GRID algorithm [36], as it did in the original approach [37]. There are three processes to calculating a SiteMap. However, to establish the active sites of 6B8Y protein, a grid is first created by the Receptor Grid Generation tool with Van der Waals residue (scaling factor of 1.0 Å and partial charge cutoff 0.25 Å), and the points are then organized into groups based on several criteria. Second, the sites are mapped on a different grid to provide files for map visualization. Finally, properties are accessed, and sites are documented in a Maestro-friendly format. An impact job is used to complete each level. The binding pocket with the highest SiteScore and druggability score (DScore) was chosen for molecular docking investigations.

SiteScore = 0.0733 $n^{1/2}$ + 0.6688 e − 0.20 p, where n is the number of site points (limited at /100), e is the enclosure score, and p is the hydrophilic score, which is set at 1.0 to restrict the impact of hydrophilicity in charged and highly polar sites [38].

DScore uses the same properties as SiteScore but different coefficients:

DScore = 0.094 sqrt $n^{1/2}$ + 0.60 e − 0.324 p

The hydrophilic score is not capped in DScore. This is one of the fundamental differences between "difficult" and "undruggable" targets and "druggable" targets [34]. Because these are independent and occasionally competing purposes, the use of different functions for binding-site identification and druggability classification is appropriate. For example, ligands that have nanomolar, and even subnanomolar, affinity for the PTP1B phosphate pocket [39]. However, these extremely active ligands are not drug-like and contain charge configurations similar to those of the natural phosphate substrate. Although such a region can bind ligands tightly, it should not be classified as druggable by the SiteMap [34].

2.6. Molecular Docking and Visualization

After the completion of extra precision (XP) molecular docking by Maestro (v12.5), every protein–ligand complex PDB structure was extracted from the docked post-viewing file for their post-docking visualization analysis of the non-bond interaction and the hydrophobicity. The Discovery Studio Visualizer (v.21) was used to perform post-docking visualization on the protein–ligand complex structures. Furthermore, the non-bonded and non-covalent bonded interactions were also carried out by the Discovery Studio Visualizer [40].

2.7. Binding Free Energy Calculation by Using Prime/MM-GBSA Approach

MMGBSA is known as the molecular mechanics-generalized Born surface area, which can be performed to calculate ligand binding free energies and ligand strain energies for a set of ligands and a single receptor. After completing the site-specific molecular docking, the MMGBSA was conducted by utilizing the Prime model of Schrödinger suite 2020-3, which analyzes the relative binding free affinity of the control and candidate ligands against the selected 6B8Y protein receptor.

2.8. Molecular Dynamics (MD) Simulations

The possible ligand compounds' binding consistency to the targeted protein AS was determined using 200 ns MD simulations [41]. The Desmond (v12.5) molecular dynamic simulation of protein–ligand complex structures was used to investigate the thermodynamic stability of receptor–ligand complexes [42]. For this framework, a pre-determined TIP3P water approach was formulated to maintain a particular volume with the orthorhombic periodic bounding box shape with a distance of 10 Å. Appropriate ions, such as O+ and 0.15 M salt (Na^+ and Cl^-), were chosen for electrically neutralizing the framework and randomly placed inside the solvent system. The system framework was reduced and relaxed by using the default protocol implemented by using force field OPLS3e within the Desmond module after the construction of the solvency protein system with a ligand complex [43]. The temperature of NPT assemblies that used the Nose–Hoover temperature combining technique and the isotropic technique was kept at 300 K and one atmospheric pressure (1.01325 bar), with 50 ps capture periods with an energy of 1.2 ps.

2.8.1. Simulation Trajectory Analysis

Schrödinger's maestro v12.5 was used to create the molecular dynamic simulation visualizations. The Simulation Interaction Diagram (SID) from Desmond modules was used to evaluate the simulation event and verify the MD simulation's quality. The root-mean-square deviation (RMSD), protein–ligand contact (P-L), and the hydrogen bond interaction were used to determine the stability of the protein–ligand complex structure.

2.8.2. RMSD Analysis

RMSD is the average distance caused by the dispossession of a single atom over time [42]. RMSD of protein structural atoms, such as Cα, backbone, sidechain, and heavier atoms, is tallied first, followed by the RMSD of protein fit ligand atoms from all time frames, which is aligned and measured against the reference time (200 ns). The *RMSD* of an MD simulation with a period of x can be determined by using the equation below (Equation (1)).

$$\mathrm{RMSD_x} = \sqrt{\frac{1}{N}\sum_{i=1}^{n}\left(r_i'(t_x)\right) - r_i\left(t_{ref}\right)^2} \quad (1)$$

N is the number of atoms chosen, t_{ref} denotes the reference time, and r' denotes the position of the chosen atom in the system x after superimposing the reference system's point.

3. Results

3.1. Compound Screening and ADME/T

The phytochemical properties of a molecule should fall within the following range, according to "Lipinski's rule of five", H-bond donors 5, H-bond acceptors 10, log P 5, and molecular weight 500 kDa. Furthermore, a substance is more likely to have poor absorption if two or more of the characteristics are not fulfilled [44]. Only 30 of the 51 phytochemicals analyzed met the criteria for further analysis (Supplementary Table S1).

TGFβR-1 structure was optimized for further investigation, and ligand molecules were eliminated based on ADME/T findings. However, 8 bioactive compounds did not display ADME/T properties, and 13 compounds did not achieve their minimum ADME/T recommended values (Supplementary Table S1), which is why we conducted our further study with the remaining 30 of 51 compounds (Supplementary Table S2).

3.2. AS Identification and Receptor Grid Generation

In an enzyme, the binding site is a specific area of the protein where amino acid residues precisely form a temporary bond with the substrate [45]. The predicted receptor domain binding sites are needed for molecular docking studies. As the 6B8Y crystal structure with ligands is unavailable in the database, these active site residues need to be predicted. After the analysis of the 6B8Y protein, five AS (AS1, AS2, AS3, AS4, and AS5) were generated (Figure 2). All the AS displayed hydrogen-bond acceptor map, hydrogen-bond donor and hydrophobic and hydrophilic map, metal-binding map, and surface map were good. The druggability of a binding site was measured by its DScore, and the higher the DScore, the better the site [35,46]. As the AS1 showed the highest DScore, this binding site was chosen for molecular docking studies and a grid was generated across the site by Glide application (Maestro v12.5). Glide (Grid-based Ligand Docking with Energetics) seeks out advantageous interactions between ligand and receptor molecules. Several different sets of fields depict the structure and features of the receptor on a grid, providing a progressively more accurate scoring of the ligand [47].

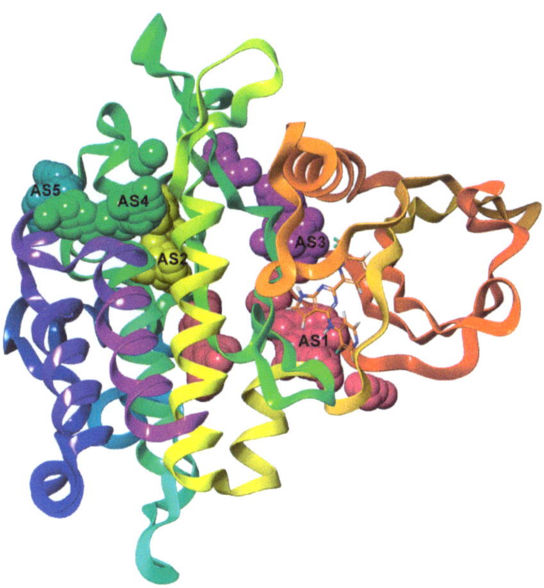

	DScore	Site Score
AS1	1.009	0.976
AS2	0.991	1.083
AS3	0.794	0.846
AS4	0.594	0.755
AS5	0.502	0.565

Figure 2. Active sites with the corresponding binding position of TGFβR-1. Ball shape with pink, yellow, purple, green, and blush color represent AS1, AS2, AS3, AS4, and AS5, respectively, with respect to their binding site position of TGFβR-1.

3.3. Molecular Docking and MMGBSA Analysis

Molecular docking is a computer-aided drug design technique, which uses certain algorithms to allocate affinity scores according to ligand positions in the target pocket. The highest binding affinity is the lowest docking score, which implies that the highest binding compound complex spends more time in contact [48].

5-Hydroxy-3,6,7,8,3′,4′-hexamethoxyflavone (C-01), (-)-Epicatechin (C-06), Resveratrol (C-09), Fisetin (C-18), and Luteolin (C-29) returned the best binding affinity score of all (Table 1). We also considered the six FDA-approved drugs of Losartan, Sitagliptin, Vildagliptin, Saxagliptin, Linagliptin, and Alogliptin as the control drugs, but Linagliptin (C-32) showed the best docking score (Supplementary Table S3) and we selected this drug as our reference drug for this study.

Table 1. List of compound codes, PubChem CID, chemical name, two-dimensional structure, and control compounds with the best binding affinity and MMGBSA score of the selected five phytochemicals.

Code	PubChem CID	Chemical Name	Chemical Structure	Docking Scores (kcal/mol)	MMGBSA Scores (kcal/mol)
C-06	72,276	(-)-Epicatechin	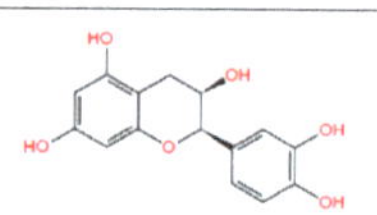	−13.585	−48.19
C-18	5,281,614	Fisetin	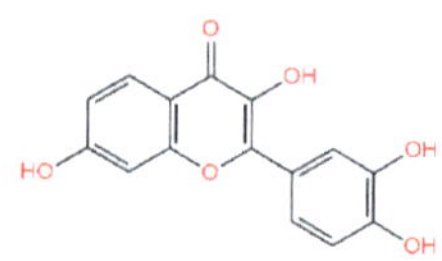	−13.177	−51.84
C-29	5,280,445	Luteolin	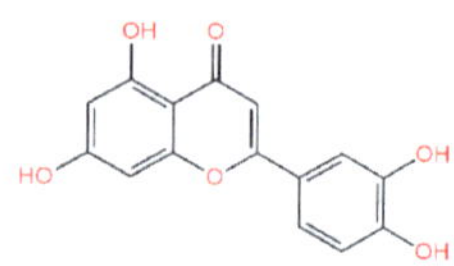	−10.506	−44.80
C-09	445,154	Resveratrol	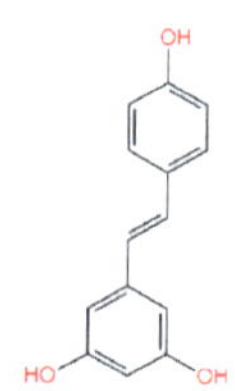	−8.552	−43.34
C-01	136,417	5-Hydroxy-3,6,7,8,3′,4′-hexamethoxyflavone	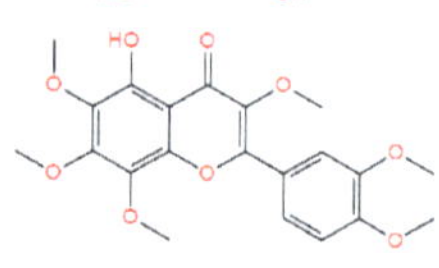	−7.808	−47.97
C-32	10,096,344	Linagliptin (control)	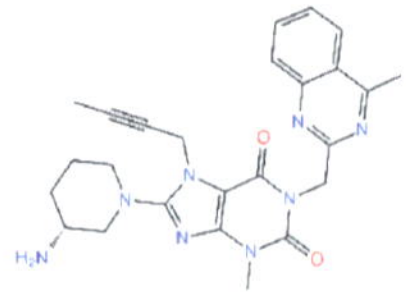	−9.074	−41.57

The 5 final selected compounds among the 31 phytochemicals (Table 1) had a docking score range from −13.0 to −7.0 kcal/mol.

Molecular docking was also evaluated using MMGBSA-free restricting vitality, which is identified with the post-scoring strategy for TGFβR-1 (PDB ID: 6B8Y) target. The docking correctness was checked by inspecting the lowest energy poses predicted by the scoring functions (Supplementary Table S4: Part 1 and 2). The greater the negative free energies of the MMGBSA binding value, the stronger the binding (Table 1). In the AS1 binding site of 6B8Y, C-18 had the highest negative binding energy of approximately 51.63 kcal/mol, C-06 had a predictive binding energy of −48.19 kcal/mol, and C-32 had a binding energy of −41.57 kcal/mol.

3.4. Analysis of Protein–Ligand Interactions

The BIOVIA Discovery Studio Visualizer tool (v21) was used to observe the interactions between the selected five ligands and the desired protein. With the TGFβR-1 protein, C-06 was found to form several conventional and carbon–hydrogen bonds. Four conventional hydrogen bonds were found to form at the positions of Asp351 (4.15 Å), Tyr249 (5.64 Å), Glu245 (4.82 Å), and His283 (4.08 Å) (Figure 3 and Table 2). Six Pi–Alkyl bonds were also found at the positions of Ala350 (536 Å), Leu260 (4.98 Å), Ile211 (4.63 Å), Ala230 (4.57 Å), Val219 (5.08 Å), and Leu340 (4.58 Å), and a Pi–Cation bond was also observed during the interaction of C-06 in the position of Lys232 (4.17 Å).

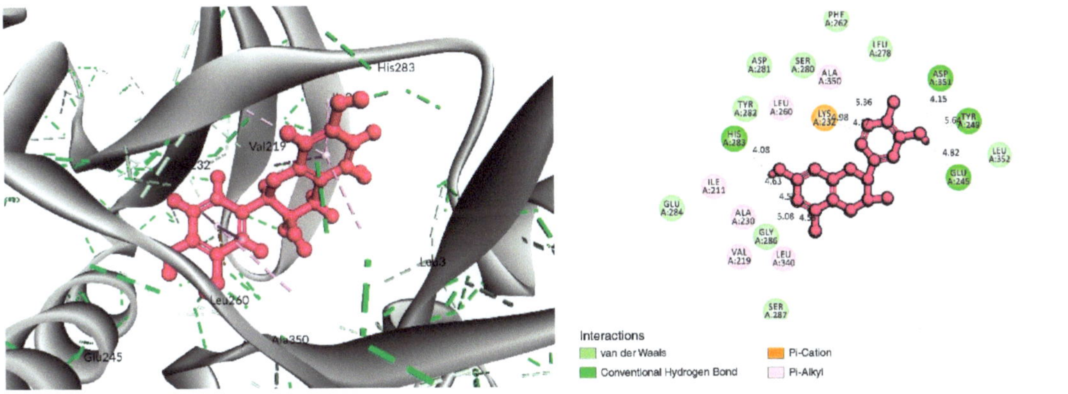

Figure 3. Interaction between Epicatechin (pink color) and 6B8Y. The **left** figure depicts the 3D complex protein–ligand interactions, while the **right** figure depicts the 2D complex protein–ligand interactions.

In the case of the C-18 phytochemical, two conventional hydrogen bonds were found at the positions of Glu245 (2.7 Å) and Ala350 (2.81 Å). Three Pi–Alkyl bonds were found at Ala230 (4.13 Å), Leu240 (4.71 Å), and Leu260 (4.92 Å). Two Pi–Sigma and a Pi-Cation bond were also found at the positions Ile211 (2.76 Å), Val219 (2.68 Å), and Lys232 (3.85 Å), respectively (Figure 4 and Table 2).

For the C-29 phytochemical, one carbon–hydrogen bond was found at Gly286 (3.61 Å), in addition to three Pi–Alkyl, two Pi–Sigma, and one Pi–Cation bond also being found at, respectively, the Ala230 (4.13), Leu340 (4.71), Leu260 (4.92 Å), Ile211 (2.76 Å), Val219 (2.68 Å), and Lys232 (3.85 Å) positions (Figure 5 and Table 2).

The interaction study of phytochemical C-09 found one Pi–Alkyl bond at the position of Ile211 (4.78 Å) (Figure 6 and Table 2). In the study of the C-01 phytochemical, there were two conventional hydrogen bonds at the positions of Lys232 (2.37 Å) and Ser280 (2.37 Å). Two carbon–hydrogen bonds were also found at the position of Ala350 (2.95 Å) and also other Pi–Alkyl bonds were found at the Ala230 (4.57 Å) position (Figure 7 and Table 2).

3.5. MD Simulations Analysis

Using MD simulations, it is possible to confirm the stability of the protein–ligand complexes in an artificial environment. To establish the binding consistency of the candidate ligand molecules to the target TGFβR-1 protein AS1, 200 ns MD simulations were performed on the protein–ligand complex structures. Remarkably detailed descriptions of these MD simulation results are provided in terms of RMSD, intramolecular hydrogen bonding (Intra HB), and protein–ligand interaction analysis (P–L contact).

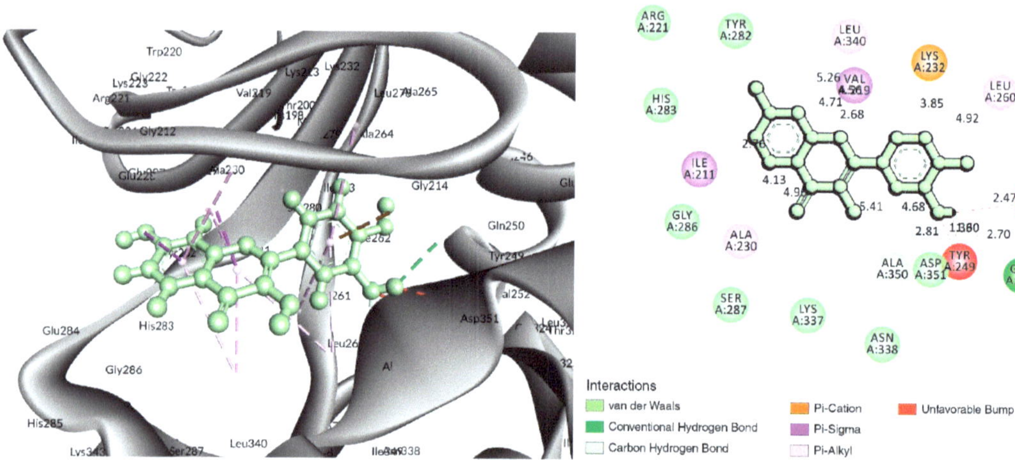

Figure 4. Interaction of 6B8Y with Fisetin (cyan color). The **left** figure depicts a 3D complex protein–ligand interaction, while the **right** figure depicts a 2D complex protein–ligand interaction.

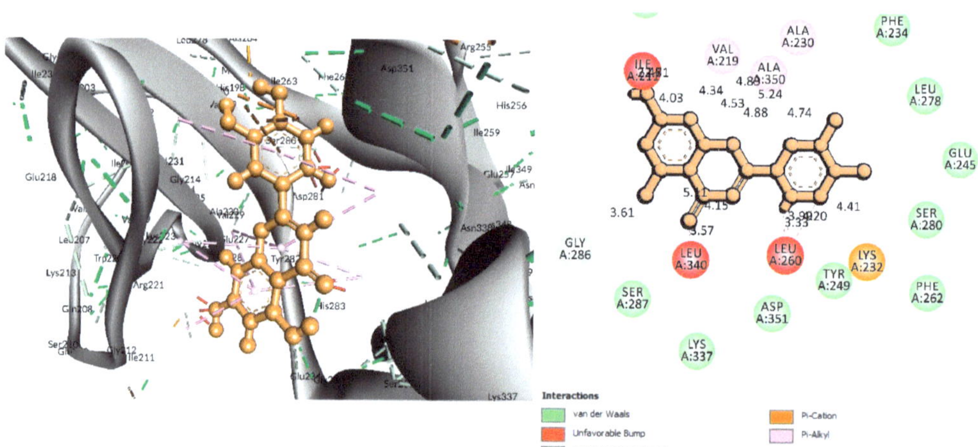

Figure 5. Interaction of 6B8Y and Luteolin (maroon color). The **left** figure depicts a 3D complex protein–ligand interaction, while the **right** figure depicts a 2D complex protein–ligand interaction.

3.5.1. RMSD Analysis

The measurement of the average displacement of atoms from one reference frame to another was conducted using RMSD. The acceptable RMSD range is from 0.01 to 3.5 Å micrometers. Figure 8 depicts the RMSD progression of a protein (left *Y*-axis) and a ligand (right *Y*-axis). The RMSD for the (-)-Epicatechin, Fisetin, Luteolin, Resveratrol, 5-Hydroxy-3,6,7,8,3′,4′-hexamethoxyflavone, and the control drug Linagliptin was determined after all protein frames were aligned on the reference frame backbone (Figure 8A–F). The RMSD of the protein found the stability of the four compounds except for the compound Resveratrol (the average value changes from the TGFβR-1 backbone to (-)-Epicatechin, Fisetin, Luteolin, and 5-Hydroxy-3,6,7,8,3′,4′-hexamethoxyflavone) within the range of 0.8–3.2 Å, where the value of Resveratrol changed from 0.6 Å, which was lower than the desired range, indicating the large conformational change of the protein. At the beginning of 0–27 ns, it was found that the fluctuation increased for (-)-Epicatechin and 5-Hydroxy-3,6,7,8,3′,4′-hexamethoxyflavone and decreasing for Fisetin and Luteolin. The state of equilibration was achieved after 30 ns for (-)-Epicatechin and 5-Hydroxy-3,6,7,8,3′,4′-hexamethoxyflavone, but the fluctuation decreased again after 90–170 ns for Fisetin and Luteolin, but maintain an average range distance of 0.8–3.2 Å. As a result, we should take into account the fact that the fluctuations will be optimized throughout the course of the long simulation run.

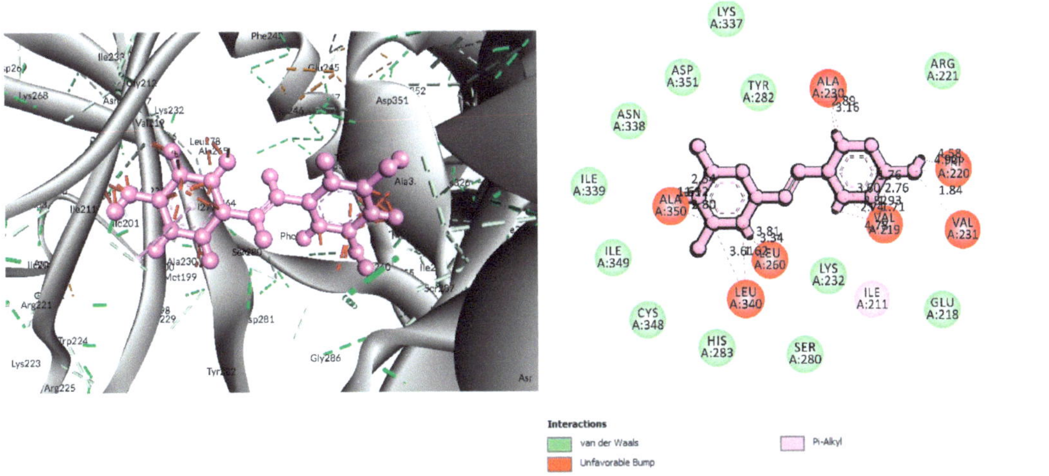

Figure 6. Interaction between 6B8Y and Resveratrol (light purple color). The **left** figure illustrates a 3D complex protein–ligand interaction, while the **right** figure represents a 2D complex protein–ligand interaction.

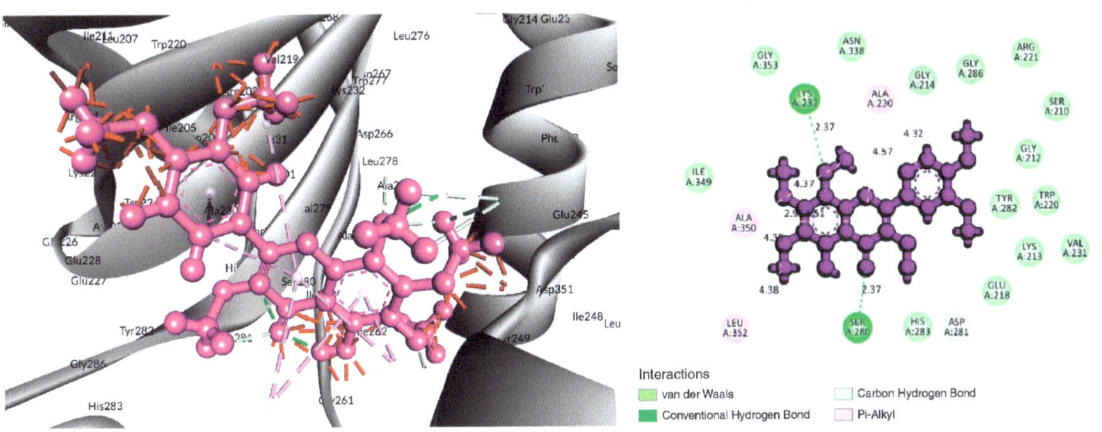

Figure 7. Interaction of 6B8Y and 5-Hydroxy-3,6,7,8,3′,4′-hexamethoxyflavone (navy-blue color). The **left** figure illustrates a 3D complex protein–ligand interaction, while the **right** figure represents a 2D complex protein–ligand interaction.

The RMSD of a ligand reflects how stable it is in relation to the protein and its binding pocket. When the protein_-ligand complex is first aligned on the reference protein backbone and then the RMSD of the ligand heavy atoms is measured, the RMSD of the ligand is presented in the plot. If the observed values are significantly greater than the RMSD of the protein, the ligand has very likely diffused away from its initial binding site [49]. In that scenario, we calculated the RMSD of compounds to determine the stability of the chosen compounds in comparison to the control compounds. Here, the observation of the compound found optimal RMSD for Resveratrol, and all other compound distances are significantly larger (>0.8 nm) than the RMSD of the control compound; therefore, the compound can diffuse away from its initial binding site.

3.5.2. Protein–Ligand Contacts

Protein interactions with the ligand may be seen throughout the 200 ns simulation. These interactions can be categorized and summarized by type, as shown in the graph above. Hydrogen bonds, hydrophobic interactions, ionic interactions, and water bridges are the four forms of protein–ligand interactions. The 'Simulation Interactions Diagram' panel can be used to look at the subcategories of each interaction type. The stacked bar charts are normalized throughout the journey. The stacked bar charts for (-)-Epicatechin indicate an interaction fraction value (IFV) of 1.1 Å at residue Asp 290, which makes contact via hydrogen and water bridge bonds, indicating that the specific interaction was maintained for over 100% of the simulated time (Figure 9A). The IFV detected a maximum of 1.75 Å (Glu 245) that was formed by the hydrogen and water bridge bond, as well as 0.8 Å at Asp 281 that was produced by the hydrogen and water bridge bond, indicating being maintained above 100% and 80%, respectively, for the compound Luteolin (Figure 9C). Furthermore, for the compound 5-Hydroxy-3,6,7,8,3′,4′-hexamethoxyflavone, the IFV value is a maximum of 1.6 Å at the position of Tyr, which was formed by a hydrogen, hydrophobic, and water bridge bond and IFV also found 1.2 Å and 1.1 Å at His 285 and Gly 286, respectively, both having been formed by a hydrogen and water bridge bond, indicating a maintenance of over 100% (Figure 9E). Compared with the three compounds and the control, the other two compounds maintained a low IFV and formed multiple hydrogens, hydrophobic, water bridge bonding, and ionic bond interactions. In the case of Fisetin, the IFV is low at the position of Asp 281 until Asp 251 but maintained an optimized IFV value from Tyr 249 to His 283 (Figure 9B). For the compound Resveratrol, the IFV is maintained very low at the position of Lys 213 and Lys 337, and the position of Ile 211 has an optimized IFV value (Figure 9D). The compound formed the minimum hydrogen bond with the desired protein, and therefore the stability of the compound should be hindered. In the case of Linagliptin, it was found to form multiple interactions with the same residue within the same atom of the ligand due to the sidechain having more than one H-bond donor feature (Figure 9F). Figure 10 shows interactions between the ligand and protein that occur for more than 30% of the simulation time for the selected compounds in a 2D format. Because some residues may have several contacts of the same type with the same ligand atom, interactions with >100% are feasible. In the Asp (290) residue, the (-)-Epicatechin displays 64% interactions from 0.00 to 200 ns of the simulation period. Fisetin has a 31% interaction in the Tyr (249) residue, while Luteolin and 5-Hydroxy-3,6,7,8,3′,4′-hexamethoxyflavone have several interactions, with the largest interaction being 98% with Glu (245) and 82% with Gly (286). Resveratrol and Linagliptin did not show any interactions over the simulation time.

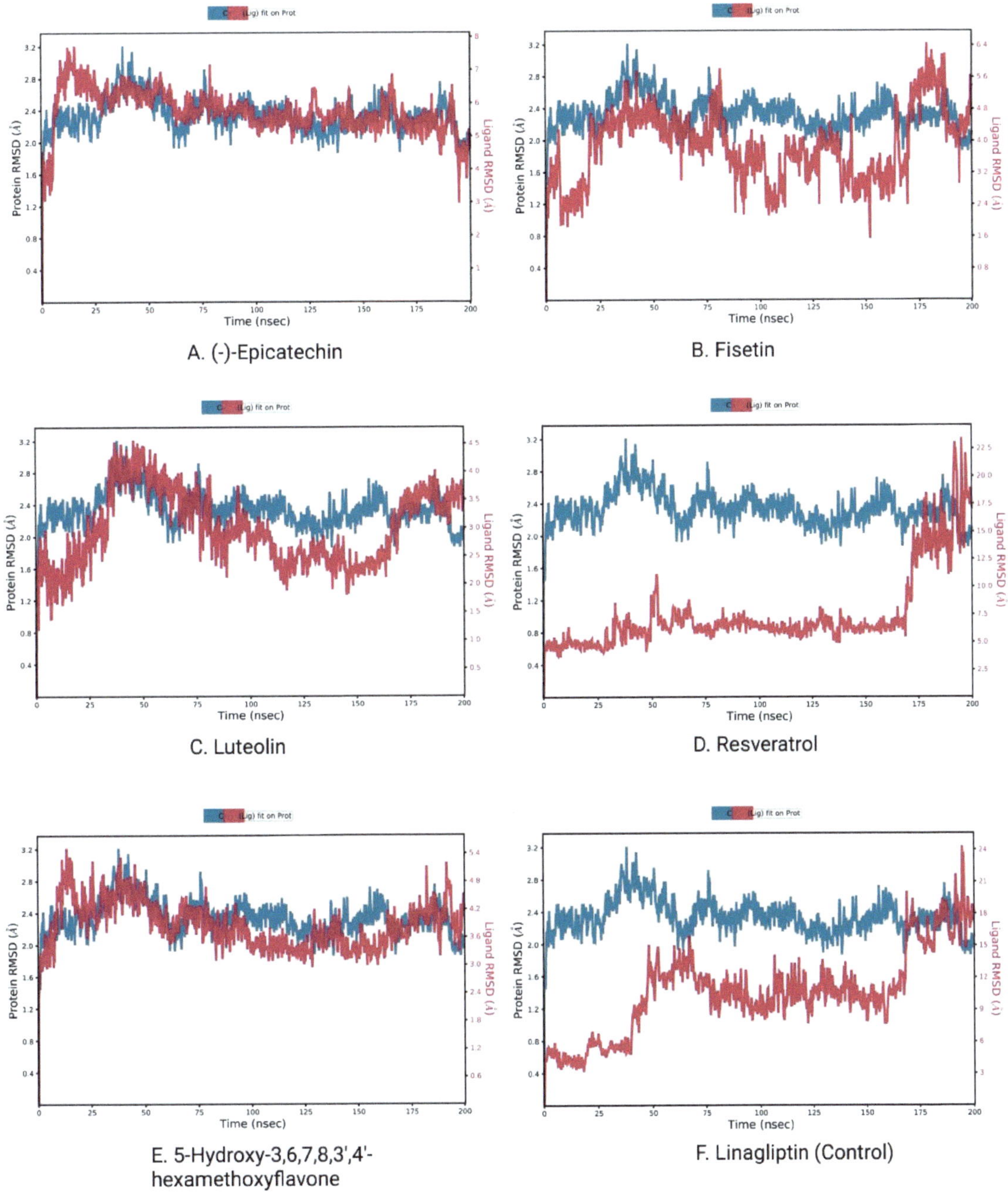

Figure 8. RMSD plots of protein–ligand interactions. (**A**) (-)-Epicatechin, (**B**) Fisetin, (**C**) Luteolin, (**D**) Resveratrol, (**E**) 5-Hydroxy 3,6,7,8,3′,4′-hexamethoxyflavone, and (**F**) Linagliptin.

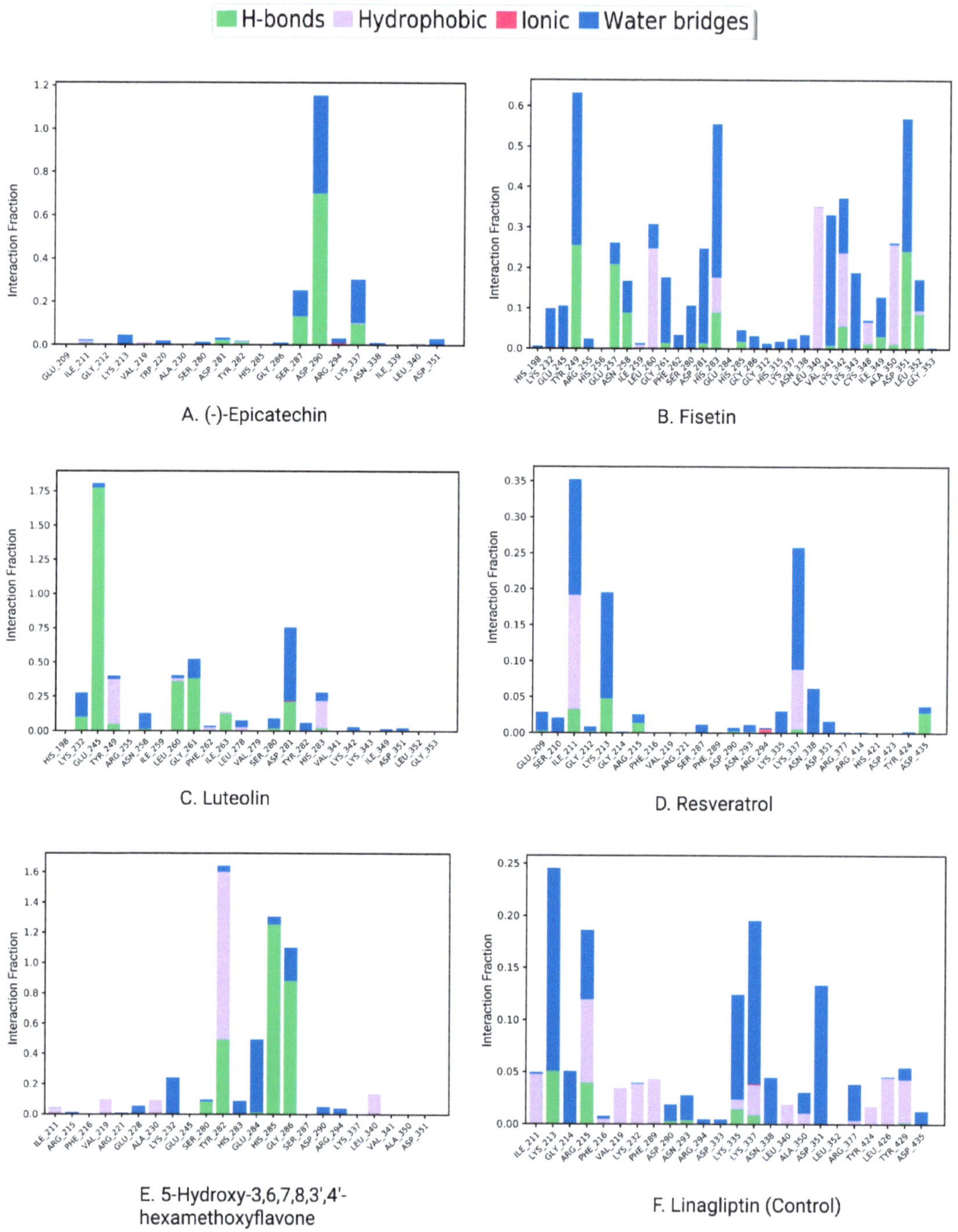

Figure 9. Protein–ligand contacts and ligand–protein contact (**right**) of the (**A**) (-)-Epicatechin, (**B**) Fisetin, (**C**) Luteolin, (**D**) Resveratrol, (**E**) 5-Hydroxy-3,6,7,8,3′,4′-hexamethoxyflavone, and (**F**) Linagliptin (control) at 200 ns of the simulation time.

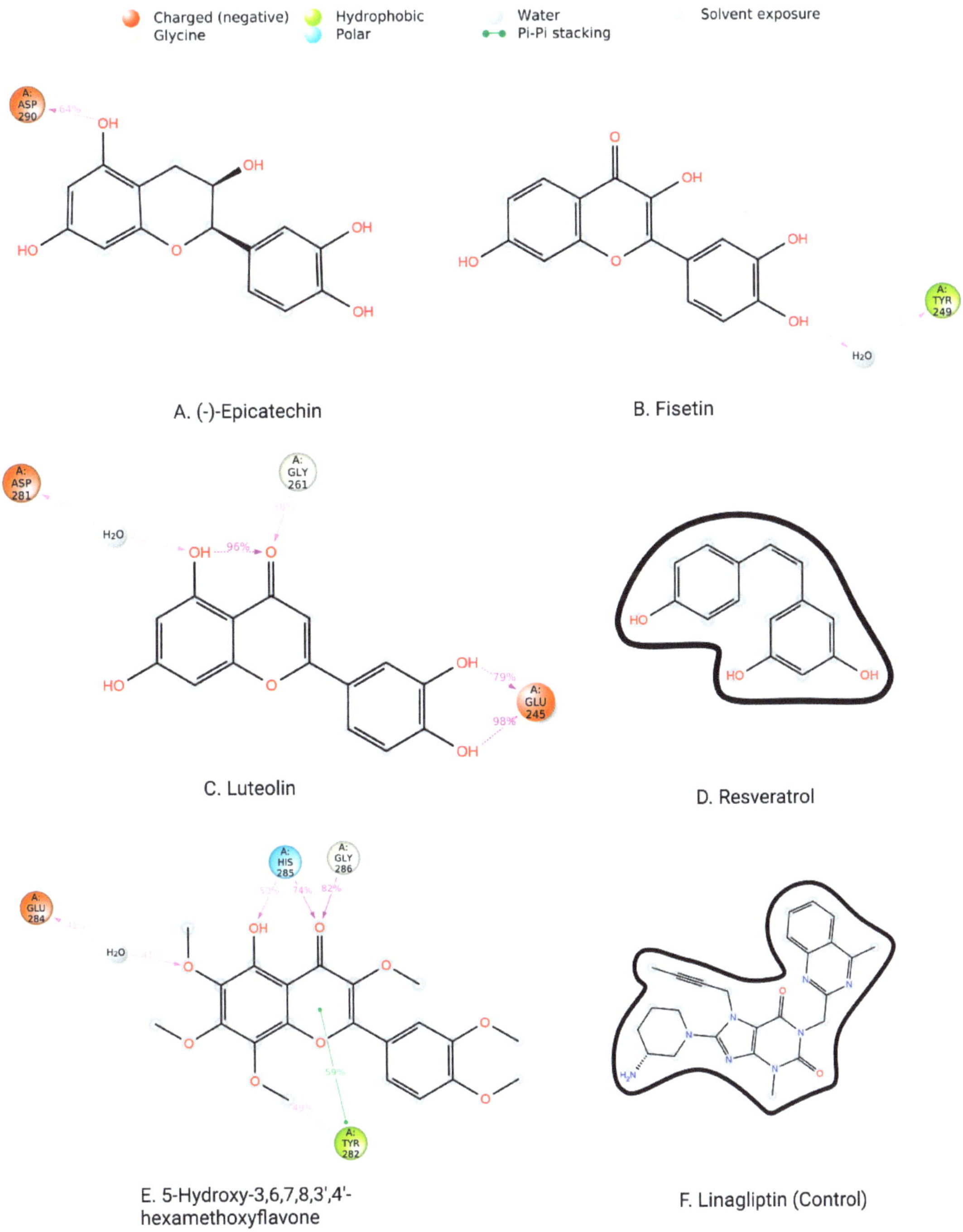

Figure 10. Two-dimensional interactions of the ligand–protein complex. (**A**) (-)-Epicatechin, (**B**) Fisetin, (**C**) Luteolin, (**D**) Resveratrol, (**E**) 5-Hydroxy-3,6,7,8,3′,4′-hexamethoxyflavone, and (**F**) Linagliptin (control).

Table 2. Bonding interactions between the selected phytochemicals with TGFβR-1.

PubChem ID	Residues	Distance(Å)	Bond Category	Bond Type
CID-72276	Asp351	4.15	Hydrogen	Conventional Hydrogen
	Tyr249	5.64	Hydrogen	Conventional Hydrogen
	Glu245	4.82	Hydrogen	Conventional Hydrogen
	His283	4.08	Hydrogen	Conventional Hydrogen
	Ala350	5.36	Hydrophobic	Pi–Alkyl
	Leu260	4.98	Hydrophobic	Pi–Alkyl
	Ile211	4.63	Hydrophobic	Pi–Alkyl
	Ala230	4.57	Hydrophobic	Pi–Alkyl
	Val219	5.08	Hydrophobic	Pi–Alkyl
	Leu340	4.58	Hydrophobic	Pi–Alkyl
	Lys232	4.17	Hydrophobic	Pi–Cation
CID-5281614	Glu245	2.7	Hydrogen	Conventional Hydrogen
	Ala350	2.81	Hydrogen	Carbon–Hydrogen
	Ala230	4.13	Hydrophobic	Pi–Alkyl
	Leu340	4.71	Hydrophobic	Pi–Alkyl
	Leu260	4.92	Hydrophobic	Pi–Alkyl
	Ile211	2.76	Hydrophobic	Pi–Sigma
	Val219	2.68	Hydrophobic	Pi–Sigma
	Lys232	3.85	Hydrophobic	Pi–Cation
CID-5280445	Gly286	3.61	Hydrogen	Carbon–Hydrogen
	Val219	4.34	Hydrophobic	Pi–Alkyl
	Ala350	4.74	Hydrophobic	Pi–Alkyl
	Ala230	5.24	Hydrophobic	Pi–Alkyl
	Lys232	4.41	Hydrophobic	Pi–Cation
CID-445154	Ile211	4.78	Hydrophobic	Pi–Alkyl
CID-136417	Lys232	2.37	Hydrogen	Conventional Hydrogen
	Ser280	2.37	Hydrogen	Conventional Hydrogen
	Ala350	2.95	Hydrogen	Carbon–Hydrogen
	Ala230	4.57	Hydrophobic	Pi–Alkyl

4. Discussion

Fibrosis is a common feature of all kinds of chronic kidney disease. TGF-β signaling plays a crucial role in cellular physiology. However, its deregulation contributes substantially to the development of renal fibrosis [50]. Pharmacological intervention to the deregulated TGF-β signaling could offer a promising approach in the management of renal fibrosis. Accumulating evidence suggests that phytochemicals, particularly flavonoids, can protect against inflammation or injury in kidney tissues [20]. However, the antifibrotic potential of flavonoids targeting TGFβR-1 in the kidney has yet to be explored. In this paper, a combined virtual screening and molecular simulation approach identified a total of five compounds that exhibited a higher binding affinity for TGFβR-1.

In recent years, In-Silico drug design has attracted attention due to its ability to accelerate the development of new drugs by analyzing the results of bioactivity profiling, molecular modeling, post-docking screening, MDS, and predictive analytics of noble compounds against various diseases [51,52]. Our study has screened 52 flavonoid compounds to evaluate their inhibitory activity against the TGF-β receptor 1 (PDB ID 6B8Y) to search for a potential drug candidate for the treatment of kidney fibrosis. Initially, molecular docking was performed to identify the best five ligand compounds based on their binding affinity score and selected one FDA-approved drug used as the control. At first, in our study, we selected 51 flavonoid compounds; however, after chemical and ADMET screening, 31 flavonoids were approved for the subsequent analysis. ADMET assessment is a cost-effective strategy for reducing drug development costs while providing "fact checks" and secondary complimentary views for high-performance imaging techniques [53,54]. Our study conducted the qikprop application of the Schrödinger package software to complete the ADMET profiling.

Molecular docking is a technique for assessing how two or more molecules will bind with the highest compositional confirmation and the lowest binding affinity. Drug candidates that delivered the most significant and stable score were selected using the Maestro application, which utilizes molecular docking to assign a score. The molecular docking study for the selected five flavonoid compounds and control drug with the TGF-β receptor 1 (PDB ID 6B8Y) reported the docking affinity of the control drug Linagliptin (PubChem CID 10096344) was −9.074 kcal/mol. Among the selected flavonoid compounds, (-)-Epicatechin (PubChem CID 72276) possessed the best binding affinity of −13.585, in which Fisetin (PubChem CID 5281614) had −13.177 and Luteolin (PubChem CID 5280445) had −10.506; all docking affinity results with their chemical structure are depicted in Table 1. Furthermore, the Discovery Studio Visualizer tool (v.21), an effective visualizer tool for drug discovery, was used to represent the post docking receptor–ligands interactions with their animated and 2D structures.

MDS is a versatile technique that analyzes biomolecular interactions and the contact between the arrangement and activity of proteins to aid in modern drug discovery and performance data from dynamic trajectory analysis [55]. Our study conducted the Desmond application of Schrödinger package software (Schrödinger Release 2020-3) to run Molecular Dynamic simulation (MDS) with the selected physiological and physicochemical parameters. This simulation trajectory of the simulation tool has also been used to perfectly analyze the root-mean-square deviation (RMSD), the radius of gyration (Rg), hydrogen bond number, and solvent accessible surface area (SASA) [56]. The root-mean-square deviation (RMSD) of the selected TGF-β receptor 1 protein backbone was used to evaluate the protein structure's reliability and identify conformational changes; the lower value indicates the most stable compounds [57]. RMSD values of less than 1.5 Å are typically indicative of greater consistency in docking since RMSD values over 1.5 Å typically indicate the average binding positions. In our study, the RMSD values of the protein–ligand interactions were within an appropriate range, namely, the average mean values of 2 (the lowest value for CAP is approximately 0.8, and maximum values of 3), suggesting a better docking position and no disruption of the protein–ligand structure (Figure 8).

On the other hand, the protein–ligand contacts, classified as the hydrogen bonds, hydrophobic interactions, ionic interactions, and water bridges, have a significant role in both protein–ligand complexes and their molecular recognition. All three protein-ligand complexes remained stable throughout the simulation trajectory, indicating that the complexes are rigid (Figure 9). Luteolin and 5-Hydroxy-3,6,7,8,3′,4′-hexamethoxyflavone were found to have strong hydrogen bonds, hydrophobic bonds, and water bridges with protein residues. Fisetin also showed strong hydrogen bonds, hydrophobic bonds, and water bridges with the protein structure. Furthermore, the other drugs had typical molecular interactions with the protein residues.

In the present In-Silico investigation, there was no available clinical research that provided clinical proof of these selected flavonoid compounds for inhibiting TGFβR-1 expression as the target for kidney fibrosis treatment. This research study concentrated on a novel approach to treat kidney fibrosis, indicating that additional wet lab and clinical studies might be necessary to authenticate these drug-like natural aromatic flavonoid compounds targeting TGFβR-1. This means that, after the validation of the activity in in vitro and in vivo modeling, these selected aromatic potential bioactive flavonoid compounds can be used as an alternative treatment option for kidney fibrosis.

5. Conclusions

With the increasing prevalence and incidence of kidney fibrosis worldwide, novel and viable therapeutic options are essential to ease the burden of this deadly disease. Notably, TGFβR-1 is one of the most important receptors in the serine/threonine protein kinase family that has been shown to contribute to EMT by activating the TGFβR-1/Smad signaling pathway leading to renal fibrosis. Considering this, in our present study, an In-Silico screening of prospective flavonoids targeting TGFβR-1 as a therapeutic approach to treat kidney fibrosis was conducted. We assembled a library of 51 flavonoids based on their pharmacokinetic properties. The virtual ADME/T analysis screened a total of 31 flavonoids with drug-like properties. In molecular docking analysis, a total of five compounds, notably Epicatechin, Fisetin, and Luteolin, exhibited higher binding affinities with the TGFβR-1 protein, which were compared to the standard drug linagliptin. In addition, these compounds maintained a stable conformational interaction with the binding sites of TGFβR-1, as shown in the molecular dynamic simulation trajectories analysis. The binding affinity and conformational interaction pattern demonstrated that these flavonoids may compete with TGF-β for TGFβR-1, thereby limiting the hyperactivation of TGF-β signaling and subsequent protection against kidney fibrosis. However, in the future, for the development of protective agents against kidney fibrosis, several practical concerns need to be addressed, including drug–drug interactions, side effects, overlapping safety issues, dosage, as well as futility restrictions, which prevent them from being used in certain situations. Therefore, subject to the successful resolution of the experimental issues, our selected flavonoid-based agents are expected to overcome all these major challenges and act as a major therapeutic option for the treatment of kidney fibrosis.

Supplementary Materials: The following supporting information can be downloaded at: https://www.mdpi.com/article/10.3390/life12111764/s1, Table S1: Compound's screening and ADMET prediction; Table S2: Final 30 screened compounds; Table S3: The Docking Score of 6 control drugs; Table S4: Part-1 Prime_mmgbsa and Part-2 Final selected Docking Score Data.

Author Contributions: This work was a collaboration among all authors. M.J.U. and M.H.R. designed outlines of the manuscript. M.H.R., P.B. and D.D. wrote the initial draft of the manuscript. M.J.U., M.A.H., T.B.E., Y.A., Y.K., M.S. and M.S.A. reviewed the scientific contents described in the manuscript. All authors have read and agreed to the published version of the manuscript.

Funding: This research was supported by Korea Basic Science Institute (National research Facilities and Equipment Center) grant funded by the Ministry of Education (2021R1A6C101A442), Republic of Korea.

Institutional Review Board Statement: Not applicable.

Informed Consent Statement: Not applicable.

Data Availability Statement: Not applicable.

Acknowledgments: We acknowledge Bioinformatics Lab, ABEx Bio-Research Center, East Azampur, Dhaka-1230, Bangladesh for providing the support to conduct this research and project guidelines. In addition, we are thankful to the Biotechnology and Genetic Engineering department of Bangabandhu Sheikh Mujibur Rahman Science and Technology University, Gopalgaj-8100, Bangladesh.

Conflicts of Interest: The authors declare no conflict of interest.

References

1. Castro, A.F.; Coresh, J. CKD surveillance using laboratory data from the population-based National Health and Nutrition Examination Survey (NHANES). *Am. J Kidney Dis.* **2009**, *53*, S46–S55. [CrossRef] [PubMed]
2. Djudjaj, S.; Boor, P. Cellular and molecular mechanisms of kidney fibrosis. *Mol. Asp. Med.* **2019**, *65*, 16–36. [CrossRef] [PubMed]
3. López-Novoa, J.M.; Martínez-Salgado, C.; Rodríguez-Peña, A.B.; López-Hernández, F.J. Common pathophysiological mechanisms of chronic kidney disease: Therapeutic perspectives. *Pharmacol. Ther.* **2010**, *128*, 61–81. [CrossRef]
4. Izuhara, Y.; Nangaku, M.; Inagi, R.; Tominaga, N.; Aizawa, T.; Kurokawa, K.; van Ypersele de Strihou, C.; Miyata, T. Renoprotective properties of angiotensin receptor blockers beyond blood pressure lowering. *J. Am. Soc. Nephrol.* **2005**, *16*, 3631–3641. [CrossRef] [PubMed]
5. Meng, X.M.; Tang, P.M.; Li, J.; Lan, H.Y. TGF-β/Smad signaling in renal fibrosis. *Front. Physiol.* **2015**, *6*, 82. [CrossRef] [PubMed]
6. Lee, S.Y.; Kim, S.I.; Choi, M.E. Therapeutic targets for treating fibrotic kidney diseases. *Transl. Res. J. Lab. Clin. Med.* **2015**, *165*, 512–530. [CrossRef]
7. Liu, Y. New insights into epithelial-mesenchymal transition in kidney fibrosis. *J. Am. Soc. Nephrol.* **2010**, *21*, 212–222. [CrossRef]
8. Ungefroren, H.; Gieseler, F.; Kaufmann, R.; Settmacher, U.; Lehnert, H.; Rauch, B.H. Signaling Crosstalk of TGF-β/ALK5 and PAR2/PAR1: A Complex Regulatory Network Controlling Fibrosis and Cancer. *Int. J. Mol. Sci.* **2018**, *19*, 1568. [CrossRef]

9. Liao, W.; Liang, P.; Liu, B.; Xu, Z.; Zhang, L.; Feng, M.; Tang, Y.; Xu, A. MicroRNA-140-5p Mediates Renal Fibrosis Through TGF-β1/Smad Signaling Pathway by Directly Targeting TGFBR1. *Front. Physiol.* **2020**, *11*, 1093. [CrossRef]
10. Qi, W.; Chen, X.; Poronnik, P.; Pollock, C.A. Transforming growth factor-beta/connective tissue growth factor axis in the kidney. *Int. J. Biochem. Cell Biol.* **2008**, *40*, 9–13. [CrossRef]
11. Wang, W.; Koka, V.; Lan, H.Y. Transforming growth factor-beta and Smad signalling in kidney diseases. *Nephrology (Carlton)* **2005**, *10*, 48–56. [CrossRef] [PubMed]
12. Hemshekhar, M.; Sunitha, K.; Santhosh, M.S.; Devaraja, S.; Kemparaju, K.; Vishwanath, B.; Niranjana, S.; Girish, K.J.P.R. An overview on genus Garcinia: Phytochemical and therapeutical aspects. *Phytochem. Rev.* **2011**, *10*, 325–351. [CrossRef]
13. Shuaib, M.; Kushwaha, P.P.; Prajapati, K.S.; Singh, A.K.; Sharma, R.; Kumar, S. Effect of Dietary Phytochemicals in Obesity and Cancer. In *Obesity and Cancer*; Springer: Berlin/Heidelberg, Germany, 2021; pp. 163–184.
14. Pagliaro, B.; Santolamazza, C.; Simonelli, F.; Rubattu, S. Phytochemical Compounds and Protection from Cardiovascular Diseases: A State of the Art. *BioMed Res. Int.* **2015**, *2015*, 918069. [CrossRef] [PubMed]
15. Castañeda, R.; Cáceres, A.; Cruz, S.M.; Aceituno, J.A.; Marroquín, E.S.; Barrios Sosa, A.C.; Strangman, W.K.; Williamson, R.T. Nephroprotective plant species used in traditional Mayan Medicine for renal-associated diseases. *J. Ethnopharmacol.* **2022**, *301*, 115755. [CrossRef]
16. Abd-Elkareem, M.; Soliman, M.; Abd El-Rahman, M.A.M.; Abou Khalil, N.S. Effect of Nigella sativa L. Seed on the Kidney of Monosodium Glutamate Challenged Rats. *Front. Pharmacol.* **2022**, *13*, 789988. [CrossRef]
17. Rahman, M.A.; Akter, S.; Dorotea, D.; Mazumder, A.; Uddin, M.N.; Hannan, M.A.; Hossen, M.J.; Ahmed, M.S.; Kim, W.; Kim, B.; et al. Renoprotective potentials of small molecule natural products targeting mitochondrial dysfunction. *Front. Pharmacol.* **2022**, *13*, 925993. [CrossRef]
18. Akter, S.; Moni, A.; Faisal, G.M.; Uddin, M.R.; Jahan, N.; Hannan, M.A.; Rahman, A.; Uddin, M.J. Renoprotective Effects of Mangiferin: Pharmacological Advances and Future Perspectives. *Int. J. Environ. Res. Public Health* **2022**, *19*, 1864. [CrossRef]
19. Akter, T.; Rahman, M.A.; Moni, A.; Apu, M.A.I.; Fariha, A.; Hannan, M.A.; Uddin, M.J. Prospects for Protective Potential of Moringa oleifera against Kidney Diseases. *Plants (Basel)* **2021**, *10*, 2818. [CrossRef]
20. Vargas, F.; Romecín, P.; García-Guillén, A.I.; Wangesteen, R.; Vargas-Tendero, P.; Paredes, M.D.; Atucha, N.M.; García-Estañ, J. Flavonoids in Kidney Health and Disease. *Front. Physiol.* **2018**, *9*, 394. [CrossRef]
21. Wu, X.; Ding, X.; Ding, Z.; Jia, P. Total Flavonoids from Leaves of Carya Cathayensis Ameliorate Renal Fibrosis via the miR-21/Smad7 Signaling Pathway. *Cell. Physiol. Biochem.* **2018**, *49*, 1551–1563. [CrossRef]
22. Chen, H.A.; Chen, C.M.; Guan, S.S.; Chiang, C.K.; Wu, C.T.; Liu, S.H. The antifibrotic and anti-inflammatory effects of icariin on the kidney in a unilateral ureteral obstruction mouse model. *Phytomedicine* **2019**, *59*, 152917. [CrossRef] [PubMed]
23. Ganbold, M.; Shimamoto, Y.; Ferdousi, F.; Tominaga, K.; Isoda, H. Antifibrotic effect of methylated quercetin derivatives on TGFβ-induced hepatic stellate cells. *Biochem. Biophys. Rep.* **2019**, *20*, 100678. [CrossRef]
24. Pan, X.; Ma, X.; Jiang, Y.; Wen, J.; Yang, L.; Chen, D.; Cao, X.; Peng, C. A Comprehensive Review of Natural Products against Liver Fibrosis: Flavonoids, Quinones, Lignans, Phenols, and Acids. *Evid. Based Complementary Altern. Med.* **2020**, *2020*, 7171498. [CrossRef] [PubMed]
25. Wang, G.G.; Lu, X.H.; Li, W.; Zhao, X.; Zhang, C. Protective Effects of Luteolin on Diabetic Nephropathy in STZ-Induced Diabetic Rats. *Evid.-Based Complementary Altern. Med. Ecam* **2011**, *2011*, 323171. [CrossRef] [PubMed]
26. Den Hartogh, D.J.; Tsiani, E. Health Benefits of Resveratrol in Kidney Disease: Evidence from In Vitro and In Vivo Studies. *Nutrients* **2019**, *11*, 1624. [CrossRef]
27. Zhang, X.; Lu, H.; Xie, S.; Wu, C.; Guo, Y.; Xiao, Y.; Zheng, S.; Zhu, H.; Zhang, Y.; Bai, Y. Resveratrol suppresses the myofibroblastic phenotype and fibrosis formation in kidneys via proliferation-related signalling pathways. *Br. J. Pharmacol.* **2019**, *176*, 4745–4759. [CrossRef]
28. Prince, P.D.; Fraga, C.G.; Galleano, M. (-)-Epicatechin administration protects kidneys against modifications induced by short-term l-NAME treatment in rats. *Food Funct.* **2020**, *11*, 318–327. [CrossRef]
29. Yao, L.; Li, L.; Li, X.; Li, H.; Zhang, Y.; Zhang, R.; Wang, J.; Mao, X. The anti-inflammatory and antifibrotic effects of Coreopsis tinctoria Nutt on high-glucose-fat diet and streptozotocin-induced diabetic renal damage in rats. *BMC Complementary Altern. Med.* **2015**, *15*, 314. [CrossRef]
30. Yao, L.; Li, J.; Li, L.; Li, X.; Zhang, R.; Zhang, Y.; Mao, X. Coreopsis tinctoria Nutt ameliorates high glucose-induced renal fibrosis and inflammation via the TGF-β1/SMADS/AMPK/NF-κB pathways. *BMC Complementary Altern. Med.* **2019**, *19*, 14. [CrossRef]
31. Lai, P.-B.; Zhang, L.; Yang, L.-Y. Quercetin Ameliorates Diabetic Nephropathy by Reducing the Expressions of Transforming Growth Factor-β1 and Connective Tissue Growth Factor in Streptozotocin-Induced Diabetic Rats. *Ren. Fail.* **2012**, *34*, 83–87. [CrossRef]
32. Harikrishnan, L.S.; Warrier, J.; Tebben, A.J.; Tonukunuru, G.; Madduri, S.R.; Baligar, V.; Mannoori, R.; Seshadri, B.; Rahaman, H.; Arunachalam, P.N.; et al. Heterobicyclic inhibitors of transforming growth factor beta receptor I (TGFβRI). *Bioorganic Med. Chem.* **2018**, *26*, 1026–1034. [CrossRef] [PubMed]
33. Xu, H.; Qu, J.; Wang, J.; Han, K.; Li, Q.; Bi, W.; Liu, R. Discovery of pulmonary fibrosis inhibitor targeting TGF-β RI in Polygonum cuspidatum by high resolution mass spectrometry with in silico strategy. *J. Pharm. Anal.* 2020, *in press*. [CrossRef]
34. Halgren, T.A. Identifying and Characterizing Binding Sites and Assessing Druggability. *J. Chem. Inf. Modeling* **2009**, *49*, 377–389. [CrossRef] [PubMed]

35. Halgren, T. New Method for Fast and Accurate Binding-site Identification and Analysis. *Chem. Biol. Drug Des.* **2007**, *69*, 146–148. [CrossRef]
36. Goodford, P.J. A computational procedure for determining energetically favorable binding sites on biologically important macromolecules. *J. Med. Chem.* **1985**, *28*, 849–857. [CrossRef]
37. Weber, A.E.; Halgren Ta Fau-Doyle, J.J.; Doyle Jj Fau-Lynch, R.J.; Lynch Rj Fau-Siegl, P.K.; Siegl Pk Fau-Parsons, W.H.; Parsons Wh Fau-Greenlee, W.J.; Greenlee Wj Fau-Patchett, A.A.; Patchett, A.A. Design and synthesis of P2-P1′-linked macrocyclic human renin inhibitors. *J. Med. Chem.* **1991**, *34*, 2692–2701. [CrossRef]
38. Friesner, R.A.; Murphy, R.B.; Repasky, M.P.; Frye, L.L.; Greenwood, J.R.; Halgren, T.A.; Sanschagrin, P.C.; Mainz, D.T. Extra Precision Glide: Docking and Scoring Incorporating a Model of Hydrophobic Enclosure for Protein−Ligand Complexes. *J. Med. Chem.* **2006**, *49*, 6177–6196. [CrossRef]
39. Thérien, M.; Skorey, K.; Fau-Zamboni, R.; Zamboni, R.; Fau-Li, C.S.; Li Cs Fau-Lau, C.K.; Lau Ck Fau-LeRiche, T.; LeRiche T Fau-Linh Truong, V.; Linh Truong, V.; Fau-Waddleton, D.; et al. Synthesis of a novel peptidic photoaffinity probe for the PTP-1B enzyme. *Bioorganic Med. Chem. Lett.* **2004**, *14*, 2319–2322. [CrossRef]
40. Hossain, R.; Al-Khafaji, K.; Khan, R.A.; Sarkar, C.; Islam, M.; Dey, D.; Jain, D.; Faria, F.; Akbor, R.; Atolani, O.J.P. Quercetin and/or Ascorbic Acid Modulatory Effect on Phenobarbital-Induced Sleeping Mice Possibly through GABAA and GABAB Receptor Interaction Pathway. *Pharmaceuticals (Basel)* **2021**, *14*, 721. [CrossRef]
41. Hoffman, J.M.; Margolis, K.G. Building community in the gut: A role for mucosal serotonin. *Nat. Rev. Gastroenterol. Hepatol.* **2020**, *17*, 6–8. [CrossRef]
42. Bharadwaj, S.; Dubey, A.; Yadava, U.; Mishra, S.K.; Kang, S.G.; Dwivedi, V.D. Exploration of natural compounds with anti-SARS-CoV-2 activity via inhibition of SARS-CoV-2 Mpro. *Brief. Bioinform.* **2021**, *22*, 1361–1377. [CrossRef] [PubMed]
43. Han, Y.; Wang, Z.; Ren, J.; Wei, Z.; Li, J. Potential inhibitors for the novel coronavirus (SARS-CoV-2). *Brief. Bioinform.* **2021**, *22*, 1225–1231. [CrossRef] [PubMed]
44. Shawky, E. Prediction of potential cancer-related molecular targets of North African plants constituents using network pharmacology-based analysis. *J. Ethnopharmacol.* **2019**, *238*, 111826. [CrossRef] [PubMed]
45. Ahammad, F.; Alam, R.; Mahmud, R.; Akhter, S.; Talukder, E.K.; Tonmoy, A.M.; Fahim, S.; Al-Ghamdi, K.; Samad, A.; Qadri, I. Pharmacoinformatics and molecular dynamics simulation-based phytochemical screening of neem plant (Azadiractha indica) against human cancer by targeting MCM7 protein. *Brief. Bioinform.* **2021**, *22*, bbab098. [CrossRef] [PubMed]
46. Fu, C.; Deng, S.; Koneski, I.; Awad, M.M.; Akram, Z.; Matinlinna, J.; Pichika, M.R.; Daood, U.; Fawzy, A.S. Multiscale in-vitro analysis of photo-activated riboflavin incorporated in an experimental universal adhesive. *J. Mech. Behav. Biomed. Mater.* **2020**, *112*, 104082. [CrossRef]
47. Friesner, R.A.; Banks, J.L.; Murphy, R.B.; Halgren, T.A.; Klicic, J.J.; Mainz, D.T.; Repasky, M.P.; Knoll, E.H.; Shelley, M.; Perry, J.K.; et al. Glide: A New Approach for Rapid, Accurate Docking and Scoring. 1. Method and Assessment of Docking Accuracy. *J. Med. Chem.* **2004**, *47*, 1739–1749. [CrossRef]
48. Sarkar, B.; Ullah, M.A.; Islam, S.S.; Rahman, M.D.H.; Araf, Y. Analysis of plant-derived phytochemicals as anti-cancer agents targeting cyclin dependent kinase-2, human topoisomerase IIa and vascular endothelial growth factor receptor-2. *J. Recept. Signal Transduct.* **2021**, *41*, 217–233. [CrossRef]
49. Lenselink, E.B.; Louvel, J.; Forti, A.F.; van Veldhoven, J.P.D.; de Vries, H.; Mulder-Krieger, T.; McRobb, F.M.; Negri, A.; Goose, J.; Abel, R.; et al. Predicting Binding Affinities for GPCR Ligands Using Free-Energy Perturbation. *ACS Omega* **2016**, *1*, 293–304. [CrossRef]
50. Meng, X.-m.; Nikolic-Paterson, D.J.; Lan, H.Y. TGF-β: The master regulator of fibrosis. *Nat. Rev. Nephrol.* **2016**, *12*, 325–338. [CrossRef]
51. Dey, D.; Paul, P.K.; Al Azad, S.; Al Mazid, M.F.; Khan, A.M.; Sharif, M.A.; Rahman, M.H. Molecular optimization, docking, and dynamic simulation profiling of selective aromatic phytochemical ligands in blocking the SARS-CoV-2 S protein attachment to ACE2 receptor: An in silico approach of targeted drug designing. *J. Adv. Vet. Anim. Res.* **2021**, *8*, 24–35. [CrossRef]
52. Jain, D.; Hossain, R.; Khan, R.A.; Dey, D.; Toma, T.R.; Islam, M.T.; Janmeda, P.; Hakeem, K.R. Computer-aided Evaluation of Anti-SARS-CoV-2 (3-chymotrypsin-like Protease and Transmembrane Protease Serine 2 Inhibitors) Activity of Cepharanthine: An In silico Approach. *Biointerface Res. Appl. Chem.* **2022**, *12*, 768–780.
53. Mannhold, R.; Kubinyi, H.; Folkers, G. *Pharmacokinetics and Metabolism in Drug Design*, 3rd ed.; John Wiley & Sons: Hoboken, NJ, USA, 2012; Volume 51.
54. Notari, R.E. Pharmacokinetics Molecular Modification: Implications in Drug Design Evaluation. *J. Pharm. Sci.* **1973**, *62*, 865–881. [CrossRef] [PubMed]
55. Sharif, M.A.; Hossen, M.S.; Shaikat, M.M.; Mashuk, F.; Haidary, T.I.E.; Dey, D.; Paul, P.K.; Al Azad, S.; Al Mazid, M.F.; Badal, M.N.U. Molecular Optimization, Docking and Dynamic Simulation Study of Selective Natural Aromatic Components to Block E2-CD81 Complex Formation in Predating Protease Inhibitor Resistant HCV Influx. *Int. J. Pharm. Res.* **2021**, *13*, 3512–3525.
56. Krieger, E.; Koraimann, G.; Vriend, G. Increasing the precision of comparative models with YASARA NOVA—A self-parameterizing force field. *Proteins Struct. Funct. Bioinform.* **2002**, *47*, 393–402. [CrossRef] [PubMed]
57. Sargsyan, K.; Grauffel, C.D.; Lim, C. How molecular size impacts RMSD applications in molecular dynamics simulations. *J. Chem. Theory Comput.* **2017**, *13*, 1518–1524. [CrossRef]

MDPI AG
Grossspeteranlage 5
4052 Basel
Switzerland
Tel.: +41 61 683 77 34

Life Editorial Office
E-mail: life@mdpi.com
www.mdpi.com/journal/life

www.ingramcontent.com/pod-product-compliance
Lightning Source LLC
Chambersburg PA
CBHW041432210926
51850CB00013B/3411
* 9 7 8 3 7 2 5 8 2 1 7 6 1 *